Mosby's
FUNDAMENTALS of
THERAPEUTIC MASSAGE

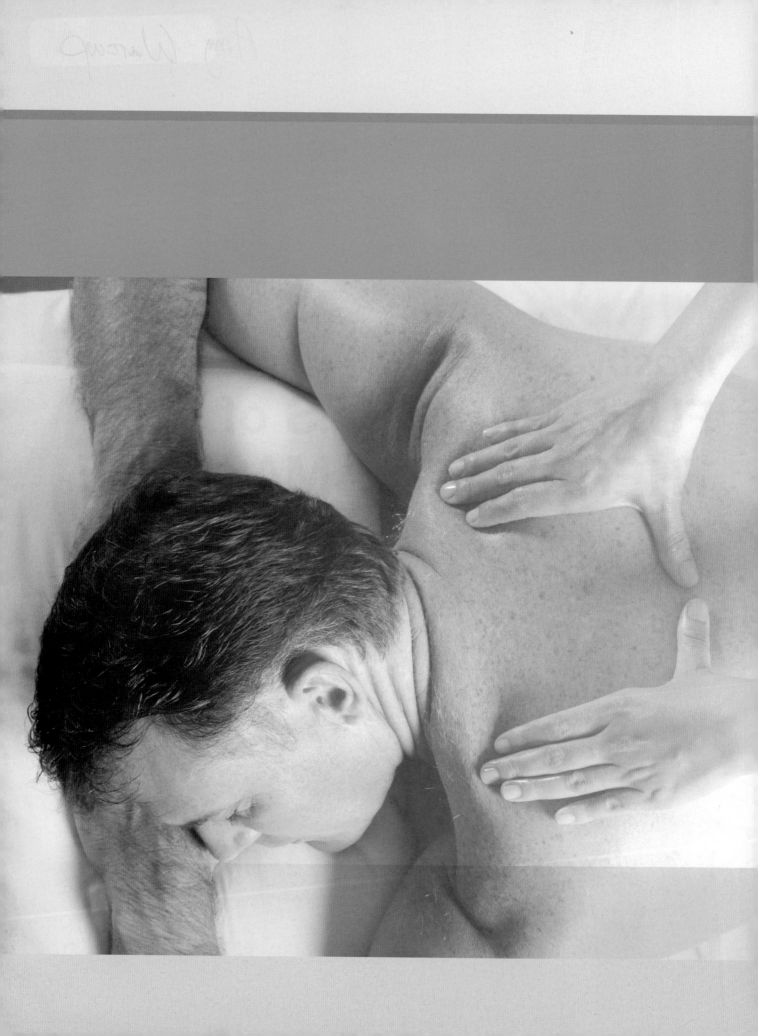

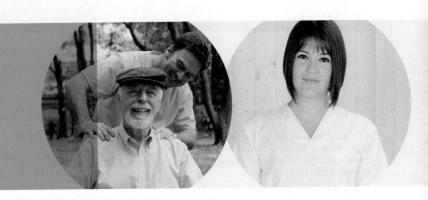

Mosby's
FUNDAMENTALS of
THERAPEUTIC MASSAGE

5th Edition

SANDY FRITZ, MS, NCTMB

Founder, Owner, Director, and Head Instructor
Health Enrichment Center
School of Therapeutic Massage and Bodywork
Lapeer, Michigan

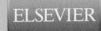

3251 Riverport Lane
Maryland Heights, Missouri 63043

MOSBY'S FUNDAMENTALS OF THERAPEUTIC MASSAGE   ISBN: 978-0-323-07740-8

Notice

Neither the Publisher nor the Author assume any responsibility for any loss or injury and/or damage to person or property arising out of or related to any use of the material contained in this book. It is the responsibility of the treating practitioner, relying on independent expertise and knowledge of the patient, to determine the best treatment and method of application for the patient.

ISBN-13: 978-0-323-07740-8

Vice President and Content Strategy Director: Linda Duncan
Executive Content Strategist: Kellie White
Content Development Specialist: Joe Gramlich
Content Coordinator: Emily Thomson
Publishing Services Manager: Julie Eddy
Project Manager: Rich Barber
Designer: Maggie Reid

Photo Credits
Cover: Tandem, Lisa F. Young
Title Page: Michael Jung

Printed in China

Last digit is the print number: 9   8   7   6   5   4   3   2   1

Contents in Brief

Reviewers

Wayne J. Albert, PhD, CK, FCSB
Professor and Dean
Faculty of Kinesiology
University of New Brunswick
Fredericton, New Brunswick
Canada

Sandra K. Anderson, BA, LMT, ABT, NCTMB
Certifications in Massage Therapy, Zen Shiatsu, and
    Thai Massage
Tucson Touch Therapies Treatment Center
Tucson, AZ

Paul V. Berry Jr., BSHA, LMT, NCTMB, PTA, NCMA
Berry's Essence LLC
Atlanta, GA

Whitney Christiano, LMT, RYT, CPT, BA
Faculty
Connecticut Center for Massage Therapy
Westport, CT

Neal Delaporta, LMT, NCTMB, CPT
Associate Director
Arlington School of Massage and Personal Training
Jacksonville, FL

Michael Garcia, RN, LMT
Chief Academic Officer
Alpha School of Massage
Jacksonville, FL

Cher Hunter, MA, LMT, NCTMB
Director, Massage Therapy Program
Community College of Baltimore County
Baltimore, MD

Christopher V. Jones, CMT, NCTMB
Member, American Massage Therapy Association
NCB Exam Committee Vice-Chair
Fitchburg, MA

Don Kelley, LMT, NCBTMB
Instructor, NMT Center, and Neuromuscular Works
Nashville, TN

Kathy Lee, LMT, BS Business Administration
Director of Career Services
Cortiva Institute
Tucson, AZ

Edward G. Mohr, MSIE, CPE, CSP, NCTM
Certified Professional Ergonomist
Certified Safety Professional, Engineering Aspects
Member, American Massage Therapy Association
Assistant Instructor, Health Enrichment Center
Lake Orion, MI

Kevin Pierce, LMT, MBA
Orlando, FL

Monica J. Reno, AAS, LMT
Massage Therapist
MVP Sportsclubs
Lady Lake, FL

Richard Schekter, MS, LMT
Core Faculty
Educating Hands School of Massage
Miami, FL

Jeffrey A. Simancek, BS, CMT, NCBTMB
Owner/Therapist
Wolf Tracks Massage Therapy
Irvine, CA

Diana L. Thompson, BA, LMP
Private Practice, Hands Heal
Seattle, WA

Jeffrey B. Wood, LMT, COTA/L, BS
Massage Therapy Program Director
Withlacoochee Technical Institute

CONTRIBUTORS

Sandra K. Anderson, BA, LMT, ABT, NCTMB
Certifications in Massage Therapy, Zen Shiatsu, and Thai
    Massage
Tucson Touch Therapies Treatment Center
Tucson, AZ

MaryAnne Hochadel, PharmD, BCPS
Managing Editor and Editor Emeritus, ELSEVIER/Gold
    Standard
Clinical Pharmacist, Bayfront Medical Center
Clinical Assistant Professor of Pharmacy Practice
University of Florida, College of Pharmacy
St. Petersburg, FL

Foreword

Education, training, and skill standards define professions. If the massage profession wishes to be more widely recognized by the general public, as well as by insurance companies, local, state and national government, and by other health care professionals, as being well educated, professional, well trained and with high standards, then it would do well to study and apply the knowledge contained in this superb, newly revised and expanded book.

The range of topics, and the depth of exploration of these—combined with the unique, practical, easy-to-follow delivery of information—makes it a universally useful resource for anyone in the manual therapy professions in general, and massage therapists in particular, and not just in their early training stages. There is much to learn for experienced therapists since the author has focused on bringing the very latest in clinical and practical research, and understanding into the text.

The first four chapters build on each other, moving from fascinating discussion of the multiple aspects of touch—the fundamental element in massage—to chapters on professionalism, ethics and standards, which go to the heart of what is essential in defining any profession in the modern world. This is followed by a laying out of protocols for the development of a professional career. The detailed evaluation of the multiple steps and stages required to achieve the launch of a successful career as a therapist are spelled out in excellent detail—with the authority of someone who has done it all.

An essential part of professional practice is the ability to accurately record what you have done, and to be able to communicate your findings and treatment interventions to the patient/client, to other health care professionals, or to those responsible for reimbursement. Chapter 4 offers the foundations for achieving this by focusing on terminology associated with the systems of the body and therapeutic methods, as well as record keeping, whether in simple SOAP notes or electronically.

Chapter 5 is among the most important chapters in the book as it eases the reader into the realm of research literacy. Knowing what evidence there is for the use of particular therapeutic approaches, in specific settings, is a vital step on the road to true professionalism—as is the need to know when not to treat a person or a condition. A part of this demands that you are able to read a research paper, or an abstract, and are able to see the key elements that might inform or modify what you do, and how you do it, in practice, as well as being able to see when research evidence may be flawed. This is a chapter to read and reread—and that advice applies to working professionals as well as students, as we move towards evidence-informed practice. Chapter 6 is a logical follow-up, since its focus is on indications and contraindications to the use of therapeutic massage—which quite naturally segues into clinical reasoning—the very heart of the clinical decision-making process. What, how and when to treat—or not ... and when to refer, and to whom!

Chapters 7 to 9 cover the detailed importance of hygiene, sanitation and safety, with that key word, safety, being the main ingredient of chapter 8. For if you wish to have a long and successful career it is vital that your own body is well cared for, with attention to good body mechanics. There is no finer teacher of this than Sandy Fritz. The number of therapists who are obliged to abandon their careers due to overuse and other results of poor use of their own bodies or hands is testament to the need for this subject to be taken very seriously. Equally important are the topics regarding massage equipment and supplies, as well as draping procedures, the veritable nuts and bolts of a clinical practice, as covered in chapter 9.

Technical skills and protocols for delivery of professional treatment—massage, manipulations and techniques, including also seated and mat massage, are all fully illustrated in color in chapter 10, followed in chapter 11 by a comprehensive focus on assessments, tests and analysis, all vital if advanced approaches are to be developed. The complementary methods associated with massage are found in chapter 12, ranging from use of water, heat, and stones to adjunctive methods such as Thai massage and shiatsu, reflexology and myofascial approaches.

Chapters 13 and 14 explore massage in a variety of settings such as spa and animal practices and adaptive massage, meaning a focus on special populations. Moving on, chapter 15 informs us on how to pay personal attention to our well-being as massage therapists—for it should be self-evident that your professional life will be more successful, and last longer, if you remain fit!

The wide range of case studies in chapter 16 allows you to tie together the mass of knowledge covered so well in the rest of the book, woven into the context of the most common problems encountered in a massage practice.

This is a really beautifully illustrated, well-thought-out and structured expansion of the previous editions of this book, with a host of new features, and the author and publishers are to be congratulated on producing it.

Leon Chaitow, ND, DO
Osteopath & Naturopath
Honorary Fellow, School of Life Sciences
University of Westminster
London

Preface

Over 35 years ago, when I was exploring a career in therapeutic massage, there were few schools. Because none of them was readily accessible to me, I taught myself. I took a course of less than 100 hours, which at least provided basic skills. The rest of my massage therapy training has come from reading a multitude of books, attending hundreds of hours of workshops, undergoing apprenticeship training, taking college courses in related subjects, teaching more than 5,000 beginning students and approximately 1,000 advanced students at my school, Health Enrichment Center School of Therapeutic Massage and Bodywork, and providing more than 35,000 massage sessions. Since the publication of the first edition, I completed my bachelor's degree at Central Michigan University and master's degree at Thomas Edison State College. Becoming a student again in the university environment had a great influence on my perspective about education, as well as on my professional development.

Educational programs between Health Enrichment Center and the Veterans Administration Hospital, hospice, and professional and collegiate sports teams continue to remind me about the importance of professional massage skills. One of the veterans we worked with spoke at a Health Enrichment Center graduation and said that because of the student massage program he has fewer bad days and more good days. What better support for massage can we get than this? I am still learning the importance of the fundamental concepts upon which all bodywork methods are based. I learn more about the elegant simplicity of massage each time I teach or do massage, and I have learned a great deal through researching and writing textbooks as well. More than ever, I am convinced that a strong understanding of the fundamental concepts of therapeutic massage and the ability to reason effectively through a decision-making process are essential for proficient professional practice. In the three-plus decades of my massage career I have experienced an evolution of massage therapy, from a fringe alternative method to the integration of massage into the maturity of evidence-based and informed practice. When I compare the first edition of this textbook to this fifth edition, it is apparent that the knowledge necessary to begin a massage therapy career has increased, yet the underlying fundamental principles remain—compassionate, beneficial application of touch to help people feel better.

WHO WILL BENEFIT FROM THIS BOOK?

The fifth edition of *Mosby's Fundamentals of Therapeutic Massage* is intended to be used by skilled therapeutic massage educators, and beginning and advanced students, in the classroom setting. It will also be used as a continuing education resource by practitioners and as a reference text for health professionals and massage and bodywork practitioners.

WHY IS THIS BOOK IMPORTANT TO THE PROFESSION OF MASSAGE THERAPY?

The changes and additions to the fifth edition reflect how much therapeutic massage has evolved as a profession over the past few years. Today, therapeutic massage is in the process of standardizing and organizing. Projects such as the Massage Therapy Body of Knowledge (MTBOK.org), an effort to unify the practice and terminology of massage and its various modalities, attest to the growing awareness among massage professionals that their success depends on clarity and an agreed-upon base of knowledge, as in other skilled fields. It is an exciting time in massage therapy, as we see more and more people turning to it as a reliable and practical form of self-care. A curriculum that is mindful of all this is a curriculum that aims high.

A well-rounded education in massage therapy includes learning all of the following: how to perform massage manipulations and bodywork techniques, understanding the anatomical and physiological underpinnings for why the methods work, and the importance of structure, intent, and purpose of touch. It is as important to touch the whole person as it is to skillfully apply techniques. The massage professional must do both. In addition, the student needs to understand the importance of sanitation, hygiene, body mechanics, research literacy, business practices, and ethics, and then apply this knowledge through effective decision-making to build a well-balanced, professional massage career. Massage therapy needs to be beneficial and meet the outcomes and results desired by the clients served to justify the cost and time spent. Massage therapists need to be able to adapt to the individual client to be successful.

The fundamentals of massage methods remain relatively simple. A well-planned school curriculum, as developed in this textbook and its instructor resources (TEACH Lesson Plan Manual and instructor resources), combined with a comprehensive science curriculum as presented in *Mosby's Essential Sciences for Therapeutic Massage* and its various ancillaries, provides a foundation for massage programs and presents information necessary for licensing and certification exams. Massage education should be competency-based, meaning all information in the educational setting is relevant to the actual professional practice of therapeutic massage. The design of this textbook combined with the extensive content on the companion DVDs and Evolve website also support various types of distance learning and web-enhanced education.

The level of knowledge in the fifth edition of this text has been increased to reflect the skills necessary to be able to work effectively in the healthcare world with supervision. While my personal love for this profession lies in humble service to the general public in the support of their wellness, and compassion and help for the daily aches and pains of life, I recognize the importance of being able to also work within the health-care and sport and fitness systems. My work over the past several years with a clinical physiologist, numerous physicians, athletic trainers, and physical therapists supports this observation. Because of the development of comprehensive textbooks, more schools will be better able to expand their curricula for those who wish to pursue therapeutic massage applications in healthcare.

Therapeutic application of massage (structured touch) is not a new phenomenon. The foundation for therapeutic massage was laid centuries ago and will not change provided the physiology of the human being remains constant. It is virtually impossible to acknowledge all those who have contributed to the knowledge base of this field. Our observations of the natural world are a good starting point for this basic knowledge. For example, animals know the value of rhythmic touch. Just watch a litter of puppies and observe the structured application of touch. The base of information goes beyond us to an innate need to rub an area that is hurting and to touch others to provide comfort, pleasure, and bonding.

ORGANIZATION

Chapters 1 through 4 focus on building a solid basis for professionalism and decision-making skills before moving into the actual physical and mental work of practicing massage. Chapter 1 begins with an exploration of touch and reveals its historical foundations. Chapter 2 introduces the clinical reasoning problem-solving model for ethical decision-making and also explains what it means to be a professional, including awareness of laws and regulations. Chapter 3 provides a newly expanded look at the business of massage, job-seeking skills, and the options of creating a career as a business owner or as an employee. Chapter 4 presents appropriate medical and massage therapy terminology to support professional record keeping and documentation. Students are exposed to a language that is understood across many disciplines and that allows professionals to communicate accurately.

Massage therapy has become an evidence-based and informed practice. Chapter 5 further explores what this means and explains the scientific basis for evidence that supports the benefits of therapeutic massage. This chapter also focuses on research literacy, empowering students to look deeper into their practice and its value. Chapter 6 begins the process of decision-making in terms of indications and contraindications to massage.

Chapters 7, 8, and 9 present information on sanitation, hygiene, safety, body mechanics, ergonomics including massage equipment and supplies, positioning and draping procedures, various massage environments, and other information ancillary to a successful massage practice.

Chapters 10 through 12 are the technical skills chapters. Each chapter builds on the previous one, beginning with the basics and expanding assessment methods to support therapeutic applications. Following is an introduction to complementary bodywork systems. As the methods and techniques of therapeutic massage and bodywork are presented, the reader learns how and why they work and when to use them

to obtain a particular physiologic response. Content in these chapters includes: palpation and differential assessment, connective tissue, myofascial and neuromuscular methods, lymphatic drainage massage, Asian and Eastern massage therapy and application, and conflict resolution. In Chapter 11, palpation assessment skills are presented as well as illustrations and text to explain gait assessment procedures and muscle firing patterns, two important areas of concern to a massage therapist. This content increases students' assessment skills to prepare them for advanced level learning.

Chapter 13 is a new chapter that focuses on three main career tracks—wellness/spa, healthcare, and athletics. Chapter 14 describes how to adapt massage to address the needs relevant to particular populations, from pregnant mothers and infants to hospice patients and people with physical impairments. Chapter 15 explores the issues of wellness and nutrition. Massage therapy is a physically taxing field of work. An MT must stay strong and healthy in order to do a good job, and to continue feeling rewarded by the work.

Finally, Chapter 16 sets the stage for putting the material and your study to work through the use of comprehensive case studies based on the clinical reasoning model, outcome-based massage, and treatment plan development. This chapter presents 20 case studies that integrate the information from both this textbook and the student's science studies, such as covered in *Mosby's Essential Sciences for Therapeutic Massage*. The case studies cover the majority of common conditions seen by massage professionals in day and destination spas, as well as in wellness, health, fitness, sport, and medical settings. If students study the process of clinical reasoning carefully, through these case examples they should be able to address almost all other conditions encountered in professional practice. The entire book focuses on developing clinical reasoning skills for this profession.

Helpful appendices are located at the end of the book. These include a pictorial skin pathology appendix, an updated appendix on indications and contraindications, as well as a basic pharmacology for massage reference written especially for this textbook by a clinical pharmacist. All three provide at-a-glance information that is supplemental to the content within the chapters of the textbook.

New activities on the companion Evolve website have been added for this edition and other resources have been updated: quiz yourself with the Certification and Licensing Exam Review Questions, review with the ExamView test bank, and enjoy interactive puzzles and games. Look for volve throughout the textbook.

AN ADAPTABLE DESIGN

The textbook can be taught in a sequential manner from chapter 1 to chapter 16, or it can be adapted to fit the order of topics within the chosen curriculum. Another approach is to cluster the chapters into units or modules such as:

- Chapters 1-4 as the professionalism and ethics unit
- Chapters 5-6 as the research literacy unit
- Chapters 7-12 build massage application skills
- Chapters 13-16 can then act as an integration unit

Another way to look at it,

- Chapters 1-6 cover the practical and critical thinking skills, which can simultaneously be taught with ...
- Chapters 7-12, so that the student learns hands-on skills with thinking skills, all in a coordinated manner.
- Chapters 13-14 can be presented as practice specialization content.

- Chapters 15-16 focus on integration of skills, such as clinical experience. Chapter 15 (as well as many of the exercises provided throughout the text) promotes introspection, understanding, and topics that are supportive to the general well-being of the therapist, and chapter 16 offers a wide variety of case studies.

Fritz Gives You the Fundamentals, and More!
Welcome to the Fifth Edition.

For content you can trust, this text delivers

CHAPTER OBJECTIVES
After completing this chapter, the student will be able to perform the following:
1. Explain the benefits of massage for animals and adapt massage for cats and dogs
2. Describe indications, cautions, and contraindications for massage and appropriately adapt massage for athletes
3. Describe and apply appropriate massage in the breast area
4. Adapt for massage during pregnancy
5. Adapt massage for infants, children, and adolescents
6. Explain the aging process and adapt massage for the geriatric population
7. Recognize acute care situations and adapt massage appropriately
8. Describe the mechanisms of chronic ○○○○○ massage for those with chronic con○○
9. Adapt massage to support clients un○○○ care
10. Adapt massage for integration into th○ settings
11. Communicate effectively and approp○ for individuals with physical impairm○
12. Communicate effectively and approp○ for individuals diagnosed with psych○

- **NEW** detailed and compentency-based chapter and section objectives

PREGNANCY
14-3

SECTION OBJECTIVES
Chapter objective covered in this section:
4. Adapt for massage during pregnancy
Using the information presented in this section, the student will be able to perform the following:
- List the three stages of pregnancy and describe the physical and emotional changes associated with each
- List common disorders of pregnancy and determine the need for referral
- Design a general massage session to meet the needs of a pregnant woman
- Teach a support person basic massage methods to use during labor

viewer to think that the applicant has a lack of interest. Also, the applicant should write down the interviewer's answers to questions about the position and the company for future reference; this is another way of showing the employer that the applicant truly wants the position.

Dressing for Success
The applicant's attire and shoes should be neat and clean. Conservative business dress is appropriate for the job, even if a uniform is usually worn. The applicant should bring a uniform and massage supplies to the interview in case the interviewer wants a demonstration massage.

For both men and women, attention to the details of one's appearance is crucial to the success of an interview. The following tips can help you present a professional appearance:
- Wear clean, polished, conservative dress shoes.
- Wear a well-groomed hairstyle.
- Make sure your fingernails are clean and trimmed.
- Wear no or minimal cologne or perfume.
- Make sure no body piercings or tattoos are visible other than conservative ear piercings.
- Make sure you have well-brushed teeth and fresh breath.
- Do not have gum, candy, or other objects in your mouth.
- Wear minimal jewelry.
- Make sure you do not have any body odor.
- If you will be performing a massage as part of the interview, bring an appropriate uniform to the interview and change before giving the massage.

Interview Questions
When the interviewer asks questions, make eye contact when you answer and be confident (Proficiency Exercise 3-3). The following are just a few questions that could be asked, for which you need to prepare answers in advance:

Closing the Interview
You should have an idea of what you will say when leaving the interview. Make sure you state the skills you have that would make this job a definite fit for you and the reasons your strengths make you right for the position. You may want to ask the interviewer if you could send some references or set up an appointment to give the person a massage. Respectfully asking when the decision will be made reinforces your desire for the position, and verifying how you should contact the employer to follow up (phone or e-mail) shows that you are considerate and polite. Finally, shake hands with the interviewer as you make a parting comment, such as, "Thank you very much for taking the time to speak with me about the [massage] position. I look forward to speaking with you again soon." After the interview, send a thank you note for the interview opportunity and again express your interest in the position. A handwritten note is the most professional way to thank the employer, but if time is an issue (e.g., the decision will be made quickly), an e-mail may be more appropriate.

SELF-EMPLOYMENT OR EMPLOYMENT BY OTHERS

SECTION OBJECTIVES
Chapter objective covered in this section:
4. The student will be able to list the pros and cons of independent and employee status.
Using the information presented in this section, the student will be able to perform the following:
- Develop the skills required for self-employment
- Develop a mission statement to use as the basis for a business plan
- Develop business goals
- Develop a personal start-up cost worksheet

- **EXTENSIVELY REVISED** Chapter 3: Business Considerations for a Career in Therapeutic Massage provides greater insight into the business of massage

Research in Plain Language

The scientific method is a model for conducting scientific research. A specific vocabulary is used during the research process. The scientific method has eight primary steps:

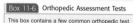

1. Defining the question

2. Locating resources and gathering information and materials

3. Forming a hypothesis (or hypotheses)

4. Planning data collection methods

5. Collecting data

6. Organizing and analyzing the data

7. Interpreting the data and drawing conclusions

8. Communicating the results

- EXTENSIVELY REVISED Chapter 5: Research Literacy and Evidence-Based Practice focuses on the expanding role students can play in learning more about the growing body of science within the massage field.

- REVISED Chapter 8: Body Mechanics takes a closer look adapting massage application based on body shape and gender. Therapeutic massage is a physically labor-intensive therapy that requires time to perform, with an emphasis on ergonomics and correct body mechanics. The fifth edition has expanded coverage of this information and new content has been evaluated by ergonomics experts.

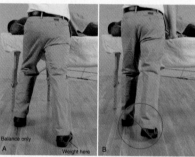

FIGURE 8-13 **A,** Maintaining alignment of the shoulder and pelvic girdle is part of stacking of the joints. **B,** During a weight transfer, the point of contact on the client and the therapist's back foot are weight bearing. The front foot is used only for balance. **C** and **D,** Weight transfer while kneeling.

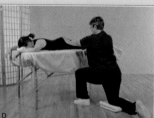

A, Correct stance. The back foot is weight bearing, and the front foot is used only for balance. **B,** Avoid standing on the ...hifts weight bearing to the front foot.

Balance only   Weight here   A   B

Box 11-6   Orthopedic Assessment Tests

This box contains a few common orthopedic test.

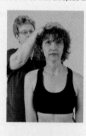

Axial Compression Test
- The client is either sitting or lying and you press down on the top of the client's head causing narrowing of the neural foramen and pressure on the facet joints, or muscle spasm.
- A positive test causes increased pain and indicates that there is some type of pressure on a nerve. *Refer client.*

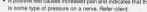

Apley's Scratch Test
- The client is seated or standing. Ask the client reach over their head with one hand to scratch their back while keeping the other hand behind the back.
- Or, tell the client to touch the opposite scapula to test range of motion of the shoulder.
- Reaching over the head allows you to assess abduction and external rotation.
- Reaching behind the back allows you to assess adduction and internal rotation.
- Compare both sides for symmetry.
- If pain or limited range of motion there may be a rotator cuff tear or shoulder impingement (there may also be a potential for adhesive capsulitis or glenohumeral osteoarthritis). *Refer client.*

Tinel's Test
- Assesses for ulnar nerve irritability.
- Assessment is performed at elbow and wrist.
- Place elbow flexion and wrist in extension.
- Tap at the cubital and/or carpal tunnel.
- A positive test produces paresthesias (numbing) or tingling along the distal course of the ulnar indicating irritability and or impingement of the ulnar nerve. *Refer client.*

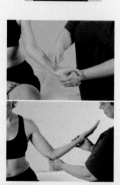

- EXTENSIVELY REVISED Chapter 11: Assessment Procedures for Developing a Care/Treatment Plan demonstrates client assessment procedures.

- **EXTENSIVELY REVISED** Chapter 13: Massage Career Tracks and Practice Settings covers the three main massage practice areas in more depth—spa, fitness and sports, and healthcare. In this fifth edition, each of these career tracks is discussed with suggestions for additional training for specialization in a specific practice focus.

- **EXTENSIVELY REVISED** • Appendix C: Basic Pharmacology for the Massage Therapist updates students on medications and their implications for massage.
- The fifth edition introduces students to the Massage Therapy Body of Knowledge (MTBOK), and this edition has been mapped to the MTBOK for instructors.
- The final chapter in this book contains 20 case studies that help the student to appreciate the complexities of a therapeutic relationship, all in a competency-based format.

Visuals that guide

- Joint range of motion

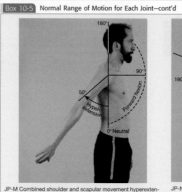

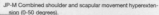

Box 10-5 Normal Range of Motion for Each Joint—cont'd

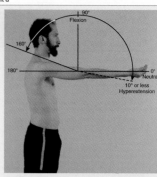

JP-M Combined shoulder and scapular movement hyperextension (0-50 degrees).

JP-N Elbow flexion (0-160 degrees); elbow extension (160- 0 degrees); elbow hyperextension (0-10 degrees).

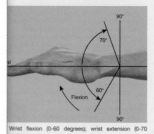

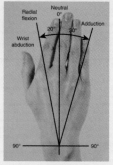

Wrist flexion (0-60 degrees); wrist extension (0-70 degrees).

JP-P Wrist abduction (0-20 degrees) Wrist adduction (0 -30 degrees)

- NEW AND UPDATED! photos sequences, including:

- Correct and incorrect body mechanics

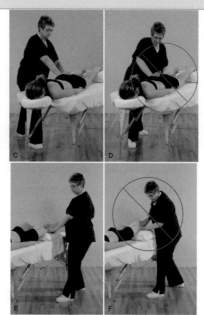

FIGURE 8-31 A, A stable low back B, Incorrect. The table is too short, and the therapist's core is unstable, as is the scapula. The arm is medially across the body, which is not lined up with the direction of the weight transfer. All of this contributes to low back strain while giving a massage. C, Using an asymmetric stance and normal knee-lock position in the weight-bearing leg protect the back. D, Incorrect. The therapist has the weight on the front foot and is standing on the toes. The elbow is bent, and the table too high. Muscle is used to apply pressure. E, Stack the joints and lean back when applying a pull to stretch an area. F, Incorrect: pulling using muscle strength instead of leaning back to stretch or traction the area.

Box 15-6 Breathing Exercises

The following breathing exercises should be taught to clients who lift their shoulders during quiet and deep inspiration. (The exercises are presented in an instructional form that addresses the client

Exercise 1 (Figures A and B)

- Breathing exercises, orthopedic tests, and more

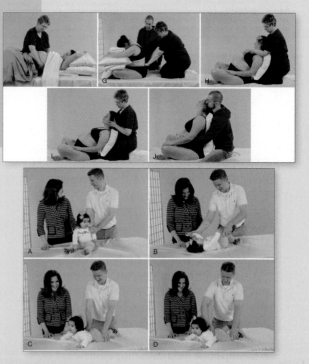

- Protocols on fluid movement and connective tissue
- Massage for expectant mothers and infants, and photo demonstration for transferring clients who use wheelchairs

- Plus, the General Massage Protocol, and protocols for seated and mat massage

Features and activities that motivate and make you think

- NEW Foot in the Door feature offers tips on how to make your way in the massage profession

- UPDATED Proficiency Exercises throughout provide students with activities to effectively engage

PROFICIENCY EXERCISE 8-2

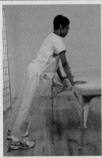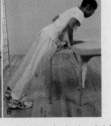

Shoulder push-ups are a good way to train the serratus anterior muscles. The idea is to push your chest away from a surface, and then lower it toward the surface, by using your shoulders, not your elbows. Massage therapists should perform this exercise by leaning against a counter, rather than prone on the floor, because the angle of the arms is similar to that used during massage.

Counter Push-Ups

1. Contract your abdomen to engage your core muscles. If you have difficulty maintaining core stability, use a belt or rope as an aid. First, maintain core stability while exhaling and then inhale normally (your abdomen should move out slightly).

Next, hold your breath and wrap the belt or r waist and fasten it. The belt or rope should tight or binding. If you lose core stability, the the belt will remind you to re-engage your c

2. Stand upright about 2 or 3 feet from t facing it.
3. Extend both arms and rest your palms on counter, keeping your elbows straight. If counter is uncomfortable, you can pad it w
4. Slowly flex your elbows and lower your c counter. Keep your feet flat on the floor.
5. Primarily use your shoulder muscles to rai up into a standing position. Repeat up to 1

24

Workbook Section

Complete these exercises and find the answers on the Evolve website. *evolve*

Short Answer

1. What is the skin's significance in touch?
2. What factors can influence an individual's experience of touch?
3. What are the forms of inappropriate professional touch?
4. What are the forms of appropriate professional touch?
5. In what way and where did massage originate? Why is this answer important?
6. What has provided the validation for massage?
7. What methods did the ancient Chinese massage system use? In what ways are the methods of today different?

Essay Questions

1. What does "touch intention" mean to you?
2. How would you describe your professional touc intention?

Matching

Match the person or information (1 to 20) with the best response (a to y).

_____ 1. Massage in the Eastern world
_____ 2. Massage in the Western world
_____ 3. Ambrose Paré
_____ 4. Per Henrik Ling
_____ 5. Followers of Johann Mezger
_____ 6. Duplicated movements
_____ 7. Active movements
_____ 8. Passive movements

- NEW boxes on MTBOK, SOAP notes, joint range of motion, research, and more
- UPDATED Workbook Sections have a new sharp look and are also available in an e-format on *evolve*

Ancillaries that are more than just extra

- New and updated activities on the Evolve Web site include interactive games, puzzles, exam and certification questions and answers, and video
- Go to www.evolvesetup.com for a demonstration on how you can start using Evolve today.
- 2 accompanying DVDs contain 3 hours of case studies, demonstrations, animated footage, and more!
- TEACH lesson plan manual for instructors is available on *evolve* *e* http://evolve.elsevier.com/fritz/fundamentals/

NOTE TO STUDENTS

As the author, my intent is to make reading this textbook an enjoyable learning experience; I hope my purpose is reflected in the conversational tone in which I have written the text. My personal conviction is that *Mosby's Fundamentals of Therapeutic Massage* effectively presents the information and reflects both the heart and the art of therapeutic massage. After all, no one cares how much you know until they know how much you care.

Sandy Fritz

Acknowledgments

My thanks to the following professionals who have influenced the content and clarity over multiple editions of this text to ensure accurate presentation of information:

Wayne Albert, PhD, CK, FCSB
Patricia J. Benjamin, PhD
Leon K. Chaitow, ND, DO
Kelly Challis
Emily Edith Safrona Cowall, Reg MT
Karen Craig, LMT, NCTMB
Peter A. Goldberg, DIPL AC (NCCA), LMT
Lucy Liben, MS, LMT
Jean E. Loving, BA, LMT
Ed Mohr, MSIE, CPE, CSP, NCTM
Karen B. Napolitano, MS
Kathleen Maison Paholsky, MS, PhD
Cherie Marilyn Sohnen-Moe, BA
Mary Margaret Tuchscherer, DC, PhD
Richard van Why
Sherri Williamson, LMT
Ed Wilson, PhD, LMT

In addition to the above-mentioned people, there are several who also deserve special recognition for their efforts in the publication of this edition in particular:

Kristen Mandava and her team, for duties and good deeds done too numerous to count

Jim Visser, for the incredible photos and for his energy and enthusiasm during the photo shoots

My son Luke, for his help and encouragement during a long week of taking many photos

Jodie Bernard, for her patience and hard work on the new artwork for this edition

Chris Roider, for his help in reorganizing the DVDs for this edition

Sandy Anderson, for being the go-to on a number of assignments for this edition

MaryAnne Hochadel, for her thorough and important update of the pharmacology appendix

And a special thank you to:

All of the individuals on my support team at Elsevier—especially Kellie White, Jennifer Watrous, Emily Thomson, Kelly Milford, Joe Gramlich, Linda Duncan, Rich Barber, Maggie Reid, Abby Hewitt, and Julie Burchett.

My staff, Roxanne, Dianne, who put up with me during this revision, and to Amy, my assistant, who worked so hard, but even more important, can read my writing.

The athletes I work with for constantly challenging me to figure out what to do with all of their assorted bumps, bruises, sprains, strains, breaks, performance stresses, and personalities.

Last, I would like to acknowledge the University of Michigan Athletic Department, the VA Hospital in Detroit, all the veterans there, and all of the residents and staff at Hospice. And to all the students I have worked with, for keeping me honest and humble.

It truly has been a team effort.

Detailed Contents

CHAPTER 15
Wellness Education, 608

CHAPTER 16
Case Studies, 630

APPENDIX A

APPENDIX B

APPENDIX C

GLOSSARY, 703

INDEX, 715

Therapeutic Massage as a Profession

CHAPTER OBJECTIVES

After completing this chapter, the student will be able to perform the following:

1. Identify personal interpretations of touch and their influence on professional interactions
2. Describe professional touch
3. Explain the rich heritage and history of therapeutic massage
4. Explain the influence of historical events and global culture on the current development of therapeutic massage

CHAPTER OUTLINE

KEY TERMS

Culture
Expressive touch
Healing
Massage
Mechanical touch
Occupation
Patterns
Profession

Professional
Professional touch
Professionalism
Service
System
Therapeutic applications
Touch technique

You are embarking on a journey that will lead you to your goal of becoming a massage professional. You are beginning an active learning process. Three important words were just used to describe how you will proceed with your education:

- *Active* means that you are participating in your education by doing something.
- *Learning* means that you are using experiences to gather and evaluate information, determining its meaning and

value. In addition, you are encoding memory (what you have learned) into a web of nerve connections that makes the information retrievable and usable.
- *Process* means that you are using an ongoing series of actions that produces a measurable and desirable outcome. In this case, the outcome is that you become a highly skilled and knowledgeable massage therapist.

Education is just as much about asking questions as it is about seeking answers. Information accumulated during an educational process, coupled with the ability to formulate insightful and productive questions, gives students the opportunity to make thoughtful decisions. Are decisions answers? Do answers come from thoughtful situational decisions? Are answers valid?

Some questions seem to have easy answers. For example, "What is the color of grass?" Quickly we jump to the answer "green"; however, is that always the correct answer? In the winter, grass is brown. Because many questions can have several answers, validity sometimes can be difficult to determine. In what way is the professional application of touch influenced by the practitioner's ability to make thoughtful decisions and to find answers that best serve the situation at a particular moment? As you read this discussion, you might get the feeling that it is written in circles instead of following a straight line. It may be confusing because one question leads back to another.

One of the many ways your brain learns is by circling around and around through the information, collecting an increased understanding with each revolution. Eventually the understanding begins to turn the circle into a spiral as comprehension leads to creative application (Figure 1-1). In straight line learning, a piece of information is presented once, then the next piece is presented, and then the next, and so on, much like driving down a road from point A to point B. Except for elementary sequential information, straight line learning is not very effective. We do not learn efficiently by experiencing something only once. Even if we go back and repeat the linear A to B sequence again and again, the brain begins to ignore the information because it is too familiar (Figure 1-2).

Repetition is absolutely necessary to learn anything. However, to keep the brain interested, the repetition somehow must be different each time. Think of a piece of music. You can hear the repetition of a melody in a few lines of music, but you can also hear where the composer has changed a note or two. You enjoy hearing the repetition of a good melody, but

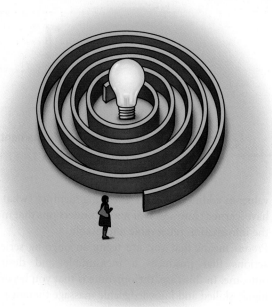

FIGURE 1-1 Spiral learning.

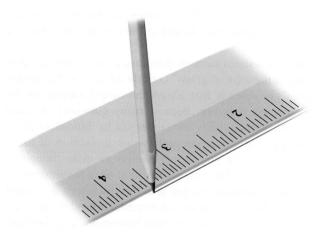

FIGURE 1-2 Straight line learning.

you also enjoy when it is changed slightly, because this prevents you from becoming bored with it. This is called *novel repetition* (Figure 1-3); that is, the same information is given over and over, but always a little differently and in a circular format. As you learn the profession of massage, this type of repetition eventually spirals into the ability to become a creative and skilled massage therapist.

In massage, which is professional, structured, therapeutic touch, education begins with questions.

- What is the significance of touch?
- What is professional touch?
- What motivates me to study therapeutic massage?
- What is therapeutic?
- How am I served by touching others?
- How does the connection with others created through touch influence the professional practice of therapeutic massage?

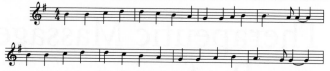

FIGURE 1-3 Novel repetition can be seen and heard in music, for example.

PROFICIENCY EXERCISE 1-1

Look up the words *truth* and *respect*, then develop your own brief definitions of each.

Truth: _____

Respect: _____

- When did touch become professional?
- Why did touch become professional?
- Do therapeutic forms of touch have to be provided by a professional?
- In what way is professional therapeutic touch different from casual touch, friendship touch, family touch, intimate touch, or erotic (sexual) touch?
- How do different individuals, social groups, or cultures view touch?
- In what way does the past affect the present and provide guidance for the future development of the profession of massage therapy?

Questions continue to arise, and the answers are not necessarily simple. As we seek to serve our clients, eventually we are faced with these questions and many others. Some of the questions mentioned previously are explored in this text, especially as they relate to the professional practice of therapeutic massage. Some are not explored directly; rather, both the questions and the answers evolve for each student as the individual's information base and experience increase and the journey through education continues. This text does not provide definitive answers to any of these questions; however, it does provide information to help you find your own answers to questions you may face.

What will your questions be? How will your answers influence those you touch? How will your answers touch you? These are huge issues to consider at the beginning of any course of study. As you begin to think about them, you might feel interested, excited, overwhelmed, or maybe even frightened as you come to realize how necessary, beneficial, complex, and powerful touch can be. Remember that understanding evolves. These important questions are posed at the beginning of this study and possibly before you have sufficient information to develop effective answers. Your awareness of these questions will help you make decisions and find answers as you progress in your study of therapeutic massage.

You will come to understand the process of developing your answers to the previously mentioned questions and many others that will arise by embracing the importance of respect, not only for yourself, but also for all those with whom you interact, both personally and professionally (Proficiency Exercise 1-1).

PROFESSIONAL TOUCH

SECTION OBJECTIVES

Chapter objective covered in this section:

1. The student will be able to identify personal interpretations of touch and their influence on professional interactions.

Using the information presented in this section, the student will be able to perform the following:

- Distinguish between professional and nonprofessional forms of touch
- List factors that influence the communication of touch

A **profession** is defined as an occupation that requires training and specialized study. An **occupation** can be defined as a productive or creative activity that serves as one's regular source of livelihood. A **professional** is a person who engages in a profession. **Professionalism** is the adherence to professional status, methods, standards, and character (see the discussion on ethics in Chapter 2).

To understand the concept of professional touch, we look at specialized training that allows a person to provide a service to another. Professionals may sell a product, but a profession usually is built around a skilled ability to provide a service, such as the professional touch of therapeutic massage. A **service** is something done for another that results in a specific outcome; for example, the car is fixed, the garden is tended, communication skills are taught, emotional problems are sorted out, bodily functions are restored, and spiritual or life paths are discovered. In return, income (livelihood) is received for that service.

When a professional relationship exists, certain agreed-upon criteria apply. The person providing the service is skilled (educated) and operates within certain standards of practice, including technical application and ethical conduct. **Professional touch** is skilled touch delivered to achieve a specific outcome, and the recipient reimburses the professional for services rendered.

The aspect of skilled or schooled touch leads to the idea of structured touch. Professional touch is not random, but purposeful. It is organized according to systems and patterns. A **system** is a group of interacting elements that functions as a complex whole. Professional touch, such as that provided by a massage practitioner, requires education in the many systems of the body; the application of massage and other forms of soft tissue methodology; and an understanding of the influence of massage on body systems. Communication and interpersonal skills, including systems of social and cultural interaction, are also part of the education of the therapeutic massage professional.

Patterns are created by the replication of structures and functions that entwine and influence each other. Patterns can be identified if we can see a big enough picture. The pattern may be missed if the focus is too small. For example, muscle tension can be identified in an individual muscle of the arm, or it can be seen as part of an interacting pattern of movement during walking. The ability to see both the individual segments or pieces and the ways the pieces interact in patterns is a necessary skill for the individual application of professional touch.

| Box 1-1 | How Massage Got Its Name |

> The term *massage* is thought to be derived from several sources. The Latin root *massa* and the Greek roots *massein* and *masso* mean "to touch, handle, squeeze, or knead." The French verb *masser* also means "to knead." The Arabic root *mass* or *mass'h* and the Sanskrit root *makeh* translate as "to press softly."

Inherent in the understanding of skilled and structured touch is the idea of therapeutic application of touch. The term **therapeutic applications** pertains to healing or curative powers. Something that is therapeutic provides the structure for beneficial change or support for current healing practices. A walk in the woods or a conversation with a compassionate friend can be therapeutic. Various bodywork modalities, medical and mental health practices, and empowering spiritual rituals can be therapeutic. **Healing** is the restoration of well-being, and therapeutic applications promote a healing environment.

Touch

Before discussing the historical perspectives of therapeutic massage (professional, structured, therapeutic touch), we need to consider the nature of touch so as to understand the role of professional touch and the evolution of therapeutic massage throughout history. It is important to look at the idea of professionalism in the physical, emotional, social, cultural and, in some instances, spiritual dimensions of touch. The roots of the word *massage* (Box 1-1) concern touch and the various applications of touch. It is important to explore the ideas behind the structure of touch. We must differentiate the therapeutic value of touch in the professional sense from forms of touch shared between people in life circumstances outside the professional environment. These themes are expanded upon throughout this chapter, and in some instances the information is further developed in future chapters.

Science of Touch

Anatomically and physiologically, touch is the collection of tactile sensations that arise from sensory stimulation, primarily of the skin but also of deeper structures of the body, such as the muscles and associated connective tissue.

The skin is an amazing organ. It has many functions, but the most notable for this discussion is its function in touch. The skin is the largest sensory organ of the body. From the outside we are always touched first on our skin, and in many ways, through the skin, we touch ourselves from the inside. Many internal somatic soft tissue structures (e.g., muscles, connective tissue) and visceral structures (e.g., the lungs, heart, and digestive organs) project sensation to the skin (see Chapter 6 for a discussion of viscerally referred pain patterns). The autonomic nervous system (see Chapter 4), which regulates the visceral and chemical homeostasis of the body, is highly responsive to skin stimulation in support of well-being. Mood (the way a person feels) often is reflected in the skin as we touch ourselves from the inside. We blush with embarrassment, flush with excitement, or grow pale with fear.

The anatomy of the skin is described in most comprehensive anatomy texts.* The anatomic parts that make up the skin—the epidermis (top layer), the dermis (inner layer), and the interlacing connective tissues of these layers—and the massive network of nerves both receive and relay information from the central nervous system. This vast network combines with the rich complex of circulatory vessels that supply the skin. Yet, even in their complexity, the anatomy and physiology of the skin cannot explain the experience of touch. In some way, the pressure, vibration, temperature, and muscle motion that move the skin enliven us with sensations and experiences of pleasure, connectedness, joy, pain, sadness, longing, and satisfaction.

We must be touched to survive. Touch is a hunger that must be fed; it is the very essence of our survival, not simply a matter of well-being. The importance of touch has been well described in the books of Ashley Montagu, particularly *Touching: The Human Significance of the Skin,* which is recommended reading for all students of therapeutic massage. Dr. Tiffany Field conducts scientific research on touch at the Touch Research Institute at the University of Miami's Miller School of Medicine, and additional research has been done at various locations (see Chapter 5). Initially much of this research was devoted to infant development, primarily in premature babies. However, Dr. Field has greatly expanded our understanding of the importance of touch by studying many different groups of people, including infants, elderly people, people currently well but under stress, and very ill people. Research supports the belief that touching in a structured way is a very important if not absolute need of all living beings.

Scientific study and technology have enabled us to describe some of the physiologic responses to touch, such as changes in the concentration of hormones, alterations in the activity of the central and peripheral nervous systems, and regulation of body rhythms (these mechanisms are discussed more extensively in later chapters). However, even this explosion of information falls short in helping us understand the experience of touch. For all its scientific interpretations, the experience of touch is much more than the sum of its parts.

The Experience of Touch

Touch often is the concrete experience of more abstract sensations. For example, something that can be seen may not necessarily be real (e.g. watching a movie), but when something can be touched, it is tangible. The concept of tangible is changing. The first edition of this textbook (1995) was available only in the traditional book format. This edition is available in both book and electronic formats. You may have one or the other or both. Is one more real than the other? Interesting question.

You will learn to listen to a client give his or her history and to observe during a physical assessment. However, not until you touch the client and feel the person will you begin to understand that individual's body. The client can sense through your touch if you understand the information the body provides. Touch is a fundamental, multilayered, and powerful form of communication, the most personalized form of communication we know.

Touch as Communication

In many ways touch is a more emotionally powerful form of communication than speech. Verbal communication uses specific words with specific meanings to relay a message. Touch communication is more ambiguous, relying on interpretation of its meaning through past experience and current circumstances. Delivering a clear, concise verbal message is difficult enough when both parties—the one delivering the message and the one receiving it—agree on the meaning of the words. How much more challenging it is to deliver a touch message in which many factors are involved in the interpretation of the message. The potential for misunderstanding increases. Often, with both verbal and touch communication, the message intended is not necessarily the one received.

The communication of touch is influenced by personal, family, and cultural contexts. Each person defines an area around himself or herself as personal space, and the distance encompassed by this personal space differs from person to person and culture to culture. Therapies of touch enter this personal space; therefore, the professional must be sensitive to the various factors that influence people's responses when their personal space is entered. Understanding each person's culture and subculture, personal experiences in that culture, and genetically predetermined tendency to have a large or a small amount of personal space often becomes mind-boggling in designing individual interactions of touch.

Cultural Influences

A **culture** is defined by the arts, beliefs, customs, institutions, and all other products of human work and thought created by a specific group of people at a particular time. To say that people of a certain culture act a certain way is stereotyping; individuals always vary. However, tendencies can be defined by culture, and this may provide a way to begin initial touch interaction until the person's uniqueness is better understood.

Culture is important; yet, it may be considered stereotypical to define a person by his or her culture. We live in a global community. We are likely to interact with people from other parts of the world. Exploring the vast diversity of cultural norms and traditions is beyond the scope of this text. However, as a professional, you are responsible for developing an understanding of the social, cultural, and spiritual ways of the client population you serve while avoiding stereotypes. You can do this in several ways. Begin by doing research at the library or on the Internet about a particular culture. In your practice, observe how clients act and model from their particular cultural background (follow the client's lead). Ask relevant and courteous questions and let your clients teach you about themselves and their culture. Most of all, be open and receptive to what your clients say and make sure you respect your clients' cultures.

---

*The anatomy and physiology of the skin are presented in detail in *Mosby's Essential Sciences for Therapeutic Massage* (2013) by Sandy Fritz.

Gender Issues

Women and men may have different concepts of the appropriateness of touch. The patterns of gender custom in touch are complex. Biology, survival behaviors, social learning, and cultural customs are some of the influences that affect the development of these patterns.

For example, women generally require a somewhat smaller and more permeable personal space for comfort. Until recently, childrearing was the responsibility primarily of women, and child care requires caregivers to enter another's personal space or allow someone to enter theirs without restriction. Men, in general, establish territories with distant boundaries. Personal space is entered by invitation, because the territory must be protected. A man's personal space often is larger and more structured, involving rules for behavior.

Although these gender trends can be viewed from biologic and survival behavior perspectives, the patterns do not necessarily hold true when cultural customs or other influences that affect gender roles or behavior patterns are factored into the equation. Stereotyping of specific behaviors as always feminine or always masculine simply is not accurate. It is important to remember that diversity of expression always exists within biologic influences and the cultural or gender rules of behavior.

Influence of Age on Touch

Age differences can be a factor in the interpretation of touch. Some may consider touching very young people appropriate but may be more cautious about touching older people. A younger person touching an elder may be acceptable, but the dynamics are different when two people of the same age touch. The touch of a young practitioner may be interpreted differently from the touch of an older practitioner, even if the skill and experience levels are equivalent.

Influence of Life Events and the Interpretation of Touch

Life events can influence the response to touch experiences. For example, people who have undergone painful and extensive medical interventions, especially at a young age, may process touch differently from those who have not had these experiences. People who have experienced touch trauma are influenced by those events, and individuals who have experienced isolation respond uniquely to touch. People who grew up with excessive touch stimulation outside the context of trauma (e.g., being part of a large family in small living quarters or being an only child with many adoring family members) may develop certain touch responses. Having a healthy, appropriate touch history also influences a person's interpretation of touch. Any of these experiences and many more affect the way a person understands another's experience of touch.

Spiritual Touch

Touch also can have a spiritual context. Many spiritual rituals incorporate touch, especially those that involve concepts of healing of the body (that which is organic), the mind (that which is of thought), or the spirit (that which is transcendent and sacred). Each person deserves respect for his or her personal truth and individual spiritual path.

Diversity and Touch

Generalities are useless in discussing cultural orientations to touch, because we cannot stereotype all people from a specific culture as holding to similar customs. The same difficulties with stereotyping occur with regard to gender, age, and life or spiritual path. Gender and age influence the interpretation of professional touch, but in just what way varies considerably.

On any given day or even at any given moment, the need, desire, interpretation, and appropriateness of touch given and received can change. These changes occur because a person is in a constant state of flux in responding and adapting to encountered events. The type of relationship between people and its duration influence touch. For example, a first-time client may not be receptive to the deeper pressure required in some applications of massage, especially if the goal of the session does not indicate this type of work. However, if 12 sessions later that same client is experiencing an altered muscle pattern in the back, he may be responsive to touch in that particular form. A client may be ticklish to light touch initially in the session, but after she relaxes somewhat, she may find light stroking pleasurable.

A person's response to and need for the delivery of touch cannot be predetermined. However, each individual, including you, has been influenced by many factors regarding the appropriate procedure for touch and ultimately the interpretation of the meaning of a touch.

As professionals, it is important that we be aware, sensitive, and open to an appreciation of the wide variety of influences that affect professional touch and also that we diligently seek an understanding of our own desires, motivations, and responses to touch After all, it is impossible to touch clients without them in turn touching us. A touch given is at the same time a touch received (Proficiency Exercise 1-2).

PROFESSIONAL CLASSIFICATIONS OF TOUCH

SECTION OBJECTIVES

Chapter objective covered in this section:
2. The student will be able to describe professional touch.
Using the information presented in this section, the student will be able to perform the following:
- Identify factors that constitute appropriate and inappropriate touch in the professional setting
- Discuss two models that illustrate professional touch

Various models have been developed for classifying touch. Touch involves many nuances, forms, and intentions. We will discuss two models for framing professional touch. Model 1 describes professional touch as inappropriate or appropriate using a platform based more on physiology and psychology. Model 2 explores a cultural perspective for understanding professional touch. Each culture and subculture has social rules for what is appropriate and inappropriate touch. Often these social rules are aspects of a particular bodywork system indigenous to that culture. Massage therapy has a

💡 PROFICIENCY EXERCISE 1-2

My Touch History

On a piece of paper, write a brief touch history of yourself. Then explain the ways your history may influence your delivery of professional touch. The following example is provided as a model.

Culture

I grew up in the United States in Michigan. I lived in a small town that was primarily Caucasian.

Subculture

My family was a blue collar, working class family.

Genetic predisposition

I am most comfortable with a large personal space and plenty of time alone.

Gender

Female

Age

Mid-50s

Life events

I experienced touch trauma from a grandfather and uncles, who would tickle me until I could not stand it.

I gave birth to three children and am a single parent.

I had a special friend who was blind.

I had unexpected open heart surgery.

My oldest son was killed in a tragic accident at age 33.

Spiritual path

I initially had an unstructured Protestant focus. I developed a specific fundamentalist path in early adulthood. I embraced many paths as truth in later years as I evolved from the practice of religion to the development of personal spirituality.

Ways my touch history may influence my delivery of professional touch

I had to learn a lot about different cultures, because my exposure to a diverse population was limited while I was growing up. I have to be careful to understand a person's culture before I approach to touch him or her. I am most comfortable with blue collar, working class people. I am more relaxed and find myself willing to spend more time when I touch someone from this population. I feel overwhelmed if I am touched too much and tend to limit initiated touch from the client. I am a woman, and I learned during my gender role development to fulfill others' needs before my own. I often overextend myself for a client instead of setting time limits. I am hypersensitive to light touch and tend to avoid giving light touch when I give a massage. I am understanding of the numerous demands on a single parent and tend to touch one in similar circumstances with sympathy instead of empathy. I have to be careful of boundaries when I touch stressed, overwhelmed single parents. I am casual when touching someone with a disability. I have experienced life-threatening illness, tragedy, and loss. This has changed my life perspective, and if I am not careful, I can discount what may seem to me to be the more minor struggles of others. I seek to understand various spiritual paths and deeply wish to respect issues of touch within each discipline. I tend to assume that one must actually make physical contact during spiritual healing and must remind myself that this is not everyone's truth.

Your Turn—Consider The Following:

Culture

Subculture

Genetic predisposition

Gender

Age

Life events

Spiritual path

Ways my touch history may influence my delivery of professional touch

---

strong historical connection to many different cultures and theoretical perspectives, such as traditional Chinese medicine (TCM), lomi lomi, and ayurveda, and these disciplines describe professional touch similarly. This chapter uses the Eastern chakra philosophy as an example of a platform for professional touch.

Model 1: Physical and Psychological Perspectives on Professional Touch

When a person is touched, energy is received and internalized. Professional touch is not overtly an act of exerting power. Although the ability to receive touch is powerful, the difference in the power base between those who give touch and those who receive it must be considered. This interplays with the appropriateness or inappropriateness of touch. Careful attention must be paid during professional touch if the issue of power is to be managed appropriately

Forms of Inappropriate Touch

Inappropriate touch in some way devalues the individual receiving the touch. This type of touch intention is often based on some sort of internal conflict in the individual doing the touching. Inappropriate touch of any kind is not to be allowed in a professional setting. The three forms of inappropriate touch in massage therapy are hostile or aggressive touch, erotic (sexual) touch, and invasive touch.

Hostile or Aggressive Touch

Hostile or aggressive touch occurs when a potential for conflict or a power struggle exists. Professionals who use touch need to be aware of the underlying energy directed toward the client to prevent this intention in the touch. The obvious is easy: if you are angry with a client, it is best not to touch at that moment. Likewise, if a client is angry with you, it is best not to touch until the energy changes. A more subtle aspect is the undercurrent of conflict. For example, the client may arrive late for the appointment, or the massage therapist may be hurried or angry about something at home. In these cases, the practitioner inadvertently may be more aggressive than necessary during the massage.

The perception that one holds power over another underlies hostile or aggressive touch. Careful attention must be paid to this idea of power in the therapeutic relationship between the professional and the client. In the professional relationship, a power difference between the professional and the client exists simply because of the knowledge base that defines the profession. Knowledge is power, and most of the time the professional knows more about the service rendered than the client does.

In body therapies such as therapeutic massage, the client's physical position often creates an environment that fosters a power differential. Clients usually lie down or are seated, and the professional is physically above the client, generating the impression of authority.

During massage we need to sustain a focus to be aware of how and where the client's body is being touched and the client's perceptions of the touch. There is a difference for clients between submitting to and enduring a massage and receiving and integrating a massage. The massage environment also can influence the perception of the massage. An environment (including the staff) that may be harsh appears hostile. A location in an area considered unsafe, or an office in which the background noise includes sirens from emergency vehicles, arguments, or gossiping will diminish the ability of the client and the therapist to relax.

Erotic (Sexual) Touch

The intention of erotic, or sexual, touch is sexual arousal and expression. The issue of erotic touch cannot be sidestepped in the study of massage therapy or any other body-oriented treatment in which touch is a primary aspect of the therapy. Complex physiologic, mental, and spiritual aspects of both the client and the practitioner influence the ideas of erotic touch.

The pleasure of being touched is inherent in many forms of massage and bodywork. Pleasure is an important therapeutic tool. In later chapters you will learn that chemicals in the body create pleasure moods, and feelings of connectedness increase during massage. These chemical responses are one of the main causes of the therapeutic benefit of massage methods. Constant attention must be paid to the appropriate understanding and interpretation of the feelings generated during professional touch so that pleasurable touch does not evolve into or become misinterpreted as erotic touch.

Not only in body-oriented therapies, but also in psychotherapy and other health care disciplines, it is not uncommon for professionals occasionally to have sexual feelings in the context of the professional environment. Professionals are people with complex, intertwined needs, desires, and means of expressing themselves. However, it is inappropriate for professionals to foster any type of erotic feelings with a client, either within the therapeutic environment or outside that environment. Erotic feelings should never be expressed with clients.

Invasive Touch

Invasive touch can be both intentional and unintentional. As a massage professional, you are responsible for understanding personal and cultural rules about where and when to touch.

Different areas of the body reflect different tactile issues. Studies show some agreement about areas of the body that are more sensitive, or "charged," in terms of emotion or erotic interpretation. The more emotionally or physically charged a body area is, the more the person may feel insecure, anxious, fearful, threatened, connected emotionally, intimate, or aroused when touched in that area.

Some body areas are considered taboo, or "do not touch" zones, in terms of professional therapeutic massage touch.

Orifices, including the anus, genitals, mouth, ears, and nose, are most taboo in most societies. The ventral, or front, surfaces of the body, including the breasts, are more charged than the dorsal surfaces. We see this pattern in massage; much of the massage session is devoted to the back of the torso and the legs while the client is lying face down, with the front of the body "protected" by the massage table. Therapeutically, this creates difficulties, because soft tissue dysfunction also occurs on the front of the body, where sensations of touch are more apt to elicit emotional responses and feelings of vulnerability.

The trunk of the body is more charged than the limbs. For this reason, a client may feel more comfortable having the legs and arms massaged than the torso. However, this does not always hold true; often the least intrusive form of touch is laying a hand on a person's upper back near the shoulder, whereas having the hands massaged can feel very intimate and connected.

The head also is an area sensitive to touch. Although children often are touched on the head and face, adults seldom are touched casually in these areas. Adults often respond emotionally to touching of the face and head.

Areas of a person's body that have experienced trauma (e.g., accidents or surgery) carry more emotional charge and therefore are more sensitive to interpretation of the appropriateness of touch.

The appropriateness or inappropriateness of touch, then, is about when, how, and with what intent we touch (Lederman, 1997).

Forms of Appropriate Touch

Nontherapeutic forms of touch that people often encounter include inadvertent touch, such as when people are jostled together in an elevator, and socially stereotyped touch, which involves highly ritualized touch that carries a consensual meaning within a culture, such as a handshake.

Therapeutic forms of touch involve touch that communicates information or that expresses feeling as part of the therapeutic relationship. This form of touch is not so much about creating a specific outcome as it is about delivering information or expressing comfort or understanding (Smith et al., 1998). Some examples of this type of touch are touching a client's shoulder to direct him to the massage room or holding a client's hand as she thanks you for the session.

Touch Technique

Touch technique is the basis of therapeutic massage methods. Touch is the tool for massage. Massage is the use of various forms of touch to achieve a specific outcome. This type of touch can be considered technical touch. In terms of touch technique, a therapeutic intent exists. The intention of touch therapy can be classified in two ways:

- Mechanical touch, which is used to achieve a specific anatomic or physiologic outcome (e.g., using massage to increase the range of motion of the shoulder)
- Expressive touch, which is used to support and convey awareness and empathy for the client as a whole person (e.g., using massage for general relaxation and pleasure

Evolve Activity 1-2

to comfort a client after a particularly hard day at work) (Lederman, 1997)

The professional's choices of the type of therapeutic intention influence the interpretation of touch. A client with a mechanical restriction in the shoulder might find a more expressive form of touch uncomfortable, because it might feel too intimate for the circumstances. Stressed, overworked clients may find a mechanical approach distant and impersonal, because they are seeking empathy and understanding along with physical changes.

As we develop as professionals, both forms of touch technique must be perfected. Mechanical touch skills increase as we learn anatomy, physiology, record keeping, and effective delivery of specific forms of massage (these topics are covered throughout the textbook). Development of the expressive form of touch technique is more complex and involves the professional's personal growth, interpersonal and communication skills, and understanding of his or her own life experiences.

Model 2: Cultural Perspectives on Professional Touch

Cultural perspectives are another way to understand the intangibles of massage and appropriate and inappropriate touch in the professional setting. Massage therapy has a strong historical connection to many different cultures and theoretical perspectives.

Chakra System

The second model describing the concepts of touch appropriateness is based on consciousness levels; this model is represented by the theory of the Eastern chakra system. Seven chakras, or energy centers, are located along the trunk of the body (Figure 1-4). This particular model demonstrates how

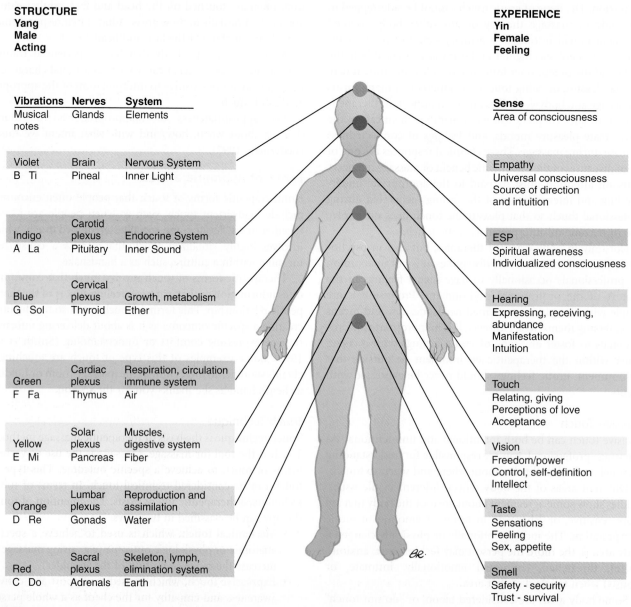

STRUCTURE
Yang
Male
Acting

Vibrations	Nerves	System
Musical notes	Glands	Elements
Violet	Brain	Nervous System
B Ti	Pineal	Inner Light
Indigo	Carotid plexus	Endocrine System
A La	Pituitary	Inner Sound
Blue	Cervical plexus	Growth, metabolism
G Sol	Thyroid	Ether
Green	Cardiac plexus	Respiration, circulation immune system
F Fa	Thymus	Air
Yellow	Solar plexus	Muscles, digestive system
E Mi	Pancreas	Fiber
Orange	Lumbar plexus	Reproduction and assimilation
D Re	Gonads	Water
Red	Sacral plexus	Skeleton, lymph, elimination system
C Do	Adrenals	Earth

EXPERIENCE
Yin
Female
Feeling

Sense
Area of consciousness
Empathy
Universal consciousness Source of direction and intuition
ESP
Spiritual awareness Individualized consciousness
Hearing
Expressing, receiving, abundance Manifestation Intuition
Touch
Relating, giving Perceptions of love Acceptance
Vision
Freedom/power Control, self-definition Intellect
Taste
Sensations Feeling Sex, appetite
Smell
Safety - security Trust - survival

FIGURE 1-4 Names and locations of major chakras.

historical, cultural, and spiritual factors dictate appropriate touch. The physical location of the chakras correlates with the autonomic nervous system plexuses. As you will learn later, the autonomic nervous system is involved with the expression of behavior. This connection begins to identify the physical (body) and emotional (mind) influence of function.

Traditionally, the base, or first, chakra pertains to survival, security, and safety. The second chakra concerns pleasure experiences of sensuality and sexuality. The third chakra involves power and control. These lower chakras are transcended by the fourth (heart) chakra, which is the center of nonjudgmental love. The heart chakra is the pivot point between the lower three chakras and the upper, more spiritual chakras. The fifth chakra is the throat center, which is concerned with communication and creativity. The sixth (brow) chakra concerns the reflection of the total or essential self. The seventh (crown) chakra reflects the transcended and spiritual self.

According to the chakra model, the intention of professional touch does not come from the lower chakra energies and needs, because the energies of these chakras can be equated with types of inappropriate touch (hostile, aggressive, and erotic), and the potential for misinterpretation and manipulation is greater. The intention of professional touch projects from the fourth through seventh chakras, which support nonjudgmental love and respect for each person's individual mode of expressing the sense of self and sacredness.

Inspiration

Inspiration can be thought of as being directed to the "right" path. The source of this direction takes many forms, but the outcome is the same—motivation. Inspiration occurs when a certain combination of ideas suddenly reveals a simple underlying pattern. When this occurs, a person typically has an intellectual, emotional, and physical response, often resulting in clarity and motivation to bring ideas into tangible form. We seem to be wired to see the pattern and make sense of it.

Inspiration is difficult to explain but simple to know because it enlivens us and creates passion and energy. Inspiration is the big picture, and in its simplicity the complicated becomes uncomplicated. It is kind of like a cookie. The cookie is the whole; the flour, sugar, eggs, butter, and vanilla are the components. There is no cookie until these components are combined and baked. Being inspired can be likened to a spiritual (not religious) experience; that is, a moment of clear knowing and understanding resulting in a deep sense of peace. More than the "aha" moment or gut feeling of intuition, inspiration is the beginning of purpose. Inspiration typically takes the form of a vision of wholeness of an end result.

Intention

Intention is knowing what you want; knowing comes from inspiration. For example, if you are shopping for a red ribbon, you eventually will find it because you are focused on it. We have all experienced a moment when we find what we are looking for; however, you have to know what it is you seek. If you have been inspired to be a massage therapist, then you will seek skills and knowledge (i.e., find a teacher and a school). The same process occurs in building a massage clientele. If you are inspired to work with a specific group, such as the military, first responders, or the elderly, you will seek what you need to build the practice.

Intuition

Intuition is the conscious awareness of the collected and integrated subconscious information that is processed through the environment, experience, and circumstances. We have all experienced an intuitive thought to give someone a call, and when we do, the person says, "I was hoping you would call." Intuition, sometimes called "gut instinct," is an important guide. The intuitive process is more concrete than it appears. Although science does not completely understand the phenomenon, there is little doubt that intuition is an aspect of survival mechanisms. With development, intuition can become a valuable source of information for important personal and professional decision making. You can experience intuition as a feeling, a gut reaction, images that recur, a dream, or an internal voice with a message. You must figure out how your inner self communicates with your conscious self.

Touch Intention During Massage

The touch intention of therapeutic massage closely fits with both models except in the area of pleasure and safety. Many seek massage because it feels good, and these pleasure needs project from the second chakra. The importance of this pleasure factor and the interpretation of the meaning of the experience for clients can blur the boundaries of the professional relationship. It is important to recognize the value of therapeutic massage in meeting nonsexual pleasure goals, because pleasure sensation supports a balance of neuroendocrine functions that affect mood.

As massage therapists, we also need to consider a client's sense of safety and security, projected from the first chakra. We can make sure a client feels secure on the massage table by demonstrating that the table is strong and stable. We need to assure clients of privacy verbally, through the use of proper draping, and a touch application that does no harm to them.

Touch intention projected from the sixth and seventh chakras also is an important consideration. Interacting professionally with the essential self (the sixth chakra) requires extensive training in mental health, which can provide expertise in the development of the essential self. Touch that influences the transcendent or spiritual self requires the discipline to walk any of the many spiritual paths. Commitment to this training prepares one to provide support that leads to understanding of the transcendent self.

Dual Roles

Professional energy focused from these areas can lead to dual roles for the massage professional. Dual or multiple roles occur when a professional operates from many bases of knowledge when interacting with clients therapeutically. The main concern with dual roles is the distribution of power in the therapeutic relationship. The more roles a professional plays with a client, the more power the professional acquires in the therapeutic relationship. A client can easily come to feel disempowered with professionals who work from dual or multiple roles. This disempowerment can manifest in various forms, including anger ("You're the expert, so you should have known"), a submissive attitude ("The professional knows best"), or excessive admiration ("No one is as gifted as you").

The development of professional expertise in more than one role requires devotion to acquiring the knowledge encompassed by several areas. As you begin to study massage therapy, you soon will realize that you could study for a lifetime just within the massage knowledge base and not absorb all the information available. Expecting a person to operate effectively as a professional in several areas may be unrealistic, because each of those areas also reflects a lifetime of experience and study.

A generalized knowledge of different areas of expertise and several forms of intervention adds to professional development. It can be helpful in fostering professional relationships with other professionals and in recognizing when a client can best be served by another discipline. However, developing expertise in several areas can become overwhelming.

Professional touch provided through therapeutic massage, coupled with an understanding of the various needs and diversity of the population we serve, is complex enough in itself. I often feel as if there is too much to know, and I can imagine the feeling of being overwhelmed that frequently besets a beginning student. It is important in professional development to honor personal and professional limits and to set appropriate personal and professional boundaries. When touch is the primary treatment method, it is even more important to understand the interpersonal dynamics of the therapeutic relationship. (Professional boundaries are discussed further in Chapter 2.)

Uniqueness of Touch

A specific touch experience is difficult to replicate, because it is extremely multifaceted. The interaction between two individuals is unique. Students often ask instructors to demonstrate a method on them so that they know how it feels. Although this is a good learning experience, it is somewhat limited in that the feeling cannot be replicated with a different touching pair.

Students or fellow practitioners may tell an instructor about a client's situation and ask for recommendations. Sometimes this is difficult for the instructor. Although instructors usually can give information about the pathology or a technical description of various methodologies, they really do not know in what way they would do a massage until they touch that particular client. If the instructor actually touches the student's client in a professional teaching session, the client's experience of the instructor's touch and the student's touch does not end up being the same, even if both use the same method. The instructor's interaction through touch is no more right than that of the student; rather, the unique quality of the touch experience makes the difference.

When an instructor demonstrates a method of massage, this touch often is developed through experience. The person receiving the massage probably notices the difference in the touch, not the method, when the student attempts to replicate the instructor's actions because the experience level is different. The confidence of experience is displayed not so much in the expert execution of the methods as in the quality of the touch in delivering those methods.

Subjective and Objective Qualities of Touch

Writing a textbook mostly involves the dispensing of objective (fact-based) information and is separate from the author's personal, subjective experiences. Each person who reads the information in a textbook incorporates the skills and information as tools and resources in his or her own experience. Most of this text is written objectively. However, ideas on the experience of touch are so subjective in interpretation and experience that presenting concepts of touch only through objective data seems impossible. The authors of the books used as references in this section have not been able to accomplish this objectification of touch, either. Something expansive and abstract about the simple, concrete experience of touch transcends technical writing. The experience of touching and being touched seems to extend beyond words and verbalization, beyond the skin, nervous system, and endocrine system, to the soul.

As this section concludes, and we begin building the foundation for using touch in a therapeutic and professional way, it seems appropriate to reflect personally on touch needs.

I know that I need to be touched, and I know what happens to me when I am not touched enough or when the touch does not satisfy me because it is not safe touch or because it is needy touch that requires me to extend energy to someone else. When those with whom I can share or experience safe touch (my close family and friends, my pets, my woods, and my massage therapist) are unavailable, I become out of sorts and moody, my back hurts, I don't sleep as well, and I find myself involved in substitute behavior, such as eating, that attempts to feed my touch hunger.

When I'm alone, on good days I experience my own sense of touch through exercise and the enjoyment of tactile sensation, such as from my flannel sheets or from listening to music. However, these forms of self-touch lack body contact with another, and often touch longings are not satisfied unless they are shared with another living being, such as holding my dogs in my lap or cuddling with my granddaughter on the couch.

On not so good days, I overeat or use other excessive and detrimental forms of sensory stimulation. The excessiveness of the behavior is somewhat like trying to be satisfied with a carrot stick when you really crave vanilla pudding. It takes lots of carrots to fill me up, but I am still not satisfied. Then, when I finally give in to the vanilla pudding, I eat the whole box instead of the indicated serving. It is because I feel starved, beyond physical need, and I am operating in realms of emotional and maybe spiritual longing. Even more, this substitution behavior never really fulfills the desire. I still feel touch-deprived and unsatisfied after the physiologic effects of the behavior (substituting food) wear off. No matter how many times I try to use them as substitutes, neither food nor exercise can replace the real need to be touched by *someone who cares.*

The desire for physical contact is an instinctive and physiologic need for well-being. Professional therapeutic touch often feeds touch hunger for people in a safe, professional environment. Massage professionals serve others by providing touch. If we are going to be able to provide this type of touch experience for others, how do we take care of our personal touch needs? What happens to you if your hunger for safe, nurturing (nutritious) touch is not met?

It is important for massage professionals to embrace the expansive, abstract experience of touch. No one really cares how much you know until they know how much you care. The concrete experience of caring most often is conveyed through touch. That knowing, or "felt sense," experienced by both the client and the practitioner often is internalized through professional touch. We must show our willingness as practitioners to be open personally to sharing the experience with the client, at the same time being professional enough to respect the client and maintain the focus of the experience for the individual. To do this, each of us who uses touch professionally must be aware of self-care, and we must develop resources and support people (and pets and plants) who touch us in a safe, respectful, and healing way (Proficiency Exercise 1-3).

PROFICIENCY EXERCISE 1-3

In the space provided, answer the following questions.
1. What do I do when I am touch hungry?

2. Who and what touches me in a safe, respectful, and healing way?

HISTORICAL PERSPECTIVES

SECTION OBJECTIVES

Chapter objective covered in this section:
3. The student will be able to explain the rich heritage and history of therapeutic massage.
Using the information presented in this section, the student will be able to perform the following:
• Trace the general progression of massage from ancient times to today

To understand professional, structured, therapeutic touch, the student must explore historical influences and the evolution of massage from its ancient foundations through projections for the future (Figure 1-5).

A knowledge of history helps massage therapists develop a sense of professional identity and pride in their profession. Historical perspectives help members of a profession identify the profession's strengths and weaknesses. As students of massage read historical books about massage, they discover that the fundamental body of knowledge has changed little over the centuries. The most prevalent concepts in massage today in fact were written about many years ago. Massage has stood the test of time, proving itself a vital, health-enhancing

technique and a rehabilitative discipline. Curre... sion is at a defining moment; it is growing in ac... in support based on valid scientific evidence. In ... beginning massage professionals will learn from our h... events.

Many people have played important roles in tracing t... historic journey of therapeutic massage and bodywork methods. Many of these resources and people are listed on the Evolve website. Specific acknowledgment must be given to Richard van Why, who compiled the Bodywork Knowledgebase, a collection of more than 100 historical books and more than 4000 research and journal articles on therapeutic massage and related methods. Much of the information in this chapter comes from this work. If it were not for van Why's diligence, much of the history of massage would be scattered in research libraries and would be unknown to us today. Another who deserves mention is Fran Tappan, a true master of massage who wrote respected textbooks that include a historical perspective about massage.

This chapter consolidates historical information about massage. Because the references used overlap extensively, text citation has been kept to a minimum. With gratitude and respect for those who have devoted their lives to compiling this history, both those mentioned and the many more who are not, let us begin the journey by looking to the past.

History of Massage

Certain animal behavior, such as the application of pressure, rubbing, and licking, indicates that massage is used instinctively to relieve pain, to respond to injury, and for comfort. Massage has always been one of the most natural and instinctive means of relieving pain and discomfort. When a person has sore, aching muscles, abdominal pain, a bruise or a wound, the impulse is to touch and rub that part of the body to obtain relief.

Touch as a method of healing appears to have numerous cultural origins (see Box 1-1). Therapeutic massage has strong roots in Chinese folk medicine, but it also has many aspects in common with other healing traditions, such as Indian herbal medicine and Persian medicine. The art of massage is believed to have been first mentioned in writing around 2000 BC (Tappan and Benjamin, 2004), and it has been discussed extensively in books since about 500 BC The historical medical literatures of Egypt, Persia, and Japan are full of references to massage. The Greek physician Hippocrates advocated massage and gymnastic exercise. Asclepiades, another eminent Greek physician, relied exclusively on massage in his practice.

Throughout history, many different systems and supporting theories for management of musculoskeletal pain and dysfunction have come and gone. In each case, the scientific thinking of the day provided the validation for massage. Over the years, scientific research has changed the philosophy of massage theory and current research continues to further define the physical effects of therapeutic massage. Trends today show an increase in popularity of massage and body-related therapies for stress reduction and chronic musculoskeletal pain.

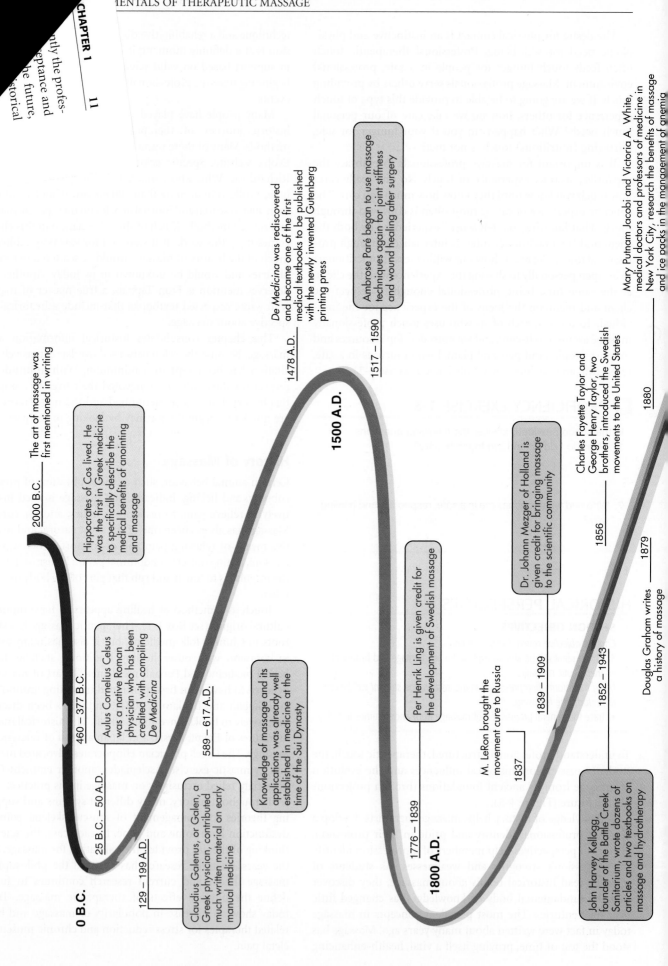

2000 B.C. — The art of massage was first mentioned in writing

460 – 377 B.C. — Hippocrates of Cos lived. He was the first in Greek medicine to specifically describe the medical benefits of anointing and massage

25 B.C. – 50 A.D. — Aulus Cornelius Celsus was a native Roman physician who has been credited with compiling *De Medicina*

129 – 199 A.D. — Claudius Galenus, or Galen, a Greek physician, contributed much written material on early manual medicine

589 – 617 A.D. — Knowledge of massage and its applications was already well established in medicine at the time of the Sui Dynasty

1478 A.D. — *De Medicina* was rediscovered and became one of the first medical textbooks to be published with the newly invented Gutenberg printing press

1517 – 1590 — Ambrose Paré began to use massage techniques again for joint stiffness and wound healing after surgery

1776 – 1839 — Per Henrik Ling is given credit for the development of Swedish massage

1837 — M. LeRon brought the movement cure to Russia

1839 – 1909 — Dr. Johann Mezger of Holland is given credit for bringing massage to the scientific community

1856 — Charles Fayette Taylor and George Henry Taylor, two brothers, introduced the Swedish movements to the United States

1852 – 1943 — John Harvey Kellogg, founder of the Battle Creek Sanitarium, wrote dozens of articles and two textbooks on massage and hydrotherapy

1879 — Douglas Graham writes a history of massage

1880 — Mary Putnam Jacobi and Victoria A. White, medical doctors and professors of medicine in New York City, research the benefits of massage and ice packs in the management of anemia

0 B.C.   0

1500 A.D.

1800 A.D.

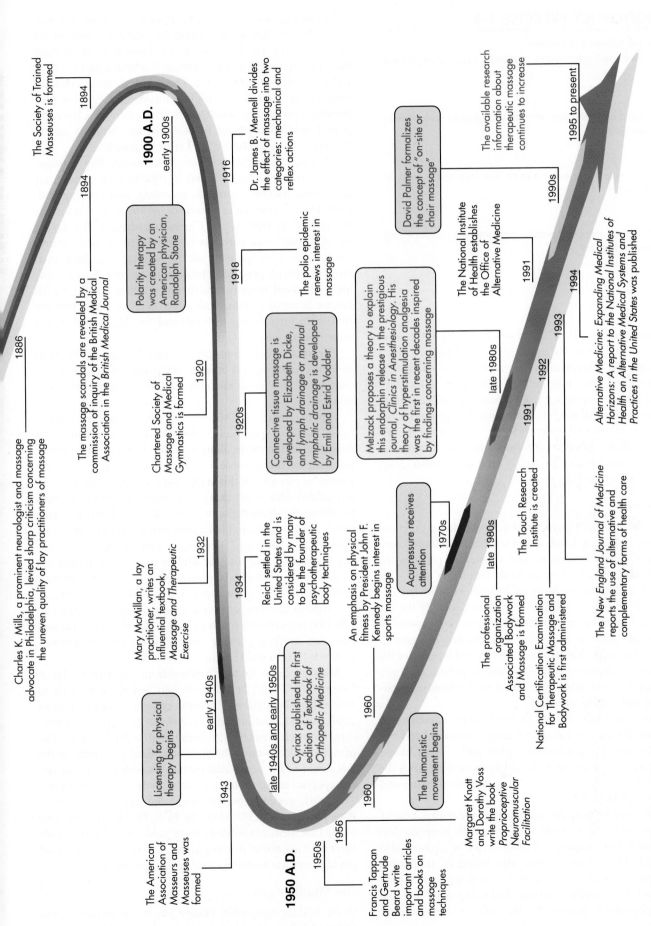

FIGURE 1-5 Historical time line of massage.

The Society of Trained Masseuses is formed — 1894

Charles K. Mills, a prominent neurologist and massage advocate in Philadelphia, levied sharp criticism concerning the uneven quality of lay practitioners of massage — 1886

The massage scandals are revealed by a commission of inquiry of the British Medical Association in the *British Medical Journal* — 1894

1900 A.D. early 1900s

Polarity therapy was created by an American physician, Randolph Stone

Dr. James B. Mennell divides the effect of massage into two categories: mechanical and reflex actions — 1916

The polio epidemic renews interest in massage — 1918

Chartered Society of Massage and Medical Gymnastics is formed — 1920

Mary McMillan, a lay practitioner, writes an influential textbook, *Massage and Therapeutic Exercise* — 1932

Connective tissue massage is developed by Elizabeth Dicke, and *lymph drainage* or *manual lymphatic drainage* is developed by Emil and Estrid Vodder — 1920s

Reich settled in the United States and is considered by many to be the founder of psychotherapeutic body techniques — 1934

The American Association of Masseurs and Masseuses was formed — early 1940s

Licensing for physical therapy begins — 1943

Cyriax published the first edition of *Textbook of Orthopedic Medicine* — late 1940s and early 1950s

An emphasis on physical fitness by President John F. Kennedy begins interest in sports massage — 1960

Acupressure receives attention — 1970s

1950 A.D. 1950s

Francis Tappan and Gertrude Beard write important articles and books on massage techniques — 1950s

Margaret Knott and Dorothy Voss write the book *Proprioceptive Neuromuscular Facilitation* — 1956

The humanistic movement begins — 1960

The professional organization Associated Bodywork and Massage is formed — late 1980s

The Touch Research Institute is created — late 1980s

National Certification Examination for Therapeutic Massage and Bodywork is first administered — 1991

Melzack proposes a theory to explain this endorphin release in the prestigious journal, *Clinics in Anesthesiology*. His theory of hyperstimulation analgesia was the first in recent decades inspired by findings concerning massage

The National Institute of Health establishes the Office of Alternative Medicine — 1991

David Palmer formalizes the concept of "on-site or chair massage" — 1990s

The available research information about therapeutic massage continues to increase — 1995 to present

The *New England Journal of Medicine* reports the use of alternative and complementary forms of health care — 1992

Alternative Medicine: Expanding Medical Horizons: A report to the National Institutes of Health on Alternative Medical Systems and Practices in the United States was published — 1994

1993

💡 PROFICIENCY EXERCISE 1-4

Answer the following questions:

1. If you were going to rename massage, what would you call it?

2. If touch is so instinctive, why do you have to go to school to learn to do it?

3. Why do you think every culture has had some form of massage?

4. What do you think is the difference between massage and manual medicine?

Manual medicine, which has always been part of the art of medicine, is the use of the hands in the treatment of injury and disease. Its therapeutic value comes from changes in soft tissue and structure rather than from surgery or pharmaceuticals (Greenman, 2003). Massage can be considered a part of manual medicine, although throughout history it also has functioned independently to promote health. Manual medicine provides the foundation for osteopathy, chiropractic, and physical therapy (Cantu and Grodin, 2001) (Proficiency Exercise 1-4).

Ancient Times

According to research reports, most ancient cultures practiced some form of healing touch. Often a ceremonial leader, such as a healer, priest, or shaman, was selected to perform the healing rituals. The healing methods frequently used were herbs, oils, and primitive forms of hydrotherapy. Archaeologists have found many prehistoric artifacts depicting the use of massage for healing and cosmetic purposes. Some speculate that massage used for pain relief incorporated concepts of counterirritation, such as scraping, cutting, and burning of the skin, as part of the process. Massage may have been used as a cleansing procedure, along with fasting and bathing, in preparation for many tribal rituals.

In China, massage has been known by three names: *anmo* and *amma*, the ancient names, meaning "press-rub," and *tuina*, of more recent origin, meaning "push-pull." These Chinese methods were administered by kneading or rubbing down the entire body with the hands and using a gentle pressure and traction on all the joints.

The practice of acupuncture involved the stimulation of specific points along the body, usually done by inserting tiny, solid needles, but massage and other forms of pressure also were used. Such practices were also found in traditional Eskimo and African medicine, in which sharp stones were used to scratch the skin's surface. Today, scientists are able to give physiologic reasons for the value of these ancient practices.

Knowledge of massage and its applications already was well established in Chinese medicine at the time of the Sui dynasty (A.D. 589-617). The Japanese came to know massage through the writings of the Chinese. Massage has been a part of life in India for almost 3000 years. The Chinese introduced the methods in India during trading forays. Like Chinese acupuncture, hatha yoga, which was developed in India, has reappeared in modern forms of body therapy, with its energy concepts of prana, chakras, and energy balance.

The ancient Egyptians left artwork showing foot massage. Before Greek athletes took part in the Olympic games, they underwent friction treatment, anointing, and rubbing with sand. The use of touch as a mode of healing is recorded in the writings of the Hebrew and Christian traditions. The "laying on of hands" was particularly prominent in first-century Christianity. Massage with oils (anointing) goes back even farther in Jewish practices. The ancient Jews practiced anointing for its ritual, hygienic, and therapeutic benefits. The Jewish culture honored rubbing with oils to such an extent that the root word for rubbing with oils and for the Messiah is the same *(ma-shi-ah)*.

The ancient Mayan people of Central America, the Incas of South America, and other native people of the American continents also used methods of joint manipulation and massage.

Hippocrates of Cos (460-377 BC) was the first physician in Greek medicine specifically to describe the medical benefits of anointing and massage, along with the chemical properties of oils used for this purpose. He called his art *anatripsis*, which means "to rub up." Of this art he said, "The physician must be acquainted with many things and assuredly with anatripsis, for things that have the same name have not always the same effects, for rubbing can bind a joint that is too loose or loosen a joint that is too hard." Hippocrates' methods survived virtually unchanged well into the Middle Ages. Many techniques similar to those methods, especially traction and stretching principles, are still in use today (Cantu and Grodin 2001).

Claudius Galenus, or Galen, another Greek physician (AD 129-199), contributed much written material on early manual medicine, including many commentaries on Hippocrates' methods (Cantu and Grodin 2001).

Massage came to the Romans from the Greeks. Julius Caesar (100-44 BC) had himself "pinched all over" daily to relieve his neuralgia and prevent epileptic attacks (Tappan 2004). Aulus Cornelius Celsus (25 BC-AD 50), a Roman physician, has been credited with compiling *De Medicina*, a series of eight books covering the body of medical knowledge of the day. Seven of the books deal extensively with prevention and therapeutics using rubbing, exercise, bathing, and anointing. This work was rediscovered during the late Middle Ages by Pope Nicholas V (1397-1455). In 1478, *De Medicina* was one of the first medical textbooks to be published with the newly invented Gutenberg printing press. It was one of the most popular medical textbooks during the Renaissance.

The Middle Ages

In the Middle Ages, while Europe was mired in superstition and feudal chaos, the Islamic countries became the intellectual center of the world. The *Canon of Medicine* is a 14-volume medical encyclopedia written by Persian scientist and physician Avicenna, (Ibn Sina, 981-1037) as he was known in the West. Avicenna's real name was Abu-Ali Husayn lbn-Abdullah Ibn-Sina. Ibn Sina completed the canon of medicine in 1025. The book was based on a combination of Islamic medicine, the writings of the Roman physician Galen, Chinese materia medica, and many other sources from the time period. The canon is considered one of the most famous books in the history of medicine and remained a medical authority up until the 18th and early 19th century. Ibn Sina described evidence-based medicine and the importance of research, both of which are important topics in the massage profession today. He is regarded as a pioneer of aromatherapy for his invention of steam distillation and extraction of essential oils (Leon 2002, Isham Ismail 2006, Masic et al, 2008).

Massage developed differently in the East and the West. In the East, as part of the Islamic empire, it represented a continuation of Greco-Roman traditions. In the West, the Greco-Roman traditions disappeared, but massage was kept alive by the common people and became part of folk culture. In this form, massage was an important part of the healing tradition of the Slavs, Finns, and Swedes. As massage was integrated into the health practices of the common people, it often was associated with supernatural experiences and observances. This association alienated massage from what little scientific approach there was during this time. Practitioners of folk medicine often were persecuted, and the Church claimed that the practitioner's healing powers came from the devil.

Not until the sixteenth century did massage regain its respectability in Europe. One of the founders of modern surgery, the French physician Ambrose Paré (1517-1590) began to use massage techniques again for joint stiffness and wound healing after surgery. In his work Paré described three types of massage strokes: gentle, medium, and vigorous. His ideas were passed down to other French physicians who believed in the value of manual therapeutics.

Nineteenth Century

Per Henrik Ling

Per Henrik Ling (1776-1839) often is credited with developing Swedish massage, but he did not invent it. The term "Swedish massage" is inaccurate; the more appropriate name is classical massage. Ling proposed an integrated program for the treatment of disease using active and passive movements; he called this program Swedish gymnastic movements. The curriculum of the Royal Central Gymnastic Institute founded by Ling in 1813 did not teach massage as we know it. Legend has it that Ling's interest in these methods was sparked by the gout in his own elbow. He developed a system that used many of the positions and movements of Swedish gymnastics, and in so doing, he healed his diseased elbow. Ling's program was based on the newly discovered knowledge of the circulation of the blood and lymph. (Interestingly, the Chinese had been using these methods for centuries.)

While teaching fencing, Ling observed that habitual movements interfered with the development of desired movements. He determined that the development of a skill depended on the mental mastery of habit; therefore, he began teaching bodily movements systematically. He developed his medical gymnastics in 1813, but his methods were bitterly opposed by the Swedish medical establishment for almost 20 years. He was not trained in medicine, and his tendency to use poetic and mystic language in his writings on gymnastics was thought to interfere with wider acceptance of his ideas. Current experts in massage would be wise to take note of Ling's experience; it is essential that massage be explained in the medical and scientific terminology of the day.

In his system, Ling divided movements into active, duplicated, and passive forms. Active movements were performed by the person's own effort; these movements correspond to what commonly is called exercise. Duplicated movements were performed by the person with the cooperation of a gymnast (therapist); they involved active effort by both parties in which the action of the one was opposed by the action of the other. Duplicated movements correspond to what today is commonly called resistive exercise. Passive movements were performed for the person by the active effort of the gymnast alone. They consisted of passive movements of the extremities, which today we call range of motion work and stretching.

Ling taught many physicians from Germany, Austria, Russia, and England, who spread his teachings to their own countries. He was recognized by his contemporaries and later followers not so much as a great innovator, but rather as a keen observer who adopted methods only after testing their effectiveness. He combined many techniques into one coherent system. By the time of Ling's death in 1839, his system had achieved worldwide recognition.

Modern Revival of Massage

Per Henrik Ling and others who practiced the Swedish movement cure deserve credit for reviving massage after the Middle Ages. Initially, nonprofessionals spoke to physicians in a language they did not share, which made communication difficult. Dr. Johann Mezger of Holland (1839-1909) is credited with bringing massage to the scientific community. He presented massage to fellow physicians as a form of medical treatment. The French terms *effleurage, pétrissage,* and *tapotement* were not used by Ling. Mezger's followers in Holland began to use these names, although historical references do not explain why French terms were chosen. So often history is confusing, and the issue of who deserves credit for what becomes clouded.

As physicians talked to one another about massage, its popularity began to grow. The physicians sought common ground between their methods and massage, both to justify their current view of massage and to expand it. Lay magazines and medical journals published manuscripts on massage. The successful experience and testimony of distinguished people, especially monarchs and diplomats, further bolstered the image of massage and increased public and medical acceptance. Many physicians were drawn to study massage because they had a strong scientific interest in its effects. They conducted animal studies and well-designed clinical trials, which further persuaded physicians of the value of the method and increased the interest of the medical community. The same situation has held true for massage in this century; it currently is bolstered by the work of Dr. Tiffany Field at the Touch Research Institute in Miami and by studies conducted under grants from the National Institutes of Health (NIH).

The Swedish movement cure quickly spread to other European countries. The first institute outside Sweden was established in Denmark. In 1837, two years before Ling's death, his disciple, M. LeRon, brought the movement cure to Russia, establishing a clinic in St. Petersburg.

Massage in the United States

In the United States the first waves of European immigration came from northern Europe, which had accepted massage earlier because of its therapeutic benefits. The immigrants produced many great writers and teachers of massage, along with eager, trusting clients.

Two brothers, Charles F. Taylor and George H. Taylor, introduced the Swedish movement system to the United States in 1856. They had learned the skills from Dr. Mathias Roth, an English physician who studied directly with Ling. Roth, also a leader in the homeopathic movement, felt that massage worked on the same principles as homeopathy: the law of similars and the concept of "like cures like."

Dr. John Harvey Kellogg (1852-1943), founder of the Battle Creek Sanitarium in Michigan, wrote dozens of articles and two textbooks on massage and hydrotherapy and edited and published a popular magazine, *Good Health.*

In his 1879 history of massage, Douglas Graham described lomi lomi, which is practiced by Hawaiians. He stated that it was used as a hygienic measure to relieve fatigue or was performed simply for the pure pleasure of it. Graham continued to write on massage and its use in almost every area of medicine until his death in the late 1920s.

In 1889 a letter from a physician in Kansas appeared in a New York medical journal. The physician said that he had thought massage was just "a novel method of therapeutics" until he had read a passage from Captain James Cook's diary of his third voyage around the world near the end of the eighteenth century. Cook had described how his pseudosciatic pain was relieved in an elegant and generous ritual by a Tahitian chief and his family, who used a type of massage method called *romee.*

Massage Scandals of the Late 1800s

In a very real sense, massage was a victim of its own success. In 1886 Dr. Charles K. Mills, a prominent Philadelphia neurologist and advocate of massage, sharply criticized the uneven quality of lay practitioners of massage and their often unsubstantiated and unethical claims. In 1889 British physicians, who were just beginning to view massage favorably because Queen Victoria supported the methods, became increasingly aware of patterns of abuse, including false claims about lay practitioners' education or skills, client stealing, and the charging of high fees. The massage scandals of 1894, revealed in the *British Medical Journal* by a British Medical Association commission of inquiry, eroded the public's and medical profession's confidence in massage as a legitimate medical art.

An inconsistent system of education, which encompassed private trade schools, hospitals, and physicians who took private students, appeared to be a major contributor to the loss of confidence in massage. Courses in technique, anatomy, physiology, and pathology varied immensely, as did the teachers' experience and capability. Some held that they could teach with minimal training in massage or directly after graduation from programs of questionable quality. Students often were encouraged to have grand expectations of career opportunities, only to find a difficult job market in which many of them were inadequately trained to compete. Richard van Why provides an example of the problem (van Why, 1992):

> Many schools used improper student recruitment tactics. The worst involved young women from poor neighborhoods, who were approached by recruiters claiming that extraordinary career opportunities awaited masseuses or medical gymnasts upon graduation from schools of professional training. The recruiters offered to defer payment of tuition until a reasonable time had elapsed after the students' graduation, so that the women could build resources to pay their living expenses and still pay the loans back. They were typically trained in short programs and then were released to a marketplace full of lay practitioners. As they found no work, they could not pay the loans back. Soon the recruiters returned, demanding payment. The women were told that if they did not pay, they would be thrown into debtors prison until they did. To work off the debt, they would have to work at a clinic attached to the school or for a friend or a colleague of a school administrator. The best of these "clinics" offered incompetently performed classical massage. The worst of the "clinics" were pretexts for houses of prostitution. In the scandals that followed in British cities and in Chicago and New York, the "massage parlor" caught on, and the lay practice of massage became associated with vice.

Another notorious abuse involved "certification," which some physicians who supported massage considered merely a receipt for money paid. Still another problem concerned advertising. The medical profession and the well-trained, classical lay practitioners of massage and medical gymnastics did not make false claims in their advertisements. Conversely, many entrepreneurs and poor massage practitioners seeking publicity to increase enrollment at their schools and attendance at their clinics did make such claims, which often flew in the face of the principles of anatomy, physiology, and pathology.

In 1894, the same year the massage scandals were revealed in Britain, eight women formed the Society of Trained Masseuses. These women envisioned massage professionals as well-trained, properly equipped masseuses serving those in need. Before this time, the quality of lay massage practitioners was inconsistent. Recognizing the need for rigorous standards, the founders modeled their standards on those used in the medical profession. They set academic prerequisites for the study of massage. Training could be given only in recognized schools, which were to be inspected regularly to ensure that standards were maintained. Only qualified instructors could teach classes. Examinations for teachers and graduates of basic massage training were conducted by a board, which included a physician. Examinations were to include both written tests and a demonstration of clinical achievement. By 1909 the society had 600 members.

Problems arose within the Society of Trained Masseuses during a period of sustained growth, and a competing association was established. This weakened both organizations. In 1920 the society assembled an advisory committee to aid reorganization and to reconcile with the opposing association. The two groups joined, becoming the Chartered Society of Massage and Medical Gymnastics. By 1939 the membership of the new organization had grown to 12,000. Certificates of competence were granted to individuals who had passed a rigorous examination. To be admitted to the Chartered Society of Massage and Medical Gymnastics, prospective members had to pledge not to accept clients unless they had been referred by a physician. Members were forbidden to advertise in the lay press. The organization worked to provide a central registry of well-trained massage practitioners and to provide referrals for inquiries from the medical profession or the public, based on location and any special needs. However, membership in the association was voluntary, and many ill-trained, unscrupulous practitioners continued to thrive.

Massage as Health Care

Massage endured even during the difficult time of the late 1800s. Institutes of massage appeared in France, Germany, and Austria by the middle of the nineteenth century. Between 1854 and 1918, the practice of massage developed from an obscure, unskilled trade to a field of medical health care from which the profession of physical therapy began. Treatments consisted of massage, mineral baths, and exercise.

Dr. David Gurevich, a Russian physician and instructor of Russian medical massage, believed that the long-standing interest in massage and its continuing development are strong proof of its usefulness and necessity. According to Dr. Gurevich, massage was practiced by ancient Slavic tribes, especially in combination with therapeutic bathing, or hydrotherapy. Beginning in the eighteenth century, many great Russian scientists and physicians (Mudroff, Manasein, Botkin, Zakharin, and others) contributed to the development of the theory and practice of massage. I. Z. Zabludovski wrote more than 100 books, textbooks, and scientific articles devoted to the methods of massage and its physiologic basis in therapy, postsurgical care, and sports.

An institute of massage and exercise was founded in Russia at the end of the nineteenth century, and many courses in massage also were started. Massage gradually progressed from an auxiliary method of therapy to an independent therapeutic method that was used effectively with other types of treatment. The practice of massage became widespread in Russia, and most medical clinics used massage therapy. Massage used with therapeutic exercises has been adapted for the management of the viscera, the nervous system, and gynecologic disorders, as well as for orthopedics, post-traumatic care, and postoperative care. Prospective students of massage must have some medical education. The change in Russia's economy in the late 1980s and early 1990s to a market system made it possible to open private massage clinics, which charge fees (Gurevich, 1992).

Historical Influence of Women

Women made early and important contributions to the development of massage and medical gymnastics, primarily in the United States. Contemporary massage has been influenced extensively by women, and 70% to 75% of practicing massage professionals today are women. Two women physicians conducted the first controlled clinical trial of the benefits of massage in the management of disease. Dr. Mary P. Jacobi and Dr. Victoria A. White were professors of medicine in New York City in 1880. Their research addressed the benefits of massage and ice packs in the management of anemia.

Broad licensing for physical therapy began in the early 1940s. Louise L. Despard's *Text-Book of Massage and Remedial Gymnastics* was one of a handful of textbooks on massage recommended in 1940 as essential reading for all students of massage by the Massage Round Table of the American Physical Therapy Association.

Mary McMillan, an English lay practitioner of massage, wrote an influential textbook, *Massage and Therapeutic Exercise*, in 1932. She had extensive experience in the field. From 1911 to 1915 she was in charge of massage and therapeutic exercise at the Greenbank Cripples Home in Liverpool, England, and from 1916 to 1918 she served as director of massage and remedial gymnastics at the Children's Hospital in Portland, Maine. During World War I she served in the military as a rehabilitation aide (Tappan and Benjamin, 2004).

In the West, Eunice Ingham formalized the system of reflexology derived from ancient Chinese roots. Dr. Janet Travell's work with myofascial pain and trigger points is unsurpassed. Bonnie Prudden popularized trigger point work. Frances Tappan's outstanding contributions to massage and physical therapy are formalized in her textbook, *Healing Massage Techniques*. Sister Kenny used massage in the treatment of polio. Ida Rolf's massage system grew to become the technique of Rolfing. Dr. Dolores Krieger has made major contributions to the more energetic approaches through her system of therapeutic touch.

Because of the extensive influence of women in massage today, it is likely that when massage history is written, many women will be listed as vital contributors to the continued development of massage.

Twentieth Century

Sigmund Freud (1856-1939), an Austrian neurologist and theorist who developed the system of psychoanalysis, experimented with the use of massage in the treatment of hysteria, a form of mental illness common in his day. This condition is characterized by a paralysis that has no physiologic basis. Freud's *Studies on Hysteria*, published in 1895, explained his methods.

Wilhelm Reich, an Austrian psychoanalyst who was a clinical assistant to Freud for 6 years, became interested in the physiologic basis of neurosis. In 1934 Reich emigrated to the United States. Many consider him the founder of psychotherapeutic body techniques. Reich gradually moved the emphasis of his therapeutic approach away from the psychological and toward the realm of the physical, the body. Reich developed many somatic techniques to dissolve what he saw as the muscular armor. Because of his controversial techniques, he came into conflict with the medical establishment and eventually was investigated by the U.S. Food and Drug Administration (FDA). He was convicted of fraudulent medical practices and died in 1957 while serving his sentence in federal prison.

Reich's earlier ideas and therapies have greatly influenced contemporary bodywork. Bioenergetics, a popular somatotherapy, evolved directly from his system. Bioenergetics was founded by Alexander Lowen, an American psychiatrist who was Reich's student for 12 years.

1900 to 1960

In the early 1900s Dr. Randolph Stone, an American physician, devised polarity therapy. Stone studied many body systems, both ancient and modern, including acupuncture, hatha yoga, osteopathy, chiropractic techniques, and reflexology. From his investigations he concluded that magnetic fields regulated and directed the physiologic systems of the body. Influenced by Eastern philosophy and medicine, Stone believed that all aspects of the universe were expressed in opposite poles (e.g., male and female, positive and negative electrical charges); therefore, he called his therapeutic method polarity.

In 1907 Edgar F. Cyriax began a distinguished publishing career that spanned almost 40 years. He was the last great proponent of Ling's Swedish movement cure, which Cyriax called mechanotherapeutics.

At the turn of the nineteenth century, the United States and England looked to Japan for innovation in the vocational rehabilitation of the blind. The British Institute for Massage by the Blind was established in 1900. Other European nations tried to develop their own models of the Japanese and British institutions but failed.

A textbook published in 1900 by Albert Hoffa and revised in 1913 by Max Bohm describes the more classic massage techniques, such as effleurage, pétrissage, tapotement, and vibration. Most therapists still learn these methods as standard massage techniques in entry level programs. However, many massage professionals of the time disregarded this type of massage, considering it too basic to be included in the realm of advanced manual therapy. Others warned against leaving behind traditional massage techniques, believing that fundamentals could not be replaced with more modern forms of bodywork.

In 1916 Dr. James B. Mennell divided the effects of massage into two categories: mechanical actions and reflex actions. Mennell showed that massage exerts a mechanical effect in four ways:

1. By aiding venous return of blood to the heart
2. By promoting lymph movement out of the tissues
3. By stretching the connective tissue (e.g., tendons and scar tissue)
4. By stimulating the stomach, small intestine, and colon

Mennell also maintained that certain forms of tactile stimulation, such as stroking and light touch, stimulated reflex arcs, causing muscles to relax or contract according to the type of stroke. He theorized that both smooth and skeletal muscles were under the control of such reflexes. Experimental research now supports the theories of Ling, Mennell, and others that massage has mechanical and reflex effects.

The polio epidemic of 1918 sparked a more widespread interest in massage, because victims and their families were desperate for any remedy that offered any promise at all. Research on the benefits of massage in preventing the complications of paralysis began at this time.

Connective tissue massage (CTM) was developed in the 1920s by German physiotherapist Elizabeth Dicke and later was expanded upon by Maria Ebner. CTM was first used because Dicke herself suffered from a prolonged illness caused by an impairment of the circulation in her right leg. As with Ling, her search for self-healing added much to the development of massage.

During this time Emil Vodder, a Danish physiologist, and his wife, Estrid, developed a technique of light massage along the course of the surface lymphatics; they called the technique lymph drainage or manual lymphatic drainage. This technique was and still is used to treat chronic lymphedema and other diseases of the lymphatic and peripheral vascular systems.

The American Association of Masseurs and Masseuses was formed in Chicago in 1943 and subsequently was renamed the American Massage Therapy Association (AMTA). Another professional organization, the International Myomassetics Federation, was formed later through the efforts of Irene Gauthier, a notable massage instructor, and others.

James H. Cyriax, the son of Edgar Cyriax, became an orthopedic surgeon at St. Thomas Hospital, a prestigious teaching institution in London. The younger Cyriax gained fame through his development of transverse friction massage. In the late 1940s and early 1950s, he published the first edition of his now classic *Textbook of Orthopedic Medicine*. His work is especially significant in the area of massage, because it recognized, categorized, and provided differential diagnoses for pathologic conditions of the body's soft tissues. The fact that pain can be caused by dysfunction of soft tissues, including periarticular connective tissue, is the foundation of soft tissue manipulation today. Cyriax also was the first to introduce the concept of end feel in the diagnosis of soft tissue lesions.

Dr. Herman Kabat researched neuromuscular concepts based on the work of neurophysiologists and Pavlov's conditioning of reflexes. Sherrington's law of successive induction provided the foundation for the development of rhythmic stabilization and slow reversal techniques. By 1951 research had begun on a new method, which was formalized in 1956 in the book *Proprioceptive Neuromuscular Facilitation*, written by Margaret Knott and Dorothy Voss (see Chapter 10).

Frances Tappan and Gertrude Beard also wrote important articles and books on massage techniques during the 1950s. Their texts are still available, and serious students of massage can benefit from reading these classic works. Frances Tappan influenced the profession of massage through interviews, conferences on the future of massage, and consultation with many leaders in the field.

1960 to the Present: the Most Recent Revival of Massage

The most recent revival of massage began around 1960 and has continued to this day. Recognition of chronic diseases that are resistant to surgical or drug treatment has increased. Neither the acute care concept nor a single-solution approach seems to work with these cases. A more complex way of envisioning and treating these diseases has had to be developed, and massage is one approach that has proven effective over time.

The humanistic movement that began during the 1960s spilled over into medicine and allied health. Concerns about "bedside manner," "genuineness," and the benefits of touch again raised the issue of the legitimacy and value of massage for its nurturing effect alone. Later, the Esalen movement and Gestalt psychology inspired psychologists and psychotherapists to explore massage and other movement therapies. Many controlled clinical studies in medicine, nursing, physical therapy, and psychology inspired more academic and clinical interest in massage.

In 1960 increased medical awareness that lack of exercise contributed to cardiovascular disease and other disorders prompted President John F. Kennedy to emphasize physical fitness, especially for children. This new interest grew into the physical fitness movement of the late 1960s and led the health sciences into a movement toward preventive medicine. The benefits of sports were rediscovered, and as a result historic literature in the field of massage was brought to light, such as Albert Baumgartner's book, *Massage in Athletics*, which discussed the relationship between massage and exercise and the value of massage in conditioning and stress control.

Acupressure received more attention than any other bodywork method during the 1970s and 1980s. The medical, physical therapy, and nursing literature examined it closely on the basis of controlled clinical trials. Through writings on nursing and rehabilitative medicine, a body of knowledge emerged on the benefits of massage in preventing and treating decubitus ulcers and in the overall management of heart rate and blood pressure in people suffering from acute and chronic manifestations of cardiovascular disease

Richard van Why has said, "It was in the field of pain research and pain management that the greatest gains for massage were made." Ronald Melzack, a professor of psychology in the anesthesiology department of McGill University Medical School and one of the initial proponents of the gate control theory of pain, published the results of several controlled clinical trials on the value of ice massage and manual massage for the relief of dental pain and low back pain. Melzack not only found these techniques effective in preventing or reducing pain, he also proposed a theory for the neural mechanisms by which they operated. Other researchers picked up on this theme and began to examine the role of massage in the liberation of endorphins, pain-killing chemicals more potent than morphine that are produced by the brain in response to certain stimuli, including massage.

In the late 1980s, in the prestigious journal *Clinics in Anesthesiology*, Melzack proposed a theory to explain endorphin release. His theory of hyperstimulation analgesia was the first

in recent decades inspired by findings concerning massage. The theory argues that certain intense sensory stimuli, such as puncture with a needle or exposure to extreme cold or pressure when applied near the site of an injury, sends a signal to the brain by a faster channel than that used by the pain signal it was attempting to treat, thereby disrupting the pain (van Why, 1992).

In 1988 the American Massage Therapy Association spearheaded a proposal for the development of a national certification process. The proposal stirred up much controversy and was hotly debated. With the participation of other professional massage and bodywork sources, the National Certification Examination for Therapeutic Massage and Bodywork was devised in 1992. Since its inception, the examination has had a positive influence on the professional development of therapeutic massage.

In the late 1980s the professional organization Associated Bodywork and Massage Professionals was formed to serve the needs of a growing and diverse group of bodywork therapists.

The 1990s saw a significant shift in the massage profession.

RECENT EVENTS AND CURRENT PROFESSIONAL TRENDS

SECTION OBJECTIVES

Chapter objective covered in this section:
4. The student will be able to explain the influence of historical events and global culture on the current development of therapeutic massage.

Using the information presented in this section, the student will be able to perform the following:
- Relate historical information to current events

In the 1990s many events took place that set the stage for the major changes that occurred in the massage profession during the first decade of the twenty-first century.

Recent Trends: 1990 to 2012

Those who have experienced the revival of massage from 1960 to the present may wonder if this success carries with it mixed blessings. Before 1985, massage professionals worked primarily in independent settings with little or no supervision. The very best of this situation was the freedom to serve clients' needs without the constraints of regulation. The worst was the lack of consistent training and the confusion among other professionals and the public about what constituted therapeutic massage.

Frustration with massage parlor regulations enacted to control prostitution and the desire of many massage professionals to enter the mainstream of public awareness pushed the massage therapy profession to begin seeking an alliance with the existing health care structure to justify the validity of massage. In some instances this movement into the existing health care world created turf battles over which profession would provide massage therapy. Both legitimate and reactionary questions and concerns were expressed by the physical therapy and nursing professions.

The public's desire for physical fitness had reached its peak during this time, and the concept of "sports massage" provided an avenue for mainstreaming massage therapy. During the 1990s the mainstream approach shifted from sports to corporate America. David Palmer can be given credit for formalizing the concepts of on-site and chair massage. These two trends allowed the public to see massage in a way much different from the preconceived notions of a "feel good" luxury of the wealthy or a front for prostitution.

As research continues to validate massage therapy and as massage evolves into a distinct professional course requiring a credible, standardized education, the turf battles in the health care system seem to be quieting down. Health care is moving in the direction of multidisciplinary teams in which many different professionals work together. As this process continues, nurses and physical therapists probably will find themselves supervising massage paraprofessionals and working as partners with more comprehensively trained massage therapists who have earned a degree.

In 1990 the AMTA established the Massage Therapy Foundation with the mission of bringing the benefits of massage therapy to the broadest spectrum of society through the generation, dissemination, and application of knowledge in this field. The foundation now is a dynamic independent organization. Current trends indicate that research will be the most important process for the future of the massage profession, and the Massage Therapy Foundation is positioned to be an ongoing leader of the massage profession.

In 1991 the Touch Research Institute at the University of Miami opened under the direction of Dr. Tiffany Field. More than any other single development in the 1990s, the research produced by the institute has moved massage into the mainstream and into accepted health care practice.

Also in 1991 the National Institutes of Health (NIH) established the Office of Alternative Medicine. Two years later, the *New England Journal of Medicine* reported on a national survey on the use of alternative and complementary forms of health care. Massage was the third most used treatment. In line with this trend, in 1994 the NIH published the report *Alternative Medicine: Expanding Medical Horizons. A Report to the National Institutes of Health on Alternative Medical Systems and Practices in the United States.*

The credibility and acceptance of natural approaches to health and illness are developing, and knowledge bases are beginning to overlap. Three areas in osteopathic medicine that currently apply to massage are muscle energy techniques, positional release and strain/counterstrain techniques, and neuromuscular techniques. The most noteworthy educator and author in these methods is Dr. Leon Chaitow. Like Ling, Chaitow is a master synthesizer of the best of many concepts. He developed a strong foundation in manual medicine working as an assistant to his uncle, Dr. Boris Chaitow, the codeveloper of neuromuscular technique along with his cousin, the legendary Dr. Stanley Lief (Chaitow, 1988). Dr. Leon Chaitow has written many books that have enriched

the body of knowledge for soft tissue methods, including therapeutic massage.

Other authors and professionals worthy of mention include Ida Rolf, developer of the Rolfing system; Dr. Milton Trager, developer of Trager; and Dr. Janet Travell, coauthor with David Simons of the most comprehensive texts written on the subject of trigger points.*

Research continued to validate the benefits of massage through the 1990s. After years of struggle for acceptance and validation, massage moved into the mainstream in the mid-1990s. Since 1995 the amount of information available on therapeutic massage has increased dramatically. Many new books are on the market, and websites for therapeutic massage have been created on the Internet. As a result of advances in technology, massage education now can be provided through a variety of formats.

In 2007 a historical research event occurred that changed our understanding of how massage supports beneficial change. The International Fascia Research Congress was held at Harvard University. The congress was conceived and organized by a multidisciplinary committee of science researchers and practicing health care professionals who share a common focus on and interest in the human body's soft connective tissue matrix. The congress meets every 2 years.

Massage Therapy Body of Knowledge and Unifying the Profession

In 2007 the massage therapy professional community began to explore the possibility of the massage therapy profession's leadership organizations working together to develop consensus around definitional and scope issues. Out of these meetings came the formation of the Massage Therapy Body of Knowledge (MTBOK) stewardship group, which was composed of representatives of six organizations: the American Massage Therapy Association (AMTA), the AMTA Council of Schools, the Associated Bodywork & Massage Professionals (ABMP), the Federation of State Massage Therapy Boards (FSMTB), the Massage Therapy Foundation (MTF), and the National Certification Board for Therapeutic Massage and Bodywork (NCBTMB).

The stewardship group defined a *body of knowledge* as, "The domain of essential information, mastery over which is the knowledge, skills and attitudes necessary to practice." The mission of the MTBOK stewards is "to develop and adopt across the massage therapy profession a living resource of competencies, standards and values that inform and guide the domains of practice, licensure, certification, education, accreditation and research," with an emphasis on articulating the foundational elements common to a massage therapy body of knowledge shared by all stakeholders in the profession (MTKOB, 2010).

---

*Travell and Simons are the authors of the two-volume text *Myofascial Pain and Dysfunction: the Trigger Point Manual.*

The foundation of the *Massage Therapy Body of Knowledge (MTBOK),* the document produced by the MTBOK stewards, consists of (1) definition of massage therapy (scope of practice, terminology, and descriptions of the therapeutic massage field) and (2) definition of the competencies of an entry-level massage therapist in terms of knowledge, skills, and abilities (KSA). The initial work was completed by mid-2010, and MTBOK projects continue. The work of the MTBOK stewards was pivotal in transforming the massage profession from a fragmented, loosely formed group into a cohesive partnership invested in the advancement of the massage therapy profession.

Certification and Licensure

In 2009 the National Certification Board for Therapeutic Massage and Bodywork began developing an advanced-level massage therapy examination with the intent of creating a formalized examination. The National Certification Advanced Practice (NCAP) exam provides a way to validate a commitment to continuing education and professional experience.

Most states now license massage therapy. The FSMTB supports its member boards in their work to ensure that the practice of massage therapy is provided to the public in a safe and effective manner by guaranteeing the provision of a valid, reliable licensing examination to determine entry-level competence. The trend toward state licensure of massage continues. Educational requirements set through state licensure average 500 to 1000 hours and show signs of increasing in the future. European and Canadian standards range from little or no training to extensive educational requirements (2200 to 3500 hours).

Schools of massage therapy have begun to work with colleges and universities to develop articulation agreements that allow graduates of their programs to complete degrees in massage. The first of these articulation agreements was reached in 1995 between the Health Enrichment Center in Lapeer, Michigan, and Siena Heights University in Adrian, Michigan, to grant both associate's and bachelor's degrees in applied science in massage therapy. The University of Westminster in England also offers bachelor's and master's degrees in complementary medicine, including massage and bodywork. Some private massage schools have increased their educational requirements to enable them to grant associate's degrees. More community colleges are developing certificate programs in therapeutic massage, and some of these programs can lead to an associate's degree in applied or general science.

As the future unfolds, committed researchers and those who apply the research to the practicalities faced by massage therapy practitioners probably will become the driving force for the advancement of massage therapy.

In 2010 the Alliance for Massage Therapy Education was established. This organization brings together directors and administrators from massage therapy schools, along with massage school teachers and those who provide continuing education seminars and advanced training in the field. All are committed to the advancement of quality education. The alliance and the Massage Therapy Foundation, working together, will ensure that massage therapy follows the path of excellence into the future.

Future of Massage

The role of massage and related bodywork methods is expanding at an accelerated rate. Massage now has enough validation to justify its use both by the public and health care professionals. An explosion of information and awareness has occurred. The future will determine the way the profession responds to the needs created by this success. Some questions we must answer to continue moving forward are:

- Will we be willing to accept research findings and let go of myths and misinformation about massage?
- Will we learn to use critical thinking skills to develop outcome-based massage sessions to achieve client goals?
- Will we learn to work together with other professionals in multidisciplinary teams?
- Will we agree on terminology about massage so that we can communicate with each other?
- Will we let go of the differences that divide us and reach for the similarities that bring us together?
- Will we commit to expertise through educational excellence, professional practice, and ethical behavior?
- Will we demand that educators and professional organizations be current, proficient, and committed to training the future generations of massage therapists?
- Will we respect our history, understand our traditions, and strive to bring those values into the future?

The massage therapy profession is changing. It is becoming more sophisticated, requiring education not only in the development of technical skills, but also in pathology, medications, record keeping, and communication skills. Professional ethics, too, is an important area. The more massage professionals work with other health care professionals, the more they need to know to be able to understand the world of health care. As we blend our world of professional touch with theirs, the exchange of information will be interesting to watch. We hope that the best of both worlds will emerge and that the lessons of the past will temper and soften the process.

More and more employment opportunities are becoming available in the area of health care. Mental health interventions that use massage are becoming more common. Some health care insurance plans and managed care systems are beginning to look at ways to include massage therapy in their covered services. Sports massage for amateur and professional athletes is becoming the norm, with massage therapists working side by side with athletic trainers and coaches.

In the wellness and personal service areas, day spas and massage franchises, such as Massage Envy, are bringing the art of pampering to the general public. The various franchised spa entities and spa industries are among the fastest-growing employers of massage professionals. Massage clinics that focus on wellness massage are becoming commonplace, as are massage professionals in the corporate setting.

Research into genetics, stress responses, neuroendocrine influences, and environmental hazards, in addition to support for the whole person in coping with a world that seems to be moving too fast, encourages the development of massage as a counterbalance to a stressful lifestyle, stressful world events, and a persistent state of ambiguity that promotes a state of

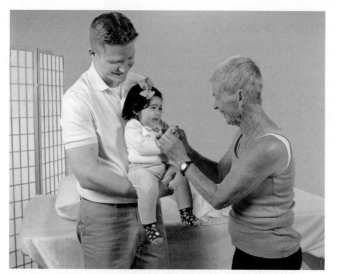

FIGURE 1-6 A bright future: teaching the next generation.

anxiety. The current trends, supported by research, seem to indicate that manual therapies are gaining recognition.

As the world becomes a global community, the ever-increasing exchange of information will enrich the knowledge base of therapeutic massage. Exploration of ancient healing methods will reveal the wisdom and scientific validity of a body/mind/spirit approach to well-being. Research has shown that various massage and bodywork methods are more alike than different. A shift has occurred from the confusing proliferation of massage and bodywork styles to understanding massage application provided to achieve outcomes such as stress and pain management, increased mobility, and enhanced performance.

Hopefully, the abundant massage and bodywork methods will continue to combine into a consolidated system of therapeutic massage without losing the rich diversity of professional expression. Terminology and education are standardizing, yet we have maintained the integrity of the individual applications of massage and bodywork. For those of you now entering the profession of massage therapy, success depends not on how many different styles of massage you know, but on your commitment to critical thinking, understanding the nature of human connection, and practice to perfect skilled application of the fundamental aspects of massage. The pressure to learn many different ways to do massage will evolve into skilled massage application based on evidence-based professional practice. The move from opinion and experience-based practice to the more objective evidence-based practice of massage is an ongoing theme in this text.

Two tracks of massage service probably will continue to standardize: wellness massage outside the health care system and medical massage within the health care system. Although very similar, these trends allow a vast diversity in the types of services available. Critical thinking skills, research literacy, experience, and empathy are the markers of career success.

The future is bright and promising, especially if we pay attention to our past and remember the words and wisdom of an old Russian physician: "massage is massage." We ourselves constitute one of the biggest threats to the future of massage.

FOOT IN THE DOOR

Laying a foundation is important as you begin the process of developing your career as a massage therapist. Your entry level education serves as this foundation. How committed are you to learning these basic skills? Sometimes students become impatient with the early material, such as fundamental draping skills, sanitation, equipment maintenance, and so forth. However, the foundation you create for yourself must be solid and sound. If you intend to be an excellent massage therapist, the process begins right now, with your commitment to your education. Then, when you graduate, you will be able to present yourself to future clients, coworkers, and employers with a self-confidence and professionalism that will help you get your foot in the door.

PROFICIENCY EXERCISE 1-5

In the space provided, answer the following questions.
1. What do you want the future of massage to bring?

2. How are you going to assist in the development of that future?

Currently the profession is fragmented, and educational standards are inconsistent. All bodywork professions must come together to work for the common good. As the massage profession moves forward and reclaims its heritage as an important health service, it is important to look back so that we can see the strengths and weaknesses of the professional journey (Figure 1-6).

Honoring those who have dedicated so much of their lives to developing the body of knowledge of therapeutic massage is also important. Many today are dedicating a significant part of their lives to the professional advancement of therapeutic massage. When the history of massage is written in the future, these names will appear with the information they have organized and contributed. We are all contributors to the future of massage, and we all will become part of its history (Proficiency Exercise 1-5).

SUMMARY

This chapter discussed the nature of touch in the professional setting and its importance. The reader should now be aware of the ways in which culture, gender, age, life events, spirituality, and diversity all influence the experience of touching and being touched. Inappropriate forms of touch were identified, and appropriate forms of professional touch were presented. An understanding of the subjective experience of touch was addressed personally.

The history of massage from ancient times to the present was explored, as were projections for the future. A time line highlighted many key dates. The foundation has been laid for the study of therapeutic massage.

References

Cantu RI, Grodin AJ: *Myofascial manipulation: theory and clinical application*, ed 2, Gaithersburg, Md, 2001, Aspen Publishers.

Chaitow L: *Soft tissue manipulation*, Rochester, Vt, 1988, Healing Arts Press.

Greenman PE: *Principles of manual medicine*, ed 3, Baltimore, 2003, Williams & Wilkins.

Gurevich D: Historical perspective, 1992 (unpublished article).

Isham Ismail Z: Glory years of Muslim medicine, *New Straits Times*, 2006. www.accessmylibrary.com/article-1G1-156711600/glory-years-muslim-medicine.html. Accessed May 7, 2010.

Lederman E: *Fundamentals of manual therapy physiology, neurology, and psychology*, New York, 1997, Churchill Livingstone.

Leon V: Aspects of Avicenna, philosophy, religion, and science, medieval philosopher/physician Abu Ali al-Husayn ibn Abdallah ibn Sina (book review), *Middle East J*, 2002.

Masic I, Dilic M, Solakovic E, et al: Why historians of medicine called Ibn al-Nafis second Avicenna, *Med Arh* 62:244–249, 2008.

MTBOK Task Force: Massage Therapy Body of Knowledge, version 1, May 15, 2010. Available from http://www.mtbok.org/downloads/MTBOK_Version_1.pdf (accessed November 2, 2011).

Rebollo Regina Andrés: The Paduan School of Medicine: medicine and philosophy in the modern era. Hist. cienc. saude-Manguinhos (serial on the Internet) June 2010, cited August 4, 2011 17(2):307–331. Available from: http://www.scielo.br/scielo.script=sci_arttext&pid=S0104-59702010000200003&lng=en. http://dx.doi.org/10.1590/S0104-59702010000200003.

Smith EWL, Clance PR, Imes S: *Touch in psychotherapy*, New York, 1998, Guilford Press.

Tappan FM, Benjamin PJ: *Tappan's handbook of healing massage techniques: classic, holistic, and emerging methods*, ed 4, 2004, Prentice Hall.

van Why RP: *History of massage and its relevance to today's practitioner, the Bodywork Knowledgebase*, New York, 1992, self-published.

Workbook Section

Short Answer

1. What is the skin's significance in touch?

2. What factors can influence an individual's experience of touch?

3. What are the forms of inappropriate professional touch?

4. What are the forms of appropriate professional touch?

5. In what way and where did massage originate? Why is this answer important?

6. What has provided the validation for massage?

7. What methods did the ancient Chinese massage system use? In what ways are the methods of today different?

8. Why was massage associated with folk medicine and connected with supernatural experiences during the Middle Ages in Europe?

9. Why is credit given to Per Henrik Ling for the development of the Swedish movement cure and Swedish massage?

10. In what way did problems with terminology interfere with the acceptance of Ling's work?

11. Who or what was one of the main contributors to the massage scandals in the late 1800s?

12. What aspect of massage remained active outside the medical establishment from the 1940s to the present?

13. What research has provided the current validation of massage?

14. In what way has massage brought the best of the East and West together?

Review Questions

Write your personal definition for each of the following words.

1. Professional

2. Structured

3. Therapeutic

4. Touch

Essay Questions

1. What does "touch intention" mean to you?

2. How would you describe your professional touch intention?

Matching

Match the person or information (1 to 25) with the best response (a to y).

_____ 1. Massage in the Eastern world
_____ 2. Massage in the Western world
_____ 3. Ambrose Paré
_____ 4. Per Henrik Ling

_____ 5. Followers of Johann Mezger

_____ 6. Duplicated movements

_____ 7. Active movements

_____ 8. Passive movements

_____ 9. Charles F. Taylor and George H. Taylor

_____ 10. Mathias Roth

_____ 11. Sister Kenny

_____ 12. Ida Rolf

_____ 13. Dr. Dolores Krieger

_____ 14. Dr. John Harvey Kellogg

_____ 15. Dr. Charles K. Mills

_____ 16. Wilhelm Reich

_____ 17. Alexander Lowen

_____ 18. Elizabeth Dicke

_____ 19. Margaret Knott and Dorothy Voss

_____ 20. Esalen and Gestalt

_____ 21. Autonomic approach

_____ 22. Mechanical approach

_____ 23. Movement approach

_____ 24. Dr. Boris Chaitow and Dr. Stanley Lief

_____ 25. Dr. Milton Trager

a. Known as exercise

b. Proposed an integrated program of active and passive movements based on Swedish gymnastics

c. An English physician who studied with Ling

d. Developed Rolfing

e. A neurologist and massage advocate who criticized the uneven quality of practitioners

f. Founded bioenergetics

g. Inspired psychotherapists to explore massage and movement therapies

h. Changes abnormal movement patterns into optimal ones

i. Used French terms such as effleurage and pétrissage

j. A continuation of Greco-Roman traditions

k. Commonly called resistive exercises

l. Cofounders of the neuromuscular technique

m. Developed the therapeutic touch–energetic approach

n. Range of motion and stretching performed by a therapist

o. A physician from Battle Creek, Michigan, who used massage and hydrotherapy

p. Attempts mechanical changes in soft tissue

q. Introduced Swedish movements in the United States

r. Used massage for joint stiffness and wound healing after surgery

s. Kept alive as part of folk culture

t. Founded psychotherapeutic body techniques

u. Developed the Trager system

v. Developed connective tissue massage

w. Wrote the first major book on proprioceptive neuromuscular facilitation

x. Used massage in the treatment of polio

y. Exerts a therapeutic effect on the autonomic nervous system

Time Line

Number the following events, activities, and people in chronologic order. For example, (e) is no. 1.

_____ a. The art of massage is first mentioned.

_____ b. Ambrose Paré uses massage to aid postsurgical recovery.

_____ c. M. LeRon introduces the Swedish movement cure in Russia.

_____ d. Julius Caesar has himself pinched all over to relieve pain.

_____ e. A cave dweller stubs his toe and instinctively rubs it.

_____ f. Per Henrik Ling develops Swedish gymnastics.

_____ g. Dr. Mary P. Jacobi and Dr. Victoria A. White research massage benefits.

_____ h. The massage scandals occur in England.

_____ i. Charles F. Taylor and George H. Taylor introduce Swedish movements in the United States.

_____ j. Galen writes on early manual medicine, supporting the methods of Hippocrates.

_____ k. Albert Hoffa publishes a textbook on classic techniques of massage.

_____ l. The polio epidemic sparks widespread interest in massage.

_____ m. Elizabeth Dicke develops connective tissue massage.

_____ n. The Royal Gymnastic Central Institute is established.

_____ o. Celsus compiles _De Medicina._

_____ p. The American Association of Masseurs and Masseuses is formed.

_____ q. Hippocrates encourages physicians to use massage.

_____ r. Dr. James H. Cyriax writes the classic _Textbook of Orthopedic Medicine._

_____ s. Dr. Charles K. Mills criticizes the uneven quality of the practice of massage.

_____ t. Margaret Knott and Dorothy Voss write _Proprioceptive Neuromuscular Facilitation._

_____ u. The National Certification Examination for Therapeutic Massage and Bodywork is developed.

_____ v. Dr. Tiffany Field researches massage.

Assess Your Competencies

Now that you have studied this chapter, you should be able to:

- Identify personal interpretations of touch and their influence on professional interactions
- Describe professional touch
- Explain the rich heritage and history of therapeutic massage
- Explain the influence of historical events and global culture on the current development of therapeutic massage

Professional Application

You are asked to present a brief lecture on the history of massage at a meeting of the local historical society. Develop a presentation outline.

2

Ethics, Professionalism, and Legal Issues

 http://evolve.elsevier.com/Fritz/fundamentals/

CHAPTER OBJECTIVES

After completing this chapter, the student will be able to perform the following:

1. Define professionalism
2. Define therapeutic massage
3. Define a scope of practice for therapeutic massage
4. Define evidence-based practice
5. Develop and explain a code of ethics and the standards of practice for therapeutic massage
6. Complete an informed consent process
7. Practice procedures to maintain client confidentiality
8. Become familiar with the Health Insurance Portability and Accountability Act (HIPAA) and its requirements and training
9. Integrate ethics into maintaining professional boundaries and the therapeutic relationship
10. Explain and demonstrate qualities of the therapeutic relationship
11. Use a problem-solving approach to ethical decision making
12. Use basic communication skills to listen effectively and deliver an I-message
13. Identify and resolve conflict in the professional setting
14. Identify legal and credentialing concerns of the massage professional
15. Identify and report unethical conduct by colleagues

CHAPTER OUTLINE

KEY TERMS

Active listening
Aspirational ethics
Clinical reasoning
Code of ethics
Confidentiality
Conflict
Countertransference
Credentials
Defensive climate

Dual role
Ethical behavior
Ethical decision making
Ethics
Evidence-based practice (EBP)
Informed consent
Initial treatment plan
Mandatory ethics
Mentoring

Needs assessment
Peer support
Power differential
Principles
Reciprocity
Reflective listening
Right of refusal

Scope of practice
Standard of care
Standards of practice
Supervision
Supportive climate
Therapeutic relationship
Transference

As a student of therapeutic massage, you must be able to define therapeutic massage, identify the types of professional services a massage practitioner legally and ethically can provide, and establish guidelines for conduct in the professional setting. This chapter cannot give specifics for all these issues, because the massage community itself is unclear in many areas, and professionalism in many ways evolves as a profession evolves. Progress has been made in the collaborative work of the various factions of the massage therapy profession, and since 2005 we have been moving steadily toward continuity and cohesiveness. Chapter 1 presented a foundation for professionalism and future trends. This chapter will help you to begin asking necessary questions intelligently and to find effective ways to answer those questions for yourself.

The professional development topics and skills addressed in this chapter include the following:

- The definition of massage
- The scope of practice for massage professionals
- Ethical conduct and standards of practice for massage professionals
- The therapeutic relationship
- Communication and conflict management skills to support professional interaction
- Professional recordkeeping to support professional achievement
- Provisions of the Health Insurance Portability and Accountability Act of 1996 (HIPAA)
- Credentialing, licensing, and other legal concerns of the massage professional
- Peer support, supervision, and mentoring

This information provides the structure for professional and ethical decision making. It can help you develop the level of professionalism essential to the successful practice of therapeutic massage.

First, we will explore the name of our profession. What do we call ourselves? You will discover that this is more complicated than it might seem at first. Then we will look at what we do; that is, study the definition of therapeutic massage. Armed with these two pieces of information, we will discuss the scope of practice for therapeutic massage and the appropriate training for the practice of this profession.

The chapter further describes professional services and the various forms of therapeutic massage services, such as wellness massage and clinical/medical/rehabilitative massage.

Ethics and professionalism have a unique language. The following definitions clarify some of the terminology used in this chapter.

- **Countertransference** is an inability on the part of the professional to separate the therapeutic relationship from

PROFICIENCY EXERCISE 2-1

Answer the following questions about professional services and the various forms of therapeutic massage services, such as wellness massage and clinical/medical/rehabilitative massage. After you have answered questions 1 through 6, write an additional question that you believe is important.

1. What is ethical conduct for the massage professional? How does one make ethical decisions?

2. What communication and recordkeeping skills are necessary to support a professional practice and fulfill legal responsibilities?

3. What are the legal requirements for practice?

4. What professional organizations represent the massage profession?

5. How does the massage professional identify and report unethical conduct in peers?

6. What is the importance of peer support, supervision, and mentoring?

7. Write your question.

personal feelings and expectations for the client; it is personalization of the professional relationship by the professional.

- A **dual role** results when scopes of practice overlap (e.g., one professional provides support in more than one area of expertise) or the personal and professional relationships overlap.
- **Ethics** is the science or study of morals, values, and principles, including the ideals of autonomy, beneficence, and justice. Ethics comprises principles of right and good conduct.
- **Ethical behavior** is right and correct conduct based on moral and cultural standards as defined by the society in which we live.
- **Ethical decision making** is the application of ethical principles and professional skills to determine appropriate behavior and resolve ethical dilemmas.
- **Informed consent** is a consumer protection process; it requires that clients be informed of the steps of treatment, that their participation be voluntary, and that they be competent to give consent. Informed consent is also an educational process that allows clients to make knowledgeable decisions about whether to receive a massage.
- **Mentoring** is a professional relationship in which an individual with experience and skill beyond those of the

person being mentored provides support, encouragement, and career expertise.

- **Peer support** is the interaction among those of similar skill and experience to encourage and maintain appropriate professional practice.
- **Principles** are basic truths or rules of conduct; they are generalizations that are accepted as true and that can be used as a basis for ethical conduct.
- The **scope of practice** is the knowledge base and practice parameters of a profession.
- **Standards of practice** are principles that serve as specific guidelines for directing professional ethical practice and quality care, including a structure for evaluating the quality of care. They are an attempt to define the parameters of quality care.
- The **standard of care** is an assessment and treatment process that a clinician (massage therapist) should follow for a certain type of clinical circumstance performed at the level at which similarly qualified practitioners manage the client's care under the same or similar circumstances.
- **Supervision** involves a person who oversees others and their professional behavior. The supervisor may be from a different discipline (e.g., a nurse) or may be a massage therapist who has more skill and experience than those supervised. Supervisors usually are in a position of authority. They are actively involved in such areas as the development and approval of treatment plans, review of clarity, scheduling, discipline, and teaching.
- A **therapeutic relationship** is created by the interpersonal structure and professional boundaries between professionals and their clients.
- **Transference** is the personalization of the professional relationship by the client.

Evolve Activity 2-1

PROFESSIONALISM AND THERAPEUTIC MASSAGE

SECTION OBJECTIVES

Chapter objective covered in this section:

1. The student will be able to define professionalism.
Using the information presented in this section, the student will be able to perform the following:
- Describe the content and impact of the Massage Therapy Body of Knowledge (MTBOK)
- Compare therapeutic massage with professional development criteria
- Describe the two professional development trends in therapeutic massage wellness and healthcare

As mentioned in Chapter 1, a very important process began with the collaborative efforts to produce the *Massage Therapy Body of Knowledge (MTBOK)*. This work was sponsored by a joint stewardship composed of the following organizations:

- Alliance for Massage Therapy Education (AFMTE)
- American Massage Therapy Association (AMTA)
- Associated Bodywork & Massage Professionals (ABMP)
- Federation of State Massage Therapy Boards (FSMTB)
- Massage Therapy Foundation (MTF)

- National Certification Board for Therapeutic Massage and Bodywork (NCBTMB)

Incorporating into their work extensive input by massage professionals, the MTBOK stewards developed a foundation that clarifies four very important elements: what is our name, who are we, what can we do, and what is our language. In the document, these elements are presented as:

- A description of the massage therapy field
- A scope of practice for massage therapy
- A description of the competencies of an entry-level massage therapist in terms of knowledge, skills, and abilities
- Terminology definitions related to the MTBOK document

According to the MTBOK, our profession is *massage therapy*, and we are *massage therapists*.

> Massage therapy is a health care and wellness profession. The practice of massage therapy involves a client/patient-centered session, intended to fulfill therapeutic goals, with the therapist being free of personal agenda. Massage therapy also meets the well researched need for touch and human connection. Massage therapy is about one human touching another with clear intention, focused attention, and the attitudes of compassion and nonjudgment (MTBOK stewards, 2010).

If we are to consider ourselves *therapists*, we must understand the implications of that title and determine how we should conduct ourselves in behaving as therapists. Other options for an occupational title exist, such as *technician* and *practitioner*, which are explored later in this chapter.

As the MTBOK states, we are professionals who use a wide variety of techniques and approaches to address the varied focuses of the client. Because the massage therapy community has determined that we are professionals, we have an obligation to conduct ourselves as professionals. The qualities of professional behavior are discussed in detail later in the chapter.

What massage therapy professionals can do is called their *scope of practice*. According to the MTBOK:

> Massage therapy is a health care and wellness profession performed in a variety of employment and practice settings. The practice of massage therapy includes assessment, treatment planning, and treatment through the manipulation of soft tissue, circulatory fluids, and energy fields, affecting and benefiting all of the body systems, for the following therapeutic purposes, including but not limited to: enhancing health and well-being, providing emotional and physical relaxation, reducing stress, improving posture, facilitating circulation, balancing energy, remediating, relieving pain, repairing and preventing injury, and rehabilitating. Massage therapy treatment includes a hands-on component as well as providing education, information, and nonstrenuous activities for the purposes of self-care and health maintenance. The hands-on component of massage therapy is accomplished by use of digits, hands, forearms, elbows, knees, and feet with or without the use of emollients, liniments, heat and cold, handheld tools, or other external apparatus (MTBOK stewards, 2010).

In developing a description of the massage therapy field and a massage therapy scope of practice statement, the MTBOK stewards focused on a description and definition that encompass the entire field of massage therapy practice as it currently exists while recognizing, respecting (and in some instances excluding) other distinct forms of touch therapy used within the broader industry of bodywork. Massage therapy is a bodywork system, but not all bodywork systems are massage. Other bodywork and somatic practices, such as shiatsu and applied kinesiology, have separately developed systems and philosophies, scopes of practice, and educational requirements.

With most of these bodywork systems, the outcomes for the client are very similar. The most common outcomes people seek from bodywork are relaxation, stress management, pain management, and support for mobility and performance. As a specific professional practice, massage therapy can achieve all of these client goals through the use of methods based on the definition of massage. Other bodywork systems, in achieving these outcomes, use different methods or have a different philosophy and specific language. Later in the text you will learn that the methods of application for most bodywork systems, including massage therapy, interact with the same physiology of the body and therefore are more alike than different.

The full scope of practice of the massage therapy profession goes beyond the minimum entry-level competency. Everyone who learns a skill needs to start at the beginning. Because you are reading this text, which is written as an entry-level textbook, you are just starting the process of achieving entry-level competency. Just as there is an entry level, there also are advanced levels of professional development that you can strive to achieve, which would allow you to practice massage therapy within the full scope of practice.

Later in the chapter we will look specifically at what is included in the scope of practice for massage therapy, what is not, and what you should be able to do upon completion of your entry-level education. Future chapters will introduce you to skills that you can add to your massage therapy skills to increase your personal scope of practice competency.

The final element addressed by the MTBOK project was an agreed-upon terminology (taxonomy). Until the release of the *Massage Therapy Body of Knowledge,* massage terminology was inconsistent and sometimes confusing and frustrating. Now we have the foundation for a language that we all can learn and understand. That terminology is used in this text.

The stewards who developed the *Massage Therapy Body of Knowledge* made a crucial contribution to the massage therapy profession. This work is considered a "living" document, which means that it can grow, it can be altered, it can be brought up-to-date, and it can lead the evolution of massage therapy. The entire document is available at www.mtbok.org; the link is provided on the Evolve website for this text.

Professionalism

Ethics and professionalism are very important to the therapeutic massage profession, as they are to all professions. In any professional practice, the ambiguity of ethics and the concreteness of professionalism and standards of practice converge to form a basis for ethical decision making. A profession is different from a job, and a professional does more

than go to work. Expanding on the definition presented in Chapter 1, we could say that a professional has the following characteristics:

- A specialized body of knowledge
- Extensive training
- An orientation toward service
- A commonly accepted code of ethics
- Legal recognition through certification or licensure by a professional organization
- Membership in a professional association

Specialized Body of Knowledge

Massage therapy methods are grounded in a specialized body of knowledge, which is presented in this textbook. Historical foundations and current research validate this body of knowledge, and the *Massage Therapy Body of Knowledge* documents it. As we discussed in Chapter 1, a lifetime of study easily could be devoted to therapeutic massage methods.

Extensive Training

Inconsistencies continue regarding the duration of massage training and the information and technical skills that should be included in that training. The *Massage Therapy Body of Knowledge* provides recommendations for knowledge, skills, and abilities applicable to entry-level education, but it does not provide recommendations for the duration of massage training and education to achieve competency for successful massage therapy practice. Professional development for therapeutic massage requires elements of standardization to allow continued progress toward professionalism.

A discrepancy also exists between current massage education and what is typically considered extensive training for professionals.

In massage therapy, two main categories of practice have emerged with five distinct practice settings:

1. Wellness
   - Spa setting
   - Massage franchise/national massage chains
   - Independent massage practice
2. Health care
   - Sports and fitness setting
   - Clinical/medical/rehabilitation setting

These categories and practice settings overlap extensively. However, categorizing information is useful when we are attempting to understand the big picture. Because massage therapy has a history of multiple practice settings, and one person can practice in multiple settings, the situation can become complex. Therefore, we start with a simple approach.

In general, the entry-level education required in the wellness categories of therapeutic massage can be considered the basic educational requirement and foundation for practice. The health care category can be considered the area in which the full scope of massage therapy practice can be achieved and therefore requires additional education and experience.

Now let's consider how those other than massage therapists view educational requirements. The National Center for Education Statistics (NCES) collects, analyzes, and reports statistics about American and international education.

| Box 2-1 | Educational Categories |

Academic majors: Formal programs of study designed to impart knowledge and skills that represent the accumulated knowledge base in a subject area. The instruction typically is designed to be comprehensive and theoretical.

Career majors: Formal programs of study designed to impart knowledge and skills that represent the relevant accumulated knowledge within the context of occupation-specific job requirements. The course of instruction typically involves less theory, more application, and a narrower focus than for an academic major. Career majors can be vocational or nonvocational.

- *Vocational career majors* consist of formal programs of study that impart the knowledge and skills required for semiskilled, skilled, technical, and paraprofessional occupations that typically require education below the baccalaureate level.
- *Nonvocational career majors* consist of formal programs of study that impart the knowledge and skills required for technical and professional occupations that typically require education at the baccalaureate level or higher.

Modified from Institute of Education Sciences: *Undergraduate enrollments in academic, career, and vocational education.* NCES 2004–018, Issue Brief.

This organization categorizes education as follows (Box 2-1) (NCES, 2004):

- Undergraduate majors are classified as either academic majors or career majors.
- Federal law defines vocational education as instruction for careers below the baccalaureate level.
- Career majors are divided into sub-baccalaureate and baccalaureate majors.
- At the baccalaureate level, career majors are considered professional (nonvocational).
- At the sub-baccalaureate level, they are considered vocational.

Where does education in massage therapy fit in? Before answering that question, let's gather more information. Career educational programs are provided at 4-year, 2-year, and less-than-2-year institutions in public, private not-for-profit, and private for-profit schools. How would you classify the school you are attending? Less-than-2-year private for-profit schools are the most common providers of personal and consumer services programs, followed by community colleges. Most massage therapy education is provided in these types of schools. Less-than-1-year certificate or diploma and associate's degrees are the most widely available credentials. Most entry-level massage education results in a diploma.

Massage therapy can be described as a career path in many different ways. Considerable inconsistency remains among federal and state governments, professional organizations, and individual massage practitioners on this issue, and it eventually must be addressed by the massage therapy profession. Perhaps an accurate description would be, "Massage therapy is a heath care service occupation that embraces professional behavior and development."

Let's return to the basic classifications of massage therapy practice:

1. Wellness
   - Spa setting
   - Massage franchise/national massage chains
   - Independent massage practice
2. Health care
   - Sports and fitness setting
   - Clinical/medical/rehabilitation setting

All of these areas provide opportunities both for entry-level practice and for advanced education and career specialization.

Entry-Level Practice

Spa Setting

The evolving spa environment encompasses a range of massage services for wellness- and pleasure-based massage; these services can overlap with sports and fitness massage and massage directly related to health care in the so-called medical spa. This text (coupled with your science studies) provides the skills necessary to develop a successful career in the spa environment, especially with supervision in the fitness-focused spa or medical spa. The spa setting also can be considered a massage specialty requiring additional education and experience. Career development in this setting usually follows the employee pathway. Chapter 13 provides specific information about the spa as a career track. Check out Chapter 3 for more information about career success as an employee.

Massage Franchise/National Massage Chains

Many massage therapy franchises have entered the massage market. This business concept is fast becoming the largest employer of massage therapists. Franchises offer a subscription-based model for clients, making massage affordable. As in the spa setting, career development follows the employee pathway. Because franchises handle all the marketing and business responsibilities, they provide an excellent entry-level opportunity; they also support employees who pursue the experience and professional development necessary for career advancement. The content of this textbook (coupled with your science studies) effectively prepares you to work in this setting.

Independent Massage Practice

The independent practice setting is the most complex, because an independent practice can be structured in many different ways. An individual may be self-employed, having a small, one-person practice, or may work as an independent contractor in another environment, such as a health club or hotel. An independent massage practice also can be developed as a massage clinic independent of the franchise system.

These career paths can serve as entry-level jobs; however, the demands of the clients and complex outcomes for the massage typically require a commitment to advanced education and experience. This textbook, coupled with science studies, can prepare you to practice massage therapy successfully in these settings if you commit to focused study and competency in the entire content presented. This means that reading the information once is not enough. You must study, review, practice, and then review some more until you have integrated the information into your massage therapy skills.

Sports and Fitness Setting

The sports and fitness career path covers a spectrum of massage outcomes, ranging from wellness to medical intervention typically (but not exclusively) based on issues related to environments that support exercise and sports performance. The importance of exercise in the management of most lifestyle-related diseases, such as diabetes, obesity, cardiovascular disease, mental illness, and many more, is well documented. Massage can support physical changes related to exercise and can help manage the discomfort related to physical activity and injury for those beginning an exercise program. Massage also can be beneficial for the extensive performance demands required of entertainers and competing athletes. Information in this text, presented in the appropriate scientific context, provides the foundation for working in this setting. However, continuing education is necessary for a practitioner to become confident and proficient in this area.

Clinical/Medical/Rehabilitation Setting

Massage provided in a health care setting is emerging as a primary avenue for massage practice. The name of this type of practice remains a little ambiguous; it currently is labeled the clinical/medical/rehabilitation career path. The term "clinical massage" is likely to become the agreed-upon title, defined as massage therapy practice that involves more extensive use of assessment, specific focused techniques, and applications with the intention of achieving clinical treatment outcomes.

The use of massage therapy in hospitals has become more common. The statistics break down as follows (AMTA, 2007):

- The number of hospitals offering complementary and alternative medicine (CAM) grew from 7.7% in 1998 to 37.3% in 2007. Of the hospitals offering CAM therapies, 70.7% offered massage therapy.
- Stress-related issues are major reasons hospitals offer massage: 71.2% of hospitals that offer massage provide it for stress reduction for patients; 69.1% provide it to staff to reduce stress.
- Other primary reasons for providing massage included:
  - Pain management
  - Pregnancy massage
  - Aid to physical therapy
  - Mobility/movement training
  - Palliative care

In 2005, 10% of massage therapists reported working in a health care environment. By 2009, that number had increased to 25%, and this trend is only expected to grow.

The common thread in clinical massage careers is integration with health care systems. This type of massage treatment may focus on stress management and prevention, management of chronic disease and pain, acute care palliation, presurgical and postsurgical care, prenatal care, elder care, and hospice care. People who receive medical care usually are called *patients*. Although all massage recipients are considered *clients*, not all clients are classified as medical patients.

This text provides the necessary foundation for general massage in the clinical/medical/rehabilitation setting, and continuing education provides the information that enables the practitioner to become confident and proficient providing this type of massage therapy (Chapter 13 describes this content in depth).

The current standard of 500 to 750 contact hours (10 to 15 credit hours) may be sufficient for basic wellness massage methods, but judging from data collected from actual job duties and current trends in licensing requirements, 1000 contact hours (20 to 24 credit hours) probably is more appropriate for supporting professional development in the wellness realm. It does not seem reasonable to expect that programs of 500 to 1000 contact hours provide sufficient time for integration of clinical reasoning methods; extensive physical assessment procedures; and the study of pathology, pharmacology, and psychology, as well as other information the massage professional needs to work effectively with other health care professionals and with complicated, multifaceted health concerns. The same can be said for sports massage or working with athletes. To work effectively with athletes, the professional must have an in-depth education in the dynamics of sports activity, the injury process, and rehabilitation.

Educational Trends

Current educational trends are moving toward the development of two professional tracks in therapeutic massage: (1) vocationally trained wellness massage service professionals and paraprofessionals in the health care area and (2) degree-holding professionals in the allied health care system.

The current model for service professionals (e.g., those working in the field of cosmetology) and for paraprofessionals (those trained to assist a professional) in health care and sports and fitness calls for 300 to 1800 contact hours (7 to 40 credit hours) of vocational training in technically based programs, after which the student is granted a certificate or diploma. Obviously, training standards vary widely.

A *professional* usually is considered to be a person who has a degree in his or her chosen field. It may be an associate's degree (usually requiring 64 credits); a bachelor's degree (usually requiring 124 credits); or a master's or doctoral degree, such as those held by teachers, physicians, athletic trainers, and mental health professionals.

Most educational models for therapeutic massage in the United States fall into the vocational services professional or paraprofessional realm. However, more massage programs have begun offering programs leading to an associate's degree or higher. Some Canadian provinces, as well as Australia, England, New Zealand, Poland, Russia, and other countries, require or offer training that meets the current definition of a professional degree. Individuals who already have professional degrees are obtaining massage therapy training and combining the two skills to function effectively in the health and athletic worlds; some examples of these combinations are nurse/massage therapist, athletic trainer/massage therapist, respiratory therapist/massage therapist, physical therapy assistant/massage therapist, occupational therapist/massage therapist, and social worker or psychologist/massage therapist.

The level of information in this text supports training programs of 500 to 1500 contact hours (10 to 34 credit hours) in the service and paraprofessional realms. The greatest employment potential for therapeutic massage probably will follow this career orientation. The training level of this text is sufficient to allow those with other degrees (i.e., nursing, athletic training) to integrate massage therapy into their professional worlds. In longer programs (i.e., those requiring more than 2000 contact hours), the information in this text can serve as the foundation on which clinical or more specific forms of therapeutic massage approaches are built.

Orientation to Service

The definition of service that best applies to this discussion is "to meet a need." An additional concept in a service orientation is that, although reimbursement is expected for services rendered, the desire to meet a need takes precedence over financial return. Observation of those who practice massage professionally and of the attitudes of current students indicates that providers of therapeutic massage definitely have an orientation toward service, sometimes to the detriment of sound business practices. Although caring for the people we serve is important, it is just as important to generate the necessary and appropriate income base to support the professional practice and a reasonably comfortable lifestyle for the professional.

Commonly Accepted Code of Ethics

A code of ethics is an agreed-upon set of behaviors developed to promote high standards of practice. As you study the rest of this chapter, you will see that although general agreement exists about what a code of ethics for massage therapy entails, no agreement has been reached on a specific code of ethics to serve the entire massage profession.

Legal Recognition Through Certification or Licensure by a Professional Organization

Currently, all U.S. states (except six at this writing), the District of Columbia, at least half of the Canadian provinces, and many other countries have formal licensing or legislated certification for massage professionals. In states that regulate massage therapy, massage therapists must meet the legal requirements to practice, which may include fulfilling a minimum number of hours of initial training and passing an examination. In states that do not regulate massage therapy, this task may fall to local municipalities. Most states that license massage therapists require a passing grade on the Massage & Bodywork Licensing Examination (MBLEx), which is administered by the FSMTB, or one of two exams provided by the NCBTMB. The exams provided by the NCBTMB provide access to licensing as well as the prerequisite to advanced level and specialty certification processes. (See the Evolve website for a list of states in which licensing is offered.)

Membership in a Professional Association

Several organizations represent the therapeutic massage profession. In addition, each of the various bodywork methods (e.g., reflexology, shiatsu, polarity) has its own professional organization. Although diversity is good for a profession and supports professional development, the lack of coherence in the field of therapeutic massage often confuses the public,

💡 **PROFICIENCY EXERCISE 2-2**

Answer the following questions, then exchange and compare your answers with others in class.
1. How would you rate massage therapy against the six criteria listed on p. 29?
2. What areas of massage therapy do you think are well developed? What areas need development?
3. What do you think is required to enable therapeutic massage to continue to evolve?
4. What can you do to contribute to this evolution?

ourselves, and other professionals. Developments in this area will be interesting to watch (Proficiency Exercise 2-2).

THE DEFINITION OF THERAPEUTIC MASSAGE

SECTION OBJECTIVES

Chapter objective covered in this section:
2. The student will be able to define therapeutic massage
Using the information presented in this section, the student will be able to perform the following:
- Describe and justify "massage therapist" as a professional name
- Develop a definition of massage
- Explain the differences between and similarities of various approaches to therapeutic massage
- Clarify the eight basic approaches to therapeutic massage
- Classify a massage method according to its fundamental physiologic basis

As mentioned previously, based on the *Massage Therapy Body of Knowledge,* a level of agreement has been reached that we are "massage therapists," and we provide "massage therapy." However, a question exists as to whether the current educational requirements support the terms "professional" and "therapist."

A technician is perceived differently from a therapist, particularly in terms of educational level. A *technician* can be defined as one who has expertise in a technical skill or process. A technician has the least training and the most limited scope of practice in a professional group.

The next educational level is the practitioner. A *practitioner* can be defined as one who practices an occupation or a profession. A practitioner operates from a greater knowledge base and within a larger scope of practice than a technician. Another term that could be used is *paraprofessional.*

A *therapist* can be defined as one who treats illness or disability. A therapist requires the highest educational background and has the broadest scope of practice.

The massage community currently does not use these designations as they are defined in this text, but the public and the health care professions often do. What is the public's perception, then, if "massage therapist" becomes our name? The confusion continues. Are we massage professionals, myomassologists, neuromuscular therapists, or soft tissue practitioners? Are we bodyworkers, and is massage a form of bodywork? Are we massage professionals, with other forms of bodywork becoming subcategories of massage? The MTBOK has

Box 2-2	Equivalent or Related Terms Recognized by the MTBOK

The *Massage Therapy Body of Knowledge* has designated the following terms as equivalent or related to the terms *massage therapy, bodywork,* and *massage therapist.*

- *Massage therapy:* Massage, therapeutic massage, body massage, myotherapy, massotherapy, body rub, massage technology, bodywork, bodywork therapy, somatic therapy or any derivation of these terms. Massage therapy may be assumed to be bodywork, but not all bodywork is massage therapy.
- *Bodywork:* A term used in complementary and integrative medicine (CIM) to describe any therapeutic, healing, or personal self-development practice; it may include massage, touch, movement, or energetic work. Massage therapy is one form of bodywork, and the terms *massage therapy* and *bodywork* frequently are used interchangeably. However, although bodywork includes all forms of massage therapy, it also includes many other types of touch and incorporates many other skills and techniques to enhance awareness of the mind/body/spirit connection.
- *Massage therapist:* Massage practitioner, massage technologist, massage technician, masseur, masseuse, myotherapist, massotherapist, bodyworker, bodywork therapist, somatic therapist, or any derivation of these terms. Massage therapists may be assumed to be bodyworkers, but not all bodyworkers are massage therapists. However, some regional regulations differentiate these terms to recognize differences in training and/or scope of practice.

Modified from Massage Therapy Body of Knowledge (MTBOK) stewards: *Massage therapy body of knowledge (MTBOK),* version 1, May 15, 2010. www.mtbok.org. Accessed March 21, 2011.

💡 PROFICIENCY EXERCISE 2-3

Justification can be defined as the act of defending a position using logical reasoning. Develop a justification statement for the validity of using the term massage therapist. The following questions can help you get started:

1. What is the current name most often used?
2. What is the definition of "therapist"?
3. What other professionals are called therapists?

helped clear up some of the confusion (Box 2-2) (Proficiency Exercise 2-3).

In Chapter 1 we began to trace the development of the term *massage*. The roots of the word *massage* mean to touch, handle, squeeze, knead, and press softly; therefore we defined *massage* as professional, structured, therapeutic touch. Over the past few years, as the popularity of therapeutic massage has grown, the profession has seen an expansion in styles and systems (Box 2-3).

The term *bodywork* has been used to cover the scope of the development of various types of hands-on modalities. As individual systems have emerged, a difference in styles has developed. However, the overlap of these methods reveals a fundamental sameness in all the work, and this core is becoming the foundation for professional standards and definitions. These similarities should not detract from the devotion, training, and expertise of the various practitioners in specific disciplines. Unification of the profession around these shared aspects should not threaten individual practice of specific disciplines.

Research indicates that the application of systematic touching for health purposes (i.e., therapeutic massage) is valid (see Chapter 5). By carefully examining any style or system of massage, the student can see that basic methods are used to stimulate sensory receptors. These methods either stimulate a rhythmic order in body functions or disrupt an existing pattern in the central nervous system control centers, resulting in a shift in nerve and chemical patterns to re-establish homeostasis (reflexive methods). The very same methods can be applied in a different way to change the consistency or position of connective tissue or to shift pressure in the vessels to facilitate blood and lymph circulation (mechanical methods). Although most of the systems have been developed over the centuries, a few new massage approaches have come into their own over the past few years (Figure 2-1).

Technology and research will most likely prove that massage methods share the same physiologic basis in their effectiveness. All massage approaches have the same basis because the people they serve have the anatomy and physiology of the human form. No one particular style of massage is better than another so long as the methods are purposefully used by a trained professional to serve the client's needs.

The massage community has made strides in standardizing terminology to prevent confusion about the various styles and systems of massage. The explanations of anatomy and physiology given in Asian styles of massage may be different from those given by Western science, but the human body is the same, and the effects of these styles are the same as those of systems developed in Polynesia, India, Europe, Africa, the United States, and around the world. Various massage systems (e.g., Swedish/classical massage, reflexology, sports massage, and body/mind integration) work through the same anatomic and physiologic mechanisms, but each has developed a language unique to that approach. The study of various systems becomes confusing only when so many different names are used for similar methods.

A core body of knowledge exists from which therapeutic massage approaches have evolved, and a skilled practitioner should be able to identify and explain any approach based on physiologic effects.

The different systems and styles presented in this text are variations on a theme. To become skilled practitioners, students learn the theme and explore the variations. Any of these systems can be explained in anatomic and physiologic terminology (Figure 2-2).

Defining Massage

A definition of massage must encompass all the methods used by various approaches. Massage cannot be considered

Box 2-3 Popular Methods of Massage

The following list of massage styles, systems, founders, and developers is not meant to be all-inclusive, because the information changes almost daily. Rather, it is meant to show the great variety of therapeutic massage approaches.

Asian

- *Amma, acupressure, shiatsu, jin shin do, do-in, hoshino, tui-na, watsu, Tibetan point holding, Thai massage*

These methods derive from traditional Chinese medicine concepts, from offshoots of this Chinese base, and from other Asian modalities (e.g., ayurveda). The efficient use of the therapist's body and the performance of these techniques on a clothed client have many benefits. The effects of compressive manipulations and stretches that focus on specific areas of the body elicit responses in the nervous, circulatory, and muscular systems and affect the energetic flows in the client's body. The philosophy of these systems is grounded in ancient concepts that have stood the test of time.

Structural and Postural Integration

- *Bindegewebs massage, Rolfing, Hellerwork, Looyen work, Pfrimmer deep muscle therapy, Soma bodywork, Bowen therapy*

These techniques focus more specifically on the connective tissue structure to influence posture and biomechanics. The approaches are systematic and are effective because they are grounded in the fundamentals of physiology and biomechanics. Practitioners of these styles must have an extensive education.

Neuromuscular

- *Neuromuscular techniques, muscle energy techniques, strain/counterstrain, orthobionomy, Trager, myotherapy, proprioceptive neuromuscular facilitation, reflexology, trigger points*

These are the European approaches based on the work of Dr. Stanley Leif and Dr. Boris Chaitow and the Western methods based on the work of Dr. Janet Travell, Dr. John Mennell, Dr. Raymond Nimmo, Dr. Lawrence Jones, Dr. Milton Trager, Eunice Ingham, William Fitzgerald, Arthur Lincoln Pauls, Bonnie Prudden, and others. Dr. Leon Chaitow has written extensively on these concepts and currently teaches in the United States and Europe. Many of the techniques are similar to those found in Rolfing, Asian methods, and Swedish massage and gymnastics. As the name implies, the approach is a nervous or reflexive method. Connective tissue also is affected. The common threads running through all the styles are the basic concepts of activation of the tonus receptor mechanism, reflex arc stimulation, positional receptors, and applications of stretching and lengthening.

Manual Lymphatic Drainage

- *Vodder lymphatic drainage*

Emil Vodder developed an excellent system that uses the anatomy and physiology of lymphatic movement with both mechanical and reflexive techniques to stimulate the flow of lymphatic fluid. Others have contributed to the understanding of lymphatic drain procedures, including Bruno Chickly and Lyle Lederman. The variations of this system sometimes are called systemic massage.

Energetic (Biofield)

- *Polarity, therapeutic touch, Reiki, zero balancing*

These systems, which are based on ancient concepts of body energy patterns, recently were formalized by Dr. Randolph Stone, Dr. Dolores Krieger, Dr. Fritz Smith, and others. Subtle energy medicine is under study by Dr. Elmer Green at the Menninger Foundation in Topeka, Kansas, and elsewhere by other researchers. Polarity and similar energetic approaches use near touch or light touch to initiate reflexive responses, often with highly effective results.

Craniosacral and Myofascial

- *Craniosacral therapy, myofascial release, soft tissue mobilization, deep tissue massage, connective tissue massage*

These systems focus more specifically on the various aspects of both mechanical and reflexive connective tissue functions. Dr. William Garner Sutherland was the first to formalize the concept of tiny movement of the cranium and dura. Dr. John Upledger and physical therapist John Barnes have expanded upon and formalized his work. Both light and deep touch are used, depending on the method. the cross-fiber friction methods of Dr. James Cyriax fall into this category.

Applied Kinesiology

- *Touch for health, applied physiology, educational kinesiology, three-in-one concepts*

Dr. George Goodheart formalized the system of applied kinesiology within the profession of chiropractic. The approach blends many techniques but works primarily with the reflexive mechanisms. A specific muscle testing procedure is used for evaluation; this process acts somewhat like a biofeedback mechanism. Some of the corrective measures use Asian meridians and acupressure; others rely on the osteopathic reflex mechanisms defined by Chapman, Bennett, and McKenzie that seem to correspond to traditional Chinese acupuncture points. Dr. John Thie and others modified these techniques for use by massage professionals and the public.

Integrated Approaches

- *Sports massage, infant massage, equine/animal massage, on-site or seated massage, prenatal massage, geriatric massage, massage for abuse survivors, Russian massage*

Many styles of massage that focus on a specific group of people use combinations of methods based on physiologic interventions. Founders and teachers of integrated methods include every massage professional who designs a massage specifically for an individual client and every devoted massage instructor who attempts to combine and explain methods to students.

---

a single skill; a more appropriate concept is a collection of skills. In addition, the definition of therapeutic massage depends on individual laws and the definition of massage included in those laws. Box 2-4 presents several definitions of massage, including the definition established by the MTBOK, a definition compiled from multiple sources, and the definition of massage therapy used by the National Center for Complementary and Alternative Medicine (NCCAM), an agency of the National Institutes of Health (NIH).

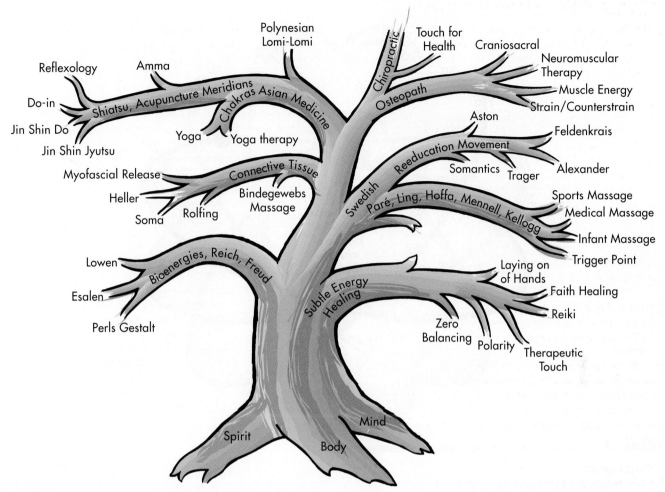

FIGURE 2-1 The therapeutic massage tree. Although massage encompasses a wide diversity in its uses and applications, all forms of therapeutic massage methods stem from the same roots.

Defining massage accurately and completely is difficult because of the many forms of massage currently practiced. An attempt is made to include items from the many definitions found in historical literature, from guidelines provided by state and local laws and professional organizations, and from individual styles and approaches to massage.

SCOPE OF PRACTICE

SECTION OBJECTIVES

Chapter objective covered in this section:

3. The student will be able to define a scope of practice for therapeutic massage.

Using the information presented in this section, the student will be able to perform the following:

- Understand the scope of practice of various health and service professionals
- Explain what constitutes the practice of medicine
- Explain the difference between medical or rehabilitative massage and wellness massage
- Develop a scope of practice for massage that respects the scope of practice of other professionals
- Explore the scope of practice presented by the MTBOK document

As mentioned earlier, the scope of practice of a profession defines the knowledge base and practice parameters of that profession. Each health and service profession has a unique information/knowledge base, yet members of many professions share a common knowledge and methodology. Because of this shared information, the lines defining a profession's scope of practice are not always clear, and overlap can occur. The scope of practice is defined and regulated by the government agency that has jurisdiction over the location of the practice. The individual practitioner is responsible for becoming fully informed about and compliant with these regulations. Practice standards, although not law, provide specific guidelines for the delivery of service and are based in well-developed ethical considerations. The NCBTMB has had standards in place for nearly 20 years; these standards have been almost universally recognized and form the basis for the peer-reviewed disciplinary process for nationally certified practitioners. The MTBOK also presented a recommendation for scope of practice for massage therapy.

Each member of a particular profession acquires a specific knowledge base and must define her personal scope of practice. A professional must be able to evaluate realistically her acquired body of knowledge and skills to determine the

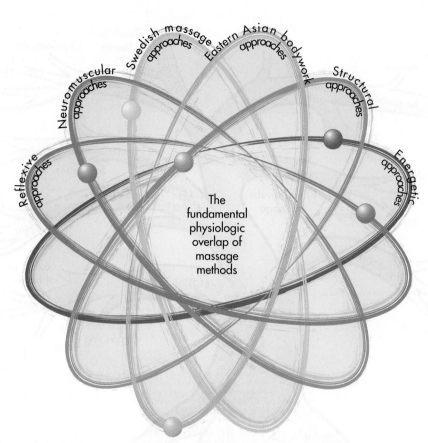

FIGURE 2-2 The fundamental physiologic overlap of massage methods.

parameters of ethical practice within the scope of practice. True professionals understand the limits of their technical skills and scopes of practice and choose to work with other professionals for the best possible outcome for the client.

Currently much of the literature defines the scope of practice of massage by what cannot be done, to prevent infringement on the scope of practice of other health and service professions (Box 2-5).

Scope of practice establishes, for example, that no one but a physician has the legal right to perform any act that falls within the parameters of a medical license. The principle underlying this is simple: a person may not dispense therapeutic or medical advice about the effect of his or her services on a specific disease, ailment, or condition unless that person has adequate training, knowledge, and experience to ensure that the advice is sound and reliable. The scope of practice authorized by a medical or surgical degree is broad and extensive. It authorizes the physician to use drugs and medical preparations and the surgeon to sever and penetrate human tissue during treatment. It further authorizes physicians to use other methods to treat disease, injuries, deformities, and other physical and mental conditions. The law grants such a broad authorization to physicians because the education and testing requirements for a physician's license ensure that the individual is qualified to act as a healer.

All the professions listed in Box 2-6 must employ people who meet educational standards far exceeding the currently accepted requirements for massage in most areas. Professionals with more education are allowed to do more within their specialized fields. Those with less education work under supervision or within a limited scope of practice. The scope of practice for therapeutic massage should complement but not infringe upon the boundaries of the work of these professionals. Hopefully, the future will allow more flexibility and overlap of professional practice for the benefit of clients.

Unique Scope of Practice Parameters for Therapeutic Massage

As mentioned previously, therapeutic massage is unique in that it can be used in two distinct professional areas: wellness and personal services, and health care and sports massage. Massage professionals are involved in various levels of care and support, each requiring more education and higher levels of competence.

Wellness and Personal Services

In the professional world of wellness services, clients seek massage for pleasure, relaxation, and general health maintenance. Wellness approaches enhance and maintain an individual's health and well-being. They usually focus on education and massage methods that encourage normal self-regulating mechanisms of the mind and body. In addition to massage skills, the massage professional must be educated and

Box 2-4 Definitions of Therapeutic Massage

Massage Therapy Body of Knowledge*

Massage therapy is a health care and wellness profession. The practice of massage therapy involves a client-centered session that is intended to fulfill therapeutic goals and in which the therapist has no personal agenda. Massage therapy also meets the well-researched need for touch and human connection. Massage therapy is about one human being touching another with clear intention, focused attention, and an attitude that is compassionate and nonjudgmental. During a session the massage therapist incorporates a wide variety of techniques and approaches to address the client's varied focuses, which may include any or all of the following:

- Treating an injury or a condition
- Relaxation
- Reducing stress
- Wellness
- Enhancing personal growth
- Encouraging awareness of the body
- Facilitating the balance and interconnection of the body, mind, and spirit

Definition Derived from Licensing, Certification, and Professional Organizations

Therapeutic massage is the scientific art and system of assessment and systematic, manual application of a technique to the superficial soft tissue of the skin, muscles, tendons, ligaments, and fascia (and to the structures that lie within the superficial tissue) using the hand, foot, knee, arm, elbow, and forearm. The manual technique involves systematic application of touch, stroking (effleurage), friction, vibration, percussion, kneading (pétrissage), stretching, compression, or passive and active joint movements within the normal physiologic range of motion. Included are adjunctive external applications of water, heat, and cold for the purposes of establishing and maintaining good physical condition and health by normalizing and improving muscle tone, promoting relaxation, stimulating circulation, and producing therapeutic effects on the respiratory and nervous systems and the subtle interactions among all body systems. These intended effects are accomplished through the physiologic, energetic, and mind/body connections in a safe, nonsexual environment that respects the client's self-determined outcome for the session.

National Center for Complementary and Alternative Medicine (NCCAM)†

The term *massage therapy* (also called *massage,* for short; *massage* also refers to an individual treatment session) covers a group of practices and techniques. More than 80 types of massage therapy exist. In all of them, the therapist presses, rubs, and otherwise manipulates the muscles and other soft tissues of the body, often varying pressure and movement. The hands and fingers most often are used for this purpose, but the forearms, elbows, or feet also may be used. Typically, the intent is to relax the soft tissues, increase the delivery of blood and oxygen to the massaged areas, warm them, and reduce pain.

*Modified from Massage Therapy Body of Knowledge (MTBOK) stewards: *Massage therapy body of knowledge (MTBOK),* version 1, May 15, 2010. www.mtbok.org. Accessed March 21, 2011.
†Modified from the National Center for Complementary and Alternative Medicine (NCCAM): *Massage therapy: an introduction.* Pub no D327, September, 2006. http://nccam.nih.gov/health/massage/massageintroduction.htm. Accessed March 21, 2011.

Box 2-5 Code of Ethics and Standards of Practice for Massage

Ethical Principles

The four basic principles that constitute the code of ethics for massage professionals are as follows:

- *Respect for the dignity of people:* Massage professionals must maintain respect for the interests, dignity, rights, and needs of all clients, staff, and colleagues.
- *Responsible caring:* Competent, quality client care must be provided at the highest standard possible.
- *Integrity in relationships:* At all times the professional must behave with integrity, honesty, and diligence in practice and duties.
- *Responsibility to society:* Massage professionals are responsible and accountable to society and must conduct themselves in a manner that maintains high ethical standards.

Standards of Practice

The principles of the code of ethics form the basis of the following standards of practice for massage professionals.

1. Respect all clients, colleagues, and health care professionals through nondiscrimination, regardless of age, gender, race, national origin, sexual orientation, religion, socioeconomic status, body type, political affiliation, state of health, personal habits, and life-coping skills.
2. Perform only those services for which the massage professional is qualified. Massage professionals must honestly represent their education, certification, professional affiliations, and other qualifications. They may apply a treatment only when a reasonable expectation exists that it will be advantageous to the client's condition. The massage professional, in consultation with the client, must continually evaluate the effectiveness of treatment.
3. Respect the scope of practice of other health care and service professionals, including physicians, chiropractors, physical therapists, podiatrists, orthopedists, psychotherapists, counselors, acupuncturists, nurses, exercise physiologists, athletic trainers, nutritionists, spiritual advisors, and cosmetologists.
4. Respect all ethical health care practitioners and work with them to promote health and healing.
5. Acknowledge the limitations of personal skills and, when necessary, refer clients to an appropriately qualified professional. The massage professional must consult with other knowledgeable professionals when:

Continued

Box 2-5 Code of Ethics and Standards of Practice for Massage—cont'd

- A client requires diagnosis and opinion beyond a therapist's capabilities of assessment
- A client's condition is beyond the massage professional's scope of practice
- A combined health care team is required

  If referral to another health care provider is necessary, it must be done with the client's informed consent.

6. Refrain from working with any individual who has a specific disease process without supervision by a licensed medical professional.

7. Be adequately educated and understand the physiologic effects of the specific massage techniques used to determine whether any application is contraindicated and to ensure that the most beneficial techniques are applied to a given individual.

8. Avoid false claims about the potential benefits of the techniques rendered and educate the public about the actual benefits of massage. Strive to maintain an evidence-based practice.

9. Acknowledge the importance and individuality of each person, including colleagues, peers, and clients.

10. Work only with the informed consent of a client and professionally disclose to the client any situation that may interfere with the massage professional's ability to provide the best care to serve the client's best interest.

11. Show respect by honoring a client's process and following all recommendations and by being present, listening, asking only pertinent questions, keeping agreements, being on time, draping properly, and customizing the massage to address the client's needs.

    Note: Draping is covered in Chapter 9. The Ontario guidelines specify the following requirements for draping (Regulated Health Professions Act, 1992):

    - It is the responsibility of the massage professional to ensure the privacy and dignity of the client and to determine whether the client feels comfortable, safe, and secure with the draping provided.
    - The client may choose to be fully draped or clothed throughout the treatment.
    - A female client's breasts are not undraped unless specified by referral from a qualified health care professional and the massage professional is working under the supervision of such a health care professional.
    - The genitals, perineum, and anus are never undraped. The client's consent is required for work on any part of the body, regardless of whether the client is fully clothed, fully draped, or partly draped.

12. Provide a safe, comfortable, and clean environment.

13. Maintain clear and honest communication with clients and keep client communications confidential.

Confidentiality is of the utmost importance. The massage professional must inform the client that the referring physician may be eligible to review the client's records and that records may be subpoenaed by the courts.

14. Conduct business in a professional and ethical manner in relation to clientele, business associates, acquaintances, government bodies, and the public.

15. Follow city, county, state, national, and international requirements.

16. Charge a fair price for the session. Gratuities are appropriate if within reasonable limits (i.e., similar to percentages for other service providers, such as 10% to 20%). A gift, gratuity, or benefit that is intended to influence a referral, decision, or treatment may not be accepted and must be returned to the giver immediately.

17. Keep accurate records and review the records with the client.

18. Never engage in any sexual conduct, sexual conversation, or any other sexual activities involving clients.

19. Avoid affiliation with any business that uses any form of sexual suggestiveness or explicit sexuality in advertising or promoting services or in the actual practice of service.

20. Practice honesty in advertising, promoting services ethically and in good taste and advertising only techniques for which the professional is certified or adequately trained.

21. Strive for professional excellence through regular assessment of personal strengths, limitations, and effectiveness and through continuing education and training.

22. Accept the responsibility to oneself, one's clients, and the profession to maintain physical, mental, and emotional well-being and to inform clients when one is not functioning at full capacity.

23. Refrain from using any mind-altering drugs, alcohol, or intoxicants before or during professional massage sessions.

24. Maintain a professional appearance and demeanor by practicing good hygiene and dressing in a professional, modest, and nonsexual manner.

25. Undergo periodic peer review.

26. Respect all pertinent reporting requirements outlined by legislation regarding abuse.

27. Report to the proper authorities any accurate knowledge and its supportive documentation regarding violations by massage professionals and other health or service professionals.

28. Avoid interests, activities, or influences that might conflict with the obligation to act in the best interest of clients and the massage therapy profession and safeguard professional integrity by recognizing potential conflicts of interest and avoiding them.

---

skilled in teaching prevention measures and encouraging a general wellness lifestyle for clients. When presenting this type of information in the educational context, the professional must make general recommendations rather than specifically tell clients what to do, because the latter can be interpreted as

diagnosing and prescribing, both of which are out of the scope of practice for massage.

In the personal services world of wellness massage, the key goal is to enhance the client's health or to provide massage for individuals who already are healthy and who want to maintain

Box 2-6 Occupational Definitions and Scopes of Practice

The scope of practice described for the following professions is derived from regulations typically established to govern these occupations. The regulations predominantly used for these descriptions are the administrative rules of the Michigan Occupational Regulations' Department of Licensing and Regulation and the Occupational Regulations section of the Michigan Public Health Code.

Acupuncture

Acupuncture is a form of primary health care based on traditional Chinese medical concepts. It uses acupuncture diagnosis and treatment, in addition to adjunctive therapies and diagnostic techniques, to promote, maintain, and restore health and prevent disease. Acupuncture includes but is not limited to insertion of acupuncture needles and application of moxibustion (medicinal herbs burned on or near the skin) to specific areas of the human body.

Athletic Training

Athletic training is the study of athletic performance, injury prevention, and rehabilitation. It includes training regimens; evaluation and assessment of injury; treatment, rehabilitation, and reconditioning of athletic injury; therapeutic exercise; and use of therapeutic modalities.

Chiropractic

Chiropractic is the discipline within the healing arts that deals with the nervous system, its relationship to the spinal column, and its interrelationship with the other body systems. Chiropractic uses radiography to detect spinal subluxation and misalignment and adjusts related bones and tissues to establish neural integrity through techniques that use the inherent recuperative powers of the body to restore and maintain health. Examples of these techniques include the use of analytic instruments, the provision of nutritional advice, and the prescribing of rehabilitative exercise. Chiropractic does not include the performance of incisive surgical procedures or any invasive procedure that requires instrumentation or the dispensing or prescription of drugs or medicine.

Cosmetology

Cosmetology is a service provided to enhance the health, condition, and appearance of the skin, hair, and nails through the use of external preparations designed to cleanse and beautify. It includes the application of beautification processes, such as makeup and skin grooming.

Dentistry

Dentistry is the discipline of diagnosis, treatment, prescription, and surgery for disease, pain, deformity, deficiency, or injury of human teeth, alveolar processes, gums, jaws, and dependent tissues. Dentistry also is concerned with preventive care and the maintenance of good oral health.

Esthetics

An esthetician is a person who works to clean and beautify the skin.

Medicine

Medicine is the diagnosis, treatment, prevention, cure, or relief of human disease, ailment, defect, complaint, or other physical or mental condition by attendance, advice, device, diagnostic test, or other means.

Naturopathy

Naturopathy is the combination of clinical nutrition, herbology, homeopathy, acupuncture, manipulation, hydrotherapy, massage, exercise, and psychological methods, including hypnotherapy and biofeedback, to maintain health. Naturopathic physicians use radiography, ultrasound, and other forms of diagnostic testing but do not perform major surgery or prescribe synthetic drugs.

Nursing

Nursing is the systematic application of substantial specialized knowledge and skill, derived from the biologic, physical, and behavioral sciences, to the care, treatment, counsel, and health education of individuals who are experiencing changes in the normal health process or who require assistance in the maintenance of health and the prevention or management of illness, injury, and disability.

Osteopathic Medicine

Osteopathic medicine is an independent school of medicine and surgery that uses full methods of diagnosis and treatment in physical and mental health and disease, including the prescription and administration of drugs and vitamins; operative surgery; obstetrics; and radiologic and electromagnetic diagnostics. Osteopathy emphasizes the interrelationship of the musculoskeletal system with other body systems.

Physical Therapy

Physical therapy is the evaluation or treatment of an individual by the use of effective physical measures, therapeutic exercise, and rehabilitative procedures, with or without devices, to prevent, correct, or alleviate a physical or mental disability. It includes treatment planning, the performance of tests and measurements, interpretation of referrals, instruction, consultative services, and supervision of personnel. Physical measures include massage, mobilization, and the application of heat, cold, air, light, water, electricity, and sound.

Podiatric Medicine

Podiatric medicine is the examination, diagnosis, and treatment of abnormal nails and superficial excrescences (abnormal outgrowths or enlargements) on the human feet, including corns, warts, callosities, bunions, and arch troubles. It also includes the medical, surgical, or mechanical treatment and physiotherapy of ailments that affect the condition of the feet. It does not include amputation of the feet or the use or administration of general anesthetics.

Psychology

Psychology is the rendering to individuals, groups, organizations, or the public service involving the application of principles, methods, and procedures of understanding, predicting, and influencing behavior for the purpose of diagnosis, assessment, prevention, amelioration, or treatment of mental or emotional disorders, disabilities, and behavioral adjustment problems. Treatment is provided by means of psychotherapy, counseling, behavior modification, hypnosis, biofeedback techniques, psychological tests, and other verbal or behavioral methods. Psychology does not include the prescription of drugs, performance of surgery, or administration of electroconvulsive therapy.

or improve their health. It also is important not to infringe upon the cosmetology scope of practice by working with cosmetic applications to the skin through the use of oils, wraps, or other preparations. The spa and massage franchise systems are major growth industries for wellness .

The wellness and personal services professional track allows the therapeutic massage professional to work most independently, with the most varied clientele (and in some instances animals), and to share the gifts of professional touch with the general population, many of whom need support in managing stress so that they do not become ill and require medical attention. Wellness services are a wonderful place for a massage professional. As the professional development of therapeutic massage progresses, care must be taken that wellness services are not abandoned.

Taking a wealth of information into account, this textbook determines the scope of practice of wellness massage to be a nonspecific approach that focuses on assessment procedures for detecting contraindications to massage, as well as the need for referral to other health care professionals, and on the development of a health-enhancing physical state for the client. The plan for the massage session is developed by combining information, desired massage outcomes, and directions from the client with the skills of the massage practitioner to provide an individualized massage session aimed at normalizing the body systems. This normalization is accomplished through the following:

- External manual stimulation of the nervous, circulatory, and respiratory systems; connective tissue; and muscles to achieve:
  - Generalized stress reduction
  - A decrease in muscle tension
  - Symptomatic relief of pain related to soft tissue dysfunction
  - Increased circulation
  - Other benefits similar to those of exercise
- Other relaxation responses produced by therapeutic massage to increase the client's well-being

Health Care and Sports Massage Services

The professional world of health care requires specific training for the skilled application of massage to promote rehabilitation and performance and to manage pathologic conditions (sports massage comes under this definition).

Currently, health care professionals do not receive extensive education in massage therapy. The time and labor-intensive therapy required for massage make it difficult for physicians, physical therapists, nurses, occupational therapists, and athletic trainers to include therapeutic massage with their other interventions and responsibilities. These considerations support the development of massage therapy as a distinct health practice and an adjunct to these other professions.

Physical therapy and athletic training are the professions most likely to be compared with the practice of rehabilitative massage, and care must be taken to respect the professional boundaries of these disciplines. This is particularly important for massage professionals with advanced training, who become qualified to work with more complicated situations involving

rehabilitation and the management of chronic conditions. Even the most comprehensive massage training programs do not compare with the extensive training of the physical therapist or other professionals, such as nurses and athletic trainers. However, this does not invalidate the expertise of the therapeutic massage professional. A higher level of education allows the massage professional to work effectively with the physician, physical therapist, or other health professional in a health care setting in which these professionals supervise an overall treatment program that includes massage.

This textbook describes the scope of practice for clinical massage delivered within the health care setting and for massage provided in conjunction with specific athletic training protocols: specifically, massage therapists develop, maintain, rehabilitate, or augment physical function; relieve or prevent physical dysfunction and pain; and enhance the well-being of the client. Methods include assessment of the soft tissue and joints, and treatment by soft tissue manipulation, hydrotherapy, remedial exercise programs, and client self-care programs.

The massage educational requirements of the Canadian provinces of Ontario and British Columbia are extensive enough to support clinical massage delivered in the health care setting and massage provided in conjunction with specific athletic training protocols. The two provinces currently require more than 2200 class hours, and that number is rising.

The information in this text can carry the student from the service world of wellness massage into the world of health care services (Figure 2-3), primarily working to manage dysfunctional conditions, such as pain and chronic disorders, and to support those who may benefit from a generalized approach to massage, such as an athlete. Chapter 16 presents a series of case studies and treatment plans that provide a model of massage applications in both professional worlds.

This text does not attempt to develop specific protocols for the precise intervention measures needed for serious illness and trauma. Massage can provide supportive care using stress and pain management for those who are ill if the massage professional is supervised by qualified medical personnel.

The distinction between wellness massage and clinical/medical/rehabilitative approaches to massage used for illness and trauma may seem subtle, but the difference is simple. Wellness massage practitioners do not work with sick or injured people unless directly supervised by licensed and qualified professionals, such as physicians, nurses, and physical therapists. Rather, they help most of the population, who are not sick but are stressed and uncomfortable, to feel better and cope with stress. This benefit of massage may help prevent more serious, stress-induced illness.

All professionals have specialized training, certain responsibilities, and positions in which they function best. Respecting each professional's strengths is the ethical thing to do. Knowing the definition and scope of practice of other health and service professionals helps the massage practitioner respect these professionals and maintain appropriate boundaries for their practices.

Normal Adaptation

Client displays resourceful functioning with good ability to respond to and recover from stress.

Massage Training

500+ hours of education.

Health Care Supervision Required?

No.

Support Professionals

Fitness trainers, cosmetologists, wellness educators, prevention and healthy lifestyle focused health care and mental health professionals.

Ineffective and Strained Adaptation

(Scope of practice encompasses Normal Adaptation)

Client displays ability to function with effort and reduced ability to respond to and recover from stress. Recovery time is increased. Client demands extraordinary function of body.

Massage Training

1000+ hours of education.

Poor Ability to Adapt

(Scope of practice encompasses technician and practitioner levels)

Client displays function breakdown — substantially reduced ability to respond and recover or extensive healing period required such as with surgery and trauma.

Massage Training

2000+ hours of education.

Health Care or Athletic Trainer Supervision Required?

Possibly. No for wellness service and mild dysfunctional patterns. Moderate to identifiable dysfunctional pattern — Yes, but indirect; attention to referral needs is important.

Support Professionals

Athletic trainers — exercise physiologist, health care and mental health professionals — spiritually based support.

Health Care Supervision Required?

Yes. Direct supervision for all clients in this category; Possibly for dysfunctional category; No for wellness clients.

Support Professionals

Entire multidisciplinary team — health care/mental health professionals — spiritually based support.

- ■ Comprehensive scope of practice for therapeutic massage
- □ Wellness personal service scope of practice for therapeutic massage
- ▨ Dysfunctional and athletic patterns scope of practice for therapeutic massage
- ▨ Illness/trauma scope of practice for therapeutic massage

FIGURE 2-3 The most expansive scope of practice for therapeutic massage is represented by the entire box (outlined in dark blue). Within this scope of practice are levels of professional function based on training and experience. The scope of practice for an entry-level position in therapeutic massage is represented by the Normal Adaptation box *(white box)*. The next higher level of professional practice, the massage practitioner, is depicted in the Ineffective and Strained Adaptation Ability box *(light violet box)*. The third and highest level of professional practice requires the most education and experience; it is depicted in the Poor or Inability to Adopt box *(light purple box)*. Note that each level encompasses the one next to it. As the model shows, the scope of practice expands with experience and education effectively with all groups.

Limits of Practice

A massage professional's ability to practice has legal limits. A scope of practice established by legislation both defines and limits the ability to practice massage. Respectful practice of therapeutic massage limits the scope of practice so that the practitioner does not encroach on the scope of practice of other professionals.

Each professional also has personal limits that affect the scope of practice. These limits involve the type and extent of the person's education, personal biases, life experiences, specific interests in terms of the type of client served, and any physical limitations, such as size and endurance levels (Proficiency Exercise 2-4).

💡 PROFICIENCY EXERCISE 2-4

1. Write a scope of practice statement for therapeutic massage that fits your level of practice upon graduation from your training program. If possible, talk with other professionals about this scope of practice and ask how it compares with their own.

2. Investigate the scope of practice defined by licensed professionals in your community for the health and service professions listed in this section. This information can be obtained from the state agency that oversees licensing and regulation.

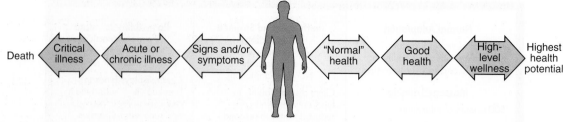

FIGURE 2-4 The illness to health continuum.
(From Chitty K, Black BP: *Professional nursing*, ed 5, St. Louis, 2007, Saunders.)

Professional limits are valid and valuable. They allow us to set and maintain boundaries that support each professional in the most successful professional practice structure. Limits of practice free us from falling into the trap of believing we must be all things to all people; we cannot be, and it is ethical to acknowledge the limits of practice and to work together with other professionals.

The client's ability to adapt also imposes limits on practice. The ability to adapt to internal and external stressors can indicate where an individual is on the illness to health continuum (Figure 2-4).

Three general categories of adaptation have been described:

- *Effective or good ability to adapt:* The client is considered generally healthy.
- *Ineffective or moderate and strained ability to adapt:* The client is considered generally to be stressed and/or chronically ill but functioning with strain, or is exposed to high or sustained levels of performance stress (e.g., competing athletes, entertainers, military on active patrol duty).
- *Poor ability or inability to adapt:* The client is considered to be at the point of breakdown. Examples of such clients include those who are suffering from acute illness or acute trauma; those who are highly stressed and not coping; those recovering from surgery; or those receiving chemotherapy or hospice care.

These adaptive categories are related to the scope of practice (see Figure 2-3).

Effective or Good Ability to Adapt

A person who is functioning well is able to be involved with work that is satisfying in both an intrinsic and extrinsic sense. For example, a woman may not love her work, but she may appreciate that the job supports her family (extrinsic value); or, she may love her work even if it does not financially provide for all wants (intrinsic value). A person responds normally when play balances work in such a way that the result is self-regulation and support for mental and physical functions.

Another example of effective adaptation is a person who can share with others or who has a passion for a mission, a cause, or a vision, be it as simple as gardening or as complex as an encompassing environmental or political cause, and who receives intimacy, support, and fulfillment from the process.

A person who can make choices to regulate and cope with exterior influences internally and who can be resourceful and flexible in life situations displays effective adaptive functioning. The ability to love and be loved supports the ability to adapt to life stressors. The supportive balance of these factors and the ability to exert an internal control to accommodate less than ideal situations, as well as to develop realistic and attainable goals and a plan to alter situations, indicate health.

Wellness approaches enhance and maintain effective adaptive capacity. Professional support can assist in the general maintenance of health through wellness support, education, and preventive care. Therapeutic massage plays a definitive role in general health maintenance. These clients use massage on a regular basis as part of a health and wellness program, comparable to the daily hygiene activities of bathing or brushing the teeth or to daily or weekly house cleaning. These clients want to maintain their current normal functioning status.

Massage professionals who provide services at the level of supportive wellness care require fundamental information about general wellness processes. Massage professionals should be able to teach general methods of stress management, including effective breathing, progressive relaxation, and quieting responses (meditation-type activities); they should be able to give general dietary recommendations; and they should emphasize the importance of appropriate exercise programs. Most people do better with the discipline required to maintain these activities when they have the support of a professional acting as a coach. A well-trained massage professional can provide this type of service.

Massage professionals need not always be supervised directly when working within a wellness scope of practice. A properly trained massage professional can recognize a client who is not functioning effectively, not recovering from the stress of daily activities, and beginning to fall into dysfunctional patterns. As the client's problems become more complicated, the support and expertise of the health or training professional become more important, and referral or supervision is indicated.

Ineffective or Moderate and Strained Ability to Adapt

People who are functioning with effort and are beginning to break down fall into this category. Physical or emotional strain may indicate the need for more focused and specific complex interventions.

Performance strain is seen in optimally functioning people who rely on fine motor skills and coordinated physical action (e.g., athletes, musicians, and dancers). This type of strain requires a more complex massage interaction than that provided for wellness and preventive care. Those who operate at a high level of stress and sustain the fight-or-flight response to cope (e.g., police, soldiers) eventually compromise their ability to adapt, leading to a maladaptive process that leads to an increased potential for illness and accident.

Those attempting to function outside their capacity strain the adaptive capacity. These individuals often are caring for elderly parents, newborn babies, or someone who is ill. They may be coping with financial strain or with grief and loss, such as the death of a child or spouse or working multiple jobs. These individuals continue to function but at a reduced level, and they show signs and symptoms of physical and emotional strain. A multidisciplinary team approach may be needed, one that uses a defined care and treatment plan to reduce the level of physical and psychological stress and to re-establish or teach internal coping methods. A massage professional who works with individuals in this category requires a broader-based education that should encompass stress response, the origin of physical and mental difficulties, methods of improving functioning, standard health care interventions, and training protocols.

Clients in this category benefit from a specifically designed care/treatment plan that includes a means of measuring the outcomes of care objectively. Realistic and attainable short- and long-term goals are developed, and time frames are set for the achievement of these goals. The general goals of the massage professional are to help the client move toward normal functioning, regain personal control of the body/mind/spirit systems, and achieve and maintain optimum health. This approach is different from that of massage used for wellness or preventive care. The methods and information provided may be the same or similar, but the focus and goals are different. Clients dealing with dysfunction or complex circumstances or who demand high levels of performance want to change where they are in life, not maintain the status quo.

Because massage temporarily helps take the edge off physical discomfort and reduces the strain of the stress response, allowing people to feel or perform better under less than desirable circumstances, massage intervention may or may not be appropriate in these circumstances. People tend to be less motivated to change if their circumstances seem tolerable. Massage may diminish the client's motivation to change, interfering with the process being worked through with other health care or training professionals. Massage can help support stress management in clients who find themselves faced with extraordinary stress loads. If the person cannot alter the situation causing the dysfunctional stress, massage can serve as a means of easing physical stress and a beneficial coping measure when combined with other medical, behavioral, and emotional coping techniques. Massage does not deal directly with the physical, emotional, or spiritual state contributing to the stress; rather, it supports the physical system so that the person can better withstand stress.

Poor Ability or Inability to Adapt

Individuals experiencing acute illness, invasive medical treatment, injury, emotional overload, or spiritual hopelessness are reaching or have reached a point where they are unable to adapt, coping mechanisms breakdown, and a marked decline occurs in the ability to function. These individuals require a comprehensive intervention process. Often little distinction can be made between dysfunction and breakdown or illness. Massage must be used very carefully during acute illnesses such as a severe infection and in various types of cancer treatment, postoperative patients, physical or emotional shock, patients receiving hospice care, and so forth. The client may have difficulty handling any additional adaptation demands created by massage. Even the most subtle forms of massage involve a controlled physiologic stress to the system that requires a physical adaptation response.

Massage therapists specifically trained to work with those experiencing these types of situations carefully monitor the response to massage and respond appropriately to any signs of adaptive strain caused by massage. A massage therapist working with individuals facing these severe situations and conditions must be part of a health care team monitored carefully and supervised by a health care professional, especially if the client is taking medications (see Appendix C). In such cases massage intervention supports health care approaches, and a comprehensive care/treatment plan is developed with massage as one of the treatment methods. Often massage is used primarily for palliative (comfort) care. The massage professional needs additional training in pathology, pharmacology, psychology, and clinical reasoning skills to be able to help integrate massage into an overall health care plan.

Body/Mind/Spirit Connection

The body, mind, and spirit share a definite link. The physical body functions involve anatomy and physiology, including the body's chemical responses. Feelings are body functions.

The cognitive process of the mind interprets physical sensations and sets physical responses in motion. Emotions seem to be the result of the interplay between body and mind. Behavior is the action that results from the physical/emotional/cognitive combination.

The spirit provides the strength, hope, faith, and love that create a reason for being. Each of these areas of functioning influences and interacts with the others.

In reality, the body, mind, and spirit cannot be separated; however, together they involve too much information to allow a professional to become an expert in all areas of human function. Professional skill levels, the parameters of the scope of practice, and avoidance of dual and multiple roles in the professional relationship artificially divide the body, mind, and spirit functioning of the person seeking assistance. This is undesirable, but often it is unavoidable. An excellent solution is for professionals to work together. A multidisciplinary, integrative approach to care is best, with professionals working together to support a comprehensive care plan that addresses all the client's needs. Most hospice programs are excellent models of multidisciplinary teams.

Determining the Limits of Practice

As a massage professional, you can determine whether you are within your scope of practice by making sure your responses to the client are from a body and massage perspective. When a client expresses distress, shares personal information, or requests specific information, first determine whether the issue is most specifically a body, mind, or spirit issue. If it is a mental or spiritual issue, use listening skills and acknowledge the situation but do not attempt to problem-solve or provide professional intervention. If the situation presented is a physical concern (i.e., affects the body), decide whether the information falls within the scope of therapeutic massage and respond accordingly.

The severity or complexity of a situation determines whether simple listening, without advice being given, is sufficient or whether a professional referral is indicated. Often the physical stress of the circumstances can be managed by massage approaches while the client seeks additional help from supportive resources and professionals who can deal more specifically with the source of the problem. Massage therapists recognize when to refer individuals to these professionals.

Health care, training, coaching, and cosmetology professionals have committed a significant part of their lives to formal schooling, licensing procedures, and continual experiential and formal education. The information they possess is specific to their professional discipline, yet also quite broad. Although massage techniques may not be common knowledge among many professionals, the importance and power of touch are. Many of these professionals understand that massage practitioners use touch skills that these other professionals may be unable to provide because of the nature of their therapeutic relationship with the client. To develop and support a cooperative, multidisciplinary philosophy of care, massage professionals must respect the dedication of the professionals with whom they work by maintaining the appropriate scope of practice for therapeutic massage.

Massage professionals benefit from being able to adapt massage therapy to various health care, training, and personal service needs; in doing so, they are best able to serve both the professionals with whom they work and the clients they serve. In a multidisciplinary team setting (e.g., the spa environment, which may employ wellness professionals, fitness and sport professionals, and medical professionals), it is important to be able to communicate effectively with any professional with whom you work; this requires you to be familiar with the language and terminology used in that profession. It is important to be able to explain massage therapy intervention in terms familiar to the professionals on the team and also to be able to explain the ways you, as a massage professional, intend to support spa, health, or training professionals in providing appropriate care.

Understanding the adaptive capacity of people and its relationship to the scope of practice of therapeutic massage helps the massage professional establish an ethical practice and begin the discovery of the therapeutic process.

EVIDENCE-BASED PRACTICE

SECTION OBJECTIVES

Chapter objective covered in this section:
4. The student will be able to define evidence-based practice.
Using the information presented in this section, the student will be able to perform the following:
- Explain the importance of an evidence-based practice as an aspect of professional behavior
- List the skills necessary to perform massage from an evidence-based and informed professional foundation

As massage therapy becomes a common part of an integrated health care system, the massage therapy profession will be expected to maintain high levels of professional practice. One area in which massage therapists must become educated is evidence-based practice. **Evidence-based practice (EBP)** is defined as "the conscientious, explicit, and judicious use of current best evidence in making decisions about the care of individual patients" (Sackett et al., 2000).

EBP requires that decisions about health care be based on the best available, current, valid, and relevant evidence. These decisions should be made by those receiving care, informed by the knowledge of those providing care, within the context of available resources.

To function in the evidence-based health care structure, you must be able to do the following:
- Find, read, and analyze research (this is called *research literacy*).
- Analyze the accuracy of clinically based evidence of massage benefit when research is not able to validate fully the massage result.
- Use clinical reasoning to apply the information to massage practice.
- Apply information derived from the clinical reasoning process to develop outcome-based massage sessions.
- Justify decisions on indications for and contraindications to massage applications for individual clients.
- Address each client in a client-centered manner, individualizing the massage for the individual client based on valid evidence.

Developing an evidence-based massage practice is a process. It is important to begin now, at the very start of your education, to use the best available research evidence, clinical reasoning, experience, and professional knowledge of the client to provide the best in massage care. Evidence-based practice is a mark of professionalism. Research literacy, clinical reasoning, and outcome-based massage application are discussed throughout this textbook, especially in Chapter 5.

Evidence in Evidence-Based Practice

Evidence can be generated from a range of sources, including but not limited to the following:
- Academic journals (e.g., the *Journal of Bodywork and Movement Therapies* and the *International Journal of Therapeutic Massage & Bodywork: Research, Education, & Practice*)
- Massage Therapy Foundation
- Research and systematic reviews of research

- The Internet (e.g., PubMed, Google Scholar, Medline)
- Data gathered from other massage therapists, especially in the form of case reports
- Knowledge gained from experienced massage therapists and other health care professionals

Once evidence has been gathered, the following questions must be answered:

- How relevant is the evidence to what we are seeking to understand or decide?
- How does the evidence represent the population that concerns us?
- How reliable and valid is the source of the evidence?

Evidence-Informed Practice

A term that is similar to evidence-based practice is *evidence-informed practice*. The original concept was evidence-based practice, meaning that quality evidence was available to support actions. However, in many disciplines, such as massage, research cannot always be related to practice. When we provide therapeutic massage for a client, we want to be as evidence-based as possible and be evidence informed when definitive evidence does not exist. Evidence-informed practice includes the following:

- Practice knowledge and experience
- The opinions of colleagues and other professionals
- Intuitive or gut feelings
- The wishes and experience of clients
- Evidence from research in massage or other, similar disciplines

You may want to use evidence to:

- Explain and justify your reasons for a decision
- Help you choose between different approaches
- Explain what the research says about massage services a client is receiving
- Raise your awareness about a condition or illness

Currently, not enough high-quality research is available for therapeutic massage practice to be considered completely evidence-based; however, the research is improving. Chapter 5 provides a glimpse into the exciting world of research. Professional and ethical behavior dictates that massage professionals must disclose to clients and others the current status of research and must not make definitive claims for methods that have not yet undergone the scrutiny of qualified researchers. Also, realizing that we will never really understand the multilayered benefits of compassionate touch is okay.

Standard of Care

As mentioned previously, a standard of care is the assessment and treatment process that a clinician (e.g., massage therapist) should follow for a certain type of clinical circumstance performed at the level at which similarly qualified practitioners manage the client's care under the same or similar circumstances. The massage therapy community, with the support of the Massage Therapy Foundation, has committed to developing best practices guidelines (i.e., a collection of standards determined and practiced by our profession). Evidence-based and informed standards will be educational for the members

of our profession and for other health care providers and the general public.

The role of Massage Therapy Foundation is to develop an inclusive process to identify evidence-based/informed practice guidelines, backed by systematic academic and peer review and clinical research when available. This process is in its infancy and will evolve over time.

ETHICS AND STANDARDS OF PRACTICE

SECTION OBJECTIVES

Chapter objective covered in this section:

5. The student will be able to develop and explain a code of ethics and the standards of practice for therapeutic massage.

Using the information presented in this section, the student will be able to perform the following:

- Develop a personal and professional code of ethics using the eight ethical principles
- Explain the standards of practice for therapeutic massage

Ethics

Culture, time, location, events, politics, religion, scientific knowledge, and many other factors affect the way we interpret behavior. Ethics defines the behavior we expect of ourselves and others and society's expectations of a profession. Simply defined, ethics is "what is right." Our society determines that a person has acted ethically when the right thing has been done. However, what is the right thing? No one individual or group has the answer. Often the best that can be offered in discussions of ethics are questions and guidelines based on principles of conduct established by a group.

Ethics has social, professional, and personal dimensions. Separating these elements is not easy in theory or in practice. We behave according to a complex and continually changing set of rules, customs, and expectations. For this reason, ethical behavior must be a dynamic process of reflection and revision.

Ethics is not just a varied collection of do's and don'ts; rather, it is a system of principles that tie together in a reasonable, coherent way to make our society and our lives as civilized and happy as possible. Conflicts and uncertainties are inevitable. For this reason, in applying ethics we must learn more than a list of guidelines, more than just what to do in this or that particular case; we must also develop a set of priorities and a way of thinking about them. To use ethics in decision making, we must be able to reason about what we have learned in order to capture the spirit of being ethical. Although morals and values ultimately are a personal concern, ethics is a reflection of one's professional and social character.

The purpose of practicing our profession ethically is to promote and maintain the welfare of the client. Laws often reflect the minimal standards necessary to protect the safety and welfare of the public, whereas codes of ethics represent the ideal standards set by a profession. Through their behavior, professionals can comply both with the law and with professional codes. If compliance with the law is the only motivation in ethical behavior, the person is said to be practicing **mandatory ethics**. If, however, the professional strives for the highest

Evolve Activity 2-2

possible benefit and welfare for the client, he or she behaves with aspirational ethics (Corey et al., 2006).

As professionals we must constantly be alert not only to gross violations of ethical principles, but also to the more subtle ethical violations that occur when the client's welfare is not the primary determining factor of professional behavior. An example of the latter is hesitating to refer a client to a more qualified massage professional because referral means the loss of a paying client. Often this type of unethical conduct goes unnoticed, yet the client's welfare is compromised. This situation is further complicated because the professional often does not recognize the breach in ethical behavior. Mentoring (career support by someone more experienced), supervision (monitoring by one with more expertise), peer support (interaction and exchange of information among fellow professionals), and meticulous objective personal reflection on professional behavior can bring to light these more subtle types of ethical violations. Professionals can monitor their own behavior by asking themselves often whether they are doing what is best for the client and whether their behavior is ethical.

Professional growth involves change in our knowledge, skills, attitudes, and beliefs. A professional code of ethics is a set of norms adopted by a professional group to direct choices and behavior in a manner consistent with professional responsibility. Many elements in the profession of massage enhance the lives of its practitioners, such as respect, authority, and prestige. In return, professionals must be willing to adjust their personal behavior for the professional good. We have to gauge our personal and professional behavior not only by what is right and good for us as individuals, but also by what is appropriate for the client and the profession as a whole.

Ethical Principles

The following eight principles guide professional ethical behavior:

1. *Respect* (esteem and regard for clients, other professionals, and oneself)
2. *Client autonomy and self-determination* (the freedom to decide and the right to sufficient information to make the decision)
3. *Veracity* (the right to the objective truth)
4. *Proportionality* (the principle that benefit must outweigh the burden of treatment)
5. *Nonmaleficence* (the principle that the profession shall do no harm and prevent harm from happening)
6. *Beneficence* (the principle that treatment should contribute to the client's well-being)
7. *Confidentiality* (respect for privacy of information)
8. *Justice* (the principle that ensures equality among clients)

These broad concepts direct the development of standards of practice.

Standards of Practice

Standards of practice provide specific guidelines and rules that form a concrete professional structure. For example, In standards of practice, the ethical principle of respect translates into professional behavior, such as maintaining the client's privacy and modesty, providing a safe environment, and being on time for appointments. The principle of client autonomy and self-determination requires informed consent and ready access for clients to their files.

Standards of practice direct quality care and provide a means of measuring the quality of care. They usually are more concrete than ethical principles.

Code of Ethics and Standards of Practice for Therapeutic Massage

Because the massage therapy profession is not yet united in terms of professional affiliation and techniques, presenting a code of ethics or providing agreed-upon standards of practice for the massage professional is difficult. Because each of the professional groups that constitute the massage profession has developed its own code of ethics and standards of practice, this text offers a comprehensive compilation of many ethical codes and standards of practice, developed through professional organizations, licensing requirements, and the standards of practice of other health professions (Box 2-5). An attempt has been made to include all points presented in the various ethical conduct codes and standards of practice statements.

INFORMED CONSENT

SECTION OBJECTIVES

Chapter objective covered in this section:
6. The student will be able to complete an informed consent process.
Using the information presented in this section, the student will be able to perform the following:
- List and explain the nine components of informed consent
- Determine whether a client can provide informed consent for a massage
- Prepare written client information materials to support the informed consent process
- Complete two different types of informed consent forms

Informed consent is a protection process for the consumer. It requires that clients understand what will occur, that they participate voluntarily, and that they be competent to give consent. Informed consent is also an educational procedure that allows clients to decide knowledgeably whether they want to receive a massage, whether they want a particular therapist to work with them, and whether the professional structure, including client rules and regulations, is acceptable to them. Informed consent supports professional ethical behavior. It reflects the ethical principle of client participation and self-determination in a client-centered approach.

Clients must be able to provide informed consent and demonstrate that they understand the information presented to them (Proficiency Exercise 2-5). Parents or guardians must provide informed consent for minors. Guardians must provide informed consent for those unable to do so (e.g., clients with dementia). Ethical decision making becomes important in "gray areas," such as when a language barrier exists and the massage professional is not sure the client understands him, or when any form of intoxication or prescription drug use is involved that alters the client's judgment.

True informed consent presents the opportunity to evaluate the options available and the risks involved in each method;

💡 PROFICIENCY EXERCISE 2-5

Gather in groups of three and write about a specific situation in which informed consent would be difficult to obtain from a client. For example, the client has diminished hearing, or you do not speak the client's language. The groups should then exchange responses and role-play some of the situations; one student acts as the massage practitioner, one as the client, and the third evaluates the way the situation was handled. Try different situations until each student has had a chance to play each role.

Box 2-7   Informed Consent

The following questions should be answered at the outset of the professional relationship:
- What are the goals of the therapeutic program?
- What services will be provided?
- What behavior is expected of the client?
- What are the risks and benefits of the process?
- What are the practitioner's qualifications?
- What are the financial considerations?
- How long is the therapy expected to last?
- What are the limitations of confidentiality?
- In what areas does the professional have mandatory reporting requirements?

---

it also requires the massage professional to include information about the inherent and potential benefits and hazards of the proposed treatment, the alternatives available, and the probable results if treatment is not provided. Clients have the legal right to choose from a range of suggested options and to receive enough information to allow them to pick the most appropriate approach for them. Credentials and personal and professional limitations that may affect the client-therapist relationship must be disclosed and validated. Clients also need information about recourse options if the outcomes of the massage are undesirable. As professionals, we are ethically bound to ensure that the client makes choices based on a solid understanding of the information presented. The professional is responsible for providing the client with this information (Box 2-7).

Intake Procedures

A comprehensive intake procedure, including an informed consent process, is necessary when defined outcomes span a series of sessions. A needs assessment, which is based on the client's history and a physical assessment, is used to devise an initial treatment plan. The initial treatment plan states the therapeutic goals, duration of the sessions, number of appointments needed to meet the agreed-upon goals, cost, general classification of intervention to be used, and an objective method for measuring progress and identifying when goals have been reached (the forms used for these procedures are presented in Chapters 4 and 11).

Single or random massage sessions usually do not necessarily require a full needs assessment or a treatment plan. Instead, possible contraindications to massage are identified. The informed consent process informs the client of the limitations of a single massage session and describes the approaches used in the single-session massage experience.

A form with all the pertinent information is signed by the client and kept in the massage practitioner's files. Maintaining a record of signed informed consent forms is an important legal issue; in many jurisdictions, touching a person without the person's consent is an action that can be prosecuted as battery.

The following is a possible sequence for obtaining informed consent.

1. The massage professional provides a general explanation of massage, supported by written information (often in the form of a brochure) about indications, benefits, contraindications, and alternative approaches that provide benefits similar to those of massage.

2. The massage professional informs the client about the scope of practice for massage; reporting measures for professional misconduct and recourse policies; the professional's training, experience, and credentials; and any limiting factors that may affect the professional relationship, including lack of training in a particular area and any special circumstances of the massage professional (e.g., hearing or vision difficulty) that may need to be considered. The client is given written information covering these topics, often in the form of a brochure, to enhance his or her understanding of this discussion.

3. The massage professional then discusses business and professional policies and procedures, including the logical consequences of noncompliance by the client. These policies include handling of payment, returned checks, additional charges, gratuities, late arrival, scheduling, sexual impropriety, draping, hygiene, sanitation, and confidentiality and limits of confidentiality. The client also is given pertinent written information about these topics, such as a professional policy statement (Box 2-8).

4. After these procedures have been followed, the client signs an informed consent form (see the sample in Box 2-10). The client should not be overwhelmed with extensive, detailed information, but it is important to provide enough information for the individual to make an informed choice. Informed consent is a continual process, and client education and involvement in the therapeutic approach are always supported and encouraged.

Needs Assessment and the Initial Care/Treatment Plan

As mentioned previously, if the client is working toward specific outcome goals that will require several appointments, a needs assessment and an initial treatment plan are completed (Box 2-9). Specific details on completing this process are provided in Chapter 4.

The process of assessing needs, identifying goals, and developing a treatment plan takes 30 minutes to 1 hour and constitutes the initial intake procedure. In complex circumstances, this process can extend over the first two or three sessions. It is appropriate to charge for the intake session, which is an important part of the professional interaction. The treatment plan may evolve or change during subsequent sessions as the

Box 2-8 **Developing a Client Brochure and Policy Statement**

A massage professional should cover the following important points in developing a client brochure and policy statement.

Type of Service
- Explain the type of massage you provide.
- Explain the benefits and limitations of this particular style of massage.
- Specify whether you specialize in working with a particular group, such as elderly people, athletes, or people with specific problems such as headaches or back pain.
- Indicate any situations or conditions with which you do not care to work, such as pregnancy or certain medical conditions. Provide a brief explanation to avoid implying discrimination; for example, "Since I do not have specific training in geriatric care, I refer clients over the age of 80."

Training and Experience
- If your state requires licensing or if you are nationally certified, provide documentation.
- State how long you have been in practice, what school you attended, whether the school was approved by any state or accrediting body, and how many classroom hours were required for graduation.
- Provide information about continuing education you have pursued.
- Provide information about any additional education (e.g., you are also an athletic trainer).
- Provide the names of any professional organizations of which you are an active member.

Appointment Policies
- Specify the length of an average session.
- Inform the client of the days you work and your hours and whether you do on-site residential or business work.
- Inform the client that the first appointment for intake will be longer than subsequent appointments; also state whether you take emergency appointments and how often you suggest that clients come for massage sessions.
- Be clear about the cancellation policy and your policy for late appointments.
- Explain to the client any change in or restriction on physical activity before or after the session.

Client and Practitioner Expectations
- Explain in detail what happens at the first massage session (i.e., paperwork, medical history, and other preliminaries).
- Make sure clients know they can partly undress or undress down to their underclothes and that they are always covered and draped during the session.
- Explain the order in which you massage (face up or face down to begin), the parts of the body on which you work and in what order, whether you use oils or creams, if a shower is available before or after the massage, and if bathing at home before the massage appointment is expected.
- Make sure the client understands whether talking is appropriate during the session and that you should be informed if anything feels uncomfortable.
- If you have low lighting and music during the session, be sure the client is comfortable with that atmosphere.

- Make sure the client understands when a reaction might be expected, such as tenderness over a trigger point when direct pressure methods are used.
- Tell clients that before the session, you will discuss with them the goals for the massage and the proposed styles and methods of massage, and that consent must be given for all massage procedures.
- Inform the client that your profession has a code of ethics and explain your policy on confidentiality.
- Let clients know that if they are uncomfortable in any way, a friend or relative may accompany them.
- Inform clients that they can stop the massage at any time and do not need to give a reason for doing so.

Fees
Make sure your fee structure is clearly defined regarding the following:
- How often you raise your fees
- Whether you have a sliding fee scale
- Whether you take only cash or will accept money orders, checks, or credit cards
- Whether you bill
- Whether you accept insurance
- How often insurance covers your services
- Different fees for variations in the length of a session
- Whether a series of sessions can be bought at a discount
- Whether you pay any referral fees for new clients

Sexual Appropriateness
- Sexual behavior by the therapist toward the client or by the client toward the therapist is always unethical and inappropriate. It is always the responsibility of the therapist or health professional to ensure that sexual misconduct does not occur.
- If a client feels that the massage therapist acted inappropriately, he or she should feel free to address this issue immediately. When necessary the client has the right to inform the massage therapist's licensing board, certification body, and professional organization.
- A person who asks someone to commit an illegal act has committed the criminal act of solicitation. If a person is looking to pay for sex and makes this request by words or gestures, the person can be arrested for solicitation of prostitution. If either the client or the massage therapist is solicited for sex for pay, this is an illegal act and the police should be called.

Recourse Policy
- Describe the policy to be followed when a client is unhappy or dissatisfied. Explain how you issue a refund (full or partial). Let the client know that if the matter is not handled satisfactorily, a professional organization or licensing board is available where complaints can be registered.
- *Note:* Some professionals send out client policy and procedure booklets before the scheduled appointment. If this is done, include a personalized cover letter asking the client to read the booklet carefully and stating that you will discuss it with him or her at the first appointment.

Needs Assessment and Development of the Initial Care or Treatment Plan

First, the client's goals and desired outcomes for the massage sessions are determined. The client agrees to proceed with the next part of the session, which consists of history taking using a client information form and a physical assessment using an assessment form (see Chapters 4 and 11). The information is evaluated to develop a care plan for the client; this is called a *needs assessment*. Care plans usually envision a series of sessions.

A care or treatment plan is developed that spells out the following:

- Specific outcomes (i.e., the therapeutic goals)
- Frequency of visits (number of appointments per week or month) and duration of visits (e.g., 30, 45, or 60 minutes)
- Estimated number of appointments needed to achieve the therapeutic goals (e.g., 10 sessions, 15 sessions, ongoing)
- General methods to be used (e.g., therapeutic massage, muscle energy methods, neuromuscular methods, trigger point techniques)
- Objective progress measurements (e.g., pain reduced on a scale of 1 to 10, 50% increase in range of motion, sleep improved by increasing 1 hour per night, episodes of tension headache reduced from four per week to one per week, feelings of relaxation maintained for 24 hours)

The client provides (informed) consent for the care or treatment plan by signing the appropriate form.

client's needs change during the therapeutic process. The initial treatment plan is the massage practitioner's best educated guess as to how the therapeutic relationship will proceed.

When massage is used in a very nonspecific way, especially if the client will be seen only once or if a series of massage sessions is not appropriate, the massage professional need not perform an extensive needs assessment or develop a comprehensive treatment plan. Instead, the practitioner should predetermine the outcome of the session by informing the client that, under these circumstances, no specific work can be done and that massage can provide a general normalizing of the body. A short history and physical assessment are done to detect any contraindications to massage. A condensed version of the client policy statement is prepared and provided in written form. The client always provides formal written consent for the massage. An example of an informed consent process is presented in Box 2-10.

CONFIDENTIALITY

SECTION OBJECTIVES

Chapter objective covered in this section:

7. The student will be able to practice procedures to maintain client confidentiality.

Using the information presented in this section, the student will be able to perform the following:

- Establish and maintain client confidentiality
- Complete a release of information form

Confidentiality is the principle that the client's information is private and belongs to the client. It is built on respect and trust. In professional terms, confidentiality concerns client information and files. Client information is never discussed with anyone other than the client without the client's written permission. During peer counseling or supervision, client confidentiality extends to the professionals we consult. Even when the client's name is withheld, a unique situation often is enough to breach confidentiality requirements.

Client files must represent information accurately and only as it relates to the service offered. Personal information about a situation that involves a muscle or skeletal complaint need not be recorded. For example, a client describes her headache and says that a coworker is disruptive and the manager does nothing about it, which she feels contributes to the tension aggravating her headache. The only part recorded in the client's file is her belief that emotional tension is contributing to the headache. Including more of the story would be considered a breach of confidentiality, because it makes a permanent record of an event that may be made public if the client's files are ordered released to the court.

Clients must be told during initial informed consent procedures that files may be ordered released to the court. Massage therapists have no professional exemptions. Clients must be made to understand these limits to confidentiality during the informed consent procedures.

Confidentiality also pertains to public recognition. Massage practitioners should not acknowledge a client in public unless the client recognizes and greets the professional first; to do so may place clients in the position of having it revealed that they were seeking professional services, a fact they may want kept private.

Clients also must be informed that confidentiality will be breached under laws that require professionals to report abuse and threat of deadly harm. If information is disclosed to you that a child, an elderly person, or a person who may be physically or mentally unable to report abuse or to protect himself is being harmed, as a professional you must report this alleged abuse to the appropriate government agencies. If a client threatens deadly harm to another person or to herself, a professional must report this information to the police or other appropriate agency. Because the massage professional is not specifically trained to identify or diagnose those who may harm themselves or others, all threats must be taken seriously. In these most difficult situations, the massage professional should seek legal counsel on ways to proceed.

To allow professionals to exchange information, the client must sign a release of information form (Box 2-11).

A copy of the release of information form is kept in the client's file, and the original is sent to the consulting professional. The use of the term "exchange information" in the form allows each professional involved to share pertinent information; otherwise, each professional must obtain a release of information form from the client to share information about that client.

Box 2-10 | Informed Consent Process

A new client arrives for a massage. (Let's assume in this case that both the client and the massage therapist are women.)

The massage professional shows the client an informational brochure explaining massage, the reasons it works, the procedures and process of massage, the benefits of massage, and the general contraindications. She asks the client to read the information. The massage professional then discusses the information with the client. In general terms the massage professional explains alternatives to massage, such as exercise and self-hypnosis, that provide benefits similar to massage.

The massage professional then tells the client about her professional background. For example, that she graduated from a state-licensed massage therapy school 2 years ago, after a training program of 1000 hours; that she has been nationally certified by the National Certification Board for Therapeutic Massage; that she has been in professional practice part time for 2 years and averages eight massages a week; and that she has taken additional training in myofascial approaches and massage for elderly people (approximately 100 hours for each). The client also is given information on methods of reporting misconduct by the massage therapist to state agencies, national professional organizations, and the police.

The massage therapist gives the client the policy and procedures booklet or statement and asks her to read it. After she has done so, the massage professional goes over the booklet with the client, point by point, so that she understands the massage therapist's rules and requirements. The massage professional makes sure to discuss the requirements to report abuse and any threat of deadly harm, in addition to the release of files by court order.

The massage professional then hands the client a consent form (such as the following example).

I, (client's name) _____, have received a copy of the policies for Massage Works operated by Sue and John Grey. I have read Massage Works' policies, and I understand them. The massage procedures, information about massage in general, general benefits of massage, contraindications to massage, and possible alternatives have been explained to me. The qualifications of the massage professional and reporting measures for misconduct have been disclosed to me.

I understand that the massage I receive is for the purpose of stress reduction and relief from muscular tension, spasm, or pain and to increase circulation. If I experience any pain or discomfort, I will immediately inform the massage practitioner so that the pressure or methods can be adjusted to my comfort level. I understand that massage professionals do not diagnose illness or disease or perform any spinal manipulations, nor do they prescribe any medical treatments, and nothing said or done during the session should be construed as such. I acknowledge that massage is not a substitute for medical examination or diagnosis and that I should see a health care provider for those services. Because massage should not be performed under certain circumstances, I agree to keep the massage practitioner updated as to any changes in my health profile, and I release the massage professional from any liability if I fail to do so.

Client's signature _____ Date _____
Therapist's signature _____ Date _____

Consent to Treat a Minor
By my signature I authorize (therapist's name) to provide therapeutic massage to my child or dependent.
Signature of Parent or Guardian _____ Date _____

For clients who will have several sessions, the next step is completion of the needs assessment and initial care or treatment plan (presented in detail in Chapter 4).

Modified Informed Consent Form for Single Session
For clients who will be seen only once (e.g., the professional is working on a cruise ship, doing sports massage at an event, or doing promotional chair massage at a health fair), the following modification in informed consent can be made.

I, (client's name) _____, have received a copy of the policies for (name of business) _____, operated by (owner) _____. I have read the rules and policies, and I understand them. The general benefits of massage and contraindications to massage have been explained to me. I have disclosed to the therapist any condition I have that would contraindicate massage. Other than to determine contraindications, I understand that no specific needs assessment has been performed. The qualifications of the massage professional and reporting measures for misconduct have been disclosed to me.

I understand that the massage I receive is for the purpose of stress reduction and relief from muscular tension, spasm, or pain and to increase circulation. If I experience any pain or discomfort, I will immediately inform the massage practitioner so that the pressure or methods can be adjusted to my comfort level. I understand that massage professionals do not diagnose illness or disease or perform any spinal manipulations, nor do they prescribe any medical treatments. I acknowledge that massage is not a substitute for medical examination or diagnosis and that I should see a health care provider for those services.

I understand that a single massage session or massage used on a random basis is limited to providing a general, nonspecific massage approach using standard massage methods and does not include any methods to address soft tissue structure or function specifically.

Client's signature _____ Date _____
Therapist's signature _____ Date _____

Consent to Treat a Minor
By my signature I authorize (therapist's name) to provide massage work to my child or dependent.
Signature of Parent or Guardian _____ Date _____

| Box 2-11 | Release of Information Form |

The following is an example of a release of information form.

I, (client's name) _____, grant permission for _____ (therapist's name), a massage practitioner, to provide or exchange information with (other professional's name) _____ about the following conditions _____ for the time frame beginning _____ and ending _____ (dates). This permission may be revoked at any time either verbally or in writing. Client's signature _____ Date _____

HEALTH INSURANCE PORTABILITY AND ACCOUNTABILITY ACT OF 1996 (HIPAA)

SECTION OBJECTIVES

Chapter objective covered in this section:

8. The student will become familiar with the Health Insurance Portability and Accountability Act (HIPAA) and its requirements and training.

Using the information presented in this section, the student will be able to perform the following:

- Explain the purpose of HIPAA and list the three primary areas it covers
- Define the chain of trust
- Store records in a HIPAA-compliant manner
- Locate additional information about HIPAA
- Describe the training for meeting HIPAA requirements

The Health Insurance Portability and Accountability Act was signed into law by President Bill Clinton on August 21, 1996. Conclusive regulations were issued on August 17, 2000, to be instituted by October 16, 2002. HIPAA requires that the transactions of all patient health care information be formatted in a standardized electronic style. In addition to protecting the privacy and security of patient information, HIPAA includes legislation on the formation of medical savings accounts, the authorization of a fraud and abuse control program, the easy transport of health insurance coverage, and the simplification of administrative terms and conditions. HIPAA encompasses three primary areas, and its privacy requirements can be broken down into three types:

- Privacy standards
- Patients' rights
- Administrative requirements

The confidentiality requirements to protect client privacy have the greatest impact on massage practice. Because massage therapists obtain a client health history, maintain client records, and may communicate with other health care professionals, including transmitting records (electronically or not), it is prudent to function in compliance with HIPAA's requirements.

Chain of Trust

If patient/client data are shared with a third party, a certain level of trust must be established to ensure that the external party to whom data are passed can guarantee that they will maintain data integrity and confidentiality; this is called the *chain of trust*. A chain of trust agreement must take the form of an approved and formal contract in which the responsibilities of the individual parties are clearly outlined (see the Evolve website for an example of a chain of trust document).

Security measures include the following:

- Obtain written consent from the client for e-mail communication that specifically relates to health records. Put a confidentiality notice on all faxes and e-mails. Avoid using this type of communication for confidential information.
- Do not leave files where they are accessible to unauthorized individuals.
- Keep appointment books private and practice management software password protected.
- Do not discuss any medical information with a third party without written authorization from the client.

Data Storage

Massage therapists also need to inform clients of how electronic client record keeping is used. This is important, because more massage therapists are using electronic practice management software that includes HIPAA-related content. A HIPAA declaration that clearly describes the process for management of a client's records must be available for the client to read and sign. This document should include the following:

- Use of the client's information
- Type of storage method used to secure the client's files
- Situations in which disclosure of information may be required
- Information on how clients can obtain copies of their records

The HIPAA notice must be posted where it is clearly visible to clients, and each client should be given a copy of this notice. All personnel involved with the client should be trained in HIPAA procedures.

Protected Health Information

HIPAA defines protected health information (PHI) as confidential, personal, identifiable health information about individuals that is created or received and is transmitted or maintained in any form. "Identifiable" means that a person reading this information could reasonably use it to identify an individual. A piece of health-related information becomes PHI if it has the following elements (among others):

- Name
- Address
- E-mail address

- Birth date (except year)
- Social Security number

The following websites present a comprehensive discussion of these terms and requirements and a complete list of HIPAA policies and procedures:

- U.S. Department of Health and Human Services, Office of Civil Rights: www.hhs.gov/ocr/hipaa
- Workgroup on Electronic Data Interchange: www.wedi.org/SNIP
- Phoenix Health: www.hipaadvisory.com
- U.S. Department of Health and Human Services, Office of the Assistant Secretary for Planning and Evaluation: http://aspe.os.dhhs.gov/admnsimp/

Training in HIPAA Requirements

Massage professionals must obtain the appropriate training for HIPAA compliance. Different work environments have different compliance procedures; therefore, employment-related compliance training is important.

HIPAA's Privacy Rule stipulates that all members of the enterprise workforce receive training that is appropriate to their organizational roles. The "workforce" includes employees, volunteers, trainees, and other individuals who work for a covered entity, regardless of whether they are paid by it. Some staff members must be trained in applying specific policies and procedures, such as providing the notice of information practices or obtaining authorizations. Others, such as those who rarely have access to PHI, may require only an overview of HIPAA's background, objectives, principles, and general regulatory requirements.

New employees who join the organization must receive training within a reasonable period. Often, the practical course is to include HIPAA privacy training in new employee orientation programs, particularly because privacy principles easily fit into discussions of the organization's mission and infrastructure. Workforce members who change jobs or receive new responsibilities must receive additional training if their new job duties include new patient privacy–related responsibilities. Further, the Privacy Rule requires retraining for each member of the covered entity's workforce whose functions are affected by a material change in policies or procedures.

Covered entities must also document that privacy training has been provided. Although members of the workforce are not required to sign a certificate after training, documenting the completion of training by each worker is useful for future verification purposes.

The privacy provisions do not prescribe the nature of the required training; the Department of Health and Human Services has left the design, approach, and specific content to the discretion of the covered entity. However, it is recommended that at the very least, the following topics be covered with all members of the workforce:

- Principles and objectives of HIPAA's Privacy Rule
- Background (e.g., what constitutes PHI)
- Need for privacy of PHI
- Overview of HIPAA privacy regulations, including penalties
- Individual's rights regarding privacy

- Individual's rights regarding control of uses and disclosure of PHI
- Individual's right to request access, accounting, and amendment
- New organizational privacy policies and procedures
- Sanction policy
- Notice of privacy practices
- Authorizations for use and disclosure
- Privacy officer's role and contact information
- Complaint policies and procedures
- Cooperating with investigations or audits
- Reporting of violations and the whistleblower policy
- The organization's commitment to patient privacy

More specialized training in detailed HIPAA requirements and internal procedural changes must be tailored for workforce groups directly affected by these requirements or changes in the course of their work (Privacy Rights Clearinghouse, 2011).

PROFESSIONAL BOUNDARIES

SECTION OBJECTIVES

Chapter objective covered in this section:

9. The student will be able to integrate ethics into maintaining professional boundaries and the therapeutic relationship.

Using the information presented in this section, the student will be able to perform the following:

- Develop strategies for maintaining professional boundaries with clients
- Explore personal prejudices, fears, and limitations that may interfere with the ability to provide the best care for a client
- Help a client recognize personal boundaries in the massage process

Needs and Wants

People have needs and wants. *Needs* sustain life; when needs are not met, people become ill and die. Needs include air, water, food, shelter, and sensory stimulation. *Wants* lead to a sense of satisfaction. Examples of wants include a certain type of car or home, a particular job, a piece of chocolate cake, or a relationship with a particular person. We all need shelter, but I want a cabin in the woods. We all need food, but I want home-baked, whole grain bread hot from the oven. We all need to be touched, but I want to be hugged by my children. When massage provides sensory stimulation in the form of touch, it meets a need for clients. A client may want only a particular professional to provide the massage to meet the need of sensory stimulation.

When a need or perceived need (want) is met for someone by another, it is very easy to feel bonded to that other person. Needs and wants often become confused in the mind of the client; therefore, the more unsettled or dysfunctional a client is, the more important it becomes to maintain boundaries in the professional relationship. This type of connection and interaction can lead to transference or countertransference (discussed later in the chapter), and it can happen with therapeutic massage. The massage professional should have a clear understanding of personal motivation in the therapy setting and a thorough understanding of professional boundaries and ways to maintain them.

Evolve Activity 2-4

| Box 2-12 | Determining a Client's Boundaries |

An effective way to determine a client's boundaries is to ask questions. For example, the massage professional might ask the client the following questions:
- Is there any part of your body that you would rather not have massaged?
- Do you prefer any particular kind of music?
- I am a smoker, and I know the smell lingers. Will that bother you? (What will you do if the client says "Yes"?)
- I have three different massage lubricants. Which would you prefer?

Boundaries

A physical boundary can be defined as the personal space within an arm's length perimeter. It also can be thought of as the personal emotional space designated by morals, values, and experience. Some people are not very good at defining personal boundaries or respecting others' boundaries. Certainly boundaries are defined by more than physical space, but for our purposes, a respect for personal boundaries simply begins with staying an arm's length away from another until invited to come closer. Personal space can be defined by extending the arm directly in front of the body and turning in a circle; the area within that space is that individual's personal space. Cultural differences may change this boundary, but for therapeutic massage, we will consider this a person's personal space range (see Touch in Chapter 1). No one should ever enter this space uninvited (i.e., without informed consent). It is important that students practice this policy while in school. They should ask whether another person may be approached, wait for the response, and act accordingly. This practice may seem silly at first, but it teaches an awareness of boundaries.

What is acceptable for us may be offensive for someone else. We may offend someone unintentionally because of differences in our personal and moral value systems. It is important for the massage therapist to help the client define a personal boundary (Box 2-12). Sometimes people who have been emotionally, physically, or sexually abused have not had the chance to define or recognize personal boundaries. Practitioners should be especially respectful in their approach and should explain professional therapeutic boundaries carefully to the client. It is just as important for those who have boundary difficulties to learn to define their own personal boundaries. Setting limits during a massage session may be a safe way to begin this process.

Once a client's boundaries have been defined, we must respect them. If a professional cannot respect a client's boundary needs, the professional should refer the client to a massage practitioner better able to deal with those needs. The massage professional should tell the client, "I will not be offended if you share with me things that you do not like about the massage. I will be happy to refer you to someone else if a different massage approach will serve you better. There are as many different ways to give a massage as there are people giving massage. I am here to help you achieve your outcomes

from massage, as long as any activity does not conflict with my professional and personal standards."

It is equally important that the client understand the therapist's personal and professional boundaries; therefore the therapist must be honest in creating a personal code of ethics and must clearly communicate the professional boundaries to the client. Boundaries are discussed with the client during the initial informed consent procedures and are included in writing in the client policy statement. (Communication skills for the professional are presented later in this chapter.)

Even when a massage professional is conscientious about establishing boundaries with the client during the initial intake procedure, those boundaries can become blurred as the professional interaction progresses, or something may occur that the professional had not considered. When this happens, the situation must be dealt with immediately; waiting only allows the problem to escalate, leading to the development of conflict.

Boundaries are difficult to define. We bring to our adulthood varying experiences that shape what we feel is correct and define our personal boundaries. As professionals we are responsible for finding the client's comfort zone. This responsibility begins with learning our personal and professional comfort zones.

Anything that prevents us from being able to touch a person in a respectful, nonjudgmental way must be considered so that we can decide whom we may best serve as massage professionals. Hindrances include personal prejudices regarding body size, color, gender, and attitude. For example, some people do not relate well to children. It is ethical for such professionals to refer children to someone else for professional care. Others may be uncomfortable with those of the opposite gender, and again, it is best to refer such clients elsewhere. We may be uncomfortable with the prospect of working with people who have certain types of diseases. If this is the case, our touch may be uncomfortable for these people. A potential client may have a behavior that drives us crazy (e.g., sniffing). The behavior interferes with our ability to be the best massage professional for that particular client.

It is important, therefore, to explore professional boundaries by looking honestly at our fears, frustrations, prejudices, biases, and personal and moral value systems. These emotions and beliefs are very personal and often deeply held. The anchors for many of these beliefs may not be easily understood at a conscious level. Acknowledging factors that define and limit our personal and professional boundaries does not necessarily involve changing or even understanding why we feel a certain way. Changing belief systems is a complex process that often requires professional help. Although personal growth is encouraged, the expectation that we can overcome all our limitations is unrealistic. Instead, it is important to recognize when our personal boundaries will affect the professional relationship, because massage professionals work very closely with their clients. We touch our clients. (The essential quality of touch communication was explored in Chapter 1.) We must be honest with ourselves and about ourselves to be able to respect the individual needs and space of our clients (Proficiency Exercise 2-6).

💡 PROFICIENCY EXERCISE 2-6

The following exercise may be the most difficult one you will have to do. On a piece of paper, write at least one page about your personal prejudices and fears about people. Be honest in listing the physical and behavioral aspects of others that you find difficult. Here are some examples:

- Old people frustrate me. I cannot make myself listen to the same stories over and over.
- I hate ragged toenails. I do not know if I can rub anyone's feet if the nails are not well trimmed.
- People who are fat are undisciplined. They should exercise more.
- People who are skinny are obsessed with their appearance and are exercise addicts.
- When someone sniffs all the time, it makes me crazy.
- I am afraid of men with mustaches because of something that happened to me when I was young.
- I am afraid of people with the human immunodeficiency virus (HIV). I do not want to catch it.
- Women are so bossy; I hate it when they tell me what to do.
- As a man, I am uncomfortable with giving another man a massage.
- I am uncomfortable working with someone who is physically disabled. I especially feel squeamish with amputations.

It is important that you be very honest with yourself. Only by accepting that we have these areas of challenge will we be able to best serve potential clients.

Right of Refusal

Clients have the right to refuse the massage practitioner's services; this is called the **right of refusal.** The client has the right to refuse or to stop treatment at any time. When this request is made during treatment, the therapist must comply even though prior consent was obtained.

Professionals also have a right of refusal. Massage professionals may refuse to massage or otherwise treat any person if a just and reasonable cause exists. Obviously, lack of appropriate knowledge or skills is a reason for refusal and referral; it is the more ambiguous situations that cause concern. The next few paragraphs provide some direction for determining what constitutes "just and reasonable cause" for refusing to provide professional massage services to a client. Massage professionals also are bound by a nondiscrimination code of conduct. You may refuse to work with anyone as long as you explain the reasons and the fact that these reasons ultimately would affect the quality of care for the client; this is called *disclosure.*

Say, for example, that a person with multiple sclerosis (MS) wants to be your client. Your mother had multiple sclerosis, and you have bitter feelings about the ways her illness interfered with your childhood. You find it difficult to be with anyone who has MS because of your memories. Here are your choices:

1. Tell the prospective client that you have limitations that prevent you from effectively working with MS and offer to refer her to a therapist who can provide the work needed. Make sure that at least three different qualified individuals are given as referrals so that the client has a choice.

2. Be very honest with the client. Explain that you are uncomfortable working with MS and that you are concerned that the way you feel may interfere with doing what is best for her. Leave out all personal details. Knowing this up front, if the client still wants to work with you, you may decide to give it a try, as long as the quality of care for the client is not compromised and you are in a space where the challenges of the interaction can be professionally addressed.

Either way, you have taken responsibility for personal attitudes, and the client has the information necessary to make an informed choice. Remember, touch tells the truth. Touching someone with whom you are uneasy is difficult, whatever the reasons. By honestly telling the person about the situation, the client can make the decision. If the professional's touch seems strained, the client may realize that it is the practitioner's issue.

A massage professional has the right to refuse to treat any area of a client's body and to terminate the professional relationship if he or she feels that the client is sexualizing the relationship or if the professional feels adversely influenced in any way by the client.

Refusal becomes more difficult when clearly defined discrimination issues are involved. This might occur if a professional limits his practice to a particular ethnic group or refuses to provide services to someone with a legally classified disability. In these cases the professional is wise to seek legal counsel to determine the extent of professional liability.

Blurred boundaries create an environment conducive to the development of ethical dilemmas. Professional boundaries are situational and must be identified and established with each client. Clear professional boundaries support an effective therapeutic process for both the client and the professional.

THE THERAPEUTIC RELATIONSHIP

SECTION OBJECTIVES

Chapter objective covered in this section:
10. Explain and demonstrate the qualities of the therapeutic relationship.
Using the information presented in this section, the student will be able to perform the following:
- Define and recognize potential transference and countertransference issues
- Explain the professional power differential
- List factors that create dual or multiple roles
- Explain to clients the feelings of intimacy that can arise between them and the massage professional
- Diffuse sexual feelings during the massage session
- Recognize and avoid sexual misconduct activities

In the therapeutic setting, specific parameters define the professional relationship between the client and the massage professional. As was explained in Chapter 1, the therapeutic relationship has an inherent **power differential,** which stems from the difference in knowledge and skills between the client and the professional. Even when services are exchanged between peer professionals, the power differential exists because

PROFICIENCY EXERCISE 2-7

Working with a partner, follow the directions provided so that each of you plays the role of strength and of vulnerability to experience the concept of the power differential.

1. The person playing the role of strength stands up. The person playing the role of vulnerability sits on the floor. The person who is standing looks down at the person sitting on the floor and says in a robust voice, "I am so strong, I am as strong as I have ever been. I am very strong." The person sitting on the floor looks up at the one standing and replies in a fragile voice, "I am so vulnerable. I have never been this vulnerable before. I am very vulnerable."

2. The two people remain in the standing and seated positions, but this time the person sitting on the floor says, "I am so strong, I am as strong as I have ever been. I am very strong." The person standing says, "I am so vulnerable. I have never been this vulnerable before. I am very vulnerable."

3. The two people change positions so that the one standing now sits on the floor, and the one sitting on the floor now stands. They then repeat the exercise.

Now, discuss what occurred. Possible experiences to explore include the following:

- Did a particular role cause discomfort?
- What was it like to be strong or vulnerable?
- How did the position influence the feelings?
- Which statement did you prefer to make?
- What position was most comfortable?
- In what way does this exercise relate to the therapeutic relationship?

Discuss what you learned about power differentials in the therapeutic relationship.

one is placed in the position of controlling the situation. This power imbalance must be minimized as much as possible without denying its existence (Proficiency Exercise 2-7).

Transference

Issues of transference and countertransference diminish the effectiveness of the therapeutic relationship. *Transference* is the personalization of the professional relationship by the client. When a person seeks out a professional, the very important issues of power, trust, and control in the therapeutic relationship become the professional's responsibility. The more disorganized a person is, the stronger is the feeling of disempowerment. Clients often seek a sense of control outside themselves to help re-establish or replace their internal sense of control. The client is in a vulnerable state when doing this.

This situation is more common with people who are ill or under considerable stress, but even a well client is vulnerable in the therapeutic setting. The reality of today's society is that although most people cannot be diagnosed as sick, most have not achieved true wellness, either. Although we ideally speak of wellness massage to help a client maintain or achieve optimum wellness, the truth is somewhat different. Unfortunately, very few people seek massage for pure pleasure and to enhance their health. Most of the clients we serve, even outside the health care setting, are not optimally well. They just are

not sick yet. Most seek massage services because they do not feel good and want to feel better.

The more disorganized, disempowered, and lacking in internal resources clients are, the more susceptible they are to transference. Transference occurs when the client sees the therapist in a personal light instead of a professional manner. This usually is a distorted view, because the professional is displaying a specific role and not letting the whole self be involved with the client. If the client becomes dependent on the professional, instead of re-establishing his or her personal functioning, unrealistic expectations may develop. Manifestations of transference include demands for more of the therapist's time, bringing the therapist personal gifts, attempting to engage the professional in personal conversation, proposals of friendship or sexual activity, and expressions of anger and blame. If the client's expectations are not met, the person may blame the professional. If the client's expectations are met, the person may project the credit to the therapist instead of acknowledging his or her own efforts. In both cases the professional takes on a superhuman image that sooner or later crumbles, often leaving the client disillusioned and disempowered.

Managing transference is a common ethical dilemma. The massage professional must understand and separate the client's appropriate, genuine feelings from the transference issues. For example, a client may be angry if the therapist continually arrives late for the appointment; this is a justified feeling, not transference. Also, the client may truly appreciate the massage therapist's skill and may express that appreciation, but this does not constitute transference unless it interferes with the boundaries of the therapeutic relationship.

The professional has the ultimate responsibility for the therapeutic relationship and the direction of the therapeutic process.

Countertransference

Countertransference is the inability of the professional to separate the therapeutic relationship from personal feelings and expectations for the client; it is the professional's personalization of the therapeutic relationship. Countertransference presents itself in feelings of attachment to the client, such as sexual feelings, excessive thinking about a client between visits, a feeling of professional inadequacy if the client does not make anticipated progress, or a sense of the client as being special; it also can manifest as favoritism, anger, or revulsion toward a client. Countertransference often is fed by the following personal needs of the therapist:

- The need to fix people
- The need to remove pain and discomfort
- The need to be perfect
- The need to have the answer
- The need to be loved

The client's problems may serve as a reflection of the professional's personal life experiences. The massage professional is wise to consider his or her own personal needs and develop a reliable sense of self-awareness. Without a high level of self-awareness on the part of the professional, the focus of the

💡 PROFICIENCY EXERCISE 2-8

1. Work with a partner. Face each other and decide who is A and who is B. A asks B the following questions, and B answers quickly. Then reverse roles.
   - When do you need to fix people?
   - When do you need to remove pain and discomfort?
   - When do you need to be involved in a dual role?
   - When do you need to be perfect?
   - When do you need to have the answer?
   - When do you need to be loved?
2. Now talk for a moment with your partner about the experience and discuss the areas in which you feel you may have the most difficulty with countertransference.
3. Go through the exercise again and substitute the word "want" for "need." Discuss the feelings that arise with the word "want" and the ways they may be different from those produced by the word "need."

massage session may shift from meeting the goals of the client to meeting the needs of the therapist. The massage therapist may begin to treat himself or herself while treating the client and lose objectivity and empathy in the therapeutic relationship (Proficiency Exercise 2-8).

Another way this can be stated is that the massage professional gives the client the kind of massage the professional would like to receive instead of the massage appropriate for the client. This situation actually occurs quite often. For example, the massage professional prefers to lie on his stomach when receiving a massage and enjoys deep work on his back. Because this position and level of pressure feel good to the massage practitioner, he may have a tendency to keep clients in the face down position and to use deep pressure on the back, even if this is not what the client would choose. Also, a massage professional may avoid using a method that she does not enjoy but that the client may like.

If the client's personal situation is similar to that of the massage practitioner, especially with regard to life challenges, the practitioner may give subconsciously based advice to the client in an attempt to solve the massage practitioner's personal problem. For example, both the professional and the client may be facing difficult marital issues, or struggling with managing menopause, or dealing with the recent loss of a parent or relocation to a new city. This dynamic can be detrimental to the client, because it breaches the professional relationship and fosters psychologically unhealthy behaviors between the massage practitioner and the client. An environment of sympathetic dependence often results, and this dynamic is a basis for countertransference.

Practitioners personalize the professional relationship when they assume too much responsibility for the outcome of the session for the client or when they project a personal situation onto the client process. Countertransference issues often reflect unresolved issues on the part of the professional. Identifying countertransference in the therapeutic relationship can point out areas the practitioner may wish to explore and resolve with a qualified professional in order to remain objective and increase effectiveness as a massage professional. The goal is not for the massage professional to be faultless before beginning practice; rather, the goal is for the therapist to be aware of personal challenges that could interfere with the therapeutic relationship and thus the therapist's ability to maintain professional boundaries.

Managing Transference and Countertransference

Transference can be expected in some form in the therapeutic relationship. As it arises, it is the massage professional's responsibility to reinforce the boundaries of the professional relationship. The practitioner should explain to clients why these feelings may occur and help them redirect the transference activity to the appropriate people or situations in the client's life. This becomes difficult when the client does not move through the transference stage toward more self-directed resources and coping strategies or when the client has extremely limited resources and coping mechanisms. Such clients may need to be referred to another professional, with appropriate disclosure for the reason for referral, to help them understand that the boundaries of the professional relationship are being breached and that the existing situation is inappropriate.

The professional is always responsible for self-monitoring for the development of countertransference issues and for seeking supervision or professional support, such as problem-solving with peers and/or a mentor or counselor, if necessary, to resolve personal issues. When the professional faces the realization that countertransference has occurred, the first step in resolving these issues has been taken. It is a breach of professional boundaries to allow countertransference issues to develop and linger or to be acted upon. In extreme cases the client may need to be referred to a different therapeutic massage professional, with appropriate disclosure on the part of the therapist, so that the client does not take the need for referral personally.

Peer support, supervision, and mentoring are important for the massage professional dealing with transference and countertransference. Seeking information from more experienced professionals, which supervision and mentoring encourage, supports professional development. Those mentoring the massage professional do not necessarily need to be massage therapists. Various health care professionals grapple with similar issues. Mental health professionals in particular must consider transference and countertransference issues frequently. If supervision and mentoring are not part of your professional practice, it may be helpful to seek out a qualified mental health professional and establish a professional relationship with that person to sort out these particular issues.

Peer support also is important. Interacting regularly with other massage practitioners creates an environment that promotes healthy work practices through both technical information and guidance on solving interpersonal dilemmas. When sharing with peers, be attentive to the confidentiality of your clients. It is important not to allow yourself to become isolated, with no regular sources of fresh information or perspectives.

Dual or Multiple Roles

A dual role exists when scopes of practice overlap and one professional provides support in more than one area of expertise or when personal relationships overlap with professional services. Dual or multiple roles develop when professionals assume more than one role in their relationship with their clients. These roles develop in many different ways. Providing massage in the professional environment for family members is a classic example of a dual role, as is providing professional services for a personal friend.

Dual and multiple roles are difficult to manage in the professional relationship and can be a breeding ground for ethical dilemmas. As soon as one professional assumes professional authority with the body and the mind, the body and the spirit, or the spirit and the mind, the therapist can be said to be assuming a dual role (or multiple roles if the authority is assumed in all three areas). In this situation the professional holds more power in the relationship than is appropriate, and the client begins to become disempowered. The power differential is increased. This allows a very dangerous power shift that supports the development of transference and countertransference. It often leads to enmeshment and dependence on the part of the client and burnout on the part of the therapist. Managing the inherent power differential of the therapeutic relationship is difficult enough without increasing the likelihood of transference and countertransference or the breach of professional boundaries by assuming dual and multiple roles.

In the professional therapeutic massage relationship, mental and spiritual issues need not be dealt with directly. The focus of massage is the body. When interacting with your client, maintain the focus of the work on the body while using attentive listening, acknowledging the client's circumstances, and always being alert to the possible need for referral. Interacting professionally in the area of the mind or spirit may breach the professional contract for services, which focuses on the body. Always recognize and appreciate the wholeness of the person while staying within the scope of massage therapy, and work with other professionals to deal with other areas so that the client remains empowered in the process of achieving wellness.

A dual role also can arise in more subtle situations. The sale of products to a client, bartering of services, excessive personal disclosure by the therapist to the client, shared social interaction, or shared professional services all create situations in which the power balance of the therapeutic relationship can become problematic. As in all ethical dilemmas, decisions about conduct are gauged against the client's welfare. The clinical reasoning process is an effective way to analyze an ethical dilemma and develop a plan to address the issue.

Massage Therapy and Intimacy

To dispel in advance any sexual innuendo associated with many of the terms used in the following paragraphs, definitions from Webster's dictionary are provided at this point for clarification (Merriam-Webster, 2002):

Intimacy: The state or fact of being intimate.

Intimate: Inmost, essential, internal, most private or personal; closely acquainted or associated; very familiar.

Essential: Intrinsic, fundamental, basic, and inherently primary.

Sensory: Connected with the reception and transmission of sense impressions (through the nervous system).

Stimulation: The act of exciting or increasing activity.

The work of a massage practitioner is sensory stimulation; therefore, by its very definition, body stimulation is sensual and may become intimate. When a person encounters the essential touch that a sensitive and confident massage practitioner provides, that person's whole system responds. For many, the closest thing to essential touch ever experienced is parenting activities and sexual interaction. Because our bodies constantly react to new situations through comparison to past experience, a client's response system understandably might interpret these feelings as sexual arousal or as maternal or paternal. Furthermore, for many adults, the only familiar routine they have for expressing these feelings is a sexual one. It is easy to see why the client might misinterpret the sensations and feelings associated with massage, confusing them with sexual responses or a parenting role.

The massage professional must understand the physiologic aspects of therapeutic massage and recognize that the same massage techniques that alleviate stress and promote relaxation also stimulate the entire sensory mechanism, which may include a sexual arousal response. Within the parameters of professional ethics, it is always considered unethical for the client or the practitioner to interact on a sexual level, whether verbally or physically. However, it is essential that both client and practitioner understand why the urges and sensations of sexuality may present themselves. A more thorough knowledge of the physiologic and psychological network leads to a better understanding of the responses by both client and practitioner. The practitioner then is better able to alter the session to maintain a proper professional relationship.

The lumbar nerve plexus (nerve bundles) and the sacral nerve plexus conduct sensory information to and from the abdominal area, the lower extremities, and the buttocks, and also to and from the genital area. Stimulation of a nerve plexus area is not confined to local perception, but rather is diffused throughout the area. For example, when the lower abdominal area is stroked, the nerve signals of the genital area also are influenced. The entire sexual arousal response is part of the relaxation response through the output from the parasympathetic autonomic nervous system. Therefore, each time a client relaxes out of the fight-or-flight responses of the sympathetic autonomic nervous system into the more relaxed response, the predisposing physiologic factors are present for sexual arousal. This reaction is possible not only for clients but also for practitioners as they begin to relax and entrain with the massage.

On a physiologic level, parasympathetic stimulation activates most of the benefits of massage for stress reduction. This neurologic state also is favorable to sexual arousal. These physical responses are all connected, but the sexual response usually is short-lived and quickly replaced by feelings of deep relaxation as the massage continues. Responses vary with each

Box 2-13 Diffusing Feelings of Sexual Arousal

1. Recognize the physiology and interrupt it; change what you are doing.
2. Be aware of your own psychological state and change it; become more alert.
3. Adjust the intent of the session to stimulate a more sympathetic output response by using stretching, compression, joint movement, and active participation by the client.
4. Change the music, lighting, and conversation and the client's position.
5. Stop working with your hands and use your forearms.
6. Explain the feelings in a professional manner using clinical terminology.

client, and the sexual response may be totally bypassed. However, physical sexual arousal may occur (e.g., engorgement of erectile tissue with blood and shifts in breathing), and the massage practitioner needs to understand both the physiology of this situation and ways to deal with it ethically (Box 2-13).

The practitioner is responsible for putting the whole issue of sexuality into perspective, understanding it clearly, and explaining the "feelings" to the client on a physiologic level. The practitioner also is responsible for monitoring the client's responses and acting appropriately to adjust the physiology and change the pattern of the massage to diffuse the sexual energy. This is easily accomplished by altering the approach of the session. It is common knowledge that sexual arousal is not purely physical and depends on both psychological and tactile responses; in these ways the practitioner can modulate the client-practitioner responses.

The Merriam-Webster dictionary defines intercourse as "connection or reciprocal action between persons or nations; the interchange of thought, feelings, products, services, communication, commerce, and association" (Webster's, 2002). Massage becomes an intercourse in the purest sense. Essential intimacy is the circle that begins to develop between practitioner and client. People want this type of intimacy; it is the type of interaction that promotes survival and health. Essential touch is vital, fundamental, and crucial to well-being. It is the touch of a litter of puppies sleeping in one big pile. It is combined with the sexual interchange between lovers. However, it does not require sexual expression to be considered essential intimacy.

Touch Intimacy

Remember that, as was explained in Chapter 1, the intention of a touch is a determining factor in the interpretation of the touch. The touch of the massage professional is not focused on sexual arousal and release, nor are we the client's parents. The psychological aspect of this topic is another matter. Here the practitioner can set the stage and monitor responses. Keep discussions light. Change the topic. This is where the interpersonal communication skills of the practitioner come into play.

The moments of intimacy must be dealt with very carefully. Misunderstanding the psychological or physiologic responses, the client may interpret them as an indication of feelings of love or that the therapist is a new best friend. Clients manifest

this response in different ways. Usually clients want to bring the professional into their lives, perhaps through invitations to lunch, a desire for more frequent sessions, or a proposal for a relationship. Do not allow this to happen. The practitioner must maintain professional space and monitor personal feelings. Keep the balance by confining the intimacy of massage to the therapy room.

Having little or no understanding of all these subtle interactions, the client cannot be blamed for wanting more attention from the massage practitioner. The moments of togetherness that are shared are special and can range from a great deal of laughter to sharing work-related experiences. The session can accomplish something as simple as relieving the day's tension or as complex as overcoming years of pain. Make no more and no less of the interaction.

Clients may look to the professional for emotional support beyond the ethical scope of practice for massage. Encourage them to find the support they require from another source. If a client needs assistance with coping skills, refer the person to someone who is qualified to help. Credit counselors, ministers, rape crisis counselors, marriage counselors, counselors for sexual dysfunction, chiropractors, physicians, and many other caregivers can provide the help clients may need. The massage practitioner's intention is to support and accept the client in a nonjudgmental manner, listen, and blend touch skills to benefit the client.

Sexual Misconduct and Sexual Harassment

Sexual misconduct is any type of sexual activity that occurs between the professional and the client. Although sexual misconduct has been relatively well defined (Box 2-14), conduct that is invasive but not blatantly sexual remains a gray area.

A joke told between friends may be totally inappropriate in the professional setting. A statement about appearance may be taken as a compliment or could be interpreted as a sexual remark. Something that is appropriate with one client may not be acceptable with another. Practitioners can find it overwhelming to try to second-guess what is appropriate for clients. The best defense against confusion is communication. Ask questions and provide clients with information about acceptable behavior in the professional setting.

Sexual harassment occurs in the work setting between peers or with supervisors. Unwelcome sexual interaction (physical or verbal) in conjunction with employment status or work environment constitutes sexual harassment. Sexual harassment is clearly defined by law, whereas sexual misconduct often is more subtle and difficult to prosecute unless clearly coerced sexual acts have been committed.

Maintaining the Professional Environment

The therapeutic relationship is a unidirectional focus in which the knowledge and skills of the professional are used to assist the client in achieving therapeutic outcomes. To preserve the unidirectional focus, certain crucial professional boundaries must be maintained. For example, it is important to maintain professional space. Box 2-15 presents some simple ways to accomplish this (see also Proficiency Exercise 2-9).

Box 2-14   Guidelines on Sexual Misconduct

Guidelines developed for practitioners in Ontario, Canada, provide the following criteria for determining what constitutes sexual misconduct.

1. The therapist will respect the integrity of each person and therefore not engage in any sexual conduct or sexual activities involving clients.
2. The therapist will not date a client.
3. The therapist will not commit any form of sexual impropriety or sexual abuse with a client.
4. Whatever the behavior of the client, it is always the responsibility of the massage therapist not to engage in sexual behavior.

Sexual Impropriety

Sexual impropriety includes the following:

- Any behavior, gestures, or expressions that are seductive or sexually demeaning to a client
- Inappropriate procedures, including but not limited to:
  - Disrobing or draping practices that reflect a lack of respect for the client's privacy
  - Deliberately watching a client dress or undress
- Inappropriate comments about or to the client, including but not limited to:
  - Sexual comments about a client's body or underclothing
  - Sexualized or sexually demeaning comments to a client

- Criticism of the client's sexual orientation
- Discussion of potential sexual performance
- Conversations about the sexual preferences or fantasies of the client or the massage therapist
- Requests to date
- Kissing of a sexual nature

Sexual Abuse

Sexual abuse includes the following:

- Therapist-client sex, whether initiated by the client or not
- Engaging in any conduct with a client that is sexual or reasonably may be interpreted as sexual, including but not limited to:
  - Genital to genital contact
  - Oral to genital contact
  - Oral to anal contact
  - Oral to oral contact (except cardiopulmonary resuscitation [CPR])
  - Oral to breast contact
  - Touching or undraping the genitals, perineum, or anus
  - Touching or undraping the breasts
  - Encouraging the client to masturbate in the presence of the massage therapist
  - Masturbation by the massage therapist while the client is present
  - Masturbation of the client by the massage therapist

Modified from Regulated Health Professions Act and the Massage Therapy Act, Ontario, Canada, 1992. www.cmto.com/regulations/mta.htm. Accessed July 10, 2011.

PROFICIENCY EXERCISE 2-9

In the space provided, list three mottos you will keep about maintaining professional space. Choose from the list in Box 2-15 or make up your own.

1.

2.

3.

PROFICIENCY EXERCISE 2-10

1. Working in groups of three, write down specific situations in which sexual misconduct or feelings of intimacy may develop. Exchange responses with other groups and role-play a situation, with one student acting as the massage practitioner, one playing the client, and the third evaluating the way the situation was handled. Try different situations until each student has had a chance to play each role.
2. Develop a "time to go" ritual and discuss it in your group.

As the therapist closes the session and leaves the client's space, it is important to change both physiology and body language. When greeting a client and providing the massage, the therapist's body language is open, inviting, connecting, and moving toward the client (Figure 2-5). When it is time to close the session, the therapist's body language moves away from the client, pulls in toward the therapist, separates, and indicates that the session is finished (Figure 2-6). Separating well from the client is a skill that gives both the client and the massage therapist a sense of closure. It often helps to establish a "time to go" ritual by always saying good-bye the same way. Clients who linger at the door may not know how to leave or may not recognize that it is time to leave. A "time to go" ritual helps considerably (Proficiency Exercise 2-10).

One example of a leaving ritual is to keep a box labeled "A thought to take with me" that contains fun, empowering quotes on note cards. Have the client pick a card from the box. Put the information for the next appointment on the back of the card, hand it to the client with a warm handshake, and say good-bye. When the session is finished, the therapist should let the client go physically and emotionally as the room is prepared for the next person.

Managing Intimacy Issues

Effectively managing intimacy issues can seem like an overwhelming task. However, do not be afraid of the special professional intimacy of therapeutic massage. Instead, educate clients by answering their questions intelligently, basing your answers on the facts of physiology, and encourage them to use this information to interact more resourcefully with others. If you begin to feel physically and emotionally receptive to a client, take steps to diffuse the response (see Box 2-13). Later, review the session to evaluate your personal

| Box 2-15 | Maintaining Professional Space |

1. At the start of a professional relationship, a formal informed consent process must be completed.
2. In most instances the time frame for working with a client should not exceed 90 minutes; 45 to 60 minutes is the norm. If more time is spent with the client, it becomes difficult for both the professional and the client to maintain the original intent and focus of the session, and the result is an environment that fosters transference and countertransference.
3. Professionals should wear clothing that sets them apart from clients; this is one of the benefits of a uniform. A name tag that identifies one as a massage therapist also is helpful. Wearing a uniform or maintaining a professional style of dress that is different from casual clothing gives visual stimulation that reflects professionalism. The clothes do not have to be white, but they must be nonrevealing and present an understated and neutral appearance. Therapists must be conscious of their appearance and make sure it is kept as nonsexual as possible.
4. The therapist should avoid assuming a dual role and multiple scopes of practice. The professional contract is for a specific type of intervention. General information about lifestyle, health, or spiritual issues can be provided, but the contract is for massage. This is a consideration even if the professional is credentialed in more than one area or discipline. Often the therapist needs to decide which professional hat to wear.
5. The professional environment should be neutral and must not indirectly imply any content other than therapeutic massage. Choices made in decorating the space or in reading material can be seen as creating an environment that fosters a dual role by promoting a specific mental, spiritual, nutritional, or exercise approach.
6. Selling products to clients can become an issue because of the perceived authority influence and power differential of the professional. Closely related products, such as self-massage tools that are made available for the client's convenience, as opposed to products sold for profit making, often present less of a problem than something like nutritional products. The client may like the services of the massage therapist but does not want to feel pressured into buying products. These situations must be managed with careful reflection, because ethical dilemmas often result from the sale of products.
7. Privacy can be preserved by using an answering machine or service and returning calls within set hours. If financially possible, have a receptionist or secretary monitor phone calls.
8. Maintain regular appointment hours. Begin and end sessions on time.
9. If you go to clients' homes, be extra cautious about entering a home alone. It is important to screen your clients carefully. The initial intake interview is a good opportunity to do this. Have the client come to your location, where you have more professional control over the screening process. Individual circumstances dictate when the following recommendations are necessary; however, remember: it is better to be safe than sorry.
   - An on-site massage session for a bedridden elderly person will have a different level of concern than a female massage therapist providing on-site massage to a single male client, or vice versa. At the very least, make sure someone always knows where you are and check in with someone periodically throughout the day. If you are anxious about doing an on-site massage session, consider referring the client to someone else or team up with a fellow massage practitioner and both perform the massage.
   - Hire someone to go with you to the client's home. This person does not need to be a massage professional. This person remains within hearing distance of the place where the massage is given and can act as a witness should the client claim inappropriate behavior by the massage professional. This person also provides protection from any type of entrapment or illicit advances against the massage practitioner. It is appropriate to charge for this protection, and it is reflected in the fee structure.
   - It is also important to use the phone when entering a home or other location where less control is available to the massage practitioner. Call a prearranged number and give an associate the name, address, and phone number of the client, the time of arrival, and the expected time of departure. Tell this person that you will call just before you leave. Leave instructions to call the authorities should you not call at the agreed time. Make sure that your client hears this conversation.
10. Think carefully before setting rules about client conduct, rescheduling, and payment methods. Make sure you are willing to enforce your policies. If you are not, do not make them. Record this information clearly and concisely and make sure the client reads it. Posting it on the wall provides additional reinforcement.
11. Do not spend personal time, such as lunch, with clients. In rare situations the professional may choose to forgo the professional relationship to develop a personal relationship. This decision can be considered a breach of professional ethics and is almost always a professional and personal mistake. The initial relationship structure was built on the basis of one who serves and one who is served. Rarely is an effective transition made to a relationship of mutual support. Both people usually end up hurt.

feelings. Was it a fleeting warm feeling? Is there just something about this particular person? Could it have been a hormonal response? Oxytocin, the bonding chemical, may be a big influence in couples bonding and parental feelings. This hormone is stimulated during skin contact such as massage. Therapists should also be aware that some women become more sexually responsive during certain times of their monthly cycle. Were you feeling alone and needing to be connected? If the problem arises from something lacking in life, empower yourself to search out the cause and change circumstances so that personal reactions are kept out of the therapy room.

Remember, as massage professionals, when we touch, we also are being touched. The exchange is unavoidable, and we also need to monitor our own feelings and expressions of intimacy. If we do not deal effectively with these responses, the feelings associated with them could become very uncomfortable. The client may react by discontinuing the massage

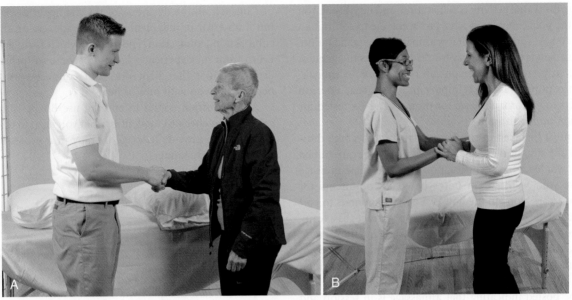

FIGURE 2-5 The body language of greeting. When greeting a client, the massage professional leans toward the person and gently draws the individual into the space of the massage session.

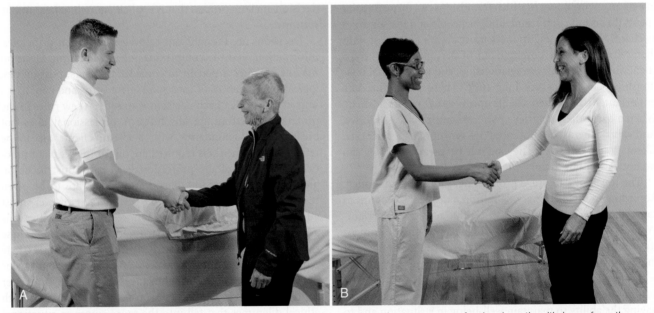

FIGURE 2-6 The body language of closure. When the massage is complete, the massage professional gently withdraws from the client by using body language that moves away from the person.

sessions, or the therapist may effectively detach from the client and possibly stop seeing the client altogether. In the latter case, the client may feel abandoned.

If a professional relationship cannot be maintained with a client, stop providing therapeutic massage and refer the client to someone else. Give an honest, simple explanation so that the client understands it was not something he or she said or did that prompted the referral. Professional ethics cannot safeguard us from being human; however, behavior becomes unethical when the problem is not acknowledged and resourceful action is not taken to solve it.

If a client refuses or is unable to change an inappropriate response to the massage, the client must be refused further treatment. Explain to the client that the situation is uncomfortable and massage therapy can no longer be provided. The dismissal must be done gently but assertively, and the client must be told the decision is final.

A client who immediately asks for sexual release is a different case. If this occurs, the massage professional explains succinctly that neither sexual release nor any other kind of sexual interaction is provided; the therapist then dismisses the person immediately and leaves the area to go to a safe place.

Asking for sexual activity is solicitation, and it is illegal. You can call the police. A person who asks someone to commit an illegal act has committed the criminal act of solicitation. When a person is looking to pay for sex and makes this request by words or gestures, the person can be arrested for solicitation of prostitution. It also is important to note that a person who offers to perform a sex act for money can be arrested for solicitation of prostitution.

Care must be taken in situations that could become difficult, and any situation in which behavior could be questioned must be avoided. One such situation concerns male massage therapists who want to do home-based appointments for women who are alone in the house. A good solution is to pair up with a female practitioner and do these massages as a team. It is important that a parent or legal guardian be in the room when massage services are given to a child under 18 years of age. A practitioner should never work behind a locked door, because this may be construed as entrapment. Instead, a sign should be posted indicating that a massage is in session and the room should not be entered without knocking.

Maintaining the delicate professional balance between client and practitioner is especially difficult with long-term clients. The nurturing approach of the massage practitioner fosters an environment in which friendships can form. Regular clients do become important, both as people and in their roles as clients. Massage practitioners must always be honest with themselves about the development of personal feelings for a client. Remember, this is a relationship, and professional relationships can last a very long time. These people become important to us. When clients move away, we miss them. When a client dies, we grieve. When clients rejoice, so do we. And when clients do not need us anymore, we celebrate. Clients touch our lives. They are our best teachers. How can we not care about them?

The touch of a massage professional should be safe touch. According to the dictionary definition, *safe* means "not apt to cause danger, harm, or hurt; to be free of risk" (Merriam-Webster, 2002). Physiologically, safe means a state of homeostasis rather than the alarm of the fight-or-flight responses of the sympathetic autonomic nervous system or the intense retreat and withdrawal responses of the parasympathetic autonomic nervous system (see Chapter 5). Being safe means having the ability to maintain well-being in a situation and to alter responses easily to cope resourcefully with the inevitable change and demands of everyday life. The therapeutic massage professional must consider everything, including personal beliefs and fears that may make touch unsafe for clients.

By using this educational experience to explore these issues, more safe places can be found for the practitioner, which will influence professional touch and make the massage environment a safe place. The essence of this work is human touch. By dealing with personal intimacy issues, not only can the massage professional provide essential touch for the client, the client also learns to establish proper boundaries. It must always be kept in mind that each individual massage practitioner represents the entire massage therapy profession. Demonstrating respect for the self demonstrates respect for the profession as a whole.

Consider all the dynamics of the therapeutic relationship, but if an error in judgment is to be made, err on the side of compassion, connection, and caring, which is no error at all. Learn from the experience. Do not become so "professionally detached" that the client does not connect with you, the person, and you with him or her.

As this section comes to an end, use Box 2-15 both as a review and a checklist to identify what you need to understand to be able to provide massage therapy in a professional and client-centered manner.

ETHICAL DECISION MAKING

SECTION OBJECTIVE

Chapter objective covered in this section:

11. The student will be able to use a problem-solving approach to ethical decision making.

Using the information presented in this section, the student will be able to perform the following:

• Implement an eight-step decision-making process

When ethical dilemmas are difficult to resolve, massage professionals are expected to engage in a conscientious decision-making process that is explicit enough to bear public scrutiny.

Decisions are thought-out responses based on principles, information, and the complexities of the situation. Decision making requires a person to consider the facts, possibilities, logical consequences of cause and effect (pros and cons), and impact on people. Each decision is unique. A few rules in the professional setting are absolutes: A professional does not breach sexual boundaries with a client; clients are to be referred when the skills required are out of the scope of practice or training of the professional; all care must focus on giving help and avoiding harm; and clients are to be given complete information about the treatment. However, most ethical dilemmas revolve around more ambiguous situations and require a thoughtful approach to decision making. These situations often are difficult to identify, and solutions may require objective input. Where does a professional go for help?

As stated previously, mentoring, supervision, and peer support are very helpful to a professional grappling with ethical dilemmas that fall into the more common situational gray areas. Recall that a mentor is usually one in the profession of therapeutic massage with a greater career experience. A mentor is concerned with the successful career growth of those they mentor. Because a mentor does not have the hire, fire, and discipline role, the relationship is more individually focused, with freedom to discuss issues without fear of inadequacy.

Supervision involves periodic review of a professional's actions by one in authority in the work setting. This can be direct supervision, in which the supervising professional actually observes the professional at work, or reflective supervision, in which the supervisor discusses the professional practice with the practitioner. Supervision can help identify potential ethical concerns and assist in ethical decision making.

Peer support provides a format for discussion, brainstorming, and reflection on the professional practice. Two or three heads are better than one in the process of ethical decision making.

Ethics is not just about answers; it is also the willingness to ask the questions and to seek help when needed. It is said that professionals do not let personal judgments interfere with professional care, but what do we do, for example, when we cannot keep our mind on our work because of a client's body odor? What do we do when a client schedules appointments more frequently than necessary because the client likes being with us? How do we handle a client who refuses to seek medical intervention when indicated? These are just a few of the many questions you may find yourself asking throughout your professional massage therapy career.

The professional may wish to ask himself or herself the following questions:

- Can I handle the professional power differential from a position of respect and empowerment for the client?
- Do I have the knowledge and skills to respond effectively to the situation?
- Am I avoiding dual or multiple roles with the client?
- Am I maintaining the boundaries of the therapeutic relationship?
- Am I within the established scope of practice for therapeutic massage?
- Am I respecting the scope of practice of other professionals?
- Do I have the highest good of the client in mind?
- Is what I am doing supporting the highest good of the profession?
- Are my professional and communication skills effective?
- Would I want anyone else to know what I am doing?

A problem may be developing if the answers to these questions become ambiguous or inconsistent. When openly answered, these questions help us recognize the need to use a problem-solving approach to make ethical decisions.

Problem-Solving Approach to Ethical Decision Making

Problem-solving to reach an effective decision is not an easy task. A generic model created from many different problem-solving methods is presented here for the purpose of ethical decision making. The model is developed from a critical thinking perspective. Critical thinking uses the scientific method as a framework for making informed and evidence-based decisions. This model is expounded on throughout the text in regard to what may be called clinical reasoning, which involves taking the client's health history, performing a physical assessment, developing a care or treatment plan, choosing methods to implement the treatment plan, and charting. Most of this information is presented in Chapter 4 with additional refinement of the material throughout this text.

Massage therapists with well-developed clinical reasoning are able to generate, implement, and evaluate approaches to care. **Clinical reasoning** involves why and how to provide massage. The difference between critical thinking and clinical reasoning is as follows: *Critical thinking* is a process that can be applied to many different situations, both in the massage therapy profession and in everyday life; *clinical reasoning* is a form of critical thinking that targets a specific therapeutic practice, such as massage therapy.

We are most comfortable believing that our decision-making abilities are comprehensive, objective, intuitive, and workable. For some this actually may be the case; however, years of teaching and self-exploration have shown that most people have never learned comprehensive decision-making skills. To complicate matters, different people, when gathering information, are naturally attracted to certain types of information and are influenced by certain types of criteria when evaluating possible solutions. Some experts believe that this attention focus is a genetic predisposition, and others believe that it is learned behavior. Regardless, most people, unless specifically trained, effectively consider only about half of the relevant and available information when making a decision. This can lead us to making decisions that do not serve us well.

A problem-solving model not only leads us through the steps we more naturally would take, but also reminds us to take note of important information we might tend to overlook when making a decision. When this process is followed diligently, it eventually becomes a habit. In the beginning the process may feel cumbersome and uncomfortable. The parts of the process that we do not understand or with which we become impatient or frustrated often are the areas on which we do not naturally focus. These are the areas, then, that need the most practice (Proficiency Exercise 2-11).

The decision-making process presented in Box 2-16 acknowledges the importance of factual data, intuitive insight, concrete and objective cause and effect, and the feelings, experiences, and influences of the people involved.

COMMUNICATION SKILLS

SECTION OBJECTIVES

Chapter objectives covered in this section:

12. The student will be able to use basic communication skills to listen effectively and deliver an I-message.
13. The student will be able to identify and resolve conflict in the professional setting.

Using the information presented in this section, the student will be able to perform the following:

- Identify a person's preferred communication pattern
- Develop and use an I-message to deliver information and listen reflectively
- Follow a suggested communication pattern for resolving ethical dilemmas and conflict
- Identify three barriers to effective communication

Communication is the act of exchanging thoughts, feelings, and behavior. Many ethical and professional dilemmas result from communication difficulties. To make ethical decisions and resolve ethical dilemmas, we must communicate effectively.

💡 PROFICIENCY EXERCISE 2-11

Be A Critical Thinker

Note: Learning this process can be difficult, but it is very important. It is okay to be confused and frustrated, but practice eventually will result in understanding. Proficiency exercises are important to do. In the beginning it is okay if you just attempt to do them. In time, they get easier. On a separate piece of paper, go through the six steps.

Decision Making Using the Problem-Solving Model with Peer Support

Identify an ethical dilemma with which you are dealing or make up a dilemma that you believe you will deal with in the future. Describe the dilemma by answering the following questions on a piece of paper.

Step 1: Identify and define the situation.

Key questions:

What is the problem?

What happened in factual terms?

What caused the situation?

What was done or is being done?

What has worked or not worked?

Who is involved and what responsibilities do they have?

Step 2: Divide into groups of four. Choose who will present the facts of his or her dilemma to the group. This presentation should not take longer than 5 minutes. Each of the other three group members will play a role in the decision-making process.

One of the three remaining group members now provides input from step 2 of the problem-solving model by suggesting possible solutions, using the following questions as a guide. For the purpose of this exercise, limit the possibilities to three or four. Spend 3 to 5 minutes on this part of the exercise and remember to stay in your role; it confuses the process when you bounce between steps 3 and 4.

Key questions:

What are the possibilities?

What does my intuition suggest?

What are the possible contributing factors?

What are possible approaches for corrective action?

What might work?

What are other ways to look at the situation?

What do the data suggest?

Provide three possible solutions to the dilemma.

Step 3: The next person uses logic to evaluate each of the possible solutions presented in step 2, using the following questions as a guide. Spend 3 to 5 minutes on this part of the

exercise. Again, stay in your role; do not work with steps 2 or 4.

Key questions:

What are the costs, resources needed, and time involved?

What is the logical progression of the pattern, contributing factors, and current behaviors?

What are the logical causes and effects of each solution identified?

What are the pros and cons of each solution suggested?

What are the consequences of not acting?

What are the consequences of acting?

Step 4: The last person evaluates each of the possible solutions generated in step 2 in terms of the people involved, using the following questions as a guide. Spend 3 to 5 minutes on this part of the exercise. Stay with the process; do not become chatty or conversational.

In terms of each possible solution being considered in step 2, what is the impact on the people involved: client, practitioner, and other professionals working with the client?

Key questions:

How does each person involved feel about the possible solutions?

Does the practitioner feel qualified to work with such situations?

Does a feeling of cooperation and agreement exist among all parties involved?

Step 5: Now, the person who originally presented the ethical problem chooses a solution and develops an implementation plan. Again, spend 3 to 5 minutes on this part of the exercise. Write the solution with the implementation plan on a piece of paper.

Step 6: Rotate the roles so that each member of the group plays all four roles. It will take 1 hour to complete the entire exercise with all participants playing all four roles. After the entire process has been completed, answer the following questions:

What was the easiest part of the process for me?

What was the hardest part of the process for me and what made it difficult?

What was the most difficult part of the process for the group?

What might help the group problem-solve more effectively?

How would I implement the process by myself without a peer support group?

Effective communication often is a difficult process for both the professional and the client. Without a direct communication approach, ethical dilemmas tend to escalate, and both parties suffer in the process. Professionals seek to establish genuine positive regard for all clients and to relate to each with sensitivity to that person's uniqueness. Professional ethics demands that when we have a feeling of criticism and negative judgment of a client, we must be aware of it and work to prevent it from interfering with our commitment to compassionate, quality care. Direct, honest communication that focuses on the concrete facts of the situation rather than the person's emotional behavior, accompanied by a gentle, respectful approach, opens the door for resolution.

As was described in Chapter 1, touch is a powerful mode of communication. The intent of professional touch may be influenced by many factors, including countertransference and the thought process of the therapist at the moment of the touch. The way touch is interpreted by the client often is influenced by the unspoken intent of the therapist; therefore, it is important to monitor thoughts and feelings while professionally communicating through touch.

Putting ethical principles into action requires some basic communication skills. Communication skills are required to retrieve information, maintain charting and client records, and provide information effectively so that the client can give informed consent. Using the following communication skills

Box 2-16   Problem-Solving Model for Decision Making

Learning how to make good professional decisions is very important; the key to this is practice, practice, practice.

Step 1: Gather the facts to identify and define the situation.
Key questions: What is the problem? What happened in factual terms?
- What are the facts?
- What has happened?
- What caused the situation?
- What was done or is being done?
- What has worked or not worked?
- Who is involved and what responsibilities do they have?

Step 2: Brainstorm possible solutions.
Key question: What might I do? or What if?
- What are the possibilities?
- What does my intuition suggest?
- What are the possible contributing factors?
- What are possible approaches for corrective action?
- What might work?
- What are other ways to look at the situation?
- What do the data suggest?

Step 3: Logically and objectively evaluate each possible solution identified in step 2; look at both sides and the pros and cons.
Note: This objective analysis of the possible solutions generated in step 2 is very important. The ability to analyze objectively is an essential skill for effective professional practice. In addition, this area of processing becomes important in dealing with conflict situations that may arise from ethical dilemmas, because the focus of this information is a process. Processes can be evaluated and altered; people's feelings usually cannot. A professional who has not developed the ability to evaluate a situation logically and objectively will have difficulty identifying where processes have broken down. Remember, change an action and people's feelings change.

   Key question: What would happen if I ... ? (Insert each brainstormed idea from step 2.)
- What are the costs, resources needed, and time involved?
- What is the logical progression of the pattern, contributing factors, and current behaviors?
- What are the logical causes and effects of each solution identified?
- What are the pros and cons of each solution suggested?
- What are the consequences of not acting?
- What are the consequences of acting?

Step 4: Evaluate the effect of each possible solution on the people involved.
Key question: How would each person involved feel if I ...? (Insert each brainstormed idea from step 2.)

- In terms of each solution being considered, what is the impact on the people involved: client, practitioner, and other professionals working with the client?
- How does each person involved feel about the possible interventions?
- Does the practitioner feel qualified to work with such situations?
- Does a feeling of cooperation and agreement exist among all parties involved?

Step 5: Choose a solution and develop an implementation plan after carefully processing steps 1 through 4.
Implementation plans are step-by-step procedures that detail what must be done to carry out the decision. For example, a solution arrived at using the previous steps might be: I will learn more about asthma so that I can work with my client better. The implementation plan would be as follows:
- Use the Internet to research asthma
- Look up asthma at the library
- Contact the local asthma support group for information
- Contact the client's physician for specific recommendations
- Talk with my friend who is a respiratory therapist
- Compile the information into a massage benefit report to develop the massage approach
- Discuss the report with my client

Step 6: Implement the plan and set a date for re-evaluation.
This is sometimes the hardest part—just doing it.

Step 7: Determine the logical consequences if the plan is not followed.
It is important to determine what will happen if one of the parties in a decision that affects more than one person does not meet his or her commitment. Make sure to document this (write it down). For example, a decision is made between a massage therapist and a chronic no-show client that the client will be charged for the full session unless she calls 24 hours in advance to cancel the appointment. Both parties agree, but the very next session, the client does not show and does not call. Because the consequence has been agreed on in advance (i.e., the client will be charged for the full session), the possibility of escalation of the conflict is diminished.

Step 8: Re-evaluate and make necessary adjustments; then implement the refined plan.
Remember, decisions are not static; re-evaluation may show you ways to alter, refine, or change them.

---

can help the professional maintain ethical practices in the therapeutic relationship.

The strongest message is delivered through the kinesthetic mode, or body language. As we express ourselves through our bodies, others visually receive the messages and feel our touch.

Congruence in what is heard, what is seen, and what is felt is important. When congruence is lacking, the kinesthetic message seems to have the strongest effect.

The tone of voice is more important than the words spoken. Tone is kinesthetic and auditory because of the

💡 PROFICIENCY EXERCISE 2-12

Write what each of the words below means to you and in what way you would behave if you were experiencing these words.

Joy

Love

Peace

Competence

Compare your list with those of three other students and identify the similarities and differences. What did you learn about the interpretation of a word?

pressure waves emitted. We hear and feel the sound waves from the tone of voice.

The words are the least effective part of the communication pattern. Words can have mixed meanings, depending on each person's definition of a particular word (Proficiency Exercise 2-12). It is important to make sure that each of the people communicating is working from the same definition of a word. For example, the massage practitioner's definition of the word disrobe may be different from the client's definition. To a massage professional, disrobe may mean to remove external clothing but keep underwear on; the client interprets the same word as meaning to take off all clothing. During the informed consent process, the massage professional may say, "It is out of my scope of practice to diagnose or treat any specific condition." The massage practitioner defines the word *treat* as meaning to provide remedial or rehabilitation procedures. The client interprets the word *treat* as any type of method used.

Preferred Communication Patterns

Each person has a preferred method of delivering and receiving information in a style that is most comfortable for that individual. This is determined by genetic predisposition and what and how the person has learned.

People who prefer the visual mode make pictures in their mind and use many descriptive words as they paint word pictures during conversation. They tend to use "see" words and want to make eye contact when conversing. Others prefer the auditory mode. These people use "hear" words during conversation and are very attentive to the tone and rhythm of speech. They often hum, talk to themselves, and listen with their eyes closed.

Some people operate primarily from the feeling, or kinesthetic, mode of communication. These people may find talking and listening fatiguing. When speaking they use a lot of body language and "feel" words. Often they find that they have to touch something or someone to understand.

Almost everyone processes visual and auditory messages through the kinesthetic mode. The most common pattern is visual/kinesthetic, and the second most common is auditory/kinesthetic. People see and feel or hear and feel.

The way information is delivered and received also depends on fundamental processing styles. Some people prefer facts and sequence, whereas others prefer concepts and ideas. Some people make decisions based primarily on processes of cause

and effect, and others structure decisions in terms of people and social structure. No one way is better than another, only different.

When providing information, it is important to deliver the message in the style the person receiving it prefers. This often requires massage professionals to communicate in a way that is different from their preferred style, and it takes practice.

Listening

Effective listening involves the development of focusing skills. You cannot listen effectively if you are distracted, planning what you will say next, or preparing your response. **Reflective listening** involves restating the information to indicate that you have received and understood the message. **Active listening** may clarify a feeling attached to the message but does not add to or change the message.

Listening does not involve giving advice, resolving the problem presented, or in any other way interjecting information about what was said. Effective listening occurs when we listen to understand instead of to respond. Understanding the message and agreeing with the content of the message are not the same thing; the basis for this confusion most likely evolved from our feeling of being most understood when someone agrees with us. Understanding can occur regardless of whether agreement exists. Much time is wasted and conflict is encouraged when people equate understanding with agreement.

For example, while studying this chapter, you, as a student, may not agree with the author's (my) position on the importance of wearing a uniform in the professional setting. Because you have a different opinion does not mean that the textbook is wrong or that you are wrong; the two positions are simply different. You can understand that I am basing my information on the existing standards of professionalism and my previous experience; however, you can choose not to follow the recommendation. I, as the author of the text, can understand that a valid case can be made for not visually creating distinction (a uniform) between the professional and the client; however, I would not agree with your decision if you decided not to wear a uniform. Sometimes this is called "agreeing to disagree," but this approach still seems to have the context of right or wrong, whereas simply being understood feels nonjudgmental and essential.

Delivering Information with I-Messages

I-messages share feelings and concerns. You-messages put a person down, blame, criticize, and provoke anger, hurt, embarrassment, and feelings of worthlessness. I-message patterns require the four components of information used in effective decision making (Box 2-17).

- Describe the behavior or problem you find bothersome (facts)
- State your feelings about the situation (impact on people)
- State the consequence (logical cause and effect)
- Request the preferred behavior or action (possibilities)

It takes practice to use the simple I-message communication pattern well (Proficiency Exercise 2-13). Just as in

Box 2-17 I-Message Pattern

The steps for creating an I-message are:
1. Describe the behavior or problem you find bothersome (facts).
2. State your feelings about the situation (impact on people).
3. State the consequence (logical cause and effect).
4. Request the preferred behavior or action (possibilities).

The pattern is:

When _____ happens, I feel _____.
The result is _____, and what I would prefer is _____.

When delivering I-messages, remain pleasant, respectful, and honest. Be aware of your body language, tone of voice, and quality of touch.

💡 PROFICIENCY EXERCISE 2-13

1. Construct an I-message about a piece of information in this chapter that you feel is important.
   Example: When I read about I-messages to enhance communication, I felt relieved. The result is that I will practice this pattern with my family, and I prefer that the communication between my family members improves.
2. Sit in a circle with at least three other people (more is better). Turn to your left and deliver your I-message to the person sitting next to you. That person repeats the I-message to you using the same format. Note what pieces are left out or how the pieces of the message become confused; or, on the other hand, note the clarity of the I-message when it is understood. Also note the preferred communication.
3. Now the person who just listened and repeated the message turns to the person on her left and delivers an I-message, which that person repeats to her. Continue this way around the circle.

problem-solving, each individual attends to certain parts of the information and ignores other parts. If you are a person who naturally attends to people's feelings and you attempt to deliver a message to someone who views the world through logical outcomes, the two of you will seem to be on different wavelengths or speaking different languages. If a message is to be understood, it must be delivered on the wavelength most easily received by the person attempting to understand.

The following exercise may help you understand the importance of delivering information the way the receiver (listener) is most apt to understand.

A father enjoys jazz music and keeps the car radio tuned to a jazz station. His daughter, a teenager, likes contemporary rock. Whenever the teenager drives her dad's car, she changes the radio station. On the few occasions the two find themselves in the car at the same time, a battle begins over which station will be on, jazz or rock. Now, if the father has something important to say to his daughter or wants to connect with her, he would be wise to put the radio on the rock station, even though he prefers jazz and may even find rock difficult

to listen to. It may be that the father can have the radio on rock only for a short time before it becomes too difficult for him and he changes to the jazz station. If he insists on jazz to begin with, his daughter will tune him out and the opportunity for connection will be lost.

To encourage effective communication, begin by identifying a person's communication pattern; that is, the words used, tone of voice, and body language. Use neutral topics to generate general discussion. During this time adjust your communication pattern to meet the person's communication style. Shift your body language, word choice, and tone to match the client's before attempting to deliver a message.

When communicating feelings, be specific. Words such as "upset" are too ambiguous; instead, use words such as afraid, angry, annoyed, discouraged, embarrassed, irritated, rejected, accepted, appreciated, capable, determined, compassionate, glad, grateful, proud, loved, and trusted. Define the words you use. Do not assume that what you mean by a word is what your listener understands it to mean.

After an I-message has been delivered, request a response using open-ended questions. Open-ended questions encourage the sharing of information and cannot be easily answered in one word. Open-ended questions begin with where, when, what, how, and which. Avoid why questions, because they encourage defensive reactions. When listening to the response, use active and reflective listening.

The I-message format also can be an effective listening tool. While listening, organize the information using the following questions:

- What happened or what are the facts?
- What feelings are being expressed?
- What was the logical outcome?
- What are the possibilities?

When listening reflectively, repeat the information as follows:

"What I heard you say was: When ____ happened, you felt ___. The result was ___, and what you prefer is ___. Did I understand correctly?"

If a person leaves out information (as commonly occurs), you will not be able to fill in that blank. In that case a clarifying question can be formed, such as, "What would you prefer?" or "What was the logical outcome of the situation?"

Conflict and Conflict Resolution

Conflict is an expressed struggle between at least two interdependent parties who perceive incompatible goals, scarce resources, and/or interference from the other party in achieving their goals. Perhaps nothing is more common than conflict. Conflict arises from a number of factors, such as:

- Varied perspectives on a situation
- Differing belief systems and values, which have arisen from the involved parties' accumulated life experience and conditioning
- Differing objectives and interests

Conflict and conflict resolution play important roles in individual and social evolution and development. Many cultures value harmony, compatibility, satisfaction, and independence. Because of these values, the tendency in the past has been to avoid conflict. Conflict arises when one or more people view the current system as not working. At least one person is sufficiently dissatisfied with the status quo to be willing to own the conflict and speak up in the hope of being able to improve the situation. Through conflict we have opportunities to do things differently in the future.

Conflict should also be recognized as existing at two levels. In addition to the typically obvious interpersonal dispute among individuals, some measure of intrapersonal conflict almost always exists within ourselves. This inner conflict may be evidenced by confusion, inconsistency, or lack of congruity.

People in conflict have both common ground and differences. Areas of common ground include:

- Overlapping interests
- Interdependence
- Points of agreement

The common ground can serve as the starting point for conflict resolution.

Conflict resolution does not necessarily resolve tensions between people. Conflict resolution may simply align matters sufficiently to allow each person to make progress toward his or her goals rather than stall in an uncertain and stressful state of disagreement.

Many people have long operated by the myth that the best way to resolve conflict is to "do battle," and the one who "wins" ends the conflict. This approach is more about power and control than conflict resolution. Doing battle and winning or losing supports a corresponding belief that every situation involves a "right" and a "wrong." If we respond to conflict this way, we have limited our awareness and understanding of the nature of conflict and of alternative means of responding to conflict, such as mediation and negotiation.

Factors and influences necessary for mediation and negotiation include the following:

- Concern about the impact of the dispute on the relationship
- Time concerns
- Expense
- Impact on affected others
- Lost opportunities
- Stress
- Lack of closure
- Uncertain compliance
- Areas of existing common ground

Types of Conflict

The decision-making process in this text presents a format for mediated and negotiated types of conflict resolution. Various types of conflict exist. If we can pinpoint the type of conflict, we are more likely to be able to resolve it.

Relationship Conflicts

Relationship conflicts, often called *personality conflicts*, occur as a result of strong negative emotions, misperceptions or stereotypes, poor communication or miscommunication, or repetitive negative behaviors. Relationship problems often lead to an unnecessary escalation in destructive conflict. Conflict resolution supports the safe and balanced expression of the perspectives and emotions of each person involved, leading to acknowledgment and understanding of that individual's point of view. Gaining a broader perspective of diversity of culture and individual operational style is very helpful. Evaluations exist for identifying different personality styles, and using these evaluation tools can be helpful. One of the most researched methods is the Myers-Briggs Type Indicator. These evaluations help individuals with opposite perspectives to interact well rather than allowing conflict to develop. The more we personalize a person's operational style, the more likely it is that conflict will develop.

EXAMPLE

Two massage therapists have worked together for 2 years. Just recently a new massage therapist has been hired. This individual prefers to eat lunch alone and remain in the massage room during breaks. Conflict develops when the original massage therapists begin to describe their new coworker as stuck up and a snob.

Data Conflicts

Data conflicts occur when people lack information necessary to make wise decisions, are misinformed, disagree on which data are relevant, interpret information differently, or have collected data differently. Some data conflicts may be unnecessary, because they are caused by poor communication between the people in conflict. Other data conflicts may be incompatibilities associated with data collection, interpretation, or communication. Most data conflicts have "data solutions," and once the information has been corrected, the conflict will resolve unless it has developed into a relationship conflict.

EXAMPLE

Conflict can occur because of a scheduling problem. Two clients arrive for their appointments at the same time. When the clients check their appointment cards, one realizes that he entered the appointment in his calendar on the wrong day.

Interest Conflicts

Interest conflicts are caused by competition over perceived incompatible needs. Conflicts of interest result when one or more people believe that in order to satisfy their needs, the needs and interests of an opponent must be sacrificed. This often occurs during times of scarcity or when it is perceived that there is not enough to go around. Interest-based conflicts may occur over such things as money, physical resources, or time; over procedural issues, such as the way a dispute is to be resolved; or over psychological issues, such as perceptions of trust and fairness and the desire for participation and respect. For an interest-based dispute to be resolved, those involved need to define and express their individual interests so that all these interests may be addressed jointly. Interest-based conflict is best resolved through maximum integration of the parties' respective interests, positive intentions, and desired experiential outcomes. A third person, such as a mediator, is often necessary to successfully resolve this type of conflict.

> **EXAMPLE**
>
> Four massage therapists have been working at the same massage franchise for a year and have had full schedules. Business has been slow for the past 3 months, and they are now competing with each other for clients.

Value Conflicts

Values give meaning to our lives. Values explain what is "just" or "unjust." Differing values need not cause conflict. People can live together in harmony with different value systems. Value disputes arise only when people attempt to force one set of values on others or lay claim to exclusive value systems that do not allow for divergent paths. It is no use to try to change values and systems during relatively short and strategic mediation interventions. However, supporting each participant's expression of his or her values and beliefs for acknowledgment by the other party can be helpful. Belief systems are more amiable to change. Values are like the ethical principles described earlier, whereas belief systems are like standards of practice. Belief systems are often superimposed on us during our developmental childhood years. We are taught what is right or wrong, good or bad. Because we learn our belief systems, we can change them through education and a willingness to be open to new possibilities.

> **EXAMPLE**
>
> A massage therapist strongly believes most health conditions can be controlled without medication. This practitioner has a new client who uses a variety of medications to manage anxiety. The massage therapist is finding it difficult to refrain from telling the client that anxiety can be managed with lifestyle changes and that medication is not necessary. The conflict is based on differing belief systems.

Ways of Dealing with Conflict

Five common methods can be used to deal with conflict. Learning about the alternative means of handling conflict gives us a wider choice of actions to use in any given situation and makes us better able to respond to the situation. Although the following methods are the common ways of increasing the chance of success, the reality is that we use each of these ways of dealing with conflict at least some of the time. We approach conflict in the way we believe will be most helpful to us. Our style for dealing with conflict changes with the circumstances. Conflict-handling behavior is not a static procedure; rather, it is a process that requires flexibility and constant evaluation to be truly productive and effective.

Denial or Withdrawal

With denial or withdrawal, a person attempts to eliminate conflict by denying that it exists and refusing to acknowledge it. Usually, the conflict does not go away, but rather grows to the point that it becomes unmanageable. When the issue and the timing are not critical and the issue is short-lived and will resolve itself, denial may be a productive way to deal with conflict. The effectiveness of this approach depends on knowing when to use denial.

Suppression or Smoothing Over

A person using suppression plays down differences and does not recognize the positive aspects of handling the conflict openly. Instead, the situation is acknowledged (unlike with denial), but it is glossed over. The source of the conflict rarely goes away. However, suppression may be used when preserving a relationship is more important than dealing with a relatively insignificant issue.

Power or Dominance

Power often is used to settle differences. It may be inherent in a person's authority or position. It may take the form of a majority (as in voting) or a persuasive minority. Power strategies result in winners and losers. The losers do not support a final decision in the same way the winners do. Future meetings of a group may be marred by the conscious or unconscious renewal of the struggle previously "settled" by the use of power. In some instances, especially when other forms of handling conflict are not effective, power strategies may be necessary. Parents often say to children, "Because I said so." This use of power works in the short term, but over time results in deeper relationship conflict.

Compromise or Negotiation

Compromise (i.e., "You give a little, I'll give a little, and we'll meet each other half way") has some serious drawbacks. Such bargaining often causes both sides to assume initial inflated positions, because they are aware that they are going to have to "give a little" and want to reduce the loss. The compromise solution may be watered down or weakened to the point that it will not be effective. There may be little real commitment by any of the parties. Still, in some cases compromise makes sense, such as when resources are limited or a speedy decision needs to be made.

Integration or Collaboration

The integration or collaboration approach suggests that all parties to the conflict recognize the interests and abilities of the others. Each individual's interests, positive intentions, and desired outcomes are thoroughly explored in an effort to solve the problems in a maximizing way. Participants are expected to modify and develop their original views as work progresses. This sounds like the ideal way to manage and resolve conflict; however, for collaboration to be successful, those involved need a nonthreatening and collectively supportive system. This process takes time, openness, and energy.

Conflict Climate: Defensive or Supportive

A defensive climate reflects the type of atmosphere characteristic of competition—an atmosphere that inhibits the mutual trust required for effective conflict management. A supportive climate reflects collaboration—an environment that leads to mutual trust and to an atmosphere conducive to managing differences. In the best case, the participants in conflict resolution come to appreciate that the apparent presenting problem does not need to limit their discussions. Participants are encouraged to express the full breadth and depth of their interests, with each participant seeking to identify a "value" that he or she can bring to the discussion and the maximized satisfaction of underlying interests and intentions.

Conflict is important. If managed well, it identifies and supports effective change. Conflict can foster avoidance, or it can expand our experiences. Making good decisions about managing and resolving conflict can pave the way for greater understanding and well-being.

During the process of resolving a conflict, written documentation should be maintained about the nature of the conflict, the type of resolution attempted, the success of the conflict resolution, and the outcome. Because conflict already exists, interpretation of the requirement for resolution can become confused. Objective documentation that is agreed upon by the parties helps maintain clarity. If the conflict cannot be resolved independently, documentation of the nature of the conflict is extremely important, in case the situation escalates to legal action.

Communicating When Dilemmas Arise

The following pattern can be used to resolve ethical dilemmas.
1. Carefully examine the facts, possibilities, logical causes and effects, and your feelings about the situation (see Box 2-16).
2. Speak with a mentor, a peer, or a supervisor about the situation in a peer review or support context.
3. Plan a time to talk about the situation with the other person or people involved.
4. Begin the conversation by identifying the problem as you see it.
5. Use the standard I-message format to provide information and professional disclosure about your inability to work with or be comfortable with the situation.

In the following example, a massage professional uses an I-message to talk with a client about the client's body odor:

"When a client seems to have a distinctive body odor that I am aware of (facts), I feel distracted from my work (impact on people). As a result, because of my inability to focus, the client does not receive the best massage (logical cause and effect). I would like to see if we can resolve this difficulty, and if I can't deal with the situation better, I may find it to your benefit to refer you to someone who is not as sensitive to odors as I am (possibilities)."

The client's body language and tone of voice may indicate embarrassment. The therapist then uses another I-message: "When I find it necessary to speak with someone about issues as personal as this (facts), I feel uncomfortable and embarrassed because I am afraid I will embarrass or hurt the person (impact on people). It is very difficult for me, but I truly want you to have the best possible care (logical cause and effect).

What information do you have that can help me (possibilities and open-ended question)?" Ending with an open-ended question encourages a problem-solving discussion.

It is essential to determine who has the problem. This can be done easily by deciding who will have to implement the solution to resolve the problem. Sometimes both parties own a part of the problem, with each needing to implement a portion of the solution for total resolution.

Continuing with the example of body odor, the therapist identifies and owns the problem by saying, "The difficulty is in my sensitivity to odors."

Next, information is gathered, and possible solutions are devised. The client continues to express embarrassment through body language and states that he was aware of the problem. He tells you that body odor has been a problem since he began taking medication for a health problem but that he had just showered before he came to the session and thought the odor was gone.

The massage practitioner responds using reflective listening: "If I understand correctly, you are taking a medication that causes the body odor (facts), and others are aware of the odor (impact on people), but you felt the odor was gone since you showered before coming to the session (logical cause and effect)."

The therapist asks, "Do you have any suggestions?" The client replies, "Could you use a scented oil or a room scent?" The client also says that he can speak to his physician and continue to shower just before coming for the session (generating possible solutions).

The therapist explains that using a scented oil may be a problem, because she has sensitive skin and that using a room scent bothers other clients. The therapist asks, "Would it bother you if I wore a mask treated with a scented oil?" The client indicates that would be fine (evaluating possible solutions in terms of logical outcomes and pros and cons, as well as people's feelings).

The therapist says, "How about if I try the mask next time you are here, and we will talk about it after the massage? If this doesn't work, we will see if we can come up with another solution. If nothing works, I will help you find a good therapist who can better serve your needs and is not so sensitive to odors." The client agrees (deciding on and implementing a plan, setting a date for re-evaluation, and agreeing on logical consequences).

After a decision has been made and agreed upon, it should be well defined and all parties should be in agreement about what will happen if the solution to the problem is not implemented effectively. The plan and the agreed-upon consequences should be written down.

The therapist closes with an I-message: "When I am able to work so well with a client about my sensitivity to odors (facts), I feel relieved (impact on people). This conversation has encouraged me to be more honest with myself and my clients (logical cause and effect). I hope that I will be able to continue to communicate effectively with you (possibilities). Thank you for being open with me."

A week later the plan is carried out, and the therapist finds that using the mask is distracting but effective. A sense of

💡 PROFICIENCY EXERCISE 2-14

In the space provided, evaluate your communication skills using the criteria presented in this section. Identify at least one area in which your communication skills currently are effective and one area that needs improvement.

Example: My communication skills generally are effective when I am not stressed. I remember to listen in a focused way and use the I-message pattern often. However, when I have many things on my mind, I become distracted, do not listen effectively, and tend to interrupt people.

Your Turn:

humor and understanding on the part of both the therapist and the client continue to support an effective solution (re-evaluate and make the necessary adjustments).

Barriers to Effective Communication

Effective communication is a skill. It can be learned. Effective communication is essential in the therapeutic relationship. Professionals diligently seek to improve their communication skills.

Time

It takes time to communicate effectively. This is why writing is sometimes a more effective form of communication. When writing, we should make time to consider the words and reflect on what is being said. The person responding to the written message also has time to reread and reflect on the message.

Old Patterns

Falling into old patterns and old conditioning limits effective communication. It is important to "know thyself," and we must recognize personal triggers to old reactionary patterns in communication (Proficiency Exercise 2-14). Sometimes we need to leave a situation and come back to it so that we can respond instead of react.

Avoidance

People generally procrastinate about addressing conflict until it is unavoidable. They avoid people who display strong emotion because it makes them feel uncomfortable.

CREDENTIALS AND LICENSING

SECTION OBJECTIVES

Chapter objective covered in this section:

14. The student will be able to identify legal and credentialing concerns of the massage professional.

Using the information presented in this section, the student will be able to perform the following:
- Describe the difference between government and private credentials
- Determine whether a credentialing program is valid
- Explain the basic roles of local and state laws and legislation and their influence on therapeutic massage

---

Box 2-18 Credentials and Regulations

Licensing
- Requires a state or provincial board of examiners
- Requires all constituents who practice the profession to be licensed
- Legally defines and limits the scope of practice for a profession
- Requires specific educational courses or an examination
- Protects the use of a title (e.g., only those licensed can use the title of massage therapist)

Government Certification
- Administered by an independent board
- Voluntary but required for anyone using the protected title (e.g., massage therapist); others can provide the service but cannot call themselves massage therapists
- Requires specific educational courses and an examination

Government Registration
(Not to be confused with private registration processes)
- Administered by the state Department of Registry or other appropriate state agency

Voluntary Verification
- Does not necessarily require a specific education, such as a school diploma; often other forms of verification of professional standards, such as years in practice, are acceptable
- Does not provide title protection

Exemptions
- Means that a practitioner is not required to comply with an existing local or state regulation
- Excuses practitioners who meet specified educational requirements from meeting current regulatory requirements
- Does not provide title protection

- Contact local, state, or provincial government agencies to obtain information about laws pertinent to the practice of therapeutic massage

Credentials

Credentials are a form of official verification, earned by completing an educational or examination process, that confirms a certain level of expertise in a given skill. Government and private professional credentialing both are used in the massage profession. Standardization of the profession has resulted in different methods of proving one's skills in order to practice therapeutic massage. The massage professional should understand the various credentialing processes and the requirements of practicing legally.

The only credentials required for the practice of therapeutic massage are those specified by government agencies (Box 2-18). All others are voluntary. Because of some confusing and difficult local laws, special legislative concerns need to be addressed by the massage professional.

Many massage organizations and training programs have developed their own types of credentials. These credentials are valid only insofar as they indicate a level of professional achievement. A school diploma, which is granted on completion of a course of study, is an example. This is a very important document for a massage professional, but it is not a legally required credential unless stipulated by the law. For instance, a massage professional may need a diploma from a state-regulated school to take licensing examinations in states that license massage therapists.

Anyone can offer private certification. Therefore, it is important to make sure that any educational program or examination you take is sanctioned and administered by a reputable, regulated provider. As an example, state-licensed schools, recognized national and state professional organizations, and classes approved for continuing education credits have had to undergo a review process that validates their educational offerings. Approval by the National Commission for Certifying Agencies (NCCA) validates certification processes.

The National Certification Examination for Therapeutic Massage and Bodywork has been available since 1992. The examination covers human anatomy, physiology, kinesiology, clinical pathology, massage and bodywork theory, assessment, adjunct techniques, business practices, and professionalism. It continues to be refined to reflect the skills and knowledge base needed to meet the current job market for massage professionals. Periodically a job analysis survey is used to upgrade and improve the examination. The examination is meant to evaluate the entry-level knowledge base and skills. The educational requirement for taking the examination is equivalent to 500 hours in class, which must cover the information base and competencies required as indicated by the most recent job survey. The question bank is developed by experts. Each examination is computer generated from the test bank, and the exams are administered regularly in convenient locations. The exam does not include a practical demonstration of skills. The questions are multiple choice. Most of the questions are not answered with a regurgitation of factual data but rather require effective decision-making skills to identify the best answer.

This examination is not a government-regulated test. It is a voluntary, privately administered examination unless an individual state decides to use it for a licensing examination. Some states have done this, and some have also required additional test components, such as a practical demonstration of skills. In the future, other reliable tests may be developed and become an option for voluntary certification or government regulation. The National Certification Board for Therapeutic Massage and Bodywork began the process of creating an advanced practice examination in 2010. This advanced certification is designed to measure professional experience and ongoing education necessary to work confidently in complex practice situations. It is based on critical thinking and clinical reasoning. In the future, the NCBTMB also may offer specialty exams. Pursuing available and recognized certification exemplifies professional development.

Passing national certification exams is a concrete means of validating professional achievement. The Evolve website provides review questions for studying for certification and licensing exams.

Laws and Legislation

The main purpose of a law or an ordinance is to protect the safety and welfare of the public. When a governing body decides to enact regulations, the regulations must meet this criterion. Laws and ordinances are not passed to protect the interests of a small group (i.e., a special interest group).

State and Local Regulation

The types of legislative controls that massage therapists most often encounter are state or provincial controls and local controls. A province is a political unit of some countries, such as Canada. It typically is a large area made up of many small local units of government. In the United States, states are the equivalent of provinces. States are further subdivided into counties, local townships, and cities.

In the United States, states that have enacted licensing laws are eligible to belong to the Federation of State Massage Therapy Boards (FSMTB). Individuals are not eligible to join this organization. The mission of the federation is to support its member boards in their work to ensure that massage therapy is provided to the public in a safe, effective manner. The *Massage Therapy Body of Knowledge* explains the federation's work as follows (MTBOK stewards, 2010):

> In carrying out this mission, the federation shall:
> - Facilitate communication among member boards and provide a forum for the exchange of information and experience
> - Provide education, services, and guidance to member boards that help them fulfill their statutory, professional, public, and ethical obligations
> - Support efforts among member boards to establish compatible requirements and cooperative procedures for the legal regulation of massage therapists, in order to facilitate professional mobility and to simplify and standardize the licensing process
> - Ensure the provision of a valid reliable licensing examination to determine entry-level competence
> - Improve the standards of massage therapy education, licensure, and practice through cooperation with entities that share this objective, including other massage therapy organizations, accrediting agencies, governmental bodies, and groups whose areas of interest may coincide with those of member boards
> - Represent the interests of its member boards in matters consistent with the scope of the bylaws

The FSMTB developed an exam specifically for state licensing of massage professions, the Massage & Bodywork Licensing Examination (commonly known as the MBLEx). Launched in 2007, this exam supports states in developing legislative guidelines for massage therapists.

Many but not all health professionals are regulated at the state level through licensing. If the government feels that a particular activity could cause harm to the public, it seeks to control and limit the individuals who can participate in the activity. (For example, physicians, nurses, chiropractors, physical therapists, dentists, builders, electricians, cosmetologists, and plumbers all are licensed.) Requirements for a knowledge base and the amount and type of education are determined. Tests, often called *boards,* are given. The scope of practice is described in the law that governs the licensed professional.

If the state does not choose to license a particular profession (occupational licensing), local governments (usually townships and cities) can choose to regulate activities within their jurisdiction. Again, local laws, usually called *ordinances,* are in place to protect the public's safety and welfare. Local governments are most concerned with what types of activities go on in their region and the way the land is used (zoning).

If the state licenses a professional, the local government does not feel the need to regulate the actual practice of the professional by setting educational standards and administering competency tests. The local government does regulate where the professional may work. This is done through zoning ordinances. Professionals such as physicians, lawyers, and accountants often are required to locate their place of business in a particular zone or area of land use. Land use usually is determined on a master plan that directs the way the local government wants to see the area grow and develop. It is important to designate areas as residential (living), industrial (manufacturing), retail business districts (commercial), professional offices (office), parks (recreational), and farming (agriculture). Without such zoning, a loud industrial operation could disturb the quiet living in a residential area. Local governments are also concerned with the safety of the buildings in their areas. Monitoring the safety of buildings is the responsibility of the building inspector.

A case has been made for licensing massage therapists as a means of protecting the public, with the profession's need for formal training in sanitation, contraindications, and necessary referrals to licensed medical personnel for suspected health problems. A case also could be made for enacting massage laws to protect the massage professional from discrimination and provide the ability to practice a professional livelihood.

Therapeutic massage is not consistently regulated by law. Each state in the United States, each province in Canada, and each country in Europe has different ways of dealing with massage regulation. Because of this inconsistency, massage professionals must carefully research the governmental controls and laws that apply in the areas where they plan to open their business.

Many old laws and local massage ordinances were written to control prostitution by preventing the practice of massage. This type of ordinance is easy to recognize because it specifies medical examinations for sexually transmitted disease and other degrading requirements. Although the situation is improving, local ordinances of this type are still found in states where the profession of massage has not yet been licensed.

Currently almost all of the United States has some type of state licensing for the professional practice of therapeutic massage. The trend continues in this direction. Licensing requirements in the European and Asian countries, Canada, New Zealand, Australia, and other countries vary to such an extent that it is impossible to cover all of that information in this chapter. Overall, licensing requirements are changing quickly.

Educational requirements that allow a person to sit for a licensing examination are increasing, and the competencies reflected in the examinations are becoming more sophisticated, reflecting the evolving professionalism of therapeutic massage. Almost all licensed states require 500 to 1000 contact hours of education (15 to 30 credits) from a state-approved school. To obtain the most current information on licensing requirements, massage therapists should contact licensed massage therapy schools or governmental licensing offices in their specific area.

In states where massage professionals must be licensed, the practitioner must still comply with local zoning ordinances and building requirements when setting up a professional practice. If the state licenses massage, the local government usually treats the massage professional like any other licensed health or service professional. The business is classified as a service, and it must be set up in the proper zoning location, usually an area of office or commercial zoning.

Local governments often discourage any type of business operation in residential areas but with special restrictions will designate what types of businesses can be operated from a home. These home occupations usually are service oriented rather than retail oriented (the sale of goods) and limit traffic to and from the home. To establish a home office, the massage therapist may need to have a special and separate area in the home, including a separate entrance. Another requirement might be that no employees other than the family in the home may be hired. Sometimes only those with a special need, such as a disability that prevents working outside the home, are eligible for a home office permit. Usually a special permit is required for a home office; each local government is different. Many massage practitioners choose to work from a home office. A massage practice is a business that fits well within these special requirements.

It is true that written tests and practical demonstrations cannot measure the massage professional's gentleness, care, nonjudgmental behavior, intuition, and touch. This does not mean that formal tests are not valid; they are. Local governments need to establish that the massage business is legitimate therapeutic massage and not a front for prostitution. State governments must protect the public's health, safety, and welfare from the unregulated practice of massage. Both units of government must protect the public from potentially dangerous acts by defining performance criteria based on education or the ability to pass a test.

Licensing, compliance with ordinances, and passing any of the nationally recognized certification examinations are important in the professional practice of massage. The bottom line is, the massage professional must comply with the existing standards of practice, both required and voluntary (Box 2-19).

If a difficult state law or local ordinance is encountered, massage therapists must work together to change the regulation. The staff at a licensed massage school is the best resource on procedures for working with local governments to change a nonsupportive massage ordinance.

Box 2-19   Steps for Complying with Licensing Requirements

1. Find out whether your state or province requires licensing. Contact the Department of Licensing and Regulation, Occupational Licensing Division, for this information. If state licensing is required, find out what educational requirements must be met to take the examination.
2. If your state does not have licensing, contact the local government for the area where you intend to work to inquire about local ordinances. Obtain a copy of the ordinances and read them carefully. Look especially for the educational, zoning, and facility requirements. Whether you live in a city, township, or similar government unit, the clerk's office is the department that usually has this information.

   Note: Even if no state or local regulation exists, attending only a licensed school or an approved training program is a good idea. Other states or local governments may require this type of education, and without it you cannot practice in their areas.
3. Shop carefully for your school of massage training. Contact the state Department of Education and confirm that the school is licensed and in compliance with state regulations.
4. Before renting, buying, or setting up your massage practice, contact the local government about zoning requirements and building codes. If you are considering a home office, check the zoning ordinances to make sure you will be in compliance. Again, your city or township officials (usually the clerk) are your best sources of information.

   Zoning permits require a public hearing. Your neighbors are notified by mail, and the hearing is advertised in the newspaper. Contact the zoning department to find out what action is required. Whether you are establishing your business in a home office or a business zone, contact the neighbors to explain your business and find out their response. Without their approval, or at least lack of opposition, you are unlikely to obtain a permit. Attend the hearing at all costs. Remember: No permit = No business. Zoning permits may require 6 to 8 weeks to complete. If you start your business without proper permits, you could be shut down at any time by government authorities.
5. Before you rent space or begin your business, contact the local government and apply for any necessary permits or business licenses. Make sure you meet all regulations. Fees can run anywhere from $25 to $500.

Reciprocity

Reciprocity is the right of exchange of privileges between governing bodies. Some states have similar licensing requirements for professionals. When this is the case, a state may accept a different state's license. This is not common for many professionals, and it is even less common for massage therapists. Individual state licensing or any type of certification does not secure the right to practice massage in any location other than that of the government issuing the license.

Regulations, standards of practice, codes of conduct, scopes of practice, and so forth are methods of setting the rules for cooperative professional relationships. All organized groups have rules that permit effective interaction between members. Respect is important, and working together as a team is essential in professional practice. Let us hope that the massage therapy profession is an example of cooperation, respect for other professions, and ethical standards of practice that provide for internal professional regulation and compliance with external governmental control.

DEALING WITH SUSPECTED UNETHICAL OR ILLEGAL BEHAVIOR

SECTION OBJECTIVE

Chapter objective covered in this section:

15. The student will be able to identify and report unethical conduct by colleagues.

Using the information presented in this section, the student will be able to perform the following:

- List and explain the four steps involved in reporting unethical behavior

💡 PROFICIENCY EXERCISE 2-15

Working in groups of three, make up and then develop a specific situation in which a colleague has acted unethically. Exchange responses with a different group and role-play to resolve the situation. One student acts as the massage practitioner, one plays the colleague, and the other evaluates the way the situation was handled. Role-play different situations until each student has had a chance to play each role. Use the problem-solving model and communication and conflict management skills during the role-playing.

Addressing unethical behavior and violations of standards of practice by colleagues can present a difficult dilemma. Everything covered in this chapter is an important consideration when dealing with inappropriate behavior by others (Proficiency Exercise 2-15). When concern develops about the conduct of a colleague, an approach that combines self-reflection, peer support, mentoring, supervision, and effective communication skills is the best way to deal with these situations.

Self-Reflection

Carefully reflect on the personal motivation causing the concern. It is important that motives for confronting a fellow professional be based on a genuine concern for the therapist and the therapist's clients, in addition to the higher good of the profession as a whole. Make sure the situation is purely one of professional ethical concern and not a reaction based on personal values or moral beliefs.

Mentoring and Peer Support

Discuss the situation with your mentor or a colleague in a peer support situation while maintaining the confidentiality of the suspected party. Explore the motives supporting your concern.

Talking with Those Involved

If others share your concern, speak directly to the colleague. Often the person is not aware of the breach of standards of practice or that the behavior appears to be unethical. Peer support and bringing the concern to the person's attention may help resolve the problem.

Formal Reporting

Depending on the seriousness of the infraction and the colleague's response, you may have to file a formal complaint through the professional organization or the legal system in your area.

Ignoring unethical behavior in colleagues is unprofessional. A willingness to be involved with profession-wide ethical concerns supports professional integrity as a whole (Corey et al., 2006). Carefully document the concerns and the process of intervention. Follow all ethical principles in these types of situations.

SUMMARY

A tremendous amount of information has been covered in this chapter. Years of experience confirm that when a massage practitioner encounters difficulty in the professional setting, the problem is seldom about a technical skill and almost always about an ethical dilemma. Wise students will review this chapter time and again during their course of study and will find support in reviewing the information periodically as they mature in their professional practice after graduation.

Decision-making skills, achieved by using the problem-solving model and by developing effective communication and conflict management skills, will prove to be some of the most valuable information in this text. Both decision making and communication are skills to be learned, and massage professionals must practice these skills to gain proficiency. And as with any skill, when you first begin to use them, you will feel awkward and uncomfortable. That's okay. You probably will have the same feeling as you practice all the new skills in this text, such as body mechanics, draping procedures, and all the massage manipulations and techniques. Practice is essential to perfect the skills required of a massage professional.

◧ FOOT IN THE DOOR

When you graduate from massage therapy education, you will be competing with others for clients, a job, and status. What will set you apart from the rest and make the future clients, employers, and others who could influence your career skills notice you? Of course your massage skills need to be excellent. However, your people skills are just as important. It is necessary to perform in an ethical and responsible manner as a massage professional. When you can communicate effectively, make responsible decisions about client care and relationships with peers and other professionals, use critical thinking skills, and conduct yourself as a professional, you will have the advantage over those who do not realize the importance of professionalism. Not only will you get your foot in the door, you will move to the head of the line.

⊝volve

http://evolve.elsevier.com/Fritz/fundamentals/
2-1 Use the electronic flashcards for this chapter to review vocabulary
2-2 Answer true or false questions on evidence-based practice
2-3 Complete a matching exercise on ethical behavior
2-4 Review HIPAA Guidelines with multiple choice questions
2-5 Play Hangman and build your vocabulary
2-6 Think it over: answer questions on professionalism
  Don't forget to study for your certification and licensure exams! Review questions, along with weblinks, can be found on the Evolve website.

References

Corey G, Corey MS, Callanan P: *Issues and ethics in the helping professions*, ed 7, Pacific Grove, Calif, 2006, Wadsworth Publishing.

Massage Therapy Body of Knowledge (MTBOK) stewards: *Massage therapy body of knowledge (MTBOK)*, version 1, May 15, 2010. www.mtbok.org. Accessed March 21, 2011.

National Center for Education Statistics: career and technical education, 1990-2005 statistical analysis report, http://nces.ed.gov/pubs2008/2008035.pdf. Accessed October 30, 2011.

Privacy Rights Clearinghouse Fact Sheet 8a: HIPAA Basics: Medical Privacy in the Electronic Age Copyright © 2003-2011 Accessed August 4, 2011.

Regulated Health Professions Act and the Massage Therapy Act, Ontario, Canada, 1992. www.cmto.com/regulations/mta.htm. Accessed July 10, 2011.

Sackett DL, Straus SE, Richardson WS, et al: *Evidence-based medicine: how to practice and teach EBM*, ed 2, New York, 2000, Churchill Livingstone.

Webster's third new international unabridged dictionary deluxe, ed 3, Springfield, Mass, 2002, Merriam-Webster.

Evolve Activity 2-6

Workbook Section

Short Answer

1. Define ethics.

2. Why is it important for a massage therapist to develop an evidence-based practice?

3. Why is it difficult to arrive at a definition for therapeutic massage?

4. Why does the massage professional need to understand the scope of practice for other professionals?

5. In what ways do massage practitioners avoid falling into a situation that could allow them to be accused of practicing medicine?

6. Why is it unethical to provide massage services to a client the practitioner does not like or with whom the practitioner is uncomfortable?

7. What is the importance of disclosure in the right of refusal?

8. Why is informed consent so important?

9. What are the implications of HIPAA and confidentiality?

10. In what way does the word *respect* relate to boundaries?

11. Determining the acts that constitute sexual misconduct is easy; however, how do you decide whether more subtle activities and feelings are a breach of the trust between client and practitioner?

12. Why might a client interpret the experience of massage as a sexual one?

13. Why is it ethical to establish rules of conduct for the client and massage therapist and to maintain professional space in the client-practitioner relationship?

14. What are the important aspects of credentialing for the massage practitioner?

15. Why does the massage professional need to understand legislative issues, local ordinances, and zoning regulations?

16. What is the main purpose of a law?

17. What are the two types of massage therapy practice?

18. What effect might the *Massage Therapy Body of Knowledge* have on the professional practice of massage?

Matching

Match the term with the best definition.

_____ 1. Applied kinesiology
_____ 2. Bodywork
_____ 3. Boundary
_____ 4. Certification
_____ 5. Coalition
_____ 6. Craniosacral and myofascial
_____ 7. Credential
_____ 8. Disclosure
_____ 9. Energetic approaches
_____ 10. Essential touch

_____ 11. Ethics

_____ 12. Exemption

_____ 13. Informed consent

_____ 14. Integrated approaches

_____ 15. Intimacy

_____ 16. License

_____ 17. Manual lymph drainage

_____ 18. Medical rehabilitative massage

_____ 19. Neuromuscular approaches

_____ 20. Asian approaches

_____ 21. Right of refusal

_____ 22. Safe touch

_____ 23. Sexual misconduct

_____ 24. Scope of practice

_____ 25. Structural and postural integration approaches

_____ 26. Therapeutic massage

_____ 27. Wellness personal service massage

_____ 28. Conflict resolution

a. A term describing all the various forms of massage, movement, and touch therapy

b. Methods of bodywork that focus on subtle body responses

c. Vital, fundamental, primary touch that is crucial to well-being

d. A voluntary credentialing process that usually requires education and training, in addition to testing administered privately or by governmental regulatory bodies

e. A tender, familiar, and understanding experience between human beings

f. A designation earned by completing a process that verifies a certain level of expertise in a given skill

g. Standards, ideals, morals, values, and principles of honorable, decent, fair, responsible, and proper conduct

h. Methods of massage that influence the movement of lymph

i. Methods of massage that evolved from the ancient Chinese systems

j. Methods of massage that influence the reflexive responses of the nervous system and its link to muscular function

k. Any sexually oriented behavior that occurs in the professional setting

l. The where, when, and how a professional may provide a service or function as a professional

m. Methods of massage derived from biomechanics, postural alignment, and the importance of the connective tissue structures

n. Personal space located within an arm's length perimeter; personal emotional space designated by morals, values, and experience

o. Combined methods of various forms of massage

p. A case in which a professional is not required to comply with an existing law because of educational or professional standing

q. Acknowledging any situation that interferes with or affects the professional relationship and informing the client of that situation

r. A scientific art and discipline involving assessment and the systematic, external application of touch to the superficial soft tissue of the skin, muscles, tendons, ligaments, and fascia and to the structures that lie in the superficial tissue; methods of touch include stroking (effleurage), friction, vibration, percussion, kneading (pétrissage), stretching, compression, passive and active joint movements within the normal physiologic range of motion, and adjunctive applications of water, heat, and cold

s. Methods of evaluation and adaptation that use an application of muscle testing, along with various forms of massage, for corrective procedures

t. Secure, respectful, considerate, sensitive, responsive, sympathetic, supportive, and empathetic contact

u. The level of professional responsibility, based on extensive education, at which the massage therapist is able to develop, maintain, rehabilitate, or augment physical function; to relieve or prevent physical dysfunction and pain; and to enhance the client's well-being; methods include assessment of the soft tissue and joints and treatment by soft tissue manipulation, hydrotherapy, remedial exercise programs, actinotherapy (light therapy), and client self-care programs

v. A type of credential required by law as a means of regulating the practice of a profession to protect the health, safety, and welfare of the public

w. Client authorization for any service from a professional, based on the premise that the massage professional has provided adequate information to enable the client to make an educated choice

x. A nonspecific approach to massage that focuses on assessment for the purposes of detecting contraindications to massage or a need for referral to other health care professionals and also for developing a health-enhancing physical state for the client

y. A group formed for a particular purpose

z. Methods of therapeutic massage that work both reflexively and mechanically with the fascial network

aa. The right of both the client and the professional to stop a session

bb. The use of mediation, negotiation, and communication skills

Standards of Practice

Put an X on the line by the situations that indicate a person who is unable to provide informed consent.

_____ a. An elderly client living alone

_____ b. A 50-year-old man taking medication for high blood pressure

_____ c. A freshman high school student

_____ d. A 30-year-old woman, the victim of a closed head injury, who communicates with a computer

_____ e. A 24-year-old developmentally disabled client

_____ f. A client who does not speak English, and no interpreter is present

_____ **g.** A client who seems to be under the influence of alcohol

_____ **h.** A 21-year-old woman in the third trimester of pregnancy

_____ **i.** A severely depressed client

_____ **j.** An elderly client with dementia

_____ **k.** A client who insists that you cure her sore knee

_____ **l.** A terminally ill hospice client

Determining Licensing Needs

List five steps in determining licensing needs.

1.

2.

3.

4.

5.

Assess Your Competencies

Now that you have studied this chapter, you should be able to:

- Define professionalism
- Define therapeutic massage
- Define a scope of practice for therapeutic massage
- Define evidence-based practice
- Develop and explain a code of ethics and the standards of practice for therapeutic massage
- Complete an informed consent process
- Practice procedures to maintain client confidentiality
- Become familiar with the Health Insurance Portability and Accountability Act (HIPAA) and its requirements and training
- Integrate ethics into maintaining professional boundaries and the therapeutic relationship
- Use a problem-solving approach to ethical decision making
- Use basic communication skills to listen effectively and deliver an I-message
- Identify and resolve conflict in the professional setting
- Identify legal and credentialing concerns of the massage professional
- Identify and report unethical conduct of colleagues

On a separate sheet of paper or on the computer, write a short summary of the content of this chapter based on the preceding list of competencies. Use a conversational tone, as if you were explaining to someone (e.g., a client, prospective employer, coworker, or other interested person) the importance of the information and skills to the development of the massage profession.

Next, in small discussion groups, share your summary with your classmates and compare the ways the information was presented. In discussing the content, look for similarities, differences, possibilities for misunderstanding of the information, and clear, concise methods of description.

Problem-Solving Scenarios

1. A new client tells you about the treatment he received during a massage in another community. Some of the information seems to conflict with the principles of the code of ethics presented in this text. The client tells you that the massage professional told him he needed to lose weight; she did not stop working on his feet when he asked her to do so; she did not explain that a trigger point area could be sore the next day; she gave him a hug at the end of the session without first asking permission; she told a joke that had some sexual innuendo; she let the drape slip while massaging his buttocks; she talked about difficulties with her children; she walked in to get a chart without knocking first while he was dressing after the session; she said that physical therapists were bad at dealing with neck pain and that she could fix his neck problem; and she did not give him a receipt when he paid for the massage.

   Which of the 28 standards of practice presented in Box 2-5 did the massage professional breach? Give the client examples of how you would practice differently.

   The following cases are situations in which intimacy issues must be explained. After reading each case, write three ways to deal with the issue. Use the clinical reasoning model to develop your answers.

2. Kathy has been a massage professional for 3 years. She has been seeing Mr. Adams for a monthly massage for 2 years. He is in the process of a divorce and begins to schedule a massage every week because of the stress. Last week he mentioned to Kathy how important the massage is for him and lightly touched her hand. Should Kathy be concerned?

3. Matt has been a massage therapist for 10 years. Recently he has been seeing a client, Jeff, who attended the same high school as Matt. Although they were only acquaintances during high school, Jeff speaks often of the good old school days. At the last appointment Jeff offered Matt an extra hockey ticket and asked if he would like to go to the game with him. How should Matt respond?

4. Mary is new to the massage therapy profession and has had only a few clients. She finds a new client very attractive and notices that she is spending extra time with that client each session. She recognizes that she is attracted to the client physically and emotionally. How should she handle the situation?

Business Considerations for a Career in Therapeutic Massage

http://evolve.elsevier.com/Fritz/fundamentals/

CHAPTER OBJECTIVES

After completing this chapter, the student will be able to perform the following:

1. Determine his or her personal motivation for pursuing a career in therapeutic massage
2. Develop an effective résumé
3. Interview effectively
4. List the pros and cons of independent and employee status
5. Explain client retention
6. Describe the process for setting fees, determining income, and doing insurance billing
7. Develop career plans
8. Identify the requirements and options for starting a business
9. Design a marketing strategy and advertising materials for a massage business
10. Develop a business management and record-keeping system
11. Develop skills to achieve employee success

CHAPTER OUTLINE

KEY TERMS

Burnout	Marketing
Career	Motivation
Employee	Self-employed
Job	Start-up costs

Success depends on the following elements:

- Intention—Goals
- Intuition—Following inner guidance
- Inspiration—Ideas that manifest the dream

These three elements provide the foundation for success.

Consider the difference between a career and a job. A **career** is commonly defined as a chosen pursuit, a life's work. A **job** is a regular activity performed for payment. Therapeutic massage can be either a job or a career. Which do you want? The answer to that question determines in large part how you proceed with your professional development. This text in general, and this chapter in particular, views therapeutic massage as a career. A career can evolve whether you are self-employed or you work for someone else. If you choose to work for someone else, your employer will take care of most of the nuts and bolts of developing and managing a business. You, as an **employee**, can concentrate on being an excellent massage therapist and supporting the business by being an excellent employee. If you choose to be **self-employed**, you must be an excellent massage therapist and also able to manage all business-related responsibilities, but you have ultimate control over how your business is managed.

Box 3-1	Business Experience

To substantiate the validity of the business information in this chapter, a brief business profile of the author is presented:

- Certificate in bookkeeping
- 30+ years as a massage practitioner
- 12 years in full-time private practice (30 to 40 clients a week)
- 18 years in part-time practice (10 to 20 clients a week)
- Professional practice locations: health club, on site (private homes, small businesses, and corporations), chiropractor's office, full-service day spa, private country club, home office, various sports, National Football League (NFL) team, amateur athletes, and professional athletes
- 6 years of professional practice with a psychologist in private practice
- Owner of a massage therapy school (director and instructor for 25 years)
- Employer of 39 associates
- Owner and manager of three commercial properties for 15 years
- Master's degree in Organizational Management and Leadership

Business-wise, for this author, "Been there, done that" fits, and the experience gained over many years has resulted in a realistic perspective on careers in therapeutic massage.

This chapter presents specific information for individuals who want to develop a massage business, but it does not attempt to be a course in small business management. The information presented here is unique to therapeutic massage. It is sufficient to guide the student toward additional learning opportunities and to generate classroom discussion (Box 3-1). The chapter takes the position that the nuts and bolts of business are no different for massage than for any other professional service business. Detailed information on topics such as marketing methods, financial record keeping, and tax requirements can be found in business textbooks and on the Internet. Resources on the business aspects of massage therapy also are available, and professional organizations often provide business information. Specifically, the textbook *Business and Professional Skills for Massage Therapists*, by the author of this text, can be helpful.

MOTIVATION

SECTION OBJECTIVES

Chapter objective covered in this section:

1. The student will be able to determine his or her personal motivation for pursuing a career in therapeutic massage.

Using the information presented in this section, the student will be able to perform the following:

- Understand the importance of motivation in successfully developing a career
- Explore personal strengths and weaknesses that would aid or impede the development of a successful career
- Develop a personal application of methods to prevent burnout

To succeed at anything, a person must be motivated. **Motivation** is an internal drive that provides the energy to do what is needed to accomplish a goal. Without the motivation to stick to the commitment, people give up during difficult times. This is especially true of small businesses with single owners, a category that includes most solely owned massage businesses.

Motivation begins with knowing what you want. Plans must be developed, but the massage professional must be willing to change them if a strategy is not working. If success is the goal, quitting cannot be an option. The following are some important points.

- *Know thyself.* No one should persist with something that goes against his or her core values, no matter how successful the process may be for someone else.
- *Follow your dream.* Success flows from desire and motivation. Desire and motivation are the driving forces for the dreams that come from deep within us to bring us joy and healing. Hard times and hard work are part of the process of building a new career. If we follow our dreams and live our purpose, the hard work provides a rewarding, intrinsic sense of satisfaction.
- *Accept that experience is the best teacher.* We learn from our mistakes as well as from our successes. Implementing plans is the only way to find out whether they work. It may become obvious over time that another approach is more advantageous, but being afraid to make mistakes will limit you as a professional.
- *Ask "What's in it for me?"* To succeed in any endeavor, we need to recognize the benefits to be gained from the process. This is an important consideration in any decision. It is not a selfish attitude; rather, it is a smart approach. People will not put energy into something that does not give them satisfaction. This concept also applies to money. Business is business, and earning money is part of any successful business operation. However, money itself is a poor source of motivation. Motivation is a deeper-felt sense that comes from the heart and soul.
- *Recognize that self-concept matters.* People have ideas about who they should be, and these often conflict with what we have been told and believe that we are. Self-esteem is very important for career success. Trying to live up to others' expectations is a bad practice. A successful career is built on who we are, not on what others want us to be. Develop your ability to use all aspects of yourself to the best advantage.
- *Believe in your product.* Understand and be able to explain the benefits of therapeutic massage. It is most acceptable to explain the benefits of massage in terms of physiologic responses that all people share. Explanations of this type are easy for most people to understand.
- *Provide a quality product.* The massage practitioner must be skilled. Clients pay for the benefits they experience from massage. Client retention is based on your ability to continue to produce those benefits. To be truly successful the practitioner must put the person, not his or her condition, first. People seek caring, nurturing, and nonjudgmental touch as much as technical skill (Figure 3-1).

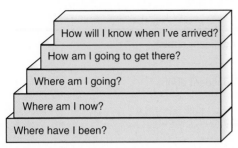

FIGURE 3-1 Job preparation. Questions to ask yourself when preparing for a job search.
(From Finkbeiner BL, Finkbeiner CA: *Practice management for the dental team,* ed 6, St Louis, 2006, Mosby.)

Seeking Help

The practitioner brings more than his or her massage skills to a career in therapeutic massage. Each professional also brings personal strengths and weaknesses, successes and failures, and experiences and learning. Using all our strengths is important. Recognizing the areas in which we are not as strong is even more important, because these limitations can influence our business activities adversely.

Business owners are wise to hire help for areas in which they may be weak. They need a diverse group of people to serve as consultants, such as a lawyer, an accountant, a skilled bookkeeper, an advertising and marketing consultant, and an adviser for business planning. Consulting these resource people need not be expensive. The local Chamber of Commerce and the Small Business Administration (SBA) offer free services. The SBA supports an organization of retired business people known as the Service Corps of Retired Executives (SCORE). The members of this organization want to help others succeed. It is essential that the massage professional talk to many people and listen to their experiences, both those who were successful and those who grappled with the consequences of their mistakes. This core information, along with the fundamentals of therapeutic massage, lays the foundation for a successful practice.

Although experts, authorities, and mentors are helpful, no single individual has all the answers or knows the whole truth. Each of us must find his or her own answers. Truth is personal, empowering, and freeing. Many motivational audio programs, books, and speakers are available that can be used for inspiration. The overlapping themes, which can be found in most of these sources, are the kernels of truth:

- Whatever we believe—with emotion and feeling—becomes our reality.
- What we do with confidence can become our self-fulfilling prophecy.
- We attract into our lives that which harmonizes with our dominant thoughts.

Burnout

When a person is burned out, motivation is lost. **Burnout** occurs when you use up your energy faster than you can replenish it. For massage therapists, this is characterized by taking better care of others than we do of ourselves. Burnout

can be a problem in most service professions. Taking care of others is a big job. If we do not take care of ourselves also, we soon have nothing to give others or ourselves. Each of us must take care of our physical needs, such as resting, eating well, getting regular massages, and paying attention to our emotional needs. Surround yourself with people who believe in you. Take care of your spiritual needs, which connect the value of what you want to accomplish with a much higher purpose. Follow the wellness guidelines presented in Chapter 15.

The actual practice of massage is simple, repetitious touch, which sometimes can get boring. It is important to keep yourself excited about the benefits of such simple applications of touch. One of the best ways to do this is to continue your education. Classes make you think and bring you together with other massage professionals. These are good opportunities to share and learn together. State-licensed massage schools and professional organizations are the best sources for massage education. Efficient body mechanics is essential to prevent physical burnout (see Chapter 8).

It also is important to get away from massage for a bit. The massage professional occasionally should take classes or vacations that have nothing to do with massage or muscles. If you commit to saving your earnings from one massage a week, you will have $500 to $1000 a year to spend on continuing education and vacations. You deserve it. Take care of yourself, and let others take care of you. Take a vacation, and burnout will be less of a problem.

After a person begins to live life—including his or her career life—with purpose, the energy to develop the career focus becomes available. Living with purpose is the key to motivation. It means drawing strength from knowing that what we have to offer is valuable. When the massage practitioner truly believes this, he or she can begin developing a business structure or seek rewarding employment (Proficiency Exercise 3-1).

THE RÉSUMÉ

SECTION OBJECTIVES

Chapter objective covered in this section:
2. The student will be able to develop an effective résumé.
Using the information presented in this section, the student will be able to perform the following:
- Describe a résumé
- Write a résumé and cover letter

A *résumé* is a compilation of professional and personal data about a person. Before we can develop a business plan and set goals or apply for employment in massage, it is important to find out who we are. A good résumé becomes part of the promotional materials we use when self-employed and is necessary to apply for a job in the massage field. The résumé should list not only massage experience but also other work experience. We are the sum total of all our experiences, and we bring that knowledge base into all work and business situations.

Many professional resources are available to help you develop your résumé. Contact the local Chamber of

💡 PROFICIENCY EXERCISE 3-1

On a separate piece of paper, explore your beliefs to find motivation for developing your career in therapeutic massage.

1. Answer the following questions:
What do I believe …

about therapeutic massage as a professional service

about my abilities as a massage professional

about myself as a person

about my future clients

2. Complete the following statement five times:
I feel confident about

I feel confident about

I feel confident about

I feel confident about

I feel confident about

3. Complete the following statement five times:
A dominant thought that influences my life is

A dominant thought that influences my life is

A dominant thought that influences my life is

A dominant thought that influences my life is

A dominant thought that influences my life is

Commerce or a nearby library branch to locate such assistance. Internet sites also can help with résumé development.

A résumé should list information about present and past employment in the following order:

1. Dates of employment
2. Companies
3. Titles held
4. Job functions

It also should list when and where you received your education. The résumé should include highlights of the scope and depth of your experience and your responsibilities at each position. It describes the knowledge you have gained and developed throughout your career that relates to the position for which you are applying; this information, in turn, prompts the interviewer to ask questions.

Cover Letters

A cover letter for your résumé is like an introduction to the hiring company. It tells them who you are, the position for which you are applying, how you found out about the position, and a brief explanation of why you should be called for an interview. In writing the cover letter, use action verbs that are descriptive and concrete, that really sell your experience, skills, and abilities. The cover letter should be one half to three fourths of a page long and should be printed on plain, white or ivory, professional-grade paper (Figure 3-2).

Developing a Résumé

The main heading of the résumé highlights your name and provides the contact information (Figure 3-3). Your name could be shown in a different, larger, or bold font that will

💡 PROFICIENCY EXERCISE 3-2

1. Draft your résumé (a sample is shown in Figure 3-3). Many computer word processing programs offer a résumé template with style options.
2. Contact your local community college, library, or public service organization and attend a class in résumé writing.

make the name on the résumé stand out. Use the same name on your references page, cover letters, and thank you letters. By creating a professional-looking letterhead, you offer a consistent image to the hiring manager (Proficiency Exercise 3-2).

Section headings are assigned to different areas of the résumé (e.g., experience, education, extracurricular activities). The résumé should be printed on the same paper as your cover letter. Microsoft provides templates for résumés, cover letters, and professional documents in some word processing programs.

A résumé can be written in many different ways. Most begin by summarizing the applicant's qualifications that pertain to the position. This section should be put at the beginning of the résumé, right under the space left after the name and contact information. The summary of your qualifications should be confined to three high-impact statements that quantify your accomplishments:

- The first statement should highlight your years of experience in the profession and industry.
- The second statement should identify the areas of expertise you want to emphasize.
- The third statement should identify personal attributes that are important to the role and the company.

Luke Fritz, MT, NCTMB
2050 Leisure Lane, Lapeer, MI 48446
(123) 456-7890 / leisurelymassage@hec.com

October 20, 20xx

Jana Larke
222 Relaxation Drive
Your Town, State 00000

Dear Ms Larke:

I am writing this letter in response to your need for an entry-level massage therapist. Given my excellent capabilities and training, I am confident you will find me an ideal candidate for this position. I would greatly appreciate your consideration. My resume is enclosed for your review.

I am trustworthy, competent, well-trained, and personable, and will dedicate myself to providing your clients with a quality massage experience. I also have advanced skills obtained from my clinical training. A graduate of the Health Enrichment School, I am currently working as a massage therapist at Sherri's Hair Salon in Lapeer. With my clinical education and relevant experience, I believe you will be very pleased with my performance.

I appreciate your time in reviewing my credentials and thank you in advance for your consideration. I look forward to speaking to you and setting up a time for an interview and demonstration of my skills. Please feel free to contact me anytime at (123) 456-7890.

Sincerely,

Luke Fritz, MT, NCTMB

FIGURE 3-2 Sample cover letter.
(From Fritz S: *Business and professional skills for massage therapists,* St Louis, 2010, Mosby.)

THE INTERVIEW

SECTION OBJECTIVES

Chapter objective covered in this section:
3. The student will be able to interview effectively.
Using the information presented in this section, the student will be able to perform the following:
- Describe an interview
- Dress appropriately for an interview
- Respond confidently to an interviewer's questions
- Follow-up appropriately after an interview

The interview allows the employer to get to know the person applying for the position. It also allows the applicant to ask questions about the company and the available position, building on the information he or she accumulated to prepare for the interview. Through the interview process, the employer develops a good sense of the applicant's communication skills, which are demonstrated when the applicant answers questions, provides feedback on possible situations, and asks questions about the position and company.

Preparing for the Interview

Communication

Some think that effective communication is one of the most important skills an employee can have. To communicate effectively during the job interview, you can research the company, the setting, and the position for which you are applying. This is a very good way to prepare for the interview.

A lack of conversation by the applicant could lead the interviewer to think that the applicant has a lack of interest. Also, the applicant should write down the interviewer's answers to questions about the position and the company for future reference; this is another way of showing the employer that the applicant truly wants the position.

Dressing for Success

The applicant's attire and shoes should be neat and clean. Conservative business dress is appropriate for the job, even if a uniform is usually worn. The applicant should bring a uniform and massage supplies to the interview in case the interviewer wants a demonstration massage.

For both men and women, attention to the details of one's appearance is crucial to the success of an interview. The following tips can help you present a professional appearance:
- Wear clean, polished, conservative dress shoes.
- Wear a well-groomed hairstyle.
- Make sure your fingernails are clean and trimmed.
- Wear no or minimal cologne or perfume.
- Make sure no body piercings or tattoos are visible other than conservative ear piercings.
- Make sure you have well-brushed teeth and fresh breath.

Quality Service
Customer Satisfaction
Welcoming and Friendly
☆☆☆☆☆

Luke Fritz, MT, NCTMB
2050 Leisure Lane, Lapeer, MI 48446
(123) 456-7890 / leisurelymassage@hec.com

Objective: To obtain a massage therapy position for an active massage practice that will enable me to use my skills and learn from others within the massage environment, while providing excellent client care.

Professional Experience:

Sherri's Hair Salon, Lapeer, MI   Massage Therapist   June 2007 – Present

Perform chair massages on a diverse population focusing on neck and shoulder techniques. Conduct open therapeutic massages to promote and generate new business. Review calendars and schedule appointments for massage therapists and hair stylists according to availability.

Provide massage services to clients using safe, appropriate, and effective massage techniques. Perform client health history and update before each session; ascertain precautions/contraindications for massage before each session. Explain procedures and applied techniques appropriate to client needs and preferences. Observe client reaction to massage and modify as necessary. Solicit feedback and respond accordingly. Document all sessions performed according to established guidelines.

Other responsibilities include maintaining client confidentiality; maintaining sensitivity to age- and gender-related issues during all client interactions; reporting any unusual client interactions to supervisor immediately; scheduling and maintaining of appointments; assisting in collection of fees; consulting with appropriate treatment staff regarding treatment plans when necessary.

Detroit Marathon, Detroit, MI   Massage Therapist   October 2007 and 2008

Perform chair massages on a diverse population focusing on neck and shoulder techniques. Provided warm-up and cool-down massage for athletes competing in the Detroit Marathon. Assessed the needs of each athlete individually and selected the appropriate treatment. Invited to be the "Official Massage Coordinator" for future Detroit Marathon events.

Health Enrichment Center, Lapeer, MI   Student Massage Therapist   August 2006-June 2007

Performed chair massages, focusing on neck and shoulder techniques.

Education: Health Enrichment Center, Massage Therapy Diploma, 720 Credit Hours, June 2007

Certification: National Certification Board for Therapeutic Massage and Bodywork

FIGURE 3-3 Sample résumé.
(From Fritz S: *Business and professional skills for massage therapists,* St Louis, 2010, Mosby.)

💡 PROFICIENCY EXERCISE 3-3

Develop a set of questions you might use to interview a massage therapist. Pair up with a fellow student and take turns practicing being the interviewer and the interviewee.

- Do not have gum, candy, or other objects in your mouth.
- Wear minimal jewelry.
- Make sure you do not have any body odor.
- If you will be performing a massage as part of the interview, bring an appropriate uniform to the interview and change before giving the massage.

Interview Questions

When the interviewer asks questions, make eye contact when you answer and be confident (Proficiency Exercise 3-3). The following are just a few questions that could be asked, for which you need to prepare answers in advance:

- What do you consider your greatest strengths and weaknesses?
- Describe a time when you were faced with problems or stresses at work that tested your coping skills. What did you do?
- How do you deal with competition? Are you a competitive person?
- What would you consider an ideal work environment?
- What are your long-range career objectives, and what steps have you taken toward realizing them?
- How well do you work with people? Do you prefer working alone or as part of a team?
- What do you think are the qualities of an effective leader?
- What do you do when people disagree with you. How do you manage conflict?

Closing the Interview

You should have an idea of what you will say when leaving the interview. Make sure you state the skills you have that would make this job a definite fit for you and the reasons your strengths make you right for the position. You may want to ask the interviewer if you could send some references or set up an appointment to give the person a massage. Respectfully asking when the decision will be made reinforces your desire for the position, and verifying how you should contact the employer to follow up (phone or e-mail) shows that you are considerate and polite. Finally, shake hands with the interviewer as you make a parting comment, such as, "Thank you very much for taking the time to speak with me about the [massage] position. I look forward to speaking with you again soon." After the interview, send a thank you note for the interview opportunity and again express your interest in the position. A handwritten note is the most professional way to thank the employer, but if time is an issue (e.g., the decision will be made quickly), an e-mail may be more appropriate.

SELF-EMPLOYMENT OR EMPLOYMENT BY OTHERS

SECTION OBJECTIVES

Chapter objective covered in this section:

4. The student will be able to list the pros and cons of independent and employee status.

Using the information presented in this section, the student will be able to perform the following:

- Determine the skills necessary for self-employment
- Apply the concepts of true earnings and real time
- Develop your personal list of pros and cons for self-employment and employee status

This chapter does what generic business texts cannot do; it shares the experience gained from walking the career path in therapeutic massage, both as an employee and as a self-employed professional. Throughout the text, you are encouraged to ask questions about your massage education, to use clinical reasoning as a problem-solving method, and to challenge information. You are urged to seek authoritative sources carefully and to compare information from many different experts. The same principles apply in the business world.

Successful self-employment requires an entrepreneurial spirit. An *entrepreneur* is a person who organizes, operates, and assumes the risk of a business venture. Not everyone is cut out for self-employment. The hours are long, and 100% commitment is required. Self-employed people must be self-starters with a broad range of professional and business skills. Some people think that self-employed individuals get to be their own boss—not so; instead of one or two bosses, every client becomes the boss.

Besides an entrepreneurial spirit, self-employment requires a deep internal commitment. During the latter part of this century, therapeutic massage has been provided primarily by self-employed massage professionals. The entrepreneurial spirit runs high in the massage/bodywork profession, but times are changing. The profession has seen a steady increase in jobs and career opportunities in the more traditional employee market, in which the massage practitioner goes to work for an individual or a company at an hourly wage or salary. More employment opportunities are opening up for

massage professionals in the personal service industry and the medical establishment. The most rapid expansion of employment opportunities is occurring in the spa setting and in the health care system. Massage professionals are working for physicians, physical therapists, mental health professionals, and other health care professionals.

The service industry is growing as well. Destination spas, which provide for extended visits, and day spas, which are places in the local area where people can "get away" for a day of pampering and massage, are very popular. The spa industry is a major source of employment for massage professionals. Full-service cosmetology businesses also offer employment opportunities.

The fitness industry is another source of employment. Many health clubs offer the services of a massage professional. The recreation industry (e.g., hotels, cruise ships, retreats, resort centers) also is an active employer of massage practitioners.

The independent massage therapy clinic offers opportunities for employment when the owner or manager of the clinic handles all business responsibilities and hires massage practitioners to do the work. Franchises and business chains are spreading quickly and also offer employment options.

You can be either self-employed or an employee, and you can either have a career or hold a job in massage. Do not think that you must be self-employed to have a career. Each of these two options has its advantages and disadvantages, and only you can decide what is an advantage and what is a disadvantage for you. For example, one person may feel that the independent decision making involved in self-employment is an advantage, whereas a person who has difficulty coming up with independent ideas would consider this a disadvantage. The key is "know thyself." If you have the commitment, drive, skill, and discipline necessary for self-employment and are willing to make the 100% commitment (and more) that it takes to build and maintain a massage therapy practice, self-employment may be the best option for you.

In determining whether self-employment is their best choice, professionals should ask themselves the following questions:

- How disciplined am I?
- Do I wait until the last minute to do a job?
- Am I on time or do I usually run late?
- Do I keep myself organized?

The very skills that make a wonderful massage therapist—intuition, sensitivity, an ability to respond to the moment—can be a source of difficulty in meeting the business requirements of planning ahead, keeping bills paid on time, carefully planning business strategy, and staying in one place long enough to carry out the business plan. If you do not have either the self-discipline or the skills necessary for self-employment, employee status may be the better choice.

Sometimes excellent massage professionals are inherently poor at business management. The intuition, spontaneous feelings, and people orientation of those entering the profession do not necessarily work in harmony with the logical, structured nature of business. Some individuals who want to develop a career in massage may find the concepts of

| Box 3-2 | Building a Business: Applying the Pregnancy and Child-Rearing Metaphor |

You might think of your education in therapeutic massage in terms of a pregnancy. It takes time (your schooling) for the baby to grow until it has developed enough to survive in an unprotected environment. This is a natural process, but it is not without its struggles and hard work. Graduation from school marks the birth of the student's professional career. Everyone is excited about the baby, but soon the parent (the new massage practitioner) realizes that for about 2 years, this new little life will require constant care, hard work, attention to detail, and very long, focused hours. A 2-year-old child seeks independence, but constant supervision is necessary until the child is about 5 years old. By age 5 the child has learned many lessons and can begin some self-care as the parent supervises from a little farther away. Each year after that, the child becomes more independent, although attention from the parent is still necessary.

Very nearly the same process unfolds with a new business.

A professional should plan to give a new business 2 years of constant attention to enable it to develop strong roots from which to grow. It will take about 5 years before attention to the business can be eased and small portions of it entrusted to another supervising person for short periods. Even then, careful attention and participation are required if a business is to remain successful. Building a business is hard work that in time reaps rewards.

developing and enforcing policy statements and determining fee structures difficult (Box 3-2). Many people have difficulty with the discipline and organization required to manage a small business. It is difficult to watch excellent massage professionals fail in their effort to serve the public because they did not recognize that they would do far better in an employee situation. It is equally disturbing to see those with the entrepreneurial spirit constrained in the structure of someone else's business dream.

True Earnings and Real Time

To earn $25,000 of net income, a self-employed massage therapist must generate about $50,000 of gross income. Based on 50 weeks of work per year and 20 massage clients per week at $50 per client, the gross receipts are $50,000 per year. Of this, 50% will be spent on overhead costs, including rent, advertising, linens, supplies, phone, mailings, and postage. The self-employed massage therapist also must consider *real time,* which is the amount of time actually put into the business. At a minimum, *for every hour spent giving a massage, at least 1 hour will be spent on business work,* such as records, clean up, advertising, and marketing. Remember, self-employed people never really leave their business. When all factors are considered, the earnings end up being about the same whether the practitioner is an hourly wage employee or the owner of his or her business.

This information is designed to provide support to those who know they would be better served by working for someone

who handles the business responsibilities. This reality check also clarifies the path of self-employment, so that if you choose this career option, you can stay grounded in realism without losing your dream.

Advantages and Disadvantages of Self-Employment

The advantages of self-employment should be considered. For example, the business income could be increased by subletting the office space (make sure any rental agreement allows for this). Likewise, after the first few years, advertising and marketing expenses decline, because you have established a repeat business with clients who return regularly for massage, and net income increases. Some feel that self-employment offers more freedom to self-direct the business structure, in addition to flexibility in scheduling work hours and long-term financial security.

Disadvantages include numerous responsibilities both for business concerns and for client services, isolation, lack of peer support and supervision if working alone, and inability to leave the business for any length of time. Income can vary, and no group benefits are available, such as insurance packages or paid vacations. Membership in professional associations can offset the benefits issue because group insurance programs are available through them.

Advantages and Disadvantages of Employment by Others

Employees who have established long-term relationships with their employers often get pay increases. For example, over a 5-year period, the massage practitioner could start at the low end ($9 per hour) and work up to $20 per hour. When choosing a career option, consider that as a therapeutic massage employee, you are not responsible for any of the business concerns and can focus most of your professional energy on client services. Employee status usually involves working with other professionals in some way, creating an environment of support and mentoring. Some businesses may offer benefits and paid vacations. Income usually is stable.

The disadvantages of being an employee might include adherence to business rules and regulations, less flexibility in work scheduling, and having to share a work space. Currently, more employment options are available, and this likely will become the dominant career status, especially in the spa and health care settings.

Many massage professionals underestimate the value of their service, whereas others overestimate themselves. When you are thinking about money and how much to charge for a service or what your wage or salary should be, it is important to realize that people usually live according to an equal exchange for services rendered or for goods received; this is called the *equity hypothesis.* It is important to charge what a massage is worth in time value. If the fee is too high, the professional does not support those stable weekly and biweekly clients who are the mainstays of a massage practitioner's client retention. However, if fees or wages are too low, the career will not generate enough income to support the practitioner.

CLIENT RETENTION

SECTION OBJECTIVES

Chapter objective covered in this section:
5. The student will be able to explain client retention.
Using the information presented in this section, the student will be able to perform the following:
- Define client retention
- Explain the relationship of client retention to career success
- Explain the importance of regular massage to clients
- List major reasons for clients to schedule regular massage sessions
- Identify problems that may arise with client retention

The key to building a successful massage practice is developing a client base that maintains a regular appointment schedule. In addition to providing exceptional massage skills, retention of clients comes from building rapport so that they look forward to coming for their massage session.

Development of a regular client base is possible with therapeutic massage, because massage benefits wear off if massage is not continued. Also, the benefits of massage are cumulative and better sustained with regular appointments.

A sustaining massage business is built on clients who receive therapeutic massage regularly. Clients who get a massage on a weekly, bimonthly, or monthly basis are the mainstay of a personal service massage business. To maintain a successful business of this type, the massage professional must provide a quality massage; offer clients consistent, personal attention; and charge affordable fees. Clients who are happy with the work are the best source of word-of-mouth advertising Retention rates are higher for educated clients.

Clients are more apt to commit to a regular schedule of massage if they:
- Notice measurable benefits
- Understand the physiologic reasons for the results of massage
- Experience a safe, professional, and ethical massage environment

Clients who maintain a regular appointment schedule typically have quantifiable and qualifiable goals they want to achieve. Long-term care/treatment plans are important for these clients. If the massage practitioner does not have the skill base to help the client achieve these goals, the client will not be satisfied and will not return for massage.

Proper marketing also is important for client retention. Clients should be asked to reschedule appointments and should be reminded of their appointment schedule by telephone or e-mail. Literature should be available that explains the benefits of regular massages.

Reality Check

If retention is a problem and at least half of first-time clients do not reschedule massage sessions at least on a monthly basis, the massage practitioner needs to evaluate his or her skills and professional interaction with those clients. Some questions to ask are:
- Were my communication skills effective?
- Did I establish rapport with the client?
- Did I look and act professionally?
- Did I offend the client?
- Did something about my appearance make the client uncomfortable?
- Was my hygiene impeccable?
- Could an offensive environmental or body odor have been a problem?
- Was the massage environment safe, clean, and comfortable?
- Did I talk too much during the massage?
- Did I use the appropriate massage methods and pressure levels?
- Did the massage I provided meet the client's goals?
- Did some sort of behavior I have make the client uncomfortable?
- Are my fees reasonable?
- Do my fees support retention?

Scrutinizing ourselves and being very honest about our massage skills, appearance, hygiene, communication skills, environment, and so forth can be difficult. However, we must perform this evaluation to support client retention. Without client retention, we do not have the opportunity for career success.

REIMBURSEMENT

SECTION OBJECTIVES

Chapter objective covered in this section:
6. The student will be able to describe the process for setting fees, determining income, and doing insurance billing.
Using the information presented in this section, the student will be able to perform the following:
- Determine criteria for massage fees in a particular geographic area
- Explain how fees charged for massage influence wages paid to massage therapists
- Explain the process of insurance reimbursement

Setting Fees

A concern for the client is how much the massage will cost. Setting fees and using incentives are great marketing tools. When you are trying to decide how much to charge for massage services, it is helpful to investigate what other massage practitioners within a 1-hour radius of your business location are charging. Consider setting your fees in the midrange of current fees in the area. Also, consider how much *you* would be willing to pay for a massage.

Incentives and coupons can be offered to generate interest in the business (Figure 3-4). However, attempting to undercut the competition by charging very low fees usually is unwise, because you will not be able to maintain the low fee structure for an extended period. Also, this is not considered an ethical business practice. The range for massage fees usually is $25 to $30 for a 30-minute massage and $40 to $60 for a full hour (Box 3-3). For sessions less than 30 minutes, the common charge is $1 per minute. These fees represent the current national average and can vary up or down, depending on the location. Typically, fees in urban areas are higher, and those in rural areas are lower.

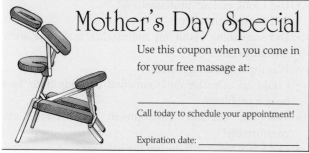

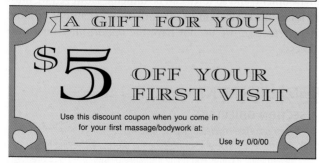

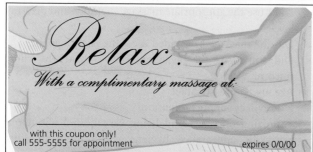

FIGURE 3-4 Sample coupons and gift certificates.

Another way to determine the fees appropriate for your area or target market is to calculate the average hourly wage of the people in your target market and multiply that by three (up to a maximum hourly fee, which usually is $75). The justification for this structure is that people may understand the value of working 3 hours a week to provide self-care.

EXAMPLE

If the employees of ABC Packing Co. make $9 per hour, the fee for a 1-hour massage would be $27. If the target market is business professionals with an average hourly wage of $25, the fee could be $75.

Using the scenarios in the Example box, if the practitioner sets a fee of $40 to $50 an hour for the packing company workers, these clients are unlikely to be able to afford weekly massage sessions, but regular every-other-week appointments are possible. If the $50 fee is set for the business professional group, weekly appointments are more likely.

Fee Discounts

Many therapeutic massage professionals or businesses give a discount to clients who schedule regular visits. This can be done in a variety of ways. One possibility is a package of massages for which the client pays in advance.

Box 3-3 Typical Fee Structure and Analysis of Income

Below is a breakdown of session lengths and client fees. Setting up a table like the one below can provide you with insight to your future earnings.

Duration of Massage Session	Low-end Fee	High-end Fee	Average
½ hr	$25	$35	$30
1 hr	$40	$60	$50
1½ hr	$60	$80	$70
1-hr on-site	$90	$150	$120

But this is only a start to figuring out how much you could be earning. You need to consider more than the time that is spent in the session—setup, possible travel, and other associated costs must be considered. It is essential to consider "real time" when calculating income. There is always time between sessions and things to attend to. Below is a breakdown of massage session lengths, "real time" required, and the income generated based on the average earnings from above.

Massage Duration	"Real Time" Required	Income Generated Based on Average Rate
½-hr massages	¾ hours (45 minutes)	$30 ($40 per hour)
1-hr massages	1¼ hours (75 minutes)	$50 ($40 per hour)
1½-hr massages	1¾ hours (105 minutes)	$70 ($40 per hour)
1-hr on-site massage	3 hours (180 min)	$120 ($40 per hour)

A massage therapist does 25 1-hr massage sessions per week at $50 per massage, which equals $1250 in gross income. 50% of the gross income is deducted for overhead expenses and taxes. This leaves $625 of net income. It takes approximately 32 hours of real time to complete 25 1-hr massage sessions. In addition, it is necessary to manage the business and take care of office and cleaning responsibilities. At a minimum this would be 8 hrs per week. The actual work week is 40 hrs per week. Hourly income would come to $15.63. The amount would result in an annual average net income (in pocket) of $32,500.

EXAMPLE

A client pays for 10 massage sessions in advance with a $5 discount for each massage. The package deal for the $50 session would be 10 massages for $450 rather than $500. Another option is to give a $5 discount to anyone who books a weekly appointment.

Reviewing Fees

It is important to review fees yearly. A good time is at the end of the year when taxes are filed (this usually happens in April, so May is a good time to raise rates). Clients should be notified at least 30 days in advance of any price changes. Also, having a full schedule of clients for 3 months is an indicator that a rate increase might be considered.

Comparing Self-Employment and Employee Incomes

Business Costs

If you intend to be self-employed, plan on spending half the gross income of your business (all income generated by business activities) on overhead expenses and setting aside one third of the net income (gross income minus business expenses) to pay income taxes. In an employee situation, these costs are the business owner's responsibility.

Always remember that each hour spent doing massage requires at least 1 hour of business management time. Giving 20 1-hour massage sessions is at least 40 hours of work if a person is self-employed.

On-Site Massage

For an on-site massage session, the practitioner travels to the client's home or business, and travel and setup time must be figured into the fee. Because the therapist is already organized to do massage, other sessions at the same location can be provided at the regular rate. If a person is housebound for health reasons, the massage therapist commonly takes this into consideration when setting the fee. The massage professional who has only an on-site business saves on rental and utility costs, which may influence the on-site fee structure. Remember that time is money, and an on-site massage takes longer than one in the office.

Hourly Wage Employment Versus Salaried Employment

Wages for employee massage professionals can be hourly, salaried, or percentage based as long as the minimum wage requirement per hour worked is paid to the employee.

An increasingly common practice is to hire massage professionals at an hourly wage. Wages per hour vary widely for massage professionals and depend on location and experience. The average pay range is $9 to $20 per hour. A beginning wage is $8 to $10 per hour. According to the U.S. Bureau of Labor Statistics, the average yearly net income for a full-time massage professional is $20,000 to $35,000. This is about $10 to $15 per hour based on a 40-hour workweek. Remember that income taxes must be paid on this amount. When practitioners work for an hourly wage, they usually are paid for the time spent at the job location, regardless of whether massage is given.

Sometimes an agreed-upon salary is offered instead of an hourly wage. Those who work for a salary are often paid on the basis of completion of certain tasks rather than the number of hours worked. A salary structure for therapeutic massage might be $400 per week based on completion of 20 massage sessions per pay period.

An hourly wage may appear to be much less than a self-employed practitioner earns. However this is not true. Hourly earnings cannot be compared with fees charged for a massage. A self-employed massage therapist may charge $50 for a 1-hour massage, but the therapist does not make $50 per hour. Self-employed massage therapists must pay overhead expenses and the calculated real time required to support the 1-hour massage fee.

Overall the actual amount in the therapist's pocket is about the same. Because the income from massage practice is about the same whether one is employed or self-employed, income potential may not be the major factor in the professional's decision on which career path to pursue.

Insurance or Third-Party Reimbursement

Personal service massage is not likely to fall under the accepted coverage of current or future health care plans. However, the possibility exists that future insurance coverage will be available for preventive health care. Some managed care systems are currently investigating options for limited coverage in this area.

As with almost all aspects of professional practice, insurance coverage has its pros and cons. The documentation requirements for collecting insurance are extensive (Figure 3-5). Most massage professionals are unable to bill the insurance company directly for reimbursement. The managed care system is affecting the ability to bill insurance directly and is reducing the number of health care providers who can bill directly.

On the other hand, some insurance companies are covering massage and providing programs in which massage providers who meet certain criteria are eligible to be listed in their members' directories. The insurance company prenegotiates a discounted fee with the massage therapist for its clients. The clients pay the massage professional the discounted fee. No billing is required. The return for the discount is the appearance of approval by the insurance company and the marketing and advertising received in the member publications.

If the massage therapist is an employee of a licensed medical professional or of a managed care corporation with access to insurance billing codes and is working under direct supervision, the massage services may be available for billing. In this situation the massage therapist receives an hourly wage or salary. The burden of collecting from the insurance company falls on the physician, chiropractor, physical therapist, dentist, psychiatrist, or corporate entity, not on the massage practitioner. However, the massage practitioner needs to be able to perform effective assessments, write appropriate treatment plans, and maintain charts.

Occasionally a client can collect from the insurance company by providing a prescription for massage from the physician and a receipt showing payment, the diagnostic code from the physician, and a description of the procedure. It is important to have the insurance company preapprove payment for therapeutic massage. This is done by having the client contact the insurance company before any massage begins. Documentation on the benefits of massage, the physician's prescription, and any other information required by the insurance company are presented for review. This usually is the client's responsibility. Based on this information, the insurance company determines whether the client will be reimbursed for the massage services and notifies the client in writing of the decision. The client pays the massage professional directly, and the massage professional provides the receipt with the physician's diagnostic code, the procedure used, and the duration of the session. Responsibility for collecting insurance reimbursement falls to the client.

1500

HEALTH INSURANCE CLAIM FORM

APPROVED BY NATIONAL UNIFORM CLAIM COMMITTEE 08/05

PICA | PICA

CARRIER

1. MEDICARE (Medicare #) | MEDICAID (Medicaid #) | TRICARE CHAMPUS (Sponsor's SSN) | CHAMPVA (Member ID#) | GROUP HEALTH PLAN (SSN or ID) | FECA BLK LUNG (SSN) | OTHER (ID)

1a. INSURED'S I.D. NUMBER (For Program in Item 1)

2. PATIENT'S NAME (Last Name, First Name, Middle Initial)

3. PATIENT'S BIRTH DATE MM DD YY SEX M F

4. INSURED'S NAME (Last Name, First Name, Middle Initial)

5. PATIENT'S ADDRESS (No., Street)

6. PATIENT RELATIONSHIP TO INSURED Self Spouse Child Other

7. INSURED'S ADDRESS (No., Street)

CITY STATE

8. PATIENT STATUS Single Married Other; Employed Full-Time Student Part-Time Student

CITY STATE

ZIP CODE TELEPHONE (Include Area Code) ( )

ZIP CODE TELEPHONE (Include Area Code) ( )

9. OTHER INSURED'S NAME (Last Name. First Name, Middle Initial)

10. IS PATIENT'S CONDITION RELATED TO:

11. INSURED'S POLICY GROUP OR FECA NUMBER

a. OTHER INSURED'S POLICY OR GROUP NUMBER

a. EMPLOYMENT? (Current or Previous) YES NO

a. INSURED'S DATE OF BIRTH MM DD YY SEX M F

b. OTHER INSURED'S DATE OF BIRTH MM DD YY SEX M F

b. AUTO ACCIDENT? YES NO PLACE (State)

b. EMPLOYER'S NAME OR SCHOOL NAME

c. EMPLOYER'S NAME OR SCHOOL NAME

c. OTHER ACCIDENT? YES NO

c. INSURANCE PLAN NAME OR PROGRAM NAME

d. INSURANCE PLAN NAME OR PROGRAM NAME

10d. RESERVED FOR LOCAL USE

d. IS THERE ANOTHER HEALTH BENEFIT PLAN? YES NO *If yes,* return to and complete item 9 a-d.

READ BACK OF FORM BEFORE COMPLETING & SIGNING THIS FORM.

12. PATIENT'S OR AUTHORIZED PERSON'S SIGNATURE I authorize the release of any medical or other information necessary to process this claim. I also request payment of government benefits either to myself or to the party who accepts assignment below.

SIGNED ____ DATE ____

13. INSURED'S OR AUTHORIZED PERSON'S SIGNATURE I authorize payment of medical benefits to the undersigned physician or supplier for services described below.

SIGNED ____

PATIENT AND INSURED INFORMATION

SECOND FOLD

14. DATE OF CURRENT: MM DD YY ◀ ILLNESS (First symptom) OR INJURY (Accident) OR PREGNANCY (LMP)

15. IF PATIENT HAS HAD SAME OR SIMILAR ILLNESS, GIVE FIRST DATE MM DD YY

16. DATES PATIENT UNABLE TO WORK IN CURRENT OCCUPATION FROM MM DD YY TO MM DD YY

17. NAME OF REFERRING PROVIDER OR OTHER SOURCE | 17a. | 17b. NPI

18. HOSPITALIZATION DATES RELATED TO CURRENT SERVICES FROM MM DD YY TO MM DD YY

19. RESERVED FOR LOCAL USE

20. OUTSIDE LAB? YES NO $ CHARGES

21. DIAGNOSIS OR NATURE OF ILLNESS OR INJURY. (Relate Items 1,2,3 or 4 to Item 24E by Line)

1. ____ . ____ 3. ____ . ____

2. ____ . ____ 4. ____ . ____

22. MEDICAID RESUBMISSION CODE ORIGINAL REF. NO.

23. PRIOR AUTHORIZATION NUMBER

24. A. DATE(S) OF SERVICE From MM DD YY To MM DD YY	B. PLACE OF SERVICE	C. EMG	D. PROCEDURES, SERVICES, OR SUPPLIES (Explain Unusual Circumstances) CPT/HCPCS MODIFIER	E. DIAGNOSIS POINTER	F. $ CHARGES	G. DAYS OR UNITS	H. EPSDT Family Plan	I. ID. QUAL.	J. RENDERING PROVIDER ID. #
1								NPI	
2								NPI	
3								NPI	
4								NPI	
5								NPI	
6								NPI	

PHYSICIAN OR SUPPLIER INFORMATION

FIRST FOLD WHCF-10-ENV / WHCF-10-ENV-SS

25. FEDERAL TAX I.D. NUMBER SSN EIN

26. PATIENT'S ACCOUNT NO.

27. ACCEPT ASSIGNMENT? (For govt. claims, see back) YES NO

28. TOTAL CHARGE $

29. AMOUNT PAID $

30. BALANCE DUE $

31. SIGNATURE OF PHYSICIAN OR SUPPLIER INCLUDING DEGREES OR CREDENTIALS (I certify that the statements on the reverse apply to this bill and are made a part thereof.)

SIGNED DATE

32. SERVICE FACILITY LOCATION INFORMATION

a. NPI b.

33. BILLING PROVIDER INFO & PH. # ( )

a. NPI b.

NUCC Instruction Manual available at: www.nucc.org

APPROVED OMB 0938-0999 FORM CMS-1500 (08/05)

A

WCMS-1500CS

FIGURE 3-5 Front **(A)** and back **(B)** of an insurance claim form.

(From Fritz S: *Business and professional skills for massage therapists,* St Louis, 2010, Mosby.)

BECAUSE THIS FORM IS USED BY VARIOUS GOVERNMENT AND PRIVATE HEALTH PROGRAMS, SEE SEPARATE INSTRUCTIONS ISSUED BY APPLICABLE PROGRAMS.

NOTICE: Any person who knowingly files a statement of claim containing any misrepresentation or any false, incomplete or misleading information may be guilty of a criminal act punishable under law and may be subject to civil penalties.

REFERS TO GOVERNMENT PROGRAMS ONLY

MEDICARE AND CHAMPUS PAYMENTS: A patient's signature requests that payment be made and authorizes release of any information necessary to process the claim and certifies that the information provided in Blocks 1 through 12 is true, accurate and complete. In the case of a Medicare claim, the patient's signature authorizes any entity to release to Medicare medical and nonmedical information, including employment status, and whether the person has employer group health insurance, liability, no-fault, worker's compensation or other insurance which is responsible to pay for the services for which the Medicare claim is made. See 42 CFR 411.24(a). If item 9 is completed, the patient's signature authorizes release of the information to the health plan or agency shown. In Medicare assigned or CHAMPUS participation cases, the physician agrees to accept the charge determination of the Medicare carrier or CHAMPUS fiscal intermediary as the full charge, and the patient is responsible only for the deductible, coinsurance and noncovered services. Coinsurance and the deductible are based upon the charge determination of the Medicare carrier or CHAMPUS fiscal intermediary if this is less than the charge submitted. CHAMPUS is not a health insurance program but makes payment for health benefits provided through certain affiliations with the Uniformed Services. Information on the patient's sponsor should be provided in those items captioned in "Insured"; i.e., items 1a, 4, 6, 7, 9, and 11.

BLACK LUNG AND FECA CLAIMS

The provider agrees to accept the amount paid by the Government as payment in full. See Black Lung and FECA instructions regarding required procedure and diagnosis coding systems.

SIGNATURE OF PHYSICIAN OR SUPPLIER (MEDICARE, CHAMPUS, FECA AND BLACK LUNG)

I certify that the services shown on this form were medically indicated and necessary for the health of the patient and were personally furnished by me or were furnished incident to my professional service by my employee under my immediate personal supervision, except as otherwise expressly permitted by Medicare or CHAMPUS regulations.

For services to be considered as "incident" to a physician's professional service, 1) they must be rendered under the physician's immediate personal supervision by his/her employee, 2) they must be an integral, although incidental part of a covered physician's service, 3) they must be of kinds commonly furnished in physician's offices, and 4) the services of nonphysicians must be included on the physician's bills.

For CHAMPUS claims, I further certify that I (or any employee) who rendered services am not an active duty member of the Uniformed Services or a civilian employee of the United States Government or a contract employee of the United States Government, either civilian or military (refer to 5 USC 5536). For Black-Lung claims, I further certify that the services performed were for a Black Lung-related disorder.

No Part B Medicare benefits may be paid unless this form is received as required by existing law and regulations (42 CFR 424.32).

NOTICE: Any one who misrepresents or falsifies essential information to receive payment from Federal funds requested by this form may upon conviction be subject to fine and imprisonment under applicable Federal laws.

NOTICE TO PATIENT ABOUT THE COLLECTION AND USE OF MEDICARE, CHAMPUS, FECA, AND BLACK LUNG INFORMATION
(PRIVACY ACT STATEMENT)

We are authorized by CMS, CHAMPUS and OWCP to ask you for information needed in the administration of the Medicare, CHAMPUS, FECA, and Black Lung programs. Authority to collect information is in section 205(a), 1862, 1872 and 1874 of the Social Security Act as amended, 42 CFR 411.24(a) and 424.5(a) (6), and 44 USC 3101;41 CFR 101 et seq and 10 USC 1079 and 1086; 5 USC 8101 et seq; and 30 USC 901 et seq; 38 USC 613; E.O. 9397.

The information we obtain to complete claims under these programs is used to identify you and to determine your eligibility. It is also used to decide if the services and supplies you received are covered by these programs and to insure that proper payment is made.

The information may also be given to other providers of services, carriers, intermediaries, medical review boards, health plans, and other organizations or Federal agencies, for the effective administration of Federal provisions that require other third parties payers to pay primary to Federal program, and as otherwise necessary to administer these programs. For example, it may be necessary to disclose information about the benefits you have used to a hospital or doctor. Additional disclosures are made through routine uses for information contained in systems of records.

FOR MEDICARE CLAIMS: See the notice modifying system No. 09-70-0501, titled, 'Carrier Medicare Claims Record,' published in the <u>Federal Register</u>, Vol. 55 No. 177, page 37549, Wed. Sept. 12, 1990, or as updated and republished.

FOR OWCP CLAIMS: Department of Labor, Privacy Act of 1974, "Republication of Notice of Systems of Records," <u>Federal Register</u> Vol. 55 No. 40, Wed Feb. 28, 1990, See ESA-5, ESA-6, ESA-12, ESA-13, ESA-30, or as updated and republished.

FOR CHAMPUS CLAIMS: <u>PRINCIPLE PURPOSE(S):</u> To evaluate eligibility for medical care provided by civilian sources and to issue payment upon establishment of eligibility and determination that the services/supplies received are authorized by law.

<u>ROUTINE USE(S):</u> Information from claims and related documents may be given to the Dept. of Veterans Affairs, the Dept. of Health and Human Services and/or the Dept. of Transportation consistent with their statutory administrative responsibilities under CHAMPUS/CHAMPVA; to the Dept. of Justice for representation of the Secretary of Defense in civil actions; to the Internal Revenue Service, private collection agencies, and consumer reporting agencies in connection with recoupment claims; and to Congressional Offices in response to inquiries made at the request of the person to whom a record pertains. Appropriate disclosures may be made to other federal, state, local, foreign government agencies, private business entities, and individual providers of care, on matters relating to entitlement, claims adjudication, fraud, program abuse, utilization review, quality assurance, peer review, program integrity, third-party liability, coordination of benefits, and civil and criminal litigation related to the operation of CHAMPUS.

<u>DISCLOSURES:</u> Voluntary; however, failure to provide information will result in delay in payment or may result in denial of claim. With the one exception discussed below, there are no penalties under these programs for refusing to supply information. However, failure to furnish information regarding the medical services rendered or the amount charged would prevent payment of claims under these programs. Failure to furnish any other information, such as name or claim number, would delay payment of the claim. Failure to provide medical information under FECA could be deemed an obstruction.

It is mandatory that you tell us if you know that another party is responsible for paying for your treatment. Section 1128B of the Social Security Act and 31 USC 3801-3812 provide penalties for withholding this information.

You should be aware that P.L. 100-503, the "Computer Matching and Privacy Protection Act of 1988", permits the government to verify information by way of computer matches.

MEDICAID PAYMENTS (PROVIDER CERTIFICATION)

I hereby agree to keep such records as are necessary to disclose fully the extent of services provided to individuals under the State's Title XIX plan and to furnish information regarding any payments claimed for providing such services as the State Agency or Dept. of Health and Human Services may request.

I further agree to accept, as payment in full, the amount paid by the Medicaid program for those claims submitted for payment under that program, with the exception of authorized deductible, coinsurance, co-payment or similar cost-sharing charge.

SIGNATURE OF PHYSICIAN (OR SUPPLIER): I certify that the services listed above were medically indicated and necessary to the health of this patient and were personally furnished by me or my employee under my personal direction.

NOTICE: This is to certify that the foregoing information is true, accurate and complete. I understand that payment and satisfaction of this claim will be from Federal and State funds, and that any false claims, statements, or documents, or concealment of a material fact, may be prosecuted under applicable Federal or State laws.

According to the Paperwork Reduction Act of 1995, no persons are required to respond to a collection of information unless it displays a valid OMB control number. The valid OMB control number for this information collection is 0938-0999. The time required to complete this information collection is estimated to average 10 minutes per response, including the time to review instructions, search existing data resources, gather the data needed, and complete and review the information collection. If you have any comments concerning the accuracy of the time estimate(s) or suggestions for improving this form, please write to: CMS, Attn: PRA Reports Clearance Officer, 7500 Security Boulevard, Baltimore, Maryland 21244-1850. This address is for comments and/or suggestions only. DO NOT MAIL COMPLETED CLAIM FORMS TO THIS ADDRESS.

B

FIGURE 3-5, cont'd

PROFICIENCY EXERCISE 3-4

1. Contact the office of a local chiropractor, physical therapist, mental health professional, or physician and talk with the billing clerk about the paperwork involved in insurance reimbursement. Ask how much the insurance company covers for various treatments.
2. Call your personal health insurance company and ask whether massage therapy is covered, what the requirements are for receiving coverage, and how much is reimbursed for a massage session.

PROFICIENCY EXERCISE 3-5

1. Investigate the fee structure for massage therapy in your area.
2. After you have determined the average fee in your area, decide how many massage sessions per month you could afford. What could you afford to pay for a massage session twice a month?
3. On a piece of paper, develop a sample incentive plan. Explain how you would track the discounts.

In some areas, licensed massage therapists may be able to bill insurance companies directly. Although this situation is not common, if you live in a jurisdiction that does allow direct billing by massage therapists, be realistic about the responsibilities required to maintain a positive working relationship with insurance companies. If you are able to bill insurance companies, contact each company individually, speak with a representative, and ask for information on the best way to work with the company.

The advisability of dealing with insurance companies is the subject of considerable controversy. Some massage professionals seem to do well with insurance reimbursement. Workers' compensation and smaller insurance companies are more apt to pay. The current widespread lack of health insurance coverage for therapeutic massage services should not discourage the new massage professional. Many health care professionals are discouraged and frustrated with the health insurance system and the limits it places on their attempts to provide their patients with quality care. Some professionals are even beginning to refuse to participate in health insurance programs; they have begun to adjust their fee schedule and are returning to a cash-for-services system (Proficiency Exercise 3-4).

Employment is available for massage professionals who want to work in the medical system, for those who want access to health insurance reimbursement, and for those who want to be independent business people providing massage services outside the medical establishment on a cash-for-services basis. Having payment options, including insurance reimbursement, is beneficial for both the client and the therapist. (See Chapter 13 for more information about massage therapy in the health care environment.)

THE BUSINESS/CAREER PLAN

SECTION OBJECTIVES

Chapter objective covered in this section:
7. The student will be able to develop career plans.
Using the information presented in this section, the student will be able to perform the following:
- Write a career mission statement
- Set career goals
- Anticipate risk
- Use the clinical reasoning model to set business goals
- Understand a business plan

Career Mission Statement

Whether you intend to be self-employed or to approach a massage career as an employee, it is important to have a plan. To make the plan workable, the professional needs to know where he or she is in the present, what his or her path has been, and what he or she has learned from accumulated experiences. When this information has become available, future plans can be made. For example:
- One career plan option is to move gradually into a new massage career by working at it part time while letting the business grow slowly (keeping your full-time job).
- Another option is to commit to the new massage business full time. If the practitioner chooses to do this and is self-employed, he or she will need to have enough money saved up to meet basic needs for about 1 year.

Either path is acceptable. You need to decide what fits you. This is the type of information that becomes formalized when you develop a business/career plan. In all business planning, the important thing is to find and fill a need. What is the massage need that you, as a practitioner, are willing to fill? The answer to this question becomes the basis of your mission statement. A mission statement expresses the intent of the business plan. To develop a mission statement, you must answer this question: What will be the main focus of my business?

An example of a mission statement might be:

My business mission is to serve the blue-collar labor population in my area by providing therapeutic massage and self-help education at a reasonable cost, with flexible appointment hours, and at an easily accessible location.

Development of your formal business plan begins while you are still in school. Education in the skills needed to carry out the mission statement is the first step of the business plan. Another part of the business plan is the development of a financial plan to support the educational process and the first year of business, which is a time when income may be low. While in school, students should use the expertise of teachers and other students to explore career options (Proficiency Exercises 3-5 and 3-6).

Goal-Setting Plan

Once the "big picture" concepts of the business/career plan are in place, smaller steps to implement the plans are identified. These are goals. Goals are important, because they provide direction and landmarks for achievement (Box 3-4).

💡 PROFICIENCY EXERCISE 3-6

Pretend that you are a successful massage practitioner 5 years from now. You have been asked to return to your massage school and speak to the business class about how you succeeded in your business. Talk into a tape recorder for 30 minutes as though you were addressing the class. Play back the tape and write down the steps you took that led to a successful business. Use these steps to develop an outline for a business plan. Then meet in groups of four students and share your outlines with one another.

Box 3-4 Guidelines for Setting Goals

1. State your goals in the present tense. Make sure you are the main character. Use the pronouns *I, me,* and *my.*
2. Make sure your goals are realistic and attainable. Can you achieve these goals using your own resources with little help from others? If the activity of a specific person is necessary to achieve your goal, rethink it. What other people may be able to be part of the goal? Avoid depending on only one other person.
3. Speak positively. Avoid words such as *should, would, could, try,* and *never.*
4. Set target deadlines for yourself; they will give you something to work toward.
5. Make sure your goals are small steps toward your ultimate plan. For example, graduating from school is too big to be a goal; it is more like a mission statement. Completing all the exercises in this chapter within 4 weeks is an attainable goal.

Goals may change over time. Goal setting can be compared to taking a trip. To stay fresh and alert during a trip, a person must stop and rest. If these stops are planned ahead of time, the journey seems shorter. The journey toward creation of a successful business is similar when attainable goals are placed along the way.

When you plan for a trip, it is important that you identify any obstacles that may be encountered. What are your financial and personal resources? It is the same with a business. Review the support available from others. Be willing to learn along the way.

Basic survival skills promote self-sufficiency in business as well as in life. A good question to ask is, "What is the worst possible thing that could happen as a result of this decision?" Think ahead to possible solutions should the worst happen and try to determine whether you could survive that experience. What would be gained? It is important to take calculated risks. If these risks are small and entered into slowly, you can change strategies if need be (Proficiency Exercise 3-7).

The clinical reasoning model used throughout this text is an invaluable tool for setting attainable goals (Box 3-5).

Business is business. If you are self-employed, all business responsibilities fall on your shoulders, including all costs. If you are an employee, it is important that you appreciate what is required of your employer.

💡 PROFICIENCY EXERCISE 3-7

Picture yourself 5 years from now enjoying a successful massage therapy business. A new student comes to you and asks how you achieved your success. You begin to tell the story of the past 5 years and all the steps it took to get where you are now. All the steps you list are possible goals. When you begin by visualizing the end result, all you have to do is identify the probable steps that got you there.

In the space provided, write down two professional goals that you identified.

Goal 1

Goal 2

Business Plan

Writing a business plan teaches you about the detail required to finance, own, operate, and succeed in business. Even if you plan to work for a business owner, developing a business plan for a "pretend" business prepares you to be a better employee, because you will understand the commitment and responsibilities required of your employer.

The Small Business Association (SBA), an independent agency of the U.S. government whose mission is to help Americans start, build, and grow businesses, is also an excellent resource for business topics. Make sure to use the extensive resources they offer.

A business plan generally consists of the following elements:

- *Executive summary:* This is the most important part of the business plan and should be devised last, once the other parts are well into development or are complete. The material from those parts helps create an executive summary that includes a mission statement, possible locations, services, market summary, number of employees, and so on. (In your case, the point of the executive summary is to demonstrate concisely the focus of your proposed massage business, your expertise, and your competitive edge in the market.)
- *Market analysis:* This section includes a description of the industry (in your case, therapeutic massage), a survey of the competition, and a description of the target market.
- *Company overview:* This section covers the way the different parts of the proposed business will work together and gives the reasons this is a recipe for success.
- *Description of management and organization of staff:* Whom the owner plans to hire and who will be in charge of certain duties and why go into this section.
- *Ownership information:* This part of the business plan reviews subjects such as the owners' names, percentage of ownership, and owner influence.
- *Funding requests:* This section explains how much money will be needed for start-up or expansion costs and the proposed uses of borrowed funds.

Box 3-5   Using the Clinical Reasoning Model to Set Goals

1. Gather facts to identify and define the situation. (This can be the mission statement.)

   Key questions:

   What is the desired outcome?

   What are the facts?

   My business mission is to serve the blue-collar labor population in my area by providing therapeutic massage and self-help education at a reasonable cost, with flexible appointment hours and at an easily accessible location.

   I will need a group of people for a client base.

2. Brainstorm possible goals.

   Key questions:

   What might I do?

   What if ...?

   What are the possibilities?

   What does my intuition suggest?

   What if I contact the XYZ manufacturing plant as a potential population?

   What if I contact the ABC packing company as a potential population?

3. Evaluate each possible goal identified in step 2 logically and objectively; look at both the pros and the cons.

   Key questions:

   What would happen if ...? (Insert each idea brainstormed in step 2.)

   What are the costs, resources needed, and time involved?

   What are the logical cause and effect of each possibility identified?

   What are the pros and cons of each goal suggested?

   What are the consequences of not acting?

   What are the consequences of acting?

   What would happen if I contacted the XYZ manufacturing plant?

   - *I would need a massage room on site.*
   - *Travel time to work would be 45 minutes.*
   - *Pro: This plant has 300 employees, a large potential client base.*
   - *Con: This plant has a history of striking.*
   - *What would happen if I contacted the ABC packing company?*

   - *I could work at my existing office site.*
   - *I am 15 minutes from work on foot.*
   - *Pro: This company is in a growth phase.*
   - *Con: This company has only 50 employees.*

4. Evaluate the effect of each possible goal on the people involved.

   Key questions:

   How would each person involved feel if ...? (Insert each idea brainstormed in step 2.)

   For each goal, what would be the impact on the people involved: client, practitioner, and other professionals working with the client?

   How does each person involved feel about the possible goals?

   Does a feeling of cooperation and agreement exist among all parties involved?

   How might people feel if I contact the XYZ manufacturing plant?

   - *This company is quite traditional. The president is sometimes resistant to change. I am socially acquainted with the plant manager, and he might like the idea.*

   How might people feel if I contact the ABC packing company?

   - *This company is very progressive in terms of human resources. I have a personality conflict with one of the vice presidents but have a good rapport with the other members of the human resources board.*

5. Choose a goal and develop an implementation plan after carefully processing steps 1 through 4.

   Based on this process, I believe the most attainable goal is to contact the ABC packing company.

6. Implement the plan and set a date for re-evaluation.

   Implementation plans are step-by-step procedures that detail what must be done to achieve the goals; these procedures can be considered subgoals.

   Steps for implementing the goal of contacting the ABC packing company:

   - *Develop a presentation packet (1 week)*
   - *Send a letter of inquiry (tomorrow)*
   - *Make an appointment for an interview (2 weeks)*

- *Financials:* This section covers the financial history of the enterprise (if applicable), in addition to short- and long-term goals and forecasts.

A resource partner with the SBA, SCORE (Service Corps of Retired Executives) is also a valuable business resource. Working and retired executives and business owners donate time and expertise as business counselors providing free advice. These mentors enjoy sharing their knowledge and want to see other entrepreneurs succeed. Both in-person and on-line counseling are available. Owners of start-up businesses can talk to a SCORE mentor as much as they need or want; no limit has been placed on any of SCORE's services. In fact, many may find long-term mentoring to be a great help.

When you complete Proficiency Exercise 3-12 later in this chapter, you will have compiled most of the information you need to create a business/career plan.

THE BUSINESS STRUCTURE

SECTION OBJECTIVES

Chapter objective covered in this section:

8. The student will be able to identify the requirements and options for starting a business.

Using the information presented in this section, the student will be able to perform the following:

- Develop an effective business name
- Determine average start-up costs, overhead expenses, and yearly income
- Negotiate lease agreements based on a flat fee or on a percentage of gross receipts
- Apply business structure concepts to either self-employment or employment by others

Regardless of the career path you follow (self-employed or employee), to be successful you must understand the fundamentals of the business structure. The foundation of a successful business is planning and implementation. Just as massage therapy is based on a few key underlying principles, so is business.

The previous section covered the structure and function of a business plan. The structure of a business plan helps to organize details, and the function supports the planning and implementation process. Now we can begin to refine the information to an individual business structure. Just as an individual has a name, so does a unique business. A business also needs resources to begin its existence, including a home and funds to support growth and success.

Business Name

Careful consideration must be given to creating a business name that clearly and concisely reflects the intention of the business. When deciding on a name for your business, you *should*:

- Create a name that appeals to you but also to the kind of clients you are trying to attract
- Create a comforting or familiar name with pleasant memories so that clients respond to the business on an emotional level
- Create a short, descriptive, concise name that is easy to pronounce and easy to remember
- Imagine how the name would look on business cards, on a website, and in advertisements,
- Determine whether a logo can be designed that reflects the intention of the name

On the other hand, when creating a business name you *should avoid*:

- Embarrassing misspellings, abbreviations, and potentially offensive undertones
- Implied associations with organizations or people with whom the business is not connected

Once you have decided on the perfect business name, you must make sure that it is secure and protected and that no other business in the area has the same name. Laws may vary from state to state, so check with the Secretary of State's office in the state in which you plan to practice to ensure compliance with regional policies.

Start-Up Costs

Start-up costs are the initial expenses required to begin a business. In addition to the start-up cost amount, you should have a minimum cash reserve equal to the amount of money needed to cover basic business and personal living expenses for 6 months to 1 year. Many people begin a business without these cash reserves and do fine. Others give up the business venture because they do not have enough money to pay bills. This situation forces them to find other jobs. Keeping a cash reserve allows you to focus on developing your business with less financial worry (Proficiency Exercise 3-8).

If you intend to look for employment, you should check out a potential employer with the Better Business Bureau, the Chamber of Commerce, and other business owners in the

PROFICIENCY EXERCISE 3-8

1. Talk with three massage practitioners and ask them what it cost to start their massage businesses.
2. Use professional massage publications and other resources to complete a sample start-up cost worksheet.

community to determine whether the business is stable and operates effectively. Otherwise, you may lose your position if your employer goes out of business.

Students are taught, when giving a massage, to keep it simple and to go slowly. The same ideas apply to business. A person beginning a massage business does not need a suite of offices. For self-employed individuals, the least expensive way to do business is to develop an on-site massage business for private homes or offices and have the business office in your home.

Starting small, with the bare essentials, keeps start-up costs below $4000.

- A basic portable table should not cost more than $500.
- Business cards and a simple brochure are needed, as are client-practitioner statements, policy and procedure booklets, receipt books, and client information forms. The total cost for these is about $500.
- A separate telephone and answering system are a good idea; together these cost about $300. A smart phone can be used as a substitute.
- Membership in one of the professional organizations also provides liability insurance; the membership and insurance usually cost less than $300.
- Linens and supplies should cost about $300.
- Opening a bank account, plus miscellaneous expenses, takes about $500.
- An expenditure of $1000 for initial advertising is reasonable.

Renting a small office can push up the start-up cost to about $6000. This includes the expenses detailed previously plus office costs, such as rent (about $1000, because renting office space often requires payment of the first and last months' rent up front) and office furniture and utility hook-ups (another $1000).

Self-Employment Status

The self-employed massage professional typically becomes affiliated with an established business (e.g., a health club, chiropractor, or full-service cosmetology business) by renting a room in that business establishment. It is important to make sure that any agreement of this type is written in contractual form and reviewed by an attorney (Figure 3-6).

A pitfall in this type of arrangement develops when the owner or manager of the business wants the massage practitioner to function as an employee but, for payment and tax purposes, to be classified as self-employed. With this arrangement, the business owner does not have to pay matching payroll taxes or benefits. However this practice is illegal and can result in huge fines from the Internal Revenue Service (IRS).

Agreement, made this_____day of_____, 20____, by and between_____, Massage Therapist, DBA, Cantonville, Maryland, and _____.

Whereas, _____Massage Therapist, DBA, is a massage therapist and an independent contractor wishing to use the facilities and services of _____ at _____ for the express purpose of the rendition of therapeutic massage services or activities related to massage therapy.

TERMS OF AGREEMENT

1. Fee for a 1-hour therapeutic massage is $55. Massage Therapist receives 75% of massage fees and _____ receives 25%. The same percentage applies regardless of the cost of the massage.
2. Fees may be adjusted only on agreement by both parties.
3. This contract is in effect through March 31. At that time either party may cancel or modify the agreement. A new contract will be issued from April 1.

The following facilities and services will be provided by the chiropractor for the massage therapist:

A. Storage for all massage supplies
B. Use of the facility and its services, i.e., telephone, bathroom, microwave, refrigerator
C. Booking and confirmation of all massage therapy appointments
D. All collection of money, whether cash or insurance
E. A room for the massage therapist to use in the rendition of therapeutic massage services or activities related to massage therapy, and _____ also furnishes electricity, heat, and cleaning for this room
F. Promotion of therapeutic massage as an enhancement to chiropractic care

The massage therapist will abide by the following conditions:

A. Bring all necessary supplies associated with therapy
B. Launder all sheets
C. Pay any and all own costs associated with being an independent contractor, i.e., liability insurance and professional membership
D. Control own hours and schedule
E. Not be held accountable for any expenses incurred by facilities or services not included in this agreement
F. Keep all tips
G. Keep all client information confidential
H. Work at facility by appointment only
I. Reconcile all accounts and pay proper percentage to chiropractor at the end of each month

Cancellation of use of facilities and services is to be in writing, giving at least 30 days' notice, thereafter releasing each party from all financial and legal obligations with the other.

Having read the terms of this agreement, _____ does hereby agree to terms and by signing does agree to use _____ facilities and services to begin on _____.

_____

Date: _____

_____

Date: _____

FIGURE 3-6 Sample facilities and services agreement written in contract form.

True self-employment status means that the professional essentially rents space from the owner. The massage business is completely independent in the way business is conducted. The business owner cannot direct the massage practitioner regarding what hours to work, what kind of work to do, or what to wear.

Facility Rental

The owner of the existing business can be paid in one of two ways. One arrangement is to pay the owner a percentage of every massage performed. This percentage varies from 10% to 50% (the average is 30%). With this arrangement, the business owner profits from every massage done and may be more likely to support your business with word-of-mouth advertising and referrals. The two businesses also commonly advertise together.

Under the other type of agreement, the practitioner pays the owner a monthly rent. Rental fees vary, depending on the business location and the area of the country. Giving a range is difficult, but most rooms in established businesses can be rented for $200 to $600 per month.

One formula for figuring rent involves calculating the percentage of the total square footage of the space.

EXAMPLE

The room you want to rent is 12 × 12 feet, or 144 square feet. The business occupies 2000 square feet. The 12 × 12 room is about 7% of the total available space. The owner pays $2800 per month for rent ($1.4/f^2 per square foot); 7% of $2800 is $196. The business owner needs to make some money to apply the business principle of making a reasonable profit. A 50% return is normal; 50% of $196 is $98. The rent for the space would be $196 plus $98, or $294 per month.

The better choice at first may be to pay a percentage for each massage. If the practitioner has a slow week or gives very few massages, he or she is not obligated to pay a monthly bill. As the business builds, the practitioner commonly ends up paying more per month with a percentage agreement than with a flat fee. If a mutually beneficial relationship is desired, a compromise can be negotiated, such as an upper limit cap on monthly rent. This is the type of information that must be included in a written legal agreement, or contract. Massage professionals should never rely on oral or handshake contracts. They should always have all business agreements in writing.

THE TARGET MARKET

SECTION OBJECTIVES

Chapter objective covered in this section:
9. The student will be able to design a marketing strategy and advertising materials for a massage business.
Using the information presented in this section, the student will be able to perform the following:
- Develop a word-of-mouth marketing plan
- Develop an informational brochure, business card, and media story
- Design a fee structure for therapeutic massage services
- Determine whether third-party insurance reimbursement is available or appropriate for the practice of therapeutic massage
- Understand Web presence

In developing a business, it is important to know the market. Many opportunities are open for the massage business, ranging from the service approaches of stress reduction massage to the allied health opportunities of working in clinical settings. The future for massage is bright. Research has provided the long-awaited verification of the benefits of massage. Educational standards continue to improve, and the profession is becoming standardized and formalized. These developments should achieve a broader acceptance of therapeutic massage and bodywork methods. As a result, more people will consider using massage as part of a health maintenance program.

Massage probably will assume a larger role in corporate stress reduction programs. Athletes will use the services of a massage practitioner more often. Pain control clinics will see its value. Both elderly and young people can benefit from the nurturing touch of the massage therapist. Opportunities for the development of the massage business will be even greater after people understand the benefits of massage. The need for consistently well-trained practitioners will increase.

There is no typical massage business. Successful massage professionals can be found practicing in many different formats. Massage professionals may be full-time employees of a chiropractor or may work part time out of their homes. A business could be developed entirely at one location or in three or four locations. A massage therapist may work one day at a local manufacturing business for the employees and the next day may do home (on-site) visits for local business people. The third day could be spent teaching a self-help massage class for the local community education program. On the fourth day, the therapist may see clients at a full-service cosmetology establishment in the morning, and that evening

💡 **PROFICIENCY EXERCISE 3-9**

Locate the phone numbers of all the service clubs in your community (e.g., Rotary International). The local phone book often lists these organizations. Send a short letter of introduction to three of the organizations offering to do a 30-minute presentation about therapeutic massage for the group. Follow up with phone calls. Arrange to do a presentation (as a student) for the group.

provide on-site massage for a local support group dealing with stress.

With all the available possibilities, the massage practitioner is wise to narrow the focus to one, two, or three specific markets to keep advertising and promotional activities manageable. Answering the following questions begins the process of narrowing and developing a target market for a therapeutic massage business:
- Where do you plan to work?
- What potential client groups or populations are available within a half-hour drive of the location?
- What type of massage or bodywork do you enjoy giving?
- What group or type of people do you want to help most?
- How are you going to reach those potential clients?
- When do you want to be available to do massage?

By the fifth year of business, the practitioner usually has established a solid focus, a narrow target market, and a consistent clientele (Proficiency Exercise 3-9).

Marketing

Marketing encompasses the advertising and other promotional activities required to sell a product or service. Advertising is a must when starting a new business, and many forms of advertising are very costly. For massage, some types of advertising work better than others (Figure 3-7).

Word of mouth is the best advertising. Meeting people and talking with them is far more effective than other forms of advertising. Having satisfied clients who tell other potential clients about you is even better. In the beginning, the massage therapist must talk with many people to develop a client base. Building a business takes time. It is important not to become discouraged, because if you want to succeed, quitting is not an option.

The massage therapist should persist in handing out business cards and brochures and giving demonstrations until the clients are found. Placing an ad and then sitting in an office waiting for clients to call does not work. Success comes by arranging to speak at service clubs and churches in the area or by volunteering to work at local events. Businesses may want to offer a stress management class. Local school districts often have adult education classes, and short classes that teach simple massage routines are popular. Charitable organizations often have auctions, which are wonderful opportunities to give away gift certificates for massage.

Being visible in the community helps to generate business. A regular base clientele of about 100 is sufficient to support a thriving therapeutic massage business. Some clients will have weekly standing appointments, others biweekly, and the rest

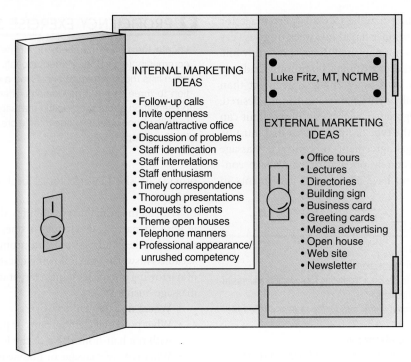

FIGURE 3-7 Internal and external marketing procedures.
(From Fritz S: *Business and professional skills for massage therapists,* St Louis, 2009, Mosby.)

💡 PROFICIENCY EXERCISE 3-10

1. Locate three different professional brochures. Evaluate them against the criteria listed in this section.
2. Develop a sample professional brochure for your future business.

will visit monthly or occasionally. It may be necessary to talk to 2000 people to find 100 clients.

The two main marketing obstacles for personal service wellness massage are:

- Convincing the public that regular massage is beneficial to a lifestyle program that focuses on managing stress and striving for wellness
- Helping would-be clients justify the fees for massage

To overcome these obstacles, it is important to provide education and an experience, such as a complimentary massage, so that potential clients understand the value of massage.

Brochure

The brochure is the primary tool for educating the public and potential clients about the services offered. It should provide the following specific information (Proficiency Exercise 3-10).

1. *The nature of the services offered.* The brochure should explain clearly that therapeutic massage is a general health service. It should state that no specific treatment of any kind is given for pre-existing physical or mental problems. It also should make clear that all specific problems of a medical, structural, psychological, or dietary nature will be referred to the appropriate licensed

professional. Written permission and supervision by a medical professional or other licensed health professional will be required in order for the massage practitioner to work with any conditions that fall within that specific scope of practice.

2. *A description of the services offered.* The brochure should give a simple explanation of the process of a massage. It should include a full description of the types of services offered and the procedures followed in rendering those services. It should explain that the client will always be properly draped or can choose to remain dressed. It should clearly state that the client may stop the session at any time and may choose not to have any area of the body touched or to have any particular technique used.

3. *The qualifications of the practitioner.* The massage professional's credentials, documenting his or her education, training, and experience, should be outlined in a manner that allows potential clients to verify the practitioner's competence. The credentials should be from a valid credentialing organization, such as a school or continuing education provider, who must maintain a record of the practitioner having completed the course.

4. *The client's financial and time investment.* The brochure must provide a realistic statement of costs and fees. It should emphasize that the effects of massage are temporary and that massage is best used as a maintenance system. The brochure should state that the massage practitioner will teach self-help to the client if requested. It also should make clear that the best results from massage are maintained when treatment is given on

a weekly or biweekly basis, and that therapeutic massage, when used only occasionally, provides only temporary effects.

5. *The client's role in health care.* The brochure should address the importance of the client's responsibility for his or her personal health care. It is important that the client realize that the massage practitioner is a facilitator in the wellness process.

Media

Media advertising is a changing environment. The best place to advertise used to be the local newspaper, but this is no longer true. With a variety of online sources, the Internet is now the main mode of advertising. Local newspapers still exist and often run stories about new and unusual businesses. Many larger papers are now delivering their product over the Internet. Media advertising (Internet, newspaper, radio, and television) is very expensive and not the best idea initially. Remember that massage is a local business. Clients typically will drive only 30 minutes to have a massage. If you are providing on-site massage service, you do not want to drive long distances. Therefore, any media marketing needs to target your local area.

When providing a story to the media, the massage professional should write his or her own draft article to prevent embarrassing mistakes. Including photographs of the professional giving a massage is a great idea. Providing the media writer, who will write the final article, with copies of other good news stories about therapeutic massage also is beneficial.

Before advertising in the *Yellow Pages* of the telephone book, which also is very expensive, the massage professional must be sure that the business location will not change for at least a year. The advertisement will be locked in for a year after the phone book has been distributed, and the contract must be paid even if the business moves. The telephone "book" is now online. It is possible to advertise in the online version and directly link to your website.

Creating a Website

The Web offers significant advantages over traditional advertising media in that it is dynamic, interactive, and relatively inexpensive. It can be used to showcase your specific skills, book appointments, and educate potential and current clients about the benefits of massage. A good website not only entices visitors, but also ensures that they keep coming back for repeat visits.

Establishing a website is an easy process. You can create your own using services offered by the professional massage organizations or hire a professional website designer. Your website should have some basic features. For example, it should:
- Load pages quickly
- Clearly identify you and your business
- Have the best template for your personality and business profile

PROFICIENCY EXERCISE 3-11

1. Locate three stories about new businesses in your area on the Internet or in the newspaper. Cut or print them out.
2. Write a media story about yourself. Include your picture.
3. Obtain three current, positive Web, magazine, or newspaper articles about therapeutic massage.
4. Design a small advertisement for your future massage business that is suitable for the Yellow Pages. Call an ad representative from your local telephone company and find out how much it would cost to run the advertisement.
5. Contact your local newspaper and ask an ad representative to help you design a display ad for your future massage business. Find out how much it would cost to run the advertisement. Repeat with Internet advertising.
6. Design the front and back of a business card.

- Be easy to navigate and read
- Have relevant content that is kept current

Make sure the website provides the name of your business and your professional name, the business's phone number and address, a link for directions, a map to your location, and brief descriptions of the types of massage skills you have. Make sure the website's directory is clear and that clients can easily find important information.

Search engine optimization (SEO) is vital for clients to find your website. You need to use keywords that apply to your business. These must be keywords that a user will enter in a search engine that make your site appear in the first page of results. Use appropriate meta-tagging for good ranking in search engines such as Google, Yahoo, and MSN. Information on these sites can help you learn about various types of optimization.

Website set-up costs and ongoing fees to maintain the website are part of business expenses. Hosting (site location) and domain (name) registration are the main costs. Domain registration costs about $10, and hosting fees can range from $10 to $25 per month. Developing a simple site is not that difficult to learn, but unless the massage professional is already skilled in website design, he or she probably would be better off hiring a professional. Various massage therapy organizations provide support for website development.

When you develop any written material or advertising, make sure you provide potential clients with the answers to these basic questions:
- Who? (You)
- What? (Therapeutic massage)
- Where? (Address and phone number)
- When? (Appointment times)
- How? (They can reach you by phone, e-mail, or Web page)

This information also should be provided on your business card. The card should be simple and direct and should not list all your credentials. It is convenient to put the information about the next appointment date on the back of the card (Proficiency Exercise 3-11).

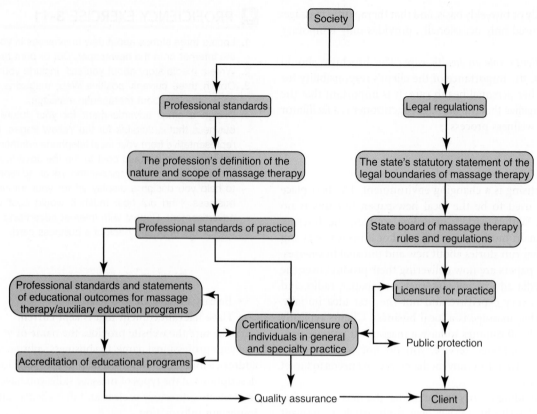

FIGURE 3-8 The pathway to licensure and quality assurance for the public.
(From Fritz S: *Business and professional skills for massage therapists,* St Louis, 2009, Mosby.)

MANAGEMENT

SECTION OBJECTIVES

Chapter objectives covered in this section:

10. The student will be able to develop a business management and record-keeping system.

Using the information presented in this section, the student will be able to perform the following:

• Use a step-by-step procedure to set up business management practices
• Set up business files
• Develop the "paper trail" required for business records
• Develop a client-practitioner agreement and statement

Management consists of all the activities required to maintain a business, particularly record keeping and financial disbursement. The KISS principle (keep it simple and specific) is an excellent concept to help organize the details of business practices. Of course, a business operation can be set up in many ways. A business consultant and an attorney usually are the best advisers. The simplest business arrangement, the sole proprietorship, is detailed in this textbook. The steps in setting up this arrangement are as follows:

1. Obtain all necessary licenses
2. Choose a business location
3. Determine the legal structure of the business
4. Register the name of the business

5. Register for tax purposes
6. Arrange for insurance
7. Open business banking accounts
8. Set up investments
9. Keep records
10. Develop a client-practitioner agreement and policy statement

(See Proficiency Exercise 3-12 at the end of this section.)

Obtaining Licenses

Massage professionals usually deal with two distinct types of licenses: professional licenses and business licenses. A professional license shows that you have achieved the skills to practice your profession. It may be issued by the state or by a local government body (see Chapter 2) and may be required for all who practice massage. Most states now license massage therapists or are in the process of developing licensure. However, difficulties occasionally arise with local licensing if state licensing is not in place. If this problem is encountered, it is important to organize a group of massage professionals and other supporters in the local community and work to change any local control that does not support massage as a profession (Figure 3-8).

If a state licenses massage practitioners, the professional usually must show proof of a certain level of education and pass some sort of licensing test. The best way to find out about licensing in any state is to contact the Department of Licensing and Regulation in the state capital. Usually the licensing department for massage is in the Occupational License Department. This agency can provide the necessary information. A business license, which is obtained from the local government, allows that government body to regulate the type and location of business operations. If a profession is licensed, the professional may need to show a copy of the license to obtain a business license. Any required forms should be filled out carefully.

Choosing a Business Location

When deciding where to locate your business, remember that each community has specific zoning regulations. These regulations protect the investment of those who own property. For example, without zoning, someone could put a junkyard next to a home. Usually the zoning that a massage business requires is general office or commercial zoning. Because of difficulties with local ordinance control of massage establishments, some restrictions may apply to locations for a massage business. To obtain this information, the practitioner should visit local government offices and ask to see the zoning ordinances.

A permit or business license may be needed. It is important that the business owner develop a good working relationship with government officials. These officials usually have a sincere concern for their communities, and the massage professional must respect this. Occasionally these officials need to be educated about therapeutic massage. Be patient, cheerful, and cooperative.

Difficulty with massage parlor ordinances has diminished substantially over the past 5 years, but the problem still exists. Hopefully, growing public awareness about therapeutic massage eventually will resolve this problem.

Determining the Legal Structure of the Business

A sole proprietorship (one-owner business) is the simplest way to set up a business. Partnerships and corporations are complicated business structures, and the need for them should be discussed with an attorney. This chapter is structured around the sole proprietorship.

Registering the Name of the Business

Registering the name of your business is known as obtaining a DBA (i.e., doing business as _____). Remember, when choosing a business name, the public's interpretation must be considered. A person who chose BODY-WORKS as a business name received calls about automotive body repair. The fee to register the name of your business is about $20, and it usually is done at the county clerk's office. The clerk will check to see whether anyone else in the county is using the name and then issue the DBA. This document may be needed to open a business checking account.

Registering for Tax Purposes

Federal, state, and local taxes must be paid. A sales tax identification number may also be needed. Information about federal taxes can be obtained from the IRS. State tax information can be obtained from the Department of the Treasury in any state. Information about local taxes can be obtained from both the county and local government offices. The IRS has many publications and counseling services that help explain the payment of business taxes. The business owner is strongly urged to seek the advice of a business attorney or certified public accountant regarding tax requirements.

One third of the gross income of a business usually is needed to cover various taxes. Gross income is the money brought into the business before any expenses have been deducted.

Tax money must be set aside every month and left untouched. One of the biggest problems new business owners have is nonpayment of taxes because the tax money was spent on overhead expenses. The best protection is to pay the government first, because the penalties are high and tax laws are difficult. A professional tax preparer can help a great deal with management of your taxes.

Arranging for Insurance

All massage practitioners need professional liability insurance, often called *malpractice insurance*. The term *malpractice* refers to professional negligence or maleficence. *Negligence* is an unintentional wrong. A negligent person fails to act in a reasonable and careful manner and consequently causes harm. *Maleficence* is causing deliberate harm. Clients expect a certain level of professional education, standards of practice, and responsibility for conduct. Unfortunately, in the highly litigious climate of today's world, the best protection against a lawsuit is insurance. Insurance reduces the risk of having a liability claim filed against you personally. To advertise this, however, only invites a lawsuit. Accurate, comprehensive records are the next best protection; anything that seems even slightly important must be documented (see Chapter 4).

The best place to obtain liability insurance is through the professional organizations. Those that have been in existence for many years are the ABMP and the AMTA. Other professional organizations for massage and bodywork professionals have been established, and careful investigation into their insurance plans is recommended. Insurance costs usually are part of the dues structure of these organizations, an arrangement that makes insurance available at a reasonable cost. Insurance also may be obtained from private companies, but it may be quite expensive.

Premise liability insurance also is needed; this is often called "trip and fall" insurance. It can be obtained through professional organizations or from a local insurance agent. Because home business offices are not covered under a homeowner's policy, additional coverage in the form of a business rider is needed. The insurance agent also can discuss fire and damage insurance on equipment.

The more complicated a business, the more comprehensive the insurance coverage must be. The sale of products requires product liability insurance. Independent contractor liability insurance protects the contractor against third-party claims from hired independent contractors, and so on. The insurance agent and the insurance representative of the professional organization can provide additional information.

Opening Business Banking Accounts

A business account can be opened at a local bank. A DBA usually is required to use a business name. All income from the business is deposited in the business account, which serves as a record of gross income. All expenses are paid from this account, which provides a record of business deductions. What is left over is called the *net income.*

If the massage professional is disciplined enough to maintain a low balance on a credit card, a business credit card is a good idea. The monthly statement is a good record of business expenses.

Income taxes are paid quarterly on the net income. A wise professional will contact a good bookkeeper or accountant to help set up the payment schedule for taxes.

After all business expenses and taxes have been covered, the massage professional may write himself or herself a paycheck (called a *draw check*). This money should be deposited in a personal account, and personal expenses can be paid from this account. Personal and business money *must not be mixed.*

Online banking has become increasingly common. When setting up business accounts, you would be wise to work with a bank representative to learn about all the available options.

Setting Up Investments

All massage professionals, whether self-employed or employed by others, should set up an individual retirement plan. After taxes have been paid, 10% of income could be invested in a long-term growth investment. A local bank or insurance company may have access to stable mutual funds. Individual retirement accounts (IRAs) also are available. Some employers offer investment plans. Money can be invested in compound interest–bearing accounts in many ways. This takes discipline, but aging is inevitable, and planning for that time now is important.

Another investment to consider is giving away one massage per week to someone who really needs it. What is given out truly does come back tenfold. Remember the equity hypothesis. This person always has something to return to the massage professional. Maybe it is only a smile of appreciation, which can be worth more than gold.

Keeping Records

All massage professionals, whether employees or self-employed, must keep accurate, comprehensive client files. The success of your professional life depends on it. Anyone who wants to manage his or her own business is advised to take some classes in small business management at a community college or to attend workshops offered by the local Chamber of Commerce. Many commercial software record-keeping systems are available. A wise course is to choose one and use it consistently. The current trend toward electronic data storage and various types of user-friendly software supports this option.

All business receipts must be saved and filed. Copies of all important documents should be stored in a location other than that of the originals. Everything must be dated. Information should be organized monthly on a spreadsheet so that when it is time for the tax preparer to do the business and personal taxes, everything can be verified. This "paper trail" is very important for a properly run business, and it must be established. Perhaps your paper trail will be an electronic trail. Make sure that backup is maintained and that hard copies of important documents are kept in a safe place.

Comprehensive client files must be kept in order (see Chapter 4). Payment records also are kept in the client files. Note whether payment was made by cash, credit card, or check. If a check is used, note the check number. If cash is paid, note the receipt number. If a monthly billing system is used, post the date the bill was sent and the date the payment was received, along with the payment form (i.e., debit or credit card or check). All credit card information should be recorded, and records must be kept current. If you must use professional liability insurance or if you are billed by a client's insurance company, the first thing the company will request is the client's records. Computer software programs are available that can manage these files for you.

Developing a Client-Practitioner Agreement and Policy Statement

It is essential to have the client read a client-practitioner agreement and policy statement (see Chapter 2). This is the document in which you set forth the professional rules for the client. People usually do quite well with information presented to them in a clear, concise, up-front way. The potential for conflict increases if the rules are not understood and agreed upon or if they are changed too often in midstream. The client-practitioner agreement and policy statement prevents conflicts by clearly stating all policies. This agreement is more comprehensive than the marketing brochure and becomes part of the informed consent process; however, it is not protection against a lawsuit. Its value is that it can:

- Clarify for the client the nature of the service rendered
- Help protect against unwarranted and unrealistic client expectations
- Serve the practitioner as a constant reinforcement of the scope and limits of his or her practice within acceptable legal parameters
- Serve as a valuable factual tool if required in court action

The agreement or policy statement should be presented in simple, easily understood language. It gives the practitioner an opportunity to define his or her practice. The practitioner-client agreement has little value if it does not accurately describe the type of service offered to the public.

⭘ PROFICIENCY EXERCISE 3-12

Using the information in this section and the following outline, develop a checklist for your personal business management plan. The first item is done as an example to get you started.

1. Obtain licenses
   - Check with the state about license requirements
   - Obtain a copy of licensing forms
   - Complete forms and return
   - Check with local government about licensing requirements for:
     - Business license
       a. Obtain copy of licensing forms
       b. Complete forms and return
     - Professional practice license or ordinance requirements
       a. Obtain copy of licensing forms
       b. Complete forms and return
2. Choose a business location
3. Establish the legal structure of the business
4. Register the name of the business
5. Register for tax purposes
6. Arrange for insurance
7. Open business banking accounts
8. Set up investments
9. Keep records
10. Develop a client-practitioner agreement and policy statement

Box 3-6	Employee "Do's" and "Don'ts"

Do
- Get to work on time
- Look and act like a professional
- Be consistent and accurate with the recording requirements of the business
- Be courteous and supportive
- Be assertive and communicate openly with your employer
- Develop a sense of commitment and loyalty to your employer
- Take your responsibilities seriously
- Improve your skills
- Own your mistakes and correct them
- Be willing to extend yourself in the short term for everyone's long-term gain
- Be a team player
- Be flexible and creative
- Use problem-solving skills to resolve potential conflict
- Commit to the job

Don't
- Gossip
- Complain without providing a viable solution
- Be dishonest
- Behave unethically
- Behave irresponsibly

HALLMARKS OF A SUCCESSFUL EMPLOYEE

SECTION OBJECTIVES

Chapter objective covered in this section:

11. The student will be able to develop skills to achieve employee success.

Using the information presented in this section, the student will be able to perform the following:
- List and describe the qualities of an excellent employee

If after reading about the responsibility of owning and managing a business you decide that you are better suited to achieving success as an employee, commit to being an excellent employee. Many employers complain about the quality and commitment of their employees. The massage/bodywork industry is no different. If you choose to be an employee, the information in this text should help you understand the commitment and responsibility required of an employer to create an environment that allows you to pursue your career as a massage professional free of business responsibilities. Study the "Do's" and "Don'ts" of a successful employee (Box 3-6) and the eight keys to employability (Box 3-7).

Recall that when applying for a therapeutic massage position, you must submit a résumé and a personal list of career expectations for the job. It is important to understand the job description, the hours that will be spent on the job, and obligations to the employer—and it is vital to get all this in writing, along with any special arrangement that may be made. This document should be signed and dated by all parties involved so that everyone has an original copy. The job interview

may include performing a massage session as a skills test (Figure 3-9).

Once you have obtained a massage therapy position, commit to career growth. You need to please the clients, improve your skills, and build relationships with people at work. In other words, you have to be an excellent employee with a good work ethic. When you do this, you invest in yourself. You develop excellent work habits one day at a time, one behavior at a time. Attitude is more than a state of mind. It's the way you look at life. Employers want friendly people with positive attitudes, and you learn to think positively about yourself by doing positive things. Make yourself valuable, and you will be valued.

SUMMARY

This chapter is full of details, regulations, requirements, obligations, paperwork, and responsibilities. Someone once said that the job is not complete until the paperwork is done. Be sure to do the paperwork and use professional help in business where necessary. Success takes time; it does not usually happen overnight. Persistence, flexibility, and determination are your keys to a successful business practice. Make your goals realistic and keep your professional dreams before you to fuel your motivation to strive for success. Define success not only by the amount of money you make, but also by the value obtained from providing professional therapeutic massage services. Take care of yourself to prevent professional burnout so that you can continue to serve your clients in this wonderful and needed profession.

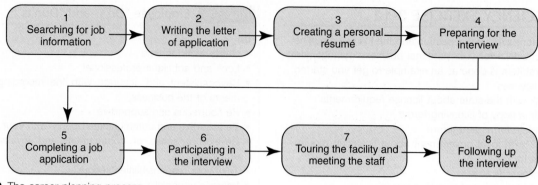

FIGURE 3-9 The career planning process.
(From Fritz S: *Business and professional skills for massage therapists,* St Louis, 2009, Mosby.)

Box 3-7   Eight Keys to Employability

1. Personal Values
Valued workers:
- Are honest
- Have good self-esteem and a positive self-image
- Have personal and career goals
- Demonstrate emotional stability
- Exhibit a good attitude
- Are self-motivated
- Do not limit themselves

2. Problem-Solving and Decision-Making Skills
Valued workers:
- Are flexible
- Are creative and innovative
- Can adapt to changing demands of a job
- Can reason and make objective decisions
- Can keep their mind on several parts of a job at a time

3. Relations with Other People
Valued workers:
- Work well with peers
- Accept authority and supervision
- Accept constructive criticism
- Are team members
- Are friendly
- Are consistent in their relations with people
- Are cooperative
- Accept assignments pleasantly
- Are tactful
- Accept all types of people
- Respect the property of other people
- Have leadership qualities

4. Communication Skills
Valued workers:
- Ask relevant questions
- Seek help when needed
- Notify supervisors of absences and the reason for the absences
- Clearly express themselves when talking
- Listen actively and communicate comprehension

5. Task-Related Skills
Valued workers:
- Complete work on time
- Can follow directions

- Are not distracting or distractible
- Work neatly and leave the work environment clean and orderly
- Care for equipment and materials
- Are accurate
- Constantly improve their performance

6. Maturity
Valued workers:
- Work well without supervision
- Are reliable and dependable
- Accept responsibility
- Don't let their personal problems interfere with their work
- Are willing to perform extra work and work overtime
- Are always prepared for work
- Show pride in their work
- Show initiative
- Remain calm and self-controlled
- Accept responsibility for their own behavior, including mistakes and successes
- Demonstrate maturity
- Evaluate their own work accurately
- Are patient and tolerant
- Use time wisely
- Are assertive when necessary
- Show self-confidence

7. Health and Safety Habits
Valued workers:
- Observe safety and sanitation rules
- Practice good personal hygiene
- Dress appropriately and are well groomed
- Are in good health
- Practice stress management

8. Commitment to the Job
Valued workers:
- Are punctual and have good attendance records
- Observe all organization policies
- Consider work more than a job
- Are interested and enthusiastic
- Obtain relevant continuing education

Modified from TTG Consultants: www.ttgconsultants.com. Accessed July 14, 2010. This information was provided courtesy of David Bowman, chairman of TTG Consultants/ Lincolnshire, a Los Angeles-based, full-service human resource consulting firm.

PROFICIENCY EXERCISE 3-13

Develop your personal lists of pros and cons for self-employment and employee status.

Self-Employment

Pros	Cons

Employee Status

Pros	Cons

Both self-employment and working for someone else are viable avenues for success. Each has its pros and cons. It is important to make good decisions about what is best for you (Proficiency Exercise 3-13). Initially, commitment to being an excellent employee can provide you with valuable experience without all the additional responsibilities of maintaining a business structure. Whatever path you choose, commit to excellence.

FOOT IN THE DOOR

The ability to manage the details of the business of massage adds to your potential for success. If your career path leads you to work as an employee, you not only will need to attend to your own business but also support those in the office or clinic who manage the business details. Stop for a moment and consider the responsibilities of the office manager, receptionist, bookkeeper, accountant, marketing manager, and those who maintain the facility. Wow! How do all the bills get paid and the floors stay clean? Think about your massage school and all the tasks that need to be done just so you can learn about massage therapy in a clean, pleasant environment.

Clients expect a well-run business. As an employee, you will want to work for a well-run business; if you decide on self-employment, you will need to maintain a well-run business. When considering what door you want your foot in, evaluate the attention the organization pays to the effectiveness of the business.

evolve

http://evolve.elsevier.com/Fritz/fundamentals/
3-1 Try a career options matching exercise
3-2 Review examples of a business card, résumé, and brochure.
3-3 Build your business vocabulary with a crossword puzzle.
3-4 Quiz yourself on sole proprietorship.
Don't forget to study for your certification and licensure exams! Review questions for this chapter can be found on the Evolve website.

Workbook Section

Short Answer

1. Why is motivation so important in building a massage business?

2. Why is it important for a massage professional to explore individual strengths and weaknesses when developing a business?

3. What is burnout and how can it be prevented?

4. Why is it important to develop a good résumé?

5. What is a business plan?

6. What are start-up costs?

7. What are the most effective marketing and advertising strategies?

8. What is the importance of a brochure?

9. How do you set fees?

10. What is real time?

11. What are the prospects of obtaining medical insurance reimbursement for personal service massage?

12. What are the three main types of business opportunities available for the massage professional?

13. What is the KISS principle and why is it important?

14. What types of insurance does the massage professional need?

15. What is the importance of record keeping?

16. Why is the client-practitioner agreement and policy statement so important?

17. Why does everyone in a business, including employees, need to understand the business's operations?

Client-Practitioner Agreement and Policy Statement

In developing a client-practitioner agreement and policy statement, you need to be specific about certain types of information. For each of the following sections, provide the information a client needs to know. When you are done, you will have a comprehensive outline to use in creating a booklet. Use Box 2-8 the text as a guide. For example, the text says to explain the type of work you provide. You should list therapeutic massage, reflexology, or whatever it is that you do. Some of the answers for this section are samples you can use to compare with your responses; others are a reiteration of the information that you will need to detail.

1. The nature of the service offered

   _____
   _____
   _____
   _____
   _____

2. Description of the service offered

   _____
   _____
   _____
   _____
   _____

3. Qualifications of the practitioner

_____
_____
_____
_____
_____

4. Client financial and time investment

_____
_____
_____
_____
_____

5. Role of the client in health care

_____
_____
_____
_____
_____

6. Types of service

_____
_____
_____
_____
_____

7. Practitioner's training and experience

_____
_____
_____
_____
_____
_____

8. Appointment policies

_____
_____
_____
_____
_____

9. Client and practitioner expectations and informed consent

_____
_____
_____
_____
_____

10. Fees

_____
_____
_____
_____
_____

11. Sexual appropriateness

_____
_____
_____
_____

12. Recourse policy

_____
_____
_____
_____
_____

Problem-Solving Scenarios

1. Tom is notified that a client is unhappy with his massage fees and is considering finding another massage professional with lower fees. What steps can Tom take to support his fee structure?

2. Marilyn is having a meeting with a client who she feels may have difficulty understanding the scope of practice of massage. How can she use the client-practitioner agreement and policy statement booklet to help establish professional boundaries and obtain informed consent?

3. Calculate real time required to learn massage. Include actual class time, travel time, homework time, and so on.

4. After graduation Terry begins a private massage practice. Business begins to build slowly but then levels off. Word-of-mouth advertising is not working as well as expected. What steps can Terry take to boost business?

Assess Your Competencies

Now that you have studied this chapter, you should be able to:
- Determine your personal motivation for pursuing a career in therapeutic massage
- Develop an effective résumé
- Interview effectively
- List the pros and cons of independent and employee status
- Explain client retention
- Describe the process for setting fees, determining income, and doing insurance billing
- Develop career plans
- Identify the responsibilities of business ownership
- Design a marketing strategy and advertising materials for a massage business
- Develop a business management and record-keeping system
- Identify the responsibilities of business ownership
- Develop skills to achieve employee success

Pretend you have been asked to present a short course on business practices. Develop a course outline based on this content. Compare with other students in small groups.

Professional Applications

1. A client calls about receiving a massage. You speak with her on the phone and offer to send her your client policies and procedures booklet. Two weeks later

you still have not heard from the prospective client. You make a follow-up telephone call, and the client has specific questions about certain aspects of the policy booklet. This client tells you that a previous massage therapist did not have all these rules. What would you do?

2. List three things that motivated you to become a massage practitioner.

3. Define the following concepts as they relate directly to you.

Know thyself

Follow your dream

Whatever we believe with emotion and feeling becomes our reality

Believe in your product

Provide a quality product

4. Develop a personal application of methods to prevent burnout. Call it the Burnout Plan or give it some other clever name. List one idea for each of the following areas.

Care of physical needs

Support person

Care of spiritual needs

Continuing education

Getaway time

5. The business structure of therapeutic massage takes many forms. Working as a massage employee is different from working as a self-employed massage professional. Choose which approach you plan to pursue and list the areas of this chapter that most directly pertain to your professional development plan.

6. List five business goals. Use the following five recommendations for goal setting (from Box 3-4) as a guide:

1. State goals in the present tense
2. Make sure your goals are realistic and attainable
3. Speak positively
4. Set target deadlines for yourself
5. Make sure your goals are small steps toward your ultimate plan

   - For each goal, *circle* any portion that meets the first recommendation.
   - *Underline* any portion that meets the second recommendation.
   - *Put a box around* any portion that meets the third recommendation.
   - *Double underline* any portion that meets the fourth recommendation.
   - *Double circle* any portion that meets the fifth recommendation.

Example:
I will (1,3) complete this exercise (2,5) within the next 30 minutes (4).

Research for Further Study

1. Compare the business procedures outlined in the text to those of another business operation; identify both similarities and differences in those procedures.

2. The statement "business is business" applies to massage. List resources in your area for further business education, such as community college courses, the Chamber of Commerce, and so forth.

Massage and Medical Terminology for Professional Record Keeping

CHAPTER 4

CHAPTER OBJECTIVES

After completing this chapter, the student will be able to perform the following:

1. Use massage terminology as presented by the Massage Therapy Body of Knowledge (MTBOK)
2. Use medical terminology to identify the three word elements used in medical terms and comprehend unfamiliar medical terms
3. Use anatomic and physiologic terminology for bones, joints, and muscles
4. Use anatomic and physiologic terminology for the nervous, cardiovascular, lymphatic, and immune systems
5. Use anatomic and physiologic terminology for the respiratory, digestive, endocrine, and integumentary systems
6. Use the information in this chapter for effective professional record keeping

CHAPTER OUTLINE

KEY TERMS

Abbreviations	Modality
Assessment	Motor tone
Body, mind, and spirit	Muscle tone
Bodywork	Nomenclature
Care or treatment plan	Patient
Charting	Physical agent
Client	Prefix
Client records	Progress or session notes
Clinical massage	Qualifiable
Contraindication	Quantifiable
Database	Root word
Deep tissue	SOAP notes
Deep tissue work/massage	Soft tissues
Discipline	Special tests
Documentation	Standards of care
Goals	Standards of practice
Indication	Suffix
Language	Taxonomy
Massage therapist	Technique
Massage therapy	Terminology
Medical massage	Therapeutic process
Mobilization	Wellness

Using agreed-upon terms to describe massage therapy has become ever more important as massage therapists increasingly interact with all types of health care professionals. In addition, a common language can help the general public better understand the purposes and benefits of massage therapy. Until the development of the *Massage Therapy Body of Knowledge (MTBOK)* in 2010, numerous terms and definitions were used to describe the same or very similar massage methods or skills. However, this confused legislators, clients, educators, students, and people in general. Fortunately, the MTBOK document has provided an example of a massage therapy language that we all can learn to speak.

The study of medical terminology provides a key to understanding the accepted language of the sciences. As massage therapy continues to move into the position of a medically valid service, the massage professional will find it increasingly important to be able to speak, write, and understand scientific language. In addition, the massage professional must be able to maintain client records accurately. The ability to record information accurately and concisely depends on correct use of terminology and an organized approach to charting procedures. This chapter provides an outline of the medical terminology most often encountered by the massage professional, particularly as it relates to charting and record-keeping procedures.

The chapter also consolidates the vast array of medical terminology, focusing on the elements specifically useful to the massage professional. You can master the information in this chapter more easily if you also use a medical terminology textbook, a medical dictionary, and the Internet. It is important to develop skills in using medical dictionaries, medication reference books, and other reference materials for several reasons. The expanding and changing knowledge base of health care makes it almost impossible for one to remember all the details required for professional practice. This chapter includes a list of the terms most often encountered by the massage professional. Definitions for these words are available in a medical terminology text or medical dictionary, and you can reinforce your learning by looking them up. Exploring medical terminology automatically provides an overview of anatomy and physiology. Although this section is not meant to replace an anatomy and physiology text, it provides a quick reference for record-keeping and charting skills.

Used with a standard anatomy and physiology textbook and class instruction, this section can help the student or professional focus on information specific to the field of massage. The recommended anatomy and physiology text is *Mosby's Essential Sciences for Therapeutic Massage: Anatomy, Physiology, Biomechanics, and Pathology,* fourth edition, by Sandy Fritz (Mosby, 2013), which was developed specifically for therapeutic massage students. However, the information in this chapter can be used with any comprehensive anatomy and physiology book.

The information presented here is especially pertinent to an understanding of massage as it relates to anatomy, physiology, pathology, and client records. Because the basis for medical terminology is scientific language, understanding this information will help massage students understand massage therapy research, in addition to articles and books on subjects related to massage. Learning the names of muscles, bones, joints, and other anatomic structures lays a firm foundation for understanding and correctly using medical terminology.

MASSAGE THERAPY TERMINOLOGY

SECTION OBJECTIVES

Chapter objective covered in this section:
1. Use massage terminology as presented by the *Massage Therapy Body of Knowledge (MTBOK)*

| Box 4-1 | **How We Communicate** |

Language is made up of socially shared rules that include the following:
- Sounds and symbols that convey meaning
- Word definitions—vocabulary
- Ability to make new words
- Agreed upon sequences of words used to communicate —grammar
- **Terminology:** language specific to a specialized knowledge; i.e. medical terminology.
- **Taxonomy:** the science of classification according to a pre-determined system
- **Nomenclature:** a system of names; a *vocabulary* is a system of names with explanations of their meanings; a *classification* is a systematic organization of things

---

Using the information presented in this section, the student will be able to perform the following:
- Define terms used in the creation of the MTBOK document

Agreement on terminology across different medical fields is important. Without a common language, we cannot communicate. For example, massage professionals must be able to communicate with their clients in a common language that both can understand. It is equally important that they be able to communicate with other health professionals.

This chapter offers a basis for agreement on terminology for the massage profession; this must occur before others in the health profession can communicate with us as a group. As mentioned in Chapter 1, Per Henrik Ling had difficulty communicating with the established authorities of his time because he did not speak their language. To receive the respect and understanding of other health professionals, we as massage professionals must explain ourselves in terms other health professionals understand and respectfully educate them in our language (Box 4-1).

Even with the MTBOK document, the terminology used in massage therapy is still inconsistent. Although similar words are used, the meanings of those words do not always coincide. The definitions for the massage therapy vocabulary in this textbook are based on traditional definitions, Canadian resources, currently available books, common knowledge, and the MTBOK document.

One of the goals of the MTBOK document is to provide a standardized nomenclature for massage therapy. More than 200 bodywork methods fall into the category of massage therapy. Fundamentally, very little difference exists among the various massage styles. As noted in Chapter 2, the fragmentation and confusion created by the splintering of massage therapy terminology is a major obstacle in the professional development of massage. The terms and definitions provided by the MTBOK document provide a common ground for a language for massage. The MTBOK document, which was crafted from a vast pool of resources, is available at www.mtbok.org. (To support classroom discussion, part of the document is presented in Box 4-2.)

Box 4-2 Terminology Defined by the *Massage Therapy Body of Knowledge (MTBOK)**

The MTBOK task force believed it was necessary to set down definitions of certain terms for the following reasons, including but not limited to:

- Assisting readers to develop a uniform approach to understanding the MTBOK document and any questions with which they may be concerned
- Helping to establish a common terminology to reduce any misunderstanding
- Clarifying commonly used terms thought to be misused in the field of massage therapy
- Defining terms for which there seems to be a lack of clarity on the way the terms are used in the field

The vocabulary presented defines how the MTBOK stewards and task force intended the meaning of the terms in the MTBOK document only. The value of this work helps the greater profession begin the process of developing a unified language.

Assessment An appraisal or evaluation of the condition of a client/patient that may be based on some or all of the following: the health and medical history, the individual's account of signs and symptoms, the primary health care provider's current diagnosis, functional data gathered from information provided on written intake forms, observation, palpation, range of motion, movement, and special tests as applicable and that help determine a person's ability to perform everyday tasks and activities of daily living.

Body, mind, and spirit The three primary, interrelated, interacting, and integrated layers that comprise a healthy, balanced, and unified human being. *Mind* includes the thoughts, feelings, and emotions (psychology) and self-awareness. *Body* refers to the three-dimensional structure and functions of the 11 systems that make up the physical body. *Spirit,* the most underlying layer of the three, is responsible for organizing, catalyzing, and enlivening both the mind and body. It includes that aspect that senses a connection to the higher or a deeper meaning in life and the fundamental vitality that animates all human life. When one or more of these layers is out of balance because of some physical, psychological, and/or spiritual reason, a human is considered to be in a state of "dis-ease." Acknowledging the mind/body/spirit connection, the massage therapy profession holds that massage therapy treatment can lead to improved health outcomes by facilitating the balance and connection of body, mind and spirit.

Bodywork A term used in complementary and integrative medicine (CIM) to describe any therapeutic, healing, or personal self-development practice, which may include massage, touch, movement, or energetic work. One form of bodywork is massage therapy, and the terms *massage therapy* and *bodywork* frequently are used interchangeably. However, although bodywork includes all forms of massage therapy, it also includes many other types of touch and incorporates many other skills and techniques to enhance awareness of the mind/body/spirit connection.

Client A recipient of a service, be it from a wellness or a health care professional, regardless of his or her health status. All patients are clients, but not all clients are patients.

Clinical massage Massage therapy practice that involves more extensive use of assessment and also the use of specific, focused techniques and applications with the intention of achieving clinical treatment or functional outcomes and

remediation of symptoms; also referred to as *treatment massage, orthopedic massage,* or medical massage.

Deep tissue The tissues beneath superficial structures that are being treated. This term is commonly misused to describe a specific technique.

Deep tissue work/massage A generic term commonly used to describe a variety of techniques to address specific deep tissues and structures, regardless of the force/pressure exerted or the level of discomfort/pain experienced during and/or resulting from the application.

Discipline An area of study with shared concepts and vocabulary (e.g., Swedish massage, sports massage, myofascial release).

Massage therapy equivalent or related terms Terms that mean the same thing as *massage;* they also include *therapeutic massage, body massage, myotherapy, massotherapy, body rub, massage technology, bodywork, bodywork therapy, somatic therapy,* or any derivation of these terms. Massage therapy may be assumed to be bodywork, but not all bodywork is massage therapy.

Massage therapist equivalent or related terms Terms that mean the same thing as *massage practitioner;* they also include *massage technologist, massage technician, masseur, masseuse, myotherapist, massotherapist, bodyworker, bodywork therapist, somatic therapist,* or any derivation of these terms. Massage therapists may be assumed to be bodyworkers, but not all bodyworkers are massage therapists. *Note:* Some regional regulations make distinctions between these terms to recognize differences in training and/or scope of practice.

Mobilization The process of making a fixed part movable or releasing stored substances, as in restoring motion to a joint, freeing an organ, or making available substances held in reserve in the body, such as glycogen or fat.

Modality A method of application or the employment of any physical agents and devices. This term is commonly misused to describe forms of massage (e.g., NMT, myofascial, Swedish).

Physical agent Tools or materials used in the application of therapeutic modalities. They consist of energy and materials applied to the client/patient to assist in the achievement of the person's therapeutic goals. Physical agents are classified as thermal (e.g., hot and cold packs), mechanical (e.g., manual traction, compression by pressurized water or compressive bandages, ultrasound), and electromagnetic (e.g., infrared heating, ultraviolet radiation, laser, transcutaneous electrical nerve stimulation [TENS]). Use of ultrasound, diathermy, ultraviolet radiation, laser, and TENS are beyond a massage therapist's scope of practice unless the therapist has separate training and certification that permits use of these agents.

Soft tissues The skin, fascia, adipose tissue, muscles, tendons, ligaments, joint capsules, cartilage, bursae, myofascial tissue, blood, blood vessels, lymph, lymph vessels, interstitial fluids, synovial fluids, cerebrospinal fluids, nerves, and periosteal tissues.

Special tests Methods used to assess for the presence of and to determine the degree of a condition in a client/patent. These assessments commonly involve specific stressing of particular structures.

Continued

Box 4-2   Terminology Defined by the *Massage Therapy Body of Knowledge (MTBOK)*—cont'd

Standards of care Treatment guidelines developed by the profession for a given condition, which identify appropriate treatment based on scientific evidence and clinical experience. In legal terms, standards of care represents the degree of prudence and caution a professional having appropriate training and experience would practice. This relates to fiduciary responsibility, scope of practice, and informed consent.

Standards of practice Standards for the practice of a profession that members of that profession or organization are expected to adopt. These standards usually include guiding principles related to professionalism, legal and ethical requirements, confidentiality, documentation, client/patient records, business practices, boundaries, hygiene, and safety.

Supportive environment An environment in which the therapist provides support and loving kindness within clear and appropriate boundaries, free from judging, enabling, caretaking, or counseling.

Technique A procedure or skill used in massage therapy, including but not limited to the following:

- *Compression:* The use of compressive force without slip. The force, which can vary in depth and pressure, commonly is applied at a 90-degree angle to the tissue and followed by a lift or release of force.
- *Friction:* Strokes that rub one surface over another with little to no surface glide, providing both compressive and shearing forces. Pressure may be superficial (light) to deep, providing friction effects between various tissue levels. Examples of friction may include warming, rolling, wringing, linear, stripping, cross-fiber, chucking, and circular. Most friction strokes are administered with little or no lubricant.
- *Gliding/stroking (effleurage):* Gliding movements that contour to the body. The pressure may be either superficial (light) or deep. Variations may include one-handed, two-handed, alternate-hand, forearm, and nerve strokes.
- *Holding:* Holding tissue without movement and with little or no force or weight in the contact.
- *Kneading (pétrissage):* Lifting, rolling, squeezing, and releasing of tissue, most commonly using rhythmic, alternating pressures. Variations may include one-handed, two-handed, alternate-hand, pulling, and skin rolling.
- *Lifting:* Strokes that entail pulling tissue up and away from its current position.
- *Movement and mobilization (stretching, traction, range of motion, and gymnastics):* Strokes that entail shortening and/or lengthening of soft tissues with movement at one or more joints. Variations include active movement (the client/patient moves structures without the therapist's help); passive movement (the therapist moves structures without the help of the client/patient); resistive movement (the client/patient moves structures against resistance provided by the therapist); and active assisted movement (the client/patient moves structures with support and assistance from the therapist).
- *Percussion (tapotement):* Alternating or simultaneous rhythmic striking movement of the hands against the body, allowing the hand to spring back after contact, controlling the impact. Hand surfaces commonly used include the ulnar surface of the hand, tips or flats of the fingers, open palm, cupped palm and back ulnar surface, knuckles, or the sides of a loosely closed fist. Technique variations may include tapping, pincement, hacking, cupping, slapping, beating, pounding, and clapping.
- *Vibration:* Shaking, quivering, trembling, swinging, oscillating, or rocking movements most commonly applied with the fingers, the full hand, or an appliance. Variations may include fine or coarse vibration, rocking, jostling, or shaking. The speed varies from slow to rapid.

Therapeutic process The capacity of the musculoskeletal system (and other body systems) to self-correct, come into balance, and achieve equilibrium through the skillful normalization of tissue tone by a massage therapist. Therapeutic processes are time dependent and may be noticed within one massage. They usually are noticeable in other body systems after several massage sessions. A therapeutic process may or may not lead to healing.

Treatment planning The documented process of determining a treatment plan to address the therapeutic goals of the client/patient. The treatment plan is based on the current condition, health history, intake interview, and the findings of assessment procedures. Assessment procedures may include postural and movement observations, palpation, objective evaluations (e.g., range of motion), and special tests. The therapist's clinical reasoning skills, scope of practice, training, and experience, in addition to the interests, concerns, and informed consent of the client/patient, influence the planning process. An integrated treatment planning process may involve working with a health care team to ensure that all health care providers for a particular client/patient understand each other's treatment goals and that these goals are complementary.

Wellness The condition of optimum physical, emotional, intellectual, spiritual, social, and vocational well-being. The concept of wellness is holistic at its core, encompassing the whole person. Several models have been developed to depict the concepts of wellness.

Modified from Massage Therapy Body of Knowledge (MTBOK) stewards: *Massage Therapy Body of Knowledge (MTBOK)*, version 1.0, section 300. www.mtbok.org. Accessed June 5, 2010.

MEDICAL TERMINOLOGY

SECTION OBJECTIVES

Chapter objective covered in this section:

2. Use medical terminology to identify the three word elements used in medical terms and to comprehend unfamiliar medical terms.

Using the information presented in this section, the student will be able to perform the following:

- Define words by breaking them down into their word elements
- Use Appendix A to identify indications for and contraindications to massage
- List and define anatomic and physiologic terms by body system
- Identify pertinent abbreviations used in health care and their meanings
- List and identify common abbreviations
- Use relevant anatomic and physiologic terminology correctly

Evolve Activity 4-1

Fundamental Word Elements

Medical terms are made up of a combination of word elements. A word can be interpreted easily by separating it into its elements: *prefix, root word,* and *suffix.*

Prefixes

A prefix is a word element placed at the beginning of a word to alter its meaning (Table 4-1). A prefix cannot stand alone; it must be combined with a root word.

Root Words

The root word provides the fundamental meaning of a term (Table 4-2). Combinations of root words, prefixes, and suffixes form medical and scientific terms. A vowel, called a *combining vowel,* often is added when two root words are combined or when a suffix is added to a root word; the combining vowel usually is *o* and occasionally *i.*

Suffixes

A suffix is a word element placed at the end of a root word to alter the meaning of the word (Table 4-3). Suffixes cannot stand alone; like prefixes, they must accompany a root word. The suffix should be the starting point for interpreting medical terms.

Root words that end in a consonant require a combining vowel. If the root word ends in a vowel and the suffix begins with a vowel, the vowel at the end of the root word is deleted.

Combining Word Elements

Word elements are the building blocks that are combined to create medical and scientific terms. Prefixes always precede root words, and suffixes always follow root words (Proficiency Exercise 4-1).

Table 4-1   **Common Prefixes**

Prefix	Meaning	Prefix	Meaning
a-, an-	Without or not	intro-	Into, within
ab-	Away from	leuk-	White
ad-	Toward	macro-	Large
ante-	Before, forward	mal-	Bad, illness, disease
anti-	Against	mega-	Large
auto-	Self	micro-	Small
bi-	Double, two	mono-	One, single
circum-	Around	neo-	New
contra-	Against, opposite	non-	Not
de-	Down, from, away from, not	para-	Abnormal
dia-	Across, through, apart	per-	By, through
dis-	Separation, away from	peri-	Around
dys-	Bad, difficult, abnormal	poly-	Many, much
ecto-	Outer, outside	post-	After, behind
en-	In, into, within	pre-	Before, in front of, prior to
endo-	Inner, inside	pro-	Before, in front of
epi-	Over, on	re-	Again
eryth-	Red	retro-	Backward
ex-	Out, out of, from, away from	semi-	Half
hemi-	Half	sub-	Under
hyper-	Excessive, too much, high	super-	Above, over, excess
hypo-	Under, decreased, less than normal	supra-	Above, over
in-	In, into, within, not	trans-	Across
inter-	Between	uni-	One
intra-	Within		

Table 4-2   **Common Root Words**

Root (Combining Vowel)	Meaning	Root (Combining Vowel)	Meaning
abdomin (o)	Abdomen	neur (o)	Nerve
aden (o)	Gland	ocul (o)	Eye
adren (o)	Adrenal gland	orth (o)	Straight, normal, correct
angi (o)	Vessel	oste (o)	Bone
arterio (o)	Artery	ot (o)	Ear
arthr (o)	Joint	ped (o)	Child, foot
broncho (o)	Bronchus, bronchi	pharyng (o)	Pharynx
card, cardi (o)	Heart	phleb (o)	Vein
cephal (o)	Head	pnea	Breathing, respiration
chondr (o)	Cartilage	pneum (o)	Lung, air, gas
col (o)	Colon	proct (o)	Rectum
cost (o)	Rib	psych (o)	Mind
crani (o)	Skull	pulm (o)	Lung
cyan (o)	Blue	py (o)	Pus
cyst (o)	Bladder, cyst	rect (o)	Rectum
cyt (o)	Cell	rhin (o)	Nose
derma	Skin	sten (o)	Narrow, constriction
duoden (o)	Duodenum	stern (o)	Sternum
encephal (o)	Brain	stomat (o)	Mouth
enter (o)	Intestines	therm (o)	Heat
fibro (o)	Fiber, fibrous	thorac (o)	Chest
gastr (o)	Stomach	thromb (o)	Clot, thrombus
gyn, gyne, gyneco	Female	thyr (o)	Thyroid
hem, hema, hemo, hemat (o)	Blood	toxic (o)	Poison, poisonous
hepat (o)	Liver	trache (o)	Trachea
hydr (o)	Water	ur (o)	Urine, urinary tract, urination
hyster (o)	Uterus	urethr (o)	Urethra
ile (o), ili (o)	Ileum	urin (o)	Urine
laryng (o)	Larynx	uter (o)	Uterus
mamm (o)	Breast, mammary gland	vas (o)	Blood vessel, vas deferens
my (o)	Muscle	ven (o)	Vein
myel (o)	Spinal cord, bone marrow	vertebr (o)	Spine, vertebrae
nephr (o)	Kidney		

Table 4-3 Common Suffixes

Suffix	Meaning
-algia	Pain
-asis	Condition, usually abnormal
-cele	Hernia, herniation, pouching
-cyte	Cell
-ectasis	Dilation, stretching
-ectomy	Excision, removal of
-emia	Blood condition
-genesis	Development, production, creation
-genic	Producing, causing
-gram	Record
-graph	Diagram, recording instrument
-graphy	Making a recording
-iasis	Condition of
-ism	Condition
-itis	Inflammation
-logy	Study of
-lysis	Destruction of, decomposition
-megaly	Enlargement
-oma	Tumor
-osis	Condition
-pathy	Disease
-penia	Lack, deficiency
-phasia	Speaking
-phobia	Exaggerated fear
-plasty	Surgical repair or reshaping
-plegia	Paralysis
-rrhage, -rrhagia	Excessive flow
-rrhea	Profuse flow, discharge
-scope	Examination instrument
-scopy	Examination using a scope
-stasis	Maintenance, maintaining a constant level
-stomy, -ostomy	Creation of an opening
-tomy, -otomy	Incision, cutting into
-uria	Condition of the urine

💡 PROFICIENCY EXERCISE 4-1

On a separate piece of paper, combine five words using the prefixes, root words, and suffixes listed in Tables 4-1 to 4-3. Define the words created. Then look up each word in a medical dictionary to verify that it exists and that you have the correct meaning and spelling.

Example

Term: Fibromyalgia

Divided into elements: *Fibro-*, fiber; *my-*, muscle; *algia-*, pain

My definition: Pain in muscle fibers

Dictionary definition: Diffuse muscle pain

Abbreviations

Abbreviations are shortened forms of words or phrases (Table 4-4). They are used primarily in written communication to save time and space. An extensive list of acceptable medical abbreviations can be found in most medical dictionaries.

Table 4-4 Common Abbreviations

Abbreviation	Meaning	Abbreviation	Meaning
abd	Abdomen	IBW	Ideal body weight
ADL	Activities of daily living	ICT	Inflammation of connective tissue
ad lib	As desired	id	The same
alt dieb	Every other day	L	Left, length, lumbar
alt hor	Alternate hours	lig	Ligament
alt noct	Alternate nights	M	Muscle, meter, myopia
AM (am, a.m.)	Morning	ML	Midline
AMA	Against medical advice	meds	Medications
ANS	Autonomic nervous system	n	Normal
approx	Approximately	NA	Nonapplicable
as tol	As tolerated	OB	Obstetrics
BM	Bowel movement	OTC	Over the counter
BP	Blood pressure	P	Pulse
Ca	Cancer	PA	Postural analysis
CC	Chief complaint	PM (pm, p.m.)	Afternoon
c/o	Complains of	PT	Physical therapy
CPR	Cardiopulmonary resuscitation	Px	Prognosis
CSF	Cerebrospinal fluid	R	Respiration, right
CVA	Cerebrovascular accident, stroke	R/O	Rule out
DM	Diabetes mellitus	ROM	Range of motion
DJD	Degenerative joint disease	Rx	Prescription
Dx	Diagnosis	SOB	Shortness of breath
ext	Extract	SP, spir	Spirit
ft	Foot or feet	Sym	Symmetric
fx	Fracture	T	Temperature
GI	Gastrointestinal	TLC	Tender loving care
GU	Genitourinary	Tx	Treatment
h (hr)	Hour	URI	Upper respiratory infection
H_2O	Water	WD	Well developed
Hx	History	WN	Well nourished

When you use abbreviations in any type of record, including charting, provide an abbreviation key either on the forms or in a conspicuous place in the file. This is especially important if you generate a specialized list of abbreviations, such as *SWM* for Swedish massage or *CTM* for connective tissue method.

Abbreviations should not be used excessively. An overabundance of abbreviations results in a passage that is difficult to read and that requires interpretation. If you are unsure whether an abbreviation is acceptable, write out the term to communicate accurately.

Do not use jargon. Jargon consists of word forms specially developed within a system or the use of existing words that have other definitions besides the dictionary meaning. For example, the word *mouse* is computer jargon for a manual device that controls a cursor. Many forms of jargon are used in the bodywork world, a problem that continues to confuse communication. In general, the words used in record keeping should be found in either a standard comprehensive dictionary or in a medical dictionary, and they should represent the definition as listed.

Sometimes jargon becomes understandable within the general community. For example, for the previous example, *mouse,* many readers immediately thought of the computer device rather than a brown, furry creature. This is an example of the way language can change. As massage becomes more generally accepted, much of our language will be standardized and lose its jargon quality. Until then, clarity and concise expression are crucial when choosing the words used for written records.

Terms Related to Diagnosis and Diseases

The massage practitioner must be able to understand medical terms related to diagnosis and various diseases. Two terms related to the diagnosis of a disease that massage professionals often encounter are *indication* and *contraindication.*

- An **indication** is a condition for which an approach would be beneficial for health enhancement, treatment of a particular condition, or support of a treatment modality other than massage.
- A **contraindication** is a condition or factor that may make an approach harmful. Contraindications may be further subdivided by severity:
  - General avoidance of application: Do not massage.
  - Regional/local avoidance of application: Perform massage but avoid a particular area.
  - Application with caution and adaptation, usually requiring supervision from appropriate medical or supervising personnel: Perform massage but carefully select the type of methods to be used, the duration of application, the frequency, and the intensity of the massage.

Terminology of Location and Position
Directional Terms

Directional terms are used to describe the way one body part relates to another. Massage professionals must be able to use directional terminology to describe the location of an area of the body accurately. The directional terms in Figure 4-1 are used most often.

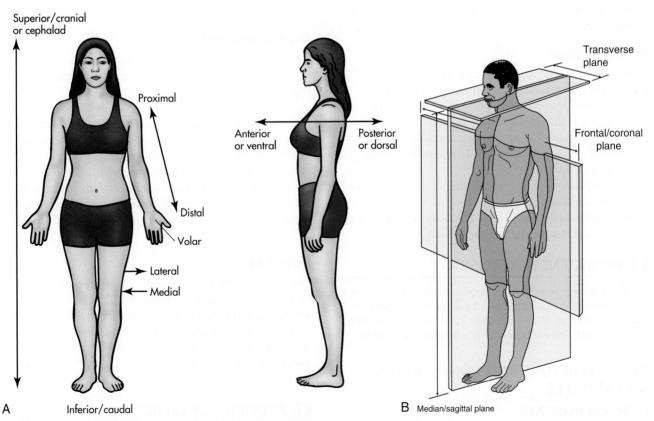

FIGURE 4-1 Anatomic position as a reference point for directional terms **(A)** and anatomic planes **(B)**.
(From Fritz S: *Mosby's essential sciences for therapeutic massage: anatomy, physiology, biomechanics, and pathology,* ed 3, St Louis, 2008, Mosby.)

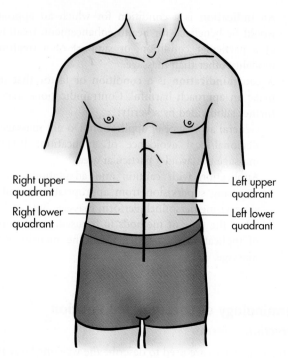

FIGURE 4-2 The quadrants of the abdomen. (From Fritz S: *Mosby's essential sciences for therapeutic massage: anatomy, physiology, biomechanics, and pathology,* ed 3, St Louis, 2008, Mosby.)

The abdomen is divided into four quadrants, and the locations of abdominal organs and the abdominal contents are described in terms of the quadrants in which they are found (Figure 4-2).

Positional Terms

Positional terms are used to describe the relationship of the body to the different planes (Proficiency Exercise 4-2):

- *Anatomic position*—The body is erect with the arms hanging at the sides and the palms facing forward.
- *Erect position*—The body is in a standing position.
- *Supine position*—The body is lying in a horizontal position, face up.
- *Prone position*—The body is lying in a horizontal position, face down.
- *Lateral recumbent position*—The body is lying horizontally on either the right or the left side.

💡 PROFICIENCY EXERCISE 4-2

1. Act out each directional and positional term by creating a movement or a pantomime or by assuming the position.
2. With a partner, place each other in the five positions listed in the text. Say each term as you position your partner.

BODY STRUCTURE AND BONES, JOINTS, AND MUSCLES

SECTION OBJECTIVES

Chapter objective covered in this section:

3. Use anatomic and physiologic terminology correctly for bones, joints, and muscles.

Using the information presented in this section, the student will be able to perform the following:

- Define and list tissues of the body
- Define organs and systems of the body
- Locate body cavities and regions of the trunk
- Describe tissues and structures of the skeletal system
- Describe joint structure and function
- Perform synovial joint movement
- Identify the structures of skeletal muscle
- Describe the functions of skeletal muscle
- Define the actions of skeletal muscles

Tissues

The structure of the body is composed of tissues. A *tissue* is a collection of specialized cells that perform a special function. *Histo* is a root word meaning "tissue." *Histology* is the study of tissue. The primary tissues of the body are the epithelial, connective, muscular, and nervous tissues (Proficiency Exercise 4-3).

💡 PROFICIENCY EXERCISE 4-3

Using a medical terminology text, anatomy and physiology textbook, or medical dictionary, look up each of the following tissue types and list its function:

connective:

epithelial:

muscular:

nervous:

Organs and Systems

An *organ* is a collection of specialized tissues. An organ has specific functions, but it does not act independently of other organs.

Organs make up systems. The body as a whole is made up of several systems. Some of the systems are concentrated in a particular part of the body (e.g., the urinary system), whereas others involve all parts of the body (e.g., the circulatory system). The body has 10 general systems (Table 4-5). Each system is made up of organs that collectively perform specific functions. (A more extensive description of these systems can be found in any good anatomy and physiology textbook.)

Body Cavities

The body cavities, which contain the organs, are divided into ventral and dorsal regions (Figure 4-3). The two dorsal cavities are the cranial cavity and the vertebral cavity. The three ventral cavities are the thoracic, abdominal, and pelvic cavities. Sometimes the abdominal and pelvic cavities are considered as one cavity (Proficiency Exercise 4-4).

💡 PROFICIENCY EXERCISE 4-4

Using clay or some other modeling compound, form the body cavities and the organs and structures they contain.

Table 4-5	Systems of the Body and Their Important Organs and Systems
System	**Important Organs**
Musculoskeletal (can be classified separately as the skeletal, articular [joints], and muscular systems)	Bones, ligaments, skeletal muscles, tendons, joints
Nervous	Brain, spinal cord, nerves, special sense organs
Cardiovascular	Heart, arteries, veins, capillaries
Lymphatic	Lymphatic vessels, lymph nodes, spleen, tonsils, thymus gland
Digestive	Mouth, tongue, teeth, salivary glands, esophagus, stomach, small and large intestines, liver, gallbladder, pancreas
Respiratory	Nasal cavity, larynx, trachea, bronchi, lungs, diaphragm, pharynx
Urinary	Kidneys, ureters, urinary bladder, urethra
Endocrine	Endocrine glands: Hypothalamus, hypophysis (pituitary), thyroid, thymus, parathyroid, pineal, adrenal, pancreas, gonads (ovary or testis)
Reproductive	*Female:* Ovaries, uterine tubes (oviducts), uterus, vagina *Male:* Testes, penis, prostate gland, seminal vesicles, spermatic ducts
Integumentary	Skin: hair, nails, sebaceous glands, sweat glands, breasts

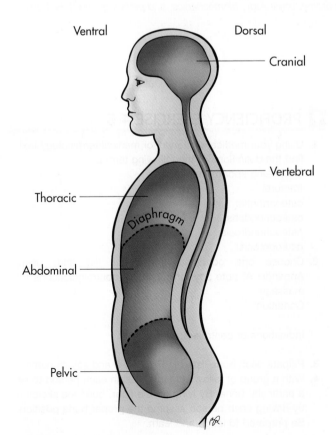

FIGURE 4-3 The body cavities.

Posterior Regions of the Trunk

The back, or posterior, surface of the trunk is divided into regions. The terms used to describe these regions are related to the names of the vertebrae in the spinal column (Figure 4-4). In descending order they are:

- Cervical region: The neck (seven cervical vertebrae)
- Thoracic region: The chest (twelve thoracic vertebrae)
- Lumbar region: The loin (five lumbar vertebrae)
- Sacral region: The sacrum (five sacral vertebrae, which are fused into one bone)
- Coccyx: The tailbone (four coccygeal vertebrae, which are fused into one bone)

Skeletal System

The skeletal system is composed of three types of tissue: bone, cartilage, and ligaments.

Bone

Bone is a dense connective tissue composed primarily of calcium and phosphate; *os-, ossa-, oste-,* and *osteo-* are all combining forms that mean "bone."

The human skeleton is composed of approximately 206 bones, and massage professionals must be familiar with most of them. Terms commonly used for some of these bones include *skull* or *cranium, cervical vertebrae, thoracic vertebrae, lumbar vertebrae, sacral vertebrae, coccygeal vertebrae, ribs, sternum, manubrium, body, xiphoid process, clavicle, scapula, humerus, ulna, radius, carpal bones, metacarpal bones, phalanges, pelvis, ilium, ischium, pubis, femur, patella, tibia, fibula, tarsal bones,* and *metatarsal bones* (see Figure 4-4; also Figure 4-5). Other terms related to bones and landmarks on bones are *malleolus, process, crest, insertion, joint, olecranon, origin, spine, trochanter,* and *tuberosity.*

Cartilage

The skeletal system includes two types of cartilage. *Hyaline cartilage,* which is very elastic, cushiony, and slippery, makes up the articular surfaces at the joints; the cartilage between the ribs and at the nose, larynx, and trachea; and the fetal skeleton. It has a pearly, bluish color. The term *hyaline* means "glass." *White fibrocartilage,* which is elastic, flexible, and tough, is interarticular fibrocartilage found in joints such as the knee. The connecting fibrocartilage is cartilage that is only slightly mobile. It is found between the vertebrae (referred to as *disks*) and between the pubic bones (the symphysis pubis).

Ligaments

A *joint* or an *articulation* is a point where the bones of the skeleton meet. Movable joints are covered by cartilage and are held together by ligaments. Ligaments are made of white fibrous tissue. They are pliant, flexible, strong, and tough (Proficiency Exercise 4-5).

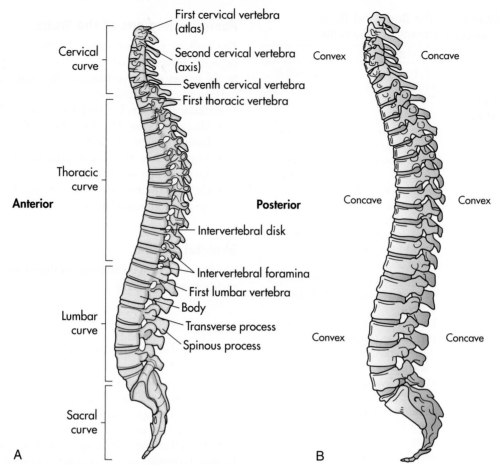

FIGURE 4-4 A, Vertebral column. **B,** The convex and concave curves of the vertebral column. (From Fritz S: *Mosby's essential sciences for therapeutic massage: anatomy, physiology, biomechanics, and pathology,* ed 3, St Louis, 2008, Mosby.)

Articular System

As mentioned, articulations are joints where two or more bones meet. The articular system concerns all of the anatomic and functional aspects of the joints.

Joints

Joints are places where bones come together, where limbs are attached, and where the motion of the skeletal system occurs. Some joints are rigid, and some allow a great degree of flexibility. The joints allow motion of the musculoskeletal system, bear weight, and hold the skeleton together.

Terms related to the articular system include *articulation, flexibility, synarthrodial, amphiarthrodial, diarthrodial, symphysis pubis, sacroiliac, symphysis, articular cartilage, articular disks, ligaments, synovial fluid,* and *tendon.*

Types of Movement Permitted by Diarthrodial Joints

Movement related to joints is described from the standard anatomic position. The types of movement permitted by diarthrodial/synovial (freely movable) joints include the following (Figure 4-6):

PROFICIENCY EXERCISE 4-5

1. Using your medical dictionary or medical terminology text, find the definitions of the following terms:
   ankylosing spondylitis:
   fracture:
   osteoarthritis:
   osteochondritis:
   osteochondrosis:
   osteoporosis:
2. Choose one condition from your list and, using Appendix A, note any indications or contraindications for massage.
   Condition:

   Indications or contraindications:

3. Palpate each bone listed in Figure 4-5 and say its name.
4. With a group of fellow students, assign each person to be a particular bone. By lying on the floor, build the skeleton by having each person assume the proper bone position. Be prepared to laugh and learn.

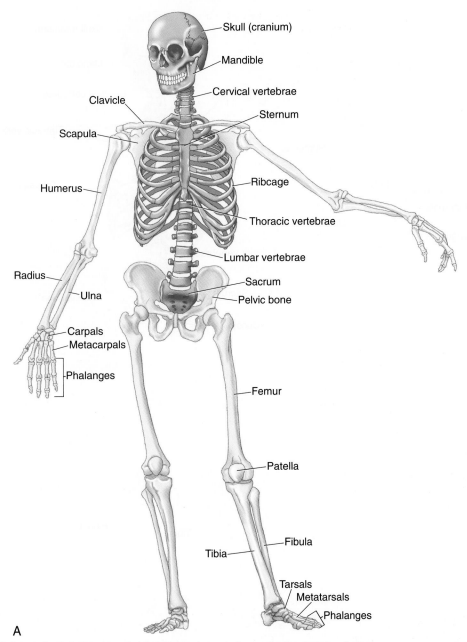

FIGURE 4-5 **The skeleton. A,** Anterior view. Axial skeleton *(green).* Appendicular skeleton *(beige).*

Continued

- Flexion: Movement that reduces the angle of a joint
- Extension: Movement that increases the angle of a joint
- Abduction: Movement away from *(ab-)* the midline
- Adduction: Movement toward *(ad-)* the midline
- Pronation: Turning of the palm downward
- Supination: Turning of the palm upward (you can hold a bowl of soup in a supinated hand)
- Eversion: Turning *(-version)* of the sole of the foot away from *(e-)* the midline (when you evert your foot, you move your little toe toward your ear)
- Inversion: Turning *(-version)* of the sole of the foot inward *(in-)*
- Plantar flexion: Movement of the plantar surface of the sole of the foot downward (plant your toes in the ground)

- Dorsiflexion: Movement of the top or dorsal surface of the foot toward the shin
- Rotation: Rolling to the side (internal rotation is rolling toward the midline; external rotation is rolling away from the midline)
- Circumduction: Making a cone; the ability to move the limb in a circular manner
- Protraction: Thrusting a part of the body forward *(pro-)*
- Retraction: Pulling a part of the body backward *(re-)*
- Elevation: Raising a part of the body
- Depression: Lowering a part of the body
- Opposition: Placing one part of the body opposite another, as in placing the tip of the thumb opposite the tips of the fingers

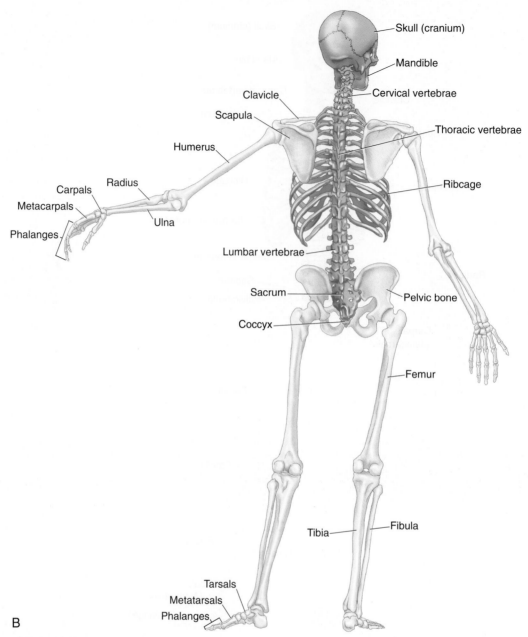

FIGURE 4-5, cont'd B, Posterior view. Axial skeleton *(green).* Appendicular skeleton *(beige).*
(From Muscolino JE: *Kinesiology: the skeletal system and muscle function,* enhanced edition, St Louis, 2007, Mosby.)

Bursae

A *bursa* is a closed sac or saclike structure. *Bursae* usually are found close to joint cavities. The lining of bursae often is similar to the synovial membrane lining of a true joint. Some bursae are continuous with the lining of a joint. The function of a bursa is to lubricate an area between skin, tendons, ligaments, or other structures and bones where friction otherwise would develop (Proficiency Exercise 4-6).

Muscular System

The muscular system is made up of contractile tissues. The three types of muscle tissue are cardiac muscle, smooth muscle, and skeletal muscle.

Many of the body's organs contain muscle tissue. Muscle tissue also makes up the muscles, which are themselves organs. Muscles give the body shape and produce movement. Muscle function is determined by the shape and location of the muscle and by the density and pliability of all the fluid, fibers, and connective tissue of the muscles; the term **muscle tone** is used to describe this aspect of muscle. The nervous system also controls how long or short a muscle is by regulating the degree of muscle fiber contraction; this is called **motor tone** (Figures 4-7 and 4-8).

Skeletal Muscle

Each skeletal muscle is made up of sections. Most muscles have two ends (proximal and distal), which are attached to other structures, and a belly. Muscles create the potential for

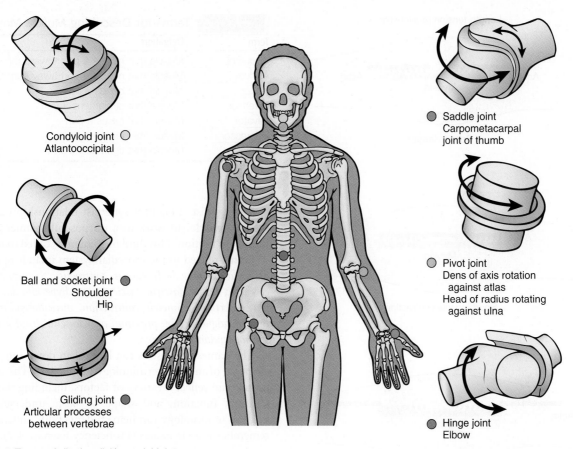

FIGURE 4-6 Types of diarthrodial/synovial joints.

💡 PROFICIENCY EXERCISE 4-6

1. Using your medical dictionary or medical terminology text, find the definitions of the following terms and write them down on a separate sheet of paper.
   ankylosis
   arthritis
   bursitis
   degenerative joint disease
   diastasis
   dislocation
   ganglion cyst
   genu valgum
   genu varum
   gout
   hallux malleus
   kyphosis
   lordosis
   rheumatoid arthritis
   scoliosis
   slipped disk
   spinal curvature
   spondylolisthesis
   sprain
   subluxation
   tendinitis
   tenosynovitis
2. Choose one condition from your list and, using Appendix A, note any indications or contraindications for massage.
3. Do a dance that incorporates each of the joint movements listed in this section. Call out the movement terms as the joint is moved.

motion by creating a pulling force. Joints allow motion to occur.

Muscles cause and permit motion by the actions of contraction and relaxation. Table 4-6 presents a list of terms used to describe the movements of different types of muscles.

Contraction is the reduction in size or shortening of a muscle. When one muscle contracts, another, opposite muscle is stretched and put in a state of tension. *Relaxation* occurs when tension is reduced, which allows the muscle to return to its resting length.

Muscles work in pairs of agonists and antagonists. *Agonists* are muscles responsible for the primary desired movement. The agonist is the prime mover, which shortens to produce movement. *Antagonists* are the muscles that oppose the action of the agonist and lengthen and control the movement produced by the agonist.

Synergists are muscles that assist the agonists by holding a part of the body steady, thereby providing leverage. In some cases synergists also produce the same action as the prime mover.

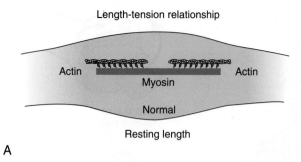

Length-tension relationship

Actin   Actin
Myosin
Normal
Resting length

A

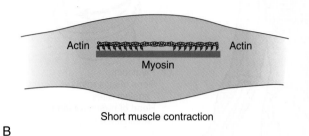

Actin   Actin
Myosin

Short muscle contraction

B

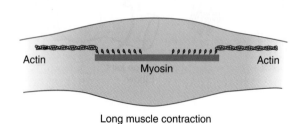

Actin   Actin
Myosin

Long muscle contraction

C

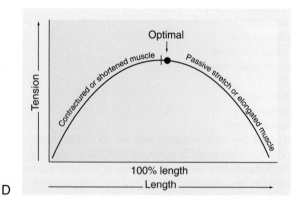

Optimal

Tension

Contracted or shortened muscle / Passive stretch or elongated muscle

100% length
Length

D

FIGURE 4-7 Length-tension relationship. **A,** Normal resting length. When a muscle is stimulated to contract, actin is in an appropriate position to attach to myosin, causing maximum contraction. **B,** Short muscle. Contraction ability is limited, because actin has no space to "crawl" and cause contraction. **C,** Long muscle. Contraction ability is limited, because actin is too far away to attach to myosin to begin contraction. **D,** Optimum length-tension relationship.
(From Fritz S: *Sports and exercise massage: comprehensive care in athletics, fitness, and rehabilitation,* St Louis, 2006, Mosby.)

Table 4-6	Terms for Describing Muscle Movement
Term	**Definition**
Adductor	Muscle that moves a part toward the midline
Abductor	Muscle that moves a part away from the midline
Flexor	Muscle that bends a part
Extensor	Muscle that straightens a part
Levator	Muscle that raises a part
Depressor	Muscle that lowers a part
Tensor	Muscle that tightens a part

Evolve Activity 4-4

The agonist-antagonist-synergist relationship permits the skeletal muscles to work in a purposeful manner and gives fluidity to motion. This fluid movement is called *coordination.*

Terms related to the muscular system include *aponeurosis, asthenia, atrophy, belly, clonus, contracture, cramp, concentric, eccentric, fascia, fascicle, fasciculation, hyperkinesia, hypertrophy, insertion, isometric contraction, musculotendinous junction, myalgia, origin, proximal attachment, distal attachment, spasm, tendon,* and *tone.*

The names of muscles can be broken down into the word elements of medical terminology (Table 4-7). The name of a muscle can reflect a variety of factors, including the muscle's location, function, and shape. A basic understanding of medical terminology can help students both understand and remember muscle names (Proficiency Exercise 4-7).

💡 PROFICIENCY EXERCISE 4-7

1. Locate a more complete list of muscles in your anatomy and physiology textbook or medical dictionary. Break down five muscle names not listed in this section into their word elements. (You will need a medical terminology book or medical dictionary or both to complete this exercise.)
   Example: Auricularis superior: *Aur-* means ear; *ar-* means pertaining to; *superior* means above or upward.
   a.
   b.
   c.
   d.
   e.
2. An excellent way to remember the names of muscles is to make up ridiculous sentences that explain listed muscle names. The crazier these sentences are, the better you will remember them. Use this memory aid as you study muscles in your anatomy and physiology classes.
   Examples
   Rectus femoris: Part of the quadriceps muscle that is straight (rectus) and lies near the femur (femoris)
   Memory aid: Attention rectus! Straighten up, and the other three of you in the quads head out to the femur.
   Flexor carpi ulnaris: Muscle that flexes (flexor) the wrist (carpi) and hand and is attached to the ulna (ulnaris)
   Memory aid: Help! There is a big carp pulling my wrist into flexion. It has my ulna in its mouth and my hand has it around the gills.

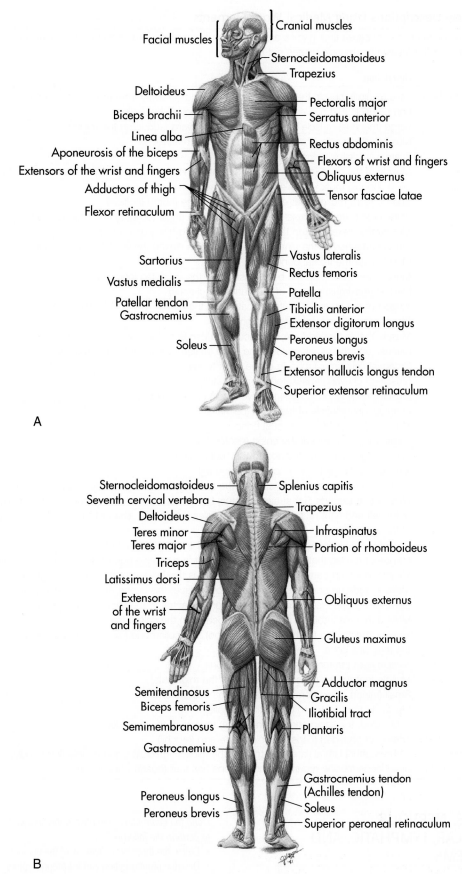

FIGURE 4-8 The muscular system. **A,** Anterior view. **B,** Posterior view.
(From LaFleur Brooks M: *Exploring medical language: a student-directed approach,* ed 5, St Louis, 2002, Mosby.)

Table 4-7   Muscle Descriptions Using Medical Word Elements

The muscles listed have been chosen because their names are made up of common word elements. After learning this list, the student should be able to figure out the meaning of muscle names not listed.

Muscle	Description
Abductor digiti minimi pedis	Little (minimi) muscle that moves the little toe (digit) away from (abductor) the midline of the foot (pedis)
Adductor longus	Long muscle that moves the leg toward (adductor) the midline
Adductor magnus	Large (magnus) muscle that moves the leg toward (adductor) the midline
Biceps brachii	Muscle with two (bi-) heads (ceps) in the arm (brachii)
Deltoid	Triangular (deltoid) muscle of the shoulder
Dilatator naris posterior	Muscle of the nose (naris) that opens (dilator) the back (posterior) portion of the nostril
Extensor hallucis longus	Long (longus) muscle that extends (extensor) the great toe (hallucis)
Extensor pollicis brevis	Short (brevis) muscle that extends (extensor) the thumb (pollicis)
External oblique	Outermost (external) muscle that extends at an angle (oblique) from the ribs to the pelvis at the iliac crest
Flexor carpi radialis	Muscle that flexes (flexor) the wrist (carpi) toward the radius (radialis)
Flexor carpi ulnaris	Muscle attached to the ulna (ulnaris) that flexes (flexor) the wrist (carpi) and hand
Frontalis	Muscle over the frontal bone
Gastrocnemius	Muscle that makes up the belly (gastroc) of the lower leg (nemius)
Gluteus maximus	Largest (maximus) muscle of the buttocks (gluteus)
Gluteus medius	Muscle of the buttocks (gluteus) that lies in the middle (medius) between the other gluteal muscles
Gracilis	Slender (gracilis) muscle of the thigh
Iliopsoas	Muscle that is formed from the iliacus and psoas major muscles; the iliacus extends from the iliac bone (iliacus), and the psoas major is the large (major) muscle of the loin (psoas)
Latissimus dorsi	Broadest (latissimus) muscle of the back (dorsi)
Masseter	Muscle of chewing (masseter) or mastication
Orbicularis oculi and oris	Muscles circling (orbicularis) the eye (oculi) or mouth (oris)
Palmaris longus	Long (longus) muscle of the palm (palmaris)
Pectineus	Muscle of the pubic (pectineus) bone
Pectoralis major	Large (major) muscle of the chest (pectoralis)
Peroneus longus	Long (longus) muscle attached to the fibula (peroneus)
Plantaris	Muscle that flexes the foot (plantaris) and leg
Pronator teres	Long round (teres) muscle that turns the palm downward into a prone (pronator) position
Rectus abdominis	Muscle that extends in a straight (rectus) line upward across the abdomen (abdominis); the center border of the left and right rectus abdominis muscles in the linea alba or the white (alba) line (linea) at the midline of the abdomen
Rectus femoris	Part of the quadriceps muscle that is straight (rectus) and lies near the femur (femoris)
Sartorius	Muscle of the leg that enables a person to sit in a cross-legged tailor's (sartorial) position
Semimembranosus	Muscle made up partly (semi-) of membranous tissue; part of the hamstring group
Semitendinosus	Muscle made up partly (semi-) of tendinous tissue; this is one of the hamstring muscles
Serratus anterior	Sawtooth-shaped (serratus) muscle in front of (anterior) the shoulder and rib cage
Soleus	Muscle that resembles a flat fish (sole) located in the calf of the leg
Sternocleidomastoid	Muscle attached to the breastbone (sterno), the collarbone (cleido), and the mastoid (mastoid) process of the temporal bone
Temporalis	Muscle over the temporal (temporalis) bone
Tensor fascia lata	Muscle that tenses (tensor) the fascia of the thigh (lata)
Teres minor	Small (minor) round (teres) muscle that moves the arm
Tibialis anterior	Muscle in front (anterior) of the tibia (tibialis)
Trapezius	Four-sided, trapezoid-shaped (trapezius) muscle of the shoulder
Triceps brachii	Three- (tri-) headed (ceps) muscle of the arm (brachii)
Vastus lateralis, medialis, intermedialis	Large (vastus) lateral (lateralis), toward the midline (medialis), and middle (intermedialis) muscles of the quadriceps muscle group; the quadriceps has four (quadri-) heads (ceps)

BODY SYSTEMS: NERVOUS, CARDIOVASCULAR, LYMPHATIC, AND IMMUNE SYSTEMS

SECTION OBJECTIVES

Chapter objective covered in this section:

4. Use anatomic and physiologic terminology correctly for the nervous, cardiovascular, lymphatic, and immune systems.

Using the information presented in this section, the student will be able to perform the following:

- Define the three basic divisions of the nervous system
- Describe proprioception and list proprioceptors
- Define reflexes
- Describe the function of the nervous system
- List and define the structures of the cardiovascular system
- Explain blood pressure

- Describe the functions of the lymphatic system
- List and describe the structures of the lymphatic system
- Locate the lymph plexuses
- Explain the main function of the immune system
- Define immunity

Nervous System

The nervous system is the most complex system in the body. The information presented here on the workings of this system is very general, although the text expands upon it where needed. Study of the nervous system is very important for the massage professional. Serious students of massage challenge themselves to study the nervous system in depth.

For purposes of study, terms related to the nervous system are presented in the following three groups:
- The central nervous system (CNS)
- The peripheral nervous system (PNS)
- The autonomic nervous system (ANS)

Central Nervous System

The CNS is the center *(central)* of all nervous control. It consists of the brain and spinal cord, which are located in the dorsal cavity (cranial and vertebral).

Peripheral Nervous System

The PNS is composed of cranial and spinal nerves. The term *nerve* refers to a bundle of nerve fibers consisting of individual nerve cells outside the spinal cord or brain. The PNS consists of the nerves that carry impulses between the CNS and muscles, glands, skin, and other organs located outside (peripheral) the CNS. The ANS is the part of the peripheral nervous system that exerts nervous control over smooth muscle, heart muscle, and glands. Individual nerve cells are called neurons. The two types of nerve cells are the sensory neurons and the motor neurons.

Spinal Nerves

The 31 pairs of spinal nerves are attached to the spinal cord along almost its entire length. They are named for the region of the spinal column through which they exit. Many of the spinal nerves are located in groups called *somatic nerve plexuses.* The term *somatic* refers to the body wall; these nerve plexuses contain nerves that are involved with the wall of the body rather than the organs in the body. A *plexus* is a network of intertwined (plexus) nerves. The major plexuses of spinal nerves are the cervical plexus, brachial plexus, lumbar plexus, and sacral plexus.

Autonomic Nervous System

The ANS is an automatic, or self-governing (self *[auto]*, governing *[nomic]*), system. It also is called the *involuntary system,* because the effects of the ANS are not usually under voluntary control. The ANS is divided in two parts: the sympathetic division and the parasympathetic division.

The sympathetic division controls the body's response to feelings *(sympath).* Because the nerves in this division come off the thoracic and lumbar segments of the spinal cord, the sympathetic division sometimes is called the *thoracolumbar division.* Actions resulting from these nerves include the fight-or-flight and fear responses. The reaction of some organs includes an increase in the heart rate, dilation of the pupils, and an increase in adrenaline secretion. A person may sometimes exhibit great strength as a result of a sympathetic response.

The nerves in the parasympathetic division come off the cranial and sacral segments of the spinal cord; therefore, this division sometimes is called the *craniosacral division.* The parasympathetic division generally causes effects opposite *(para-)* those caused by the sympathetic system. These effects include constriction of the pupils, the return of the heart rate to normal, and stimulation of the lacrimal glands to produce tears.

The intertwined *(plexus)* nerves of the ANS are called the *autonomic plexuses.* Examples of these are the cardiac plexus (the intertwined nerves of the heart *[cardiac]*) and the celiac plexus (the intertwined nerves of the organs of the abdomen *[celiac]*). The celiac plexus sometimes is called the *solar plexus* because of the sunray *(solar)* fashion in which the nerves exit the plexus.

Proprioception

Proprioception is the kinesthetic sense. Sensory receptors receive information about position, rate of movement, contraction, tension, and stretch of tissues through distortion of and pressure on the sensory receptor. After proprioceptive sensory information is processed in the CNS, motor impulses carry the response message back to the muscles. The muscles then contract or relax to restore or change posture, movement, or position. Proprioception maintains motor tone in muscle.

Terms related to proprioception include *mechanoreceptor, Golgi tendon organ, joint kinesthetic receptors, kinesthetic,* and *muscle spindle cells.*

Reflex

A *reflex* is an involuntary body response to a stimulus. Important reflexes stimulated by massage are crossed-extension, extensor thrust, flexor withdrawal, gait, intersegmental, monosynaptic, nociceptive, optical righting, ocular pelvic, pilomotor, psychogalvanic, postural, proprioceptive, righting, startle, stretch, tendon, tonic neck, vasomotor, and visceromotor reflexes.

Function of the Nervous System

The function of the nervous system is to receive impressions from the external environment, organize the information, and provide appropriate responses. In other words, the nervous system allows the body to react to outside influences (environment). Outside information enters the nervous system through nerve endings in the skin and in special sense organs. These nerve endings are referred to as *receptors.*

Nerve endings in the skin are sensitive to pain, touch, pressure, vibration, and temperature. Special sense nerve endings are responsible for taste, smell, vision, hearing, and sense of position and movement. Sensations from the environment are picked up by these receptors and sent to the CNS by way of the PNS. The CNS sorts out the information and

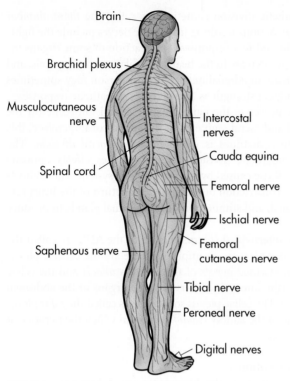

FIGURE 4-9 A simplified view of the nervous system. (Modified from LaFleur Brooks M: *Exploring medical language: a student-directed approach*, ed 5, St. Louis, 2002, Mosby.)

Labels: Brain, Brachial plexus, Musculocutaneous nerve, Spinal cord, Saphenous nerve, Intercostal nerves, Cauda equina, Femoral nerve, Ischial nerve, Femoral cutaneous nerve, Tibial nerve, Peroneal nerve, Digital nerves

PROFICIENCY EXERCISE 4-8

1. On a separate piece of paper, list five of the disease conditions of the nervous system described in the indications and contraindications section in Appendix A.
2. Choose one condition from your list and, using Appendix A, note any indications or contraindications for massage.
3. Choose one of the reflexes and look it up in a medical dictionary. Define the term and then write down how you think that reflex is implicated during massage.

Example

Reflex: Psychogalvanic

Definition: *Psycho-* relates to the mind and *galvanic* pertains to electricity.

Implication: This reflex involves changes in electrical activity in the body connected with mind processes or thoughts. In the galvanic skin response, changes in electrical activity are related to the activity of the sweat glands. Massage stimulates both the skin and electrical activity in the body, which in turn may influence the mind.

sends back a message, again by way of the PNS. Information is transferred from one nerve to another by chemicals called *neurotransmitters.*

The nervous system and neurotransmitters, along with the endocrine system, also maintain the internal environment, or the balance of the many activities in the body (homeostasis). Although the divisions of the nervous system may be treated independently, they do not function independently (Figure 4-9).

Terms Related to Nerves

Afferent nerves are nerves that carry (*ferent*) messages to (*af-,* variation of *ad-*) the CNS; they also are known as *sensory nerves* because they pick up and transmit sensation (*sen*) (Proficiency Exercise 4-8).

Efferent nerves are nerves that carry (*ferent*) messages away from (*ef-,* variation of *ex-*) the brain, resulting in motion (*motor*). They also are known as *motor nerves.*

Cranial nerves are the 12 pairs of nerves that arise from the brainstem in the cranium or skull (*cranial*).

Spinal nerves are the 31 pairs of nerves that branch off the spinal cord.

A *ganglion* is a mass of nerve cell bodies located outside the CNS (the plural form is *ganglia*). *Neuro* is the root word meaning "nerve."

Cardiovascular System

The cardiovascular system consists of two parts, the heart and the blood vessels (Figure 4-10). The *heart* is a four-chambered pump. *Arteries* are tubes (vessels) that deliver oxygenated

blood to the body. They carry blood under pressure and are located relatively deep in the body. *Veins* are vessels that return the blood to the heart. They are located in more superficial areas and therefore are easier to palpate. Veins have a valve system that prevents the backflow of blood. Breakdown of a valve may result in a varicose vein. *Capillaries* are very small, thin vessels (usually one cell thick) that allow the exchange of blood gasses and nutrients. Blood vessels *vasoconstrict* (become smaller inside) and *vasodilate* (become larger inside).

Blood pressure is a measurement of the pressure exerted by the circulating volume of blood on the walls of the arteries, veins, and heart chambers. Blood pressure is maintained by the complex interaction of the homeostatic mechanisms of the body. Normal blood pressure varies according to age, size, and gender, but the average is approximately 120 mm Hg during systole and 70 mm Hg in diastole. High blood pressure is called *hypertension,* and low blood pressure is called *hypotension.*

Blood is composed of blood cells, platelets, and a clear, yellow fluid called *plasma.* The main functions of blood are to transport oxygen and nutrients to the cells and to remove carbon dioxide and other waste products. The amount of blood in muscle tissue influences the muscle tone. If muscle tissue contains too much blood, it is said to be *congested,* and methods to encourage blood flow are used.

Terms and combining forms that relate to the cardiovascular system include *angio-, artery, arteriole, blood pressure, bruise, capillary, edema, phleb-, vasoconstriction, vasodilation, vein,* and *venule* (Proficiency Exercise 4-9).

Lymphatic System

The lymphatic system is responsible for several functions, such as the following:

- It returns vital substances, such as plasma protein, to the bloodstream from the tissues of the body. The fluid around the cells in tissues is called *interstitial fluid.*
- It helps maintain fluid balance by draining fluid from body tissues.

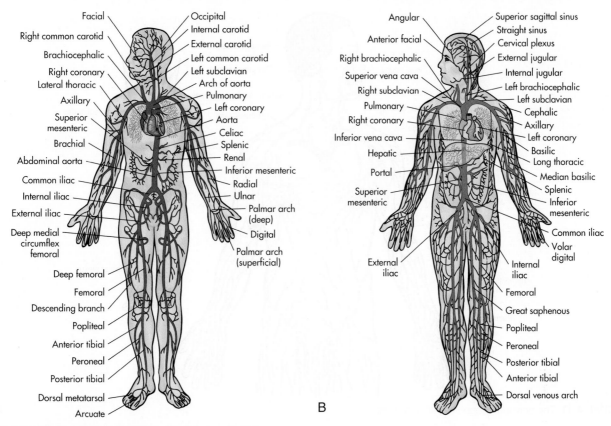

FIGURE 4-10 The systemic circulation. **A,** Arteries. **B,** Veins.
(Modified from Seidel HM et al: *Mosby's guide to physical examination*, ed 5, St. Louis, 2003, Mosby.)

💡 PROFICIENCY EXERCISE 4-9

1. List five of the disease conditions of the cardiovascular system described in the indications and contraindications section in Appendix A.
2. Choose one condition from your list and, using Appendix A, note any indications or contraindications for massage.
3. Look up the medication classification *anticoagulant* in Appendix C and in a pharmacology reference text or online. List the contraindications and side effects of these medications. Also describe possible contraindications to massage for a client or patient taking an anticoagulant medication.
4. Choose a partner and draw the major arteries and veins on the body with washable markers. Target those on the arms and legs. Use red for arteries and blue for veins. Note that you can almost trace the veins because they are located near the surface of the body.

- It aids the body's defense against disease-producing substances.
- It aids the absorption of fats from the digestive system.

The lymphatic system is a network of channels and nodes in which a substance called *lymph* travels (Figure 4-11). Lymph is a clear, watery fluid similar to plasma. The system collects and drains fluid from around tissue cells from different areas of the body and carries it through the lymphatic channels back to the venous system. There it is deposited, mixed with venous blood, and recirculated.

Lymphatic capillaries are found near and parallel to the veins that carry blood to the heart. The ends of the lymphatic capillaries meet to form larger lymph vessels. The lymph

Table 4-8	Types of Lymph Nodes
Nodes	**Description**
Parotid	Nodes around (para-) or in front of the ear (otid)
Occipital	Nodes over the occipital bone at the back of the head
Superficial cervical	Nodes close to the surface (superficial) of the neck (cervic)
Subclavicular	Nodes under (sub-) the collarbone (clavicular)
Hypogastric	Nodes in the area beneath (hypo-) the stomach (gastric)
Facial	Nodes draining the tissue in the face
Deep cervical	Deeply (deep) situated nodes in the neck (cervic)
Axillary (superficial)	Nodes in the armpit (axilla)
Mediastinal	Nodes in the mediastinal section of the thoracic cavity
Cubital	Nodes of the elbow (cubit)
Para-aortic	Nodes around (para-) the aorta (aortic)
Deep inguinal	Deeply (deep) situated nodes in the groin (inguin)
Superficial inguinal	Nodes in the groin (inguin) close to the surface (superficial)
Popliteal	Nodes in back of the knee (popliteal)

vessels in the right chest, head, and right arm join the right lymphatic duct, which drains into the right subclavian vein. The lymph vessels from all other parts of the body join to meet the thoracic duct, which drains into the left subclavian vein.

Lymph nodes are distributed throughout the lymphatic system (Table 4-8). Lymph nodes are small bodies present in the path of the lymph channels that act as filters for lymph

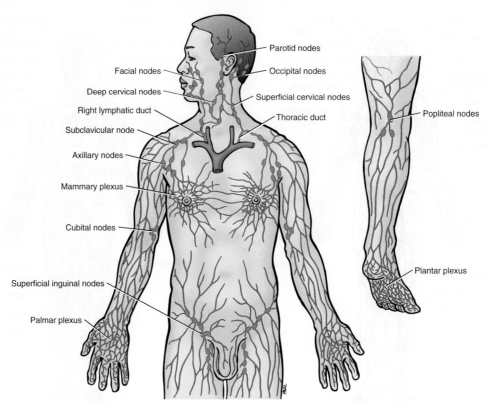

FIGURE 4-11 The principal lymph vessels and nodes.

🔎 PROFICIENCY EXERCISE 4-10

1. List five of the disease conditions of the lymphatic and immune systems described in the indications and contraindications section in Appendix A.
   a.
   b.
   c.
   d.
   e.
2. Choose one condition from your list and, using Appendix A, note any indications or contraindications for massage.
   Condition:

   _____

   _____

   Indications or contraindications:

   _____

   _____

before it returns to the bloodstream. The main locations of the more superficial lymph nodes are the cervical area, axillary region, and groin or inguinal area.

Plexuses of lymph channels are found throughout the body. They include the following:

- Mammary plexus (lymphatic vessels around the breasts)
- Palmar plexus (lymphatic vessels in the palm *[palmar]* of the hand)
- Plantar plexus (lymphatic vessels in the sole *[plantar]* of the foot)

If soft tissue has too much interstitial fluid around the cells or if the lymph vessels are full of fluid that is moving slowly or is stagnant, the tissue is said to be *infused* or *edematous.*

Excess fluid in muscle tissue contributes to problems with muscle tone.

Immune System

The human body is able to resist organisms or toxins that tend to damage its tissues and organs. This ability is called *immunity* (Table 4-9). As a massage professional, you should explore the immune system in much greater depth. Use your anatomy and physiology textbook as a place to begin, but do not stop there. Exciting new research is being published in professional journals (Proficiency Exercise 4-10).

BODY SYSTEMS: RESPIRATORY, DIGESTIVE, ENDOCRINE, AND INTEGUMENTARY SYSTEMS

SECTION OBJECTIVES

Chapter objective covered in this section:

5. Use anatomic and physiologic terminology correctly for the respiratory, digestive, endocrine, and integumentary systems.

Using the information presented in this section, the student will be able to perform the following:

- Describe the function of the respiratory system
- Explain the phases of respiration
- Describe the structures and functions of the digestive system
- Define the endocrine system
- List the structures of the integumentary system
- Describe each of the three tissue layers of the skin
- Define sebaceous and sweat glands
- Explain the importance of studying medical terminology

Table 4-9	Selected Terms Related to Immunity
Term	**Meaning**
Acquired immunity	Resistance (immunity) to a particular disease developed by people who have acquired the disease
Acquired immunodeficiency	A group of symptoms (syndrome) caused by the transmission (acquired) of a virus that causes a breakdown (deficiency) of the immune system (AIDS)
Active immunity	Resistance (immunity) in which the antibodies produced by the body currently exist
Allergy	A state of hypersensitivity to a particular substance; the immune system overreacts (over [hyper-], reacts [sensitive]) to foreign substances, and physical changes occur
Antigen	A substance that stimulates the immune response
Susceptible	An individual who is capable (-ible) of acquiring (suscept) a particular disease

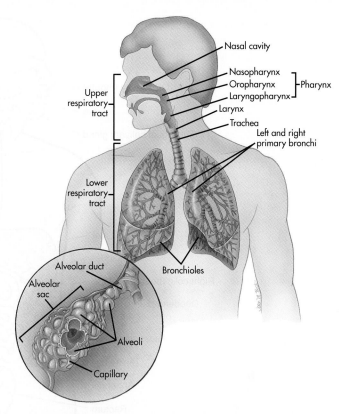

FIGURE 4-12 The structural plan of the respiratory system. The inset shows the alveolar sacs, where oxygen and carbon dioxide are exchanged through the walls of the grapelike alveoli. Capillaries surround the alveoli.
(From Thibodeau GA, Patton KT: *Anatomy and physiology,* ed 6, St Louis, 2009, Mosby.)

Respiratory System

4-5

The respiratory system supplies oxygen to and removes carbon dioxide from the cells of the body (Figure 4-12). Respiration is divided into two phases, external respiration and internal respiration. *External respiration* involves the absorption of oxygen from the air by the lungs and the transport of carbon dioxide from the lungs back into the air. *Internal respiration* involves the exchange of oxygen and carbon dioxide in the cells of the body. The mechanisms of breathing and their relationship to massage are discussed in future chapters.

Terms and combining forms related to the respiratory system include *alveoli, lungs, nares, nostrils, olfactory cells, pneumo-, rhino-,* and *trachea* (Proficiency Exercise 4-11).

💡 PROFICIENCY EXERCISE 4-11

1. List five of the disease conditions of the respiratory system described in the indications and contraindications section in Appendix A.
   a.
   b.
   c.
   d.
   e.
2. Choose one condition from your list and, using Appendix A, note any indications or contraindications for massage.
   Condition:

   _____

   _____

   Indications or contraindications:

   _____

   _____

Digestive System

Anatomically, the digestive system can be loosely described as a long, muscular tube that travels through the body (Figure 4-13). The organs of the digestive system transport food through this muscular tube. The wavelike contraction of the smooth muscles of the digestive tube is called *peristalsis.* Accessory organs carry out functions directly related to digestion and are connected to the system by means of ducts. It is important for massage professionals to understand the flow of contents through the large intestine, because methods of massage can be used to enhance this process. Refer to your anatomy and physiology textbook to learn more about the digestive process (Proficiency Exercise 4-12).

Endocrine System

The endocrine system is composed of glands that produce hormones, which are secreted directly into the bloodstream to stimulate cells in a specific way or to set a body function into action (Figure 4-14). The endocrine system is complex and important, because it serves as a control and regulation system for the body. As with the nervous system, the massage professional should commit to an in-depth study of the endocrine system, its relationship to the nervous system, and the connection to the mind/body processes. Information from research on the mind/body phenomenon is being released too

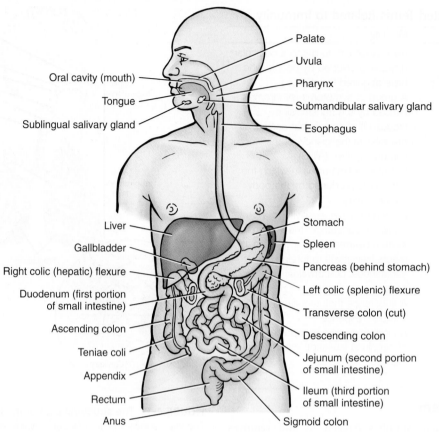

Palate
Uvula
Oral cavity (mouth)
Pharynx
Tongue
Submandibular salivary gland
Sublingual salivary gland
Esophagus

Liver
Stomach
Gallbladder
Spleen
Right colic (hepatic) flexure
Pancreas (behind stomach)
Duodenum (first portion of small intestine)
Left colic (splenic) flexure
Ascending colon
Transverse colon (cut)
Teniae coli
Descending colon
Appendix
Jejunum (second portion of small intestine)
Rectum
Ileum (third portion of small intestine)
Anus
Sigmoid colon

FIGURE 4-13 The organs of the digestive system and some associated structures.

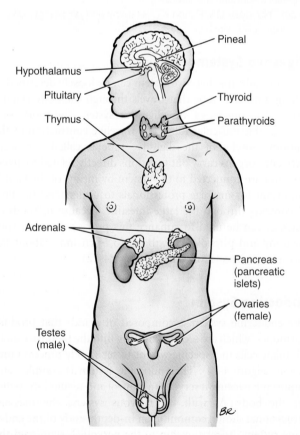

Pineal
Hypothalamus
Pituitary
Thyroid
Thymus
Parathyroids

Adrenals
Pancreas (pancreatic islets)
Ovaries (female)
Testes (male)

FIGURE 4-14 The locations of the major endocrine glands.

💡 PROFICIENCY EXERCISE 4-12

1. List five of the disease conditions of the digestive system described in the indications and contraindications section in Appendix A.
   a.
   b.
   c.
   d.
   e.
2. Choose one condition from your list and, using Appendix A, note any indications or contraindications for massage. Condition:

   _____

   Indications or contraindications:

   _____

   _____

quickly to remain current in any textbook. The massage professional must read medical and scientific research reports to keep up-to-date. The implications for massage are important, because the effects of massage are related to the nervous system and endocrine body control functions (Proficiency Exercise 4-13).

Integumentary System

The integumentary system consists of the skin and its appendages, including the hair and nails.

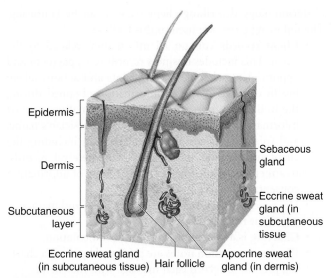

FIGURE 4-15 The structure of the skin.
(From Jarvis C: *Physical examination and health assessment,* Philadelphia, 1992, WB Saunders.)

💡 PROFICIENCY EXERCISE 4-13

1. List three of the disease conditions of the endocrine system described in the indications and contraindications section in Appendix A.
   a.
   b.
   c.
2. Choose one condition from your list and, using Appendix A, note any indications or contraindications for massage.
   Condition:

   _____

   _____

   Indications or contraindications:

   _____

   _____

Skin

The skin is the largest organ of the body. It is composed of three layers of tissue: the epidermis, the dermis, and the subcutaneous tissue (Figure 4-15). The *epidermis* is the outer layer of skin, which contains many layers of tissue and melanocytes, the cells that give skin color. The *dermis,* or dermal layer, lies directly under the epidermis and is often called the *true skin.* It is composed of connective tissue. Embedded in the dermis are the blood vessels, lymphatic vessels, hair follicles, and sweat glands. *Subcutaneous tissue* attaches the dermis to the underlying structures. This fatty tissue contains varying amounts of adipose tissue and acts as insulation for the body.

The functions of the fascial network of the skin are protection; control and maintenance of body temperature; detection of the sensations of touch, temperature, pain, and pressure; secretion of sweat and sebum; and production of vitamin D when the skin is exposed to the sun.

Many disease signs (particularly color changes) may first be noticed in the skin. Terms relating to skin color

changes include *cyanosis* (bluish), *erythema* (red), *jaundice* (yellow-orange), and *pallor* (a decrease in color) (Proficiency Exercise 4-14).

Sebaceous Glands

Sebaceous glands are located in the skin. They secrete an oily substance, called *sebum,* that gives the skin and hair a glossy appearance. Most of these glands open into the walls of hair follicles. Other sebaceous glands are located at the corners of the mouth and around the external sex organs that open directly on the surface of the skin.

Sweat Glands

The function of sweat glands, which are found in most areas of the body, is to cool the body. The most abundant type of sweat gland is the eccrine sweat gland. The palms of the hands and soles of the feet contain large numbers of eccrine sweat glands. Sweat from these glands is odorless. Another type of sweat gland is the apocrine sweat gland, which is connected to hair follicles in the armpits and the pubic area and is found at the navel and nipples. Secretions from these sweat glands increase in response to sexual stimulation. These secretions lubricate the genital area, and their mild odor plays a part in sexual arousal.

💡 PROFICIENCY EXERCISE 4-14

1. Using Appendix A, list at least three skin conditions that could be contagious.
   a.
   b.
   c.
2. Choose one condition from your list and, using Appendix A, note any indications or contraindications for massage.
   Condition:

   _____

   _____

   Indications or contraindications:

   _____

   _____

Terminology as a Continuing Study

The study of medical terminology, anatomy, physiology, and pathology must be an ongoing process for the massage professional, who needs this base to understand the research, books, and journal articles that relate to massage, record keeping, and charting. This base also is required if the massage professional is to communicate effectively with other health care professionals.

Many clients are not familiar with medical terms; therefore, it is important to use the language patterns of the people with whom you speak. In many cases, using technical terms with a client is not appropriate; using big words and technical language is not necessary when presenting yourself to the general public. The massage professional must speak two languages and must be able to translate effectively back and forth between them.

When you speak with health care professionals and researchers who use this special language of the sciences, it is important that you ask questions about any term you do not understand. Acting as though you understand what is being said when you do not will not help you increase your knowledge and skills, and it is unprofessional. The development of this language base has prepared the student to begin the process of maintaining records and charting.

RECORD KEEPING

SECTION OBJECTIVES

Chapter objective covered in this section:

4. The student will be able to use the information in this chapter for effective professional record keeping.

Using the information presented in this section, the student will be able to perform the following:

- Implement the clinical reasoning/problem-solving/decision-making model for charting purposes
- Use a problem- or goal-oriented charting process
- Complete a client intake process using sample forms
- Chart using a SOAP note format
- List the pros and cons of computerized record keeping

Accurate, comprehensive documentation is becoming increasingly important for massage professionals. Massage has adopted and adapted documentation methods used by the medical profession (Box 4-3).

Terminology describing client records can be confusing. The following terms are used in this textbook.

- **Client records** contain all information related to the client. This includes business records (e.g., payment and appointment schedules); complaints and actions taken; health care records (e.g., information obtained during the initial visit, relevant insurance information, contact information in case of an emergency, physician's name, and so forth); needs assessment records, including the client history and initial assessment; referral records; treatment plan; informed consent; release of information consent; and all session notes.
- **Documentation** is the process of creating and maintaining client records.
- **Charting** is a systematic form of documentation.
- **Progress or session notes** are produced by using a charting process to record each massage with the client.

Problem-Oriented Medical Record

In the 1960s Dr. Lawrence Weed developed a method of record keeping that is organized around the problems of the client or **patient.** (Remember, in massage therapy, all patients are clients, but not all clients are patients. This text uses the term *client* for general discussion purposes and *patient* where that term is more appropriate.) This type of documentation is known as the *problem-oriented medical record (POMR) system.* A critical thinking process is used to collect information and organize it according to a system known as the *SOAP format.*

| Box 4-3 | Documentation Rules for Medical Records and Health Care Professionals |

Medical records must be maintained in a specific way:

- Each page of the record must identify the patient by name and by the clinical record number of the hospital, clinic, or private physician.
- Each entry in the record must include the date and time the entry was made and the signature and credential of the individual making the entry.
- No blank spaces should be left between entries.
- All entries should be written in ink or produced on a printer or typewriter or recorded appropriately in electronic format.
- The record must not be altered in any way. Erasures, use of correction fluid, and marked-out areas are not appropriate. Errors should be corrected in a manner that allows the reader to see and understand the error. Errors are corrected as follows:
  1. A single line is drawn through the error, and the legibility of the previous entry is checked.
  2. The correct information is inserted.
  3. The correction is dated and initialed by the person recording the data.
  4. If space is inadequate to allow the correction to be made legibly at the error, a note should be made indicating where the corrected entry can be found; this cross-reference should be dated and initialed. The correct information is entered in the proper chronologic order for the date the error was discovered and corrected.
  5. If something is spilled on the pages of a chart, they should not be discarded. The pages should be copied,

and the original and copied sheets then should be put together in the chart. "COPIED" is written on the copied pages.

- All information should be recorded as soon as possible. Memories can fade, and important facts can be omitted.
- Abbreviations should be used sparingly, and only those approved by the organization are appropriate. The same abbreviation can have different meanings, which can be misleading. Writing out the information is always better than using abbreviations that can be misinterpreted.
- All writing must be legible. Because the patient record is used by so many other clinicians and practitioners in providing care, it is important to the quality of patient care that the record be legible. An electronic format can be helpful with this issue.
- All entries must be consistent with one another. The assessment must agree with the diagnostic testing, or an explanation must be given as to the reason it does not.
- Entries should be factual accounts.
- All information given to the patient before any procedure should be recorded. This ensures and verifies that the patient was properly informed of the benefits and risks before he or she gave consent for the procedure.
- Telephone contacts with the patient should be entered into the record immediately.
- Some method of organizing entries (e.g., the SOAP format) must be used to ensure that the entries are comprehensive and reflect the thought processes involved when decisions were made about the patient's care.

"SOAP" stands for *subjective, objective, assessment/analysis,* and *plan.*

Subjective Data

The chief complaint (main problem) and history portion of the record represents subjective information collected from the client or a significant other and from previous records. For each problem, the applicable parts of a traditional history (present illness, past medical history, personal/social history, family history, and review of systems) are summarized in a paragraph placed directly under the subjective heading.

Objective Data

The objective data, which include the findings from the physical examination and the results of any tests, follow the list of problems. The physical examination usually is recorded in the traditional format; that is, the results are listed by the parts of the body. After the initial assessment, this section includes any changes in the physical findings and the results of any tests or treatment.

Assessment/Analysis

The assessment/analysis section presents the conclusions reached based on the subjective and objective data. During the process of reaching conclusions, critical thinking becomes clinical reasoning.

Plan

The next section is the plan for that particular problem. A plan consists of three parts: the diagnosis (Dx), the treatment (Rx), and patient education.

- In this case, *diagnosis* means the diagnostic tests needed to identify the cause or to follow the case.
- Treatment can include special therapy, drugs, radiation, chemotherapy, and other modalities, including massage.
- Patient education is the information the patient is given about the problem.

Organizing patient data in this way shows exactly what the medical caregiver is thinking. Each problem can be followed easily through the record. This saves valuable time for the caregiver and enables others to take over the patient's care if necessary. The documentation process is based on a clinical reasoning pattern.

The massage profession began informally using the SOAP format in the 1980s. In 1993 a book called *The Hands Heal: Documentation for Massage Therapy: A Guide to S.O.A.P. Charting,* by Diana L. Thompson, was published. Since then, the SOAP charting process has become the most used documentation method for therapeutic massage. Because diagnosis and prescribing are out of the scope of practice for massage therapy, the SOAP process has been modified over time to better fit the practice of therapeutic massage; however, it retains its roots in the POMR.

Progress/Session Notes

Progress (or session) notes chart each visit by the client. These notes should follow a systematic method of organizing the information for decision making (e.g., the SOAP method).

This helps massage therapists organize their thinking and justify their actions. The basic plan of SOAP is easily modified to other charting styles. Computer record keeping soon will be required in medical environments; therefore, massage students should learn basic computer skills.

Following the documentation rules in Box 4-3 will result in a record that is accurate, timely, specific, objective, concise, comprehensive, logical, and legible. All entries must be consistent with one another. The assessment must agree with the diagnostic testing, or the discrepancy must be explained. Records created in this way reflect the thought processes of the health care providers (including massage therapists). Not only is such a record the best defense in case of a lawsuit, but it also results in the best care for the client or patient.

Good record-keeping skills equip the massage therapist to communicate with other health care personnel. They also help create an accurate record of specified treatment goals, the methods of massage, and the effectiveness of treatment.

Confidentiality of Medical Records

A patient's right to privacy traditionally has imposed an ethical responsibility on the people involved in the patient's care. Many different people may see and treat a patient during the provision of health care, and each of them needs particular information. Protecting the patient's right to privacy while keeping all caregivers informed can present a dilemma. Passage of the Health Insurance Portability and Accountability Act (HIPAA) in 1996 substantially strengthened the patient's right to privacy.

HIPAA's Privacy Rule includes standards that protect a patient's individually identifiable data; this type of data is considered protected health information (PHI). Generally speaking, PHI covers information that identifies a patient and his or her health status. The Privacy Rule applies to health plans, health care clearinghouses, and other health care providers. It covers a broad range of information. Protections apply to the information in many different formats, including electronic files (Internet, Intranet, private networks, and data moved from one location to another by disk, magnetic tape, or compact disk), paper records, and verbal information.

Most health care providers, and certainly hospitals, have policies and procedures governing the release of any information about a patient. Massage therapists must be aware of those policies. Policies on the release of information generally include provisions such as the following:

- A requirement for the patient's consent to the release of any information to any outside entity; any exceptions are outlined.
- Special considerations for the release of information on sensitive conditions, such as alcohol, drug, or psychiatric diagnoses, and conditions related to infection with the human immunodeficiency virus (HIV).
- Required data elements for a proper consent form and specification of how long the form is valid.
- Identification of those who can release information to outside parties.
- Appropriate fees or charges for copies that may be requested.

Other issues should be addressed in separate policies. For example, individuals by title who may release information to the media could be the subject of one such policy. Another policy could indicate what information hospital employees may disclose to telephone callers regarding the condition of the patient during hospitalization.

To ensure compliance, health care providers have implemented policies and procedures that adhere to HIPAA regulations. The massage therapist in the medical environment should be specifically trained in the HIPAA procedures in place in the medical environment. This must be in-house training. If it is not offered as part of the orientation training, massage therapists should request specific information on the ways in which they are expected to comply with these regulations.

All states have laws about which diseases, conditions, and events must be reported to appropriate agencies. Such incidents include births, deaths, gunshot wounds, communicable diseases, and evidence of child and elder abuse. When reporting is required by law, confidentiality is no longer an issue. Reporting such incidents to anyone other than the responsible agency, however, is a breach of confidentiality.

Documentation in the Massage Therapy Practice

Maintenance of a written record of the professional relationship with massage therapy clients is essential. The informed consent procedure and the legal implications of documentation were presented in Chapter 2. The decision-making skills that also were introduced in that chapter will continue to be developed throughout the text. Ethical decisions are only one type of decision made in professional practice. Clinical decisions using clinical reasoning involve the client's concerns and the methods to use to achieve clients' goals, as well as business decisions. This discussion focuses on clinical decision making and the records necessary for maintaining a written account of the professional interaction. Clinical decision making is discussed in further detail in other chapters. Chapter 3 more thoroughly discussed business records, and Chapter 16 provides examples of case studies.

Client record keeping involves the creation of a written or an electronic record of intake procedures, including informed consent and needs assessments (including the history and physical assessment); obtaining permission for the release of information (if communication among health professionals is anticipated); and the ongoing process of recording each session, which is called *charting*. Clients have the right to see their file, receive a copy of the file, and have any information contained in the file explained to them.

At this point, you, as students, will find it difficult to complete a needs assessment and to devise an initial treatment plan, because you are still developing the assessment skills and technical skills required to perform these procedures. The same is true of charting. Even so, it is important that you understand the mechanics of the record keeping and charting process so that as your technical skills improve, your ability to perform record-keeping procedures also develops (Box 4-4).

Box 4-4   SOAP in the Massage Practice

The SOAP note has four parts:

Subjective data: The client's explanation of his or her goals for massage and information about the current and past conditions, pain, complaints, reactions, and so forth.

Objective data: The information obtained through physical assessment and observations and also the massage techniques used.

Assessment: (Think of this as an analysis.) Evaluation of the condition, based on the subjective and objective information, using clinical reasoning skills. It involves thinking about the data gathered and deciding on the main issues, the contributing factors, and possible courses of action. It also includes the information from a postmassage evaluation of the results of the massage interventions.

Plan: The details of implementation of the course of treatment chosen, including the frequency of the massage sessions, methods, client education, referrals, need for additional information, and so forth.

Clinical Reasoning and Charting

As the volume of knowledge increases and as soft tissue methods, such as massage, are integrated into health care systems, the ability to think or reason through an intervention process and justify the effectiveness of a therapeutic intervention is becoming increasingly important. Therapeutic massage practitioners must be able to gather information effectively, analyze that information to make decisions about the type and appropriateness of a therapeutic intervention, and evaluate and justify the benefits derived from the intervention. Charting is the process of keeping a written record of these professional interactions. Effective charting is more than writing down what happens during a session; it is a clinical reasoning methodology that emphasizes a problem-solving approach to client care. As noted at the beginning of this chapter, you must have a comprehensive knowledge base of massage terms, medical terms, abbreviations, and anatomy and physiology in both normal and diseased states to be able to reason clinically and chart effectively.

Effective assessment, analysis, and decision making are essential to meeting the needs of each client. Routines or recipe-type applications of therapeutic massage often are limited and ineffective, because each person's presenting circumstances and outcome goals are so varied. Effective clinical reasoning skills are the mark of an experienced professional. As with all skills, clinical reasoning can be learned (Box 4-5).

Goals and Problems

Massage sessions are goal oriented. **Goals** describe desired outcomes. Decisions must be made regarding which goals are obtainable and the way the goals will be achieved. Problems indicate limits in functions. Goals support desired function. Consider the following example:

- Description of the problem: Client has disturbed sleep pattern because of multiple physical and emotional stressors.

Box 4-5 Methods of Organized Thinking

Organized thinking is based on four primary elements:
- **Database:** The client's past and present health status.
- **Goals/problems list:** The list of massage-related health goals and current and past problems.
- **Initial plan:** The massage therapy plan devised to help achieve goals and overcome health problems.
- **Progress notes:** The ongoing description of each massage session using a logical method (style) of charting.

Charting Methods

Three commonly used charting methods are SOAP, SOAPIER, and PIE.

SOAP Method

The SOAP method is used for problem-oriented charts.

    S—Subjective (what the client tells you)
    O—Objective (what you observe, see, assess, and measure)
    A—Assessment/analyze (what you think is going on based on your data)
    P—Plan (what you are going to do)

SOAPIER Method

    S—Subjective (what the client tells you)
    O—Objective (what you observe, see, assess, and measure)
    A—Assessment/analyze (what you think is going on based on your data)
    P—Plan (what you are going to do)
    I—Intervention (specific methods used)
    E—Evaluation (response to interventions)
    R—Revision (changes in treatment)

PIE Method

The PIE method, which is similar to SOAP charting, also is a problem-oriented method.

    P—Problem (what is bothering client or what is the intended outcome for massage)
    I—Intervention (what type and how massage was used)
    E—Evaluation (what worked and what did not work)

- Goal: Reduce physical stress symptoms to support more effective sleep.

Two primary reasons for developing treatment and care plans are to set achievable goals and to outline a general plan for the way the goals will be reached. Achievable goals often relate to day-to-day activities (functional goals), either personal or work related.

It is important to develop measurable, activity-based goals that are meaningful to the client, such as improvement in the ability to perform activities of daily living.

Quantifiable and Qualifiable Goals

Goals must be **quantifiable**; that is, they must be measurable in terms of objective criteria, such as time, frequency, rating on a 1 to 10 scale, a measurable increase or decrease in the ability to perform an activity, or a measurable increase or decrease in a sensation, such as relaxation or pain.

Goals also must be **qualifiable**. Massage therapists must determine measures by which they will know when a goal has been achieved. One such measure might be an activity that the client will be able to do that he or she is unable to do now.

PROFICIENCY EXERCISE 4-15

Following the examples given in this section of the text, write three quantifiable and qualifiable goals you might set for yourself in therapeutic massage.

1.
2.
3.

The following are examples of quantifiable and qualifiable goals (Proficiency Exercise 4-15):

- Client will be able to manage independently (qualified) daily hygiene activities of bathing and dressing with a pain level of 5 on a scale of 1 to 10 (quantified), with 10 being unable to function without severe pain.
- Client will be able to work at the computer for 1 hour (quantified) without pain (qualified).
- Client will be able to incorporate a 30-minute walking program (quantified) without stiffness in left knee (qualified).
- Client will be able to fall asleep within 15 minutes (quantified) and sleep uninterrupted for 7 hours (qualified).
- Client will be able to increase duration of breath exhale to reduce sympathetic arousal (quantified), allowing her to drive car to and from market (qualified).
- Client will be able to meditate for 15 minutes (quantified) without racing thoughts (qualified).
- Client will be able to use massage to relax for 1 hour each week (quantified) to enjoy family more by being able to participate in a family outing after each massage (qualified).

Intake Procedures

Before massage therapists begin working with a client, it is important that they gather information on which to build the professional interaction, establish client goals, and develop a plan for achieving those goals. This is called a *database*.

Database

A **database** consists of all the information available that contributes to therapeutic interaction. It is created with information obtained from a history-taking interview with the client and other people who may have pertinent information, a physical assessment, previous records, and health care treatment orders. Information obtained during the history and assessment process becomes the needs assessment and provides the basis for the development of a treatment or care plan, identification of contraindications to therapy, and assessment of the need for referral.

To gather the information, the professional must have effective communication skills. The same communication skills learned for ethical decision making in Chapter 2 are applied in this process. The I-message pattern can be altered slightly to develop effective, open-ended questions that support data collection.

The four basic questions are:

1. Will you please explain the situation or tell me what happened?

2. How did/do you feel about the situation?
3. What has been the result of the situation in terms of costs, limitations, and changes in activity or performance?
4. How would you prefer the situation to be or what would you like to occur?

Note: The answer to the last question can easily become the basis for the functionally oriented treatment goal.

History

The history interview provides information about the client's health history, the reason for contact, a descriptive profile of the person, a history of the current condition, a history of past illness and health, and a history of any family illnesses. It is important to gather information about any prescription medication, herbs, or vitamins the client may be using (see Appendix C for more information on pharmacology). The history also contains an account of the client's current health practices (Figure 4-16).

Physical Assessment

The physical assessment findings make up the second part of the database. Assessment procedures identify both noneffective functioning and deviations from the norm. The extent and depth of this assessment vary from setting to setting, practitioner to practitioner, and client to client. Practitioners of therapeutic massage generally use some sort of visual assessment process that looks for bilateral symmetry and deviations. Functional assessment looks for restricted, exaggerated, painful, or otherwise altered movement patterns. Palpation is used to identify changes in tissue texture and temperature, locate energy changes, and identify areas of tenderness. Various manual tests may be used to differentiate soft tissue problems from such other problems as joint dysfunction and muscle function (Figure 4-17).

Analysis of Data

After the information has been collected, it is analyzed. The analysis is a critical thinking and clinical reasoning process. It is a very important process that follows the same model as that for decision making. Effective decision making depends on both thorough collection and effective analysis of data. The following are the steps of the analysis process.

1. Review the facts and information collected.
     Questions that help with this process include the following:
   - What are the facts?
   - What is considered normal or balanced function?
   - What has happened? (Spell out events.)
   - What caused the imbalance? (Can it be identified?)
   - What was done or is being done?
   - What has worked or not worked?
2. Brainstorm the possibilities.
     Questions that help with this process include the following:
   - What are the possibilities? (What could it all mean?)
   - What does my intuition suggest?
   - What are the possible patterns of dysfunction?

   - What are the possible contributing factors?
   - What are possible interventions?
   - What might work?
   - What are other ways to look at the situation?
   - What do the data suggest?
3. Consider the logical outcome of each possibility.
     Questions that help with this process include the following:
   - What is the logical progression of the symptom pattern, contributing factors, and current behaviors?
   - What is the logical cause and effect of each intervention identified?
   - What are the pros and cons of each intervention suggested?
   - What are the consequences of not acting?
   - What are the consequences of acting?
4. Consider how people involved would be affected by each possibility.
     Questions that help identify these effects are the following:
   - In terms of each intervention considered, what is the impact on the people involved (i.e., client, practitioner, and other professionals working with the client)?
   - How does each person involved feel about the possible interventions?
   - Is the practitioner within his or her scope of practice to work with such situations?
   - Is the practitioner qualified to work with such situations?
   - Does the practitioner feel qualified to work with such situations?
   - Does a feeling of cooperation and agreement exist among all parties involved?

Identification of Problems and Goals

Problems are identified based on a conclusion or decision resulting from examination, investigation, and analysis of the data collected. A problem is defined as anything that causes concern to the client or caregiver, including physical abnormalities, physiologic disturbances, and socioeconomic or spiritually based problems. Realistic and attainable massage-based outcome goals are established. A decision then is made about an intervention or care or treatment plan.

Not all therapeutic goals are related to problems. Clients commonly use massage for health maintenance, stress management, and fulfillment of pleasure needs. The same analysis process is used to best determine the methods and approach to meet the goals of these clients.

Care or Treatment Plan

After the analysis is complete and problems and goals have been identified, a decision must be made about the **care or treatment plan.** Anytime a decision must be made about the care plan, the massage practitioner should return to the problem-solving model, which includes consideration of the facts, possibilities, logical outcomes, and impact on others involved.

CLIENT INTAKE AND HEALTH HISTORY FORM

Name: _____ Date: _____

Address: _____ City: _____ State: _____ Zip: _____

Phone: (day) _____ (eve) _____ Date of Birth: _____

Occupation: _____ Employer: _____

Referred by: _____ Physician: _____

Previous experience with massage:

_____

Primary reason for appointment / areas of pain or tension:

_____

Emergency contact—name and number: _____

Please mark (X) for all conditions that apply now. Put a (P) for past conditions, an (F) for family history of illness.

Pain Scale: minor-1   2   3   4   5   6   7   8   9   severe-10

_____ headaches, migraines	_____ chronic pain	_____ fatigue
_____ vision problems, contact lenses	_____ muscle or joint pain	_____ tension, stress
_____ hearing problems, deafness	_____ muscle, bone injuries	_____ depression
_____ injuries to face or head	_____ numbness or tingling	_____ sleep difficulties
_____ sinus problems	_____ sprains, strains	_____ allergies, sensitivities
_____ dental bridges, braces	_____ arthritis, tendinitis	_____ rashes, athlete's foot
_____ jaw pain, TMJ problems	_____ cancer, tumors	_____ infectious diseases
_____ asthma or lung conditions	_____ spinal column disorders	_____ blood clots
_____ constipation, diarrhea	_____ diabetes	_____ varicose veins
_____ hernia	_____ pregnancy	_____ high/low blood pressure
_____ birth control, IUD	_____ heart, circulatory problems	
_____ abdominal or digestive problems	_____ other medical conditions not listed	

Explain any areas noted above:

_____

_____

Current medications, including aspirin, ibuprofen, herbs, supplements, etc.:

_____

_____

Surgeries: _____

Accidents: _____

Please list all forms and frequency of stress reduction activities, hobbies, exercise, or sports participation:

_____

_____

FIGURE 4-16 A sample history form. This information is provided by the client. To complete the form correctly, ask relevant questions to gather data.

MASSAGE ASSESSMENT/PHYSICAL OBSERVATION/PALPATION AND GAIT

PRE
POST

Client Name:_____   Date:_____

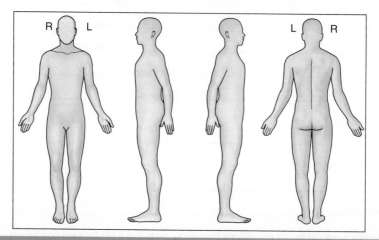

OBSERVATION & PALPATION		
ALIGNMENT	**RIBS**	**SCAPULA**
Chin in line with nose, sternal notch, navel	Even	Even
Other:	Springy	Move freely
HEAD	Other:	Other:
Tilted (L)	**ABDOMEN**	**CLAVICLES**
Tilted (R)	Firm and pliable	Level
Rotated (L)	Hard areas	Other:
Rotated (R)	Other:	**ARMS**
EYES	**WAIST**	Hang evenly (internal) (external)
Level	Level	(L) rotated ☐ medial ☐ lateral
Equally set in socket	Other:	(R) rotated ☐ medial ☐ lateral
Other:	**SPINE CURVES**	**ELBOWS**
EARS	Normal	Even
Level	Other:	Other:
Other:	**GLUTEAL MUSCLE MASS**	**WRISTS**
SHOULDERS	Even	Even
Level	Other:	Other:
(R) high / (L) low	**ILIAC CREST**	**FINGERTIPS**
(L) high / (R) low	Level	Even
(L) rounded forward	Other:	Other:
(R) rounded forward	**KNEES**	**PATELLA**
Muscle development even	Even/symmetrical	(L) ☐ movable ☐ rigid
Other:	Other:	(R) ☐ movable ☐ rigid

FIGURE 4-17 A sample physical assessment form. This information is obtained by observing (looking and feeling) and measuring. To complete the form correctly, you should identify what is the same on the two sides of the body and what is different. Have the client color symptoms on the figures.

The care or treatment plan is not an exact protocol set in stone, but rather a flexible guide (the professional's best educated guess). The plan may evolve over the first three or four sessions, and it may be altered, including changes in the therapeutic goals. The development of the care or treatment plan is the end of the intake process (Figure 4-18).

As the plan is implemented, it is recorded sequentially, session by session, in some form of charting process, such as

SOAP notes. The plan is re-evaluated and adjusted as necessary.

SOAP Notes

Charting is the process of producing an ongoing record of each client session. As was mentioned previously, commonly used methods of charting are based on the problem-oriented

ANKLES		TRUNK		LEGS	
Even		Remains vertical		Swing freely at hip	
Other:		Other:		Other:	
FEET		**SHOULDERS**		**KNEES**	
Mobile		Remain level		Flex and extend freely through stance and swing phase	
Other:		Rotate during walking		Other:	
ARCHES		Other:		**FEET**	
Even		**ARMS**		Heel strikes first at start of stance	
Other:		Motion is opposite leg swing		Plantar flexed at push-off	
TOES		Motion is even (L) and (R)		Foot clears floor during swing phase	
Straight		Other:		Other:	
Other:		(L) swings freely		**STEP**	
SKIN		(R) swings freely		Length is even	
Moves freely and resilient		Other:		Timing is even	
Pulls/restricted		**HIPS**		Other:	
Puffy/baggy		Remain level		**OVERALL**	
Other:		Other:		Rhythmic	
HEAD		Rotate during walking		Other:	
Remains steady/eyes forward		Other:			
Other:					

FIGURE 4-17, cont'd

medical record system. The POMR system involves a problem-solving and clinical reasoning analysis process. Therefore after one method has been learned, adapting to any of the other charting methods is relatively easy. The most important skill involved is the ability to reason logically and comprehensively through a therapeutic interaction. A charting process can provide the structure necessary to think through a process effectively and develop a written record of the process.

The charting process includes recording any therapeutic action taken, its effectiveness, and its outcome progressively from session to session. Effective charting requires an organized approach to recording the information that relates to the facts, possibilities, logical consequences of cause and effect, and impact on involved people, an approach similar to that used for the development of the initial care or treatment plan. This process again is a direct application of the decision-making model. While charting, a practitioner gathers and records subjective and objective information, records the methods used, and analyzes the effectiveness of the process. The plan for further sessions is then indicated and noted.

Although many different charting processes exist, massage professionals seem to be using the standardized SOAP model. This is a helpful choice in terms of learning because the four-part model correlates with the clinical-reasoning/decision-making model.

SOAP notes or similar charting methods are used to document all massage sessions.

After the initial intake and care/treatment plan development, subsequent visits require a modified and shortened subjective and objective assessment process to determine goals for each individual massage session. When a massage is given to the client after the intake session, specific treatment goals for the particular session are developed. Information from the history pertinent to the first session is transferred to *S* in SOAP notes. Physical assessment information pertinent to this session is transferred to *O* in SOAP notes.

When using SOAP note charting, the massage practitioner should use the following format (Thompson, 2005):

S stands for subjective data recorded from the client's point of view. Subjective information usually includes the following:
- Key goals that are quantified and qualified
- Activities that are affected by the situation; often stated as what can no longer be done or what increase in performance is desired
- The methods or activities currently used in adjunctive treatment

O stands for objective data acquired from inspection and palpation. A list of assessment procedures and interventions used during the session is recorded. Objective information usually includes the following:
- Significant physical assessment findings
- Intervention modalities and locations used (limit specifics to interventions used to work toward treatment goals)
- General approach used, such as general massage focus, connective tissue focus, Swedish massage focus, neuromuscular focus, or circulatory focus
- If not recorded elsewhere, the duration of the session

A stands for analysis or assessment of the subjective and objective data. It includes an analysis of the effectiveness of the intervention and action taken, with a summary of the most pertinent data recorded.

CARE/TREATMENT PLAN

Client Name:_____

Choose One: ☐ Original plan   ☐ Reassessment date_____

Short-term client goals:
Quantitative:_____
Qualitative:_____

Long-term client goals:
Quantitative:_____
Qualitative:_____

Therapist objectives:

_____

_____

1) Frequency, 2) length, and 3) duration of visits:
1) _____   2) _____   3) _____

Progress measurements to be used: (Ex.— pain scale, range of motion, increased ability to perform function)

_____

_____

Dates of reassessment:

_____

Categories of massage methods to be used: (Ex.— general constitutional, stress reduction, circulatory, lymphatic, neuromuscular, connective tissue, neurochemical, etc.)

_____

_____

Additional notes:

_____

_____

_____

Client Signature:_____   Date:_____

Therapist Signature:_____   Date:_____

FIGURE 4-18 A sample form for a care or treatment plan.

(*Note:* Traditionally in SOAP charting, the *A* stands for assessment. However, observation of many students indicates that they confuse physical assessment information recorded in the objective data with assessment in the SOAP model, which is actually an analysis of the data and effectiveness of the interventions. Therefore this text uses the idea of analysis for the A section of SOAP charting.) Analysis of information includes the following:

• Changes, whether subjective (i.e., related to the client's experience, such as "pain reduced" or "feel relaxed") or objective (i.e., measurable, such as "flexion of elbow increased by 15 degrees"). If no change occurs or if the condition worsens, record this also.

• Analysis of which methods were effective or not effective, such as "Trigger point methods most effective in increase of flexion of elbow," "Client indicated she responded best to rhythmic rocking for relaxation," "Tense-and-relax methods not effective in reducing pain in shoulder." Also indicate whether it is unclear which methods were effective: "Range of motion in neck increased 25%, but it is unclear which methods brought about the change."

SESSION NOTES
SOAP CHARTING FORM

Client Name: _____ Date: _____
Manage Therapist Name: _____

S ubjective

CLIENT STATUS
- **Information from client, referral source, or reference books:**
1) Current conditions/changes from last session: _____
_____
_____
_____

O bjective

2) Information from <u>assessment</u> (physical, gait, palpation, muscle testing):
_____
_____

CONTENT OF SESSION
- **Generate goal (possibilities) from analysis of information in <u>client status</u>.**
1) Goals worked on this session. (Base information on client status this session and goals previously established in Treatment Plan):
_____
_____

What was <u>done</u> this session:
_____
_____
_____

A nalysis

RESULTS
- **Analyze results of session in relationship to what was done and how this relates to the session goals. (This is based on <u>cause</u> and <u>effect</u> of methods used and the effects on the persons involved.)**
1) What worked/what didn't: (Based on measurable and objective Post Assessment)
_____
_____
_____

P lan

PLAN: Plans for next session, what client will work on, what next massage will reassess and continue to assess: _____
_____
_____

CLIENT COMMENTS:
_____

Time In: _____ Time Out: _____

Therapist signature: _____

FIGURE 4-19 A SOAP charting form modified for student learning. To complete the form correctly, you should: answer the questions based on what happened during the massage.

The *A* (analysis/assessment) section of the SOAP charting process is very important. It is, in fact, the most important area in terms of determining future intervention procedures and communicating process information to other caregivers and insurance companies.

The A portion of the SOAP note is where the actual process of decision making is recorded. Decision making occurs during every step of the charting process; however, in the other areas of charting, only the decision is recorded, not the way the decision was made. Obviously a condensed version of the more detailed process is written down in the chart, but the components of the process (facts, possibilities, logical outcomes, impact on people) are evident in the *A* portion of the SOAP note.

P stands for plan, including the methodology for future intervention. The progress of the sessions is developed and recorded. Plan information usually includes the following:

- Frequency of appointments
- Continuation of a step-by-step process as it unfolds session by session to achieve treatment plan goals
- Client self-care
- Referrals

A sample SOAP charting form is presented in Figure 4-19; it has been modified for use by the beginning student. An example of SOAP charting is presented in Box 4-6.

Individual session goals need to be in line with the initial care/treatment plan agreed to in the informed consent process. If the goals are radically different, the client needs to sign an addendum to the informed consent form. Minor changes can be reflected in the SOAP notes or session charting procedure.

To maintain the integrity of client charts, make sure that any abbreviations used are universally understood, or write out the word. Use a black pen or type the notes. Make sure handwritten notes are readable. Never erase or white-out a correction. Draw a single line through any error and make

Box 4-6   Example of SOAP Charting in Therapeutic Massage

In this example, a massage therapist uses SOAP charting for a new client who complains of frequent headaches. The SOAP format has been modified slightly to help students complete the documentation process.

S (Subjective)

Client reports tension headache and indicates with hand placement that the major concentration of pain is at the occiput and upper cervical area with a secondary pain pattern at the temples. Client reports that on a pain scale of 0 to 10, the headache is a 7.

O (Objective)

Both shoulders are observed to be elevated, with increased elevation on the right. Range of motion of the neck appears to be generally limited to the left. Palpation of the upper back muscles elicited some pain behaviors, including pulling away, grimacing, and verbal indications of pain. The upper trapezius muscles seem to be warm but without indications of inflammation, suggesting tension in the muscles.

Approach used (what I did)

* *General massage focus:* Stress reduction with specific focus on shoulder and neck tension using positional release and lengthening
* *Basic methods used:* Gliding, compression, rocking, and passive joint movement

Postassessment

After the massage session, a postassessment is done. The client is asked how he or she feels and what is different from before the session. The client is asked what methods used seemed to be most beneficial. One or two of the methods identified are then modified for client self-care and are taught to the client.

After the massage and postassessment, the *A* (assessment/analysis) part of the chart is recorded.

A (Analysis/Assessment)

Appears as if the client may be experiencing changes in soft tissue structures leading to the described headache. Post massage, client indicates a reduction in headache by 50% (pain rating of 3), less tension in the shoulders, and increased range of motion of the neck to the left. Pain behaviors related to the upper back are not occurring, but the client still indicates tenderness in the area during palpation. Upper trapezius area is still warm, with exaggerated vasomotor response (reddening) and itching after massage, indicating possible connective tissue involvement in this area. Client now can look over the left shoulder, which he could not do without a catch before the massage. The shoulders are observed to be level within 1 inch, indicating a change in the right shoulder tension pattern. The methods that were most effective were compression and positional release. Rocking methods were ineffective, and the client reported an increase in head pain when rocking was used. *Note:* Make sure client's feet stay warm.

P (Plan)

Client selected self-help consisting of towel compression to the head and flexion/extension range of motion of the arms and shoulders. Client scheduled an appointment for 2 weeks and will monitor response to massage. Expect three to four sessions before beginning specific connective tissue work on the shoulder area. Client was advised to contact his personal physician and report that he has begun to receive massage.

Note: The interventions used and the plan recorded in SOAP charting need to reflect the original treatment plan developed during the intake procedure.

---

the correction above or next to the error. It is important to share the charting notes with the client regularly and to explain them to him or her.

Computer-Based Patient Record and Electronic Health Record

Paper records are becoming a thing of the past. They are difficult to access, often lack information, and can be available only in a single location for a single use. The paper record has changed very little over the past 50 years, whereas the expectations for use of the data it contains have changed significantly.

Technology has improved over the past decades, allowing the design and implementation of electronic record-keeping systems (Box 4-7). Automated record-keeping systems have a variety of names, such as *computer-based patient record (CPR), electronic patient record (EPR), computerized medical record,* and *electronic health record (EHR).*

Regardless of whether the record-keeping system is electronic or paper, high-quality client care depends on massage therapists' expertise in collecting information and their ability to interpret it (see Box 4-6).

Box 4-7   Pros and Cons of Computerized Record Keeping

Pros

* All parts of the record are legible.
* The date and time are recorded automatically.
* Abbreviations, specific terms, and formats are standardized by the facility.
* Less space is needed for record storage (computerization does not eliminate paper records, but it does significantly reduce the amount of paper needed).
* The members of a health care team are able to coordinate care.
* Searching for a particular item is quicker.

Cons

* Use of a computerized system involves a significant learning curve.
* Information and systems are not yet uniform, which makes integration difficult.
* Care must be taken to ensure that computer screens cannot be seen by unauthorized individuals.
* A password is required, which must never be shared and must be changed frequently.

⬚ FOOT IN THE DOOR

The language you use and the records you keep will influence and impress both clients and employers. If you want an advantage in the career world, perfect your vocabulary, writing skills, intake skills, and critical thinking skills. The discipline of these systems helps organize your internal and external self. An organized person stands out in the interview process. Your ability to understand terminology and maintain professional records will help you communicate and work with health care professionals. If you want to practice massage therapy in the health care setting, you will not be able to get your foot in the door without these skills. The spa and wellness industries, also, expect massage therapists to speak and document professionally.

SUMMARY

Record-keeping and documentation skills, in addition to a knowledge of the necessary language base for keeping records effectively, are important aspects of professional development. The ability to communicate clearly in both the written and spoken forms fosters understanding and accurate exchange of information. Consider record keeping as writing the client's professional interaction story. Realize that reflection on the healing journey provided by reading this story allows both you and your client, and any other authorized individuals, to appreciate the process and to remember and replicate the steps in achieving goals that honor the effort put forth by all concerned.

ⓔvolve

http://evolve.elsevier.com/Fritz/fundamentals/
4-1 Categorize roots, prefixes, and suffixes to build your medical vocabulary.

4-2 Medical terminology flashcards are available for further study

4-3 Complete a crossword puzzle on terminology from this chapter

4-4 Review vocabulary with an audio spelling activity

Don't forget to study for your certification and licensure exams! Review questions, along with weblinks, can be found on the Evolve website.

Reference

Thompson DL: *Hands heal: documentation for massage therapy: a guide for SOAP charting*, Philadelphia, 2005, Lippincott Williams & Wilkins.

Workbook Section

Short Answer

1. What are the three word elements and how are they used?

2. What are abbreviations? Provide guidelines for their use.

3. Explain what is meant by *quantifiable* and *qualifiable* functional goals.

4. What is the difference between an intake procedure and charting?

5. What are the four steps in the analysis of data acquired during the intake process and how does analysis relate to the development of a care or treatment plan?

6. Explain the four parts of the SOAP charting process.

7. What is required to maintain the integrity of charts when writing in them?

Matching I

Match the term to the best definition.

_____ 1. Abbreviation
_____ 2. Combining vowel
_____ 3. Prefix
_____ 4. Root
_____ 5. Suffix
_____ 6. Word element

a. A vowel added between two roots or a root and a suffix to facilitate pronunciation
b. A word element that gives the fundamental meaning of the word
c. A word element placed at the beginning of a word to alter the meaning of the word
d. A reduced form of a word or phrase
e. A part of a word
f. A word element placed at the end of a root to alter the meaning of the word

Matching II

Match each of the following word elements to its proper meaning. Then indicate its type; that is, whether it is a prefix (p), a root word (r), or a suffix (s). Remember that some of the root words may not have a vowel at the end because vowels are added only when combined with a suffix.

Word Element	Meaning	Type
1. ab	_____	_____
2. ad	_____	_____
3. algia	_____	_____
4. arthro	_____	_____
5. chondr	_____	_____
6. circum	_____	_____
7. contra	_____	_____
8. cost	_____	_____
9. de	_____	_____
10. dia	_____	_____
11. dis	_____	_____
12. dys	_____	_____
13. epi	_____	_____
14. fibr	_____	_____
15. genesis	_____	_____
16. genic	_____	_____
17. gram	_____	_____
18. graph	_____	_____
19. graphy	_____	_____
20. hyper	_____	_____
21. inter	_____	_____
22. intra	_____	_____
23. intro	_____	_____
24. ism	_____	_____
25. it is	_____	_____
26. myo	_____	_____
27. myel	_____	_____
28. neuro	_____	_____
29. orth	_____	_____
30. osis	_____	_____
31. osteo	_____	_____
32. pathy	_____	_____
33. plegia	_____	_____
34. post	_____	_____
35. stasis	_____	_____
36. sterno	_____	_____
37. sub	_____	_____
38. supra	_____	_____
39. therm	_____	_____
40. thoraco	_____	_____

a. Toward
b. Over, on, upon
c. Producing, causing
d. A diagram, a recording instrument
e. Excessive, too much, high
f. Around
g. Against, opposite
h. Joint
i. Record
j. A condition
k. Away from
l. Nerve
m. Condition
n. Making a recording
o. Paralysis
p. Maintenance, maintaining a constant level
q. Development, production, creation
r. Pain
s. Above, over
t. Disease
u. Chest
v. Fiber, fibrous
w. Cartilage
x. Under
y. Heat
z. Rib
aa. Bad, difficult, abnormal
bb. Within
cc. Down, from, away from, not
dd. Across, through, apart
ee. Inflammation
ff. Spinal cord, bone marrow
gg. Separation, away from
hh. Between
ii. Into, within
jj. Straight, normal, correct
kk. Bone
ll. After, behind
mm. Sternum
nn. Muscle

Matching III

Match the lymph nodes and plexuses to their correct description.

_____ 1. Parotid
_____ 2. Occipital
_____ 3. Superficial cervical
_____ 4. Subclavicular
_____ 5. Hypogastric
_____ 6. Facial
_____ 7. Deep cervical
_____ 8. Axillary
_____ 9. Mediastinal
_____ 10. Cubital
_____ 11. Para-aortic
_____ 12. Deep inguinal
_____ 13. Superficial inguinal
_____ 14. Popliteal
_____ 15. Mammary plexus
_____ 16. Palmar plexus
_____ 17. Plantar plexus

a. Deeply situated nodes in the groin
b. Nodes in the groin close to the surface
c. Nodes under the collarbone
d. Nodes draining the tissue in the face
e. Lymphatic vessels in the sole of the foot (plantar)
f. Lymphatic vessels in the palm of the hand (palmar)
g. Nodes around or in front of the ear
h. Nodes over the bone at the back of the head
i. Nodes in the area beneath the stomach
j. Nodes around the aorta
k. Deeply situated nodes in the neck
l. Lymphatic vessels around the breasts
m. Nodes in the armpit
n. Nodes of the elbow
o. Nodes close to the surface of the neck
p. Nodes in back of the knee
q. Nodes in the mediastinal section of the thoracic cavity

Assess Your Competencies

Now that you have studied this chapter, you should be able to:
- Use massage terminology as presented by the *Massage Therapy Body of Knowledge (MTBOK)*
- Use medical terminology to identify the three word elements used in medical terms and comprehend unfamiliar medical terms
- Use anatomic and physiologic terminology correctly
- Use the information in this chapter for effective professional record keeping

On a separate sheet of paper or on the computer, write a short summary of the content of this chapter based on the preceding list of competencies. Use a conversational tone, as if you were explaining to someone (e.g., a client, prospective employer, coworker, or other interested person) the importance of the information and skills to the development of the massage profession.

Next, in small discussion groups, share your summary with your classmates and compare the ways the information was presented. In discussing the content, look for similarities, differences, possibilities for misunderstanding of the information, and clear, concise methods of description.

Problem-Solving Scenarios

Six new clients came to your office this week. Each had filled out a client history form ahead of time, providing you with the following information on medical conditions that have been diagnosed and treated by their physicians. In the following list, break down each of the italicized medical terms into its word parts to define the various conditions.

Dermatitis of the hands

Neuropathy in the left leg

Hypothyroidism

Dyspnea

Hemangioma

Polyarthritis

Myocarditis

Hydronephrosis

Research for Further Study

List three resource books or Internet sites you could use for further study of medical terminology. Include the title, publisher, and type of reference.

Record-Keeping Exercise

Complete the forms in Figures 4-16 through 4-19, using the clinical reasoning process and yourself as the client. When you complete the SOAP form, make up a massage session that would be applicable to your personal situation as reflected on the intake forms.

Note: Before you do this exercise, you might want to make copies of the blank forms to use during practice sessions. Also, remember that these are sample forms, which are presented as a guide for learning and for the development of your own professional forms.

Research Literacy and Evidence-Based Practice

http://evolve.elsevier.com/Fritz/fundamentals/

CHAPTER OBJECTIVES

After completing this chapter, the student will be able to perform the following:

1. Define research literacy
2. Use levels of evidence guidelines to categorize research
3. Cite current research that validates the underlying physiologic mechanisms of therapeutic massage
4. Describe the fundamentals of the Western scientific process
5. Interpret a research paper
6. Relate the concepts of physics to the experience of touch and massage therapy
7. Explain the effects of therapeutic massage in physiologic terms

CHAPTER OUTLINE

KEY TERMS

Absolute risk
Attunement
Breathing pattern disorder
Centering
Circulation
Compression
Connective tissue
Conservation withdrawal
Cortisol
Counterirritation
Dopamine
Dynorphins
Electromyography (EMG)
Endocannabinoids
Endorphins
Enkephalins
Entrainment
Entrapment
Epinephrine/adrenaline
Ethics
Evidence-based practice
Experiment

Gate control theory
General adaptation syndrome
Growth hormone
Harmonics
Heart rate variability
Hormones
Hyperstimulation analgesia
Hypothesis
Informed consent
Intuition
Joint kinesthetic receptors
Law
Mechanical effects
Muscle spindles
Neurotransmitter
Norepinephrine/ noradrenaline
Oxytocin
Parasympathetic patterns
Placebo effect
Reflexive effects
Relative risk

Research literacy
Resonance
Resonator
Science
Scientific method
Serotonin
Stress

Sympathetic autonomic
    nervous system (ANS)
Tendon organs
Tensegrity
Toughening (hardening)
Trigger point
Vibration

STUDENT NOTE: This chapter is long and sometimes complex. However, it is crucial to your development as a massage professional. You will find it helpful to keep a medical dictionary and an anatomy and physiology textbook, such as *Mosby's Essential Sciences for Therapeutic Massage,* at hand to use as references while studying this chapter. You can also use electronic sources, such as the Internet. This chapter contains many technical terms, and you may need to read and study it more than once to fully understand the information presented. The Evolve website has links that can help you.

As discussed in Chapter 2, claims made for massage benefits must be based on valid evidence. An important source of this evidence is scientific research. The *American Heritage Dictionary* defines science as, "the intellectual process of using all mental and physical resources available to better understand, explain, and predict both normal and unusual natural phenomena." The scientific approach to understanding anything involves observation, measurement of things that can be tested, accumulation of data, and analysis of the findings. The scientific approach, therefore, is different from an intuitive approach.

Intuition is knowing something without using a conscious process of thinking. Other terms for intuition are *feelings, inspiration, instinct, revelation, impulse,* and *idea.* The term *intuition* is not used in this textbook to mean a psychic or extrasensory experience; rather, it means the ability to act purposefully on subconsciously perceived information. Intuition is the ability to bring subconscious information into conscious awareness. Developing intuitive skills assists the massage therapist in the assessment process and in adapting massage for each client. Through experience, massage therapists just "know" when a certain area of the client's body needs to be worked, and they can sense when the area is complete and needs no more work.

Biofeedback works on a similar principle. Using equipment that detects the heart rate, blood pressure, and skin temperature, a person can monitor and adjust involuntary, or subconscious, responses.

Centering is the ability to pay attention to a specific area of focus. Centering skills allow us to screen sensation and concentrate. Learning to pay attention to quiet, subtle information amid all the loud, exaggerated stimulation that can blast our sensory receptors every day takes practice. When we are centered, intuition is more apparent. Also, the ability to center oneself is a crucial aspect of developing intuition.

Scientific and intuitive approaches are equally important. Renowned researcher Hans Selye, in a lecture titled "Stress without Distress: Evolution of the Concept," emphasized the importance of both science and intuition. Unless there is first an idea (intuition), Dr. Selye said, there is nothing to research, and without research (science), an idea does not develop

💡 **PROFICIENCY EXERCISE 5-1**

Give your explanation of Dr. Selye's statement: "If there is not first an idea, there is nothing to research. Without research, an idea does not develop form and usefulness. One does not function without the other."

form and usefulness. One does not function without the other (Proficiency Exercise 5-1).

You may hear or read that massage is an art, not a science. In reality, massage is both. Art is craft, skill, technique, and talent. Perfecting your artistic approach to massage involves disciplined and ongoing practice. As you begin learning about massage application, you must spend considerable time practicing before the art of massage application becomes evident. Talent is defined as some sort of natural, innate ability. Although some may have a talent for massage, massage therapy is a learned art. Diligent practice, along with desire, passion, and compassion, will help you become an excellent massage therapist.

Recognizing how important intuition is in the art of the massage profession is important. However, realizing how scientific research validates massage therapy is equally important. This validation separates fact from mere speculation about massage and related bodywork methods.

Sometimes beginning students of massage may find scientific justification intimidating. However, it is important to develop an understanding of this knowledge at the beginning of the educational process, because it is one of the foundations of our profession. This firm foundation in the anatomic and physiologic explanations of the reasons massage works enables us to trust our intuition while designing a massage based on the information we receive from the client during assessment procedures. Therefore, the purpose of this chapter is to help you understand the physiologic basis for the effectiveness of therapeutic massage.

Massage therapy is an evidence-based and evidence-informed practice. Evidence includes everything that is used to determine or demonstrate the truth of a claim. For example, if we are going to state that massage therapy is beneficial, then we need to support that assertion. Many types of evidence exist; the two most valid are well-conducted scientific research (evidence-based) and supported expert clinical experience (evidence-informed). As we search for evidence, we must remain objective and willing to collect all the relevant research available, not just the information that supports massage.

When making informed decisions about the value and approach of massage, we need to consider all the evidence from scientific research, both supportive and nonsupportive. We also must consider other forms of valid evidence, such as collective clinical experience, historical and cultural foundations, and consistency of client experience. Although scientific research is not the only form of valid evidence, it is a very important part of an evidence-based massage practice. Most of us will not actually conduct formal research in a research laboratory. All of us, however, need to be research users and evaluators to make sure we are the most informed massage therapists possible (Box 5-1). This is the major focus of this chapter.

We Can All Be Researchers

All massage therapists can serve as researchers and contributors to the massage body of evidence by collecting information and writing case reports. The Massage Therapy Foundation, which has established research contests for both students and practitioners, provides the following guidelines for students who want to produce a case report.

Case Report Guidelines and Case Report Structure
Students must report on independent clinical interventions on one client with guidance from a case report supervisor and a clinic supervisor. This includes doing a literature review on the presenting condition or client goal; creating and implementing a treatment plan in accordance with the literature, the needs of the client, and the students' expertise; writing up the results; discussing the implications of the outcomes; and offering suggestions for future study. Also:

- Students must conduct a minimum of five massage therapy sessions with the participating client.
- It is highly recommended that massage therapy be the only new intervention in the client's treatment plan.
- Patient confidentiality and the security of health information must be maintained. No personal identification of the student or client may be included in the report.

The Case Report
A well-written scientific report explains the scientist's goal for doing an experiment, the experimental design and execution, and the meaning of the results. A beautifully conducted study loses much of its value if it is not presented in a succinct and coherent manner. Therefore, scientific papers are written in a style that is intended to be clear and concise. Their purpose is to inform an audience about an important issue and to document the particular approach used to investigate that issue.

The following eight sections should be included in the report.

1. **Cover page:** The cover page contains the title and the author's name, contact information, mailing address, e-mail address, and signature.
2. **Acknowledgments:** This section recognizes any individuals other than the author who helped substantially with the work, including any mentors or contributors. (The cover page and acknowledgments are removed from the submitted papers for the process of blind review.)
3. **Abstract/keywords:** An abstract is a condensed version of the paper (200-word limit). It should have the following subsections:
   - Background and objectives for the study
   - Methods used for any interventions, evaluation techniques, and measurement tools
   - Results obtained
   - Conclusion from the study
   Frequently, readers of a scientific journal read only the abstract, choosing to read the full text only of papers that are most relevant to them. For this reason, and because abstracts frequently are made available by various Internet abstracting services, this section is an important summary of the study
   Keywords: Citation indexes use keywords (or phrases) to help people search for relevant articles. Authors therefore should list four or five keywords that

define their study. These words or phrases should not include words used in the title.

4. **Introduction:** In this section the author should build a case for conducting the study. Enough background information should be provided on the condition studied to enable a reader to understand the topic. Findings of previously published studies must be presented to help explain the reasons the current study is of scientific interest. This is called a *literature review.* No results or data from the study should be in this section. The last sentence or sentences of the introduction should state the study objective and/or hypothesis: the research question. This should make a smooth transition from the introduction section to the methods section. Appropriate use of citations from the literature review are emphasized in the scoring process. References must include at least some of the academic books, professional journals, and peer-reviewed journals. Students are expected to use reputable biomedical and massage therapy databases as part of their literature search strategy. Use of sources that are not peer-reviewed should be kept to a minimum.

5. **Methods:** This section, which comprises two parts, provides all the methodological details necessary for another scientist to duplicate the work. The two parts are the client profile and the treatment plan. It is safe to assume that readers have the same basic skills as the author but do not know the specific details of the study. This section should be a narrative of the steps in the study, but not a list of instructions one might find in a cookbook. An important part of writing a scientific paper is deciding which information should be condensed and what needs to be described in detail.

- *Client profile:* This part should contain a detailed account of the subject. This may include a presentation of the subject's medical history and diagnosis (including the discipline of the professional who arrived at the diagnosis), prior treatments, findings from a massage assessment, findings from other health care providers, and any contraindications to the use of massage. The client should have a condition that is modifiable by massage. The student should include a description of the client's desired outcomes.
- *Treatment plan:* This part should describe the massage/bodywork procedures used and the way the subject's progress was monitored. The author should provide specific details on the massage/bodywork techniques, including the duration of treatment, type of stroke, body regions worked, number of treatments, and so on.
  - A crucial component of the treatment plan is the author's rationale for the particular massage/bodywork technique or techniques used. Treatment choices must be supported with reference to the available literature, massage texts/instructional handbooks, and safe practice guidelines. If there are no direct references to massage therapy for the condition, the student should indicate why the treatment approach was chosen based on an understanding of how the condition typically

Continued

Box 5-1   We Can All Be Researchers—cont'd

presents and how it presents in the client. References from other disciplines (e.g., physical therapy, occupational therapy) also may be helpful.

- Students should avoid using trademarked names of modalities and traditional French names for strokes; instead, simply provide a description of the work. For example, "longitudinal stroking" is more appropriate than "effleurage."
- A description of the plan for assessing progress should also be presented in the treatment plan. Any instrument used to assess progress (e.g., questionnaire, Visual Analog Scale, ergometer, goniometer) should be presented and its use described in moderate detail. Also, the frequency of assessment, the number of trials (if appropriate), and the time tested (in relation to treatment) are important factors. A reader of this section should be able to visualize how a subject's progress was assessed.
- A summary of any methodological changes that occurred during the course of the treatment plan, along with the rationalization for these changes, should be included.

6. **Results:** This section presents the results of the experiment but should not attempt to interpret their meaning. Data should be presented in an organized and easily understandable manner; raw data should not be presented. Authors are encouraged to succinctly present study findings in either a table or graph format. However, data should be presented only once. If a table or figure is presented, it should be titled as such and have a caption (and legend, if necessary) so the reader can

quickly understand what is being presented. The written portion of the report must refer to any table or figure, if presented.

7. **Discussion:** The discussion section provides an opportunity to summarize and evaluate the outcomes of the treatment process. It is also important to integrate the findings from the study into the body of literature that currently exists on the topic. Therefore, this section should:
   - Summarize the outcomes and effectiveness of treatment
   - Relate the study findings back to the objective/hypothesis
   - Place the results in context of published findings (using sources previously cited as well as other sources)
   - Explain the reasons obtained results may differ from what others have found
   - Speculate on whether the treatment had an effect
     The author should also note problems with the methods, explain any anomalies in the data, and suggest future research directions that are based on the results of the study.

8. **References:** Although no specific point value is awarded for the references section, the strength of a report depends partly on the citations referenced. Therefore, students are strongly encouraged, in preparing the report, to use citations from the primary research literature (e.g., peer-reviewed journal articles) rather than secondary sources (e.g., Internet websites).

Modified from the Massage Therapy Foundation. www.massagetherapyfoundation.org. Accessed February 8, 2011.

Author Support: I know that reading information written in a technical style can be tedious and confusing if you are not familiar with it. Writing in a technical and scientific style also can be tedious. However, research is conducted and presented in a specific way for good reasons. One very important reason is consistency in the way the research is conducted. That consistency is reflected in the way the paper that describes the process and outcomes of the research is presented. Professional trends indicate that the ability to find, critique, and apply research is becoming a vital skill for massage therapists. Once you get used to the style and terminology, research can be really exciting.

Throughout the next sections of the text, explanations of some of the terminology are provided in parentheses to help you understand the content. However, it is important that you develop the habit of learning the meanings of words you do not know, so continue to *look them up*. This is how you build your professional vocabulary.

RESEARCH LITERACY

SECTION OBJECTIVES

Chapter objective covered in this section:

1. The student will be able to define research literacy.
2. The student will be able to define the levels of evidence guidelines to categorize research

Using the information presented in this section, the student will be able to perform the following:

- Describe evidence-based practice
- Use the Cochrane Reviews to find systematic reviews for massage therapy–based research

Research literacy (or *scientific literacy*) is the knowledge and understanding of scientific concepts and processes required for personal and professional decision making. When we are research literate, we can find, read, and understand the research and use critical thinking to determine the validity of the information presented by the paper. Learning to be a critical thinker (see Chapter 2) is the first step in becoming research literate. Critical thinking and the scientific method are very similar.

Developing an inquiry-based approach to life also is important. This means that we learn to ask relevant questions. Relevant questions evolve from mindfulness and intuition. For example, "Why and how does massage help reduce uncomfortable stress responses?" Only when we have relevant questions can we begin the research process. Scientifically based research methods are a way to seek answers to those questions.

A research-literature search discovers information from researchers who designed and conducted a study to look for answers to some of the same questions we might have. Because most of us will not perform complex research studies (although we can all be researchers if we do case reports), we need to find and examine other people's research on questions that are the same or similar to ours. Part of reading research articles involves making sure the research was conducted properly and that the information is scientifically valid and not just opinion.

Valid Research

Effective outcomes from massage applications are achieved when massage methods interact with physiologic processes. Because massage has demonstrable physiologic effects, those effects can be studied through the scientific method. The **scientific method** is a means of objectively researching a concept to determine whether it is valid. Research begins with a **hypothesis** (i.e., "If this happens, then that will happen."). The hypothesis must then be tested; this usually is accomplished through an **experiment**. Interpretation of the data collected during the experiment is expressed in statistical form; therefore, the reader must be able to interpret terms used in statistical reporting. This requirement sometimes makes reading research papers difficult for the general public. However, you do not have to be an expert in statistics; you simply must understand what the statistical terms mean. Usually the statistical results are presented in a chart or graph, which is helpful.

The experiment must follow accepted design measures so that others can replicate it to see whether they get the same result. The results of the experiment should either prove or disprove the hypothesis. Often the results of the research generate more questions, leading to more research. Different types of experiments are performed in research.

- *Randomized controlled trials* involve a randomization procedure in which each subject has an equal chance of being assigned to an intervention group that actually receives the treatment or a control group that receives a fake treatment. Randomization helps prevent researchers from knowingly or unknowingly creating bias in the outcomes. Randomized controlled trials are the "gold standard" for establishing the effects of a treatment.
- *Cohort studies,* also called *prospective* or *longitudinal studies,* use observation as the research method. The interventions are not manipulated; rather, the researchers select and follow a large population of people who have the same condition and/or are receiving a specific intervention over a period of time. The progression and results of treatment are compared with a group not affected by the condition.
- *Outcomes research* involves a larger group of individuals who receive the same intervention. They are evaluated for outcomes after the intervention is complete.
- A *case series* is a collection of comprehensive reports that follow the research method on a series of clients with the same condition who are receiving the same intervention.
- A *case report* involves a report on the intervention and outcome for a single client.

Box 5-2 **Guidelines for Levels of Evidence: ABC System**

> **Level A:** Well-done, random controlled studies (RCT) with 100 or more subjects
> **Level B:** Well-conducted case-control study; poorly controlled or uncontrolled observations studies with high potential for bias; or RCT with one or more major, or three or more minor, methodological flaws or case series or case reports
> **Level C:** Expert opinion

Modified from Rich NC: Levels of evidence, *J Womens Health Phys Ther* 29:19, 2005.

Evidence-based practice, as explained in Chapter 2, is "the conscientious, explicit, and judicious use of current best evidence in making decisions about the care of individual patients" (Sackett et al., 2000). It comprises interventions for which consistent scientific and clinical evidence shows improved client outcomes. The best evidence to determine whether an intervention, such as massage, actually causes the outcome is the double-blind, random controlled clinical trial. It consists of the randomized assignment of subjects or participants in a double-blind design, in which neither the investigators nor the study subjects know the actual treatment group in which the subjects are placed. This type of trial also uses a control group, in which no intervention is used, and a sham group, in which a fictional treatment is provided. This type of trial is difficult to design for massage therapy research. One of the biggest challenges is devising fake or fictional massage. However, progress is being made, and more quality research should be forthcoming in the future.

Evidence can be classified into different levels. Professional journals that publish research are introducing guidelines and instructing authors to label the strength of evidence of their research in terms of rating scales. In addition, multiple methods are used to categorize research. The simplest method is the ABC method (Box 5-2).

Systematic Review and Meta-Analysis

Systematic reviews and meta-analyses combine multiple research studies that are similar in design. A systematic review usually is restricted to random controlled studies, which are considered valid evidence if they are well done. A group of reviewers searches the available literature databases by entering common terminologies into the databases and retrieving copies of all the articles written on a specific topic. After all the research has been collected, the reviewers use critical thinking methods to evaluate the validity of each study and then synthesize the results. The final product reports on properly completed, meaningful research that is relevant to practitioners and clinicians.

A meta-analysis is a type of systematic review that uses statistical methods to combine and analyze multiple investigations. Two important sources of systematic reviews that involve massage are the Cochrane Database of Systematic Reviews (commonly called the Cochrane Reviews) and the Database of Abstracts of Reviews of Effects.

Box 5-3   Cochrane Reviews Relevant to Massage Therapy

The Cochrane Reviews consolidate research findings and provide plain language explanations of those findings. The Cochrane Collaboration is an international network that helps health care providers, policy makers, patients, and their advocates make well-informed, evidence-based decisions.

A *systematic review* is a high-level overview of primary research on a particular research question. Evidence-based clinical practice, such as massage therapy, is an approach to decision making in which the clinician uses the best evidence available. The Cochrane Collaboration has more than 100 systematic reviews relevant to massage therapy, such as massage and touch for dementia; massage for people with human immunodeficiency virus (HIV) infection and acquired immunodeficiency syndrome (AIDS); and massage for low back pain. The Cochrane Reviews are available at www2.cochrane.org/reviews.

- *Cochrane Database of Systematic Reviews (CDSR)* is a great resource for looking up health care reviews. The review databases are created by professional review groups and are peer reviewed (Box 5-3).
- *Database of Abstracts of Reviews of Effects (DARE)* contains 15,000 abstracts of systematic reviews, including more than 6000 quality-assessed reviews and details of all Cochrane Reviews and protocols. The database focuses on the effects of interventions used in health and social care. DARE is prepared by the National Health Service's Centre for Reviews and Dissemination (NHS CDR) at the University of York, England.

As the massage profession evolves and more research becomes available, it is important to search for and use first interventions that have been shown to have a statistically significant treatment effect with well-controlled research studies. As more of this type of evidence becomes available, all of us in the massage profession must examine some of the "myths" that arose before valid evidence was available. Most of the myths began as well-intentioned, educated guesses. Valid research indicates that some of those educated guesses are accurate, but many are not. For example, not many years ago, cancer was considered an absolute contraindication to massage; now, research has shown that massage therapy has many benefits for those undergoing cancer treatment.

We all need to develop an inquiring mind; therefore, practice asking your instructors relevant questions. Remember, it is not the instructor's job to know all the answers. Instead, work together to find the evidence. If no systematic reviews or meta-analyses are available, consider using other types of guidance, such as the opinions of multiple experts (Box 5-4).

A number of questions have arisen in the massage profession regarding the emphasis on evidence-based practices, such as the following:
- What should be done when there are different levels of evidence or changes in evidence?
- What are the limits of evidence?
- What should be done when no scientific evidence exists for a massage approach?

Box 5-4   Quality of Evidence

The U.S. Preventive Services Task Force (USPSTF), established by the Department of Health and Human Services, is a multidisciplinary team of primary care experts that uses a systematic, evidence-based approach to focus on preventive services in the clinical setting. The task force specifically bases its recommendation on a balanced evaluation of the benefits and potential for harm of a preventive service.

Quality of Evidence
The task force grades the quality of the overall evidence for a service on a three-point scale:
- *Good:* Evidence includes consistent results from well-designed, well-conducted studies in representative populations that directly assess effects on health outcomes.
- *Fair:* Evidence is sufficient to determine effects on health outcomes, but the strength of the evidence is limited by the number, quality, or consistency of the individual studies; the generalizability to routine practice; or the indirect nature of the evidence on health outcomes.
- *Poor:* Evidence is insufficient to assess the effects on health outcomes because of limited number or power of studies, important flaws in their design or conduct, gaps in the chain of evidence, or lack of information on important health outcomes.

Strength of Recommendations
The task force grades its recommendations as A, B, C, D, or I, depending on the strength of the evidence and the magnitude of net benefit (benefits minus harms).
- **A:** The task force strongly recommends that clinicians provide the service to eligible patients. The task force found good evidence that the service improves important health outcomes and concludes that benefits substantially outweigh harm.
- **B:** The task force recommends that clinicians provide this service to eligible patients. The task force found at least fair evidence that the service improves important health outcomes and concludes that benefits outweigh harm.
- **C:** The task force makes no recommendation for or against routine provision of the service. The task force found at least fair evidence that the service can improve health outcomes but concludes that the balance of benefit and harm is too close to justify a general recommendation.
- **D:** The task force recommends against routinely providing the service to asymptomatic patients. The task force found at least fair evidence that the service is ineffective or that harm outweighs benefits.
- **I:** The task force concludes that the evidence is insufficient to recommend for or against routinely providing the service. Evidence that the service is effective is lacking, of poor quality, or conflicting and the balance of benefits and harm cannot be determined.

Modified from U.S. Preventive Services Task Force Ratings: *Grade definitions—guide to clinical preventive services*, ed 3, Periodic updates, 2000-2003, Rockville, MD, Agency for Healthcare Research and Quality. Rockville, Md, http://www.ahrq.gov/clinic/3rduspstf/ratings.htm. Accessed February 2, 2009.

- What if an intervention, such as massage therapy, cannot be easily researched in double-blind, random controlled studies?
- What if studies produce conflicting evidence?

Research evidence often is complicated by differences in the design, quality, and number of studies performed on any single intervention. Often the results are inconsistent. With the increase in the types and quality of research being done in massage therapy, the evidence is changing quickly, and this increases the demand on massage therapists to stay current. For example, this textbook was based on the most current research available at the time. However, a textbook usually is revised only every 3 to 5 years; consequently, some of the information it contains already may be outdated. For these reasons, you must learn how to ask relevant questions and find the evidence for yourself.

As the massage profession moves toward evidence-based practices, we must be honest about the quality of the evidence for therapeutic massage. Currently the evidence is limited and of less than optimum quality. As a profession we must acknowledge this while still striving to determine the best practices for massage. In some situations, essentially no research exists on certain types of bodywork and claimed benefits. This does not mean these types of bodywork are of no value or that they are not valid. It means that we do not know, and that is okay. The emphasis on evidence-based practices should create pressure to develop and test these interventions to fill the need for informed rather than opinion-based massage therapy practice. When we do not know whether a massage method is valid, but the potential exists for benefit with little chance of harm, then informed decision making, by the massage therapist and the client together, determines whether including the method in the massage session is appropriate. Mysteries will always remain, but we are professionally obligated to know the research available and to admit when we do not know the answers.

Most health care professionals use evidence-based best practices. Massage therapists have a lot of support as they search for evidence related to a massage therapy practice. For example, the mission of the Agency for Healthcare Research and Quality (AHRQ) is to improve the quality, safety, efficiency, and effectiveness of health care for all Americans. Information from AHRQ's research helps people make more informed decisions and improves the quality of health care services. The Evolve website provides a link to the AHRQ website, which offers extensive resources for investigating evidence-based practice in health care disciplines, including massage therapy.

Technologic advances have allowed researchers to see more deeply into the human experience than ever before. We are on the verge of understanding the more mysterious and hidden workings of the body. Only a growing body of research and data replication that establishes the positive biochemical and behavioral reaction to touch will convince the scientific community that massage is therapeutic. Fortunately, this type of research is now being done, and the health care professions and the public are responding by seeking massage therapy services. Validation through scientific research has opened these doors.

CURRENT RESEARCH

SECTION OBJECTIVES

Chapter objective covered in this section:
3. The student will be able to cite current research that validates the underlying physiologic mechanisms of therapeutic massage.
Using the information presented in this section, the student will be able to perform the following:
- Use search engines and databases to locate research related to massage therapy
- Categorize and review current research related to massage therapy

Now that you have an idea of the importance of research to support an evidence-based and evidence-informed massage practice, we can explore the current research specific to massage therapy. As a result of growing interest, and through funding provided by the National Institutes of Health (NIH) Research Centers, research on the benefits of massage is increasing in the United States. Similar research is underway in other parts of the world, such as Canada, Europe, Australia, New Zealand, Japan, and China. These studies continue to validate the benefits of therapeutic massage applications for various conditions. The data are beginning to identify patterns of the underlying physiologic mechanisms that massage addresses.

Research results now are available to anyone who wants to understand the underlying physiologic mechanisms of therapeutic massage benefits, and they continue to support the value of therapeutic massage. In 2002, the Massage Therapy Foundation's comprehensive database for therapeutic massage research became available on the foundation's website. Other websites for research include PubMed, Medline, and Google Scholar. This chapter does not attempt to list individual research results, but rather consolidates the research into categories and physiologic processes. The Evolve website for this chapter provides weblinks to research papers.

The Touch Research Institute (TRI) of the University of Miami School of Medicine, directed by Tiffany Field, PhD, deserves credit for supporting the current commitment to the understanding of massage therapy. Dr. Field believes that the clinical health care system will come to incorporate touch therapy in the same way it incorporated relaxation therapy, exercise, and diet (Field, 2000). Since 1992 the studies that have been published by or are under way at the TRI cover a broad range of subjects and conditions, and they show that massage affects many aspects of human physiology and experience. These research findings are available on the TRI website.as well as the Evolve website.

In 2000 Dr. Field noted the need for further investigation:

Across studies, decreases were noted in anxiety, depression, stress hormones (cortisol), and catecholamines. Increased parasympathetic activity may be the underlying mechanism for these changes. The pressure stimulation associated with touch increases vagal activity, which in turn lowers physiologic arousal and stress hormones such as cortisol. Appropriate application of pressure is critical, because light stroking is generally aversive (much like a tickle stimulus) and does not produce these effects. Decreased cortisol levels in turn lead to enhanced immune function. Parasympathetic activity is also associated with increased alertness and better performance on cognitive tasks. Given that most diseases are exacerbated by stress and given that massage therapy alleviates stress, receiving massages should probably be high on the health priority list, along with diet and exercise (Field, 2000).

Research is ongoing, and more is needed to replicate findings on the benefits of massage and to investigate the underlying psychological mechanisms. In general, the quality of massage-related research is considered less than optimal, and those conducting research need to be more diligent in the research process. Past research needs to be revisited and results verified. For example, Christopher Moyer studied the effects of massage on cortisol levels and concluded that cortisol may not be directly affected by massage, but rather that a reduction in perceived anxiety may lead to changes in cortisol levels (Moyer, 2011).

Until the quality of research improves, the quantity increases, and the underlying mechanisms are understood, the general public and the health care community are less likely to wholly incorporate these therapies into general practice. In addition to studies on mechanisms of effect, the massage community needs research involving treatment comparison studies to determine the best massage techniques for different conditions and the arousing versus the calming effects of different treatments. As these studies progress, the massage professional should evolve from a method approach (e.g., Swedish/classic massage, deep tissue massage, Rolfing, shiatsu) to an orientation toward desired physiologic outcomes achieved by using variations in pressure, speed, rhythm, direction, and duration (Field, 2000).

Research Findings

The summary of massage research that follows is based on an Internet search using the terms *massage, massage therapy, manual therapy,* and *manual lymph drainage.* The search process for this text involved mainly Internet sources, such as ScienceDirect, PubMed, and Google Scholar. Studies dating from 2000 are included, and research conducted from 2005 to the present was the main focus. Representative studies, especially systematic reviews and meta-analyses, were analyzed, and the findings of some of these reports appear in this content. Because research is an evolving process, the studies and conclusions presented can be either confirmed or questioned based on the results of future research. Therefore, the massage professional must remain current on advances in the understanding of the benefits of massage.

Before we investigate the research, it is important to remember that the specific massage methods these researchers and clinicians applied during the study are not the most important factor; rather, their commitment to research and to intelligent, informed application is the key.

General Massage Benefits and Safety

Research findings are mixed regarding the efficacy of massage. *Efficacy* is the ability to produce an effect. In general, massage in and of itself was not found to be a definitive treatment for various conditions; rather, it was found to be supportive of many other interventions, either enhancing effects or

managing side effects of other treatments. This means that typically massage would be a beneficial part of a wellness or health care treatment program, but it should not be expected to provide optimum outcomes if used as the only therapeutic intervention.

For any treatment, safety (i.e., do no harm) is a primary concern. If harm is possible, the benefits of receiving massage must exceed the potential for harm. A summary of a review of massage safety by Ernst et al. (2006) concludes that massage is generally safe. Massage is not entirely risk-free, and massage therapists need to be aware of the possibility of harm. However, serious adverse effects are rare. Most adverse effects from massage have been associated with aggressive types of massage or massage delivered by untrained individuals. In addition, such effects have been associated mostly with massage techniques other than "Swedish" (classic) massage. Adverse effects also may result when massage interferes with various types of implants, such as stents, ports, prostheses, and so on. In the *Journal of Vascular and Interventional Radiology,* Haskal (2008) reported a case in which a stent placed in a lower limb to treat peripheral artery disease migrated to the right atrium after 3 years. Open heart surgery was required to remove the embedded stent fragments. The dislodgement and migration of the stent were attributed to deep tissue massage of the thigh. Although such cases are rare, it is important to pay attention to adverse effects caused by massage.

The reasons massage works remain elusive, but recurring findings indicate the possibility of physiologic mechanisms. A study by Field et al. (2005) is particularly relevant, because it focuses on serotonin, a neurotransmitter associated with the body's pain modulation mechanisms. In other studies, Diego et al. (2004) and Diego and Field (2009) found that massage must be applied with sufficient compressive force to stimulate the antiarousal response and that light massage tends to stimulate the **sympathetic autonomic nervous system (ANS)** response.

Massage therapy appears to affect anxiety levels. The therapeutic relationship established between the massage therapist and the client is similar to the developments that occur in psychotherapy, in which treatment is based on communication and the therapeutic relationship. Some researchers believe that the effects of massage may stem from a therapeutic relationship (Moyer et al., 2004; Fellowes et al., 2004). Whether massage directly affects neurochemicals that influence mood and behavior is unclear, but research in touch has shown promising results. Because massage is a touch therapy, we can at least wonder whether the effects seen in these studies also relate to massage. For example, a study by Holt-Lunstad et al. (2008) investigated whether a support intervention ("warm touch," meaning warm, compassionate touch) influenced physiologic stress systems linked to important health outcomes. They concluded that increasing warm touch among couples had a beneficial influence on multiple stress-sensitive systems and that significant increases occurred in the subjects' oxytocin level. The latter finding is significant, because the hormone oxytocin is involved in pair bonding and parental bonding, both of which support positive health states. In addition, husbands in the intervention group had significantly lower post-treatment 24-hour systolic blood pressures than did those in the control group.

Serotonin is another important neurochemical related to stress levels. A study conducted in the Netherlands by Bakermans-Kranenburg and van Ijzendoorn (2008) explored the relationship of oxytocin and serotonin to "sensitive parenting." Animal studies suggest that oxytocin plays an important role in parenting and social interactions with offspring. Evidence indicates that serotonin may be important because of its influence on mood and the release of oxytocin. The researchers found a genetic influence in parents; those with a possibly less efficient response to oxytocin and serotonin showed lower levels of sensitive responsiveness to their toddlers.

A study by Henoch et al. (2010) investigated the relational and behavioral effect of soft skin massage on children with severe developmental disabilities. Soft skin massage was found to contribute to greater closeness and social interaction between the children and their caregivers; it also improved the children's communication skills. The children became more aware of their bodies and increased their bodily activities, which fostered a sense of well-being.

Correlation of **stress**, anxiety, depression, and pain is common. *Correlation* means that a relationship exists between elements, but it does not mean that one of the elements causes the other. Therefore, although stress, anxiety, depression, and pain often are found together, whether any one of them causes any of the others is unclear. Regardless, the four conditions often respond to the same applications of massage. For example, using a massage-like intervention, Lund et al. (2002) found a relationship between pain perception and oxytocin levels. (Remember that oxytocin is related to feelings of connectedness and bonding.) Although most studies on oxytocin involve touch, massage therapists can intelligently speculate that massage would have similar responses, because massage is a pleasurable touch.

The results of a study by Frey Law et al. (2008) suggest that massage can reduce myalgia symptoms by about 25% to 50%, depending on the technique used to measure pain. This study is a good example of a well-designed research project. It was a double-blind, randomized controlled trial that studied the effects of massage on pressure/pain thresholds (PPTs) and perceived pain. The researchers used delayed onset muscle soreness (DOMS) as a model of myalgia (muscle pain). They randomly assigned participants to a no-treatment control, superficial touch, or deep tissue massage group. At visit 1, a specific type of wrist exercise was performed; this caused DOMS 48 hours later, which was assessed at visit 2. The pain was assessed using visual analog scales (VAS); pressure was applied to cause pain, which was measured at baseline, after exercise, before treatment, and after treatment. The results of the study showed that deep massage reduced pain (48.4% DOMS reversal) during muscle stretch. Mechanical hyperalgesia (increased pain response to pressure) was reduced (27.5% reversal) in both the deep massage and superficial touch groups compared to the control group. The control group, which did not receive any massage, had an increased pain perception of 38.4%. Resting pain did not vary between treatment groups.

If we analyze the study by Frey Law et al., we can conclude that both deep and light pressure massage reduce the sensation of pain and that deep pressure massage helps reduce pain when stretching sore muscles. However, when no activity was involved, massage did not reduce the sensation of pain. To help you think about ways this information can be used in a massage practice, consider the scenario in the Example box.

> **EXAMPLE**
>
> A client did a lot of yard work and is sore and achy. He feels stiff, and stretching is painful. Based on the information in the Frey Law study, massage most likely will be beneficial if a variety of pressures are used, and deeper pressure massage is used to target areas that hurt when the client stretches. It might be important to explain to the client that he may still feel achy, but he should be able to move more easily.

Massage is not always the best way to manage symptoms. Hanley et al. (2003) found that, despite a very strong patient preference for therapeutic massage, it did not show any benefits over a relaxation tape in controlling postoperative pain. These researchers found that although massage was effective for managing pain and anxiety, it was no more effective than other relaxation interventions. An important point, however, is that the patients *liked* massage; this is a crucial factor in compliance with treatment. Müller-Oerlinghausen et al. (2007) concluded that slow-stroke massage is a suitable intervention for depression, along with other treatment, and is readily accepted by very ill patients. The same study found that massage reduced distress in oncology patients regardless of gender, age, ethnicity, or cancer type.

Other studies have shown that massage therapy enhances the treatment course of hospitalized oncology patients. Currin and Meister (2008) and Billhult et al. (2007) found that therapeutic massage showed potential benefits for reducing the chemotherapy and radiation side effects of breast cancer treatment and for improving perceived quality of life and overall functioning.

Key Points

The research studies discussed in this section, as well as other studies (see the Evolve website), provide evidence that massage therapy:

- May play a role in reducing detrimental stress-related symptoms
- Is pleasurable
- Appears to manage some muscle-type pain
- Supports social bonding
- Likely improves the perception of quality of life in individuals who enjoy massage
- Typically is safe when provided in a conservative and general manner with sufficient pain-free pressure

Mechanical Effects Related to Massage Benefit

The benefits of massage appear to be related to the application of mechanical forces to soft tissue. As you will learn in Chapter 10, massage methods involve the application of mechanical forces such as compression and tension. Possible results of these methods include the following:

- Altered pliability of connective tissue
- Stimulation of nerve endings in the fasciae
- Changes in local circulation
- Changes in the motor tone of muscles

According to Langevin and Sherman (2007), pain-related fear related to movement leads to a cycle of decreased movement, connective tissue remodeling, inflammation, and nervous system sensitization, all of which result in a further decrease in mobility. The mechanisms of a variety of treatments, including massage, may reverse these abnormalities by applying mechanical forces to soft tissues. Based on a tensegrity principle (everything is connected, like a spider web; see the following section), direct or indirect connections between fasciae seem to allow the transfer of tension over long distances. Massage applied to deform (change the shape) and stretch the soft tissue has an effect on the electrical and mechanical activities of muscles that are not being massaged but that are indirectly connected to the massaged tissue. Massage therapy appears to influence muscle motor tone not only through direct massage of the tissue, but also through indirect effects on another distant soft tissue structure (Kassolik et al., 2009).

The Tensegrity Principle

Tensegrity is an architectural principle developed in 1948 by R. Buckminster Fuller. The tensegrity principle is the foundation of the geodesic dome. A tensegrity system is characterized by a continuous tensional network (e.g., tendons, ligaments, and fascial structures) that is connected by a discontinuous set of compressive elements, or struts (e.g., bones). A tensegrity structure forms a stable yet dynamic system that interacts efficiently and resiliently with forces acting upon it (Figure 5-1). Attaching tendons and muscles to the bones results in a

three-dimensional tensegrity network that supports and moves the body. Tensegrity of the body explains how inflexibility or shortening in one tissue influences the structure and movement of other parts (Figures 5-2 and 5-3) (Chen and Ingber, 1999; Oschman, 2002).

These concepts are useful for massage practitioners who work with athletes and other performers in whom flexible and well-organized fascia and myofascial relationships enhance performance and reduce the incidence of injuries. Because the living tensegrity network is both a mechanical and a vibratory network, restrictions in one part have both structural and energetic consequences for the entire organism.

Myofascial System

According to Day et al. (2009), the myofascial system is a three-dimensional continuum; this means that we cannot truly separate muscle or any other type of tissue from the surrounding fascia or the body as a whole (i.e., there is no such thing as an individual muscle). Dr. Carla Stecco and Dr. Antonio Stecco have done extensive research into the anatomy and histology of the fascia through dissection of unembalmed cadavers (Stecco, 2006, 2007). Their work has provided a biomechanical model that helps decipher the role of fascia in musculoskeletal disorders.

Everything moves in the body, and parts must slide over and around other parts. Slippery fluid secreted by the body allows structures to slide. In muscle or myofascia, part of the fascia is anchored to bone (or another structure), and part is free to slide. If tissues cannot slide as they are supposed to, inflammation and reduced range of motion and strength can result. Fascia is formed by crimped/wavy collagen fibers and elastic fibers arranged in distinct layers; the fibers are aligned in a different direction in each layer. These fibers are embedded in a gelatin-like structure called *ground substance*. Fascia can be stretched because of the wavy nature of the fiber structure and the elastic fibers, which allows the fascia to return to its original resting state. Subcutaneous fascia (tissue containing body fat that is located under the skin but on top of muscle) forms a very elastic sliding membrane that is essential for thermal regulation, metabolic exchanges, and protection of vessels and nerves. Deep fascia is stiffer and thinner (resembling duct tape) than subcutaneous fascia. Deep fascia surrounds and compartmentalizes the muscles and forms the structures that attach soft tissues to bone. This type of fascia also forms a complex latticework of connective tissue, resembling struts, crossbeams, and guy wires, that helps maintain the structural integrity and function of the body.

Researchers think that the richly innervated fascia could be maintained in a taut resting state, called *fascial tone,* as a result of the different muscular fibers that pull on it (somewhat like a trampoline). This resting state enables the free nerve endings and receptors in the fascial tissue to sense any variation in the shape of the fascia (and therefore any movement of the body) whenever it occurs (Schleip et al, 2005); (Stecco et al., 2007a). Deep fascia is designed to sense and assist in organizing movements. Whenever a body part moves in any direction, a myofascial, tensional rearrangement occurs within the corresponding fascia. Sensory nerve receptors embedded in the

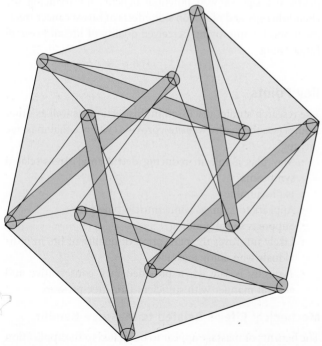

FIGURE 5-1 An abstract image of a cell that is kept together by tensegrity.

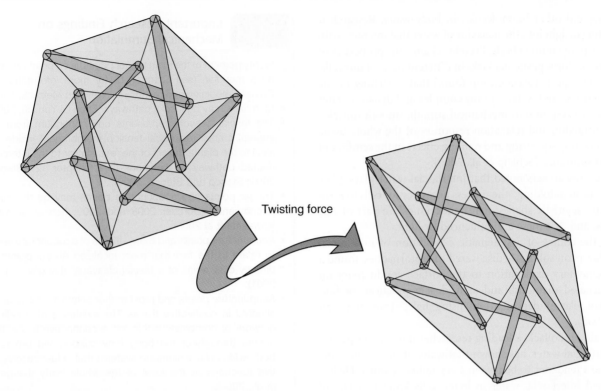

FIGURE 5-2 Demonstration of the cell reacting to a twisting force.

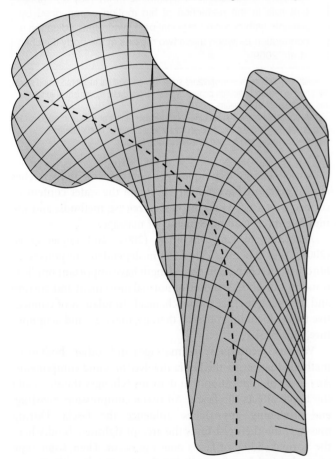

FIGURE 5-3 The head of the femur is a tensegrity structure, because it uses both compression and tension-resisting elements to support weight.
(Modified from Oschman JL: *Energy medicine: the scientific basis,* London, 2000, Churchill Livingstone.)

fascia are stimulated, producing accurate directional information that is sent to the central nervous system (CNS). Changes in the gliding of the fascia (e.g., too loose, too tight, or twisted) cause altered movement and thus tissue adaptation.

The Steccos sought to identify specific, localized areas of fascia affected by specific, limited movements. That is, identification of a limited or painful movement implicated a specific point on the fascia. Then, through appropriate manipulation of that precise part of the fascia, movement could be restored (Stecco, 2004; Stecco and Stecco, 2009). The method the Steccos used in their studies involved deep kneading of muscular fascia at specific points called *centers of coordination* and *centers of fusion,* along myofascial sequences, diagonals, and spirals. This method is called the *fascial manipulation technique* (Pedrelli et al., 2009). The fascial manipulation technique is based on principles similar to those that underlie other connective tissue–based methods, such as myofascial release (discussed in detail in Chapter 12).

In 2003 Robert Schleip, director of the Fascia Research Project at the University of Ulm in Germany, and research director of the European Rolfing Association, found that fascia is embedded with sensory receptors called *mechanoreceptors* (Schleip, 2003, 2004; Langevin, 2005). These receptors make fascia a sensory organ, which has free nerve endings that respond to mechanical force stimulation. Massage is a form of mechanical force stimulation. Schleip et al. (2006) found that when connective tissues are out of balance, resulting in soft tissue strain, mechanoreceptors in the fascia can trigger changes in the autonomic nervous system.

Mechanical Stimulation and Interfascial Water

The physical properties of the water in our bodies are different from those of ordinary water because of the presence of proteins and other biomolecules in body water. Research is providing insight into the behavior of water that interacts with proteins in the human body. Proteins change the properties of water to perform particular tasks in different parts of our cells.

The European Fascia Group found that stretching of the fascia squeezes out water, causing complex and dynamic water changes. In response to mechanical stimuli, smooth muscle–like contraction and relaxation responses of the whole tissue occur, creating squeezing and refilling effects in the semiliquid ground substance (Schleip et al., 2006).

Other researchers noted that interfascial water plays a key role in "protein folding," the process necessary for cells to form their characteristic shapes; that nanocrystals are part of this process; and that these are influenced by light.

"In the course of a systematic exploration of interfascial water layers on solids, we discovered microtornadoes, found a complementary explanation to the surface conductivity on hydrogenated diamond, and arrived at a practical method to repair elastin degeneration, using light" (Sommer and Zhu, 2008).

Gerald H. Pollack, a leading researcher into the properties of interfascial water, has shown that water at times can demonstrate a tendency to behave in a crystalline manner. He has discussed interfascial water in living cells known as *vicinal* (crystalline) *water*. Interfascial water exhibits structural organizations that differ from those of common bulk water. Vicinal water seems to be influenced by structural properties that make up the cell. Pollack uses the example of water in the temporomandibular joint:

The combined data from three different methods lead to the conclusion that all or almost all of the water in the intact disc is bound water and does not have properties consistent with free or bulk water.

If you want to understand what happens in any system—be it biological, or physical, or chemical, or oceanographic, or atmospheric, or whatever—it doesn't matter; in anything involving water, you really have to know the behavior of this special kind of gel/liquid crystalline-like water, which dominates (Pollack et al., 2006).

Klingler and Schleip (2004) showed that the water content of fascia partly determines its stiffness and that stretching or compression of fascia (as occurs during almost all manual therapies) causes the extrusion of water (like squeezing a sponge), making the tissues more pliable and supple. Eventually the water is taken up again and the stiffness returns, but in the meantime structures can be mobilized and stretched more effectively and comfortably than when they were densely packed with water.

Klingler et al. (2004) measured wet and dry fresh human fascia. They found that during an isometric stretch, water is extruded, and the fascia refills during a subsequent rest period. As water is extruded during stretching, the longitudinal arrangement of the collagen fibers relaxes temporarily. If the strain is moderate and no microinjuries occur, water soaks back into the tissue until it swells, becoming stiffer than before. This research suggests that tissue response to manual therapy may relate to the spongelike squeezing and refilling effects in the semiliquid ground substance of connective tissue.

Box 5-5	Important Research Findings on Mechanical Stimulation

- Eighty percent of the main trigger points lie on points located on a meridian (see Chapter 12 for more information on Chinese medicine and meridians) (Wall and Melzack, 1990).
- Meridians may be fascial pathways (Zhen Ci Yan Jiu, 2009).
- The fascial network represents one continuum from the internal cranial reciprocal tension membranes* inside the skull to the plantar fascia of the feet, similar to the interconnected pathway of meridians (see Chapter 12) (Stecco, 2004; Stecco and Stecco, 2009).
- Trigger points and acupuncture points may be the same phenomenon (Dorcher 2008 and 2009; Itoh et al 2007; Kawakita et al 2006).
- Acupuncture points and many effects of acupuncture seem to relate to the fact that most localized Ah shi points lie directly over areas of a fascial cleavage† (Langevin et al., 2001).
- Acupuncture points and most trigger points are structurally situated in connective tissue. The existence of a cellular network of fibroblasts within loose connective tissue that occurs throughout the body may support yet unknown body-wide cellular signaling systems that influence integrative functions at the level of the whole body (Langevin et al., 2004).
- Temporomandibular joint dysfunction may play an important role in the restriction of hip motion experienced by patients with complex regional pain syndrome, indicating a connection between these two regions of the body (Fischer et al., 2009).

Cranial reciprocal tension membranes are a network of dural membranes and spinal dura held in reciprocal tension (tensegrity) that create cyclic movement of inhalation and exhalation of the cranium.
†*Ah shi points* are areas that become spontaneously tender or painful in response to local problems. *Fascial cleavage* is an area where sheets of fascia diverge to separate, surround, and support different muscle bundles.

Muscle energy technique–type contractions and stretches almost certainly have similar effects on the water content of connective tissue, as do myofascial release methods, and the multiple force–loading elements of massage.

According to Langevin et al. (2004) and Engler et al. (2006) the dynamic, cytoskeleton-dependent responses of fibroblasts to changes in tissue length have important implications for our understanding of normal movement and posture and for therapies that use mechanical stimulation of connective tissue, including physical therapy, massage, and acupuncture (Box 5-5).

Various techniques in massage and other bodywork methods that target the fascia involve the same components. Any form of application that deforms (changes the shape of) the tissue affects the fascia. All tissue compression, twisting, and stretching approaches influence the fascia. During massage, the therapist finds the area of tightness/bind where the normal sliding of fascia does not occur. Then, some type of mechanical force is applied to that area to allow the tissues to normalize by becoming more pliable; through a change in the water content; by sending signals to adjacent and distant areas of the body; and likely through many more mechanisms waiting to be identified through research.

Key Points

- The benefits of massage may occur when we normalize tissues that are tense, tight, deformed, twisted, or compressed by introducing mechanical forces (e.g., pulling, pressing, bending, and twisting) into body tissues using massage, stretching, mobilizing, and so on.
- The fascia is everywhere, connecting everything so that the body functions as a single, integrated unit instead of individual parts. We still do not know the specific massage applications that best influence the fascia.
- Focused tension (stretching) of the tissues currently appears to be the most effective mechanical force for influencing the fascia.
- We think that the force applied during massage must move the tissue until it binds, at which point just a bit more force is applied and then held.
- The currently accepted range for how long force should be applied is 15 seconds to 3 minutes.
- How often force should be applied has not yet been determined definitively. Expert opinion ranges from daily to weekly. However, these opinions may be related more to the way massage is practiced, following the "best to get a massage once a week" axiom.

Fluid Movement—Blood and Lymph

Circulation

Massage also affects the **circulation**, although the research on this point is sparse. Castro-Sánchez et al. (2009) found that connective tissue massage improved blood circulation in the lower limbs of people with stage I or stage IIa type 2 diabetes and that it may be useful for slowing the progression of peripheral artery disease. A different study led by Castro-Sánchez (2010) indicated that a combined program of exercise and massage improved arterial blood pressure in individuals with type 2 diabetes who had peripheral arterial disease. Walton (2008) investigated the use of myofascial release techniques in the treatment of primary Raynaud's phenomenon. This researcher found that releasing restricted fascia with myofascial techniques may influence the duration and severity of the vasospastic episodes that occur with this condition.

Massage also may reduce blood flow in tissues. Wiltshire et al. (2010) found that massage may impair tissue recovery after strenuous exercise by mechanically impeding blood flow.

Exercise and Lactic Acid

Another area of research that may have implications for massage involves exercise and lactic acid. Lactic acid does not actually exist as an acid in the body; rather, it occurs as *lactate*. The belief that lactic acid causes stiffness after a sporting event, such as a marathon, and that massage can flush it out is a myth. Another misconception is that lactate acidifies the blood, causing fatigue and the burning sensation felt during prolonged exercise. Lactate actually is an important fuel that the muscles use during prolonged exercise. It is released from the muscle and converted in the liver to glucose, which serves as an energy source. Therefore, rather than cause fatigue, it

actually helps delay a drop in the blood glucose concentration, a condition called *hypoglycemia* (Bosch, 2006).

Postexercise stiffness, properly called *delayed onset muscle soreness,* is due mostly to damage to the muscle, not to an accumulation of lactic acid or lactate crystals in the muscle. After unaccustomed exercise, which results in DOMS, the levels of the enzyme creatine kinase increase, indicating that muscle damage has occurred. This type of tissue damage occurs in the form of tiny microscopic tears in the muscle. Hydroxyproline, an amino acid produced during the breakdown of collagen, also is present, indicating disruption of the connective tissue in and around the muscle structures. Postexercise stiffness, therefore, is the result of muscle damage and the breakdown of connective tissue.

Inflammation occurs as part of the normal healing, process. Signs of inflammation are heat, redness, swelling, and pain. One theory is that inflamed and swollen muscle fibers press on pain receptors (imagine an overfilled water balloon) and alert the brain to register pain. Another theory suggests that cells called *phagocytes* come to clean up the damaged tissue but in turn further damage the tissue, leading to pain. Still another theory is that free radicals (molecules that are highly reactive and harmful in the body) produced by the inflammatory cells aggravate the already existing damage, causing pain.

Most likely a combination of these factors contributes to the pain of DOMS. A possibly helpful use of massage for this condition may involve applications that target lymphatic drainage, thereby reducing the increased fluid pressure in the tissue stemming from the swelling caused by the inflammatory response. Theoretically, pain and stiffness thus should diminish. However, this hypothesis remains unproven.

Olszewski et al. (2009) and Zainuddin et al. (2005) found that massage was effective at alleviating DOMS by approximately 30% through the effect of reduced swelling. They also found that massage treatment had important effects on plasma creatine kinase activity, citing a significantly lower peak value at 4 days after exercise. Despite these changes, massage application had no effect on muscle function.

In a different study, Bakowski et al. (2008) found that massage administered 30 minutes after exercise could have a beneficial influence on DOMS by reducing soreness but that it did not affect muscle swelling or range of motion. Massage applied too aggressively actually can interfere with the recovery process, because it may cause more tissue damage, which triggers an inflammatory response and more swelling.

Studies justifying the use of massage for lymphatic movement are few in number. In lymphedema caused by damage to or removal of collecting trunks, lymph is present only in the subepidermal lymphatics (those just under the skin), whereas the bulk of stagnant tissue fluid accumulates in the subcutaneous tissue and above and beneath muscular fascia. These facts should be useful for designing pneumatic rhythmic pumping devices that wrap around an edematous limb and for providing effective manual lymphatic drainage, in terms of sites of massage and the level of applied external pressures. Manual lymphatic drainage after treadmill exercise was associated with a faster decrease in serum levels of muscle enzymes. This may indicate improved regenerative processes for structural damage and muscle cell integrity (Schillinger et al., 2006). Torres Lacomba et al. (2010) reporteaged that physiotherapy (exercise and manual lymphatic drainage) could be effective in preventing secondary lymphedema in women for at least 1 year after breast cancer surgery involving dissection of axillary lymph nodes.

Giampietro et al. (2009) summed up the evidence for the effects of massage on lymph movement by commenting that manual lymphatic drainage techniques remain a clinical art founded on hypotheses, theory, and preliminary evidence.

Key Points

- Based on current research, it is difficult to state confidently that massage influences the movement of body fluids, even though research seems to support the theory that massage affects the water content of fascia.
- The main component of body fluid is water. It seems reasonable to expect that the mechanical forces applied during massage at least affect the fluid in a particular area while the tissue is massaged.
- Squeezing and compressing fluid in tissue (massage) should help the body move and process the various body fluids. However, more research is needed before a specific massage effect on blood and lymphatic movement can be stated with confidence.
- The use of methods thought to influence blood and lymph movement is appropriate. However, massage professionals must explain to clients that although the methods appear to be clinically effective, research as yet is unable to prove the outcomes.

Research Related to Massage, Tissue Healing, and Musculoskeletal Pain

Research provides varying levels of evidence for the benefits of massage therapy for different chronic pain conditions (Tsao, 2007). Existing research provides good support for the analgesic (reduces pain sensations) effects of massage for nonspecific low back pain. Massage therapy appears to be effective for treatment of chronic back pain for up to 6 months. Interestingly, the researchers found no significant difference between relaxation and structural massage in terms of relieving disability or symptoms (Furlan et al, 2008; Cherkin et al, 2011) Only modest, preliminary support has been found for the use of massage in the treatment of mixed chronic pain conditions, headache pain, shoulder pain, neck pain, and carpal tunnel syndrome.

Recent studies suggest that cyclic stretching of fibroblasts contributes to the antifibrotic processes of wound healing by reducing the production of connective tissue growth factor (CTGF) (Kanazawa et al., 2009). This finding may support the use of massage to manage scar tissue formation and promote pliability in scar tissue.

Ho et al. (2009) studied the use of massage therapy for adhesive capsulitis (AC), shoulder impingement syndrome, and nonspecific shoulder pain or dysfunction. For shoulder impingement syndrome, they found no clear evidence suggesting benefits of massage therapy over those of other interventions. Also, massage was not shown to be more effective than other conservative interventions for adhesive capsulitis. However, compared with no treatment, massage and mobilizations-with-movement methods may be useful for short-term outcomes in shoulder dysfunction. In another study, Sherman et al. (2009) determined that massage is safe and may have clinical benefits for treating chronic neck pain, at least in the short term.

A study by Toro-Velasco et al. (2009) found that a single session of manual therapy (massage is a type of manual therapy) produced a decrease in tension, anger status, and perceived pain and pressure pain thresholds in patients with chronic tension-type headache. In addition, an immediate increase in heart rate variability was seen. Heart rate variability (HRV) is a physiologic phenomenon in which the interval between heart beats varies. Increased HRV is the result of a good balance in the ongoing sympathetic and parasympathetic influences on the heart. Generally, greater HRV exists when a person is relaxed and breathing in a regular or slow pattern.

Arroyo-Morales et al. (2008) used electromyography (EMG) to evaluate and record the electrical activity of skeletal muscles. They found that massage is beneficial when applied as a passive recovery technique after a high-intensity exercise protocol. This means that the muscles relax, and a psychological state of relaxation occurs. However, this same response may cause a short-term loss of muscle strength or a change in the muscle fiber tension-length relationship, resulting in alterations of muscle function.

Kassolik et al. (2009) conducted research to determine whether massage on one part of the body influences other parts of the body. They concluded that both an electrical and a mechanical response occurred in muscle connected indirectly by structural elements with the muscle being massaged. This finding supports the research findings on tensegrity discussed earlier.

Key Points

Research supports massage as a means of managing anxiety related to pain and a means of altering mood, the pain threshold, and the perception of pain. We now can expand upon what we had learned about massage earlier; we can say that massage:

- Appears to reduce stress
- Is pleasurable
- Improves the perceived quality of life
- Changes the shape of the fascia
- May influence the entire body even if only one area is massaged
- May help move fluids around
- Is safe when provided in a conservative and general manner with sufficient pain-free pressure

Overall it appears that a general full body massage can directly and indirectly influence many structures and functions to help the person adapt and cope and to help restore function. We may not be able to identify the results of individual, specific applications, because massage encompasses many different elements. Benefits can be derived from the quiet, nurturing presence of the massage therapist, the duration of the massage, the massage environment, and the unlimited variations in methods, pressure, speed, and so forth. A well-performed, full body massage is somewhat like a tasty cookie—the ingredients are all mixed together in the right proportions, baked at the correct temperature for the right amount of time, and served in a relaxing environment with time to enjoy the pleasure.

Remember that additional links and studies are provided for you on the Evolve website. Practice doing an Internet search yourself. (Box 5-6 presents information on PubMed.)

THE RESEARCH PROCESS

SECTION OBJECTIVES

Chapter objectives covered in this section:
4. The student will be able to describe the fundamentals of the Western scientific process.
5. Interpret a research paper.
Using the information presented in this section, the student will be able to perform the following:
• List the components of the scientific method
• Describe basic types of research
• Critically read a research paper

This section focuses on preparing you to become a consumer of research. Students interested in a more detailed discussion of research methods should consult the textbook *Research Methods for Massage and Holistic Therapies,* by Glenn Hymel. This section provides a brief survey of the process of conducting research. In addition, it teaches you how to read research papers critically so that you can make two important determinations: (1) whether the research is valid and (2) how the research influences massage application.

The scientific method is an excellent model for logical thinking. As a massage professional, logical thinking is a skill you use every day, whether to design a treatment plan or to determine what information from a research paper is valid and useful and what is not. Understanding the research process can help you make successful decisions in many aspects of your life. You may even become interested in writing a case report for the Massage Therapy Foundation case report contest (see Box 5-1).

Definition and Origin of Research

At its most basic, research can be defined as a process in which researchers explore one or more areas of interest (called *factors* or *variables*) by analyzing numeric and/or verbal data (*collected information*) to advance the understanding of that subject. For example, a researcher might undertake the task of characterizing the percentage of adults surveyed nationwide who have used therapeutic massage as a form of complementary and alternative health care. Researchers might also explore massage as an intervention for chronic low back pain. They might develop a detailed interview process to document a client's individual experience and perception of therapeutic massage over a designated period as an intervention for chronic low back pain. Research could explore the relationship, if any, between aquatic massage therapy and increased range of motion for clients recovering from bilateral hip replacement surgery. In another case, a massage therapist could complete an exhaustive review and synthesis of what the professional literature has to say about therapeutic massage as a viable intervention for clients suffering from fibromyalgia. All of these examples describe different types of research processes.

Ethics in Research

Research involves several very important concerns related to ethics and the ethical conduct of research. Informed consent, confidentiality, the ability to exit the study at any time without prejudice, and debriefing are some of the ethical issues researchers must face, for the obvious reason that the advancement of science must not occur at the expense of the safety and well-being of research participants.

Research in Plain Language

The scientific method is a model for conducting scientific research. A specific vocabulary is used during the research process. The scientific method has eight primary steps:

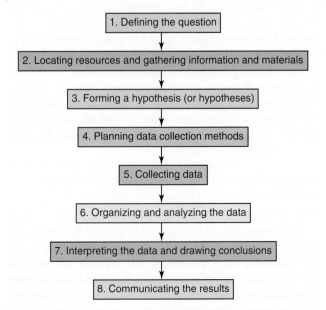

1. Defining the question
2. Locating resources and gathering information and materials
3. Forming a hypothesis (or hypotheses)
4. Planning data collection methods
5. Collecting data
6. Organizing and analyzing the data
7. Interpreting the data and drawing conclusions
8. Communicating the results

Defining the Question

All research begins with a basic question: What do I want to know? Examples of research questions might include the following:

1. Does using essential oils in combination with massage increase arterial circulation to the extremities better than massage alone?
2. How long should a hamstring stretch be maintained during massage to affect the pliability of the associated connective tissue?
3. How much pressure (compressive force) is required to influence lymphatic flow in a healthy subject?

This first step of the scientific method involves narrowing down possible topics and then choosing the question that will be the focus of the research. The research question must be specific. For example, in the preceding example question 1, the topics of essentials oils, massage, and arterial circulation are too broad. A better question would be: Does using lavender essential oil in combination with compression massage to the soles of the feet increase arterial circulation to the feet better than compression massage to the soles of the feet without lavender essential oil?

To develop a research question, the researchers must identify five specific goals:

1. What they want to know
2. The reason for asking the question
3. What the answer will tell them
4. How the information can be beneficial
5. Whether the question can be answered through research

Continuing with our previous example, the researchers want to know whether combining lavender oil with massage is better than massage alone for increasing circulation to the feet (goal 1). The reason for asking the question is to determine whether better results can be obtained in supporting circulation to the feet if lavender oil is used with massage (goal 2). The results (answer) will determine whether including lavender oil in compression massage of the feet is worth the expense and effort (goal 3). If using lavender oil with compression massage does increase arterial circulation better than massage alone, then clients with circulation problems in the feet would get better results (goal 4). An experiment could be conducted in which one group received massage with lavender oil and another group received massage without lavender oil; or, a group of people could be massaged one day without lavender oil and 2 days later with lavender oil. In both types of experiments, measurement tools are available for determining any changes in circulation; therefore, research could answer the question (goal 5).

Locating Resources and Gathering Information and Materials

After defining the research question, the researchers must educate themselves on the topic to be studied by reading the existing literature and talking to experts. With regard to the question about using lavender oil with massage, the researchers would learn about essential oils in general and lavender oil specifically, in addition to cardiovascular functioning specifically, arterial functioning in the extremities, massage in general, and compression methods specifically. They also would search through any pertinent research that had already been done. They would talk to an aromatherapist, a person who combines massage and essential oils, and other professionals who would be able to provide information. Having learned as much as possible about the various aspects of the research question, the researchers then would develop a hypothesis.

Forming a Hypothesis

Based on their knowledge of the topic, the researchers should be able to make an educated guess as to what may happen at the end of the experiment. The hypothesis is important, because it will be compared to the factual information gained from the experiment. The researchers then can determine whether the hypothesis was correct. Note that the research is still valuable even if the hypothesis is inaccurate at the conclusion of the research process.

An example of a hypothesis could be: Using lavender essential oil during foot massage increases peripheral circulation.

Planning Data Collection Methods

The fourth step of the scientific method involves drawing up a specific, detailed plan for conducting the research. The procedure should be clear enough that other researchers could follow it exactly. During this planning phase, the following must be determined:

- What steps are necessary to find the answer to the research question (i.e., to test the hypothesis)?
- What data need to be collected?
- How will the data be collected?
- What equipment, supplies, facilities, assistants, text subjects, support people, and so on will be required?
- What is the reference point (control) with which the data will be compared?
- How many samples, sites, tests, and so on are required?
- What variables will be manipulated and in what ways?
- What record-keeping techniques will be used (e.g., data sheet, journal)?
- How will data collection techniques be organized?
- What are the sequential steps to the research?
- What are the schedule, time line, and time expenditure?
- What are the financial obligations?

To complete this fourth step, the researchers must decide on the type of research design to use.

Types of Scientific Research

Basically, two types of research are used for scientific studies, observational research and experimental research.

Observational Research

Although observational research may be used in the laboratory, it is primarily conducted in a natural setting to study the relationship between a specific factor and some aspect of health or illness. For this reason, observational research may suggest an association, but it cannot be used to determine cause and effect. An example of observational research would be a study focusing on whether males or females receive massage more frequently.

Compared to experimental studies, observational research designs are very simple. Fundamentally, the research team simply observes the target groups or processes and uses statistical methods to determine whether an association exists. However, this approach gives rise to many problems. The results of the research may confuse the true effect of a variable and the possible effects of other factors in the environment. For example, an observational study may indicate that women receive massage 50% more often than men, but it cannot determine the reasons for this difference. Observational research, therefore, often is followed by experimental studies that can validate cause and effect.

The most frequently used type of observational research is the *epidemiologic study,* which is considered the basic science of public health. Usually focused on the study of large groups (sometimes tens of thousands or hundreds of thousands of people), epidemiology attempts to identify possible factors that increase the risk or probability of a disease or behavior in groups of people. Through one type of epidemiologic research, the *analytic study,* scientists observe certain behaviors (e.g., receiving massage) and track whether certain outcomes occur (e.g., the gender differences in massage frequency). Another type of epidemiologic research, the *descriptive study,* involves the collection of information to characterize and summarize a behavior, health event, or problem. For example, a descriptive study may examine the massage frequency associated with such factors as the time of day, the gender of the massage therapist, or the age of the client.

Scientists also use several other methods to conduct epidemiologic studies, and all of these methods have a number of significant limitations. One type of study design, the *cross-sectional study,* is basically the same as a survey. In this type of study, the researcher defines the population to be studied and then collects information from members of the group about their behavior. Because the data represent a point in time, this is like taking a snapshot of the population. Cross-sectional studies are good for examining the relationship between a variable and a behavior (e.g., receiving massage) or a disease (e.g., the flu) but not for determining cause and effect, which requires the collection of data over time.

In a *cohort study,* researchers select the study population according to the group members' exposure, regardless of the health outcome being studied or whether the group has the disease. The researchers then determine the outcomes of interest and compare the results on the basis of the individuals' exposures. Cohort studies often are referred to as *prospective studies,* because they follow the study population forward in time, from suspected cause to effect. An example of a cohort study would be defining a group of people on the basis of massage received weekly and following them for 5 years to see whether they showed a reduced tendency for muscle tension headache.

Another option is the *case control study,* in which the research team works backward, from the effect to the suspected cause. For this reason, case control studies often are referred to as *retrospective studies.* Participants are selected on the basis of the presence or absence of the disease or outcome in question; therefore, the study involves one group of people who have the behavior or problem (case subjects) and one group of people who do not (controls). These groups are compared to determine the presence of specific exposures or risk factors. An example of a case control study would involve forming a group of people with tension headache and another group without it and then comparing the two groups for their history of receiving massage.

Regardless of the method used, the important point to understand about the results of observational studies is that they are observations of associations and nothing more. They can tell us what but not why. By conducting observational studies, researchers can add valuable information to the existing literature on a particular topic, which helps them design future research studies, including clinical trials.

Experimental Research

Basic research generates data by investigating biochemical substances or biologic processes. It often is conducted to confirm observations or to determine the way a particular process works. For example, an experiment might be conducted to examine how massage for 20 minutes on the head, hands, and feet helps promote falling asleep in less than 15 minutes after going to bed.

Basic research often is conducted in test tubes *(in vitro)* or with animals *(in vivo).* Research with animals is an important tool for determining how humans may react when exposed to particular substances. However, it is important to note that, because of differences in physiology and the fact that animals are routinely exposed to levels of compounds far higher than those humans typically encounter, one cannot assume that results from animal studies can be generalized to humans. Therapeutic massage is extremely difficult to test in vitro, although various studies based on fascia tissue samples may be possible.

For experimental research, study subjects, whether human or animal, are selected according to relevant characteristics and are then randomly assigned to an *experimental group* (i.e., the group that will receive the treatment or intervention) or a *control group* (i.e., the group that does not receive the treatment). Random assignment ensures that factors that may affect the outcome of the study *(variables)* are distributed equally among the groups and therefore cannot lead to differences in the effect of a treatment. As a result, any differences in results between the groups can be attributed to the treatment. However, controlled experimental research can be flawed; therefore, it is important to know how the study was designed and conducted.

The most significant type of experimental research is the *clinical trial,* which uses human subjects to evaluate the effectiveness and safety of a nutrient treatment by monitoring its effect on large groups of people. Clinical trials generally are conducted by independent researchers or by researchers affiliated with a hospital or university medical program or private industry. These studies may be small, involving a limited number of participants, or they may be large intervention trials that attempt to discover the outcome of treatments on entire populations. The more participants in the study, the greater the likelihood that the results can be replicated in the general population.

Besides the size of the study, another other critical factor is the way the research was designed. As mentioned previously, scientists place the most value on the double-blind, placebo-controlled study that uses random assignment of subjects to experimental and control groups. Considered the gold standard of clinical research studies, the double-blind, placebo-controlled study provides dependable findings that are free of bias introduced by either the subject or the researcher. In this type of study, neither the subject nor the researcher knows whether the test substance or a placebo has been administered. For the results to be valid and to ensure that the subject cannot violate the blinding, the placebo and the test substance must be virtually identical (i.e., look, smell, and taste similar). Blinding for massage is very difficult; what can be used as a placebo for massage? A possible blinding approach might be a study in which all participants received the same massage routine, but some received trigger point therapy on four specific points related to low back pain and other participants did not. Blinding is one of the hurdles researchers must overcome in conducting massage-based research.

To conduct a clinical trial, researchers must follow a series of steps, or phases, each of which is designed to answer a separate research question. The NIH defines the four phases of a clinical trial as follows:

- Phase I: Researchers test a new treatment or intervention in a small group of people for the first time to evaluate its safety, determine a safe dosage range, and identify side effects.
- Phase II: The treatment is given to a larger group of people to determine whether it is effective and to further evaluate its safety.
- Phase III: The treatment is given to large groups of people so that the researchers can confirm its effectiveness, monitor for side effects, compare it to commonly used treatments, and collect information that will allow the drug or treatment to be used safely.
- Phase IV: Studies are done after the treatment has been marketed to gather information about its effect in various populations and any side effects associated with long-term use.

Obviously the findings of a phase III study are more significant for the public than those of a phase I or phase II study, which requires further investigation. Preliminary findings may make for interesting reading, but it is important for the public to recognize that the study represents only an initial step in the research process and its findings must be confirmed through additional studies.

A *meta-analysis* is performed to reconcile differences among studies or to consolidate relevant findings across studies. As mentioned earlier, a meta-analysis is a statistical method of combining results from separate studies to derive overall conclusions about a question or hypothesis. This method is most appropriate for examining studies that investigate the same question and use similar methods to measure relevant variables. For example, using meta-analysis, Moyer et al. examined the available massage literature to determine whether consistent, identifiable benefits for massage could be found. They concluded that, "This meta-analysis supports the general conclusion that [massage therapy] is effective. Thirty-seven studies yielded a statistically significant overall effect as

well as six specific effects out of nine that were examined." The authors also found that although individual studies showed inconsistent results, pooling of data from similar studies showed benefits from massage for trait anxiety (an ongoing predisposition to anxiety over time) and depression (Moyer, 2011).

Meta-analysis has limitations. Data from flawed studies may be included, or the analysis may include data from studies that used different methods to measure variables, resulting in a comparison of apples and oranges.

Collecting Data

Researchers must collect all the information (data) that could affect the answer to the research question. The following criteria are useful in this process:

- All relevant data must be recorded.
- Researchers must keep track of the step-by-step process.
- Objectivity must be maintained in the data collection.

Organizing and Analyzing the Data

In the sixth step of the scientific method, the researchers pull together the data collected and examine them more closely. The information is compared and contrasted. The data are:

- Organized and summarized
- Presented graphically (e.g., bar graphs, tables, pie charts, line graphs) so that others can see the results clearly
- Tested to determine whether the results are significant

Interpreting the Data and Drawing Conclusions

The researchers analyze the data and determine their conclusions, such as the following:

- What alternative hypotheses might explain these results?
- Were all relevant data, including extremes, or "oddball" data, analyzed?
- How might the sampling or data collection methods have affected these results?
- What answer do the results provide to the original question?
- How do the results compare to what was expected to happen (the hypothesis)?
- What can be concluded from the results? How do the conclusions affect the community or the "big picture" (implications)?

Communicating the Results

In the final step of the scientific method, the research and its findings are presented to the public. Important questions that must be considered in this process include the following:

- Who is the audience? (Who wants to read the research?)
- What is the best way to communicate the information (e.g., written report, oral or poster presentation, video)?
- What visual aids will help the audience clearly understand this research?

All of the following components of the research must be addressed:

- An introduction to the research question, the purpose of the research, and why it is interesting or matters
- A description of methods used to collect data

- The results
- The conclusions
- Questions raised by the research (Ginorio, nd)

Reading and Interpreting a Research Paper*

The reader (consumer) of research must review the methodology of a study to make sure the objective of the analysis is clearly stated and that the researchers explain the limitations of their findings so that the results can be put into context. Besides knowing the limitations of the different types of studies, those who read research papers also must understand the way the study was conducted. Some important factors are:

- The setting of the study (e.g., clinic, laboratory, or population)
- How variables were controlled (How did the researchers adjust for specific subject qualities or outside influences that could affect the results?)
- The sample size
- The number of study groups
- The treatment or variables observed (e.g., a vitamin supplement, a specific diet, massage)
- The length of the study
- How the data were collected
- How and by what statistical procedures the data were analyzed

One of the most significant factors in the evaluation of a study's findings is the study design, especially the randomness of the selection of the study's participants. If the subjects were selected randomly, the study results are more predictive of the population. If the only participants in the study were volunteers who belonged to an interest group or a media organization, greater potential exists for bias in the study.

Another important factor is the sample size. Although a small sample does not mean that the study is flawed, the conclusions that can be drawn clearly have limitations. For this reason, federal agencies, such as the U.S. Food and Drug Administration (FDA), require multiple studies involving large numbers of subjects before approving a new treatment or intervention.

In interpreting a study's findings, the reader also must understand the statistical significance. When conducting both observational and experimental research, scientists use statistical measures to convey the existence and strength of relationships. However, although statistics presents the findings in an organized fashion, they do not provide information about cause and effect. Moreover, a statistically significant finding does not guarantee that the research is without bias or confounding factors that could make the statistical value irrelevant. Statistical significance is only part of the picture; to get the whole picture, the reader must consider the context of the study and the findings of other research on the subject.

A primary challenge in interpreting the findings of a research study for the public is communicating the potential risk. Those who use research must understand the difference between *relative risk* and *absolute risk* and must use these distinctions in explaining the findings of a study.

Absolute risk is the chance a person will develop a specific disease or potential injury over a specified period. For example, a woman's lifetime absolute risk of breast cancer is 1 in 8; that is, one woman in nine will develop breast cancer at some point in her life.

Relative risk puts the chance in comparative terms by describing the outcome rate for people exposed to the factor in question compared with the outcome rate for those not exposed to the factor. In most cases, the absolute risk is a far more relevant statistic for the public.

For example, suppose a study shows that people who get a massage once a week are 50% less likely to develop sacroiliac (SI) joint dysfunction in the next 3 years than people who get a massage only once a month. The relative risk is that a person who does not get a massage once a week will face a 50% greater likelihood of developing SI joint dysfunction. Yet the absolute risk for an individual who does not get a massage once a week may be only 1%. In this case, the relative risk makes the massage intervention seem more important than it really is. Therefore, it is important to consider both the relative risk and the absolute risk when discussing study results.

As the research on massage increases and as current literature is interpreted, it is important for massage therapists to acquire adequate information on a study's original purpose, research design, and methods of data collection and analysis. Massage therapists also must have an understanding of the limitations of specific types of research and must recognize when a study is preliminary or when the findings differ from previous research.

Most important, proper interpretation of a new study's findings requires that the potential risk/benefit be put into perspective. It also requires clarification of cause and effect, which can be demonstrated only through rigorous experimental studies, not epidemiologic research.

Framework for Reading a Research Article: Structure, Function, and Implied Criteria for Evaluation

The structure, or "anatomy," of an empiric research article is a rather standard feature of this form of scientific or technical writing. Because the intent is to enhance communication among professionals across various disciplines and professions, a research report has six major sections (with subsections) that serve specific purposes; they are analogous to the "physiology" of the research report:

1. Preliminary section
2. Introduction
3. Method
4. Results
5. Discussion
6. Conclusion

Examining the structure and function of a research article can help the reader identify several criteria or standards that might be used to determine whether the report provides appropriate information. The availability of appropriate

---

*The information in this section has been modified from *Research Methods for Massage and Holistic Therapies,* by Glenn M. Hymel (Mosby, 2005).

information in the report allows the reader to evaluate the research effort's potential for advancing the knowledge base and thus the evidence-based practice of massage therapists.

Preliminary Section (Title and Abstract)

The first section of a research article contains the title and an abstract of the study. Although fairly self-explanatory, the title of a study must be formulated so that a potential reader (e.g., a person scanning a list of studies by bibliographic citation only) can accurately determine the type of study, the major variables involved, and the participants who were the focal point of the researchers' efforts.

In the abstract, or summary, the author synthesizes as efficiently as possible the main body of the report (i.e., the introduction, method, results, and discussion sections). A well-written abstract gives the reader a precise idea of what the study found, allowing the person to decide whether to read the entire report.

Introduction

The introduction provides the context for the rest of the report. It has five subsections: (1) a general review of the literature; (2) a specific review of the literature; (3) a purpose statement, which identifies the research question; (4) the rationale for the study's research hypothesis; and (5) a statement of the research hypothesis.

The first subsection, the general review of the literature, identifies the broader context of the study's major research problem area. This addresses at a general level earlier researchers and authors who have contributed to the research problem area.

The second subsection, the specific review of the literature, provides a more detailed treatment of related sources in the professional literature. This subsection allows the reader to become considerably more familiar with earlier literature that informs the current study.

The two literature review subsections serve a dual purpose:

(1) They establish in the reader's mind the researchers' familiarity with the existing sources of information in the research problem area.

(2) They inform the reader of the information and insight needed to better comprehend the current research report.

The third subsection, the purpose statement, must have the research question either implied or, more preferably, stated. It represents the reason the study was performed. This subsection communicates to the reader what is truly the starting point in the study, because in any research endeavor, the many decisions are based precisely on the research question. The research question is never formulated in a vacuum. The researchers must have read relevant literature to identify the question they are asking. At the same time, the researchers must have had at least the beginnings of a research question to know exactly where in the literature they must search.

The fourth subsection, the rationale for the research hypothesis, relies on and may even extend the preceding literature review subsections. The authors of a research report must rely on the available research literature in a given problem area to justify what becomes their study's research hypothesis. The research hypothesis is basically the predicted answer to the study's research question. It is not an "educated guess" but a predicted answer to the research question based on concepts, theories, and/or existing empiric research from the professional literature. The rationale for the research hypothesis, then, should be presented immediately before the actual statement of the hypothesis. In this way, a context is already in place that clarifies the reasons the researchers predict a certain answer to the study's question. The rationale usually is only implied, but the preferred approach is to clearly identify it for the reader's benefit.

The final subsection of the introduction is the statement of the research hypothesis. Sometimes authors fail to provide a clear statement of what they anticipate, with justification, will be the outcome of the study (i.e., the answer to the study's research question). Many authors tend to allow the research hypothesis simply to be implied. The major advantage of a clear statement of the hypothesis is that it alerts the reader to several critical features of the study, including the research category, strategy, and method used; the variables investigated and their predicted relationship; the participants studied; and the context or setting of the study. Knowledge of a study's research hypothesis sets the stage for the study's methodology, the next major section in the research article.

Method

Just as the name suggests, the method section of the research report provides a detailed account of the methodology used to carry out the study. It identifies the various research procedures used at different stages and explains them in such detail that the study can be replicated by others. This section also gives the reader as complete a basis as possible for determining whether the implementation of the study justifies (or in any way compromises) the results and conclusions reached.

To accomplish these tasks, the method section must describe how the participants were chosen, the instruments used to measure variables, and the procedures by which the study was actually implemented. Standard subsections that constitute the method section are (1) participants and sampling procedures; (2) research method and design; (3) variables investigated; and (4) instrumentation. These four subsections allow the authors to specify precisely what was done in carrying out the study. Readers should keep in mind that the labeling of these subsections can vary slightly across different studies; the important point is to make sure the method section addresses the issues of participants, measuring instruments, and procedures.

The first subsection, typically labeled participants and sampling procedures, describes the characteristics of the study participants and the activities used to select and assign them. The researchers identify and justify the inclusion and exclusion criteria used to determine who did and who did not qualify as study participants. In addition, the researchers must state the extent to which they used random selection of sample participants from an accessible population and random assignment of subjects to comparison groups. If the researchers used procedures other than random selection and random assignment, they must specify the alternatives chosen. These issues are critical when determining whether a study is valid. The participants and sampling procedures subsection also should specify the ethical provisions of the study that ensured the protection of participants, the overall integrity of the study, and prior approval from the appropriate institutional review board (IRB). An IRB is a federally mandated committee that provides oversight for all research activities with the aim to protect the rights and welfare of the human subjects recruited to participate in research.

The second subsection focuses on the research method and design.

The third subsection addresses the variables investigated in the study. Although this is not the first time the variables are mentioned in the report, this is where the researchers describe the variables as specifically as possible. In this subsection the reader can learn all the details of how the researchers identified, defined, characterized, controlled, manipulated, and measured the study's variables.

The final subsection of the methods section is instrumentation. Although this refers primarily to measuring instruments used to generate numeric or verbal data or both, this subsection also may specify the type or model of equipment or apparatuses that played a role in the study. Technical factors, such as the validity and reliability of instruments, are crucial and therefore are prominent features of the information provided in this subsection.

Results

The results section provides the reader with a full accounting of the outcomes or results of the data analysis performed in the study.

Discussion

The final section of the report's main body is the discussion of the study's findings. This section provides the researchers with the opportunity to do the following:

- Reflect on the manner in which the study was conducted, including its limitations and delimitations (boundaries)
- Elaborate on the interpretation of the study's findings that was begun in the results section
- Acknowledge the significance of the study's results and their relationship to earlier research findings in the problem area investigated
- Theorize as to the reason or reasons the results were obtained (i.e., which intervening variables may have come into play)
- Suggest areas of further research that would be a logical sequence to the current study

Conclusion (References and Other Material)

The concluding section of the research report begins with a list of the bibliographic citations for each of the sources cited in the research report. This list constitutes the references, and it is very important not only because it gives detailed credit to sources used in the study, but also because it provides the reader with the information necessary to access the sources cited. In addition to this list, research reports often include information in appendices, authors' notes, and footnotes.

💡 PROFICIENCY EXERCISE 5-2

Choose one of the links to a full text article provided on the Evolve website for this chapter. Then use the information from Dr. Hymel's "Criteria for Critiquing a Research Article" to assess the quality of the research.

Criteria for Critiquing a Research Article

The sections and subsections of a research report provide the foundation for identifying certain criteria that can be used to evaluate the merits of a report. They also provide an organizational framework for systematically working through the process of reflecting on the contents of a report. The following lists of specific questions can help you evaluate the designated sections and subsections of a research article (Proficiency Exercise 5-2).

Preliminary Section

1. Does the title of the study provide a basis for identifying the type of study, major variables, and participants?
2. Does the abstract summarize the main body of the report (i.e., the introduction, method, results, and discussion sections)? Does it focus on the research question, research hypothesis, participants, research method and design, major variables, instruments, statistical techniques, principal findings, and conclusions?

Introduction

1. Does it contain professional literature that has bearing on the study reported? Does it provide an overview of the research problem area and more specific coverage of individual studies?
2. Is the purpose of the study clearly identified by the research question?
3. Is a rationale or justification, based on various features of the professional literature, presented as a context or framework for the study's research hypothesis?
4. Do the authors state the study's research hypothesis in such a way that the predicted answer to the study's research question is clear and unambiguous?

Method

1. Are the study's participants clearly characterized, along with the inclusion and exclusion criteria used to choose them?
2. Did the researchers justify the number of participants constituting the sample size.
3. Was an accessible population of potential participants acknowledged, along with an indication of how the sample was derived from such a population, whether through random selection or some other procedure?
4. Did the authors specify the manner in which the participants were assigned to the two or more comparison groups, whether through random assignment or some other means?
5. Was any clarification provided as to how the ethical aspects of the study were governed, particularly with regard to protection of the participants, the overall integrity of the research, and prior approval of the study by an IRB?

6. Were the study's variables detailed in a comprehensive fashion so that their manipulation and measurement could be replicated?
7. Did the authors clearly specify the equipment and instruments used to manipulate and measure the variables and did they provide documentation of the technical factors?

Results

1. Were the data analysis techniques used identified and justified?
2. Were the results of the study communicated?
3. Were tables and figures used appropriately to present the data analyses in a comprehensible manner?

Discussion

1. Did the researchers reflect on the manner in which the study was designed and conducted with regard to any limitations and/or delimitations (i.e., intentional or unintentional boundaries)?
2. Did the authors elaborate on the interpretation of the study's findings beyond the interpretation that was begun in the results section?
3. Did the researchers address the significance of the study and its findings, particularly as they relate to earlier studies in the problem area investigated?
4. Were possible intervening variables addressed that might explain the reason or reasons the results were obtained?
5. Were recommendations made regarding follow-up studies that might fully or partly replicate or at least augment the current study?

Conclusion

1. Does the list of references accurately reflect each of the sources cited in the research report and is the list presented in a consistent bibliographic citation style?
2. Does the research report contain any appendices that provide more detailed information than that given earlier in the article?
3. Is any information provided, in the form of authors' notes, that gives insight into the funding support for the study?
4. Are any footnotes provided that elaborate on one or more aspects of the study and that would have been misplaced or distracting if embedded in the main body of the report?

TOUCH, MASSAGE THERAPY, AND PHYSICS

SECTION OBJECTIVES

Chapter objective covered in this section:

6. The student will be able to relate the concepts of physics to the experience of touch and massage therapy.

Using the information presented in this section, the student will be able to perform the following:

• Define physics
• Explain how basic terminology and principles of physics relate to massage application and outcomes

During appropriate therapeutic interactions, a bond forms between the therapist and the client. Many different terms,

such as *unity, connection,* or even *in the zone,* can be used to describe this intangible experience. Terms to describe this bond are even found in an area of "hard" science—physics, which may surprise some students of massage therapy.

People generally think of physics in terms of nuclear reactions, mechanical devices, or astronomy. In fact, physics is the scientific study of matter, energy, force, and motion and the ways they interact. In even broader terms, physics is the general analysis of nature, which we study to understand how the universe functions. Because all living beings are part of nature, principles of physics apply to us, which means that these principles are involved in massage therapy. Therefore, studying basic physics terminology and principles can help you better understand massage application and outcomes.

Matter, force, and motion are tangible aspects of massage therapy. For example, *matter* is the human body; *force* is the effort used to perform techniques, and *motion* is the actual application of techniques. Motion also is involved in the way the body moves. *Energy* is the source of the force of the effort used to perform techniques and also the life force of the body. In this sense, energy can be both *intangible* (as in the production of adenosine triphosphate [ATP], which is needed to generate force) and *tangible* (as in the way energy is detected and used by a practitioner of shiatsu).

Other common terms from physics that are used to describe physical phenomena experienced during massage are *entrainment, resonance, tensegrity,* and *attunement.* A further understanding of these four concepts can help us understand the massage experience. Although these phenomena are largely intuitive and intangible, research is showing that they are scientifically valid.

Entrainment

Entrainment is a physical phenomenon that occurs when rhythms synchronize. The rhythm of a drumbeat combined with the beat-keeping motion of the drummer's body provides a good example of this phenomenon. Your organs, most notably your heart, provide rhythms with which other organs and organ systems synchronize. Your body and its organ systems have internal rhythms that keep you functioning.

Entrainment appears to be an underlying benefit of many bodywork disciplines, including massage. Centering activities that focus the massage therapist's attention on the client enhance entrainment. When the massage therapist is centered and grounded so that his or her attention is focused solely on the client, the therapist's body rhythms (e.g., heartbeat) tend to synchronize with the client's. When body rhythms are synchronized, the people involved feel a sense of moving and working together rather than of opposing each other. Therefore, entrainment strengthens the bond that forms in the therapeutic treatment and increases the likelihood of a successful massage outcome.

If a practitioner focuses intentions of empathy and compassion before beginning a massage, this can lead to a strong response called *resonance,* which results in entrainment and the experience of connectedness (Yakita et al., 2001; McPartland et al., 2005; Roenneberg et al., 2005; Mirskya et al., 2009).

Resonance

Resonance has two distinct yet interrelated meanings. According to the *Massage Therapy Body of Knowledge (MTBOK):*

Resonance involves the alignment of psychobiological states between a client/patient and a therapist. Each person responds to the other's body language, nonverbal signals, tone of voice, facial expression, eye gaze, bodily motion, and touch. These nonverbal signals reveal unconscious shifts in the state of mind of the patient or therapist. Resonating with these expressions requires that the therapist feel his or her own feelings through interoceptive self-awareness and not merely understanding them conceptually.

In short, this means that the therapist and the client are in sync.

In physics, resonance is the tendency of an object to move back and forth or up and down. This motion generally is called *oscillation*. Oscillation can be easily seen (e.g., the motion of a swing on a playground) or impossible to see with the naked eye (e.g., electrons in an electrical circuit oscillating on an atomic level). At the cellular level, all components oscillate; this means that all cells have resonance.

Scientists have discovered cells in connective tissue that oscillate; these cells are considered biologic oscillators. One function of these oscillating cells is to influence body rhythms that affect parts of the brain that determine pain perception, mood, and rhythm cycles, such as the sleep/wake cycle (McPartland, 2008).

Entrainment, therefore, begins on the cellular level. Body rhythms are affected by biologic oscillators. In turn, the body rhythms of the therapist affect the body rhythms of the client, and vice versa.

Resonators

A device or system that has resonance or shows resonant behavior is a **resonator**. Resonance frequencies are the frequencies at which a resonator oscillates, and they can be either electromagnetic or mechanical. Resonators are used either to generate waves of specific frequencies or to select specific frequencies from a signal. For example, musical instruments use mechanical resonators, which are acoustic, that produce sound waves of specific tones. Music often is used with massage to create physiologic outcomes. We even say that a certain type of music resonates with us.

Is the body a resonator? Magnetic resonance imaging (MRI), a diagnostic tool, uses resonance from the body to create images. The images are derived from the energy released by molecules transitioning from a high-energy state to a low-energy state in response to magnetic fields. This exchange of energy is called *resonance* (hence the name *magnetic resonance imaging*). A computer interprets the data and creates images that display the different resonance characteristics of different tissue types. Ultrasound technology also is based on mechanical vibration and frequency response. Based on the working process of an MRI, the body apparently exhibits resonance.

Crystals as Resonators

The quartz crystal is the most common mechanical resonator in nature. Crystalline material performs two functions: (1) it acts as a good resonator, keeping the resonant frequency constant; and (2) its piezoelectric property converts mechanical vibrations into an oscillating voltage. The piezoelectric properties of quartz crystals give them an electric potential upon application of mechanical stress. The resonant frequency of a crystal oscillator is changed by mechanically loading it so that it changes shape.

Liquid crystals exist somewhere between the solid and liquid phases. Their molecules are shaped to align together in certain directions. Because of the molecular shape, order, and direction of the molecules, liquid crystals can be manipulated with mechanical, magnetic, or electrical forces. Liquid crystals are temperature-sensitive; they turn solid when cold and liquid when hot. Since the late 1980s, researchers have known that connective tissue and other structures in the body display the properties of liquid crystals. Today we can actually see the liquid crystal structure through special imaging methods that use **harmonics**. The properties of connective tissues as a liquid crystal are influencing research into tissue regeneration, the growth of replacement organs and tissues, and bioengineering and nanotechnology; they also are changing the way we understand the effects of massage therapy (Deniset-Besseau et al., 2009).

Massage mechanically loads the tissues of the body. Fascia (discussed earlier), a type of connective tissue found extensively throughout the body, is a liquid crystal that is piezoelectric in nature. Mechanically loading the tissue stimulates the liquid crystal structure to release electrons. This energy release influences the fascial ground substance to shift from a gel or stiff state to a more liquid or pliable state. Simply stated, massage can make the client feel less stiff and more pliable. Practice sensing this by playing with clay. It is stiff and cold when you start squeezing and pressing it, but after a time it becomes warm, soft, and pliable.

Tensegrity

Tensegrity (also called *tensional integrity*) is the balance between the tension (pulling force) components and the compression (pushing force) components of a structure. When pull equals push, a structure is strong yet flexible. The concept has applications in the body. In biologic structures, such as muscles and bones or rigid and elastic cell membranes, a balance exists between tensioned and compressed parts. For example, the myofascial-skeletal system is a synergy of muscle, fascia, and bone; the muscle fascial unit provides pull, and the bones provide the push force. The body, from the cells all the way up to the organs, follows the principles of tensegrity (Cai et al., 2010).

Remarkably, tensegrity may even explain how all the physics phenomena we discussed are so perfectly coordinated in a living creature. Deoxyribonucleic acid (DNA), nuclei, cytoskeletal filaments, membrane ion channels, and entire living cells and tissues show characteristic resonant frequencies.

Very simply, the property of tensional integrity provides a way to distribute forces to all interconnected elements while "tuning" the whole system mechanically as one (Mammoto and Ingber, 2010).

Attunement

Attunement means to bring into a harmonious or responsive relationship. In massage therapy, *rapport* is another term that can be used to describe the concept of attunement.

We have already discussed oscillators as entrainment sources. One level of attunement is based on entrainment. Scientists have discovered cells in the brain, called *mirror neurons,* that support human connection. Mirror neurons play a major role in the imitation necessary for learning and the ability to empathize with others. An important aspect of the professional relationship is understanding the condition of another person while remaining nonjudgmental. Vittorio Gallese, who identified mirror neurons, describes *intentional attunement* as a state that generates a peculiar quality of familiarity with other individuals (Gallese et al., 2005, 2007).

The amygdala is the part of the brain that underlies empathy and allows for emotional attunement. Facial expressions, voices, gestures, and body movements transmit emotions. Humans especially tend to subconsciously mimic and model the facial expressions, vocalizations, postures, and movements of others, especially when an interdependent or survival relationship exists. Understanding the communication of body language processed by mirror neurons is a fundamental aspect of attunement. With this mechanism we do not just see an action, an emotion, or a sensation in another; we feel what one would feel during a similar action and are able to determine the intentions and emotions behind that action.

To summarize, tensegrity is integral to resonance, resonance is part of entrainment, and entrainment is essential to attunement. The therapeutic relationship is grounded in all these concepts.

WHY MASSAGE IS EFFECTIVE—TRANSLATING EVIDENCE INTO PRACTICAL APPLICATION

SECTION OBJECTIVES

Chapter objective covered in this section:
7. The student will be able to explain the effects of therapeutic massage in physiologic terms.
Using the information presented in this section, the student will be able to perform the following:
• Identify and categorize massage methods as reflexive or mechanical
• Explain the anatomic and physiologic influences of massage

We have discussed the importance of valid evidence and the relationship between science and art. We also have learned about the research process, summarized current research applicable to massage therapy, and learned how to read a research paper to determine whether it is relevant and accurate. Your "inquiring mind" may be overwhelmed by now, especially if all this is new information for you. The crucial

point, though, is to be able to apply the information to the actual massage process.

The manual techniques of massage are physiologically specific and well defined by the following:
• Mode of application (i.e., rubbing, pulling, pressing, touching)
• Speed (sustained or slow, rhythmic, staccato, or fast)
• Intensity and depth of pressure of touch (light touch, deep touch, or a combination of the two)
• Part of the therapist's body used to apply the techniques (fingers, hands, forearms, knees, or foot).

The techniques of therapeutic massage and other types and styles of bodywork are merely variations of the fundamental application of manual manipulations. The benefits of the techniques are simply the result of basic physiologic effects. It is helpful to have a method to categorize information into similar bundles. By doing this, we can take many pieces of information and sort it into manageable sizes. This process helps with the clinical reasoning process used to make sense of information and to make decisions about what to do with the data. The problem with this method is that most things do not clearly fit into one category or another, and often the result is not entirely accurate. However, as long as we understand this, we can make use of the process.

These latter sections of the chapter consolidate the known and suspected benefits of massage and the mechanisms of action into a format that is usable in the practical application of massage. To really appreciate these sections, we first had to understand the process of finding and evaluating research to determine whether the evidence is relevant and justifiable. Now we can proceed with the practical application of the evidence in massage therapy practice.

Physiologic Effects

The fundamental concepts that explain the effects of therapeutic massage can be divided into two general categories, mechanical effects and reflexive effects.
• **Mechanical effects** occur when various types of mechanical force (tension, bending, shear, torsion, and compression) are applied directly to the body and directly affect the soft tissue through techniques that normalize the connective tissue or move body fluids and intestinal contents. Myofascial tissue (muscle and its associated connective tissues) and fluid content determine the density and pliability of a muscle structure (i.e., muscle tone). Mechanical methods primarily influence muscle tone.
• **Reflexive effects** occur when various mechanical forces are introduced into body tissues during massage with the intent to stimulate the nervous system, the endocrine system, and the chemicals of the body. A reflex is an involuntary response to a stimulus, and massage can be the source of the stimulus.

The problem with this simple categorization is that the mechanism by which massage produces an effect cannot always be clearly identified. According to Dr. Philip E. Greenman, the effects of massage occur through the interrelationships of the peripheral nervous and central nervous systems (and their reflex patterns and multiple pathways), the autonomic nervous system, and neuroendocrine control (Greenman, 2003). Dr. John Yates (1990) has said, "It appears far more reasonable just to recognize that massage produces effects that are due to a combination of mechanical, neural, chemical, and psychological factors and to identify these wherever possible rather than to attempt to use them as a basis for classifying those effects."

To understand the basis of research findings, we must understand the mechanisms by which massage applications achieve benefits. This understanding is grounded in the study of functional anatomy and physiology as they relate to therapeutic massage. The recommended text for this purpose is *Mosby's Essential Sciences for Therapeutic Massage: Anatomy, Physiology, Biomechanics, and Pathology,* by Sandy Fritz.

The anatomic and physiologic areas most targeted by massage are the following:

- Nervous/neuroendocrine system (the central, autonomic, and somatic nervous systems, in addition to neurochemicals and hormones)
- Circulation
- Connective tissue
- Energy systems (biofields)

TRANSLATING EVIDENCE INTO PRACTICAL APPLICATION: NERVOUS/NEUROENDOCRINE SYSTEM

SECTION OBJECTIVES

Chapter objective covered in this section:

7. The student will be able to explain the effects of therapeutic massage in physiologic terms.

Using the information presented in this section, the student will be able to perform the following:

- Explain the anatomic and physiologic influences of massage on the neuroendocrine system

Effects of Massage on the Nervous System

The body's responses to massage and its effects on the nervous system are primarily reflexive.

Briefly, the nervous system is divided into the central nervous system (CNS), which consists of the brain and the spinal cord and its coverings, and the peripheral nervous system (PNS), which consists of nerves and ganglions (Figure 5-4). The PNS is further divided into the autonomic and somatic divisions. The autonomic nervous system (ANS) division is subdivided into the sympathetic and parasympathetic systems. The sympathetic system is responsible for functions that expend energy in response to emergency or arousal situations. The parasympathetic system is more restorative and normalizing and returns the body to a nonalarm state. The somatic division of the PNS is made up of the peripheral nerve fiber innervations of the body wall (e.g., muscles, joints, and other structures).

The nervous system responds to therapeutic massage methods through stimulation of sensory receptors. Feedback loops are activated that intervene and adjust various homeostatic processes. The sensory stimulation from massage

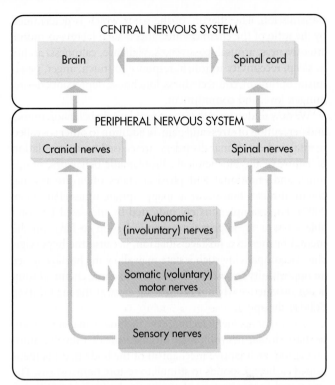

FIGURE 5-4 The divisions of the nervous system. (From Thibodeau GA, Patton KT: *The human body in health and disease,* ed 3, St Louis, 2002, Mosby.)

disrupts the existing pattern in the CNS control centers; this results in a shift of motor impulses, most often in the PNS, that re-establishes homeostasis. Usually both the somatic and autonomic divisions of the PNS are influenced as balance is restored.

Neuroendocrine Interactions

To understand the benefits of massage, as defined in current research, it is important to understand the functions of some of the neuroendocrine chemicals.

The endocrine system is regulated through the influence of the nervous system, and the endocrine system in turn influences the nervous system; this is a feedback loop, similar to the thermostat on a furnace. The feedback system and autoregulation (maintenance of internal homeostasis) are interlinked with all body functions. The controls for initiation of a reaction come through the nervous system and the endocrine system. Neuroendocrine chemicals are the communication transmitters of these control systems. A neuroendocrine chemical in the synapse of the nerve is called a **neurotransmitter**. A neuroendocrine chemical carried in the bloodstream is called a **hormone**. *Neuropeptide* is another term used to describe some of these substances.

The neuroendocrine substances carry messages that regulate physiologic functions. Neuroendocrine regulation is a continuous, ever-changing chemical mix that fluctuates with each external and internal demand on the body to respond, adapt, or maintain a functional degree of homeostasis. The immune system also produces and responds to these communication substances. The substances that make up this "chemical soup" remain the same, but the proportion and ratio change with each regulating function or message transmission. The "flavor" of the soup, which is determined by the ratio of the chemical mix, affects such factors as mood, attentiveness, arousal, passiveness, vigilance, calmness, ability to sleep, receptivity to touch, response to touch, anger, pessimism, optimism, connectedness, loneliness, depression, desire, hunger, love, and commitment.

We now understand that most problems in behavior, mood, and perception of stress and pain, in addition to other so-called mental and emotional disorders, are caused by dysregulation or failure of the biochemicals. Problematic behaviors, symptoms, and emotional and physical states often are normal chemical mixes that occur at inappropriate times (Patterson, 2007). For example, anxiety indicated by increased irresolvable stress is an appropriate chemical soup to have on the mental burner in a hostage situation, because the hypervigilance accompanying such a state may allow the hostage to see an opportunity for escape. However, this same chemical soup is not productive when it is bubbling away at the mall during holiday shopping.

Stress management techniques (including massage) seem to share similar neurobiologic mechanisms that involve autoregulation, an adaptive mechanism of the body that (as mentioned earlier) responds to stimuli to restore homeostasis. The emotional limbic system of the brain determines whether a situation is safe or unsafe. Neurochemicals such as dopamine, endogenous opiates, endocannabinoids, oxytocin, serotonin, and others are secreted. (These neurochemicals are discussed in more detail later in this section.) Based on self-care and stress research findings, it is reasonable to conclude that the body has the capacity to heal itself using natural or innate health-regulating systems.

Early Endorphin Research

In 1969 researchers observed that pain could be eliminated in rats without the use of anesthesia by stimulating the periaqueductal gray matter in the brainstem. Other important discoveries soon confirmed this finding. The work of Dr. Candice Pert and others led to the discovery of the endogenous (made by the body) endorphin and nonendorphin pain-inhibiting systems of the CNS (Asplund, 2003). The body produces several endogenous, opiate-like compounds, including enkephalin and beta endorphins (beta endorphin is a fragment of the pituitary hormone beta lipotropin). These peptides attach to opiate receptors (as does morphine) and, in most cases, relieve pain, especially chronic pain, and produce euphoria. This finding supports the validity of acupuncture.

Acupuncture Studies and Implications for Massage

Acupuncture is an ancient healing art that involves much more than the insertion of needles into the body. Only the most fundamental concepts of acupuncture have been studied scientifically, but that research has revealed physiologic mechanisms affected by the method. Agreement has not been reached on what acupuncture points are, but the points used in acupuncture have anatomic components. The traditional acupuncture points correspond to nerves that are close to the surface of the body. Most of the points fall into fascial cleavage areas over neurovascular bundles (areas of nerves and vessels),

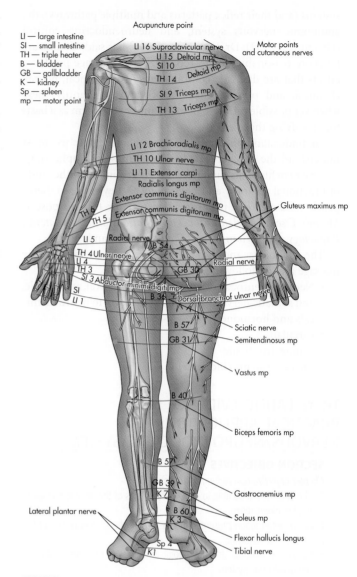

FIGURE 5-5 A comparison of traditional acupuncture points, motor points, and cutaneous nerves of the arms and legs.

motor points (places where nerves innervate muscles), the focal meeting of superficial nerves in the sagittal plane, superficial nerves or nerve plexuses, and muscle-tendon junctions at the Golgi tendons (Figure 5-5) (Gunn, 1992; Langevin and Yandow, 2002).

Rather than needles, acupressure uses specific pinpoint compression over the same points. Some evidence indicates that acupuncture exerts its analgesic effect by causing the release of enkephalins, and this analgesia is said to be blocked by the morphine antagonist naloxone. In addition, a component of stress analgesia seems to arise from endogenous opiates, because in experimental animals some forms of stress analgesia are blocked by naloxone.

Acupuncture and acupressure seem to work by taking advantage of the body's natural inhibitory influences, which normally can block pain pathways. For example, it has been established that sensory pain fibers release a neurotransmitter called *substance P*, which increases the transmission of pain impulses. Enkephalin blocks the release of substance P, thereby inhibiting pain transmission to the brain. The effects of these and other neurotransmitters released during massage may explain and validate the use of sensory stimulation methods to treat chronic pain, anxiety, and depression (McKeon et al., 2006).

The effect of acupuncture or acupressure is delayed until the enkephalin level rises to inhibitory levels. It usually takes about 15 minutes for the blood level of enkephalin to begin to rise. The implication for massage is that the pain-inhibiting effects do not occur immediately. Massage practitioners should keep this in mind with regard to the intensity and duration of applications as they work.

Influence of Massage on Neuroendocrine Substances

Much of the research on massage, especially that done at the Touch Research Institute, revolves around shifts brought about by massage in the proportion and ratio of the chemicals that make up the body's "chemical soup" (Medina et al., 2006).

Some of the main neuroendocrine chemicals influenced by massage are:

- Dopamine
- Serotonin
- Epinephrine/adrenaline
- Norepinephrine/noradrenaline
- Enkephalins, endorphins, and dynorphins
- Endocannabinoids
- Oxytocin
- Cortisol
- Growth hormone

Indications for massage are explored in greater depth in Chapter 6. The following information is intended to help the student understand the current research findings that point toward neuroendocrine chemicals as a big piece of the "why massage works" puzzle.

Dopamine

Dopamine influences motor activity that involves movement (especially learned, fine movement, such as handwriting), conscious selection (the ability to focus attention), and mood in terms of inspiration, possibility intuition, joy, and enthusiasm. Dopamine is involved in pleasure states, seeking behavior to achieve pleasure states, and the internal record system. Low levels of dopamine result in the opposite effects, such as lack of motor control, clumsiness, inability to focus attention, and boredom.

Massage increases the available level of dopamine in the body and can explain the pleasure and satisfaction experienced during massage.

Serotonin

Serotonin allows a person to maintain context-appropriate behavior; that is, to do the appropriate thing at the appropriate time. It regulates mood in terms of appropriate emotions, attention to thoughts, and calming, quieting, comforting effects; it also subdues irritability and regulates drive states so that we can suppress the urge to talk, touch, and be involved in power struggles. For example, when someone tells you to

"get a grip," they are saying that you could use a good boost in serotonin.

Serotonin also is involved in satiety; adequate levels reduce the sense of hunger and craving, such as for food or sex. In addition, it modulates the sleep/wake cycle. A low serotonin level has been implicated in depression, eating disorders, pain disorders, and obsessive-compulsive disorders.

Massage seems to increase the available level of serotonin. A balancing effect occurs between dopamine and serotonin, much like agonist and antagonist muscles. Massage may support the optimum ratio of these chemicals.

Epinephrine/Adrenaline and Norepinephrine/Noradrenaline

The terms epinephrine and adrenaline, and norepinephrine and noradrenaline, are used interchangeably in scientific texts. Epinephrine activates arousal mechanisms in the body, whereas norepinephrine functions more in the brain. These are the activation, arousal, alertness, and alarm chemicals of the fight-or-flight response and of all sympathetic arousal functions and behaviors. If the levels of these chemicals are too high or if the chemicals are released at an inappropriate time, the person feels as though something very important is demanding attention, or the person reacts with the basic survival drives of fight or flight (hypervigilance and hyperactivity). The person might have a disturbed sleep pattern, particularly a lack of rapid eye movement (REM) sleep, which is restorative sleep. With low levels of epinephrine and norepinephrine, a person is sluggish, drowsy, fatigued, and underaroused.

Massage seems to have a regulating effect on epinephrine and norepinephrine through stimulation or inhibition of the sympathetic nervous system or stimulation or inhibition of the parasympathetic nervous system. This generalized balancing function of massage seems to recalibrate the appropriate adrenaline and noradrenaline levels. Depending on the response of the ANS, massage can just as easily wake up a person and relieve fatigue as it can calm down a person who is angry and pacing the floor. It should be noted that initially, touch stimulates the sympathetic nervous system, whereas it seems to take 15 minutes or so of sustained stimulation to begin to engage the parasympathetic functions. Therefore, it makes sense that a 15-minute chair massage tends to increase production of epinephrine and norepinephrine, which can help corporate workers become more attentive, whereas a 1-hour slow, rhythmic massage engages the parasympathetic functions, reducing epinephrine and norepinephrine levels and encouraging a good night's sleep.

Enkephalins, Endorphins, and Dynorphins

Enkephalins, endorphins, and dynorphins (endogenous opiates) are mood lifters that support satiety and modulate pain. Massage appears to increases the available levels of these chemicals.

Endocannabinoids

Endocannabinoids are a group of neuromodulatory chemicals involved in a variety of physiologic processes, including appetite, pain sensation, mood, memory, motor coordination, blood pressure regulation, and combating cancer. Endocannabinoids, which are endogenous, stimulate the same receptors as cannabis. Endocannabinoids are synthesized on demand, but the question is, what triggers the process? This question must be answered before we can theorize about how massage would interact with these chemicals.

The endocannabinoid system modulates anxiety-like behaviors and stress adaptation. Most research studies suggest that acute stress triggers the release of the endocannabinoid chemicals, which then bind to cells' receptors. This causes changes in cell function, which causes changes in emotional behavior, reversing the stress response. The endocannabinoid system functions as a neuromodulator of the CNS.

Researchers at the University of Georgia Neuroscience and Behavior Program demonstrated that brains in rats release endocannabinoids as a response to painful stimuli (Rahn, Hohmann, 2009). The researchers reported an increase in the concentration of endocannabinoids 2 minutes after the introduction of painful stimuli and again 15 minutes later. Endogenous opioids are well known to suppress pain. The so-called runner's high may be more directly related to endocannabinoids than to endorphins.

Cacao, the main ingredient in chocolate, contains a number of compounds that are believed to improve mood by interacting with endocannabinoid receptors in the brain. Unlike with marijuana, cacao stimulation of the endocannabinoid system is triggered by an increase in the body's natural endocannabinoid receptors, resulting in a natural, even boost in mood. A foreign compound, such as THC (found in marijuana), floods the receptors, often overloading the system and creating the potential for adverse effects.

Cacao also improves mood by stimulating the release of endorphins, the body's own opiates. Endorphins are compounds produced naturally by the body that relieve pain and produce feelings of well-being. A strong interaction seems to occur among endorphins, dopamine, and endocannabinoids, but research has not clarified the nature of this relationship.

Massage therapy can be applied to stimulate the "good hurt" sensation that triggers endorphin action and also, possibly, endocannabinoids. New research has shown that endogenous cannabinoids also function as stress-induced analgesics (Hohmann et al., 2005). Recent research supports the theory that cacao exerts its effect on mood by stimulating endocannabinoid receptors and the release of endorphins. Increased levels of endocannabinoids are associated with relaxation and pain reduction. Whether massage works in a similar way would be an interesting research topic.

Oxytocin

The hormone **oxytocin** has been implicated in pair or couple bonding, parental bonding, feelings of attachment, and care taking, along with its more clinical functions during pregnancy, delivery, and lactation.

Massage tends to increase the available level of oxytocin, which could explain the connected and intimate feeling of massage.

Cortisol

Cortisol and other glucocorticoids are stress hormones produced by the adrenal glands during prolonged stress. Elevated levels of these hormones indicate increased sympathetic arousal. Cortisol and other glucocorticoids have been implicated in many stress-related symptoms and diseases, including suppressed immunity states, sleep disturbances, inappropriate inflammatory response, and increases in the level of substance P.

Massage has been shown to reduce levels of cortisol and substance P, although researchers disagree to some extent whether these finding are accurate (Moyer et al, 2011).

Growth Hormone

Growth hormone promotes cell division and in adults has been implicated in the functions of tissue repair and regeneration. This hormone is necessary for healing and is most active during sleep.

Massage increases the availability of growth hormone indirectly by encouraging sleep and reducing the level of cortisol.

Combined Neuroendocrine Influences

Massage balances the blood levels of serotonin, dopamine, endorphins, and possibly endocannabinoids; this in turn facilitates the production of natural killer cells in the immune system and regulates mood. This response indicates that including massage in the treatment program for viral conditions, some forms of cancer, and mood disturbances would be beneficial. Oxytocin tends to increase feelings of connectedness. At the same time, massage reduces cortisol and regulates epinephrine and norepinephrine, facilitating the action of growth hormone.

It is easy to understand the reasons massage is beneficial for so many conditions and how it indirectly influences many others. Consider the following scenarios as examples of what may occur:

- A lonely, depressed person feels more alive after a massage (increase in serotonin and oxytocin; decrease in cortisol).
- A child with attention deficit/hyperactivity disorder (ADHD) can do her homework after a 15-minute massage (increase in dopamine and noradrenaline).
- A person suffering from chronic pain functions better after a massage (increase in endorphin, serotonin, and oxytocin).
- A smoker trying to quit can forestall a craving for a cigarette after a massage (increase in noradrenaline, dopamine, serotonin, endocannabinoids, and endorphin).
- A person who has had surgery heals faster with massage (decrease in cortisol and adrenaline; increase in restorative sleep through pain reduction; increase in endorphin and serotonin, resulting in greater availability of growth hormone).
- An individual infected with the human immunodeficiency virus (HIV) may have a stronger immune response after massage (increase in serotonin, dopamine, and endorphin; decrease in cortisol).

- A couple may relate better to their newborn after learning to give the infant a massage (increase in serotonin and oxytocin; decrease in cortisol).

We may never fully understand the effects of massage on the integrated neuroendocrine mechanism; however, we do know that people who enjoy massage feel better.

TRANSLATING EVIDENCE INTO PRACTICAL APPLICATION: AUTONOMIC NERVOUS SYSTEM

SECTION OBJECTIVES

Chapter objective covered in this section:

7. The student will be able to explain the effects of therapeutic massage in physiologic terms.

Using the information presented in this section, the student will be able to perform the following:

- Explain the anatomic and physiologic influences of massage on the autonomic nervous system

Autonomic Influences

The ANS is best known for regulating the sympathetic fight-flight-fear and excitation response, and the parasympathetic relaxation and restorative response (Table 5-1). The sympathetic and parasympathetic systems work together to maintain homeostasis through a feedback loop system. These systems both affect and are affected by the endocrine glands. Specific muscle patterns are associated with both systems. Arm, leg, and jaw muscles may be tight during the sympathetic response (the attack posture), whereas postural muscles often tighten with the parasympathetic response (Figure 5-6). Excessive sympathetic output causes most of the stress-related diseases physicians see, such as headaches, gastrointestinal difficulties, high blood pressure, anxiety, muscle tension and aches, and sexual dysfunction.

Recently the ANS has been reclassified into three divisions: the sympathetic nervous system, the parasympathetic nervous system, and the enteric nervous system. The enteric nervous system controls gastrointestinal motility and secretions. It is a meshwork of nerve fibers, including the vagus nerve, that innervate the viscera, gastrointestinal (GI) tract, pancreas, and gallbladder. It has its own sensory and motor reflexes, which are independent of the CNS. A link exists between the mind and the gut. Digestion works best when we feel safe and are relaxed. In addition, the act of eating is relaxing. Consider the calming effect that sucking on a bottle or pacifier has on an infant or that eating a nice meal has on adults. Research suggests that when the enteric nervous system is out of balance, not only do inappropriate weight gain or loss and diseases of the digestive system occur, but mood and outlook on life also are affected.

The ANS is regulated by several centers in the brain, particularly the cerebral cortex, hypothalamus, and medulla oblongata. The hypothalamus largely controls the ANS. It receives impulses from the visceral (organ) sensory fibers and from some somatic (muscle and joint) sensory fibers. The hypothalamus plays an important role in the body/mind

Table 5-1	Functions of the Autonomic Nervous System	
Component	Sympathetic Control	Parasympathetic Control
Viscera		
Heart	Accelerates heartbeat	Slows heartbeat
Smooth Muscle		
Most blood vessels	Constricts blood vessels	None
Blood vessels of skeletal muscle	None	Dilates blood vessels
Digestive tract	Decreases peristalsis; inhibits defecation	Increases peristalsis
Anal sphincter	Stimulates (closes sphincter)	Inhibits (opens sphincter for defecation)
Urinary bladder	Inhibits (relaxes bladder)	Stimulates (contracts bladder)
Urinary sphincters	Stimulates (closes sphincters)	Inhibits (opens sphincters for urination)
Iris	Stimulates radial fibers (dilation of pupil)	Stimulates circular fibers (constriction of pupil)
Ciliary muscles	Inhibits (accommodates for far vision; flattening of lens)	Stimulates (accommodates for near vision; bulging of lens)
Hair (pilomotor muscles)	Stimulates (goose bumps)	None
Glands		
Adrenal medulla	Increases secretion of epinephrine	None
Sweat glands	Increases secretion of sweat	None
Digestive glands	Decreases secretion of digestive juices	Increases secretion of digestive juices

connection (Schillinger et al., 2006). It is one of the main components of the limbic system.

The limbic system is a group of brain structures, activated by emotional behavior and arousal, that influences the endocrine and autonomic systems. Limbic responses are reflected in a general alteration of mood and in feelings of well-being or distress. A property of limbic neural circuits is their prolonged after-discharge following stimulation; this may explain why emotional responses generally are extended and outlast the stimuli that initiate them.

Research indicates that the cerebellum, the limbic pain and pleasure centers, and the various relay centers are all part of one circuit (Schillinger et al, 2006). The cerebellum controls both conscious and subconscious movements of skeletal muscle, input from proprioceptors, and feedback loops.

The effects of massage can be processed through the ANS. These effects, which are primarily reflexive, can influence the following:

- Sympathetic activation and stress
- Parasympathetic patterns and conservation withdrawal
- Entrainment
- Body/mind interaction

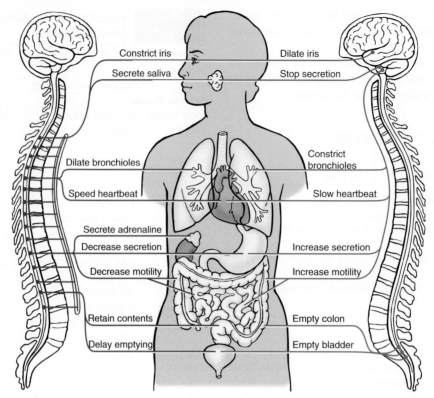

FIGURE 5-6 Innervation of the major target organs by the autonomic nervous system.

- Toughening (hardening)
- Placebo effect

Sympathetic Activation and Stress

Hans Selye called the body's response to stress the **general adaptation syndrome,** which he suggested can be divided into three stages:

1. *Alarm reaction:* Also called the *fight-or-flight response,* this is the body's initial reaction to a perceived stressor.
2. *Resistance reaction:* Through the secretion of regulating hormones, this reaction allows the body to continue fighting a stressor long after the effects of the alarm reaction have dissipated.
3. *Exhaustion reaction:* This reaction occurs if the stress response continues without relief.

Selye's general adaptation syndrome responses are commonly called *sympathetic activation* or *sympathetic dominance.* Activation of the sympathetic nervous system usually results in sensations that people call *stress.* Excessive stress can cause body-wide distress.

The question is, which comes first—the emotion or the release of the hormones? Science has discovered that it is rather like the chicken and the egg problem. Intense emotion, such as fear, rage, and anxiety, plays a part in activating the fight-or-flight response. The hormones epinephrine and norepinephrine are released in response to stimulation, and the alarm reaction begins. This is the stage of "do or die," or "make it happen or get away." The body provides energy for action. The alarm reaction lasts 15 to 30 minutes. When this fight-or-flight response occurs, the blood pressure increases, muscles tense, digestion and elimination shut down, circulation patterns shift, and glycogen is mobilized.

Long-term stress (i.e., stress that cannot be resolved by fleeing or fighting) may also trigger the release of cortisol, a cortisone manufactured by the body. Long-term high blood levels of cortisol cause side effects similar to those of the drug cortisone, including fluid retention, hypertension, muscle weakness, osteoporosis, breakdown of connective tissue, nonproductive inflammation, peptic ulcer, impaired wound healing, vertigo, headache, reduced ability to deal with stress, hypersensitivity, weight gain, nausea, fatigue, and psychic disturbances. This is a phase of enduring circumstances that are less than ideal and of constant vigilance in a world perceived as unsafe and hostile.

When the body can no longer tolerate the effects of stress, the exhaustion phase begins. In long-term sympathetic stress, tension builds until the body basically wears out. Cardiovascular, upper respiratory, and GI problems tend to develop. The body begins to break down. This is the stage in which burnout occurs.

In our society most of us do not physically fight or flee from stressors, although the chemical reactions commanding these actions may be activated several times a day. So what happens to the chemicals? We each find our own way to dissipate them, such as yelling at our family or driving aggressively. Most of us would like to find more appropriate ways to release the chemicals. Moderate exercise is one of the best ways to burn up fight-or-flight chemicals (see Chapter 15).

Massage research studies have supported the premise that the application of massage reduces sympathetic arousal.

Parasympathetic Patterns and Conservation Withdrawal

Because parasympathetic patterns are restorative, physical activity is curtailed and digestion and elimination increase. Peace and calmness are results of parasympathetic influence. When we become fatigued, parasympathetic functions signal the body to rest. Chronic fatigue syndrome is a good example of a parasympathetic reaction to stress. More drastically, depression can manifest with parasympathetic dysfunction.

Conservation withdrawal is another factor to be considered in a discussion of the parasympathetic patterns. In animals, conservation withdrawal is similar to "playing possum" or hibernation; in human beings it may arise as a result of intense negative experiences, such as abuse, neglect, or starvation. To a lesser degree, conservation withdrawal patterns play a part in depression.

A massage that is more stimulating may help draw a client out of withdrawal patterns. All sensations, including touch, initially stimulate, whether they are received through visual, audio, or kinesthetic processes. Stimulation that is quick and unexpected arouses sympathetic functions. More commonly, massage encourages parasympathetic dominance and vagus nerve stimulation to counter the effects of sympathetic over-arousal (Cassileth and Vickers, 2004).

Entrainment

Entrainment, mentioned earlier, is an important reflexive effect that seems to be processed through the ANS. To entrain means to drag with. Entrainment is the coordination or synchronization of rhythms. In the body, biologic oscillators such as the heart and the thalamus regulate the rhythmic occurrence of certain biochemical, physiologic, and behavioral events, such as sleep, hunger, and so forth. Synchronization of the heart rate, respiratory rate, and thalamus activity supports the entrainment process, and the other, more subtle body rhythms follow. Synchronization of the rhythms of the heart, respiration, and digestion promotes balance, or homeostasis, which supports a healthy body. A balance between the sympathetic and parasympathetic divisions of the ANS influences the heart and the vascular systems, modulating the heart rate and blood pressure. Nasal reflexes, which are stimulated by the movement of air through the nose, rhythmically interact with the heart, lungs, and diaphragm. Therefore, the entire body is affected, because biologic rhythms are interconnected.

The body also entrains to external rhythms (Szirmai, 2010). Any activity that uses a repetitive motion or sound quiets or excites the nervous system (depending on the speed and pace of the rhythm) through entrainment and thereby alters the physiologic process of the body. Sometimes the body rhythms are disrupted. Music with disharmony and discord can be disruptive, as can multiple rhythms out of sync in the same environment, such as a shopping mall with flashing lights, many different types of music played at one time, and the humming of machinery. People often become fatigued or out of sorts in these disharmonic environments.

The body most easily entrains to natural rhythms, such as the sounds of a babbling brook, ocean waves, or the rustling of leaves in the breeze. Studies have shown that the rhythmic

physiologic patterns of a dog's or cat's breathing or heart rate can be beneficial to the elderly. Music with a regular 4/4 beat at 60 beats per minute or slower tends to order rhythms and calm the body. A tempo faster than 60 beats per minute seems to excite physiologically, but if the rhythm is even, the body can achieve a focused, alert state. Many forms of classical music provide resourceful entrainment rhythms. Music therapy is one of the main sources of entrainment research (Wang et al., 2002). Music is a common addition to massage and provides an external entrainment rhythm for the practitioner and the client.

When a person experiences positive emotional states, the biologic rhythms naturally tend to begin to oscillate together, or entrain. Body entrainment processes also can be enhanced by techniques that shift the consciousness to the breathing patterns and heart rate. Most meditation processes or relaxation methods create an environment for entrainment by reducing external influences and focusing on internal rhythms, such as breathing. Many disciplines quiet the mind and body during meditation; yoga, for example, focuses attention on breathing, whereas Qigong focuses on the point below the navel. These systems center attention on body areas with known biologic oscillators. The location of the chakra system correlates with biologic oscillators. The rhythmic patterns of singing, chanting, and movement in our religious and social rituals interact with biologic patterns, resulting in a calming or exciting organization or disruption of body rhythms.

Many years of research will be required before we understand the magnitude of the influences that affect our body rhythms. Current research focuses on the possibility that disease processes result from disruptions in body rhythms and on the effects of work environments that directly disturb or alter natural body rhythms.

Influence of Massage on Entrainment

To encourage entrainment, massage is provided in a quiet, rhythmic manner. The rhythmic application of massage and the proximity of a centered, compassionate professional's breathing rate and heart rate can support restorative entrainment if body rhythms are out of sync. A focused, centered professional introduces his or her own ordered rhythms as part of the environment; these rhythms serve as an additional external influence that enables the client's body rhythms to synchronize. When synchronization occurs, homeostatic mechanisms seem to work more efficiently.

Body/Mind Interaction

The body/mind link is best understood in association with the ANS. An altered state of consciousness is any state of awareness that differs from the normal awareness of a conscious person. Altered states of consciousness are a factor in body/mind interactions. Consciousness can be altered in many ways, such as by medications or foods that change chemical processes, by repetitive activities or sounds (entrainment), or by a trance state. For centuries many cultures and religions have explored altered states of consciousness and have used them readily in defensive actions, in healing, and in controlling pain. Meditation, tai chi, and yoga are examples of ancient methods used to achieve altered states of consciousness. We can achieve a similar result by gardening, drawing, knitting, rocking in a rocking chair, or playing a musical instrument.

Both the practitioner and the client can achieve an altered state of consciousness during a massage session. After the altered state has been achieved, it must be maintained for at least 15 minutes for the person to reap the most therapeutic benefit.

State-Dependent Memory

Another aspect of the body/mind connection with the ANS is state-dependent memory. Triggering of a pattern of movement or a particular pressure sensation related to pleasurable sensation or caused by trauma or learned habit sometimes is enough to enable a person to achieve a particular altered state of consciousness, whether pleasurable or distressing. This results in a release of the chemical codes of the emotions involved in the initial memory encoding. Emotional input registers in the body through the ANS and the endocrine system. As described previously, a definite chemical factor is involved in the arousal of emotions based on the body's production of endorphins, enkephalins, epinephrine, norepinephrine, dopamine, serotonin, oxytocin, and other hormones and neurotransmitters. If these chemicals are released into the bloodstream during bodywork, the individual may once again feel the chemical arousal of an emotion, perhaps triggering a memory.

The adrenal hormones that interplay with the sympathetic responses are intimately involved with short-term memory. Depletion of norepinephrine reduces memory storage, and elevation of the hormone increases it. The "state" in state-dependent memory is either a sympathetic or a parasympathetic nervous system function coupled with a unique neuroendocrine chemical mix. If a person has an experience while in one of these states, the memory is encoded (stored in that state). Research shows that memory is accessible to an individual only when the particular body chemistry and function are similar to those of the experience as it first happened (Pert, 1997).

Because of its effects on the ANS, massage can stimulate these state-dependent memory patterns. This can be useful in allowing the client to resolve a past experience that was irresolvable when it occurred. Often professional counseling is necessary to help the person sort out a memory pattern that is distressing and nonproductive and to develop strategies for resolution, integration, and coping. These activities are outside the scope of practice for therapeutic massage; however, combined with effective counseling by trained professionals, massage can be a very beneficial part of an overall treatment plan. Exciting research is underway on state-dependent learning in sympathetic and parasympathetic patterns of function (Proficiency Exercise 5-3).

Toughening (Hardening)

The autonomic reaction to massage can be explained by a concept known as toughening (or hardening), which is the reaction to repeated exposure to stimuli that elicit arousal responses. The planned presentation of stimuli teaches the

💡 PROFICIENCY EXERCISE 5-3

1. In what way do you think the following day-to-day activities depend on the ANS?
  - A person eats when tired but not hungry.
  - The driver of a car does not have to stop to use the restroom, although the children in the back seat do. When the driver of the car tells the children that they are not going to stop to use the restroom and that they have to wait, the children start fighting.
  - A person's stomach starts growling half an hour after a boring lecture begins.
  - Watching a scary movie makes a person feel like doing something exciting and active.

2. Give two other daily experiences that are influenced by the ANS.

body to manage more efficiently with sympathetic stress responses. Forms of passive toughening, such as repeated exposure to cold shock, have been found to increase an individual's tolerance to stress. During exposure to the cold, two hormones of the adrenal medulla, epinephrine and norepinephrine, are released into the bloodstream.

Although massage is not as severe as cold shock, the increase in autonomic functioning and its passive nature may indeed be characterized as a form of passive toughening (Knott et al., 2005). As with exercise, massage methods that require the client's active participation help dissipate sympathetic stress hormones (sympathoadrenal response), allowing the system to re-establish homeostasis.

Placebo Effect

Throughout history people have known that treatment in itself influences the course of a disease, even if the treatment is not specific. This placebo effect probably is caused by several mechanisms, most of which are not yet clearly understood. Suggestions from the environment, the attitude of the person giving the placebo, and the patient's confidence in the treatment's effectiveness all act together to produce the placebo effect. Some studies have reported a success rate of 70% to 90% using placebos.

The gentle, caring attention focused on the client during therapeutic massage may work as a powerful placebo effect.

Influence of Massage on the Autonomic Nervous System

Because of its generalized effect on the ANS and associated functions, massage can cause changes in mood and excitement levels and can induce the relaxation and restorative response. Massage seems to be a gentle modulator, producing feelings of general well-being and comfort. However, this does not always mean that the client responds to the massage by becoming very relaxed. The most common response is a sense that "the edge is off," or the person has a less urgent or intense emotional state.

The client may be better able to control his or her emotional state rather than being controlled by it. This ability to self-regulate is very important in the physiologic process of maintaining homeostasis. Another name for self-regulation is *internal control*. We tend to feel more at ease when we feel a sense of internal control.

Initially massage stimulates sympathetic functions. This really surprises students who think that they are giving a relaxation massage. The increase in autonomic sympathetic arousal is followed by a decrease if the massage is slowed and sustained with sufficient pleasurable pressure. To encourage more of a sympathetic response, participation in muscle energy techniques is helpful (see Chapter 10). Compression in a fast-paced massage style also stimulates sympathetic responses and may lift depression temporarily.

Slow, repetitive stroking, broad-based compression, or rhythmic movement initiates relaxation responses. Rhythmic bodywork creates a trancelike effect. Sufficient pressure applied with a compressive force to the tissues supports serotonin functions.

Point holding, such as acupressure or reflexology (see Chapter 12), releases the body's own painkillers and mood-altering chemicals from the entire endorphin class. These chemicals stimulate the parasympathetic responses of relaxation, restoration, and contentment. Acupressure causes sympathetic inhibition (Hodge et al., 2007). These methods of bodywork depend on the creation of a moderate, controlled pain to relieve pain. A greater pain or stress stimulus than the perception of the existing pain is required to generate the endorphin response. When the release of substance P triggers pain, enkephalins are released, suppressing the pain signal. A negative feedback system activates the release of serotonin and opiates, which inhibit pain. Therapeutic massage methods can be used to create a controlled, noxious (pain) stimulation that triggers this cycle. Clients often refer to this noxious stimulation as good pain.

Breathing is a powerful way to interact with the ANS. Chest breathing and hyperventilation are common components of increased sympathetic stimulation. For the body to deal with stress, the muscular patterns of breathing must be normalized (see Chapter 15). Most meditation breathing patterns, singing, and chanting are ways to normalize those patterns through entrainment.

Altering the muscles so that they are more or less tense or changing the consistency of the connective tissue affects the ANS through the feedback loop, which in turn affects the powerful body/mind phenomenon.

TRANSLATING EVIDENCE INTO PRACTICAL APPLICATION: SOMATIC NERVOUS SYSTEM

SECTION OBJECTIVES

Chapter objective covered in this section:

7. The student will be able to explain the effects of therapeutic massage in physiologic terms.

Using the information presented in this section, the student will be able to perform the following:

- Explain the anatomic and physiologic influences of massage on the somatic nervous system

The effects of massage can be processed through the somatic division of the PNS. The somatic division controls movement and muscle contraction and relaxation patterns, in addition to the motor tone of muscles. The length-tension relationship of a muscle is maintained through somatic influence. The length-tension relationship is how long or short the muscle fibers are and how this affects both the contraction ability and resting length of the muscle. A muscle that is either too short or too long cannot contract effectively. The effects of massage on the length-tension relationship are primarily reflexive.

Somatic effects are produced by means of the following:
- Neuromuscular mechanisms
- Hyperstimulation analgesia
- Counterirritation
- Reduction of impingement (entrapment and compression)

Neuromuscular Mechanisms

The prefix *neuro-* refers to the nervous system; *muscular* refers to the muscles. The neuromuscular effect refers to the control of the muscles through signals from the nervous system and the response of the muscles to those signals.

Nerve cells stimulate muscles to contract or to relax (release a contraction). Specialized nerve receptors called *proprioceptors* (or *mechanoreceptors*) provide a constant monitoring and protective function. Proprioceptors receive and transmit information about body position, muscle tension, static tone, degree of stretch, joint position and activity, and speed and direction of movement and equilibrium.

Dysfunction of soft tissue (muscle and connective tissue) usually occurs as a result of proprioceptive hyperactivity or hypoactivity. Proprioceptive hyperactivity causes tense or spastic muscles and hypoactivity of opposing muscle groups. Put simply, a tight muscle area results in (or from) an inhibited (weakened) muscle area and vice versa.

The three main types of proprioceptors are muscle spindles, tendon organs, and joint kinesthetic receptors.

- Muscle spindles are found primarily in the belly of the muscle; they respond to both sudden and prolonged stretches.
- Tendon organs are found in the tendon and musculotendinous junction; they respond to tension at the tendon. Articular (joint) ligaments, which have receptors similar to tendon organs, adjust reflex inhibition of the adjacent muscle when excessive strain is placed on the joints.
- Joint kinesthetic receptors are found in the capsules of joints; they respond to pressure and to acceleration and deceleration of joint movement. The two main types of joint kinesthetic receptors are type II cutaneous mechanoreceptors and pacinian (lamellated) corpuscles.

Somatic Reflexes

Stimulation of nervous system receptors is interpreted and processed through the somatic reflex arcs. Reflexes are fast, predictable, automatic responses to a change in the

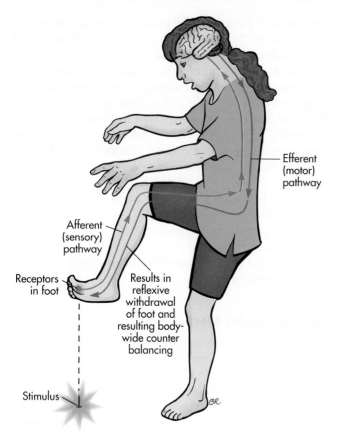

Efferent (motor) pathway

Afferent (sensory) pathway

Receptors in foot

Results in reflexive withdrawal of foot and resulting body-wide counter balancing

Stimulus

FIGURE 5-7 Reflex response—localized stimulation of a few specific receptors leads to many outgoing impulses, which affect a large number of muscles.

environment that help maintain homeostasis (Figure 5-7). The stimulation of therapeutic massage constitutes a change in the environment, and the body is called on to restore homeostasis. The reflexes most often stimulated are the stretch reflex, tendon reflex, flexor reflex, and crossed-extensor reflex.

Stretch Reflex

The stretch reflex operates as a feedback mechanism to control muscle length by causing muscle contraction. It is activated by the muscle spindles, which sense muscle stretching. In response to massage methods that stretch muscles, a muscle spindle produces nerve impulses that stimulate a somatic sensory neuron in the posterior root of the spinal nerve. When the motor nerve impulse reaches the stretched muscle, a muscle action potential is generated, which causes the muscle to contract. Muscle contraction stops spindle cell discharge. The muscle stretch stimulates the stretch reflex, resulting in shortening of the muscle. The sensitivity of the muscle spindle in response to stretching influences the level of muscle tone throughout the body.

Therapeutic massage methods can make use of this reflex to stimulate inhibited muscle patterns by stretching the muscles and initiating the stretch reflex. An awareness of this reflex response is important in all stretches that are intended to lengthen and relax the muscles; in these circumstances the reflex must be avoided. Often this system of reflexes becomes hyperactive, resulting in an increase in muscle tension. Massage

techniques that use isometric and isotonic muscle contraction to relax and lengthen muscles are helpful for normalizing short muscles and associated soft tissue.

Tendon Reflex

The tendon reflex operates as a feedback mechanism to control muscle tension by causing muscle relaxation. This reflex is mediated by the tendon organs, which detect and respond to changes in muscle tension caused by the pull of muscular contraction.

The most common massage technique used to stimulate the tendon reflex is postisometric relaxation (see Chapter 10). This technique increases tension at the tendon. The tendon organ is stimulated, which sends a signal along a sensory neuron. In the spinal cord the sensory neuron synapses with an inhibitory association neuron, which inhibits motor neurons that innervate the muscle associated with the tendon organ. This inhibition causes the muscle to relax. The sensory neuron from the tendon organ also stimulates an association neuron in the spinal cord. The association neuron synapses with a motor neuron, controlling antagonistic muscles and causing them to contract. To simplify, when one muscle contracts, its antagonist, or opposing muscle group, inhibits. This is called *reciprocal innervation.* Massage practitioners can use reciprocal innervation to avoid the stretch reflex response and prepare a muscle for lengthening and stretching.

Recently Ballantyne et al. (2003) questioned the validity of the effects of proprioceptive neuromuscular facilitation (PNF) and muscle energy techniques (MET) based on the tendon reflex. They found that these methods are effective, but a different physiology appears to be involved; specifically, strong research evidence indicates that increased tolerance to the sensation of stretch is the main mechanism.

Flexor and Crossed-Extensor Reflexes

The flexor (withdrawal) and crossed-extensor reflexes are polysynaptic reflex arcs. Stimulation of these reflexes affects both sides of the body through a series of intersegmental reflex arcs, which usually are linked in a pattern that includes postural muscles and muscle action in the limbs. A single sensory neuron can activate several motor neurons. The flexor reflex is involved in movement away from a stimulus, such as pulling away from a hot stove burner. The crossed-extensor reflex is involved in maintaining balance, such as staying upright when tripping over something. Synchronized control over the muscles that are contracting and those that are inhibited is achieved through contralateral reflex arcs, or reflex arcs on both sides of the body. Similar reflex patterns interact to coordinate movement; these are called *gait reflexes.* Others are involved with posture, such as the ocular pelvic reflex and righting reflexes.

By creating a noxious signal (i.e., pain or an unpleasant sensation), therapeutic massage can stimulate a withdrawal response to stimulate opposite-side patterns of tension or weakness. This is a powerful response, because withdrawal reflexes take priority over all other reflex activity occurring at the moment. If the massage application is so painful that the body tightens to guard against the noxious sensation, the effectiveness of the massage is lost. These reflex patterns also explain why tension patterns seldom occur only on one side of the body. The linked patterns of the various reflexes explain why dysfunctional patterns of groups of muscles often are identified on both sides of the body and not just where the dysfunction exists.

Influence of Massage on Neuromuscular Mechanisms

When working with the neuromuscular mechanism in massage, the massage therapist must keep in mind that the basic premises are (1) to substitute a different neurologic signal stimulation to support a normal muscle resting length through lengthening and stretching or strengthening of muscles and connective tissue, and (2) to re-educate the muscles involved (e.g., take the joint through its increased range of motion).

Movement, stretch, and pressure methods of massage focus on the activities of the muscles, tendons, joints, and ligaments to stimulate the proprioceptors. Massage methods can stimulate the resetting of unproductive reflex actions.

The effects of therapeutic massage depend heavily on the reflex mechanism. The effectiveness of the techniques depends on how efficiently the receptors for these reflexes are stimulated. The targeted receptor must be accessed with the appropriate technique and intensity so that the stimulated reflex can function appropriately.

Various neurologic laws come into play to help explain the effects of therapeutic massage on the somatic nervous system (Box 5-7). (A *law* is a scientific statement that is uniformly true for a whole class of natural occurrences.) A degree of controversy exists about the validity of some of these laws, primarily Pflüger's laws; however, the neurologic laws are worth considering as we attempt to understand the physiologic effects of massage.

Box 5-7   Laws of Neurology and Their Implications for Massage

Arndt-Schulz Law

Weak stimuli activate physiologic processes; very strong stimuli inhibit them (St John, 1990).

Implication for massage: To encourage a specific response, use gentler methods. To shut off a response, use deeper methods.

Bell's Law

Anterior spinal nerve roots are motor roots, and posterior spinal nerve roots are sensory roots (Thomas, 2006).

Implication for massage: Massage along the spine is a strong sensory stimulation.

Bowditch's (All or None) Law

The weakest stimulus capable of producing a response produces the maximum response contraction in cardiac and skeletal muscle and nerves (Anderson et al., 2005).

Implication for massage: Techniques need not be extremely intense to produce a response; all that is needed is enough sensory stimulation to begin the process.

Cannon's Law of Denervation

When autonomic effectors are partly or completely separated from their normal nerve connections, they become more sensitive to the action of chemical substances (DeGroot and Chusid, 2002).

This denervation supersensitivity involves injured nerves, which respond to all sensory stimulation regardless of whether the stimulation is specific to that nerve. Denervation supersensitivity is a universal phenomenon that affects muscles, nerves, salivary glands, sudorific glands, autonomic ganglion cells, spinal neurons, and even neurons in the cortex. Changes in muscle structure and biochemistry also occur, as does progressive destruction of the contractile elements of fibers.

Furthermore, unlike normal muscle fibers, which resist innervation from foreign nerves, degenerated muscle fibers accept contacts from other motor nerves, preganglionic autonomic fibers, and even sensory nerves.

Implication for massage: An injured area may hyperreact to all sensory stimulation, even after healing. If a person has a cold or is stressed at work or cannot sleep, previously injured areas may flare up.

Hilton's Law

A nerve trunk that supplies a joint also supplies the muscles of the joint and the skin over the insertions of such muscles (Thomas, 2006).

Implication for massage: Determining whether pain originates from the joint itself, the muscles around the joint, or the skin over the joint can be difficult; stimulation of each area affects all parts.

Hooke's Law

The stress used to stretch or compress a body is proportional to the strain experienced, as long as the elastic limits of the body have not been exceeded (DeGroot and Chusid, 2002).

Implication for massage: Methods that lengthen the tissue must be intense enough to match the existing shortening but must not exceed it.

Law of Facilitation

When an impulse has passed through a certain set of neurons to the exclusion of others one time, it will tend to take the same course on a future occasion, and each time it traverses this path, the resistance will be reduced (St John, 1990).

Implication for massage: The body likes sameness, which produces habitual patterns. After a pattern has been established, less stimulation is required to activate the response.

Continued

Box 5-7   Laws of Neurology and Their Implications for Massage—cont'd

Law of Specificity of Nervous Energy

Excitation of a receptor always gives rise to the same sensation, regardless of the nature of the stimulus (Thomas, 2006).

Implication for massage: Whatever the method used, if a sensory receptor is activated, it will respond in a specific way.

Newton's Law

When two bodies interact, the force exerted by the first on the second is equal in magnitude and opposite in direction to the force exerted by the second on the first.

Implication for massage: This law explains various aspects of pressure delivery during massage. When two bodies interact (the massage therapist and the client), the force extended by the first (the massage therapist) on the second (the client) is equal in magnitude and opposite in direction (i.e., the client's body will push back). The point where they meet is a point of balance. This is especially important in body mechanics and with regard to the way tissue binds in response to pressure.

Pflüger's Laws

Law of Generalization

When an irritation becomes very intense, it is propagated in the medulla oblongata, which becomes a focus from which stimuli radiate to all parts of the cord, causing a general contraction of all muscles in the body (St John, 1990).

Implication for massage: This response must be avoided if possible. It is important to keep invasive massage measures (e.g., frictioning) below the intensity level that causes a general body response.

Law of Intensity

Reflex movements usually are more intense on the side of irritation; at times the movements of the opposite side equal the movements in intensity, but they usually are less pronounced (St John, 1990).

Implication for massage: See Law of Symmetry.

Law of Radiation

If excitation continues to increase, it is propagated upward, and reactions take place through centrifugal nerves coming from the higher cord segments (St John, 1990).

Implication for massage: See Law of Symmetry.

Law of Symmetry

If stimulation is increased sufficiently, a motor reaction is manifested not only on the irritated side but also in similar muscles on the opposite side of the body (St John, 1990).

Implication for massage: By using increasing levels of massage intensity, a bilateral effect can be created, even if only one side of the body is massaged. This is especially useful for massage applications to painful areas. By massaging the unaffected side, the painful areas can be addressed without receiving direct massage work.

Law of Unilaterality

If a mild irritation is applied to one or more sensory nerves, movement will take place usually on one side only and on the side that has been irritated (St John, 1990).

Implication for massage: Light stimulation remains fairly localized in response to massage.

Weber's Law

The increase in stimulus necessary to produce the smallest perceptible increase in sensation bears a constant ratio to the strength of the stimulus already acting (Thomas, 2006).

Implication for massage: To change a sensory perception, the intensity of a massage method must match and then just exceed the existing sensation.

Wolf's Law

Biologic systems (including soft and hard tissues) deform in relation to the lines of force imposed on them.

Implication for massage: Massage is the application of mechanical force. Massage therefore deforms tissue, changing its shape.

Vestibular Apparatus and Cerebellum

The vestibular apparatus is a complex system composed of sensors in the inner ear (vestibular labyrinth), upper neck (cervical proprioception), eyes (visual motion and three-dimensional orientation), and body (somatic proprioception). These sensors send messages to several areas of the brain (brainstem, cerebellum, parietal and temporal cortices), where they are analyzed. The messages affect the eyes (vestibulo-ocular reflexes), neck (vestibulocollic reflexes), and balance (vestibulospinal reflexes); at the same time, they keep individuals aware of where they are and how they are moving through the world (visuospatial orientation).

The vestibular apparatus and the cerebellum are interrelated. The output from the cerebellum goes to the motor cortex and brainstem. Stimulating the cerebellum by altering muscle tone, position, and vestibular balance stimulates the hypothalamus to adjust ANS functions to restore homeostasis.

Influence of Massage on the Vestibular Apparatus and Cerebellum

The techniques that most strongly affect the vestibular apparatus and therefore the cerebellum are those that incorporate rhythmic rocking into the application of massage. Rocking produces movement at the neck and head that influences the sense of equilibrium. Rocking stimulates the inner ear balance mechanisms, including the vestibular nuclear complex and the labyrinthine righting reflexes, to keep the head level. Pressure on the sides of the body may stimulate the body righting reflex. Stimulation of these reflexes produces a body-wide effect involving stimulation of muscle contraction patterns, which pass throughout the body.

Massage alters the body's positional sense and the position of the eyes in response to postural change; it also initiates specific movement patterns that change sensory input from muscles, tendons, joints, and the skin and stimulates various vestibular reflexes. This feedback information, which adjusts and coordinates movement, is relayed directly to the motor cortex and the cerebellum, allowing the body to integrate the sensory data and adjust to a more efficient homeostatic balance.

Hyperstimulation Analgesia

In 1965 Melzack and Wall proposed the gate control theory of pain transmission (see Chapter 6). Although some aspects of the original theory have been modified over the past 40 years, the basic premise remains the same. According to this theory, a gating mechanism functions at the level of the spinal cord; that is, pain impulses pass through a "gate" to reach the lateral spinothalamic system. Painful impulses are transmitted by large-diameter and small-diameter nerve fibers. Stimulation of large-diameter fibers prevents the small-diameter fibers from transmitting signals. Stimulation (e.g., rubbing, massaging) of large-diameter fibers helps suppress the sensation of pain, especially sharp pain.

The skin over the entire body is supplied by spinal nerves that carry somatic sensory nerve impulses to the spinal cord. Each spinal nerve serves a specific segment of the skin, called a *dermatome*. Dermatomes, which can be affected by massage techniques that stimulate the skin, may account for hyperstimulation analgesia. The reduction of pain through stimulation (hyperstimulation analgesia) produced by massage and acupuncture has been used for many years (Gunn, 1992). In recent years transcutaneous electrical nerve stimulation (TENS) has become a popular method of producing hyperstimulation analgesia.

Massage and the Production of Hyperstimulation Analgesia

Stimulation of the PNS may produce analgesia by using some type of stimulation to mask pain sensation. Evidence suggests that the development of analgesia depends on the stimulation of specific points in the muscle that correspond to certain types of muscle receptors. These same points correspond with many traditional acupuncture points (see Figure 5-2) If massage stimulates these points with sufficient intensity, the large-diameter fibers can be stimulated and the gating mechanism at the spinal cord and hyperstimulation analgesia may be activated.

Tactile stimulation produced by massage travels through the large-diameter fibers. These fibers also carry a faster signal. In essence, massage sensations win the race to the brain, and the pain sensations are blocked because the gate is closed. Many parents and small children seem to know this instinctively. They rub an injured spot, thus activating large-diameter fibers. Stimulating techniques, such as percussion or vibration of painful areas to activate stimulation-produced analgesia (hyperstimulation analgesia), also are effective.

Counterirritation

Taber's Cyclopedic Medical Dictionary defines counterirritation as superficial irritation that relieves some irritation of deeper structures (Thomas, 2006). Counterirritation may be

explained by the gate control theory. Inhibition in central sensory pathways, produced by rubbing or shaking an area, may explain counterirritation. Noxious stimuli suppress nociceptive (pain) impulses. Changing the perception of pain by introducing a different pain signal is akin to stepping on a person's foot to relieve the pain in the thumb just hit by a hammer.

Inhibition of central sensory pathways may explain the effect of counterirritants. Stimulation of the skin over an area of pain or dysfunction produces some relief from the pain. Various analgesic rubs and creams contain chemicals (e.g., capsaicin) that are intended to produce this kind of counterirritation.

Massage and the Production of Counterirritation

All methods of massage can be used to produce counterirritation. Many people have learned from practical experience that touching or shaking an injured area diminishes the pain of the injury. Any massage method that introduces a controlled sensory stimulation intense enough to be interpreted by the client as a good pain can create counterirritation. Massage therapy in many forms stimulates the skin over an area of discomfort. Techniques that result in reddening of the skin and underlying tissue (histamine response) are effective. Compression and movement methods require the body to attend to a different signal and temporarily ignore the original discomfort (Proficiency Exercise 5-4).

Trigger Points

No one is quite sure exactly what a trigger point is. Many terms, including myalgia, myositis, fibrositis, fibromyalgia, myofibrositis, fibromyositis, fasciitis, myofascitis, rheumatism, fibrositic nodule, and myogelosis, seem to describe the myofascial trigger point (Chaitow, 2006). For the purposes of this text, a trigger point is an area of local nerve facilitation in the muscle or associated connective tissue that creates small areas of shortening or microspasm. These points are sensitive to pressure and, when stimulated, can become the site of painful sensation. Dr. Janet Travell spent much of her professional career researching and developing a treatment for myofascial trigger points.

Opinions differ on whether trigger points are more a neuromuscular or a connective tissue phenomenon. Fortunately, the kinds of pathophysiologic mechanisms responsible for the development of trigger points are becoming clear, and the different mechanisms may explain why some therapeutic approaches are so effective and others have limited benefit for this condition.

Muscles and associated structures with trigger points feel abnormal when palpated and have a reduced range of motion because of the increased tension of the palpable taut band that is associated with the trigger points. This palpable increase in muscle tension is commonly mistaken for muscle spasm. Muscle spasm is clearly marked by motor unit activity, which can be identified electromyographically; taut bands, on the other hand, show no motor unit activity at rest. The fluid around the trigger point is more acidic that the surrounding area.

The increased tension of the palpable taut band is the result of regional shortening of the sarcomeres of involved muscle fibers in the taut band. In the region of a motor endplate, the sarcomeres in the area are hypercontracted; the remaining sarcomeres of an involved muscle fiber are noticeably stretched to compensate for the missing length of the shortened sarcomeres. Because of the nature of actin (the springlike molecule that holds the myosin molecules in place), the maximally contracted sarcomeres would tend to become stuck in this shortened position. The effect of these shortened sarcomeres is one likely source of increased resting tension in an involved muscle fiber.

Effect of Massage on Trigger Points

Travell, Simons, and others suggest that the effects of massage on myofascial trigger points are the result of stimulation of proprioceptive nerve endings, changes in sarcomere length, release of enkephalin, stretching of musculotendinous structures that initiate reflex muscle relaxation through the Golgi tendon organ and spindle receptors, connective tissue changes, and increased circulation (Travell and Simons, 1992; Baldry, 2005; Chaitow, 2006). Various massage methods, including pressure, positioning, and lengthening, provide this stimulation. (Trigger points are discussed in detail in Chapter 12.)

Nerve Impingement (Entrapment, Compression)

Soft tissue often impinges upon a nerve, a condition commonly called *pinched nerve.* Tissues that can bind include skin, fascia, muscles, ligaments, joint structures, and bones. Short muscles and stiff, dense connective tissue (fascia) often impinge upon major and minor nerves, causing discomfort.

Entrapment and compression are technically different dysfunctions. **Entrapment** results when soft tissue (e.g., muscles and ligaments) exerts inappropriate pressure on nerves. **Compression** occurs when hard tissue (e.g., bone) exerts inappropriate pressure on nerves.

Regardless of the source of impingement, the symptoms are similar. However, the therapeutic interventions are different. Soft tissue approaches are beneficial for entrapment but less so for compression.

Effect of Massage on Nerve Impingement

Because of the structural arrangement of the body, impingement often occurs at major nerve plexuses (Figure 5-8). The specific nerve root, trunk, or division affected determines the condition, such as thoracic outlet syndrome, sciatica, or carpal tunnel syndrome. Therapeutic massage techniques

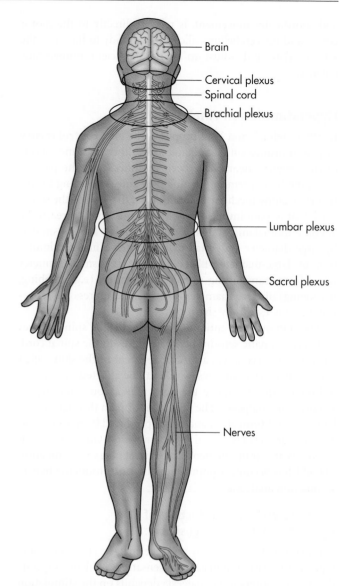

FIGURE 5-8 Major nerve plexuses.

work in many ways to reduce pressure on nerves. The main ways are to (1) reflexively change the motor tone pattern and lengthen the muscles, (2) mechanically stretch and soften connective tissue, and (3) interrupt the pain-spasm-pain cycle caused by protective muscle spasm that occurs in response to pain.

Effect of Massage on the Somatic Nervous System

Massage methods directly stimulate the reflex mechanisms of the somatic functions. Often the ANS and the endocrine system are influenced by secondary reflex activity in response to homeostatic changes caused by somatic stimulation during massage. All massage methods can be effective. The specific result depends on precise communication with the somatic sensory receptor, and the massage application needs to mimic the stimuli recognized by the targeted sensory receptor.

TRANSLATING EVIDENCE INTO PRACTICAL APPLICATION: CIRCULATION

SECTION OBJECTIVES

Chapter objective covered in this section:

7. The student will be able to explain the effects of therapeutic massage in physiologic terms.

Using the information presented in this section, the student will be able to perform the following:

- Explain the anatomic and physiologic influences of massage on the circulation

Three to five basic types of circulation have been recognized. All anatomy texts recognize arterial, venous, and lymphatic circulation. The other two types discussed in this text are respiratory and cerebrospinal fluid (CSF) circulation. All five depend on the pumping action of the skeletal muscles as they contract and relax. Arterial flow has the additional pumping action provided by the heart and smooth muscle tissue in the arteries. The lymphatic system has its own rhythmic pumping action. The implication is that some of the benefits of massage may be a result of its influence on this rhythm (Oschman, 1997; Lancaster and Crow, 2006).

These circulatory functions are both directly linked and interdependent. For example, the carbon dioxide level of the CSF affects the respiratory center in the medulla, helping to control breathing. Application of a mechanical device that produces a rhythmic massage in a proximal direction reduces edema, increases lymphatic movement from the tissues to the blood, and improves blood circulation. The massage practitioner must know the anatomy and physiology of the blood and lymph circulations to understand the effect of massage on these systems.

Circulation enhancement is fairly straightforward. Although more body fluids are moved by a 5-minute walk than by a 50-minute massage, for those unable to walk or even get out of bed, manual facilitation of the movement of body fluids can be a significant therapeutic option.

Arterial Flow

Arteries carry blood under pressure from the heart as a result of the pumping action of the heart muscle. The arteries themselves also have a muscular component that contracts rhythmically, facilitating arterial flow. An increase in arterial flow is beneficial in any situation in which an increase in oxygenated blood is desirable. Such situations include sluggish circulation in a sedentary person or increased demand in an athlete (see Chapter 12).

Massage application that creates direct compression into the area of an artery effectively crimps the artery, much like crimping a hose, and allows some back pressure to build up. When the pressure is released, the blood rushes through like water released from a dam. Arteries are accessible to compressive pressure on the soft medial areas of the arms and legs. Compressions should begin proximal to the heart to take advantage of the force of the heart pumping and move in a distal direction. Heavy pressure or sustained compression is not necessary; rather, moderate pressure is used in the right location to pump rhythmically at the client's current heart rate as the practitioner moves distally toward the fingers or toes.

Venous Return Flow

Venous return flow largely depends on contraction of the muscles against the veins. Back flow of blood is prevented by valves. Veins usually run more superficially than arteries. Because of the valve system in the veins and the fact that the blood is intended to flow back toward the heart, strokes to encourage venous flow move toward the heart.

Massage applications using short, pumping, gliding strokes are most effective in enhancing this flow. Passive and active joint movements also encourage the muscles to contract against the deeper vessels, assisting venous blood flow. If this is not possible for the client, slow, meticulous mechanical work is required to drain the area. Placing the limb above the heart, allowing gravity to assist, is beneficial (see Chapter 12).

Lymphatic Drainage

As described in Chapter 4, the lymphatic system consists of the tissues and organs that produce, store, and carry white blood cells that fight infection and other diseases. This system includes the bone marrow, spleen, thymus, lymph nodes, and lymphatic vessels. The lymphatic vessels are a network of thin tubes that carry white blood cells and lymph, a colorless fluid containing oxygen, proteins, glucose, and lymphocytes. As do blood vessels, lymphatic vessels branch into all the tissues of the body. The lymphatic system plays an important role in controlling the movement of fluid throughout the body.

The lymphatic system controls the flow of lymph. Lymph is derived from interstitial fluid or fluid that surrounds cells. Once interstitial fluid enters the lymphatic capillaries, it is called *lymph*. Lymphatic capillaries merge into small lymphatic vessels, which then merge into larger ones; along these larger lymphatic vessels are situated the lymph nodes. Lymph nodes are kidney bean–shaped tissues found in grapelike clusters in several locations in the body. They are sites of immune system activation and immune cell proliferation (growth). Once the lymph nodes have filtered lymph, the lymph drains into even larger vessels called *trunks*. All the trunks of the body drain into one of two ducts, the left lymphatic (thoracic) duct and the right lymphatic duct; these ducts return lymph to the bloodstream. The fluid in this extensive network flows throughout the body, much like the blood supply.

The massage procedures for lymphatic drainage are similar to those for venous return. Because lymph vessels open into tissue space, surface work that pulls gently on the skin is performed over the entire affected body region rather than focused over only the major veins. Pumping of jointed areas with passive joint movement seems to assist the movement of lymph through the areas of lymph node filtration. Deep breathing assists lymph movement in the thorax and abdomen. Unless the massage therapist is using manual lymphatic drainage as a specific therapeutic intervention (i.e., in cases of a pathologic condition of the lymphatic system), precision in the specific flow patterns does not seem necessary. It is important to note that the lower abdomen (from the umbilicus down) drains into the inguinal area and eventually into the thoracic duct and that the right side (right arm and head) drains into the right lymphatic duct. Both major vessels dump into the vena cava (see Chapter 12).

Respiration

The muscular mechanism for inhalation and exhalation is designed like a simple bellows (a device that is expanded to draw air in and compressed to force air out). Inhalation and exhalation depend on unrestricted movement of the musculoskeletal components of the thorax. The muscles of respiration include the scalenes, intercostals, serratus anterior diaphragm, abdominals, pelvic floor muscles, and lower leg muscles (which surprises many people). This can be demonstrated by contracting any of these muscle groups and attempting to take a deep breath; you will note that the ability to breathe is restricted. Disruption of function in any of these groups inhibits complete and easy breathing. Often subclinical overbreathing, called *breathing pattern disorder,* occurs, which causes many physical symptoms (Box 5-8).

Physiologists define *hyperventilation* as abnormally deep or rapid breathing in excess of physical demands. Dyspneic fear (no air) is a core factor in the cause of panic attacks, which result in rapid breathing.

All massage approaches that restore mobility to the thorax and the muscles of respiration affect the ability to breathe. Particularly with breathing pattern disorder, breathing retraining often is ineffective, because the mobility of the respiratory mechanism is disrupted. Often massage can restore the normal function of the soft tissue involved with breathing, which enables breathing retraining to become effective.

Cerebrospinal Fluid Circulation

CSF cools, nourishes, and protects the brain and nerves and influences breathing through carbon dioxide levels. The movement of CSF involves a pumping rhythm that some contend can be palpated. Entrainment has been implicated as a factor, as has lymphatic undulation (Oschman, 1997). More research must be done before the anatomic and physiologic mechanisms of this phenomenon can be understood scientifically.

Craniosacral therapy techniques specifically target CSF circulation (Figure 5-9). General massage also may influence this mechanism indirectly.

Box 5-8	Breathing Pattern Disorder

Breathing pattern disorder is a complex set of behaviors that leads to overbreathing despite the absence of a pathologic condition. It is considered a *functional syndrome;* that is, because all the parts are working effectively, a specific pathologic condition does not exist. Instead, the breathing pattern is inappropriate for the situation, producing confused signals to the central nervous system and resulting in a chain of events.

Increased ventilation is a common component of the fight-or-flight response. However, when the breathing rate increases but the body's actions and movements are restricted or do not increase accordingly, the person is breathing in excess of the metabolic need. Blood levels of carbon dioxide (CO_2) fall, and symptoms may occur. Because the person exhales too much CO_2 too quickly, the blood becomes more acidic. These biochemical changes can cause many of the following signs and symptoms:

- *Cardiovascular effects:* Palpitations, missed beats, tachycardia, sharp or dull atypical chest pain, "angina," vasomotor instability, cold extremities, Raynaud's phenomenon, blotchy flushing of the blush area, and capillary vasoconstriction (face, arms, hands)
- *Neurologic effects:* Dizziness; unsteadiness or instability; a sensation of faintness or giddiness (in rare cases, actual fainting); visual disturbance (blurred or tunnel vision); headache (often migraine); paresthesia (numbness, uselessness, heaviness, pins and needles, burning, limbs feeling out of proportion or as if they "don't belong"), commonly of the hands, feet, or face but sometimes of the scalp or whole body; intolerance of light or noise; and enlarged pupils (needing to wear dark glasses on a dull day)
- *Respiratory effects:* Shortness of breath, typically after exertion; irritable cough; tightness or oppression of chest;

difficulty breathing; "asthma"; air hunger; inability to take a satisfying breath; excessive sighing, yawning, and sniffing
- *Gastrointestinal effects:* Difficulty swallowing, dry mouth and throat, acid regurgitation, heartburn, hiatal hernia, nausea, flatulence, belching, air swallowing, abdominal discomfort, and bloating
- *Muscular effects:* Cramps, muscle pain (particularly in the occipital area, neck, shoulders, and between the scapulae; less commonly in the lower back and limbs), tremors, twitching, weakness, stiffness, or tetany (seizing up)
- *Psychological effects:* Tension, anxiety, "unreal" feelings, depersonalization, feeling "out of body," hallucinations, fear of insanity, panic, phobias, and agoraphobia
- *General effects:* Feelings of weakness; exhaustion; impaired concentration, memory, and performance; disturbed sleep, including nightmares; emotional sweating (axillae, palms, and sometimes the whole body); and confused mental state
- *Cerebrovascular constriction:* This condition, a primary response to breathing pattern disorder, can reduce the oxygen available to the brain by about one half. Among the resulting symptoms are dizziness, blurring of consciousness, and, possibly, because of a decrease in cortical inhibition, tearfulness and emotional instability.

Other effects of breathing pattern disorder for which massage therapists should watch are generalized body tension and chronic inability to relax. In addition, individuals with a tendency for breathing pattern disorder are particularly prone to spasm (tetany) in muscles involved in the "attack posture"; they hunch the shoulders, thrust the head and neck forward, scowl, and clench the teeth.

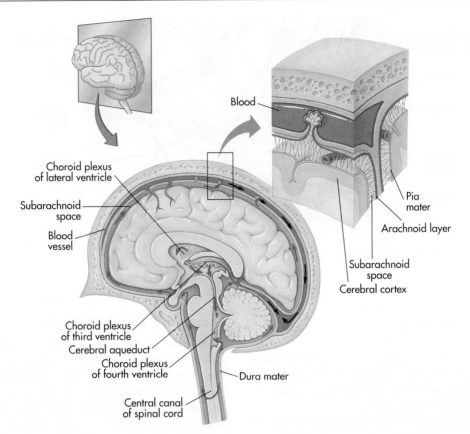

FIGURE 5-9 The flow of cerebrospinal fluid (CSF). Filtration of the blood by the choroid plexus of each ventricle produces the CSF, which flows inferiorly through the lateral ventricles, the interventricular foramen, the third ventricle, the cerebral aqueduct, the fourth ventricle, and the subarachnoid space into the blood.
(From Thibodeau GA, Patton KT: *The human body in health and disease,* ed 3, St Louis, 2002, Mosby.)

Effect of Massage on Circulation

Increased blood flow on a local level is achieved by compression of tissues, which empties capillary beds, lowers venous pressure, and increases capillary blood flow, which is quickly counteracted by autoregulation. Massage stimulates the release of vasodilators, especially histamine. Blood flow changes also may be induced through the autonomic vascular reflexes. This type of increase in blood flow has a body-wide effect. Compression against arteries mechanically influences internal blood pressure receptors in the arteries. As discussed previously, blood and lymph circulation are affected by massage. In addition, massage and other forms of bodywork mimic and assist the pumping action of the muscles and respiratory pump, influencing breathing and possibly the movement of CSF.

TRANSLATING EVIDENCE INTO PRACTICAL APPLICATION: CONNECTIVE TISSUE

SECTION OBJECTIVES

Chapter objective covered in this section:

7. The student will be able to explain the effects of therapeutic massage in physiologic terms.

Using the information presented in this section, the student will be able to perform the following:

• Explain the anatomic and physiologic influences of massage on connective tissue

Connective tissue, the structural component of the body, is the most abundant body tissue. Its functions include support, structure, space, stabilization, and scar formation. It assumes many forms and shapes, from fluid blood to dense bone. The pliability of connective tissue, which is based on its water-binding components, is significant in effective connective tissue support and function. Connective tissue is adaptive and responsive to a variety of influences, such as injury, immobilization, overuse (increased demand), and underuse (decreased demand).

Connective tissue is made up of various fibers and cells in a gelatinous ground substance. In bone this ground substance is impregnated with minerals that harden the bone. The combination of the fibers and the cells that produce the fibers and the ground substance is called the *connective tissue matrix* (Figure 5-10).

During ANS sympathetic arousal, the ground substance thickens to provide protection from impact trauma. Enzyme action reverses this process during parasympathetic dominance. Healing of damaged body tissues requires the formation of connective tissue. The inflammatory response is one process that generates the healing process. Sometimes more tissue than is needed forms, and adhesions develop. An adhesion is a binding of connective tissue to structures not directly involved with the area of injury. Fascia (discussed earlier) is a type of connective tissue that forms in sheets. It is embedded

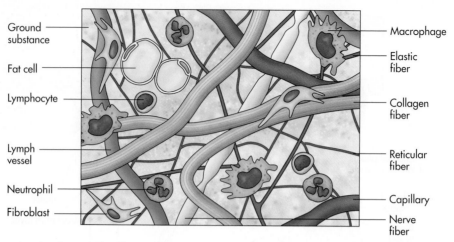

Ground substance

Fat cell

Lymphocyte

Lymph vessel

Neutrophil

Fibroblast

Macrophage

Elastic fiber

Collagen fiber

Reticular fiber

Capillary

Nerve fiber

FIGURE 5-10 The components of connective tissue.

with smooth muscle bundles that contribute to fascial tone (tautness).

In areas of acute (active) dysfunction, connective tissue initially may not play a role in the dysfunctional pattern. Connective tissue dysfunction usually is suspected as a factor in disorders that last longer than 12 weeks.

With overuse, additional connective tissue forms to provide stabilization to the musculoskeletal areas involved. When the soft tissue problem is chronic, the connective tissue becomes fibrotic and involves areas surrounding the dysfunctional area. After this has occurred, either the connective tissue thickens or thins, or it dries out or becomes waterlogged.

Ligaments and tendons may fail to support joint stabilization, or the connective tissue may bind, restricting movement and function.

Piezoelectricity is an electrical current produced by applying pressure to certain crystals (e.g., mica, quartz, or Rochelle salt). Collagen fibers of connective tissue have a piezoelectric property. The piezoelectric phenomenon in some way affects the connective tissue properties. With its piezoelectric properties, the collagen portion of connective tissue may be the link to energy-related forms of bodywork.

As discussed earlier, our understanding of the function of fascia in the body is increasing with information about smooth muscle type structures, innervations, mechanotransduction (the process by which cells convert mechanical stimulus into chemical activity), water movement, and tensegrity. Fascia plays an important role in the support and function of our bodies, because it surrounds and attaches to all structures. In the normal healthy state, the fascia is relaxed, wavy, and slippery, which gives it the ability to stretch and move without restriction. If fascia loses its pliability or is not slippery, it becomes tight, restricted, and a source of tension to the rest of the body. Fascial restrictions pull, twist, and create pressure, causing all kinds of symptoms that produce pain, headache, or restriction of motion. Fascial restrictions affect our flexibility and stability and are a determining factor in our ability to withstand stress and perform daily activities.

Connective Tissue Methods

Connective tissue massage was formalized in 1929 by Elizabeth Dicke, a German physiotherapist. Dr. James Cyriax contributed extensively to this methodology through his research on deep transverse friction massage. Fibrotic tissue responds well to the specific approaches of connective tissue massage (see Chapter 12). Studies indicate that massage may reduce the formation of adhesions and the scarring that often results from soft tissue injury. Similar approaches for the fascial or connective tissue component of muscles are called *myofascial techniques.* Connective tissue methods are primarily mechanical.

Connective tissue methods primarily affect the body structure. Methods that directly address the connective tissue do so by mechanically changing the consistency and pliability of the connective tissue, usually by softening it, and by creating physical space in the body. Mechanical dysfunctions call for more direct methods and depend on an actual physiologic change in the area. Cross-fiber frictioning (see Chapters 10 and 12) and inhibitory (direct) pressure approaches (see Chapter 10) are examples of mechanical massage methods. Mechanical force influences the smooth muscle bundles in fascia.

Effects of Massage on Connective Tissues

Massage methods most often affect the superficial and deep fascial sheaths, the ligaments, and the tendons. Three basic approaches are used:

- Methods that address the ground substance, which is *thixotropic* (i.e., the substance liquefies on agitation and reverts to gel when standing). Ground substance is also a *colloid.* A colloid is a system of solids in a liquid medium that resists abrupt pressure but yields to slow, sustained pressure.
- Methods that address the fibers within the ground substance; the fibers are collagenous (ropelike), elastic (rubber band–like), or reticular (meshlike).
- Methods that influence fascial tone through direct stimulus of muscle bundles in the fascia and indirectly through influence of the nervous system.

Methods that primarily affect the ground substance have a quality of slow, sustained pressure and agitation. The shearing, bending, and torsion forces and tensile stretch applied during massage add energy to the matrix and soften it. Most massage methods can soften the ground substance as long as the application is not abrupt. Abrupt tapotement and compression (see Chapter 10) are less effective than slow, gliding methods that have a drag quality. Kneading and skin rolling (see Chapter 10) that incorporate a slow pulling action also are effective. Parasympathetic activation helps create connective tissue pliability by causing smooth muscle contraction and a chemical response.

The fiber component is affected by methods that elongate the fibers past the elastic range (i.e., past the normal give) into the plastic range (i.e., past the bind or point of restriction). This creates either a freeing and unraveling of fibers or a small therapeutic (beneficial and controlled) inflammatory response that signals for change in the fibers. Transverse friction (see Chapter 12) also creates therapeutic inflammation.

Massage that provides for a gentle, sustained pull on the fascial component stimulates smooth muscle bundles and cutaneovisceral (skin to organ) reflexes, and together with autonomic reflex pathways and endocrine responses produces body-wide reactions to connective tissue massage. Connective tissue massage helps harmonize the relationship between the sympathetic and parasympathetic divisions of the ANS. It also helps normalize the circulation between organs and organ systems and other tissues. Locally, it improves the blood supply of the surface tissues in the area treated, especially in the particular connective tissue element. Connective tissue applications using massage methods are addressed specifically in Chapter 12.

TRANSLATING EVIDENCE INTO PRACTICAL APPLICATION: ENERGY SYSTEMS (BIOFIELDS)

SECTION OBJECTIVES

Chapter objective covered in this section:

7. The student will be able to explain the effects of therapeutic massage in physiologic terms.

Using the information presented in this section, the student will be able to perform the following:

- Explain the anatomic and physiologic influences of massage on energy systems (biofields)

Both styles of massage, mechanical and reflexive, influence the energy component of the body by stimulating electrochemical, electromagnetic, and piezoelectric fields. These electrical fields exist. Animal behavior studies have shown that the platypus detects a living food source by sensing the weak electrical field around its prey (Alcock, 2001).

Technology just recently has enabled researchers to measure this subtle component of the body. Consequently, the validity of the effectiveness of any method based on the reaction of the electrochemical, electromagnetic, or piezoelectric component of the body is controversial. The terms *subtle energy* or *biofield therapies* cover a wide range of techniques that affect the subtle electrical fields of the body.

The laws of physics dictate that when electrical currents flow through tissues, magnetic fields must be created in the surrounding region. Early in the twentieth century, it was discovered that the various organs in the body produce electrical fields that can be detected on the skin. Instruments to detect these fields, such as electrocardiography (ECG) and electroencephalography (EEG), were developed in the 1950s. Today, the superconducting quantum interference device (SQUID) magnetometer is used in medical research laboratories around the world to map the biomagnetic fields produced by various organs; this has led to new clinical tools, such as magnetocardiography and magnetoencephalography.

Sensitive photometers and thermographic imaging techniques have enabled scientists to map the patterns of light and heat emitted by cells, tissues, organs, and the whole body. Spectroscopic methods reveal the roles of energy fields in molecular processes, including hormone-receptor, antibody-antigen, and allergic interactions. Spectroscopy provides the basis for pharmacology, homeopathy, aromatherapy, and herbal medicines.

Cell biologists are recognizing that nuclear, cytoplasmic, and extracellular matrices form a continuous and interconnected communication system that plays a key role in the integration of functions, including injury repair and defense against disease. Tensegrity concepts explain the various forms of energy absorbed and conducted throughout the framework of the body, affecting all cells. Of all the discoveries discussed here, the most exciting for the massage profession is the discovery of the biomagnetic fields emitted by the hands of various types of therapists.

Amplification

Amplification is the building of stronger and more coherent biomagnetic fields. Magnetic brain waves associated with the sensory and motor cortex become stronger when an action is practiced again and again, such as occurs when a person rehearses with a musical instrument. Similar changes may occur with repeated practice of various "hands on" therapies.

Although more research is needed, the most logical explanation for amplification is that the waves of electrical and magnetic activity from the brain are amplified as they pass through the peripheral tissues. Crystalline components of the living matrix, such as the collagen arrays in tendons, ligaments, and bones and the arrays of lipids in cell membranes, probably act as coherent, resonant molecular broadcasting systems. Vibrating molecules throughout the body may become cooperatively entrained with the brain rhythms. As more and more molecules in the crystalline living matrix become vibrationally entrained, the fields become stronger.

Bodywork, including massage and other repetitive practices (e.g., yoga, Qigong, tai chi, meditation, and therapeutic touch), may gradually lead to more structural coherence (crystallinity) in the tissues, facilitating both the detection and radiation of energy fields (Oschman, 2000).

Connective Tissues and Body Energy

The role of the connective tissue as a body-wide signaling network has been recognized by ancient cultures. It also has been recently studied by authors such as Helenne Langevin, who made the connection between the connective tissue planes and the meridians (Langevin et al., 2004; Langevin, 2006). The major stimulus for bone and cartilage formation is a piezoelectric signal generated when the bone or cartilage is subjected to tension or compression. This knowledge is widely used today in orthopedics (Oschman, 2008; Smit, 2008). The concept of body energy, therefore, is not new and has been scientifically studied since the 1940s (Box 5-9) (Szent-Györgyi, 1941a,1941b).

The connective tissues form a mechanical three-dimensional network or matrix continuum, extending throughout the body, even into the innermost parts of each cell. All movement, of the body as a whole or of its smallest parts, is created by tensions carried through the connective tissue structure. The living matrix is the continuous molecular fabric of the organism, consisting of fascia, the other connective tissues, extracellular matrices, integrins, cytoskeletons, nuclear matrices, and DNA. The extracellular, cellular, and nuclear biopolymers or ground substances constitute a body-wide reservoir of charge that can maintain electrical homeostasis and "inflammatory preparedness" throughout the organism (Oschman, 2009).

Each force introduced to or generated by the body causes the crystalline lattice of the connective tissues to generate piezobioelectric signals that are precisely characteristic of those tensions, compressions, and movements. Stimulation of a piezomaterial causes either generation of electrical currents or a vibration. The connective tissue fabric is a semiconducting communication network that can carry bioelectronic signals between every part of the body.

Nervous System as an Energy System

The nervous system is an energy system in the body. Researchers study its operation by measuring electrical fields generated during the transmission of nerve impulses. Because electrical currents always give rise to magnetic fields, the nervous system also is a source of some of the biomagnetic fields in and around an organism. Moreover, the nervous system regulates all muscular movements and therefore is one of the keys to the conversion of thoughts into energetic actions.

Neurophysiologists, who focus most of their attention on the "classic" nervous system (composed of the neurons that conduct information from place to place as electrical impulses), maintain that all functions of the nervous system result from the activities of the neurons. Hence integration of brain function, memory, and even consciousness has been assumed to arise from the interconnectivity of the neurons. This is a partial view, because it neglects another energetic and informational system consisting of the perineural connective tissue system, which constitutes more than half of the cells in the brain (the prefix *peri-* means about, around, encircling, or enclosing). Perineural cells surround each neuron in the brain and follow each peripheral nerve to its termination.

Perineural System

Robert O. Becker was a pioneer in the exploration of the functions of the perineural system and its relationship with the semiconducting matrix that forms and surrounds it. To document the properties of this system, Becker refers to a "dual nervous system" consisting of the classic digital nerve network, which controls movement and body function, and the perineural analog network, which regulates wound healing and tissue repair. Dr. Becker also was a pioneer in the field of regeneration and its relationship to electrical currents in living things. He found clues to the healing process in the long-discarded theory of the eighteenth-century vitalists, that electricity is vital to the life process. Becker, an orthopedic surgeon, explored the relationship between human physiology and electricity. For 30 years he investigated the healing of bone, organs, and nerve tissue. He proved that electrical stimulation

---

| Box 5-9 | Body Energy Is Not a New Idea |

What is life? This is the main problem of biology. Many have asked this question, but nobody has answered it. Science is based on the experience that nature answers intelligent questions intelligently, so if she is silent, there may be something wrong about the question.

Think boldly, don't be afraid of making mistakes, don't miss small details, keep your eyes open, and be modest in everything except your aims.

—Albert Szent-Györgyi

Albert Imre Szent-Györgyi (1893-1986), a Hungarian-born biochemist, was the first to isolate vitamin C, and his research on biologic oxidation provided the basis for an understanding of the Krebs citric acid cycle. His discoveries about the biochemical nature of muscular contraction revolutionized the field of muscle research. His later career was devoted to research in "submolecular" biology, applying quantum physics to biologic processes. He was especially interested in cancer and was one of the first to explore the connections between free radicals and cancer. Szent-Györgyi won the Nobel Prize in 1937 for Physiology or Medicine for his work in biologic oxidation and vitamin C, and the Lasker Award in Basic Medical Research in 1954 for contributions to an understanding of cardiovascular disease through basic muscle research.

Albert Szent-Györgyi proposed that electrons can propagate through crystalline structures both within and between molecules, forming semiconducting currents entirely separate from the movement of ions, previously assumed to be the only possible basis for bioelectricity. Said Szent-Györgyi in 1941, "The study of crystals and metals, however, has revealed the existence of a different state of matter. If a great number of atoms is arranged with regularity in close proximity, as for instance, in a crystal lattice, the terms of the single valency electrons may fuse into common bands. The electrons in this band cease to belong to one or two atoms only, and belong to the whole system."

From U.S. National Library of Medicine, 8600 Rockville Pike, Bethesda, Md 20894, National Institutes of Health, Department of Health & Human Services. http://profiles.nlm.nih.gov/WG/ Profiles in Science National Library of Medicine's Profiles in Science® accessed August 9, 2011.

with direct current can promote healing in bone and other tissue. He went on to prove that some body parts can even be encouraged to regenerate.

Anticipatory Fields

Pulses of electrical and magnetic energy, called *anticipatory fields,* begin in the brain before any movement occurs. Anticipatory fields are an important phenomenon, and they are being investigated for their application in training for athletic events, dance, theater, music, and so on. A benefit is derived from mental rehearsals or internal imaging without the individual physically doing anything. Many athletes, performers, and therapists of various kinds have described the profound experience of being totally prepared, present, and focused. In such a state, sometimes referred to as being "in the zone," extraordinary accomplishments take place. Many therapeutic schools emphasize the importance of this phenomenon but call it *intention;* that is, the practitioner decides in advance the goals he or she wants to attain for a particular client. This approach is based on the frequent experience that a vivid image of expectations facilitates change in that direction. Intention also seems to be all the more effective when the client participates, as in directed movement therapies or image-based cancer treatments.

The effectiveness of various kinds of hands-on bodywork may derive from the entrainment of electrical and magnetic rhythms from therapist to client, and the anticipatory fields may be an important component of this entrainment.

Healing Energies

On the basis of the information presented thus far, we can begin to form a picture of the energy systems in the living body. Current knowledge about the roles of electrical, magnetic, elastic, acoustic, thermal, gravitational, and photonic energies in living systems shows that, most likely, no single "life force" or "healing energy" exists. Rather, the living body seems to have many energy systems, and there seem to be many ways of influencing those systems. The concepts of "living state" and "health" encompass all of these systems, both known and unknown, functioning collectively and synergistically. The debate over whether such a thing as a healing energy or a life force exists is being replaced by study of the ways biologic energy fields, structures, and functions interact.

The scientific discoveries in energy systems is complemented by a long history of experiential evidence and clinical techniques developed by therapists of various modalities. The growing popularity of bodywork and energy and movement therapies is leading us to a synthesis of ideas that will benefit all.

The research summarized thus far points to a remarkable model that may explain the unusual emissions of Qi, or "healing energy," and other phenomena observed in a wide variety of energy therapies. These practices seem to have in common periodic entrainments of brain waves, whole body biomagnetic emissions, and resonances in the earth's atmosphere. The result may be whole body collective oscillation entrained with geophysical fields. Brain electrical activity (measured by EEG) and the biomagnetic emissions from the body (measured with magnetometers) seem to be linked to the healing response.

Scientific consensus has gone from a certainty that weak environmental energies can have no influence on living systems to agreement that such influences are extremely important and deserving of intense study to determine the precise mechanisms involved. Collectively, the discoveries of modern researchers tell a story of biologic sensitivity that coincides with the daily experiences of energy therapists ranging from medical doctors using imaging techniques to massage therapists, acupuncturists, polarity therapists, Reiki practitioners, herbalists, aroma therapists, and so on.

Evidence for Energy Methods

Healing energy studies overall are of medium quality and generally meet minimum standards for validity of inferences. Biofield therapies show strong evidence for reducing pain intensity in pain populations and moderate evidence for reducing pain intensity in hospitalized and cancer populations. Moderate evidence exists for reduction of negative behavioral symptoms in dementia and for decreasing anxiety for hospitalized patients. Evidence supports the effects of biofield therapies in improving fatigue and quality of life in cancer patients, for improving comprehensive pain outcomes and effects in pain patients, and for reducing anxiety in cardiovascular patients. As always, further high-quality studies are needed in this area (Engebretson and Wardell, 2007; So et al., 2007; Fazzino et al., 2010; Jain and Mills, 2010).

Having an open mind to the potential of energy-based healing methods does not require us to abandon our sophisticated understandings of physiology, biochemistry, or molecular biology. The definition of living matter is being expanded, not replaced. Nerve impulses and chemical messengers are contained within the individual, whereas energy fields radiate indefinitely into space and therefore affect others who are nearby. For millennia, energy therapists have had a practical appreciation of these phenomena, which are finally open to scientific research.

In her book, *Molecules of Emotion: Why You Feel the Way You Feel,* Dr. Candace Pert speculated on how energy healers may use their own energy fields to trigger receptors in the bodies of their patients. Receptors on the cell surface are the primary sites of action of low-frequency electromagnetic fields. It is at the receptor that cellular responses are triggered by hormones, growth factors, neurotransmitters, taste and smell molecules, pheromones, light, and a variety of other electromagnetic signals. Dr. Pert called for basic research into this promising area. Her careful research on neuropeptides can be integrated with the emerging understanding of electromagnetics in the living body to give us a much clearer picture both of the human body in health and disease and of the biophysics of emotions.

Certainly for a culture that has become accustomed to having large numbers of tasks handled by invisible currents flowing through chips in computers and its television sets adjusted by invisible beams from remote control devices, it is not unreasonable to look at the ways our bodies are regulated and coordinated by invisible energies. The principles of physics discussed here offer potential for understanding how conscious healing intention works and the ways the power of subtle energies might be harnessed for health enhancement.

The lack of sufficient Western scientific validation of the ancient energy flows of Chi, prana, meridians, chakras, auras, or whatever else they may be called causes us to represent this area of bodywork to the public carefully. Until our technology can prove the validity of energy techniques, remember the wisdom of Hippocrates, "Do no harm," and also Bernie Siegal's belief, "There is no false hope." It is important to represent subtle techniques simply, professionally, and without false expectations and mysticism. Additional training is required to learn to use the subtle energy approaches purposefully. It also is important not to discount the stimulation of the powerful placebo effect. If touch can activate it, why not use it? It will be exciting to watch science "discover" the validity of more and more of the ancient energy concepts.

Effect of Massage on Body Energy

As previously discussed, sufficient research exists to demonstrate that methods using "energy" have an effect through ANS activity and endocrine responses in regard to entrainment, motor nerve points, and the piezoelectric properties of connective tissue fibers. Acupuncture points and meridians can be correlated directly with the nerve tracts and motor nerve points; chakras are located over nerve plexuses and biologic oscillators.

Therapeutic massage stimulates the nervous system and applies pressure to the connective tissues to produce a measurable electrical current by means of the piezoelectric properties of the connective tissue and the deformation of tensegrity structures. The generalized therapeutic approach of massage seems to have a normalizing effect on the body's energetic processes.

SUMMARY

Therapeutic massage methods are simple and appear to be effective in producing responses mediated through the nervous system, the interaction with the endocrine system, the connective tissue, and the circulatory system. Massage is beneficial for anxiety, depression, and chronic pain as part of an overall treatment protocol. Most forms of musculoskeletal pain and discomfort respond to massage at least temporarily. General daily stress responds well to massage. Armed with an understanding of the physiologic effects of massage, massage professionals hopefully will be able to collaborate with medical, scientific, and trained personnel in the use of these very old and effective methods. When provided by trained professionals, therapeutic massage can be beneficial in conservative treatment plans for chronic pain and stress-induced disease before more invasive measures are attempted.

Therapeutic massage can play an important role in prevention programs by providing a natural mechanism for stimulating the body to adjust to the stress of daily life and to restore the natural homeostatic balance. Additional information can be obtained by locating and studying the references in this

☐ FOOT IN THE DOOR

The trend in massage therapy toward evidence-informed and evidence-based professional practice means that massage students must become *research literate*; that is, they must be able to translate research findings into practical applications. To remain current you must read research reports regularly. Even after your massage therapy career is well under way, you must review your information base often to make sure it is up-to-date on current trends and that you understand the new and emerging evidence of massage therapy benefits and practice. Research is continually revealing new evidence of ways massage benefits the body. If you do not stay current, you could find yourself providing inaccurate information during an interview, a discussion with a client, or when documenting in clients' records. Providing inaccurate information will keep your foot out of the door for sure. Maintain your creditability by remaining accurate and informed.

chapter. Application of the techniques that bring about the physiologic effects is discussed in more detail in Chapters 10, 11, and 12.

Most clients say they get a massage because it feels good and helps them feel better. Researching "good" and "better" scientifically is difficult. Massage professionals can provide the services of this art, confident that the reasons massage works and feels good are grounded in sound scientific research. Intuition and intent are necessary aspects of the professional application of massage. Clients care about how much you know, but they care more about how much you care and about how good they feel after a massage.

The massage profession needs more research. Therefore, the massage profession needs to cooperate with researchers and appreciate the work involved in doing research. The scientific community and the public need quality research studies to strengthen their belief in massage so that they can justify receiving or recommending it. The massage profession needs the public and the scientific community to support massage. Whatever the massage or bodywork system used, the beneficial effects of therapeutic massage are elicited from the client's physiology as it adjusts to the external sensory information supplied by massage and responds to the compressive forces of massage and the nurturing, confident, compassionate, mindful, and centered presence of the massage therapist.

℮volve

http://evolve.elsevier.com/Fritz/fundamentals/
5-1 Learn about valid research methods with a fill-in-the-blank activity.
5-2 Review the scientific method.
5-3 Identify the parts of a research paper.
5-4 Study up on the physics of massage.
5-5 Label sympathetic and parasympathetic responses.
5-6 Based on photographs, identify which type of reflex is occurring in each photo.
Don't forget to study for your certification and licensure exams! Review questions, along with weblinks, can be found on the Evolve website.

References

Alcock J: *Animal behavior: an evaluatory approach*, ed 7, Sunderland, Mass, 2001, Sinauer.

Anderson K, Anderson LE, Glanze WD, editors: *Mosby's medical, nursing, and allied health dictionary*, ed 6, St Louis, 2005, Mosby.

Arroyo-Morales M, et al: Psychophysiological effects of massage—myofascial release after exercise: a randomized sham-control study, *J Altern Complement Med* 14:1223, 2008.

Asplund R: Manual lymph drainage therapy using light massage for fibromyalgia sufferers: a pilot study, *Phys Ther* 7:192, 2003.

Bakermans-Kranenburg MJ, van Jzendoorn MH: Oxytocin receptor (OXTR) and serotonin transporter (5-HTT) genes associated with observed parenting, *Am Pain Soc* 9:714, 2008.

Bakowski P, Musielak B, Sip P, Bieganski G: Effects of massage on delayed-onset muscle soreness, *Chir Narzadow Ruchu Ortop Pol* 73:261, 2008.

Baldry PE: *Acupuncture, trigger points and musculoskeletal pain*, ed 3, New York, 2005, Churchill Livingstone.

Ballantyne B, Fryer G, McLaughlin P: The effect of muscle energy technique on hamstring extensibility: the mechanism of altered flexibility, *J Osteopath Med* 6:59, 2003.

Billhult A, Bergbom I, Stener-Victorin E: Massage relieves nausea in women with breast cancer who are undergoing chemotherapy, *J Altern Complement Med* 13:53, 2007. Online at www.liebertonline.com/doi/abs/10.1089/acm.2006.6049.

Bosch AN: Exercise science and coaching: correcting common misunderstandings about endurance exercise, *Int J Sports Sci Coach* 1:77–87, March 2006.

Cai Y, et al: Cytoskeletal coherence requires myosin-IIA contractility, *J Cell Sci* 123(3):413–423, 2010.

Cassileth BR, Vickers AJ: Massage therapy for symptom control: outcome study at a major cancer center, *J Pain Symptom Manage* 28:244, 2004.

Castro-Sánchez AM, et al: Connective tissue reflex massage for type 2 diabetic patients with peripheral arterial disease: randomized controlled trial, *Evid Based Complement Alternat Med* Nov 23, 2009.

Castro-Sánchez AM, et al: Efficacy of a massage and exercise programme on the ankle-brachial index and blood pressure in patients with diabetes mellitus type 2 and peripheral arterial disease: a randomized clinical trial, *Med Clin (Barc)* 134(3):107–110, 2010.

Chaitow LND: *Muscle energy techniques*, ed 3, Edinburgh, 2006, Churchill Livingstone.

Chen CS, Ingber DE: Tensegrity and mechanoregulation: from skeleton to cytoskeleton, *Osteoarthr Cartil* 7:81, 1999.

Cherkin DC: A comparison of the effects of two types of massage and usual care on chronic low back pain: a randomized, controlled trial, *Ann Intern Med* 155:1–9, 2011.

Currin J, Meister EA: A hospital-based intervention using massage to reduce distress among oncology patients, *Cancer Nurs* 31:214, 2008. Online at www.ncbi.nlm.nih.gov/pubmed/18453878.

Day JA, Stecco C, Stecco A: Application of fascial manipulation technique in chronic shoulder pain: anatomical basis and clinical implications, *J Bodyw Mov Ther* 13:128, 2009.

DeGroot J, Chusid JG: *Correlative neuroanatomy*, ed 25, San Mateo, Calif, 2002, McGraw-Hill.

Deniset-Besseau A, et al: Measurement of the second-order hyperpolarizability of the collagen triple helix and determination of its physical origin, *J Phys Chem* 113:13437–13445, 2009.

Diego MA, Field T: Moderate pressure massage elicits a parasympathetic nervous system response, *Int J Neurosci* 119:630, 2009. Online at www.ncbi.nlm.nih.gov/pubmed/19283590.

Diego MA, Field T, Sanders C, Hernandez-Reif M: Massage therapy of moderate and light pressure and vibrator effects on EEG and heart rate, *Int J Neurosci* 114:31, 2004. Online at www.ncbi.nlm.nih.gov/pubmed/14660065.

Dorsher PT: Myofascial referred-pain data provide physiologic evidence of acupuncture meridians, *J Pain* 10(7):723–731, 2009.

Dorsher PT: Can classical acupuncture points and trigger points be compared in the treatment of pain disorders? Birch's analysis revisited, *J Altern Complement Med* 14(4):353–359, 2008.

Engebretson J, Wardell DW: Energy-based modalities, *Nurs Clin North Am* 42:243, 2007.

Engler AJ, et al: Matrix elasticity directs stem cell lineage specification, *Cell* 126:677–689, 2006. (doi:10.1016/j.cell.2006.06.044)

Ernst E, Pittler M, Wider B: *The desktop guide to complementary and alternative medicine: an evidence-based approach*, ed 2, St Louis, 2006, Mosby.

Fazzino DL, Griffin MT, McNulty RS, Fitzpatrick JJ: Energy healing and pain: a review of the literature, *Holist Nurs Pract* 24:79, 2010.

Fellowes D, Barnes K, Wilkinson S: Aromatherapy and massage for symptom relief in patients with cancer, *Cochrane Database Syst Rev* 4:CD002287, 2004. Online at www.ncbi.nlm.nih.gov/pubmed/15106172.

Field T: *Touch therapy*, Edinburgh, 2000, Churchill Livingstone.

Field T et al: Cortisol decreases and serotonin and dopamine increase following massage therapy, *Int J Neurosci* 115:1397, 2005. Online at www.ncbi.nlm.nih.gov/pubmed/16162447.

Fischer MJ, Riedlinger K, Gutenbrunner C, Bernateck M: Influence of the temporomandibular joint on range of motion of the hip joint in patients with complex regional pain syndrome, *J Manip Physiol Ther* 32:364, 2009.

Frey Law LA, et al: Massage reduces pain perception and hyperalgesia in experimental muscle pain: a randomized, controlled trial, *J Pain* 9:714, 2008.

Furlan AD, Imamura M, Dryden T, Irvin E: Massage for low back pain, *Cochrane Database Syst Rev* 4:CD001929, 2008.

Gallese V, et al: Being like me: Self-other identity, mirror neurons and empathy. In *Perspectives on imitation: From Cognitive Neuroscience to Social Science*, Cambridge, 2005, MIT Press.

Gallese V: Before and below "theory of mind": embodied simulation and the neural correlates of social cognition, *Philos Trans R Soc Lond B Biol Sci* 362:659–669, 2007.

Giampietro L, et al: Systematic review of efficacy for manual lymphatic drainage techniques, *J Man Manip Ther* 17(3):80–89, 2009. Online at www.ncbi.nlm.nih.gov/pmc/articles/PMC2755111.

Ginorio A (principal investigator): Rural girls in science: meeting the challenge through a comprehensive approach, a program funded by National Science Foundation Project HRD-94500053. http://depts.washington.edu/rural/RURAL/design/scimethod.html (accessed August 16, 2011).

Greenman PE: *Principles of manual medicine*, ed 3, Philadelphia, 2003, Lippincott Williams & Wilkins.

Gunn CC: *Reprints on pain, acupuncture and related subjects*, Seattle, 1992, University of Washington.

Hanley J, Stirling P, Brown C: Randomised controlled trial of therapeutic massage in the management of stress, *Br J Gen Pract* 53:20, 2003. Online at www.ncbi.nlm.nih.gov/pubmed/12564272.

Haskal ZJ: Massage-induced delayed venous stent migration, *J Vasc Interv Radiol* 19:945, 2008. Online at www.ncbi.nlm.nih.gov/pubmed/18503913.

Henoch I, et al: Soft skin massage for children with severe developmental disabilities: caregivers' experiences, *Scand J Disability Res* 12(4):221–232, 2010.

Ho CY, Sole G, Munn J: The effectiveness of manual therapy in the management of musculoskeletal disorders of the shoulder: a systematic review, *Man Ther* 14:463, 2009.

Hodge LM, King HH, Williams AG et al: Abdominal lymphatic pump treatment increases leukocyte count flux in thoracic duct lymph, *Lymph Res Biol* 5:127, 2007.

Hohmann AG et al: An endocannabinoid mechanism for stress-induced analgesia, *Nature* 435:1108, 2005.

Holt-Lunstad J, Birmingham WA, Light KC: Influence of a "warm touch" support enhancement intervention among married couples on ambulatory blood pressure, oxytocin, alpha amylase, and cortisol, *Psychosom Med* 70:976, 2008. Online at www.ncbi.nlm.nih.gov/pubmed/18842740.

Itoh K, et al: Randomised trial of trigger point acupuncture compared with other acupuncture for treatment of chronic neck pain, *Complement Ther Med* 15(3):172–179, 2007.

Jain S, Mills PJ: Biofield therapies: helpful or full of hype? A best evidence synthesis, *Int J Behav Med* 17:1, 2010.

Kanazawa Y, et al: Cyclical cell stretching of skin-derived fibroblasts downregulates connective tissue growth factor (CTGF), *Connect Tissue Res* 50:323, 2009.

Kassolik K, et al: Tensegrity principle in massage demonstrated by electro- and mechanomyography, *J Bodyw Mov Ther* 13:164, 2009.

Kawakita K, et al: How do acupuncture and moxibustion act? Focusing on the progress in Japanese acupuncture research, *J Pharmacol Sci* 100(5):443–459, 2006.

Klingler W, Schleip R, Zorn A: *European Fascia Research Project report*, Fifth World Congress on Low Back and Pelvic Pain, Melbourne, November, 2004.

Knott EM, Tune JD, Stoll ST, Downey HF: Increased lymphatic flow in the thoracic duct during manipulative intervention, *J Am Osteopath Assoc* 105:447, 2005.

Lancaster DG, Crow WT: Osteopathic manipulative treatment of a 26-year-old woman with Bell's palsy, *J Am Osteopath Assoc* 106:285, 2006.

Langevin HM: Connective tissue: a bodywide signaling network? *Med Hypotheses* 66:1074, 2006.

Langevin HM, Bouffard N, Badger G et al: Dynamic fibroblast cytoskeletal response to subcutaneous tissue stretch ex vivo and in vivo, *Am J Physiol Cell Physiol* 288:C747, 2005.

Langevin HM, Churchill D, Cipolla M: Mechanical signaling through connective tissue: a mechanism for the therapeutic effect of acupuncture, *FASEB J* 15:2275, 2001.

Langevin HM, Cornbrooks CJ, Taatjes DJ: Fibroblasts form a bodywide cellular network, *Histochem Cell Biol* 122:7, 2004.

Langevin HM, Sherman KJ: Pathophysiological model for chronic low back pain integrating connective tissue and nervous system mechanisms, *Med Hypotheses* 68:74, 2007.

Langevin HM, Yandow JA: Relationship of acupuncture points and meridians to connective tissue planes, *Anat Rec* 269:257, 2002.

Lund I, et al: Repeated massage-like stimulation induces long-term effects on nociception: contribution of oxytocinergic mechanisms, *Eur J Neurosci* 16:330, 2002.

Mammoto T, Ingber DE: Mechanical control of tissue and organ development, *Development* 137(9):1407–1420, 2010. http://www.ncbi.nlm.nih.gov/pubmed/20388652

McKeon PO, Medina JM, Hertel J: Hierarchy of evidence-based clinical research in sports medicine, *Athl Ther Today* 11:42, 2006.

McPartland JM, et al: Cannabimimetic effects of osteopathic manipulative treatment, *J Am Osteopath Assoc* 105:283, 2005.

McPartland JM: The endocannabinoid system: an osteopathic perspective, *J Am Osteopath Assoc* 108(10):586–600, 2008. http://www.jaoa.org/cgi/content/full/108/10/586.

Medina JM, McKeon PO, Hertel J: Rating the levels of evidence in sports medicine research, *Athl Ther Today* 11:38, 2006.

Mirskya HP, Liub AC, Welshb DK et al: A model of the cell-autonomous mammalian circadian clock. *Proc Natl Acad Sci USA* 106:11107, 2009. Online at www.pnas.org/content/106/27/11107.full.

Moyer CA et al: Does massage therapy reduce cortisol? A comprehensive quantitative review, *J Bodywork Mov Ther* 15(1):3–14, 2011.

Moyer CA, Rounds J, Hannum JW: Meta-analysis of massage therapy research, *Psychol Bull* 1:30, 2004.

Müller-Oerlinghausen B, Berg C, Droll W: The efficacy of slow stroke massage in depression, *Psychiatr Prax* 34(Suppl 3):S305, 2007. Online at www.ncbi.nlm.nih.gov/pubmed/17786889.

Olszewski WL, et al: Where do lymph and tissue fluid accumulate in lymphedema of the lower limbs caused by obliteration of lymphatic collectors? *Lymphology* 42:105, 2009.

Oschman JL: What is healing energy? III. Silent pulses, *J Bodyw Mov Ther* 1:179, 1997.

Oschman JL: *Energy medicine: the scientific basic*, Edinburgh, 2000, Churchill Livingstone.

Oschman JL: Clinical aspects of biological fields: an introduction for health care professionals, *J Bodyw Mov Ther* 6:117, 2002.

Oschman JL: Perspective: assume a spherical cow—the role of free or mobile electrons in bodywork, energetic and movement therapies, *J Bodyw Mov Ther* 12:40, 2008.

Oschman JL: Charge transfer in the living matrix, *J Bodyw Mov Ther* 13:215, 2009.

Patterson MM: Mechanisms of change: animal models in osteopathic research, *J Am Osteopath Assoc* 107:593, 2007.

Pedrelli A, Stecco C, Day JA: Treating patellar tendinopathy with fascial manipulation, *J Bodyw Mov Ther* 13:73, 2009.

Pert CB: *Molecules of emotion: why you feel the way you feel*, New York, 1997, Scribner.

Pollack GH, Cameron IL, Wheatley DN, editors: *Water and the cell*, The Netherlands, 2006, Springer.

Rahn EJ, Hohmann AG: *Cannabinoids as pharmacotherapies for neuropathic pain: from the bench to the bedside*, University of Georgia, Athens, Georgia, 2009, Neuroscience and Behavior Program, Department of Psychology. http://www.ncbi.nlm.nih.gov/pmc/articles/PMC2755639/.

Roenneberg T, et al: Demasking biological oscillators: properties and principles of entrainment exemplified by the *Neurospora* circadian clock, *Proc Natl Acad Sci USA* 102:7742, 2005.

Sackett DL, et al: *Evidence-based medicine: how to practice and teach EBM*, ed 2, New York, 2000, Churchill-Livingstone.

Schleip R: Fascial plasticity: a new neurobiological explanation, *J Bodyw Mov Ther* 7(1):11, 7(2):104, 2003.

Schleip R, Klingler W, Lehmann-Horn F: Active fascial contractility: fascia may be able to actively contract in a smooth muscle-like manner and thereby influence musculoskeletal dynamics, *Med Hypotheses* 65:273–277, 2005.

Schleip R, Klingler W, Lehmann-Horn F: Active contraction of the thoracolumbar fascia—Indications of anew factor in low back pain research with implications for manual therapy. In Vleeming A, Mooney V, Hodges P, editors: *The proceedings of the Fifth Interdisciplinary World Congress on Low Back and Pelvic Pain*, Melbourne, 2004.

Schleip R, Zorn A, Else MJ, Klinger W: *The European fascia research project report*. (2006). www.somatics.de/FasciaResearch/ReportIASIyearbook06.htm. Accessed September 16, 2009.

Schillinger A, et al: Effect of manual lymph drainage on the course of serum levels of muscle enzymes after treadmill exercise, *Am J Phys Med Rehabil* 85:516, 2006.

Sherman KJ, et al: Randomized trial of therapeutic massage for chronic neck pain, *Clin J Pain* 25:233, 2009.

Smit AA: *Movement and the matrix: the importance of biomechanical signals in matrix remodeling*, Baden-Baden, Germany, 2008, Verlegt durch: International Academy for Homotoxicology Gmbh.

So PS, Jiang Y, Qin Y: Energy-based modalities, *Nurs Clin North Am* 42:243, 2007.

Sommer AP, Zhu D: From microtornadoes to facial rejuvenation: implication of interfascial water layers, *Cryst Growth Des* 8:3889, 2008.

St John P: *Workshop notes: seminar I, St John Neuromuscular Therapy Seminars*, Largo, Fla, 1990, self-published.

Stecco C, et al: Histological characteristics of the deep fascia of the upper limb, *Ital J Anat Embryol* 111:105, 2006.

Stecco C, et al: Anatomy of the deep fascia of the upper limb. II. Study of innervation, *Morphologie* 91:38, 2007a.

Stecco C, et al: Tendinous muscular insertions onto the deep fascia of the upper limb. I. Anatomical study, *Morphologie* 91:29, 2007b.

Stecco L: *Fascial manipulation for musculoskeletal pain*, Padova, Italy, 2004, Piccin.

Stecco L, Stecco C: *Fascial manipulation: practical part*, Padova, Italy, 2009, Piccin.

Szent-Györgyi A: The study of energy-levels in biochemistry, *Nature* 148:157, 1941a.

Szent-Györgyi A: Towards a new biochemistry? *Science* 93:609, 1941b.

Szirmai I: How does the brain create rhythms? *Ideggyogy Sz* 63(1–2):13–23, 2010.

Thomas CL: *Taber's cyclopedic medical dictionary*, ed 20, Philadelphia, 2006, FA Davis.

Toro-Velasco C, et al: Short-term effects of manual therapy on heart rate variability, mood state, and pressure/pain sensitivity in patients with chronic tension–type headache: a pilot study, *J Manip Physiol Ther* 32(7):528–535, 2009.

Torres Lacomba M, et al: Effectiveness of early physiotherapy to prevent lymphoedema after surgery for breast cancer: randomised, single blinded, clinical trial, *Br Med J* 340:b5396, 2010. Online at www.ncbi.nlm.nih.gov/pubmed/20068255?dopt= Abstract.

Travell JG, Simons DG: *Myofascial pain and dysfunction: the trigger point manual, vol 2, The lower extremities*, Philadelphia, 1992, Lippincott Williams & Wilkins.

Tsao JCI: Effectiveness of massage therapy for chronic, nonmalignant pain: a review, *Evid Based Complement Alternat Med* 4:165, 2007.

Wall P, Melzack R: *Textbook of pain*, ed 2, Edinburgh, 1990, Churchill Livingstone.

Walton A: Efficacy of myofascial release techniques in the treatment of primary Raynaud's phenomenon, *J Bodyw Mov Ther* 12:274, 2008.

Wang SM, Kulkarni L, Dolev J, Kain ZN: Music and preoperative anxiety: a randomized, controlled study, *Anesth Analg* 94:1489, 2002. Online at www.medscape.com/medline/abstract/12032013.

Wiltshire EV, et al: Massage impairs postexercise muscle blood flow and "lactic acid" removal, *Med Sci Sports Exer* 42:1062, 2010.

Yakita K, et al: Molecular mechanisms of the biological clock in cultured fibroblasts, *Science* 292:278, 2001.

Yates J: *Physiological effects of therapeutic massage and their application to treatment*, Vancouver, BC, 1990, Massage Therapists Association of British Columbia.

Zainuddin Z, Newton M, Sacco P, Nosaka K: Effects of massage on delayed-onset muscle soreness, swelling, and recovery of muscle function, *J Athl Train* 40:174, 2005.

Zhen Ci Yan Jiu: Advances in the study on the role of connective tissue in the mechanical signal transduction of acupuncture 34(2):136–139, 2009 (article in Chinese). www.ncbi.nih.gov.pubmed/1968573

Workbook Section

Short Answer

1. What are the sources of evidence to support evidence-based massage practice?

2. What is a case report?

3. Define research literacy.

4. What are the five basic physiologic effects of massage?

5. In what way do chronic problems affect the connective tissue?

6. What are the five types of circulation?

7. What three words describe the sympathetic ANS functions?

8. What words describe the parasympathetic functions?

9. What is the importance of state-dependent memory to the massage therapist?

10. What is hyperstimulation analgesia?

11. How does massage promote the body's ability to maintain self-regulation and structural and functional balance?

12. Why is it easy to validate massage?

13. Why are research and its replication to verify the positive biochemical and behavioral responses to touch important?

14. Is it possible to separate the somatic, emotional, and cognitive elements in the response to massage? Is it possible to separate the mechanical, neural, chemical, and psychological effects?

15. How does the gate control theory explain hyperstimulation analgesia and counterirritation?

16. What role does massage play in relieving nerve impingement?

17. Why are reflexes important to the understanding of the reasons massage works?

18. How does massage interact with the powerful body/mind phenomenon?

19. How does massage stimulate the release of neurotransmitters, endorphins, and enkephalins?

20. What seem to be the effects of massage on myofascial trigger points?

21. In what ways does massage encourage circulation?

22. What are the possible physiologic mechanisms that support energy methods?

Matching I

Match the term with the best definition.

_____ **1.** Autoregulation
_____ **2.** Body/mind
_____ **3.** Centering
_____ **4.** Cognitive
_____ **5.** Counterirritation
_____ **6.** Endogenous
_____ **7.** Endorphins
_____ **8.** Feedback
_____ **9.** Gate control theory
_____ **10.** Toughening (hardening)
_____ **11.** Hyperstimulation analgesia
_____ **12.** Intuition
_____ **13.** Law
_____ **14.** Nerve impingement
_____ **15.** Noxious stimulation
_____ **16.** Placebo
_____ **17.** Reflex
_____ **18.** Science
_____ **19.** Somatic
_____ **20.** Subtle energies
_____ **21.** Randomized controlled trial
_____ **22.** Cohort studies
_____ **23.** Evidence-based practices
_____ **24.** Level C evidence
_____ **25.** Systematic reviews

a. The ability to focus on a specific circumstance by screening sensation
b. Superficial stimulation that relieves deeper sensation by stimulating different sensory signals
c. Weak electrical fields that are said to surround and run through the body
d. An involuntary response to a stimulus; the response is specific, predictable, adaptive, and purposeful
e. The interaction between thought and physiology connected to the limbic system, the hypothalamic influence of the ANS, and the endocrine system
f. A controlled pain sensation; "good pain"
g. A scientific statement found to be true for a whole class of natural occurrences
h. A method of teaching the body to deal with stress
i. A method of autoregulation to maintain internal homeostasis that interlinks body functions
j. Made in the body
k. One of the endogenous opioid peptides that have morphine-like analgesic properties, behavioral effects, and neurotransmitter and neuromodulator functions
l. Reduction of perception of a sensation by stimulation of large-diameter nerve fibers
m. Awareness with perception, reasoning, judgment, intuition, and memory

n. Knowing something by using subconscious information
o. The hypothesis that painful stimuli can be prevented from reaching higher levels of the CNS by stimulating larger sensory nerves
p. Pressure against a nerve by skin, fascia, muscles, ligaments, and joints
q. A treatment for an illness that influences the course of the disease even if it is not specifically validated
r. Pertaining to the body
s. The intellectual process of understanding through observation, measurement, accumulation of data, and analysis of the findings
t. Control of homeostasis by alteration of tissue or function
u. A process that combines multiple research studies that are similar in design into meaningful research useful to practitioners
v. A process in which researchers select and follow a large population of people who have the same condition
w. Expert opinion
x. Interventions for which consistent scientific and clinical support exists showing that they improve client outcomes
y. A type of research design in which each subject has an equal chance of being assigned to an intervention group or a control group

Matching II

Match the scientific laws affecting massage with their descriptions.

_____ **a.** Hilton's law
_____ **b.** Law of unilaterality
_____ **c.** Law of facilitation
_____ **d.** Hooke's law
_____ **e.** Law of generalization
_____ **f.** Arndt-Schulz law
_____ **g.** Bowditch's (all or none) law
_____ **h.** Bell's law
_____ **i.** Law of specificity of nervous energy
_____ **j.** Weber's law
_____ **k.** Law of symmetry
_____ **l.** Law of intensity
_____ **m.** Law of radiation
_____ **n.** Cannon's law of denervation

1. The weakest stimulus capable of producing a response produces the maximum response contraction in cardiac and skeletal muscle and nerves.
2. Anterior spinal nerve roots are motor roots, and posterior spinal nerve roots are sensory roots.
3. When an impulse has passed once through a certain set of neurons to the exclusion of others, it tends to take the same course on a future occasion, and each time it traverses this path, the resistance is smaller.
4. The stress used to stretch or compress a body is proportional to the strain experienced, as long as the elastic limits of the body have not been exceeded.

5. Excitation of a receptor always gives rise to the same sensation, regardless of the nature of the stimulus.
6. The increase in stimulus necessary to produce the smallest perceptible increase in sensation bears a constant ratio to the strength of the stimulus already acting.
7. A nerve trunk that supplies a joint also supplies the muscles of the joint and the skin over the insertions of such muscles.
8. If a mild irritation is applied to one or more sensory nerves, movement usually occurs only on one side, the side that is irritated.
9. If stimulation is increased sufficiently, a motor reaction is manifested not only on the side of irritation, but also in similar muscles on the opposite side of the body.
10. Reflex movements usually are more intense on the side of irritation; at times the movements of the opposite side equal them in intensity, but they usually are less pronounced.
11. If excitation continues to increase, it is propagated upward, and reactions take place through centrifugal nerves coming from the higher cord segments.
12. When an irritation becomes very intense, it is propagated in the medulla oblongata, which becomes a focus from which stimuli radiate to all parts of the cord, causing a general contraction of all muscles in the body.
13. Weak stimuli activate physiologic processes; very strong stimuli inhibit them.
14. When autonomic effectors are partly or completely separated from their normal nerve connections, they become more sensitive to the action of chemical substances.

Matching III

Match the visceral functions with their sympathetic or parasympathetic controls. Column 1 lists the visceral functions. Choose the best match from the Control List and place the corresponding letter in column 2. In column 3, put either "S" for sympathetic or "P" for parasympathetic, depending on the control response.

Column 1	Column 2	Column 3	Control List
1. Heart muscle			a. Increases the secretion of digestive juices
2. Digestive tract			
3. Skeletal muscle blood vessels			
4. Smooth muscle blood vessels			b. Increases the secretion of sweat
5. Urinary bladder			c. Slows the heartbeat
6. Iris			d. Constricts blood vessels
7. Pilomotor muscles			e. Relaxes the bladder
8. Adrenal medulla			f. Increases peristalsis

Column 1	Column 2	Column 3	Control List
9. Sweat glands			g. Dilates blood vessels
10. Digestive glands			h. Increases the secretion of epinephrine
			i. Stimulates goose bumps
			j. Constricts the pupil

Labeling

Label the major nerve plexuses and more.

Brachial plexus
Brain
Cervical plexus   Sacral plexus
Lumbar plexus   Spinal cord
Nerves

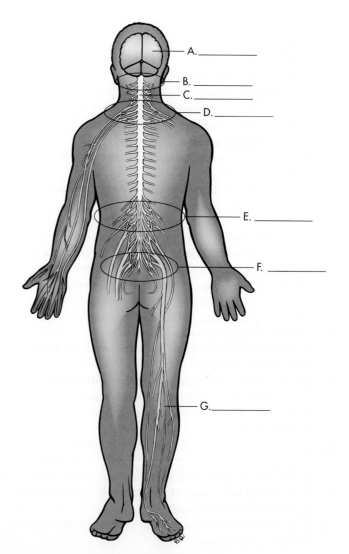

A. _____
B. _____
C. _____
D. _____
E. _____
F. _____
G. _____

Assess Your Competencies

Now that you have studied this chapter, you should be able to:
- Define research literacy
- Use levels of evidence guidelines to categorize research
- Cite current research that validates the underlying physiologic mechanisms of therapeutic massage
- Interpret a research paper
- Describe the fundamentals of the Western scientific process
- Relate the concepts of physics to the experience of touch and massage therapy
- Explain the effects of therapeutic massage in physiologic terms
- Use the Internet to do research
- Classify massage methods into basic concepts

On a separate sheet of paper or on the computer, write a short summary of the content of this chapter based on the preceding list of competencies. Use a conversational tone, as if you were explaining to someone (e.g., a client, prospective employer, coworker, or other interested person) the importance of the information and skills to the development of the massage profession.

Next, in small discussion groups, share your summary with your classmates and compare the ways the information was presented. In discussing the content, look for similarities, differences, possibilities for misunderstanding of the information, and clear, concise methods of description.

Problem-Solving Scenarios

1. A physician refers a client to you for basic relaxation massage to ease chronic pain of undetermined cause. Using the information presented in this chapter, list at least four principal reasons massage could benefit the client.

2. After a series of massages, a client finds that her anxiety and impatience have diminished. How would you explain this using the current research evidence?

3. A client brings in a research article about the use of massage for a specific condition, but he does not understand what it means. What steps would you take to explain it to him?

Professional Applications

1. Make a list of your daily experiences with ANS functions. Make a second list of ANS functions you encounter while performing massage.

2. Read through the various therapeutic massage journals. Find one or two articles on bodywork and classify the information presented according to the following effects:

   a. Mechanical or reflexive

   b. Nervous system primarily affected; benefits primarily somatic, visceral, peripheral, central, or autonomic, connective tissue, or circulatory

   c. Stimulation of chemicals (i.e., hormones) and neurotransmitters

   d. Sensory receptor responsible for responding to the stimulation

3. Design a possible research study. Develop an idea (a hypothesis), narrow the topic, then decide what measurements will be used. Identify possible outcomes. Identify other factors that may influence the outcome. Look at other research studies for examples of research design. Locate resources on ways to develop a research study.

4. Complete a case report.

Endangerment site
General adaptation syndrome
  (GAS)
Health
Homeostasis
Impingement syndromes
Indication
Inflammatory response
Malignant tumors
Medications
Metastasis
Pain-spasm-pain cycle

Palliative care
Pathology
Peak performance
Referral
Referred pain
Signs
Suffering
Symptoms
Syndrome
Synergistic
Therapeutic change
Trauma

KEY TERMS

Acute
Antagonistic
Benign tumors
Caution
Chronic

Communicable diseases
Compensation
Condition management
Contraindication
Dysfunction

INDICATIONS FOR MASSAGE

SECTION OBJECTIVES

Chapter objective covered in this section:
1. The student will be able to define the terms *indication* and
   contraindication.
*Using the information presented in this section, the student will be able
to perform the following:*
* Explain the difference between objective and subjective massage
  benefits
* Explain the benefits of massage to others

Massage professionals must be able to identify indications
and contraindications for therapeutic massage. An **indication**
is a condition for which an approach would be beneficial
for health enhancement, treatment of a particular disorder,
or support of a treatment modality other than massage. A
contraindication is a condition for which an approach
could be harmful. The three types of contraindications are
as follows:
* General avoidance of application—No massage techniques may be performed.
* Regional/local avoidance of application—Massage may
  be performed, but a particular area must be avoided.
* Application with caution (a **caution** is a condition that
  requires the massage therapist to adapt the massage
  process so that the client's safety is maintained)—Massage may be performed, but the practitioner must take
  extra care in determining the methods to be used, the
  duration of the massage, the depth and intensity of pressure, and the frequency of application.

Indications for massage are based on the massage's objective and subjective health-enhancing benefits. Some results of massage can be measured (objective), whereas others are assumed effective based on experience (subjective). The effects of massage are both physical and mental. Physical effects are objective and can be measured physically through some type of observation. Mental effects are subjective perceptions that are reported by the client (Proficiency Exercise 6-1).

💡 PROFICIENCY EXERCISE 6-1

On a separate piece of paper, write two dialogs that explain the benefits of massage. Direct one discussion to a group of health care professionals such as physicians, chiropractors, nurses, physical therapists, and psychologists; direct the other discussion to a group of business professionals, factory workers, construction workers, food service workers, and athletes.

Choose one: Physicians, chiropractors, nurses, physical therapists, psychologists

Type of health professional:

Choose one: Business professionals, factory workers, construction workers, food service workers, athletes

Type of group:

APPROACHES TO CARE

SECTION OBJECTIVES

Chapter objective covered in this section:
2. The student will be able to define therapeutic change, condition management, and palliative care as therapeutic approaches.
Using the information presented in this section, the student will be able to perform the following:
* Explain the concepts of therapeutic change, condition management, and palliative care
* Implement a clinical reasoning process to determine the type of care most beneficial for the client

The benefits of massage occur as a result of therapeutic change, condition management, and palliative care. This section explains each of these approaches.

Therapeutic Change

Therapeutic change is a beneficial alteration in the client's physical, mental, and/or spiritual state that results from a therapeutic massage process. Any change process, including beneficial change, requires energy and resource expenditure on the part of the client. The decision whether to implement a therapeutic change process requires assessment of the client's ability to expend the energy required for active change and the availability of the support and resources often necessary during a change process.

To facilitate a change process, the practitioner must have the appropriate knowledge and skills (current or acquired)

and often a network of support from other professionals. The client must have the motivation and resources (e.g., information, money, time, social support, and coping mechanisms) to complete a change process. Careful assessment helps identify whether a change process program holds a likely chance for success. If resources are insufficient or nonexistent or if the existing situation supports some sort of coping mechanism or allows for some sort of benefit (secondary gain) for the client, the person may not be motivated to commit to the change process.

If the conditions are not suitable for active change, other interventions can be developed. Many clients lead complex lives, and although change often is indicated, it may not be realistically possible at a particular time or under a current set of circumstances.

When the likelihood of a successful change outcome is not good, condition management and palliative care can be offered instead. These approaches reduce suffering and allow clients to be more effective at addressing life's demands within their current set of circumstances. An example of therapeutic change would be addressing scar tissue adhesions. Methodically using methods that introduce therapeutic inflammation and encourage increased pliability in the client's tissue may be helpful. However, the methods used to produce these changes can be uncomfortable and require frequent massage sessions over a long period. If the client is unable to commit to this type of intervention, it may be better to approach the situation in a more conservative manner, such as condition management or palliative care.

Condition Management

Condition management is the use of massage methods to support clients who are not able to undergo a therapeutic change process but who want to live their life to the fullest within an existing set of circumstances. Condition management is beneficial when a client is dealing with a chronic health condition or a set of life circumstances that creates chronic stress, such as caring for an ailing parent or child, having a stressful work environment, dealing with strain in a relationship, or having ongoing financial strain. Condition management also is beneficial when changing a situation is not a viable possibility (e.g., amputation, diabetes, job-related repetitive strain) or when the time frame for changing a situation needs to be postponed (e.g., pregnancy, chemotherapy, graduation from school, end of season for an athlete).

On a physical level, massage can offer benefits by managing the existing physical compensation patterns and sometimes by slowing the progression of chronic conditions or preventing a situation from becoming worse. On an emotional level, massage can assist in the management of physical stress symptoms, allowing the person to cope better with life stresses that cannot be altered.

Condition management accounts for the largest client base for therapeutic massage. Many people find themselves in undesirable or unchanging circumstances and search for ways to cope with, but not necessarily change, the existing conditions while remaining productive. Most of us can relate to the importance of being able to remain resourceful and responsive to life events. Although the ideal is to make changes when life is not as we would like it to be, we all know that sometimes this is not possible for many reasons. Therapeutic massage offers support, acceptance, compassion, and a short-term respite.

Palliative Care

To *palliate* is to soothe or to relieve. Massage can be soothing and can provide comfort, whether the client seeks relaxation to meet pleasure needs, to cope with some type of chronic pain, or to make the transition from life to death.

In a health care context, palliative care attempts to relieve or reduce the intensity of uncomfortable symptoms, but it does not try to produce a cure. Palliative care is provided when the client's condition is most likely going to worsen and degenerative processes will continue (e.g., terminal illness, dementia). It involves massage approaches that reduce suffering.

Because the term *suffering* is inherently subjective and multifaceted, completely understanding the client's experience often is difficult. Suffering can be defined as an overall impairment in quality of life. Many times suffering overshadows the client's ability to create or participate in meaningful experiences or to experience pleasure. Some say we may not have a choice whether to experience pain, be it physical, emotional, or spiritual, but we can choose to suffer or not. Often, pain management does not alleviate suffering, because dealing with only the physical aspects of pain does not take into account that suffering also can be mental and spiritual issues.

Palliative care is also appropriate when the condition should not be changed or the person does not desire a specific outcome other than pleasure and relaxation. Providing massage to a woman during labor, receiving a massage while on vacation, supporting an athlete during training for an event, providing massage at a public event such as a health fair, giving a massage to someone just before surgery, and providing massage to a wedding party the day before the event are all examples of the appropriate use of palliative care.

Massage approaches are very effective for palliative care. The pleasurable experience of touch and human connection, when presented through massage, may be one of the greatest therapeutic gifts our profession offers.

Determining the Type and Timing of an Approach

Some questions that can help a massage therapist determine the most effective approach to use, when to use it, and when to change it include the following:
- When is change appropriate?
- When is change not desirable and condition management and palliative support more appropriate?
- How does the massage professional determine what type of care is appropriate: therapeutic change, condition management, or palliative care?
- How does the massage professional know when transitions occur in types of care (i.e., therapeutic change to

💡 PROFICIENCY EXERCISE 6-2

Metaphor
A metaphor is a figure of speech in which a word or a phrase describing one thing is used to express likeness to another thing. For example:
- "Cleaning the house" could be a metaphor for "offering palliative and management care, reducing suffering, and encouraging better coping in the existing situation"
- "Remodeling the house" could be a metaphor for "a process of active change"

For both the professional and the client, list the differences between "cleaning the house" and "remodeling the house" in terms of skill levels, cost, time, materials, difficulties, disruption in daily living, and other factors.
Example
Cleaning the house
Professional—Ongoing service
Client—Ongoing appointments
Remodeling the house
Professional—Defined number of appointments with a specific outcome
Client—Commitment to a specific set of appointments

Your Turn
List three differences in each area.
   Cleaning the house
   Professional
1.
2.
3.
   Client
1.
2.
3.

   Remodeling the house
   Professional
1.
2.
3.
   Client
1.
2.
3.

condition management, or condition management to palliative care)?

Palliative care can progress to condition management, and with the gradual restoration of energy, the client may even progress to a therapeutic change process. Eventually a therapeutic change process ends or transforms, and condition management, such as stress management, becomes the professional focus once again (Proficiency Exercise 6-2).

Chapter 1 presented information about professional touch. Chapter 2 described professional behavior and introduced the clinical reasoning process. Chapter 4 presented a detailed look at intake procedures, which includes a client history, physical assessment, and methods to develop this information into a care/treatment plan. The clinical reasoning process was related to the procedures for client intake and documentation.

💡 PROFICIENCY EXERCISE 6-3

Student Note: *These problem-solving activities can seem overwhelming. However, it is important to understand how to do them, and the only way to learn is to practice. Whenever you encounter these exercises in the book, attempt to do them. Don't worry about whether you are correct or not; just practice the process.*

After reading the following client case situations, decide whether you would introduce therapeutic change, condition management, or palliative care. Explain your reasons for the decision using the clinical reasoning model. An example of a massage therapist thinking through a case study is provided. Only the result of the process would actually be communicated to the client. Read through the example case study; then for case studies 1, 2, and 3, write down your answers to the questions on a separate piece of paper.

Example Case Study

A male client, age 47, is experiencing fatigue and neck and shoulder pain. He is a cross-country truck driver. He is married, has three children, and has the normal financial obligations of a house payment, car payment, and other responsibilities. One child just started college, and the client is somewhat concerned about the tuition expenses. He likes his job and is content with his family and social life. He can't seem to understand why he is tired or why his shoulder hurts. He can think of no reason for the pain other than the strain of the driving position and the long work hours. This pain never bothered him before. He went to the doctor for a physical examination, and nothing out of the ordinary was identified. The physician thinks that an old football injury involving his shoulder, coupled with some age-related changes, is responsible. The doctor also thinks that the pain in the shoulder might be interfering with the client's sleep and might be a cause of fatigue. The doctor recommends an over-the-counter antiinflammatory agent and painkiller, such as aspirin, and suggests that massage might help. The doctor also recommends that the client cut back on his work hours and relax more. Aspirin helps the shoulder pain but upsets the client's stomach. He does not want to cut back on work hours. He is seeking help for shoulder pain and would like more physical energy.

1. Identify the facts.

Questions that can help with this process include the following:

- What is considered normal or balanced function?
  Answer: The ability to work pain free with reasonable stamina at a job one enjoys.
- What has happened? (Spell out events.)
  Answer: Nothing substantial has occurred to account for the changes other than age-related influences and a previous football injury.

- What caused the imbalance? (Can it be identified?)
  Answer: A previous injury, long work hours, a static seated position with the arms elevated on the steering wheel and repetitive looking to the left during driving.
- What was done or is being done?
  Answer: Treatment with aspirin.
- What has worked or not worked?
  Answer: Aspirin has benefits but upsets the client's stomach. The client has chosen to maintain his current work schedule.

2. Brainstorm the possibilities.

Questions that help with this process include the following:

- What are the possibilities? (What could it all mean?)
  Answer:
  - The fatigue and pain could be a result of age-related changes and the previous injury, coupled with repetitive use; this in turn could interfere with sleep, as suggested by the doctor.
  - The condition could be related more to emotional stress caused by financial concerns.
  - The client may have an undiagnosed health condition that is not sufficiently evident to allow a definitive diagnosis.
- What is my intuition suggesting?
  Answer: I think we likely are dealing with a combination of the doctor's diagnosis and unexpressed emotional stress over financial concerns, particularly the tuition costs for the child in college.
- What are the possible patterns of dysfunction?
  Answer: The static driving position may be aggravating the old football injury.
- What are the possible contributing factors?
  Answer: Worry, postural distortion from the static position, and age-related tissue changes, because the body becomes somewhat less flexible with age and lack of exercise.
- What are possible interventions?
  Answer: A job change, a stretching program, massage therapy, short-term mental health support, treatment with a different medication that does not upset the client's stomach.
- What might work?
  Answer: Massage and a stretching program
- What are other ways to look at the situation?
  Answer: The client does not seem to want to use medications, does not want to change his job, and does not seem to think that there is anything wrong with his emotional or social life. Maybe if the financial situation were different, the stress load would be low enough so

Continued

Chapter 5 described the importance of research and compared the scientific method to the process of clinical reasoning and logical thinking. In this chapter, the clinical reasoning model provides a decision-making process for analyzing whether therapeutic changes or methods to maintain or support an existing state are the best approach. The ability to analyze data collected during assessment procedures is crucial for making decisions about which massage therapy intervention to use and whether the desired outcome is a therapeutic change process, condition management, or palliative care. The massage therapist must consider these factors to develop a plan that best serves the client (Proficiency Exercise 6-3).

💡 PROFICIENCY EXERCISE 6-3—cont'd

that his energy levels would increase and he could ignore the pain. Maybe a financial advisor would be helpful or maybe his wife could get a job.

- What do the data suggest?

  Answer: Emotional stress seems to be a factor. The data seem to suggest that an age-related process and a previous injury are aggravated by repetitive job strain and a static seated position.

3. Consider the logical outcomes of each possibility.

Questions that can help determine outcomes include the following:

- What is the logical progression of the symptom pattern, contributing factors, and current behaviors?

  Answer: If the pain remains or worsens and sleep continues to be interrupted so that fatigue worsens, the immune system could be compromised and other disease processes might develop. The client eventually may be unable to work. His mood would be altered, which would affect family and social relationships.

- What are the pros and cons and the logical effect of each intervention suggested?

  Answer:

  - Job change—would remove repetitive strain on the shoulder and eliminate static seated position; drastic change in lifestyle, finances, and work environment.
  - Stretching program—would increase flexibility and counterbalance the static seated position; could make the situation worse if the stretching is too aggressive, not progressive, and intermittent instead of used daily; program is self-initiated and once learned would not incur any ongoing costs; does not require a regular appointment schedule (helpful because client is frequently on the road); requires discipline to do the stretches.
  - Massage therapy—would help alleviate pain symptoms and support better sleep; does not require extensive self-discipline other than making regular appointments; would incur a financial obligation; would support a daily stretching program; would reduce the use of medication.
  - Short-term mental health support—would not require extensive self-discipline other than making regular appointments; would incur a financial obligation; does not address the physical condition but does address emotional strain.
  - Requesting that the physician consider treatment with a medication that does not upset the client's stomach—would help alleviate pain symptoms and support better sleep; does not require extensive self-discipline; would incur a small financial obligation; does not need regular appointment schedule (helpful because client frequently is on the road); possible side effects and development of dependency on the medication.
  - Consultation with a financial advisor—would help client achieve better control of finances, eliminating the basis for worry and emotional stress; does not address physical conditions, long work hours, or job stress.
  - Wife getting a job—would eliminate financial burden; could create stress in the marriage; requires action on the part of a person other than the client; does not address physical conditions, long work hours, or job stress.

- What are the consequences of not acting?

  Answer: The situation could stabilize and resolve itself, or the condition could become more problematic, requiring more drastic intervention measures in the future.

- What are the consequences of acting?

  Answer: The problem would remain stable or improve. The client would be better able to cope with the current situation.

4. Identify the effect of each possibility on the people involved.

Questions that can help identify possible effects include the following:

- For each intervention considered, what would be the impact on the people involved: client, practitioner, and other professionals working with the client?

  Answer:

  - Job change—Client is not supportive; wife may or may not like idea.
  - Stretching program—Client does not like to fuss with himself and avoids activities having to do with self-care.
  - Massage therapy—Client is open to idea but nervous; wife, doctor, and massage practitioner are supportive.
  - Short-term mental health support—Client and wife are not open to this possibility at this time; they do not think that this is an emotional problem. Massage practitioner is hesitant about the client being unwilling to seek mental health services and does think emotion is involved (worry over finances) and would like client to remain open to this possibility.
  - Treatment with a medication that does not upset the client's stomach—Client does not like to take medication, and the doctor is unwilling to prescribe at this time until other measures have been explored.
  - Consultation with a financial advisor—Client and wife think this is a good idea and will pursue this possibility.
  - Wife getting a job—Not an option at this time.

- How does each person involved feel about the possible interventions?

  Answer:

  - Job change—None are supportive.
  - Stretching program—Client is ambivalent; massage practitioner and wife are supportive.
  - Massage therapy—All are supportive.
  - Short-term mental health support—Massage therapist is supportive; client and wife are not supportive.
  - Treatment with a medication that does not upset the client's stomach—Doctor and client are not supportive.
  - Consultation with a financial advisor—Client and wife are supportive.
  - Wife getting a job—Not an option.

- Is the practitioner within his or her scope of practice to work with such situations?

  Answer: Yes

- Is the practitioner qualified to work with such situations?

  Answer: Yes

- Does the practitioner feel qualified to work with such situations?

  Answer: The practitioner is concerned about the client's ambivalence toward a stretching program and his lack

PROFICIENCY EXERCISE **6-3**—cont'd

of interest in a mental health referral. These concerns raise questions for the practitioner about the ability to work effectively with the client's physical problems when other causal factors may exist.
- Does a feeling of cooperation and agreement exist among all parties involved?
  Answer: A degree of cooperation exists, as does some resistance. All agree on the benefit of massage therapy.

5. Result of the process.
Based on this analysis of the information provided, the massage practitioner would recommend a condition management program rather than a therapeutic change process, for the following reasons:
- Causal factors are involved that the client may not be able to address during a change process.
- The client is resistant to the idea of an exercise or a stretching program that would interfere with his driving schedule.

Case Study 1
A 17-year-old volleyball player is in training for a playoff tournament in 4 weeks. She has been somewhat sore after practice and anxious about the playoffs. Her game is a bit "off," which is adding to her anxiety. Both her coach and her parents think that massage would be helpful to her. She is in good health and takes no medications, but she does have an erratic eating pattern and recently has been drinking soda with caffeine in it. She also has been working with visualization and progressive relaxation before sleeping. She thinks these methods help her sleep better.

1. Identify the facts.
Questions that can help with this process include the following:
- What is considered normal or balanced function?

- What has happened? (Spell out events.)

- What caused the imbalance? (Can it be identified?)

- What was done or is being done?

- What has worked or not worked?

2. Brainstorm the possibilities.
Questions that can help with this process include the following:
- What are the possibilities? (What could it all mean?)

- What is my intuition suggesting?

- What are the possible patterns of dysfunction?

- What are the possible contributing factors?

- What are possible interventions?

- What might work?

- What are other ways to look at the situation?

- What do the data suggest?

3. Consider the logical outcomes of each possibility.
Questions that can help determine outcomes include the following:
- What is the logical progression of the symptom pattern, contributing factors, and current behaviors?

- What are the pros and cons and the logical effect of each intervention suggested?

- What are the consequences of not acting?

- What are the consequences of acting?

4. Identify the effect of each possibility on the people involved.
Questions that can help identify effects include the following:
- For each intervention considered, what would be the impact on the people involved: client, practitioner, and other professionals working with the client?

- How does each person involved feel about the possible interventions?

- Is the practitioner within his or her scope of practice to work with such situations?

- Is the practitioner qualified to work with such situations?

- Does the practitioner feel qualified to work with such situations?

- Does a feeling of cooperation and agreement exist among all parties involved?

5. Result of the process.
Based on this analysis of the information provided, the massage practitioner would recommend _____, for the following reasons:

Case Study 2
A 39-year-old premenopausal woman was divorced 2 years ago. Her only child just graduated from high school and has joined the military. She has a supportive circle of friends and is financially stable and secure in her job. She was in a car accident 3 years ago and suffered a whiplash injury, which was treated successfully with physical therapy. However, she still has some residual stiffness in her neck. Currently she is experiencing mood swings and headaches, and she recently visited her doctor because of them. Her doctor recommended stress management and moderate exercise. She says that she wants to feel more in control of her body and wants to be able to self-manage the mood swings and headaches. She is not opposed to hormone therapy for menopause but would like to see if she can manage without it. She is seeking massage as part of her lifestyle self-care program and is motivated.

Continued

💡 PROFICIENCY EXERCISE 6-3—cont'd

1. Identify the facts.

Questions that can help with this process include the following:

- What is considered normal or balanced function?

- What has happened? (Spell out events.)

- What caused the imbalance? (Can it be identified?)

- What was done or is being done?

- What has worked or not worked?

2. Brainstorm the possibilities.

Questions that can help with this process include the following:

- What are the possibilities? (What could it all mean?)

- What is my intuition suggesting?

- What are the possible patterns of dysfunction?

- What are the possible contributing factors?

- What are possible interventions?

- What might work?

- What are other ways to look at the situation?

- What do the data suggest?

3. Consider the logical outcomes of each possibility.

Questions that can help determine outcomes include the following:

- What is the logical progression of the symptom pattern, contributing factors, and current behaviors?

- What are the pros and cons and the logical effect of each intervention suggested?

- What are the consequences of not acting?

- What are the consequences of acting?

4. Identify the effect of each possibility on the people involved.

Questions that can help identify effects include the following:

- For each intervention considered, what would be the impact on the people involved: client, practitioner, and other professionals working with the client?

- How does each person involved feel about the possible interventions?

- Is the practitioner within his or her scope of practice to work with such situations?

- Is the practitioner qualified to work with such situations?

- Does the practitioner feel qualified to work with such situations?

- Does a feeling of cooperation and agreement exist among all parties involved?

5. Result of the process.

Based on this analysis of the information provided, the massage practitioner would recommend _____, for the following reasons:

Case Study 3

A 26-year-old man with asthma is experiencing an increase in symptoms. Medication is effective in treating the asthma. He was recently married and has just moved to a new city because of a job transfer. His wife is 3 months pregnant. He takes good care of himself and is careful with his diet. However, his exercise regimen was disrupted by the move, and he has not re-established a regular exercise program. His respiratory therapist has recommended massage, because she believes that the increased stress is a possible cause of the increase in the severity of the asthma.

1. Identify the facts.

Questions that can help with this process include the following:

- What is considered normal or balanced function?

- What has happened? (Spell out events.)

- What caused the imbalance? (Can it be identified?)

- What was done or is being done?

- What has worked or not worked?

2. Brainstorm the possibilities.

Questions that can help with this process include the following:

- What are the possibilities? (What could it all mean?)

- What is my intuition suggesting?

- What are the possible patterns of dysfunction?

- What are the possible contributing factors?

- What are possible interventions?

- What might work?

- What are other ways to look at the situation?

- What do the data suggest?

3. Consider the logical outcomes of each possibility.

Questions that can help determine outcomes include the following:

- What is the logical progression of the symptom pattern, contributing factors, and current behaviors?

☉ PROFICIENCY EXERCISE 6-3—cont'd

- What are the pros and cons and the logical effect of each intervention suggested?

- What are the consequences of not acting?

- What are the consequences of acting?

4. Identify the effect of each possibility on the people involved.

Questions that can help identify effects include the following:

- For each intervention considered, what would be the impact on the people involved: client, practitioner, and other professionals working with the client?

- How does each person involved feel about the possible interventions?

- Is the practitioner within his or her scope of practice to work with such situations?

- Is the practitioner qualified to work with such situations?

- Does the practitioner feel qualified to work with such situations?

- Does a feeling of cooperation and agreement exist among all parties involved?

5. Result of the process.

Based on this analysis of the information provided, the massage practitioner would recommend _____, for the following reasons:

PATHOLOGY

SECTION OBJECTIVES

Chapter objective covered in this section:

3. The student will be able to define pathology and explain the causes of disease.

Using the information presented in this section, the student will be able to perform the following:

- Define the terms *health, dysfunction,* and *pathology*
- Explain the disease process including risk factors for the development of pathologic conditions
- Recognize a client condition that should be evaluated by a primary health care provider
- List the mechanisms and risk factors that predispose people to disease processes
- Explain the stress response, inflammatory response, and pain response
- Explain the mechanisms of pain and evaluate pain for referral purposes
- Identify indications for massage therapy and justify those indications

Pathology is the study of disease. To practice safely, massage practitioners need a basic understanding of pathologic processes. The body is designed for health. A sequence of events must occur for disease to develop. **Trauma** is an abrupt shock or injury to the body or psyche; like disease, trauma requires the body to heal.

The diagnosis of disorders is not a function of a massage professional. However, to refer clients appropriately to a health care professional, the massage practitioner must be able to recognize when the client's condition represents an irregularity that should be evaluated by the person's primary health care provider. When working with a referral and under proper supervision, the massage professional also must be able to alter the application of massage if any disease process or trauma is present so that the client receives the benefits of massage without harm.

Massage students should have both a general awareness of the types of disorders that occur in each major body system and more specific knowledge of the signs and symptoms of selected disorders that could endanger the health of either the client or the practitioner (see Appendix A for specific contraindications to massage). The massage professional also needs a basic understanding of pharmacology and the possible interactions between **medications** and massage (see Appendix C for specific information on these interactions).

A massage practitioner is not a physician or a mental health professional and is not expected to know the symptoms of all diseases; however, resources for locating specific information needed must be available . The massage practitioner also should have a current medical dictionary and comprehensive pathology reference available to research unfamiliar terms and pathologic conditions. Internet search programs also are helpful. (Helpful and reliable links are available on the Evolve website.)

To understand disease, we first must understand the definition of health. **Health** is optimal functioning with freedom from disease or abnormal processes. Health is influenced by many factors, including inherited (genetic) and acquired conditions. Lifestyle, activity level, rest, loving relationships, exercise, a balanced diet, empowering beliefs and attitudes, self-esteem, authentic personality, and freedom from self-hindering patterns all support health. When a state of health no longer exists or is interrupted, dysfunction begins.

Dysfunction is the in-between state of "not healthy" but also "not sick" (i.e., experiencing disease). Unfortunately, many people experience dysfunctional states. Western medicine has a difficult time identifying and dealing with dysfunctions, because these are prepathologic states that often are not revealed by current diagnostic methods. An actual pathologic condition usually needs to exist before medical tests and diagnostic methods can detect a disease state.

Recent prevention methods, many modeled after more "Eastern" or "holistic" approaches, are beginning to address the states of dysfunction. Many ancient healing methods are more focused on the process of dysfunction, introducing restorative methods before a system breaks down into a disease process. When used in the prepathologic state of dysfunction, these methods of mind/body medicine, stress management, and prevention are very effective. They are less effective when applied to an active pathologic process, although they remain an important part of the total healing program. Often more aggressive approaches are required to reverse the pathologic condition and allow healing to begin.

Peak performance is defined as maximum conditioning and functioning in a particular action. Although most associated with athletes or entertainers such as dancers, peak performance also can occur in more mental actions, such as studying for school or dealing with a demanding workload or with family issues. Peak performance also can pertain to massage professionals who keep themselves in the best shape possible for performing treatments in their massage practices. Maximum use of body functions and resources becomes energy-consuming and stressful to the body. During peak performance, the body does not hold back energy expenditure, and all available resources are used. If the person's lifestyle does not support recuperation time or if anatomic or physiologic limits are exceeded, injury or depletion commonly occurs, and illness results (Goodman and Fuller, 2008).

Disease

Homeostasis is the relative constancy of the body's internal environment. If homeostasis is disturbed, as occurs in a disease process, a variety of feedback mechanisms usually attempt to return the body to normal. A disease condition exists when homeostasis cannot be restored easily. In **acute** conditions, the body recovers its homeostatic balance quickly. In **chronic** diseases, a normal state of balance may never be restored, and compensation develops. Compensation is the process of counterbalancing a defect in body structure or function.

A pathologic condition is seldom caused by one thing; rather, a series of events usually occurs. For example, the flu is caused by the influenza virus, but not everyone exposed to the virus gets the flu. Consider the situation of a person who gets the flu and another who does not. The person who has the flu smokes, had a minor car accident 2 weeks ago, is experiencing a short-term financial setback, and got into an argument with a coworker 3 days before the onset of the flu. The person who does not have the flu has not experienced anything out of the ordinary for the past 3 months, exercises moderately, and follows a fairly supportive dietary plan with lots of fruits and vegetables. Stress and lifestyle habits, therefore, are contributing factors in the breakdown of the body's healing mechanisms.

Functioning Limits

The body has anatomic and physiologic functioning limits. The heart can beat only so fast, the endocrine glands can secrete only a maximum amount of hormones, and the skeletal muscles can lift only so much weight or jump so high. However, extraordinary events push the body's limits of functioning. Athletes and new parents, for example, often function at maximum body limits, or peak performance.

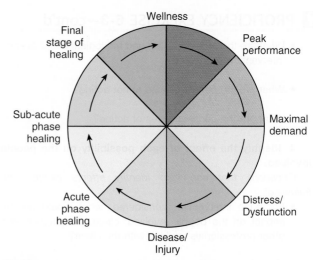

FIGURE 6-1 The health–wellness–injury–illness continuum.

Under normal conditions the body functions within a margin of safety. Normal physiologic mechanisms inhibit the tendency to function at the body's limits. We usually do not run as fast as we can, work as long as we could, or exert all of our energy to complete a task. Instead, the body signals fatigue, pain, or strain before the anatomic or physiologic limits are reached, and we back off. This very important protective mechanism allows us to live within a healthy range of energy expenditure while keeping functioning energy reserves in place in case of an emergency or extraordinary demand (Figure 6-1). Each time we tap into this reserve, the body tends to work to restore what was used and, if possible, to add a little more to the reserve (Box 6-1).

Dysfunction occurs when the reserve runs low because restorative mechanisms are unable to function effectively or when the body begins to limit function in an attempt to maintain higher energy reserves.

Massage professionals serve many people at the beginning of dysfunctional patterns; that is, when the client does not feel his or her best but is not yet sick. Monitoring clients to make sure the dysfunctional patterns do not progress is important. Early intervention and referral to appropriate health care professionals are important for identifying potential problems; this gives clients the opportunity to take appropriate measures for preventing these problems from developing. Massage also can support the restorative process to help maintain peak performance. The benefits of massage are most effectively focused on helping people stay within the healthy range of functioning.

Development of Pathologic Conditions

As mentioned previously, homeostasis is the relative constancy of the body's internal environment.

Therapeutic massage has widespread effects on the physiologic functions of the body. Therefore, the massage professional must learn about pathologic conditions, contraindications, and endangerment sites. Obtaining a consensus

Box 6-1 Examples of Dysfunction Related to Functional Limits

Dysfunction Related to Low Reserves

A new mother with a fussy baby is unable to get restorative sleep; this continues for 6 months. The mother gets a cold that lingers. The infant is prone to recurring ear infections over the next 3 years, which continues to disturb the mother's sleep pattern. In addition, the mother's diet begins to consist mostly of snack foods. The mother begins first to have headaches, then neck and shoulder pain, and then low back pain. Finally, 5 years after the birth, just as the child begins school, the mother develops chronic fatigue syndrome with fibromyalgia.

Massage intervention early in the process may help support restorative sleep, especially if help with the baby is provided. Massage and other similar stress management systems could at least slow the progression of dysfunction. After the headaches appear, massage could be used to manage the pain and reduce the muscle tension patterns in an attempt to support innate body healing and restorative mechanisms. After chronic fatigue symptoms begin with fibromyalgia pain, a multidisciplinary team and lifestyle approach are necessary to reverse the pathologic condition.

Dysfunction Related to Attempts to Maintain a Higher Energy Reserve

If a person who plays tennis overstretches the shoulder while reaching for a serve, the body senses a danger of harm to the joint. Neurologic sensors may reset muscle patterns, limiting range of motion slightly to prevent this. Physiologically, protective space has been formed in the body reserves even though range of motion has been sacrificed. If this continues, eventually the limited range of motion interferes with the ability to play tennis. Dysfunction occurs. If the dysfunction is perpetuated and the body compensates for it over time, a pathologic condition usually develops. The person could end up with a condition called "frozen shoulder," in which movement is significantly limited.

Massage intervention just after the first event, coupled with a more conservative playing style or improved playing form, might reverse the process, and dysfunction would not develop. Intervention applied at the point when range-of-motion limits were first observed likely would still be effective in reversing the dysfunctional process. However, the intervention plan would be more complex and time-consuming. Interventions introduced after a pathologic process has begun are complex, sometimes aggressive, and occasionally too late to support repair and restoration of function.

on such information is difficult, however, because all sources do not agree on all points.

Illness

Clients can become ill or suffer injury, and risk factors can increase the potential for illness or injury. Illness occurs when a body process breaks down. A person whose immune system did not effectively fight off a cold virus becomes ill with a cold.

Chronic fatigue syndrome, ulcers, cancer, and multiple sclerosis are all examples of illnesses.

Injury

Injury occurs when tissue is damaged. Cuts, bruises, burns, contusions, fractured bones, sprains, and strains are examples of injuries. Illness tends to indicate general cautions and contraindications, whereas injury more often creates regional cautions and contraindications.

Inflammation is a factor in both illness and injury, because healing for both involves appropriate activation of the inflammatory response system. Healing an injury is taxing on the body and strains its restorative abilities. If an injured person is not in a state of health to begin with, the stress of the injury frequently compromises the immune system, and the person then becomes susceptible to illness.

Therapeutic massage is indicated for both illness and injury. Massage techniques for illness involve very general application of massage to support the body's healing responses (e.g., stress management, pain control, restorative sleep). This approach to massage, sometimes called *general constitutional application,* is used to reduce the stress load so that the body can heal.

Massage for injury incorporates aspects of general constitutional massage, because healing is necessary for tissue repair. In addition, lymphatic drainage can be used to control edema. Gliding methods are used to approximate (bring close together) the ends of some types of tissue injuries, such as minor muscle tears and strains. Hyperstimulation analgesia and counterirritation reduce acute pain. Methods to increase circulation to the area support tissue formation. Connective tissue applications are used to manage scar tissue formation.

Because many diseases and injuries have similar symptoms, determining the specific underlying causes of a pathology can be difficult. The massage professional must refer clients to qualified, licensed health care providers for a specific diagnosis.

Disease or injury conditions usually are diagnosed or identified by signs and symptoms. **Signs** are objective abnormalities that can be seen or measured by someone other than the patient. **Symptoms** are the subjective abnormalities felt only by the patient. A **syndrome** is a group of different signs and symptoms, usually arising from a common cause. A disease is classified as acute when signs and symptoms develop quickly, last a short time, and then disappear. Diseases that develop slowly and last for a long time (sometimes for life) are classified as chronic.

Communicable diseases can be transmitted from one person to another. The study of communicable diseases is an important process for the massage professional (see Chapter 7).

Risk Factors

Certain predisposing conditions may make the development of a disease or some types of injury more likely. Usually called *risk factors,* these conditions may put an individual at risk for developing a disease, but they do not actually cause the disease. Examples of risk factors include genetic factors, age, lifestyle, environmental factors, pre-existing conditions, and stress.

Genetic Factors

Several types of genetic risk factors can play a role in illness. An inherited trait may put a person at a greater than normal risk for developing a specific disease. For example, a genetic link has been established to a specific form of breast cancer. A family history of disease processes and causes of death usually can reveal possible genetic traits. Steps can be taken to support the body against the genetic tendency for a disease process. Careful monitoring by the physician allows early detection and treatment. In addition, the individual can make beneficial changes in diet and lifestyle to reduce risk.

Age

Biologic and behavioral factors increase the risk of developing certain diseases or injuries at certain ages. For example, musculoskeletal problems are common between the ages of 30 and 50 years.

Lifestyle

The way we live, work, and play can put us at risk for some diseases or injuries. Some researchers believe that the high-fat, low-fiber diet common among people in developed nations increases their risk of developing certain types of cancer and cardiovascular diseases. Smoking cigarettes, drinking excessive alcohol, and not getting enough exercise are all lifestyle risks. Some athletes face an increased risk; playing hockey, for example, predisposes one to bruises, sprains, and broken bones.

Environmental Factors

Some environmental conditions put people at greater risk of contracting certain diseases. For example, living in an area with high concentrations of air pollution may increase a person's risk of developing respiratory problems. Snow and ice predispose people to injury from falls.

Pre-existing Conditions

A primary (pre-existing) condition can put a person at risk of developing a secondary condition. For example, a viral infection can compromise the immune system, making the person more susceptible to bacterial infection.

Stress

Stress can be defined as any substantial change in routine or any activity that forces the body to adapt. Stress places demands on physical, mental, and emotional resources. Research has shown that as stresses accumulate, especially if the stress is long term, the individual becomes increasingly susceptible to physical illness, mental and emotional problems, and accidental injuries.

General Adaptation Syndrome

As discussed in Chapter 5, Dr. Hans Selye, a pioneer in stress research, labeled the body's response to stress the **general adaptation syndrome (GAS).** The GAS describes the way the body mobilizes different defense mechanisms when threatened by harmful stimuli (actual or perceived). The syndrome has three stages: (1) alarm, or the fight-or-flight response, which is the body's initial reaction to the perceived stressor; (2) the resistance reaction, in which the secretion of regulating hormones allows the body to continue fighting or to endure a stressor long after the effects of the alarm reaction have dissipated; and (3) exhaustion, which occurs if the stress response continues without relief.

In generalized stress conditions, the hypothalamus acts on the anterior pituitary gland to cause the release of adrenocorticotropic hormone (ACTH), which stimulates the adrenal cortex to secrete glucocorticoid. In addition, the sympathetic division of the autonomic nervous system (ANS) is stimulated by the adrenal medulla, resulting in the release of epinephrine and norepinephrine to assist the body in responding to the stressful stimulus. Unfortunately, during periods of prolonged stress, glucocorticosteroids (cortisol) may have harmful side effects, including a diminished immune response, altered blood glucose levels, altered protein and fat metabolism, and decreased resistance to stress.

Considering the variety and number of organs and glands innervated by the ANS, it is no wonder that autonomic disorders have varied and broad consequences. This is especially true of stress-induced diseases. A prolonged or excessive physiologic response to stress, the fight-or-flight response, can disrupt normal functioning throughout the body. Stress has been cited as an indirect cause or an important risk factor in many conditions.

PATHOLOGIC CONDITIONS AND INDICATIONS FOR MASSAGE

SECTION OBJECTIVES

Chapter objective covered in this section:
4. The student will be able to develop a basic understanding of pathology and use the knowledge to determine the indications and contraindications for massage.

Using the information presented in this section, the student will be able to perform the following:
- Describe the inflammatory response and pain response
- Explain the mechanisms of pain and evaluate pain for referral purposes
- Identify and justify indications for massage therapy regarding impingement syndromes and psychological dysfunctions

Massage has been shown to be especially beneficial for chronic inflammation, pain management, impingement syndromes, and psychological dysfunctions. It is especially effective for anxiety disorders related to the ANS that manifest with physical symptoms (called *somatization*). Inflammation and pain are signs and symptoms of many pathologic conditions. A common source of soft tissue pain is impingement syndrome, in which nerves are compressed, causing pain to radiate. A common response to pain is an increase in anxiety. The indications for massage often are based on the beneficial effects of massage that target the body's ability to resolve inflammation, manage pain, reduce pressure on nerves, and soothe anxiety.

Inflammatory Response

Inflammation may occur as a response to any tissue injury, and the inflammatory response is an active and important part of the healing process. The inflammatory response is a combination of processes that attempts to minimize injury to tissues and promote healing, thus maintaining homeostasis. Inflammation also may accompany specific immune system reactions. Acute inflammation occurs during the onset of injury or illness and is an essential aspect of the healing process. Chronic inflammation is an inflammatory process that occurs or persists without a beneficial outcome and thus becomes a disease-producing process. The signs and symptoms of inflammation include heat and redness, and swelling and pain.

- *Heat* and *redness:* When tissue cells are damaged, they release inflammatory mediators, such as histamine, prostaglandins, and compounds called *kinins.* Some inflammatory mediators cause the blood vessels to dilate, increasing the blood volume available to the tissue. The increased blood volume produces the redness and heat of inflammation. This response is important, because it allows immune system cells (white blood cells) in the blood to travel quickly and easily to the site of injury.
- *Swelling* and *pain:* Some inflammatory mediators increase the permeability of blood vessel walls. When water (plasma fluid) leaks out of the vessel, tissue swelling (edema) results. The pressure caused by edema triggers pain receptors. The fluid that accumulates in inflamed tissue (inflammatory exudate) has the beneficial effect of diluting the irritant. Inflammatory exudate is removed slowly by the lymphatic system. Bacteria and damaged cells are held in the lymph nodes and are destroyed by white blood cells. Occasionally lymph nodes enlarge when they process a large amount of infectious material.

Sometimes the inflammatory response is more intense or prolonged than desirable. Inflammation can be suppressed by antihistamines, which block the action of histamine, and by antiinflammatories such as aspirin, which disrupts the body's synthesis of prostaglandins.

Tissue Repair

The processes of inflammation triggers tissue repair. Tissue repair is the replacement of dead cells with living cells. In a type of tissue repair called *regeneration,* the new cells are similar to those they replace. Another type of tissue repair is *replacement.* In replacement the new cells are formed from connective tissue and are different from those they replace, resulting in a scar. Often, fibrous connective tissue replaces the damaged tissue, resulting in a condition called *fibrosis.* Most tissue repairs are a combination of regeneration and replacement. A goal in the healing process is to promote regeneration and keep replacement to a minimum. Massage has been shown to slow the formation of scar tissue and to keep scar tissue pliable when it does form.

Inflammatory Disease

Productive local inflammation occurs in a limited area, such as in a small cut that becomes infected. Productive systemic inflammation occurs when the irritant spreads throughout the body or when inflammatory mediators cause changes throughout the body.

As mentioned earlier, inflammation that is persistent without benefit is considered chronic inflammation. Conditions involving chronic inflammation are classified as inflammatory diseases (Table 6-1). Inflammatory conditions such as arthritis, inflammatory bowel disease, asthma, eczema, and chronic bronchitis are among the most common.

Indications for Massage

Generally, acute inflammatory conditions indicate cautions for massage application. Local areas of inflammation typically are avoided during the acute inflammatory phase, especially if infection is present. A systemic acute inflammatory response related to infection typically involves fever, although not always. Productive fever supports healing and indicates that adaptive capacity is strained. Massage typically (but not always) is avoided during the acute phase of disease.

Massage is indicated with cautions when local acute inflammation is present. The area of inflammation is avoided, and if the area is related to injury susceptible to infection, diligence

TABLE 6-1	Diseases Related to Chronic Inflammation

Many seemingly unrelated diseases have a common link—inflammation. This is a partial list of common medical problems associated with chronic inflammation.

Disease or Disorder	Mechanism
Allergy	Mediators induce autoimmune reactions.
Alzheimer's disease	Chronic inflammation destroys brain cells.
Anemia	Mediators disrupt erythropoietin production.
Aortic valve stenosis	Chronic inflammation damages heart valves.
Arthritis	Inflammatory mediators destroy joint cartilage and synovial fluid.
Asthma	Mediators close the airways.
Cancer	Chronic inflammation causes most cancers.
Cardiovascular disease	Inflammation contributes to the formation of plaque in blood vessels.
Congestive heart failure	Chronic inflammation causes wasting of the heart muscle.
Fibromyalgia	Mediators are elevated in fibromyalgia.
Fibrosis	Mediators attack traumatized tissue.
Heart attack	Chronic inflammation contributes to coronary atherosclerosis.
Kidney failure	Mediators restrict circulation and damage nephrons.
Lupus	Mediators induce an autoimmune attack.
Pancreatitis	Mediators induce pancreatic cell injury.
Psoriasis	Mediators induce dermatitis.
Stroke	Chronic inflammation promotes thromboembolic events.
Surgical complications	Mediators prevent healing.

for sanitation and infection control is necessary. An example of this situation is massage application after surgery.

If the acute inflammation is systemic, the individual is ill. Palliative massage may support restorative sleep. However, it is very important to avoid any approach that adds any more adaptive strain than the client can manage. When in doubt—don't massage. Wait until the person is feeling better or has received clearance for massage from his or her health care provider.

Therapeutic massage seems to be beneficial in cases of prolonged chronic inflammation. A number of theories have been proposed to explain this, including the following:
- The stimulation from massage activates a release of the body's own antiinflammatory agents.
- Certain types of massage increase the inflammatory process (therapeutic inflammation) to a small degree, triggering the body to complete the process.
- Massage may facilitate dilution and removal of the irritant by increasing lymphatic flow.
- Massage supports parasympathetic function.

Therapeutic Inflammation

Because the inflammatory response is part of a healing process, deliberate creation of inflammation can generate or stimulate healing mechanisms. Certain methods of massage can be used to create a controlled, localized area of therapeutic inflammation. Deep frictioning techniques and connective tissue stretching methods are the most common approaches. In some healing practices, such as moxibustion, the skin is burned to create inflammation. Acupuncture also may create very small localized areas of inflammation to generate healing mechanisms. These methods are most beneficial in resolving connective tissue dysfunction, particularly fibrotic changes of muscle tissue and areas of scar tissue adhesion.

The benefit derived from the use of therapeutic inflammation depends on the body's ability to generate healing processes. If healing mechanisms are suppressed, methods that create therapeutic inflammation should not be used. Therapeutic inflammation is not used when sleep disturbance, compromised immune function, a high stress load, or systemic or localized inflammation is already present. This method also is contraindicated if the client has any condition marked by impaired repair and restorative functions (e.g., fibromyalgia) unless massage application is carefully supervised as part of a total treatment program.

A client's use of antiinflammatory medications is another factor that must be considered. If a person is taking such medications, either the steroidal or nonsteroidal type, the effectiveness of therapeutic inflammation is negated or reduced and restorative mechanisms are inhibited. Any methods that create inflammation must be avoided when these medications are used.

Pain

Pain provides information about stimuli that can damage tissue; it therefore often enables us to protect ourselves from greater damage. Pain often initiates a person's search for medical assistance. The individual's subjective description and indication of the location of the pain help pinpoint the underlying cause of trauma or disease.

Massage professionals especially need to understand the mechanisms of pain. Chapter 5 presents reasons massage is beneficial for symptomatic reduction of pain perception. In this section, we consider the types of pain and the ways massage may be indicated or contraindicated for pain. Understanding the various types of pain helps the massage practitioner recognize when to refer the client to a physician.

Mosby's Medical, Nursing, and Allied Health Dictionary defines pain as "an unpleasant sensation caused by noxious stimulation of the sensory nerve endings. It is a subjective feeling and an individual response to the cause" (Anderson et al., 2008). Pain is a complex, private, abstract experience that is difficult to explain or describe. It is the main symptom or complaint that causes people to seek health care. Effective management of pain is a major challenge. Defining pain in descriptive and measurable terms is not easy, because pain has physiologic, psychological, and social aspects. Massage professionals need to recognize that pain is what the client says it is, and it exists when the client says it does.

Pain Sensations

Four distinct processes are involved in pain sensation: transduction, transmission, modulation, and perception. Pain transduction is the process by which noxious stimuli lead to electrical activity in the pain receptors. Pain transmission involves the process of transmitting pain impulses from the site of transduction over peripheral sensory nerves to the spinal cord and the brain. Pain modulation involves neural activity through descending neural pathways from the brain that can influence pain transmission at the level of the spinal cord. Modulation also involves the chemical factors that produce or enhance activity in the primary afferent pain receptors. Pain perception is the subjective experience of pain by the person that is somehow produced by the neural activity of pain transmission.

The receptors for pain, called *nociceptors*, are simply the branching ends of the dendrites of certain sensory neurons. Pain receptors are found in almost every tissue of the body and may respond to any type of stimulus. When stimuli for other sensations, such as touch, pressure, heat, and cold, reach a certain intensity, they also stimulate the sensation of pain. Injured tissue may release prostaglandins, making peripheral nociceptors more sensitive to the normal pain response (hyperalgesia). Aspirin and other nonsteroidal antiinflammatory drugs (NSAIDs) inhibit the action of prostaglandins and reduce pain.

Excessive stimulation of a sensory organ causes pain. Additional stimuli for pain receptors include excessive distention or dilation of a structure, prolonged muscular contractions, muscle spasms, inadequate blood flow to tissues, or the presence of certain chemical substances. Because of their sensitivity to all stimuli, pain receptors perform a protective function by identifying changes that may endanger the body.

Pain receptors adapt only slightly or not at all. *Adaptation* is the decrease or disappearance of the perception of a sensation even though the stimulus is still present. (An example is the way we get used to our clothes soon after dressing.) If adaptation to pain occurred, pain would cease to be sensed, and irreparable damage could result.

Pain sensation is carried on two types of nerve fibers: large, myelinated A fibers, and small, nonmyelinated C fibers. A and C nerve fibers can be distinguished by the two types of pain they elicit: fast pain and slow pain.

Fast pain signals are transmitted to the spinal cord by the A nerve fibers and are felt within 0.1 second. Fast pain usually is local and specific and has a prickling, sharp, or electrical quality. Fast pain is elicited in response to mechanical or thermal stimuli on the skin surface but is not felt in deeper tissues of the body. Slow pain is transmitted by the C fibers and is felt 1 second after a noxious stimulus.

Slow pain is less well localized and has a burning, throbbing, or aching quality. Slow pain may be elicited by mechanical, thermal, or chemical stimuli in the skin or most deep tissues or organs and usually is associated with tissue damage.

Because of this double system of pain innervation, tissue injury often occurs as two distinct pain sensations: an early, sharp pain (transmitted by A nerve fibers), followed by a dull, burning, somewhat prolonged pain (transmitted by C nerve fibers).

Sensory impulses for pain are conducted by the central nervous system (CNS) along spinal and cranial nerves to the thalamus. From there the impulses may be relayed primarily to the parietal lobe of the brain. Recognition of the type and intensity of most pain ultimately is localized in the cerebral cortex of the brain. Pain is called a *thalamic sense,* because it is probably brought to the consciousness in the thalamus. Neurons in the thalamus carry the pain impulses to the primary somatosensory cortex, where the sensory aspects of pain are identified by location, nature, and intensity.

This system of pain transmission through the thalamus influences the expression of pain in terms of tolerance, behavior, and sympathetic autonomic responses, especially in relation to chronic pain, because of the associated autonomic responses, emotional behavior, and lowered pain thresholds that often occur.

An understanding of the pain pathways is important, because massage application can modulate pain transmission. Individuals perceive painful stimuli in different ways. Specific areas in the brain itself control or influence pain perception: the hypothalamus and limbic structures serve as the emotional center of pain perception, and the frontal cortex provides the rational interpretation and responses to pain. The CNS has a variety of mechanisms for modulating or suppressing nociceptive pain stimuli. Sensory input to the spinal cord also may be influenced by neurotransmitters or neuromodulators. Neurotransmitters are neurochemicals that inhibit or stimulate activity at postsynaptic membranes. Substance P, a neuropeptide, is a pain-specific neurotransmitter present in the dorsal horn of the spinal cord (at the "gate," as proposed by the gate control theory), among other sites. Other CNS neurotransmitters involved in pain transmission include acetylcholine, norepinephrine, epinephrine, dopamine, and serotonin.

Serotonin inhibits dorsal horn nociceptor neurons, thereby modulating pain transmission. In addition to serotonin, neurotransmitters such as norepinephrine and endogenous opioid peptides (i.e., endorphins), are implicated in pain modulation. Opioid peptides, known as *neuromodulators* (pain reducers), are naturally occurring compounds that have morphine-like qualities. Massage influences these neurochemicals (see Chapter 5).

The point where a stimulus is perceived as painful, known as the *pain threshold,* varies somewhat from person to person. One factor that affects the pain threshold is perceptual dominance, in which the pain felt in one area of the body diminishes or obliterates the pain felt in another area. Not until the most severe pain is diminished does the person perceive or acknowledge the other pain. This mechanism is often activated with massage application that produces a "good hurt."

Pain tolerance is the duration or intensity of pain that a person can endure before acknowledging the pain and seeking relief. Pain tolerance is more variable from one person to another than is the pain threshold. A person's tolerance to pain is influenced by a variety of factors, including personality type, psychological state at the onset of pain, previous experiences, sociocultural background, and the meaning of the pain to that person (e.g., the ways in which it affects the person's lifestyle). Factors that reduce pain tolerance include repeated exposure to pain, fatigue, sleep deprivation, and stress. Warmth, cold, distraction, alcohol consumption, hypnosis, and strong religious beliefs or faith increase pain tolerance (Price and Wilson, 2002).

The origins of pain can be divided into two types, somatic and visceral. Somatic pain arises from stimulation of receptors in the skin (superficial somatic pain) or from stimulation of receptors in skeletal muscles, joints, tendons, and fascia (deep somatic pain). Visceral pain results from stimulation of receptors in the viscera (internal organs).

The ability of the cerebral cortex to locate the origin of pain is related to past experience. In most instances of somatic pain and in some instances of visceral pain, the cortex accurately projects the pain back to the stimulated area.

Pain usually is classified as acute, chronic, intractable, phantom, or referred.

Acute Pain

Acute pain is either a symptom of a disease condition or a temporary aspect of medical treatment. It acts as a warning signal, because it can activate the sympathetic nervous system. Acute pain usually is temporary, of sudden onset, and easily localized. The client frequently can describe the pain, which often subsides with or without treatment. During acute pain, arousal of the sympathetic ANS occurs.

Chronic Pain

Chronic pain is a major health problem for approximately 25% of the population. Chronic pain is pain that persists or recurs for indefinite periods, usually for longer than 3 to 6 months. It frequently has an obscure onset, and the character and quality of the pain change over time. Anxiety, sleep disturbances, and depression are common. Chronic pain usually is diffuse and poorly localized and often requires the efforts of a multidisciplinary health care team, which may include a massage therapist, for effective management.

Intractable Pain

Chronic pain that persists even when treatment is provided or that exists without demonstrable disease is called *intractable pain*. Intractable pain represents the greatest challenge to all health care providers. Massage may provide short, temporary, symptomatic relief of this type of pain. This is accomplished by flooding the sensory receptors with sensation, distracting the client temporarily from the perception of pain.

Phantom Pain

Phantom pain is a type of pain frequently experienced by clients who have had a limb amputated. These clients experience pain or other sensations in the area of the amputated extremity as if the limb were still there. This pain probably occurs because the remaining proximal portions of the sensory nerves that previously received impulses from the limb are stimulated by the trauma of the amputation. Stimuli from these nerves are interpreted by the brain as coming from the nonexistent (phantom) limb.

Referred Pain

Pain may be felt in a surface area far from the stimulated organ; this is called **referred pain.** In general, the area or areas to which the pain is referred and the visceral organ involved receive their innervations from the same segment of the spinal cord. Figure 6-2 shows the cutaneous regions to which visceral pain may be referred. A client who has a recurring pain pattern

that resembles the patterns on the chart should be referred to a physician for a more specific diagnosis.

As already stated, irritation of the viscera frequently produces pain that is felt not in the viscera but in some somatic structure that may be located at a considerable distance. Such pain is said to be *referred* to the somatic structure. Deep somatic pain also may be referred, but superficial pain is not. When visceral pain is both local and referred, it sometimes seems to spread (radiate) from the local to the distant site. Visceral pain, like deep somatic pain, initiates reflex contraction of nearby skeletal muscle. Because somatic pain is much more common than visceral pain, the brain has "learned" to project the pain to the somatic area.

A knowledge of referred pain and the common sites of pain referral from each of the visceral organs is very important to massage therapists and other health care professionals. However, sites of reference are not invariable; unusual reference sites occur with considerable frequency. Heart pain, for instance, may be experienced as purely abdominal, or it may be referred to the right arm or even the neck. Any client with a referred or unexplained pain pattern should be referred to a physician, especially if the pattern is similar to visceral referred pain patterns (see Figure 6-2). When pain is referred, it usually is referred to a structure that developed from the same embryonic segment or dermatome as the structure in which the pain originates (Figure 6-3).

Evaluation of Pain

Because pain is a primary indicator in many disease processes, massage practitioners must have a basic evaluation protocol for pain so that they can determine when to refer their clients

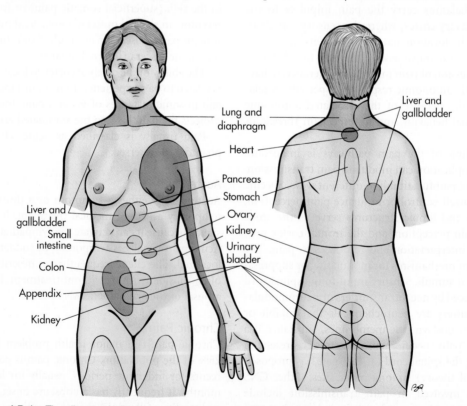

FIGURE 6-2 Referred Pain. The diagram indicates cutaneous areas to which visceral pain may be referred. If pain is encountered in these areas during a massage, the massage practitioner should refer the client to a physician for diagnosis to rule out visceral dysfunction.

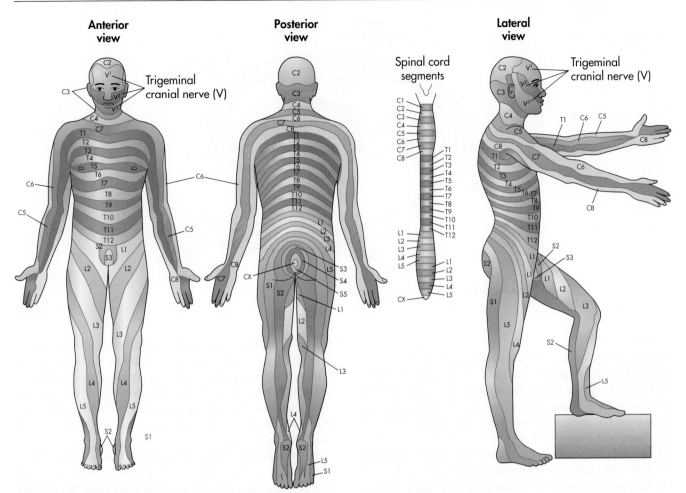

FIGURE 6-3 Dermatomes. Segmental dermatome distribution of spinal nerves to the front, back, and side of the body. *C,* Cervical segments; *T,* thoracic segments; *L,* lumbar segments; *S,* sacral segments; *CX,* coccygeal segments. (From Thibodeau GA, Patton KT: *The human body in health and disease,* ed 4, St Louis, 2010, Mosby.)

to the appropriate health care provider. The following guidelines for evaluating pain can help in this process:

Location of Pain
- *Localized pain* is confined to the site of origin of the pain.
- *Projected pain* typically is a result of proximal nerve compression. This pain is perceived in the tissue supplied by the nerve.
- *Radiating pain* is diffuse pain around the site of origin that is not well localized.
- *Referred pain* is felt in an area distant from the site of the painful stimulus.

Types of Pain
- *Pricking or bright pain:* This type of pain is experienced when the skin is cut or jabbed with a sharp object. It is short-lived but intense and easily localized.
- *Burning pain:* This type is slower to develop, lasts longer, and is less accurately localized. It is experienced when the skin is burned. It often stimulates cardiac and respiratory activity.
- *Aching pain:* Aching pain occurs when the visceral organs are stimulated. It is constant, not well localized, and often is referred to areas of the body far from where the damage is

occurring. This type of pain is important, because it may be a sign of a life-threatening disorder of a vital organ.
- *Deep pain:* The main difference between superficial and deep sensibility is the different nature of the pain evoked by noxious stimuli. Unlike superficial pain, deep pain is poorly localized, nauseating, and frequently associated with sweating and changes in blood pressure. This type of pain initiates reflex contraction of nearby skeletal muscles. This reflex contraction is similar to the muscle spasm associated with injuries to bones, tendons, and joints. The steadily contracting muscles become ischemic, and ischemia stimulates the pain receptors in the muscles. The pain, in turn, initiates more spasms, creating a vicious cycle called the **pain-spasm-pain cycle** (Figure 6-4).
- *Muscle pain:* If a muscle with an adequate blood supply contracts rhythmically, pain does not usually result. However, if the blood supply to a muscle is occluded (cut off), contraction soon causes pain. The pain persists after the contraction until blood flow is re-established. If a muscle with a normal blood supply is made to contract continuously without periods of relaxation, it also begins to ache, because the maintained contraction compresses the blood vessels supplying the muscle.

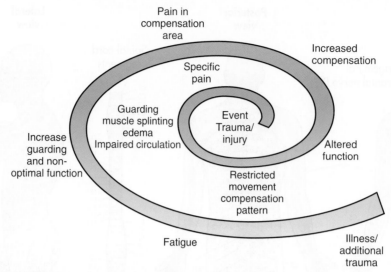

FIGURE 6-4 Pain-spasm-pain cycle.

Pain Assessment

Massage professionals gather subjective information by asking the client about symptoms associated with the pain. Practitioners should provide ample opportunity to discuss with the client what the pain means to that person by asking about its impact on the client's lifestyle. They also should document pain treatment methods the client has used in the past and the effectiveness of those methods. Direct observation of nonverbal and verbal behavior may provide additional clues to the client's pain experience. Nonverbal behaviors such as grimacing, flinching, tearing, abnormal gait or posture, muscle tension, and guarding of the body are common indicators of pain. Verbal and emotional signals indicating pain may include crying, moaning, groaning, irritability, sadness, and changes in voice tone.

Gender and cultural differences affect the types of displays people use to express pain. As described previously, acute pain often activates a sympathetic response, resulting in increases in the heart and respiratory rates and blood pressure, pallor, flushing, sweating, and pupil dilation. Very brief, intense pain may be followed by a rebound parasympathetic response, such as nausea and dizziness.

The massage practitioner should inspect and palpate the painful area to test the range of motion of involved joints, to determine whether muscle guarding is present, and to identify trigger points and other tender points of pain and areas of decreased sensation or increased sensitivity.

Indications for Massage

Pain is a complex problem with physical, psychological, social, and financial components. Subjective measurements of pain intensity are more reliable than observable ones. Pain scales, such as a 1 to 10 scale, are helpful for measuring necessary pain perception. Only the client can determine the degree of severity. Pain is rarely the same at all times. It is felt and perceived differently over time and differs with various precipitating and aggravating factors. Pain can range from excruciating to mild and may be difficult for the client to verbalize. Pain

can be alleviated in many ways. The massage professional, as part of a health care team, can contribute valuable manual therapy in various pain conditions using direct tissue manipulation and reflex stimulation of the nervous system and the circulation. As a therapeutic intervention, massage may help reduce the need for pain medication, thus reducing the side effects of medication.

All medications, including over-the-counter (OTC) drugs (i.e., those available without a prescription), have some side effects. Obviously, with clients in extreme pain, the massage therapy must be monitored by a physician or other appropriate health care professional. Most people experience pain in less severe forms occasionally throughout life. Massage may provide temporary symptomatic relief of moderate pain brought on by daily stress, replacing OTC pain medications or reducing their use.

Acute pain and chronic pain are managed somewhat differently; therefore, distinguishing between the two is important. Intervention for acute pain is less invasive and focuses on supporting a current healing process. Chronic pain is managed either with symptomatic relief or with a more aggressive rehabilitation approach that incorporates a therapeutic change process.

Impingement Syndromes

The two types of nerve **impingement syndromes** are compression and entrapment. As explained in Chapter 5, *compression* is pressure on a nerve by a bony structure, and *entrapment* is pressure on a nerve from soft tissue. Massage is beneficial for entrapment and can manage some symptoms of nerve compression, even though the direct causal factor is not addressed.

Cervical Plexus

The cervical plexus is formed by the upper four cervical nerves. The phrenic nerve is part of this plexus. It innervates the diaphragm, and any disruption to this nerve affects breathing. Many cutaneous (skin) branches of the cervical plexus transmit sensory impulses from the skin of the neck, ear, and shoulder. The motor branches innervate muscles of the anterior neck.

If the impingement is on the cervical plexus, the person experiences headaches, neck pain, and breathing difficulties. The muscles most responsible for pressure on the cervical plexus are the suboccipital and sternocleidomastoid muscles. Shortened connective tissues at the cranial base also can press on these nerves.

Brachial Plexus

The brachial plexus is situated partly in the neck and partly in nerves that innervate the upper limb. Any imbalance that brings pressure on this complex of nerves results in shoulder pain, chest pain, arm pain, wrist pain, or hand pain.

The muscles most often responsible for impingement on the brachial plexus are the scalenes, pectoralis minor, and subclavius. Muscles of the arm occasionally impinge on branches of the brachial plexus. Brachial plexus impingement is responsible for thoracic outlet symptoms, which often are misdiagnosed as carpal tunnel syndrome. Whiplash injury involves the brachial plexus.

Lumbar Plexus

Impingement on the lumbar plexus nerve may give rise to low back discomfort with a belt distribution of pain, in addition to pain in the lower abdomen, genitals, thigh, and medial lower leg. The main soft tissue structures that impinge on the lumbar plexus are the quadratus lumborum muscles and the associated fascia.

Sacral Plexus

The sacral plexus has approximately a dozen named branches. Almost half of these serve the buttock and lower limb; the others innervate pelvic structures. The main branch is the sciatic nerve. Impingement of this nerve by the piriformis muscle gives rise to sciatica. Ligaments that stabilize the sacroiliac joint can affect the sacral plexus. Pressure on the sacral plexus can cause gluteal pain, leg pain, genital pain, and foot pain.

Indications for Massage

Massage methods can soften, lengthen, and stretch connective tissues that may impinge on nerves. They also can normalize muscle tension patterns, restoring a more normal resting length to shortened muscles, thereby reducing pressure on nerves.

Psychological Dysfunctions

Science has validated the body/mind link in terms of health and disease. Many risk factors for the development of physical (body) pathologic conditions are mentally (mind) influenced, such as stress levels and lifestyle choices. The same is true for mental health and pathologic conditions of the mind. A person's physical state has a strong influence on mental functioning. Usually when people feel well physically, they also feel well mentally. The reverse, too, is often the case; feeling bad mentally results in physical dysfunctions. Neurochemicals such as serotonin and dopamine exert a strong influence on a person's mental state.

The major mental health dysfunctions that affect Western society are trauma and post-traumatic stress disorder, pain and fatigue syndromes, anxiety and depressive disorders, and stress-related illness.

Trauma is defined as (1) physical injury caused by violent or disruptive action or by a toxic substance or (2) psychic injury resulting from a severe emotional shock, either short term or long term.

Post-traumatic stress disorder (PTSD), as defined by the *Diagnostic and Statistical Manual of Mental Disorders (DSM-IV)*, includes flashback memory experiences, state-dependent memory, somatization, anxiety, irritability, sleep disturbance, concentration difficulties, times of melancholy or depression, grief, fear, worry, anger, and avoidance behavior. Post-traumatic stress disorder can have long-term effects.

Pain and fatigue syndromes are defined as multicausal and often chronic nonproductive patterns that interfere with well-being, activities of daily living, and productivity. Some conditions currently included in this category are fibromyalgia, chronic fatigue syndrome, Epstein-Barr viral infection, sympathetic reflex dystrophy, headache, arthritis, chronic cancer pain, neuropathy, low back syndrome, idiopathic pain, somatization disorder, and intractable pain syndrome. Acute pain can be a factor, as can acute "episodes" of chronic conditions.

Anxiety and depressive disorders are characterized by anxiety and depression. *Anxiety* is an uneasy feeling usually connected with increased sympathetic arousal responses. *Depression* is characterized by a decrease of vital functional activity and mood disturbances of exaggerated emptiness, hopelessness, and melancholy or unbridled periods of high energy with no purpose or outcome. Anxiety and depressive disorders commonly are seen with fatigue and pain syndromes. Panic behavior, phobias, and a sense of impending doom, along with the sense of being overwhelmed and hopeless, are common with these disorders. Mood swings, breathing pattern disorder, sleep disturbance, concentration difficulties, memory disturbances, outbursts of anger, fatigue, changes in habits of daily living, appetite, and activity levels are symptoms of these disorders.

Stress-related illness is defined as an increased stress load or reduced ability to adapt that depletes the reserve capacity of individuals, increasing their vulnerability to health problems. Stress-related illness can encompass the previously mentioned conditions as the primary cause of dysfunction or as the result of the stress of the dysfunction. Excessive stress sometimes manifests as cardiovascular problems, including hypertension; digestive difficulties, including heartburn, ulcer, and bowel syndromes; respiratory illness and susceptibility to bacterial and viral illness; endocrine dysfunction, particularly adrenal or thyroid dysfunction and delayed or reduced cellular repair; sleep disorders; and breathing pattern disorder, just to mention a few conditions (Proficiency Exercises 6-4 and 6-5).

PROFICIENCY EXERCISE 6-4

Student Note: *Take a crack at another case study. Follow the example case study and then give it a try. Remember, the more you practice, the more you will understand the process and the easier it will become.*

Read the case study presented under Your Turn. Then use the clinical reasoning model (presented in the example case study) to develop a statement validating the indication for the use of therapeutic massage. Answer the questions on a separate piece of paper.

Example Case Study

The client is a 46-year-old woman who works 6 to 8 hours a day on the computer. She is experiencing mind fatigue and midback tension with pain. Her left arm tingles during sleep and wakes her up. She has a chronic compressed disk at L4. Currently she is involved in a large writing project and has a deadline to meet. Her exercise and stretching program has become sporadic. She also finds herself regularly driving for 3 and 4 hours at a time, which aggravates the nerve impingement in her low back. What are the indications for massage?

1. Identify the facts.

Questions that can help with this process include the following:

- What is considered normal or balanced function?
  Answer: Regular movement without prolonged static positions.
- What has happened? (Spell out events.)
  Answer: Client's workload and a deadline are requiring more time at the computer. Long periods are required in the car. The client's exercise and stretching program has been interrupted.
- What caused the imbalance? (Can it be identified?)
  Answer: Static seated position with the arm held in fixed position.
- What was done or is being done?
  Answer: Exercise and stretching, but this pattern has been interrupted.
- What has worked or not worked?
  Answer: Exercise and stretching have helped, but this program has been interrupted.

2. Brainstorm the possibilities.

Questions that can help with this process include the following:

- What are the possibilities? (What could it all mean?)
  Answer:
  - Muscles could be shortening in the front, changing the posture and straining the back muscles.
  - Something may be interfering with circulation.
  - Nerves could be impinged.
  - Pain and increased tension could be contributing to mind fatigue.
- What is my intuition suggesting?
  Answer: The client is tired, overworked, and sitting in one position too long.
- What are the possible patterns of dysfunction?
  Answer: The existing back disk dysfunction could be causing compensation, which is being aggravated by the ongoing static seated position. A fixed position of the shoulder while driving or at the computer may cause muscle tension that is causing impingement on a nerve.

Stress from the deadline for the project is interfering with sleep.

- What are the possible contributing factors?
  Answer: Pre-existing back injury, age, improper posture at the computer, or an ergonomically incorrect chair
- What are possible interventions?
  Answer: Massage, stretching, exercise, progressive relaxation, changing the position of equipment.
- What might work?
  Answer: A combination of the possible interventions might be beneficial.
- What are other ways to look at the situation?
  Answer: The client has an excessive workload and is using equipment that is positioned to aggravate the problem.
- What do the data suggest?
  Answer: Multiple causal factors

3. Consider the logical outcomes of each possibility.

Questions that can help determine outcomes include the following:

- What is the logical progression of the symptom pattern, contributing factors, and current behaviors?
  Answer: If the condition remains unchanged, the symptoms are likely to worsen. Possibly, after the client has met her deadline, the main causal factor will be eliminated and the condition may reverse itself.
- What are the pros and cons and the logical effect of each intervention suggested?
  Answer:
  - Massage—reduces muscle tension, supports sleep; requires time away from work; effects may be short term. Massage may provide temporary relief until the condition changes.
  - Stretching—can be done throughout the day; would not require time away from job; effects are short-lived. Stretching would temporarily relieve the tension pattern and provide a counterbalancing activity to the static seated position.
  - Exercise—reduces muscle tension, supports sleep, clears mind fatigue; requires time away from work; effects may be short term. Exercise may provide temporary relief until the condition changes while supporting ongoing health maintenance.
  - Progressive relaxation—supports sleep and helps relieve muscle tension; can be done throughout the day; would not require time away from job; effects are short-lived. Progressive relaxation would provide some symptomatic relief.
  - Changing position of equipment—would address a possible causal factor; would not require any other energy expenditure; would not address emotional stress or physical symptoms. If equipment position is a causal factor, a change may eliminate a source of the problem.
- What are the consequences of not acting?
  Answer: The situation may worsen, or it may resolve after the writing project has been completed.
- What are the consequences of acting?
  Answer: Symptoms and further compensation patterns may be managed.

4. Identify the effect of each possibility on the people involved.

Questions that can help identify effects include the following:

💡 PROFICIENCY EXERCISE 6-4—cont'd

- For each intervention considered, what would be the impact on the people involved: client, practitioner, and other professionals working with the client.
  Answer:
  - Massage—pleasurable but time consuming for client
  - Stretching—can be incorporated into daily activities and is pleasurable for client
  - Exercise—client may avoid and can be perceived as time consuming
  - Progressive relaxation—client may use for supporting sleep and does not involve extensive time commitment, so she may enjoy
  - Changing position of equipment—may be confusing for the client but has potential for being beneficial
- How does each person involved feel about the possible interventions?
  Answer:
  - Massage—Client is supportive, massage therapist is supportive.
  - Stretching—Client is supportive.
  - Exercise—Client is supportive.
  - Progressive relaxation—Client does not feel that benefits are sufficient to justify time spent.
  - Changing position of equipment—Client is supportive.
- Is the practitioner within his or her scope of practice to work with such situations?
  Answer: Yes
- Is the practitioner qualified to work with such situations?
  Answer: Yes, with cautions for disk compression.
- Does the practitioner feel qualified to work with such situations?
  Answer: Yes
- Does a feeling of cooperation and agreement exist among all parties involved?
  Answer: Yes

5. Result of the process.
Based on this analysis of the information provided, the massage practitioner would recommend massage, stretching, exercise, and an equipment change, for the following reasons:

- The condition is short term until the writing project has been finished.
- The client has previously used stretching and exercise and needs encouragement to begin to use those methods again.
- Minor changes in the position of the computer may offer benefits.
- Massage is indicated to support sleep and address the general stress, the possible minor nerve impingement, the muscle tension from the static position, and management of muscle pain.

Your Turn
Case Study
The client is an 81-year-old man who is in good health for his age. His wife died 18 months ago after a long illness. He is active in his church and works in his garden. He fell 6 months ago but recovered nicely. Lately his age-related aches and pains are bothering him more, especially in his knees. This is interfering with his activities. He has mild hypertension and is taking medication for the condition. Currently the hypertension is under control. He takes aspirin for his arthritis as needed. No problems were detected during his last physical. What are the indications for massage?

1. Identify the facts.
Questions that can help with this process include the following:
- What is considered normal or balanced function?

- What has happened? (Spell out events.)

- What caused the imbalance? (Can it be identified?)

- What was done or is being done?

- What has worked or not worked?

2. Brainstorm the possibilities.
Questions that can help with this process include the following:
- What are the possibilities? (What could it all mean?)

- What is my intuition suggesting?

- What are the possible patterns of dysfunction?

- What are the possible contributing factors?

- What are possible interventions?

- What might work?

- What are other ways to look at the situation?

- What do the data suggest?

3. Consider the logical outcomes of each possibility.
Questions that can help determine outcomes include the following:
- What is the logical progression of the symptom pattern, contributing factors, and current behaviors?

- What are the pros and cons and the logical effect of each intervention suggested?

- What are the consequences of not acting?

- What are the consequences of acting?

4. Identify the effect of each possibility on the people involved.
Questions that can help identify effects include the following:
- For each intervention considered, what would be the impact on the people involved: client, practitioner, and other professionals working with the client?

Continued

💡 PROFICIENCY EXERCISE 6-4—cont'd

- How does each person involved feel about the possible interventions?

- Is the practitioner within his or her scope of practice to work with such situations?

- Is the practitioner qualified to work with such situations?

- Does the practitioner feel qualified to work with such situations?

- Does a feeling of cooperation and agreement exist among all parties involved?

5. Result of the process.

Based on this analysis of the information provided, the massage practitioner would recommend _____, for the following reasons:

💡 PROFICIENCY EXERCISE 6-5

1. Do a self-evaluation and list all your predisposing risk factors for disease in the space provided.
2. Pick one risk factor. Research a wellness plan to provide support for your body to prevent or reduce the likelihood of your developing the pathologic condition. Summarize the condition.

Indications for Massage

Massage intervention has a strong physiologic effect through the comfort of compassionate touch, in addition to a physical influence on mental state through the effect on the ANS and neurochemicals. Therefore, people experiencing mental health problems may benefit from massage. Management of pain is an important factor if the client is experiencing pain. Because therapeutic massage often can offer symptomatic relief from chronic pain, the helplessness that accompanies these difficulties may dissipate as the person realizes that management methods exist. Soothing of any ANS hyperactivity or hypoactivity provides a sense of inner balance. Normalization of the breathing mechanism allows the client to breathe without restriction and can reduce the tendency for breathing pattern disorder, which feeds anxiety and panic.

Therapeutic massage can provide intervention on a physical level to restore a more normal function to the body, which supports appropriate interventions by qualified mental health professionals. Certainly strong and appropriate indications exist for the use of massage therapy in the restoration of mental health, but caution is indicated in terms of the establishment of dual roles and boundary difficulties. It is very important to work with mental health providers in these situations.

CONTRAINDICATIONS TO MASSAGE THERAPY

SECTION OBJECTIVES

Chapter objective covered in this section:

5. The student will be able to identify contraindications to massage and develop massage adaptations to support any cautions identified.

Using the information presented in this section, the student will be able to perform the following:

- Evaluate a client's status to determine whether massage is contraindicated
- Interpret the reference list of indications and contraindications in Appendix A
- Interpret the basic pharmacology information in Appendix C
- Recognize the warning signs of cancer
- List the endangerment sites for massage
- Effectively refer a client to a primary health care provider

As mentioned earlier in this chapter, a contraindication is any condition that renders a particular treatment improper or undesirable or that raises cautions concerning treatment, requiring supervision. Contraindications to massage are the responsibility of both physicians and massage practitioners. The massage professional is not expected to diagnose any condition but should learn the client's particular condition by taking a thorough history and completing a physical assessment. The massage professional must be able to recognize indications and contraindications for therapeutic massage based on this information.

In general, massage is indicated for musculoskeletal discomfort, circulation enhancement, relaxation, stress reduction, and pain control and also for situations in which analgesics, antiinflammatory drugs, muscle relaxants, and blood pressure, antianxiety, and antidepressant medications may be prescribed. Therapeutic massage, appropriately provided, can support the use of these medications, manage some side effects, and in mild cases may be able to replace them.

The general effects of stress and pain reduction and increased circulation, in addition to the physical comfort derived from therapeutic massage, complement most other medical and mental health treatment modalities. However, when other therapies, including medication, are used, the physician must be able to evaluate accurately the effectiveness of each treatment the client is receiving. If the physician is unaware that the client is receiving massage, the effects of other therapies may be misinterpreted.

Clients with any vague or unexplainable symptoms of fatigue, muscle weakness, and general aches and pains should be immediately referred to a physician. Many disease processes share these symptoms. This recommendation may seem overly cautious, but in the early stages of some very serious illnesses, the symptoms are not well defined. If the physician is able to detect a disease process early in its development, often a more successful outcome is possible. A specific diagnosis is essential for effective treatment. Massage should be avoided in all infectious diseases suggested by fever, nausea, and lethargy until a diagnosis has been made and recommendations from a physician can be followed.

Massage practitioners should not rely on lists of specific contraindications, but rather should use a set of medical and therapeutic guidelines pertinent to clinical applications and recent research developments. Unfortunately, such guidelines are not consistent in current literature.

Contraindications are unique to each client and to each region of the body. The ability to reason clinically is essential to making appropriate decisions about the advisability of, modifications to, or avoidance of massage interventions. It is important to understand when to refer a client for diagnosis and when to obtain assistance in modifying the approach to the massage session so that it will best serve the client. A medical professional (including mental health and athletic training) must always be consulted if any doubt exists concerning the advisability of therapy. When in doubt, refer!

Contraindications can be divided into regional and general types, and each type can involve avoidance or application with caution and appropriate massage adaptations.

- *Regional contraindications* relate to a specific area of the body. For our purposes, a regional contraindication means that massage may be provided but not to the problematic area. However, the client should be referred to a physician, who can make a diagnosis and rule out underlying conditions.
- *General contraindications* require a physician's evaluation to rule out serious underlying conditions before any massage is indicated. Mental health dysfunctions fall into this category.

Cautions

As mentioned earlier, a caution is a condition that requires the massage therapist to adapt the massage process so that the client's safety is maintained. Common adaptations required by cautions include the type of massage lubricant used, depth of pressure, duration of the massage, client positioning, avoidance of a type of massage application, and so forth. Consider the following examples:

- An elderly female client has osteoporosis and thinning skin. Both of these conditions are cautions for massage application. Adaptation of the massage to benefit this client would include careful monitoring of the depth of pressure and using enough lubricant to reduce friction on the skin.
- A middle-aged male client has plantar fasciitis. Two days ago he received a cortisone injection at the site of inflammation. The caution is the site of the injection; the area needs to be avoided.
- Therapeutic massage often is beneficial for clients receiving treatment for a specific medical or mental health condition and for clients involved in a training program, such as a dancer or gymnast. However, caution is indicated because of the demands these circumstances place on the client's body, and the massage application must be adapted according to the client's situation.

If a physician recommends massage, he or she must help the massage therapist develop a comprehensive treatment plan that includes appropriate cautions.

Medications

The massage professional needs to be aware of any medications the client takes. Massage therapists should have a current edition of *Mosby's Drug Consult, Physicians' Desk Reference, Medical Economics,* or a similar drug reference book so that all medications listed on the client information form can be researched. Internet programs for researching medications also are available. In addition, clients may be able to provide information about each medication they take.

In general, a medication is prescribed to do one of the following:

- Stimulate a body process
- Inhibit a body process
- Replace a chemical in the body

Therapeutic massage also can stimulate, inhibit, and replace body functions. When the medication and massage stimulate the same process, the effects are synergistic, and the result can be too much stimulation. If the medication and massage inhibit the same process, the result again is synergistic, but this time with too much inhibition. If the medication stimulates an effect and massage inhibits the same effect, massage can be antagonistic to the medication. Although massage seldom interacts substantially with a medication that replaces a body chemical, it is important to be aware of possible synergistic or inhibitory effects.

Massage often can be used to manage undesirable side effects of medications. In particular, medications that stimulate sympathetic ANS function can cause uncomfortable side effects, such as digestive upset, constipation, anxiety or restlessness, and sleep disruption. The mild inhibitory effects of massage resulting from stimulation of parasympathetic activity sometimes can provide short-term relief of the undesirable effects of the medication without interfering with its desired action. Especially in these instances, caution is required, as is close monitoring by the primary care physician. For example, a side effect of some medications is anxiety. Massage may help the client by reducing anxiety, or it may be the cause of an adverse reaction. If the physician is using the client's level of anxiety to monitor the correct medication dosage and if anxiety levels are lowered through massage, the medication dosage may appear to be too high.

Massage professionals should be able to assess the effects of medications and should be aware of the ways massage may influence these effects. Massage practitioners need to be especially knowledgeable about antiinflammatory drugs, muscle relaxants, anticoagulants (blood thinners), analgesics (pain modulators), and other medications that alter sensation, muscle tone, standard reflex reactions, cardiovascular function, kidney or liver function, or personality. They also should be aware of the effects of OTC medications, herbs, and vitamins. If a client takes medication, it is important to have the physician confirm the advisability of therapeutic massage. Appendix C presents information on basic pharmacology and a list of common medications and possible interactions with massage.

Box 6-2 Warning Signs of Cancer

- Sores that do not heal
- Unusual bleeding
- A change in the appearance or size of a wart or mole
- A lump or thickening in any tissue
- Persistent hoarseness or cough
- Chronic indigestion
- A change in bowel or bladder function

Tumors and Cancer

Benign tumors remain localized within the tissue from which they arise and usually grow very slowly. Malignant tumors (cancer) tend to spread to other regions of the body. The cells migrate by way of lymphatic or blood vessels; this manner of spread is called metastasis. Cells that do not metastasize also can spread by growing rapidly and extending the tumor into nearby tissues. Malignant tumors may replace part of a vital organ with abnormal tissue, which is a life-threatening situation.

Early detection of cancer is important, because cancer is most treatable in the early stages of primary tumor development, before metastasis and the development of secondary tumors. Box 6-2 presents the warning signs of cancer, as summarized by oncologists (cancer specialists). The massage practitioner may be the first to recognize these early warning signs in a client.

Although it is important to refer the client for proper evaluation so that it can be determined whether cancer is developing, the massage practitioner must never suggest to the client that cancer is evident. Instead, the practitioner should simply point out changes and explain the importance of having them evaluated by a qualified professional.

Massage is not necessarily contraindicated for people with cancer. Current research indicates that massage can support the immune system's battle with cancer cells and manage the side effects of treatment. However, massage must be used as part of the entire treatment program and supervised by qualified medical personnel. As with any stressful condition, the massage practitioner must not overtax the system of a client with cancer; instead, massage must be used as a general support to the body's healing mechanisms.

Endangerment Sites

An endangerment site is an area on the body where it is possible to do damage. When the massage therapist is working over an endangerment site, avoidance or light pressure is indicated to prevent damage. Endangerment sites include areas in which nerves and blood vessels surface close to the skin and are not well protected by muscle or connective tissue. Deep, sustained pressure in these areas can damage the vessels and nerves; however, surface gliding with light pressure is appropriate. Areas containing fragile bony projections that could be broken off also are considered endangerment sites; surface gliding with light pressure also is appropriate in these areas. The kidney area is considered an endangerment site, because the kidneys are loosely suspended in fat and connective tissue.

PROFICIENCY EXERCISE 6-6

Locate all of the following endangerment sites on a fellow student:
- Brachial artery
- Basilic vein
- Cubital (anterior) area of the median nerve, radial and ulnar arteries, and median cubital vein
- Deep stripping over a vein in a direction away from the heart (contraindicated because of possible damage to the valve system)
- Knees (application of lateral pressure)
- Ankle area (some acupuncture authorities consider this to be an endangerment site for pregnant women)

Heavy pounding is contraindicated in that area; however, other massage methods are appropriate. The areas shown in Figure 6-5 are commonly considered endangerment sites for the massage therapist (Proficiency Exercise 6-6). Other endangerment sites include the following:
- Eyes
- Area inferior to the ear (fascial nerve, styloid process, external carotid artery)
- Posterior cervical area (spinous processes, cervical plexus)
- Lymph nodes
- Medial brachium (between the biceps and triceps)
- Musculocutaneous, median, and ulnar nerves

Referral

Referral is a method by which a client is sent to a health care professional for diagnosis and treatment of a disease. Massage professionals may pick up subtle changes in the tissue before the client consciously recognizes that something is out of balance. When this happens, the client should be referred to a qualified professional for a specific diagnosis.

Massage practitioners should become familiar with the health professionals in their area, including medical doctors, osteopathic doctors, podiatrists, chiropractors, physical therapists, occupational therapists, psychologists, licensed counselors, athletic trainers, exercise physiologists, and dentists. Some health care providers offer alternative therapies, such as acupuncture and homeopathy. Because clients trust the massage practitioner, the practitioner should take the time to get to know a health professional before referring a client to him or her. This can be done by calling the professional's office and making an appointment for a short visit, during which the professional's feelings about massage could be discussed. Information about massage should be left for reference.

Clients must always be referred to their personal health care professionals. The massage therapist should make no attempt to direct them to different health care professionals. If the client does not have a doctor, chiropractor, or counselor, a list of professionals who have been contacted and educated about therapeutic massage should be provided.

When referral is indicated, the massage practitioner should simply tell the client the reason for recommending referral to a health care professional, explaining that the observed set of

Evolve Activity 6-2   Evolve Activity 6-3

signs or symptoms should be evaluated by someone with more specialized training (Box 6-3). No specific condition should be named. The client should be given the massage professional's business card or brochure to give to the health care professional to facilitate contact. The client must sign a release of information before information can be exchanged between professionals.

If the massage therapist believes that referral of a client for diagnosis is necessary, the therapist needs some sort of written permission from the doctor to continue to see the client. The client should obtain the written documentation and bring it to the next massage session. This information is kept in the client's file. If the doctor or other health care professional has given any specific directions or recommendations, they must be followed exactly.

Massage therapy must never interfere with or contradict the physician's care plan, nor should the massage therapist assume the role of counselor. If the health care professional must be contacted directly, the massage professional should always work through the receptionist. Leave whatever information is needed with the front desk; if the doctor believes that speaking with the massage therapist directly is important, he or she will call.

The reason for referral and the date of referral must be noted on the client's record, along with the signs and symptoms. If the client responds in any unusual way, such as by panicking or refusing to go to the doctor, this must be indicated in the client's record. The written permission for continuation of massage from the health professional must be placed in the client's file.

Most disease processes present with a few basic symptoms (see Appendix A). A client should always be referred for diagnosis if the symptoms listed in Box 6-4 do not have a logical explanation (e.g., if the client has been up late or working long hours, naturally he or she will show the symptom of fatigue). Massage practitioners should use common sense tempered with accurate information and caution (Proficiency Exercises 6-7 and 6-8).

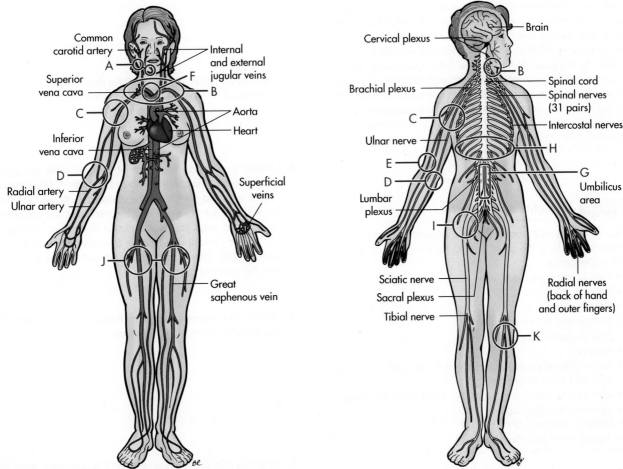

FIGURE 6-5 Endangerment sites of the nervous system and the cardiovascular system. *A,* Anterior triangle of the neck—carotid artery, jugular vein, and vagus nerve, which are located deep to the sternocleidomastoid muscle. *B,* Posterior triangle of the neck—specifically the nerves of the brachial plexus, the brachiocephalic artery and vein superior to the clavicle, and the subclavian arteries and vein. *C,* Axillary area—brachial artery, axillary vein and artery, cephalic vein, and nerves of the brachial plexus. *D,* Medial epicondyle of the humerus—ulnar nerve; also the radial and ulnar arteries. *E,* Lateral epicondyle—radial nerve. *F,* Area of the sternal notch and anterior throat—nerves and vessels to the thyroid gland and the vagus nerve. *G,* Umbilicus area—to either side; descending aorta and abdominal aorta. *H,* Twelfth rib, dorsal body—location of the kidney. *I,* Sciatic notch—sciatic nerve (the sciatic nerve passes out of the pelvis through the greater sciatic foramen, under cover of the piriformis muscle). *J,* Inguinal triangle located lateral and inferior to the pubis—medial to the sartorius, external iliac artery, femoral artery, great saphenous vein, femoral vein, and femoral nerve. *K,* Popliteal fossa—popliteal artery and vein and tibial nerve.

Box 6-3 Example of a Referral by a Massage Therapist

Sandy, a veteran massage practitioner, has been seeing a client, Ms. Jones, every other week for massage for about 1 year. Ms. Jones has a mole on her left shoulder. At the previous two visits, Sandy noticed that the mole had started to change shape and looked different, and she thinks these signs should be evaluated by a health care professional with more specific training. She says to Ms. Jones, "The mole you have on your left shoulder looks a little different to me. Have you noticed any change? It's important to have your doctor look at any changes in a mole. Will you please make an appointment with your personal physician to have the mole examined? Have your doctor give you a written statement that you were seen and that massage may be continued, along with any special instructions. It's important for you to do this before we schedule the next massage. After I determine that it's a good idea to refer a client to a doctor, and I put that on your record, I will need written verification from the doctor to see you again."

If the client does not have a personal physician, Sandy could say, "I have talked with various health care professionals in our area and have developed a referral list. I am sure one of the doctors listed will be able to help you, or you can ask a family member or friend for a recommendation."

Ms. Jones says, "What do you think the change in the mole means?" Sandy replies, "I'm trained to notice changes in the body and indicators that I should refer a client. However, I'm not trained to diagnose any specific condition; that's the role of a physician. You need to have the mole checked by someone with much more training in this area."

Box 6-4 Indications for Referral

If any of the following conditions are present and cannot be explained logically, the client should be referred to a health care professional:

- Pain (local, sharp, dull, achy, deep, superficial)
- Fatigue
- Inflammation
- Lumps and tissue changes
- Rashes and changes in the skin
- Edema
- Mood alterations (e.g., depression or anxiety)
- Infection (local or general)
- Changes in habits (e.g., appetite, elimination, or sleep)
- Bleeding and bruising
- Nausea, vomiting, and diarrhea
- Temperature (hot [fever] or cold)

💡 PROFICIENCY EXERCISE 6-7

1. Using the reference section in Appendix A, list five regional contraindications to massage that you have encountered (or that you think you may encounter) with clients.
   a.

   b.

   c.

   d.

   e.

2. List the five general contraindications you think you will encounter most often.
   a.

   b.

   c.

   d.

   e.

3. Using Appendix A, list two specific disease conditions that correspond to the seven warning signs listed in Box 6-2.
   a.

   b.

4. Choose a condition from each of the categories in Appendix A. Pretend that clients display symptoms of that condition or use role playing in the classroom, having a fellow student act out the signs and symptoms of the condition. Write down what you would notice about each condition that would prompt you to refer the client to a health care professional. Also write down or act out a referral process with the pretend client.

5. Choose two medications from Appendix C and describe the possible interactions with massage.
   a.

   b.

6. On a separate piece of paper or on the computer, write the names of health care providers in your area whom you would like to include in a referral list. Because these providers would need to support your work, set up a plan to meet and interview each one. Prepare a list of questions you should ask and information you must provide about your skills. Include at least three professionals in each category of your referral list so that the client has a choice. If time permits, contact these people while you are still a student.

PROFICIENCY EXERCISE 6-8

Student Note: *Keep practicing the clinical reasoning process. Keep working at answering the questions. It's okay to be frustrated; just keep practicing. Remember, many times there's no correct answer—just (in your opinion) an effective decision to be made.*

After reading the case study, use the clinical reasoning model to identify whether contraindications exist for the use of therapeutic massage and whether referral is necessary. If you determine that referral is necessary, list the reasons for it.

Case Study

A 32-year-old woman wants to try massage for stress management and for pain management for headaches. A coworker had recommended massage therapy. Over the past 3 months, the client has been increasingly unable to maintain her work schedule, and work time missed is increasing to the point where her job is in jeopardy. She is a production line worker in a small plastics factory. The work environment has adequate ventilation but requires repetitive movement of the arms. She is getting afternoon headaches almost daily. She has been moody and temperamental, which is unusual for her. Her weight has risen by 15 pounds over the past year. She exercises sporadically and crash-diets. She is single and has no children, but she has close family ties in a nearby town. Her last physical examination was 5 years ago, and at that point no problems were identified. Her menstrual cycle is somewhat erratic, and she had episodes of heavy bleeding during her last two periods. She is prone to hay fever and is currently self-medicating with an OTC antihistamine. She takes aspirin for the headaches and also a multivitamin tablet. She takes no other medications. She thinks the cause of her problems is job stress, but she does not feel that a job change is possible at this time.

1. Identify the facts.

Questions that can help with this process include the following:

- What is considered normal or balanced function?

- What has happened? (Spell out events.)

- What caused the imbalance? (Can it be identified?)

- What was done or is being done?

- What has worked or not worked?

2. Brainstorm the possibilities.

Questions that can help with this process include the following:

- What are the possibilities? (What could it all mean?)

- What is my intuition suggesting?

- What are the possible patterns of dysfunction?

- What are the possible contributing factors?

- What are possible interventions?

- What might work?

- What are other ways to look at the situation?

- What do the data suggest?

3. Consider the logical outcomes of each possibility.

Questions that can help determine outcomes include the following:

- What is the logical progression of the symptom pattern, contributing factors, and current behaviors?

- What are the pros and cons and the logical effect of each intervention suggested?

- What are the consequences of not acting?

- What are the consequences of acting?

4. Identify the effect of each possibility on the people involved.

Questions that can help identify effects include the following:

- For each intervention considered, what would be the impact on the people involved: client, practitioner, and other professionals working with the client?

- How does each person involved feel about the possible interventions?

- Is the practitioner within his or her scope of practice to work with such situations?

- Is the practitioner qualified to work with such situations?

- Does the practitioner feel qualified to work with such situations?

- Does a feeling of cooperation and agreement exist among all parties involved?

5. Result of the process.

Based on this analysis of the information provided, the massage practitioner would recommend _____, for the following reasons:

⊡ FOOT IN THE DOOR

If you want to get your foot in the door and boost your chances of career success, you must learn how to think and justify the results of that thinking. Clients, employers, and health care professionals who refer clients expect you to know when massage can help or harm and why. Results that meet goals ensure career success. No recipes or checklists are used for massage application. Each client requires individualized and adaptive massage application. You can get your foot in the door by looking and acting professional, being business savvy, using medical terminology correctly, having good documentation skills, and being able to look up and analyze research. However, you won't be kept in the practice if you cannot develop and implement appropriate and effective massage care.

SUMMARY

Indications for massage are based on the physiologic effects that provide the benefits of massage. Massage is beneficial for most people; however, contraindications do exist. Responsible massage professionals always refer a client for diagnosis and treatment by a qualified health professional, without delay, as soon as they notice any condition that may suggest an underlying physical or mental health problem. After the condition has been diagnosed and appropriate treatment has been established, the massage professional may provide massage under the supervision of a medical professional. Massage may prove beneficial and supportive to the interventions of the health care professional and may enhance the healing process by temporarily reducing pain, relaxing the client, reducing stress responses, increasing circulation, and much more. In addition, the one-on-one contact given by the massage professional may provide support and compassionate touch during a difficult time, thereby reducing the feelings of frustration, isolation, anxiety, and depression that often accompany illness or periods of stress.

⊖volve

http://evolve.elsevier.com/Fritz/fundamentals/

6-1 Review pathological condition terminology

6-2 Categorize several pathologies into "indicated" or "contraindicated" columns.

6-3 Read two pathology-related case studies—one on shingles and one on eczema—and answer true/false questions at the end.

6-4 Complete a vocabulary-building exercise with terms from this chapter.

6-5 Indications and contraindications: know them well enough to Beat the Clock!

Don't forget to study for your certification and licensure exams! Review questions, along with weblinks, can be found on the Evolve website.

References

Anderson K, Anderson LE, Glanze WE: *Mosby's medical, nursing, and allied health dictionary*, ed 8, St Louis, 2008, Mosby.

Goodman C, Fuller K: *Pathology: implications for the physical therapist*, ed 3, St Louis, 2008, Saunders.

Price SA, Wilson LM: *Pathophysiology: clinical concepts of disease processes*, ed 6, St Louis, 2002, Mosby.

Workbook Section

Short Answer

1. What is an indication for a massage?

2. What is a contraindication to a massage?

3. Name and define three approaches to care.

4. Define health.

5. What is dysfunction as defined in this text and how is massage beneficial in dysfunctional situations?

6. How do acute and chronic conditions affect homeostasis?

7. Why would a massage practitioner need to be aware of risk factors?

8. Why does the massage practitioner need to understand tumor pathology?

9. Why does the massage therapist need to understand the inflammatory response?

10. Define therapeutic inflammation.

11. Under what conditions should therapeutic inflammation not be used?

12. Why is pain difficult to describe?

13. What would the benefits of massage be for acute pain, chronic pain, and intractable pain?

14. What is the difference between localized pain, radiating pain, referred pain, and projected pain?

15. What is the difference between somatic and visceral pain?

16. Why is a knowledge of referred pain patterns important?

17. What role do dermatomes play in the pain pattern?

18. What is phantom pain?

19. What is the difference between entrapment and compression impingement and when is massage most indicated?

20. What are endangerment sites?

21. What are some important warning signs that indicate the client should be referred to a physician for specific diagnosis?

22. What resource materials should massage practitioners have available to help them understand medications and terminology?

23. Why should the massage therapist understand the actions of medications?

24. How do you refer a client to a health care professional?

25. How can the student best make use of Appendix C, which provides information on massage interactions with medications?

Matching I

Match the term to the best definition.

_____ **1.** Acute pain
_____ **2.** Chronic diseases
_____ **3.** Chronic pain
_____ **4.** Contraindication
_____ **5.** Disease
_____ **6.** Endangerment site
_____ **7.** General contraindications
_____ **8.** Health
_____ **9.** Homeostasis
_____ **10.** Indication
_____ **11.** Inflammatory response
_____ **12.** Intractable
_____ **13.** Metastasis
_____ **14.** Pain
_____ **15.** Pain-spasm-pain cycle
_____ **16.** Pathology
_____ **17.** Phantom pain
_____ **18.** Referral
_____ **19.** Referred pain
_____ **20.** Regeneration
_____ **21.** Regional contraindications
_____ **22.** Risk factors
_____ **23.** Signs
_____ **24.** Somatic pain
_____ **25.** Stress
_____ **26.** Symptoms
_____ **27.** Syndrome
_____ **28.** Visceral pain

a. Tumor cell migration by way of lymphatic or blood vessels

b. An unpleasant sensory and emotional experience associated with actual or perceived tissue damage or described in terms of such damage

c. A warning signal that activates the sympathetic nervous system; it can be a symptom of a disease or a temporary aspect of medical treatment; it usually is temporary, of sudden onset, and easily localized

d. Dynamic equilibrium of the internal environment of the body through the processes of feedback and regulation

e. Diseases that develop slowly and last for a long time

f. Pain arising from stimulation of receptors in the skin or skeletal muscles, joints, tendons, and fascia

g. Any substantial change in routine or any activity that requires the body to adapt, including changes for the better and for the worse

h. A diffuse, poorly localized discomfort that persists or recurs for indefinite periods, usually for more than 6 months

i. Subjective abnormalities felt only by the patient

j. A collection of different signs and symptoms, usually having a common cause, that present a clear picture of a pathologic condition

k. Pain that results from stimulation of receptors in the internal organs

l. An abnormality in a body function that threatens well-being

m. A healing process in which new cells are similar to those they replace

n. A method for sending a client to a health care professional for specific diagnosis and treatment of a disease

o. A therapeutic application that promotes health or assists in a healing process

p. Any condition that renders a particular treatment improper or undesirable

q. A normal mechanism that usually speeds recovery from an infection or injury characterized by pain, heat, redness, and swelling

r. Physical, mental, and social well-being, not merely the absence of disease

s. The study of disease

t. A kind of pain frequently experienced by patients who have had a limb amputated

u. A steady contraction of muscles that causes them to become ischemic, which stimulates the pain receptors in the muscles; the pain, in turn, initiates more spasms, setting up a vicious cycle

v. Chronic pain that persists even when treatment is provided or that exists without demonstrable disease

w. An area of the body where nerves and blood vessels surface close to the skin and are not well protected by muscle or connective tissue; deep, sustained pressure into these areas could damage these vessels and nerves

x. Findings that require a physician's evaluation to rule out serious underlying conditions before any massage is indicated

y. Contraindications that relate to a specific area of the body

z. Predisposing conditions that may make a person more likely to develop a disease than some other person

aa. Objective abnormalities that can be seen or measured by someone other than the client

bb. Pain felt in an area different from the source of the pain

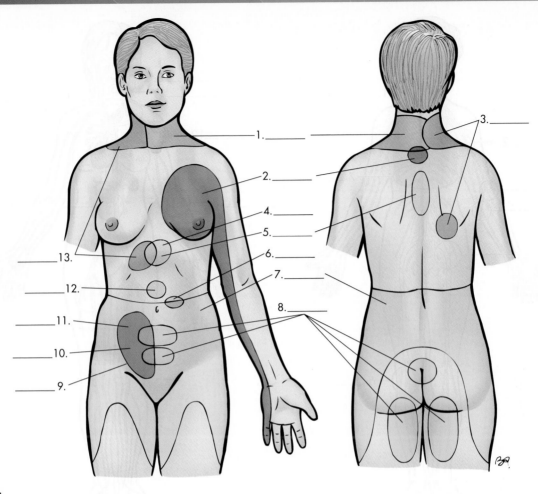

FIGURE 6-6

Matching II

Match the correct terms with the primary responses 1 or 2.

1. Heat and redness
2. Swelling and pain

_____ **a.** Release of histamine, prostaglandins, and kinins
_____ **b.** Increased permeability of vessel walls
_____ **c.** Enlargement of lymph nodes
_____ **d.** Dilation of blood vessels
_____ **e.** Triggering of pain receptors by pressure from edema
_____ **f.** Irritant diluted through excess fluid
_____ **g.** Destruction of bacteria by white blood cells
_____ **h.** Increase in blood volume

Labeling I

Label the endangerment sites in Figure 6-6 with the corresponding letter or letters from the following list (terms may be used more than once).

A. Urinary bladder
B. Colon
C. Appendix
D. Heart

E. Lung and diaphragm
F. Liver and gallbladder
G. Ovary
H. Pancreas
I. Small intestine
J. Kidney
K. Stomach

Labeling II

Label the endangerment sites in Figure 6-7 with the corresponding letter or letters from the following list (terms may be used more than once).

A. Anterior triangle of neck
B. Posterior triangle of neck
C. Axillary nerve
D. Ulnar nerve
E. Radial nerve
F. Vagus nerve, nerves and vessels to thyroid gland
G. Abdominal and descending aorta
H. Kidney
I. Sciatic nerve
J. Inguinal triangle

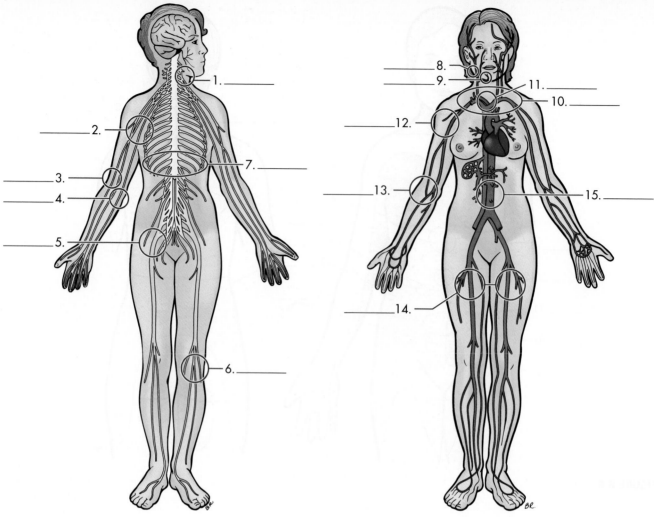

FIGURE 6-7

K. Tibial nerve, popliteal artery and nerve
L. Kidney

Risk Factors

1. List all the risk factors for developing disease. Then, in separate columns, list your personal risk factors and the risk factors of two friends.

2. When interviewing a client or doing a massage, how would you determine whether the person has any of the possible warning signs of cancer? Using the following list, explain how or when you would discover the warning sign if the client did not reveal it.
   - Sores that do not heal
   - Unusual bleeding
   - A change in a wart or mole
   - A lump or thickening in any tissue
   - Persistent hoarseness or cough
   - Chronic indigestion
   - A change in bowel or bladder function

   Example answer: Sores that do not heal—Noticed during proper draping techniques; skin on body has open wounds.

Assess Your Competencies

Now that you have studied this chapter, you should be able to:
- Define the terms *indication* and *contraindication*
- Define therapeutic change, condition management, and palliative care as therapeutic approaches
- Develop a basic understanding of pathology and use the knowledge to determine indications and contraindications for massage
- Identify contraindications to massage and develop massage adaptations to support any cautions identified
- Explain the stress response, inflammatory response, and pain response
- Identify indications for massage therapy and justify those indications
- Use a clinical reasoning model to determine the appropriate intervention process
- Determine when to refer clients to licensed medical professionals

On a separate sheet of paper or on the computer, write a short summary of the content of this chapter based on the preceding list of competencies. Use a conversational tone, as if you were explaining to someone (e.g., a client, prospective employer, coworker, or other interested person) the importance of the information and skills to the development of the massage profession.

Next, in small discussion groups, share your summary with your classmates and compare the ways the information was presented. In discussing the content, look for similarities, differences, possibilities for misunderstanding of the information, and clear, concise methods of description.

Problem-Solving Exercise

You just ran into a friend you have not seen in 5 years. Your friend is now a college professor who teaches anatomy and physiology. When you mention that you are studying massage, your friend says, "It sounds interesting, but I don't think I'd ever need one." Take 5 minutes to list all the reasons you think your friend might need a massage.

CHAPTER 7

Hygiene, Sanitation, and Safety

 http://evolve.elsevier.com/Fritz/fundamentals/

CHAPTER OBJECTIVES

After completing this chapter, the student will be able to perform the following:

1. Identify and implement effective health and personal hygiene practices
2. Explain the major disease-causing agents and implement Standard Precautions
3. Provide information about human immunodeficiency virus infection, hepatitis, tuberculosis, and other contagious conditions
4. Describe measures for ensuring a hazard-free massage environment

CHAPTER OUTLINE

KEY TERMS

Acquired immunodeficiency syndrome (AIDS)
Aseptic technique
Bacteria
Environmental contact
Fungi
Hepatitis
Human immunodeficiency virus (HIV)
Methicillin-resistant *Staphylococcus aureus*, (MRSA)
Opportunistic invasion
Pathogenic animals
Person-to-person contact
Protozoa
Sanitation
Severe acute respiratory syndrome (SARS)
Standard Precautions
Tuberculosis (TB)
Viruses

This chapter discusses hygiene and sanitation practices in a professional setting. The information may seem mere common sense, but specific skills are needed to practice massage in a way that protects the safety of both the client and the massage professional. Many local and state laws governing massage deal extensively with sanitary procedures. The Oregon health code requirements, which have been used as a model for part of this chapter, are both typical and well defined (Oregon Board of Massage Technicians, 2006).

The primary importance of sanitation is to prevent the spread of contagious diseases. Diseases caused by "germs" (viruses, bacteria, fungi, and parasites) are considered contagious. Some contagious diseases are rare; others are becoming more common.

Parasitic infection is more common than many realize. Children are especially vulnerable, but adults also can have parasites. Many parasites are microscopic protozoa.

Until recently, tuberculosis, a bacterial disease, was considered to be under control; however, the incidence of the disease has begun to rise, and strains resistant to current medications have emerged. Various streptococcal bacteria also are becoming resistant to the antibiotics currently available. The common cold and influenza viruses constantly mutate, thwarting scientific development of any sort of consistent vaccine.

The key, then, is prevention. Contagious diseases are best controlled by sanitary practices before infection occurs.

Considerable concern, misinformation, and misunderstanding have arisen about the spread of hepatitis, the human immunodeficiency virus (HIV), and acquired immunodeficiency syndrome (AIDS), in addition to certain other viruses. Intense education of the public through the media about HIV and AIDS has dispelled some of the misunderstanding about these conditions. Better care and research developments are beginning to move the prognosis of HIV infection to that of a chronic disease.

The infection rate for hepatitis is increasing alarmingly, which poses a significant health danger. Currently, concern is rising about the global spread of infectious diseases caused by several viruses, including the various forms of the influenza virus. An extensive section of this chapter is devoted to these topics to provide accurate information about hepatitis, HIV, AIDS, and other contagious diseases and also to explain in detail the massage practitioner's responsibilities.

Because new information about the spread and control of contagious diseases becomes available almost daily, it is important that massage practitioners keep themselves well informed. As information develops, the federal Centers for Disease Control and Prevention (CDC) adjusts its standards and guidelines for prevention of the transmission of communicable diseases. Massage practitioners are responsible for updating themselves semiannually on changes in the CDC's recommendations and for following the most recent standards and guidelines. (Helpful links are provided on the Evolve website for this chapter.)

In addition to a sanitary environment, the massage professional must provide a safe environment. The prevention of accidents and fire for both the client and the professional is an important consideration. The massage professional is well served by becoming certified in first aid and cardiopulmonary resuscitation (CPR) through the Red Cross or a similar organization.

Let's begin with the personal care of the massage practitioner. It is important that we take care of ourselves, not only so that we function at our best, but also because, as wellness and health professionals, we set an example for our clients. Clients notice the way we look and act, as well as our energy and vitality levels. Clients respect professionals who care for themselves, because the professional thus models self-care for clients. The ethical principle of respect (see Chapter 2) is reflected in the way we care for ourselves and for our clients.

PERSONAL HEALTH, HYGIENE, AND APPEARANCE

SECTION OBJECTIVES

Chapter objective covered in this section:

1. The student will be able to identify and implement effective health and personal hygiene practices.

Using the information presented in this section, the student will be able to perform the following:

- Identify the basic hygiene procedures important to a professional environment

One of the best ways to control disease is to stay healthy. If our bodies are strong and our immune systems are functioning properly, we do not become sick easily. If injured, we heal better if we are healthy. Diet, sleep, rest, body mechanics (the way we use our bodies), exercise, and lifestyle all must be considered in the overall health picture, in addition to actively practicing prevention. It also is important to keep to a schedule of regular physical checkups, because early detection of disease leads to more successful treatment.

Smoking

Smoking is considered one of the leading causes of disease. It is directly linked to cardiovascular disease, and it is the leading cause of lung cancer (Thibodeau and Patton, 2007). Exposure to secondhand smoke has been found to cause cancer and other health problems in nonsmokers. Besides its dangerous health effects, smoking is offensive to many people. Smoke odors linger in the air and on the hands, hair, and clothing. Many nonsmokers find this smell offensive, and the smell of smoke can cause reactions in sensitive individuals. Because the massage professional works physically close to the client, any smoke odors from the professional are reason for concern. Ideally, the massage practitioner should seek to quit smoking both for personal and professional reasons.

Massage professionals who smoke should inform clients, when they make appointments, that the practitioner smokes. If the client is bothered by smoke odors, referral to a different massage professional is appropriate. Massage professionals who smoke should never smoke in the massage therapy room, even when clients are not present, because the smell of smoke lingers in carpets, draperies, and furniture. If the practitioner must smoke during business hours, it should be done outside, away from any access doors or windows. After smoking the practitioner should wash the hands carefully, brush the teeth, and use mouthwash before performing a treatment.

Alcohol and Drugs

Alcohol and drugs interfere with the ability to function as a massage professional. Because these substances affect thinking, feeling, behavior, and functioning, and it is extremely unethical, the practitioner must never be under the influence of alcohol or illegal drugs when working with a client. A massage professional should wait at least 8 hours after the last alcoholic drink before working with a client, because it takes this long for the direct effects of alcohol to wear off. The indirect effects last for the next 24 hours. In this condition, often called a *hangover,* the body is exhausted and toxic; it is not a good condition to be in while giving a massage. Clients should be referred or rescheduled if the professional's ability to function is affected. Any prescription or over-the-counter medications that affect mental or physical abilities must be considered carefully, because use of these substances by the massage professional can place the client at risk.

Hygiene

The massage professional must pay careful attention to personal hygiene (Figure 7-1). Preventing breath and body odor without using chemical cover-ups is essential. Massage professionals should not wear perfume, aftershave, or perfumed hair products, because many clients are sensitive to these odors.

Massage professionals should bathe or shower at the start of each workday. The armpits, genitals, and feet should be washed carefully with soap or a similar cleaning agent. Female professionals must be especially mindful of odor during menstruation.

Because breath odor is offensive, careful brushing and flossing of the teeth and scraping of the tongue after each meal are important. Any food that may cause breath odor should be avoided during work hours. Gum chewing is unprofessional and irritating to many people and is ineffective in combating breath odors. Breath mints may help, but they are no substitute for good dental hygiene.

Hair should be kept clean. Chemicals such as hair spray or gel must be avoided, because they may cause an allergic reaction in chemically sensitive clients. The hair must not fall onto

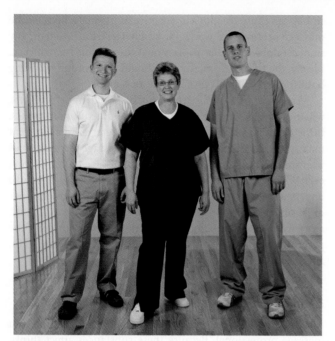

FIGURE 7-1 Properly groomed massage professionals.

the professional's face or drag on the client. If it is long, it should be kept pulled back.

Proper care of the hands is especially important. To avoid hurting the client while performing massage, practitioners should keep their nails short and well manicured, and nails should not extend past the tips of the fingers. Fingernails can harbor bacteria and other pathogens. Care must be taken to keep the space under the nails clean, which is best accomplished with a nailbrush. Any hangnails, breaks, or cracks in the skin of the hands must be kept clean and covered during a massage. Intact, strong skin is the professional's first line of defense against infection. Nail polish and synthetic nails promote the growth of bacteria, and hand jewelry can harbor pathogens; these should not be worn while the practitioner gives a massage.

Massage uniforms should be loose and made of cotton or a cotton blend. Because body temperature increases while the professional gives a massage, clothing must "breathe" and absorb and evaporate perspiration. Sleeves should be above the elbow, but the uniform should not be sleeveless. All clothing should be opaque and modest. T-shirts and shorts usually are inappropriate. If skirts or shorts are worn, they should be knee length or longer; loose pants are preferable.

White clothing is not necessary or even desirable, because it shows lubricant stains more than colored clothing does. Clothing should be laundered with detergent in hot water. If clothing comes in contact with a client's bodily fluids, it needs to be laundered in detergent and a disinfectant, such as bleach. The uniform must be able to withstand this type of laundering. If perspiration is heavy or if the clothing becomes stained, the practitioner may need to change clothes. A spare uniform should be kept available. Underclothing must be changed daily, more often if perspiration is heavy. Some professionals use uniforms called *scrubs*. Scrubs meet all the previously mentioned criteria, are inexpensive, and are easy to obtain.

The practitioner should wear clean, comfortable shoes while giving a massage. Going barefoot or wearing only socks is neither sanitary nor professional. Changing socks daily helps prevent foot odor.

Makeup should be modest, and heavy makeup is never appropriate. Male practitioners must keep facial hair shaved or neatly trimmed.

Jewelry of all types creates sanitation and safety hazards and should not be worn while giving a massage. Necklaces, bracelets, and hair jewelry can become tangled or can drag on the client, and jewelry of all types, including piercings, can harbor pathogens and collect debris, creating a sanitation hazard.

If the client or professional is ill and if any concern exists that the condition might be contagious, the massage professional should refer or reschedule the client until the condition changes (Proficiency Exercise 7-1).

SANITATION

SECTION OBJECTIVES

Chapter objective covered in this section:
2. The student will be able to explain the major disease-causing agents and implement Standard Precautions
Using the information presented in this section, the student will be able to perform the following:
- Identify the transmission routes for disease-causing pathogens
- Describe methods for preventing and controlling disease
- Give specific recommendations for sanitary practices for massage businesses
- Demonstrate Standard Precautions during massage
- Implement sanitation practices, including Standard Precautions, to prevent and control the spread of disease

Sanitary massage methods promote conditions that are conducive to health. This means that pathogenic organisms must be eliminated or controlled. Pathogens are spread by direct contact, through blood or other body fluids, or by airborne transmission.

Pathogenic Organisms

Pathogenic organisms cause disease. They include viruses, bacteria, fungi, protozoa, and pathogenic animals.

Viruses

Viruses invade cells and insert their own genetic code into the host cell's genetic code. They use the host cell's nutrients and organelles to produce more virus particles. By bursting the cell membrane, the new virus particles escape to infect other cells.

Bacteria

Bacteria are primitive cells that have no nuclei. They cause disease in one of three ways: (1) by secreting toxic substances that damage human tissues; (2) by becoming parasites inside human cells; or (3) by forming colonies in the body that disrupt normal function. Because bacteria can produce resistant forms, called *spores*, under adverse conditions, pathogenic bacteria are difficult for the human body to destroy.

Fungi

Fungi are a group of simple parasitic organisms that are similar to plants but have no chlorophyll (green pigment). Most pathogenic fungi live on the skin or mucous membranes (e.g., athlete's foot, vaginal yeast infections). Yeasts are small, single-celled fungi, and molds are large, multicellular fungi. Because fungal, or mycotic, infections can be resistant to treatment, they can become quite serious.

Protozoa and Pathogenic Animals

Protozoa are one-celled organisms that are larger than bacteria. They can infest human fluids and cause disease by parasitizing (living off) or directly destroying cells. **Pathogenic animals**, sometimes called *metazoa*, are large, multicellular organisms. Most are worms that feed off human tissue or cause other diseases.

Many of these pathogens cause skin diseases when the pathogen commonly is spread through direct contact. Because massage professionals spend much time working directly with skin, they would be wise to learn to recognize these various skin conditions. Most anatomy, physiology, and pathology textbooks have color plates showing different skin diseases (see Appendix B for color illustrations showing examples of skin disorders).

Intact skin (skin integrity) prevents infection and various skin diseases, whereas abrasions and cuts breach the protective layer of the skin. Therefore, it is important that the massage professional obtain additional information about pathologic skin conditions.

Disease Prevention and Control

The key to preventing many diseases caused by pathogenic organisms is to prevent the organisms from entering the body. This sounds simple enough, but often it is difficult to accomplish. Three primary means by which pathogens can spread are environmental contact, opportunistic invasion, and person-to-person contact.

- **Environmental contact.** Many pathogens are found in the environment; that is, in food, water, and soil and on various surfaces. Diseases caused by environmental pathogens often can be prevented by avoiding contact with certain materials and by following safe sanitation practices.
- **Opportunistic invasion.** Some potentially pathogenic organisms are found on the skin and mucous membranes of nearly everyone. These organisms do not cause disease until they have the opportunity to do so. Preventing opportunistic infection involves avoiding conditions that promote infection. Changes in pH (acidity), moisture, temperature, or other characteristics of the skin and mucous membranes often promote these infections. Aseptic treatment and cleansing of wounds can prevent them.
- **Person-to-person contact.** Small pathogens often can be transmitted in the air from one person to another. Direct contact with an infected person or with materials handled by the infected person is a familiar mode of transmission. The rhinovirus that causes the common cold often is transmitted in these ways. Some viruses, such as the hepatitis B virus (HBV), are transmitted when infected blood, semen, or other body fluids enter the bloodstream.

Aseptic Technique

Aseptic technique kills or disables pathogens on surfaces before they can be transmitted (Table 7-1).

Most sanitation conditions for massage require disinfection. Occasionally protective apparel is necessary. In rare instances, use of a mask, gown, and gloves may be appropriate to protect the massage professional or the client. These cases are discussed later in the chapter.

Hand Washing

Proper hand washing is the single most effective deterrent to the spread of disease (Figure 7-2). The hands must be washed before and after each massage, after blowing the nose or coughing into the hands, and after using the toilet. The hands and forearms must be washed in hot, running water for at least 15 seconds to remove any infectious organisms. Soap or another antiseptic hand-washing product must be used, and a clean towel is used to dry the hands and forearms. Faucets and door handles are contaminated and should not be touched after washing the hands. The towel should be used to turn off the water and open the door. Because frequent hand washing may dry and chap the skin, using a lotion after washing helps replace natural oils. Using the clean towel to hold the lotion bottle helps prevent contamination of the hands.

Table 7-1	Common Aseptic Techniques for Preventing the Spread of Pathogens	
Method	**Action**	**Example**
Sterilization	Destroys all organisms by means of heat	Pressurized steam bath, extreme temperature, irradiation
Disinfection	Destroys most or all pathogens (but not necessarily all microbes) on inanimate objects	Chemicals (e.g., iodine, chlorine, alcohol, soap)
Isolation	Separates potentially infectious people or materials from uninfected individuals	Quarantining infected patients; wearing protective apparel while giving treatments; and sanitary transport, storage, and disposal of body fluids, tissues, and other materials

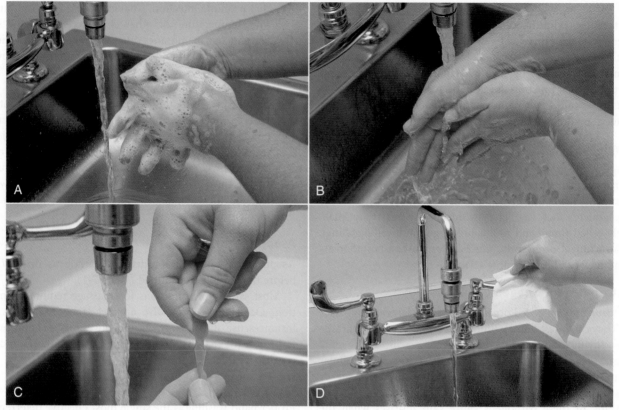

FIGURE 7-2 Hand-washing technique. A, Create a lather with the soap. Interlace your fingers to wash between them, keeping your hands pointed down. **B,** Rinse the hands well, keeping your fingers pointed down. **C,** Use the blunt edge of an orangewood stick to clean under your fingernails. **D,** After drying your hands, use a dry paper towel to turn off the water.
(From Zakus SM: *Mosby's clinical skills for medical assistants,* ed 4, St Louis, 2001, Mosby.)

💡 PROFICIENCY EXERCISE 7-2

Contact your local health department for information on disease control, health practices, and sanitation requirements.

Suggested Sanitation Requirements

Box 7-1 provides a summary of sanitation procedures that all massage professionals should observe. State and local laws may mandate additional procedures, and the professional should be aware of these (Proficiency Exercise 7-2).

Indications for the Use of Standard Precautions by the Massage Professional

Under normal circumstances the massage professional does not come in contact with a client's blood, body fluids, or body substances (e.g., urine, feces, and vomit). However, in rare cases an accident may occur in which such contact is possible. The best recommendation is always to make Standard Precautions part of the professional practice (Box 7-2). Gloves are not necessary for most massage sessions unless the skin of the massage practitioner's hands or any skin area of the client has a rash, cut, abrasion, infection, or any other condition that would allow the transmission of fluids. A mask may be appropriate if transmission of an airborne pathogen, such as the flu virus, is a concern. In most cases use of a mask protects the client from the massage professional's pathogens; therefore, a mask is used with clients who have any form of immune suppression, including excessive stress, which makes the client more susceptible to infection.

Required Use of Standard Precautions

With additional training and under medical supervision, massage professionals may work with clients who have a contagious condition. In these cases, a knowledge of Standard Precautions is essential. However, it is wise to remember the importance of the massage professional's gentle, nurturing touch. The human connection becomes difficult through layers of protective coverings.

Massage therapists must always keep in mind that their normal germs can be very dangerous for any immune-suppressed client, and Standard Precautions must be used to protect the client from viruses and bacteria. Extra effort is required to follow Standard Precautions, but this extra effort should not hinder the safety of either client or practitioner.

Clients considered contagious may feel isolated and "unclean." We do not want to make such clients feel ashamed and guilty for having a contagious disease. Many of them desperately need to be touched in a supportive, nonjudgmental way. It is the pathogen that is undesirable, not the client. All clients must be treated with respect, dignity, and kindness.

Box 7-1 Sanitation Practices for Massage Professionals

The following are based on the Oregon model for massage sanitation practices.

- Massage professionals must clean and wash their hands and forearms or feet thoroughly with an antibacterial/antiviral agent before touching each client. Any professional known to be infected with any communicable disease or to be a carrier of such disease or who has an infected wound or open lesion on any exposed portions of the body is excluded from practicing massage until the communicable condition is alleviated.
- The professional must wear clean clothing. If at all possible, lockers or closets for personnel should be maintained apart from the massage room for the storage of personal clothing and effects.
- All doors and windows opening to the outside must be tight fitting and must ensure the exclusion of flies, insects, rodents, or other vermin. All floors, walks, and furniture must be kept clean, well maintained, and in good repair.
- All rooms in which massage is practiced must meet the following requirements: (1) heating must be adequate to maintain a room air temperature of 75° F; (2) ventilation must be sufficient to remove objectionable odors; and (3) lighting fixtures must be capable of producing a minimum of 5 foot-candles of light at floor level; this level of lighting should be used during cleaning.
- All sewage and liquid waste must be disposed of in a municipal sewage system or approved septic system. All interior water distribution piping should be installed and maintained in conformity with the state plumbing code. The water supply must be adequate, deemed safe by the health department, and sanitary. Drinking fountains of an approved type or individual paper drinking cups should be provided for the convenience of employees and clients.
- Every massage business must have a sanitary toilet facility with an adequate supply of hot and cold water under pressure, and it must be conveniently located for use by employees and clients. Bathroom doors must be tight fitting, and the rooms must be kept clean, in good repair, and free of flies, insects, and vermin. A supply of soap in a covered dispenser and single-use sanitary towels in a dispenser must be provided at each lavatory installation, as well as a covered waste receptacle for proper disposal; a supply of toilet paper on a dispenser must be available for each toilet.

- Lavatory and toilet rooms must be equipped with fly-tight containers for garbage and refuse. These containers should be easily cleanable, well maintained, and in good repair. Any refuse must be disposed of in a sanitary manner.
- Massage lubricants, including but not limited to oil, alcohol, powders, and lotions, should be dispensed from suitable containers, to be used and stored in such a manner as to prevent contamination. The bulk lubricant must not come in contact with the massage professional. It should be poured, squeezed, or shaken into a separate container or the massage professional's hand. Any unused lubricant that comes into contact with the client or massage professional must be discarded.
- The use of unclean linen is prohibited. Only freshly laundered sheets and linens should be used for massage. All single-service materials and clean linens should be stored at least 4 inches off the floor on shelves or in compartments or cabinets used for that purpose only. All soiled linens must be placed in a covered receptacle immediately and kept there until washed in detergent and an antiviral cleaning agent (e.g., a 10% bleach solution, or one part bleach to nine parts water) in a washing machine that provides a hot water temperature of at least 140° F.
- Massage tables must be covered with impervious material that is cleanable and must be kept clean and in good repair. Equipment that comes in contact with the client must be cleaned thoroughly with soap or other suitable detergent and water, followed by adequate sanitation procedures before use with each individual client (a 10% bleach solution, made up daily, is recommended). All equipment must be clean, well maintained, and in good repair.
- When cleaning the massage area, observe the following rules:
  - Do not shake linen. Dust with a damp cloth to minimize the movement of dust.
  - Clean from the cleanest area to the dirtiest; this prevents soiling of a clean area.
  - Clean away from your body and uniform. If you dust, brush, or wipe toward yourself, microorganisms are transmitted to your skin, hair, and uniform.
  - Store used linens in a closed bag or container while in the massage room or during transport.
  - Floors are dirty; any object that falls on the floor should not be used on or for a client.

Modified from Oregon Board of Massage Technicians: *Sanitation requirements for the state of Oregon,* Oregon Administrative Rules, November 2006.

The professional must remember to touch the person and not the disease, to see and listen to the person rather than the disease. These are *people* who are sick—not sick people.

The massage professional may need to wear gloves if a client is infected with a contagious, transmittable disease or if a client is in an immunosuppressed state, such as might occur with chemotherapy, and must be protected from germs. In these situations the massage therapist will be working under the supervision of a medical professional, and it is important to follow all of his or her directions carefully.

If massage professionals work in a health care setting, such as a hospital, an extended care facility, or a rehabilitation center, it is essential that they follow the posted standard

precautionary procedures for that facility. Most often special training is provided. If this is not the case and the massage professional is concerned in any way about the application of required sanitation procedures, he or she should speak directly to the supervisor.

Possible Exposure to Contaminants and Body Fluids

Any persons whose job may cause them to come in contact with blood or other body substances, such as vomit, urine, or feces, should wear single-use, disposable gloves (Figure 7-3). Such contact conceivably could happen during a massage. The most common blood exposure is to menstrual blood, an incident that can occur if the client's protective product is

Box 7-2   Standard Precautions

Standard Precautions, established by the Centers for Disease Control and Prevention (CDC), synthesize the major features of Universal Precautions (blood and body fluids), which are designed to reduce the risk of transmission of blood-borne pathogens, and body substance isolation, which is designed to reduce the risk of transmission of pathogens from moist body substances. Standard Precautions apply to (1) blood; (2) all body fluids, secretions, and excretions except sweat, regardless of whether they contain visible blood; (3) nonintact skin; and (4) mucous membranes. Standard Precautions are designed to reduce the risk of transmission of microorganisms from both recognized and unrecognized sources of infection in hospitals.

Hand Washing and Gloving

Many consider hand washing the single most important measure for reducing the risk of transmitting organisms from one person to another or from one site to another on the same patient. Washing your hands as promptly and thoroughly as possible between clients is very important. In addition to hand washing, gloves play an important role in reducing the risk of transmission of microorganisms.

Gloves are worn for two important reasons: (1) to provide a protective barrier and (2) to reduce the likelihood that microorganisms on the massage practitioner's hands will be transmitted to clients. Wearing gloves does not replace the need for hand washing, because gloves may have small, unapparent defects or may be torn during use, and hands can become contaminated during the removal of gloves. Gloves must be changed and the old ones discarded after each use.

A mask provides protection against the spread of infectious, large-particle droplets that are transmitted by close contact and that generally travel only short distances (up to 3 feet) from infected patients who are coughing or sneezing. Massage professionals occasionally use masks.

Gowns and Protective Apparel

Various types of gowns and protective apparel are worn to provide barrier protection and to reduce the opportunity for transmission of microorganisms in medical settings.

Immunocompromised Clients

Standard Precautions, or the equivalent, are used for the care of all clients.

Hand Washing

1. Wash the hands after touching blood, body fluids, secretions, excretions, and contaminated items, regardless of whether gloves are worn. Wash the hands immediately after removing gloves, between client contacts, and when otherwise indicated to prevent the transfer of microorganisms to other clients or environments. It may be necessary to wash the hands between tasks and procedures on the same client to prevent cross-contamination of different body sites.
2. Use a plain (nonantimicrobial) soap for routine hand washing.
3. Use an antimicrobial agent or a waterless antiseptic agent if hand washing is not possible.

Gloves

1. Wear gloves (clean, nonsterile gloves are adequate) when touching blood, body fluids, secretions, excretions, and contaminated items. Put on clean gloves just before touching mucous membranes and nonintact skin.
2. Change gloves between tasks and procedures on the same client after contact with material that may contain a high concentration of microorganisms.
3. Remove gloves promptly after use, before touching uncontaminated items and environmental surfaces, and before going to another client; wash hands immediately to avoid transferring microorganisms to other clients or environments.

Mask, Eye Protection, and Face Shield

Wear a mask and eye protection or a face shield to protect the mucous membranes of the eyes, nose, and mouth during procedures and client care activities that are likely to generate splashes or sprays of blood, body fluids, secretions, and excretions.

Gown

Wear a gown (a clean, nonsterile gown is adequate) to protect skin and to prevent soiling of clothing during procedures and client care activities that are likely to generate splashes or sprays of blood, body fluids, secretions, or excretions. Select a gown that is appropriate for the activity and the amount of fluid likely to be encountered. Remove a soiled gown as promptly as possible and wash the hands to prevent the transfer of microorganisms to other clients or environments.

Modified from the Centers for Disease Control and Prevention, National Center for Infectious Diseases. Available at http://www.cdc.gov/hicpac/2007IP/2007isolationPrecautions.html (accessed August 24, 2011).

inadequate. In rare cases men who have a history of premature ejaculation could be stimulated indirectly by the general massage and ejaculate or leak fluid. An incontinent client could leak urine or feces, or a client could suddenly become sick and vomit. Standard Precautions should be followed during any cleanup.

Approved Cleaning Solutions

The CDC has recognized the following three levels of solutions and products that destroy HIV, HBV, and other viral organisms. These recommendations should be followed in every practice.

- *High-level sanitation:* Products labeled "sterilant/disinfectant glutaraldehyde—air dry"; massage professionals do not need to practice high-level sanitation techniques under normal conditions.
- *Medium-level sanitation:* Bleach solution—one part bleach to nine parts water (10% solution), made up daily or a hospital disinfectant labeled "tuberculocidal" (Proficiency Exercise 7-3).
- *Low-level sanitation:* Hot, soapy water (with air drying) or a hospital disinfectant effective against viruses and bacteria. Hands are to be washed in hot, soapy water or with surgical soap.

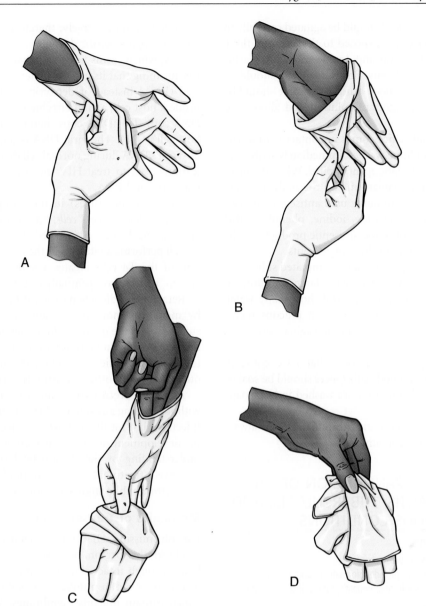

FIGURE 7-3 Procedure for Removing Gloves. A, Grasp the glove below the cuff. **B,** Pull the glove down over the hand, turning the glove inside out. **C,** Insert the fingers of the ungloved hand into the other glove. **D,** Pull the glove down and over the hand, turning the glove inside out.
(Modified from Sorrentino SA: *Mosby's textbook for nursing assistants,* ed 5, St Louis, 2000, Mosby.)

💡 PROFICIENCY EXERCISE 7-3

Obtain a 1-quart spray bottle. Using a permanent marker, mark the bottle so that it is divided into 10 equal portions. This bottle now can be used as a dispenser for a 10% bleach solution: fill the bottle to the first line with bleach; then fill it to the top line with water. Make sure to put the cap on tightly and then shake the bottle to mix the solution.

Medium- and low-level sanitation are adequate for most therapeutic massage practices. Cleanup of a body fluid spill might require high-level procedures. Massage professionals should update their information on recommended sanitary practices at least every 6 months. The CDC provides current information.

Cleanup Procedures Using Standard Precautions

Latex gloves should be worn during the cleanup process. If the massage professional is allergic to latex, gloves made of vinyl or nitrile rubber can be worn instead.

Bleach is the preferred cleaning agent. A 10% bleach solution (one part bleach to nine parts water) should be used to clean up spills of body fluids. A bleach and water solution should be prepared daily, and any leftover solution should be discarded at the end of the day. If blood or body fluid seepage is excessive, a stronger mixture of bleach should be used.

The spill should be surrounded with solution and then mopped or wiped up, with the professional working slowly and carefully inward to avoid splashes or aerosols (airborne particles). Stronger bleach solutions should be used if excessive amounts of blood or other substances are present. Afterward, the mop head or cloth should be soaked in the bleach solution. The mop head should be agitated carefully to ensure that all its surfaces are exposed to the cleaning fluid. All linens should be rolled away and double-bagged in plastic, separate from other soiled linens. The outside bag should be marked "contaminated with body fluids." The table should be washed with a strong disinfectant solution and allowed to air dry.

If a contaminated substance comes in contact with a person's skin, the skin should be washed immediately with soap and hot water and an antiseptic agent applied. When disinfectants are used to kill microorganisms on the body, they are referred to as *antiseptics.* Commonly used antiseptics are isopropyl alcohol, hydrogen peroxide, iodine, phenol, methyl salicylate, and thymol. Most of the antiseptic products on the market contain one or more of these ingredients.

If an open wound is exposed to a contaminated substance, it should be flushed immediately with large amounts of hydrogen peroxide and then washed with hot, soapy water. Hydrogen peroxide should not be used on mucous membranes or in any body orifice (e.g., mouth, vagina, anus, eyes, or urethra).

Any massage equipment and tools that have come in contact with blood or other body substances should be soaked in 10% bleach solution before they are washed in hot, soapy water.

All surfaces, including those in bathrooms, should always be cleaned as if they were contaminated.

PREVENTING THE TRANSMISSION OF HIV INFECTION, HEPATITIS, TUBERCULOSIS, AND OTHER CONTAGIOUS CONDITIONS

SECTION OBJECTIVES

Chapter objective covered in this section:
3. The student will be able to provide information about human immunodeficiency virus infection, hepatitis, tuberculosis, and other contagious conditions.

Using the information presented in this section, the student will be able to perform the following:
- Define AIDS in detail
- Identify behavior that could result in the transmission of HIV or HBV infection and other contagious conditions

HIV and AIDS

A *syndrome* is a group of clinical symptoms that constitute a disease or abnormal condition. *Clinical* means reported or observed symptoms not discovered by laboratory tests. An individual need not have all the symptoms of a particular disease or condition to have a syndrome. Syndromes may be caused by many different things, but with AIDS, the cause is a dysfunction in the body's immune system, one of the body's primary defenses against disease.

The diseases of AIDS are caused by pathogens we encounter every day. In fact, some of these pathogens live permanently in small numbers inside the human body. A healthy immune system is able to keep these pathogens in check. However, when the immune system weakens, these pathogens

are able to multiply freely; therefore, the diseases they cause are called *opportunistic diseases.*

HIV, which seems to be responsible for AIDS, is a retrovirus, meaning that its genetic material is carried in ribonucleic acid (RNA) instead of deoxyribonucleic acid (DNA). Once inside a host cell, a viral enzyme reads the RNA and makes a DNA copy. This DNA copy then becomes integrated into the host cell's DNA. The viral DNA is duplicated along with the host cell's DNA during normal cell division. Some of the medications used to treat HIV infection target the enzyme that reads the viral RNA.

HIV replicates (lives) in the group of white blood cells called *lymphocytes,* or *T cells.* Among the T cells, HIV's favorite target is the T4 cell. Also called the *helper/inducer T cell,* the T4 cell performs a vital job in the immune system. HIV infection of the T4 cells creates a defect in the body's immune system, which may eventually result in AIDS.

Retroviruses die when exposed to heat. They can be killed by many common disinfectants, and they usually do not survive well if the tissue or blood they are in dries up. However, retroviruses have a high mutation rate and consequently tend to evolve very quickly into new strains. HIV shares this and other traits with other known retroviruses.

As a group, retroviruses can live in the host for a long time without causing any sign of illness. In most animals, retroviral infections last for life. Long-term infection with HIV without the development of AIDS is becoming more common. Better understanding of the disease by health care professionals, improved treatment, increased public education, and less stress from public stigma support this process.

Mechanics of Transmission

For transmission, HIV must travel from inside one person to inside another person. Because viruses are unable to enter the body through intact skin, they must enter through an open wound or one of a number of possible body openings, all of which contain mucous membranes. *Mucous membranes* are thin tissues that protect most openings and passages in the human body. They are found in the mouth, inside the eyelids, in the nose and air passages leading to the lungs, in the stomach, along the digestive tract, in the vagina, in the anus, and inside the eye and the opening of the penis. These membranes secrete mucus, which contains antipathogenic chemicals and keeps the surrounding tissues moist. From the surface of a mucous membrane, many viruses can travel through the membrane and enter the tiny blood vessels inside. The mucous membranes of the eyes and mouth often are doorways for highly infectious viruses, such as the flu virus.

HIV can be found in any body fluid or substance. The presence of HIV in a substance does not necessarily indicate that the substance is capable of transmitting the infection. The concentration of HIV (i.e., the number of viral particles per unit of volume) determines its infectivity. If a substance has a high concentration of HIV, it is more likely to transmit the virus.

In theory, all body fluids are capable of transmitting disease; in reality, the substances most likely to transmit HIV seem to be blood, semen, and pre-ejaculate fluid; cervical and vaginal secretions; and perhaps feces. Despite much research, a clear-cut case of saliva causing transmission has not been found. A pregnant woman can transmit the virus to her unborn child. The concentration of HIV in mother's milk and in saliva, urine, and tears typically is low. Theoretically these are infectious substances that could transmit HIV infection; however, no cases have been reported in which contact with these secretions caused HIV infection. Sweat cannot transmit HIV.

HIV Survival Outside the Host

If HIV is present in a substance that leaves the body, the viral particles can remain infectious until the substance dries up. Depending on the circumstances, this could be a matter of minutes or hours. If the substance stays moist, the viral particles can survive much longer. For example, in water and blood solutions (10% blood, 90% saline), HIV can survive at room temperature for 2 weeks. In refrigerated blood, such as that used for transfusions, HIV can survive indefinitely.

The public has a widespread fear that AIDS can be contracted through casual contact, such as shaking hands, being in the same room with an individual infected with HIV, touching doorknobs, or sharing bathroom facilities. However, the fear is far greater than the risk. Diseases spread by casual contact invariably are spread through saliva or sputum, and they exist in the saliva or sputum in very high concentrations. The concentration of HIV in saliva and sputum is very low, if it exists in these substances at all. After 25 years of documentation of the AIDS epidemic, there are no known cases of AIDS or HIV infection being transmitted by casual social contact, not even among people living in the same household. In some cases household members have even shared toothbrushes with infected housemates without contracting the virus.

To date no medical or health care workers have contracted HIV from casual contact. The contact between the massage professional and the client falls under this classification, because we touch only the skin, which is not a transmission route.

Hepatitis

Hepatitis is an inflammatory process, an infection of the liver caused by a virus. It is classified as type A, B, C, D, E, or G.
- *Hepatitis A,* caused by the hepatitis A virus (HAV), is a less serious form and usually is transmitted by fecal contamination of food and water.
- *Hepatitis B* is a potentially fatal disease caused by the hepatitis B virus (HBV), which is transmitted through routes similar to those for HIV. HBV is 100 times more contagious than HIV, and it is estimated that more than 1 million people in the United States are carriers of HBV. Two types of vaccine are available for preventing the transmission of HBV.
- *Hepatitis C* accounts for 86% of new cases of hepatitis each year.
- The *hepatitis D* virus (HDV) infects only those who have hepatitis B, and its symptoms are more severe than other forms of hepatitis. Vaccines do not appear to be effective for HDV.

- *Hepatitis E* is transmitted through food and water contaminated by fecal material.
- *Hepatitis G* is a sexually transmitted virus (McCance and Huether, 2005).

Following Standard Precautions prevents the spread of hepatitis. It is important to be cautious of all behaviors in which body fluids are contacted or unsanitary conditions may be present that may allow the transmission of HIV and the hepatitis viruses (Proficiency Exercise 7-4).

Tuberculosis

Tuberculosis (TB) is an infection caused by a bacterium that usually affects the lungs but may invade other body systems. It is estimated that approximately 1.86 billion people, more than one third of the world's population, are infected with TB. Transmission occurs via airborne droplets that are produced when an infected person coughs, sneezes, or talks. TB also can be spread through contaminated food.

In many infected individuals, tuberculosis is asymptomatic. In others, symptoms develop so gradually that they are not noticed until the disease is advanced. However, symptoms can appear in immunosuppressed individuals within weeks of exposure to the bacillus. Symptoms include fatigue, weight loss, lethargy, anorexia (loss of appetite), and a low-grade fever that usually occurs in the afternoon. A cough that produces a mucus matter that contains pus (purulent sputum) develops slowly and becomes more frequent over several weeks or months. Night sweats and general anxiety often are present. Because these are common signs and symptoms of all chronic infections, referral is necessary for diagnosis. Difficulty breathing, chest pain, and coughing up blood or bloody sputum may also occur as the disease progresses.

Tuberculosis is diagnosed by a positive tuberculin skin test (PPD), sputum culture, and chest x-ray film. A positive tuberculin skin test indicates that an individual has been infected and has produced antibodies against the bacillus. By itself the positive skin test does not indicate the presence of an active disease. Treatment consists of antibiotic therapy to control active or dormant tuberculosis and to prevent transmission. Massage professionals should be tested yearly because of their contact with the public.

Severe Acute Respiratory Syndrome

Severe acute respiratory syndrome (SARS) is a respiratory illness that has been reported in Asia, North America, and Europe. In general, SARS begins with a fever over 100.4° F (38° C). Other symptoms may include headache, an overall feeling of discomfort, and body aches. Some people also experience mild respiratory symptoms. After 2 to 7 days, SARS patients may develop a dry cough and have trouble breathing. SARS appears to spread primarily through close person-to-person contact. Most cases of SARS have involved people who cared for or lived with someone with SARS or who had direct contact with infectious material (e.g., respiratory secretions) from a person with SARS.

Potential ways SARS can be spread include touching the skin of other people or touching objects that are contaminated with infectious droplets and then touching the eyes, nose, or mouth. Droplet contamination occurs when someone who is sick with SARS coughs or sneezes droplets onto themselves, other people, or nearby surfaces. SARS may be spread more broadly through the air or in other currently unknown ways. Most U.S. cases of SARS have occurred among travelers returning from other parts of the world that were experiencing a SARS outbreak. A small number of cases resulted from spread of the disease to close contacts, such as family members and health care workers (CDC, 2005).

The transmission of SARS to health care workers has resulted from close contact with sick people before recommended infection control precautions were put into use. The CDC has issued interim infection control recommendations for health care settings and for the management of exposure to SARS in health care and other institutional settings.

Although SARS is not commonly contracted by health care workers, it is essential that massage professionals strictly follow Standard Precautions (see Box 7-2) to reduce the spread of such diseases. The practitioner also is responsible for consistently checking the CDC website for updates on all diseases.

Methicillin-Resistant *Staphylococcus aureus*

Methicillin-resistant *Staphylococcus aureus* (MRSA) can be categorized according to where the infection was acquired: hospital-acquired MRSA (HA-MRSA) or community-associated MRSA (CA-MRSA).

MRSA is a potentially dangerous type of staphylococcal bacterium that is resistant to certain antibiotics and that may cause skin and other infections. MRSA is spread through direct contact with an infected person or by sharing personal items, such as towels or razors that have touched infected skin.

Most staphylococcal (or "staph") skin infections, including MRSA, appear as a bump or an infected area on the skin. Some signs may include:

- Redness
- Swelling
- Pain
- Warmth to the touch
- Pus or other drainage
- An accompanying fever

Treatment for MRSA skin infections may involve drainage of the lesion by a health care professional and, in some cases, antibiotic therapy.

PREMISE AND FIRE SAFETY

SECTION OBJECTIVES

Chapter objective covered in this section:

4. The student will be able to describe measures for ensuring a hazard-free massage environment.

Using the information presented in this section, the student will be able to perform the following:

- Recognize and avoid fire and safety hazards
- Complete an accident report

A massage professional's facility must be kept free of hazards. Some clients will need additional assistance to prevent falls or other injury. The following safety rules are guidelines for creating a hazard-free massage environment.

- Infants and young children should not be left unattended. Parents or guardians should always be present during massage for minors.
- Women in the last trimester of a pregnancy should not be left in the massage room alone and may need assistance getting on and off the massage table; they also may need help in rolling over.
- Elderly individuals may be less steady on their feet and should not be left in the massage room unattended.
- Any client whose mobility is impaired, including those with visual impairments, may need assistance getting on and off the massage table. People with disabilities should be asked what assistance they need, and their instructions should be followed carefully.
- Preventing falls is very important. The massage professional should observe the following rules to prevent falls.
  - Provide barrier-free access
  - Provide good lighting (never perform a massage in a dark room)
  - Do not use throw rugs; they may slip or tangle in the feet
  - Avoid slippery tile floors
  - Keep floors and walkways uncluttered
  - Keep electrical and phone cords out of traffic areas
  - Regularly check all massage equipment to make sure it is sturdy and in good repair
  - Make sure all outside entrances are free of clutter and hazards caused by ice, snow, or rain

If an accident occurs, all information about the accident must be written down. An insurance company will need the following information:

- Where and when the accident occurred
- Detailed information about the accident
- Names and addresses of the person or people involved in the accident
- Names of any witnesses to the accident
- Names of manufacturers, if equipment is involved

Most accidents can be prevented. Knowing the common safety hazards, recognizing which clients need extra assistance, and using common sense are all necessary to promote safety.

Fire prevention also is essential (Proficiency Exercise 7-5). The massage professional should observe the following rules to prevent fires:

PROFICIENCY EXERCISE 7-5

1. Contact your local fire marshal and learn more about fire prevention.
2. Draw up a fire escape route and emergency plan for your massage business.
3. Contact the local building and safety inspector and find out more about accident prevention.
4. Contact a local insurance agent. Find out about the requirements for reporting accidents to the insurance company and also the insurance plan recommended for this type of protection.
5. Take basic and advanced first aid classes and learn cardiopulmonary resuscitation (CPR).

FOOT IN THE DOOR

The foot you put in the door needs to be clean; it also needs to be wearing a nonskid shoe for safety purposes. To maintain a successful massage practice, you must be clean, scent free, well groomed, and professionally dressed. You also must meticulously follow the rules of sanitation to ensure not only your own safety, but also that of your clients and coworkers. Sanitation is not an option. Both your massage methods and your environment must be safe. When evaluating a possible job location, find out whether others in the practice maintain professional hygiene, sanitation, and safety. You will not be successful in an environment that is dirty and unsafe. You may not even want your foot in that door! Instead, make sure to put your foot in a door that opens to a clean, neat, fresh, sanitary, and safe environment.

Evolve Activity 7-3

- Provide a nonsmoking environment. In places where smoking is allowed, make sure proper ashtrays are used. Empty ashtrays only into a metal container that is partly filled with sand or water.
- Regularly check all electrical cords and equipment to make sure they are in good condition. Do not plug more than two cords into an electrical outlet.
- Never use candles, incense, or any open flame.
- Routinely check three or four times a year that the massage area is equipped with a working smoke detector and fire extinguisher.

SUMMARY

The information in this chapter can help you establish a safe, professional practice. Massage professionals should review these procedures regularly to maintain the attention to detail that ensures a safe, sanitary massage environment for our clients. It is our responsibility to act reliably in emergencies. As massage professionals, we must understand the use of Standard Precautions and fire and premise safety measures to serve our clients in a health-promoting and hazard-free manner.

ⓔvolve

http://evolve.elsevier.com/Fritz/fundamentals/

7-1 The Evolve Web site has a video demonstration of proper hand-washing procedures

7-2 Total recall: Play a memory game with abbreviations for contagious conditions

7-3 Review chapter vocabulary with a matching exercise

Don't forget to study for your certification and licensure exams! Review questions, along with weblinks, can be found on the Evolve website.

References

Centers for Disease Control and Prevention: *Fact sheet: basic information about SARS.* May 3, 2005. www/cdc/ncidod/sars/factsheet.htm. Accessed August 3, 2010.

McCance K, Huether S: *Pathophysiology: the biologic basis for disease in adults and children,* ed 5, St Louis, 2005, Mosby.

Oregon Board of Massage Technicians: Sanitation requirements for the state of Oregon, *Oregon Administrative Rules,* November, 2006.

Thibodeau GA, Patton K: *Anatomy and physiology,* ed 6, St Louis, 2007, Mosby.

Workbook Section

Short Answer

1. Why is the massage professional's hygiene so important?

2. What odors may be offensive or a health risk to clients?

3. Why does the use of alcohol and certain drugs interfere with the ability to function as an effective massage professional?

4. Why should the massage professional study pathogenic organisms?

5. Why is the integrity of the skin so important?

6. What are the main ways diseases caused by pathogenic organisms are spread?

7. What are aseptic techniques?

8. What are the main concepts presented in the section on sanitation requirements?

9. What is the main goal of Standard Precautions?

10. Why should the massage professional have some knowledge of hepatitis, HIV, AIDS, SARS, and MRSA?

11. What single sanitation method is most effective in controlling the spread of disease?

12. What are the main precautions necessary for preventing falls and accidents?

13. What are the main ways to prevent a fire?

14. Why should the massage professional study emergency care and CPR?

Matching I

Match the term to the best definition. You may need to use your anatomy and physiology text or a medical dictionary to complete this exercise.

_____ 1. AIDS
_____ 2. Centers for Disease Control and Prevention
_____ 3. Disinfection
_____ 4. HIV
_____ 5. Sanitation
_____ 6. Sterilization
_____ 7. Standard Precautions

a. Human immunodeficiency virus
b. The formulation and application of measures to promote and establish conditions favorable to health, especially public health
c. Procedures developed by the CDC to prevent the spread of contagious disease
d. The process by which all microorganisms are destroyed
e. Acquired immunodeficiency syndrome
f. The process by which pathogens are destroyed
g. A division of the U.S. Public Health Service that investigates and controls diseases with epidemic potential

Matching II

Match the ways pathogens can be spread or controlled with the proper description.

_____ **1.** Pressurized steam bath, extreme temperature, or irradiation

_____ **2.** Chemicals such as iodine, chlorine, alcohol, and soap

_____ **3.** Quarantine of affected individuals; protective apparel worn while giving treatments

_____ **4.** Pathogens found in the environment, such as in food, water, and soil and on assorted surfaces

_____ **5.** Disease that does not develop until the pathogens have the opportunity

_____ **6.** Transferal of pathogens from one person to another

_____ **7.** Killing or disabling of pathogens on surfaces before they can spread to other people

a. Aseptic technique

b. Person-to-person contact

c. Opportunistic invasion

d. Environmental contact

e. Isolation

f. Disinfection

g. Sterilization

Assess Your Competencies

Now that you have studied this chapter, you should be able to:

- Identify and implement effective health and personal hygiene practices
- Explain the major disease-causing agents
- Provide information about human immunodeficiency virus infection, acquired immunodeficiency syndrome, hepatitis, and MRSA
- Describe measures for ensuring a hazard-free massage environment
- Describe methods for preventing and controlling disease
- Give specific recommendations for sanitary practices for massage businesses
- Implement Standard Precautions

On a separate sheet of paper or on the computer, write a short summary of the content of this chapter based on the preceding list of competencies. Use a conversational tone, as if you were explaining to someone (e.g., a client, prospective employer, coworker, or other interested person) the importance of the information and skills to the development of the massage profession.

Next, in small discussion groups, share your summary with your classmates and compare the ways the information was presented. In discussing the content, look for similarities, differences, possibilities for misunderstanding of the information, and clear, concise methods of description.

Professional Activity

List 20 suggested sanitation requirements developed from the Oregon model.

1.
2.
3.
4.
5.
6.
7.
8.
9.
10.
11.
12.
13.
14.
15.
16.
17.
18.
19.
20.

Professional Application

Completing an Accident Report

It is a fact of life that accidents happen daily. When they involve personal injury or property damage, information is needed so that the involved parties and any insurance companies can recognize and repair the damage. A massage practitioner, like any other business person, may be called on to fill out an insurance report. This exercise presents a practice story about an accident. The story is followed by some standard questions, and the correct answers are supplied so that you can see how the information should be presented. (The following scenario is intended to be humorous.)

This afternoon you had a new client. He is the contortionist from the traveling circus, which is in town for the next week. He brought along his wife, who works with him, to observe your techniques so that she can help him as they travel. Unfortunately, some interesting things happened. You sit for a few minutes to recollect the events, and this is what you remember:

You had completed the massage with Mr. Gummy and had just asked him to roll over when you noticed that the table had started swaying. Ms. Gummy, who is an acrobat, was doing a handstand on Mr. Gummy's shoulders. Your table was sturdy enough, but because of the lubricant on your client's shoulders, his wife slid off and out the window. She was able to catch herself on the awning of the store below your office, but in doing so she bent the frame and tore the canvas. No one was injured, but the other tenant called emergency services, so reports had to be filed.

Because your immediate supervisor was not available, you had to complete the accident report yourself. Using your narrative, fill out the following information for the police and insurance companies.

1. State where and when the accident occurred.

2. Provide detailed information about the accident.

3. Give the names and addresses of the person or people involved in the accident.

4. Give the names of any witnesses to the accident.

5. Give the names of manufacturers, if equipment was involved.

6. Describe all property damage.

7. Detail any injuries to the people involved.

Body Mechanics

 http://evolve.elsevier.com/Fritz/fundamentals/

CHAPTER OBJECTIVES

After completing this chapter, the student will be able to perform the following:

1. Interpret biomechanical research related to massage application
2. Create an ergonomically effective massage environment
3. Use basic biomechanical principles to develop effective body mechanics
4. Determine appropriate pressure, drag, and duration application while applying massage methods
5. Alter ergonomic and biomechanical principles based on gender
6. Identify and correct nonoptimal massage application that causes pain and discomfort for the massage therapist

CHAPTER OUTLINE

KEY TERMS

Asymmetric standing	Drag
Balance	Ergonomics
Balance point	Friction
Biomechanics	Leverage
Center of gravity	Pressure
Compressive force	Traction

This chapter is very important to your success as a massage therapist. You want to be able to provide an effective, pleasurable massage for the client without harming yourself in the process. You want to generate enough income to meet your financial goals, which directly depends on whether clients value the massage you provide and how many quality massage sessions you are able to do each day.

Massage is physical, labor-intensive work, so the ability to work for 8 full hours a day is important. To generate an income sufficient to meet moderate living expenses, you must be able to give 20 to 25 sessions a week (see Chapter 3). Some massage therapists may choose to work fewer hours. However, for those who work full time, knowing the best ways to work is beneficial. Therefore, this chapter presents information on ergonomics and biomechanics that can enable a massage therapist to complete 25 massage sessions over a typical 5-day period. The goal is five 1-hour massage sessions a day, 5 days a week. Not only do you need to be able to work at this level, you need to be able to do it without hurting yourself. Effective body mechanics allow the massage practitioner's body to be used in a careful, efficient, and deliberate way. Proper body mechanics involve good posture, stability, balance, leverage, and use of the strongest and largest muscles to perform the work.

There is no single correct way to use the human body efficiently, and the recommendations in this chapter are effective methods. Three important things the massage practitioner must learn and remember are to remain relaxed, to stay comfortable, and to avoid straining when doing massage. If the practitioner looks and feels as if he or she is working hard while giving a massage, something is wrong with the body mechanics. With proper body mechanics, the practitioner looks and feels relaxed and graceful while giving a massage.

Think of the body as a mechanical device. The action of muscles and bones is the result of leverage, and levers operate according to mechanical laws. All mechanical devices are subject to wear during use; however, the advantage of the human body is that it is made up of living tissue that has the ability to heal. Therefore, an understanding of the biomechanical principles of the body helps to prevent injury and also to restore function when injury occurs.

Fatigue, muscle strain, and injury, including overuse syndromes, can result from improper use and positioning of the massage practitioner's body while giving a massage. In this chapter students learn methods of working more efficiently so that providing 8 hours of massage in a day does not cause dysfunction or pain. Efficient use of the body helps prevent burnout. These topics are explored throughout this chapter and in Chapter 10 as you learn to perform a massage.

The information in this chapter has been taken from standard ergonomics recommendations for service professions, from personal observation, and from the author's professional and teaching experience.

The delivery of therapeutic massage makes unique postural and physical demands. For most professionals, body mechanics focus on lifting or exerting a force in an upward direction, such as when a nurse lifts a patient from the bed to a chair. Other aspects of body mechanics apply to dynamic movement, such as for dancing and participating in athletics or the martial arts. In massage, in contrast, most of the effort exerted is a sustained, restrained, and somewhat static movement, with pressure focused downward and forward to deliver compressive and tension force. The massage practitioner makes extensive use of the forearms, wrists, hands, fingers, thumbs, knees, and foot to deliver compressive force. Because of this difference, the standard recommendations provided to most professionals for safe use of the body are of little help to massage practitioners. In fact, attempting to modify these forms of body mechanics may result in injury to the massage professional.

Massage professionals need to consider their body types and musculoskeletal limitations. The suggestions in this chapter can help most students develop the best personal body mechanics style for them as individuals. If you use effective body mechanics, you will not injure yourself or be any more fatigued than is expected after a full day of work. If your body mechanics are effective, the client experiences a quality massage. If you do not use your body in a biomechanically correct way, the massage pressure is uneven, too light or too deep, poky (painful), and generally uncomfortable for both the client and you. Make sure to view the DVD segment for this chapter and practice.

RESEARCH: EFFICACY OF BODY MECHANICS IN MASSAGE THERAPISTS

SECTION OBJECTIVES

Chapter objective covered in this section:

1. The student will be able to interpret biomechanical research related to massage application.

Using the information presented in this section, the student will be able to perform the following:

- Relate research to the recommendations for body mechanics while applying massage

Two basic factors of body mechanics are important for the massage therapist: ergonomics and biomechanics. **Ergonomics** focuses on the design of equipment, the work environment, and the workload with the goal of reducing musculoskeletal stress on the body. **Biomechanics** focuses on the body motions and the muscular forces used to complete tasks. For massage therapists, the major ergonomic issues are the height and width of the massage table and the amount of space around the table, all of which must support ease of massage application. The number of massage sessions or hours performed each day or each week also is a factor. The major biomechanical concerns are improper use of body areas that cannot be sustained in a stable position (i.e., the thumb, shoulder, low back, and knee).

Little ergonomic or biomechanical research has been done in the area of massage therapy. However, a few studies have been conducted that are directly related to massage therapy, and studies that apply to physical therapists can be considered to a certain extent. Ideally, the massage therapy community will conduct comprehensive studies on the ergonomics (environment and equipment) and biomechanics (use of the human body) needed for occupational safety, career longevity, and success in the future (Box 8-1).

Research Outcomes

One study specifically concerned with massage therapy involved a survey of 161 visually impaired massage practitioners in Taiwan. In this study, Jang et al. (2006) found that work-related musculoskeletal disorders (WMSDs) occurred in about 71.4% of those surveyed. The prevalence rates for injury were as follows:

- Finger or thumb—50.3%
- Shoulder—31.7%
- Wrist—28.6%
- Neck—25.5%
- Arm or elbow—23.6%
- Forearm—20.5%
- Back—19.3%

A study by Buck et al. (2007) investigated the postural and low-back demands of performing a standard, 45-minute massage using a massage table or a massage chair. The researchers reported that nonneutral wrist, shoulder, and trunk postures placed the therapists at risk for soft tissue injury. When using a massage table, the massage therapists spent significantly more time in mild trunk flexion (more than 10 degrees of flexion). Spinal loading increases when the trunk is bent forward from the upright position. Takahashi et al. (2006) reported a two-fold increase in L4/5 compression at 10 degree trunk flexion and a 3.5 increase at 30 degrees of flexion demonstrating that even small postural changes from the upright standing position magnify spinal loading and increase the potential for back pain. When using a massage chair, therapists spent significantly more time in severe radial deviation (>30 degrees of radial deviation) and mild shoulder flexion (x > 20 degrees of flexion). Using the chair placed increased strain on the therapist's anterior deltoid, and using a table increased strain on the lumbar erector spinae muscle group. The study found that massage therapists adopted trunk and wrist postures that would increase the risk of upper extremity injury while using either the massage chair or table. Ergonomic strategies that are used to minimize this source of

| Box 8-1 | Basic Concepts of Body Mechanics |

- *Biomechanics* is the understanding of the motion and forces produced by the human body.
- *Work* is the result of a force acting through a distance.
- *Power* relates to the time element and the work accomplished.
- *Applied force* is the energy or effort provided to perform work. Applied force has many forms, such as the power of an electric motor or the push from human hands.
- *Muscle contraction* is work and reflects the consumption of mechanical energy. Using muscles to generate applied force during massage application is fatiguing.
- *Joint structures* are designed to adapt to external and internal forces as long as these forces are not excessive and sustained.
- *Joint stress* is defined as the mechanical force that develops in a joint.
- The *closed packed position* is the most stable joint position (where movement normally halts). During massage application, some joints are placed in this stable position.
- According to Newton's basic laws, for every force, an opposite force is created. For example, downward pressure evokes an equal opposing upward push. A twisting force in one direction must be followed by an equal twisting force in the opposite direction. A force allowing a part to slide downward must be resisted by an adequate upward force. A force that tends to bend a structure along its axis must be resisted by an equal force to prevent such bending. Pressure always results in compression stress, and a pull produces tensile stress. Pressure causing compression moves into tissue. A pull on the same tissue is an action directly opposite of the compression.
- A force directed against a structure so that the parts slide against each other produces a shearing stress. Both parts may be movable, with the parts sliding in opposite directions, or one part may be fixed. Incorrect application of massage causes compression and shearing stress to the massage therapist's joints.
- Spinal bending involves the actions of tension, compression, and torsion (twisting). It is important that the massage therapist avoid bending over or twisting while performing massage.
- The cumulative effects of constant or repeated small stresses over a long period can cause the same difficulties as severe sudden stress. This means that even if an action, such as applying a massage method, does not cause pain while performed, performing this same action over and over incorrectly eventually leads to difficulty.
- With good postural body mechanics, the massage therapist can apply force to the client's tissue with the least amount of muscular effort, thus encouraging longer endurance with less strain on any one part.

loading include table height adjustment and altered positioning of the client's body.

A survey done in Australia in 2008 found that most massage therapists were women (79%), who worked in the industry 3 to 5 years (Terra Rosa, 2008). (Later in this chapter you will learn that women massage therapists often need a higher table than men massage therapists.) Most therapists worked only 10 to 20 hours a week, far fewer than the number of hours generally accepted as full time. Seventy percent of the respondents indicated that they had received training in posture and self-care, and 90% currently were involved in self-care. Regardless, a high number reported pain in the wrist and thumb (69%), neck (59%), shoulder (54%), and lower back (26%). The most troublesome problem appeared to be wrist pain; 42% of the respondents indicated daily to weekly pain that affected their work. The survey number was small, but the data collected are consistent with the findings of other surveys.

Multiple studies of physical therapy (physiotherapy) and occupational therapy have identified an unacceptable prevalence of low back and thumb pain in these professionals (Cromie et al., 2000; Snodgrass et al, 2003; Buckingham et al., 2007; Campo et al., 2008; Hu et al., 2009). The main causes of the discomfort are use of the thumb to apply pressure, awkward postures, and a heavy workload. Cromie et al. (2000) found that more than 90% of these professionals experienced work-related musculoskeletal disorders.

In a survey of more than 500 massage therapists across Canada, Albert et al. (2008) found a high prevalence of musculoskeletal pain in all areas of the upper extremity. A high prevalence of injury also was seen, even though most of the respondents indicated that they had received proper training in body mechanics and self-care. Pain and discomfort were most often reported in the wrist and thumb (83%), followed by the lower back (65%) and the neck and shoulders (64%).

Most of those surveyed indicated that they had received proper training in massage therapy school. However, the injury rate would seem to indicate that the training they received was not effective at preventing injury. Either the skills taught were ineffective and based on flawed information, or the massage therapists were not implementing what they have been taught.

Taken together, the studies clearly show that even with the best biomechanics, the thumb cannot withstand the strain placed on it during manual therapy. We must provide massage with minimal use of the thumb and never use the thumb to generate pressure (Figure 8-1).

A study by E.G. Mohr, a certified engineer and ergonomist, found that the economic viability (ability to make money) of the manual therapy practitioner depended on the number of massages or treatments that could be given in a day or a week (Mohr, 2010). Fatigue or injuries can have a major impact on income potential and ultimately may cause the practitioner to quit the profession and seek other, less physically demanding employment.

Manual therapy practitioners in general, and massage therapists in particular, can use a wide variety of body postures in providing treatments. Mohr suggests that an optimum method exists for applying a variety of mechanical forces during a massage; this maximizes the benefit to the client while minimizing the strain and effort required by the practitioner. (Mohr reviewed the body mechanics presented in this chapter.)

Albert et al. (2006) have performed a number of studies on the biomechanics of massage therapists. Collectively these

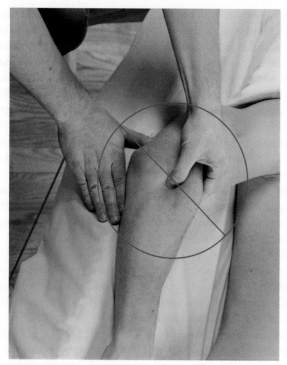

FIGURE 8-1 Avoid using the thumb while giving a massage.

studies found that massage therapists assume nonneutral trunk, neck, and arm postures for a significant part of the massage, placing the therapist at risk of cumulative musculoskeletal disorders. Although the amount of pressure on the therapists' lower back was considered to be in the safe range in the short term, the cumulative compression and shearing fell into the problematic range. Gliding methods intended to access the entire back in long strokes, muscle stripping, and kneading required severe nonneutral posture of the trunk for less than 10% of the activity time. However, over a typical workload, the cumulative effects of using these long gliding methods were significant. On average, during 50% of the massage, the trunk was required to be flexed away from neutral. Deviation from neutral also was required of the arms for 70% of the massage, and of the shoulders and neck for 60% of the massage. This is significant, because most of the massage time was spent performing these techniques. Activities such as static touch and wringing required the largest percentage of time in nonneutral neck postures, but fortunately these techniques were performed for short periods (1 minute). The findings of these studies indicated that the body mechanics used by the subjects did not support long-term practice as a massage therapist. Effective body mechanics require attention to ergonomics and biomechanics.

ERGONOMICS AND BIOMECHANICS

SECTION OBJECTIVES

Chapter objectives covered in this section:

2. The student will be able to create an ergonomically effective massage environment.
3. The student will use basic biomechanical principles to develop effective body mechanics.

4. The student will be able to determine appropriate pressure, drag, and duration application while applying massage methods.

Using the information presented in this section, the student will be able to perform the following:

- Apply principles of ergonomics and biomechanics to massage therapy
- Use massage equipment in an ergonomically effective manner
- Explain how massage application applies mechanical force to the client's body
- Demonstrate the application of compressive force when providing massage
- Implement body mechanics principles while doing massage
- Apply a variety of pressure levels during massage
- Modify massage application using drag and duration

Practical application of ergonomics and body mechanics involves integrating the information discussed earlier into the actual performance of a massage. It is one thing to understand the principles, and quite another to actually do what has been described. In this section, we will learn how to "do."

Applying Ergonomics

Physical ergonomics in general deals with the human body's responses to physical and physiologic loads. The following are primary topics addressed by physical ergonomics that apply to massage therapists (Barnett and Liber, 2006).

- Manual materials handling, workstation layout, job demands, and risk factors (e.g., repetition, vibration, force, and awkward or static posture), as they relate to musculoskeletal disorders and repetitive strain injury.
- Work activities, which should allow workers to adopt several different postures, all equally healthy and safe. Muscular force should be exerted by the largest appropriate muscle groups available.
- Human push capability (weight transfer to apply compressive force), which involves strength, weight, weight distribution, push angle, footwear/floor friction, and the friction between the upper body and the pushed object.

Ergonomically, the workstation is the primary focus. Massage therapists have an uncomplicated work environment: a massage area and equipment such as a massage table and a massage mat or chair (or both). Improper workstation design, including the width and height of the massage table and the size of the massage room, can lead to poor posture and body mechanics, resulting in an increase in musculoskeletal injuries.

Massage Area

The massage area encompasses the open space around the massage table, mat, or chair. This space must be large enough to allow the therapist to move easily around the equipment. A space 12 × 12 feet is ideal, but other dimensions will work. The area should not be smaller than 9 × 9 feet. If the area is cluttered, too small, or an odd shape (e.g., narrow), the therapist must alter his or her stance, and smooth movement around the client becomes more difficult, whether the person is on a massage table or mat or in a massage chair.

The floor of the massage area must be nonslip to ensure safety and to allow the therapist's feet to obtain a grip on the floor. Massage therapists should wear nonslip shoes.

Proper airflow, temperature, lighting, and noise levels are other ergonomic factors that promote the well-being of both the massage therapist and the client. The ideal massage area is quiet and has windows to allow natural light and fresh air, adjustable heat and air conditioning, circulating airflow, and lighting that can be adjusted from bright to dim. Most massage therapists work in conditions that are less than ideal; however, it is important to strive for the healthiest and most ergonomically correct work space possible.

Massage Equipment

Massage Table

Massage therapists typically work in the standing position. Therefore, the width and height of the massage table determine the postures the therapist uses. Massage therapists are at higher risk of cumulative episodes of pain in the low back and upper extremities if they are required to maintain awkward, static postures for the duration of a massage treatment. The massage table can cause these awkward postures in three main ways:

- If the table is too low, the therapist may be required to slouch and bend over. In this case, the table should be raised.
- If the table is too high, the therapist may have to elevate the shoulders, use lateral flexion and twisting of the torso, and stand on the toes. The solution is to lower the table.
- If the table is too wide (or the massage stroke is too long), the therapist must reach. The solution is to use a narrower table, shorten the strokes, and step forward and perpendicular to the massage table.

Ideally the table height could be varied according to the technique used and the client's size. However, for now, this seldom is actually possible. Although electric-lift adjustable massage tables are becoming more common, they are not portable. Many textbooks state that the proper working height of a table is equal to the distance from the floor to a point between the therapist's wrist and the tips of the extended fingers (or about the middle of the hand) when the arm is hanging at the side of the body. However, some suggest that occasionally the optimum height may be as low as the therapist's knees or as high as the waist (Figure 8-2).

According to the Canadian study by Albert et al. (2006) mentioned earlier, the average fingertip height is 38% of a person's stature. Interestingly, the massage therapists in this study all chose table heights that were 40% to 43% of their standing height, which would be between the fingertips and wrist, as suggested in their training manuals. The study found that on average, trunk postures were divided 50/50 between the neutral position category and the mild posture distortion category; the shoulder and neck were in neutral postures for 30% and 40% of the time, respectively. Obviously, these table heights resulted in an inappropriate workstation.

Punnett et al. (1991) found that the risk of back disorders increased significantly with time worked in nonneutral postures and that the risk increased further when a nonneutral posture (meaning some sort of twisting) was used in more than one of the principal axes at a time.

The posture categories reported in the study by Albert et al. (2006) mirrored those of Punnett, and the significant working time in a mild trunk flexion reported for the massage therapists is reason for concern. The trunk postures required of the massage therapists in this study would result in significant cumulative loads for a 45-minute massage. These findings indicate that the massage therapists were flexing forward to do massage; therefore, the massage table was too low, and raising the height of the table would be logical. The massage table must be kept at a comfortable height, which depends on the practitioner's height, the client's size (thick or thin), and the style of massage used (Box 8-2).

Box 8-2 Massage Equipment Ergonomics

Working with a Massage Table

- As a general rule, the table height should be one half the practitioner's height. Therefore, if the practitioner is 5 feet, 6 inches tall (66 inches), the table should be approximately 33 inches high.
- Depending on the therapist's torso, arm, and leg length ratios, the correct height for the table will be 2 to 3 inches higher or lower. An individual with long arms may need a shorter table than a person with short arms. A person with a short torso, short arms, and long legs often needs a taller table.
- Typically a woman needs a taller table than a man of the same height.
- A table 24 to 28 inches wide provides adequate space for the client to lie down comfortably, but it is not so wide that the therapist must reach for the client in the middle of the table.
- The knees and hips are used to lift portable tables. The therapist should not bend forward at the waist. Some tables have shoulder straps, wheel bases, and other devices to aid in transport by redistributing the weight load.
- Consistently carrying the table on only one side of the body may be harmful. Alternate carrying arms; for example, carry in with the left arm, carry out with the right.

Working on a Floor Mat

- Body mechanics similar to those used for working with a table apply for working on a mat on the floor. The notable difference is that the center of gravity is lower, necessitating greater core strength.
- Movement around the client is different when the person is on a floor mat rather than a massage table. The weight-bearing balance points on the floor are from the knees instead of the feet.
- Padding on the knees may be required. Knee pads are available.
- The mat must be large enough so that the massage therapist can keep his or her knees on the mat while doing the massage.

Working with a Massage Chair

- Specially designed massage chairs help with positioning the client so that compression can be applied correctly.

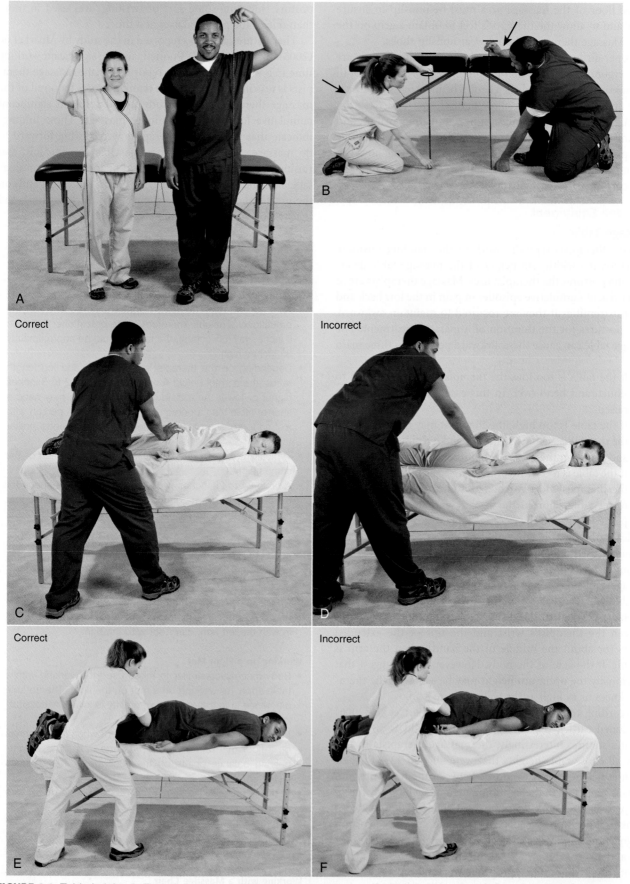

FIGURE 8-2 Table height. **A,** The practitioner's height is measured with a cord and then the cord is folded in half. **B,** At first the table height is set according to half of the practitioner's height, then adjusted slightly higher or lower if necessary for comfort. **C,** Table at correct height. **D,** Incorrect height—table too low. **E,** Efficient body mechanics with table at appropriate height. **F,** Incorrect height—table too high.

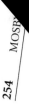
Box 8-3	Causes of Muscle Injury

Four theories have been proposed to explain how people incur muscle injuries.

Multivariate interaction theory: The combined effects of an individual's genetics, body type, and psychosocial makeup, along with occupational biomechanical hazards, lead to injury.

Differential fatigue theory: Different muscles are loaded differently, depending on the motion, and this may not occur in proportion to the muscles' capacity; therefore, they fatigue more quickly (e.g., the thumbs compared to the trunk or smaller muscles of the back), causing injury.

Cumulative load theory: Cumulative submaximum loads result in injury as a result of the cumulative loading of the muscle, which reduces the tolerance of the soft tissues to handle the load.

Overexertion theory: Exertion exceeds the tolerance limit, and musculoskeletal injury occurs.

In terms of providing massage, this means that the therapist engages several body parts to deliver a massage treatment, but muscles are not equal in strength and endurance capabilities. Different body parts will fatigue more quickly than others. Over a prolonged period, a change in technique may be initiated to accommodate the fatigued body segments, placing higher stress on some joints.

Awkward posture is associated with an increased risk for injury, and the more a joint deviates from the neutral position, the greater the risk of injury (Box 8-3). Every joint in the body has a neutral position, in which joint spaces are even and symmetric (Box 8-4). The muscles around a joint in neutral position are neither short nor long, but rather at their neutral physiologic resting lengths. Joint stability is provided with the least amount of muscle activity and maximizing stability provided by joint shape, joint capsule, ligaments, and normal co-contraction of the muscles around the joint.

Massage therapists need to consider all these factors to prevent injury and have a long, prosperous massage career (Box 8-5).

Biomechanics: Center of Gravity and Leaning

The basic concept of the style of body mechanics presented in this text is that **compressive force** should be applied to the client's soft tissue by shifting body weight and moving the center of gravity forward. The average position of an object's weight distribution is called the **center of gravity.** Your center of gravity is closest to the area where most of the weight is located in your body; this usually is somewhere around the navel when you are standing upright with your feet about shoulder width apart. In biomechanics, **balance** is the ability to maintain the body's center of gravity within the base of support. When the center of gravity is moved outside a base of support created by your feet on the floor, the center of gravity is supported by another support structure, such as the client's body (Figure 8-3).

The point of contact between the practitioner and the client is the **balance point;** the practitioner would fall forward

Box 8-4	Neutral Posture

Neutral posture is the resting position body is in neutral posture, little or n exerted on nerves, tendons, muscl posture also is the position in whic resting length. One of the jobs of workstations and processes that allc remain in neutral position as much as possible. The following guidelines describe neutral position for body areas.

Neck
The head is balanced on the spinal column. It is not tilted forward, back, or to either side. It is not rotated to the left or right.

Back
The spine naturally assumes an S-shaped curve. It is not rotated or twisted or tilted left or right. The trunk is not bent forward (flexion) or backward (extension).

Shoulders
The shoulders are in a resting position, neither hunched up nor pulled down, and are not pulled forward or back.

Upper Arms
The upper arms hang straight down the sides of the body.

Forearms
The forearms rest with the thumbs up. They are not in pronation or supination. This positioning is especially important when using the forearm to apply massage.

Elbows
The elbows are in a neutral position when the angle between the forearm and the upper arm is close to a right angle (90 degrees). This position is important when bending the elbow to perform massage with the forearm. When the arm is straight and the elbow is in extension, the elbow must be stabilized in the closed packed position for efficient force transmission. Logically, it is best to use the forearm position with the elbow in neutral position for most massage applications.

Wrists
The wrists are in line with the forearms. They are neither bent up (extension) nor bent down (flexion). They are not bent toward the thumbs (radial deviation) or toward the little fingers (ulnar deviation).

Fingers (Waterfall Position)
The fingers are gently curved as if placed on a large ball. They are not spread apart, fully straightened (extended), or tightly curled (flexed).

Lower Body
Seated and standing postures involve deviations from neutral posture. Neutral posture is the flexed fetal position (i.e., hip and knee joints flexed).

Modified from Warren N, Morse TF: *Neutral posture.* ErgoCenter, University of Connecticut Health Center. http://oehc.uchc.edu/ergo_neutralposture.asp. Accessed June 10, 2011.

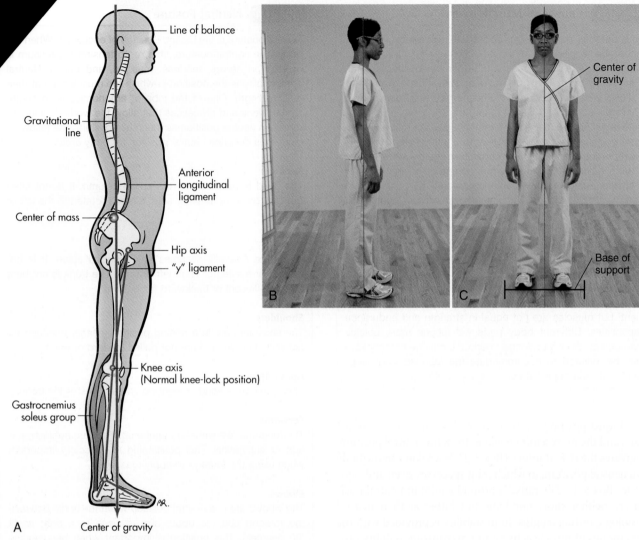

FIGURE 8-3 A, Relaxed standing posture that supports the gravitational line with normal knee-lock position in the last 15 degrees of extension. The gravitational force line falls behind the hip joint, in front of the knee joint, and in front of the ankle joint. The only muscle group used for balance is the gastrocnemius-soleus group. The relaxed stance involves leaning on the "y" (iliofemoral) ligament, the anterior longitudinal ligament, and the posterior knee ligaments. **B,** Center of gravity standing. **C,** Center of gravity at the midsection and base of support at the feet.

| Box 8-5 | OSHA's Ergonomics Recommendations |

The Occupational Safety and Health Administration (OSHA) has performed numerous studies of body mechanics and ergonomics for various occupations. The following are some of OSHA's consistent recommendations.

- Any posture significantly different from "neutral" is considered to be at risk for musculoskeletal distress. "Neutral" is considered to be the position about halfway through the available range of motion for the joint.
- The number and severity of torso flexions should be limited. Generally, torso flexion should be limited to 6 to 10 degrees from vertical.
- The head should be vertical and should not tilt forward more than about 15 degrees.
- Awkward postures should be avoided, including torso bending, twisting, and reaching.

- The arms should hang normally at the sides of the body and should not reach forward farther than 16 to 18 inches. When reaching, the hands should be maintained vertically between the waist and midchest.
- Midrange working postures should be maintained by sitting or standing upright and not bending the joints into extreme positions. The neck, back, arms, and wrists should be kept within a range of neutral positions.
- When standing, the weight should be shifted from one leg to the other.
- The most stable position of the knee is extension.
- Work should not be performed at too low or too high a height.

Modified from the National Institute for Occupational Safety and Health (NIOSH). www.osha.gov/ergonomics/guidelines/retailgrocery/retailgrocery.html. Accessed November 17, 2011.

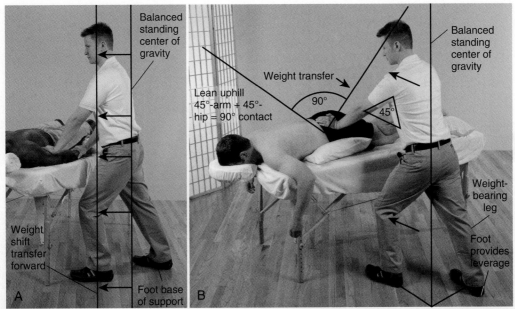

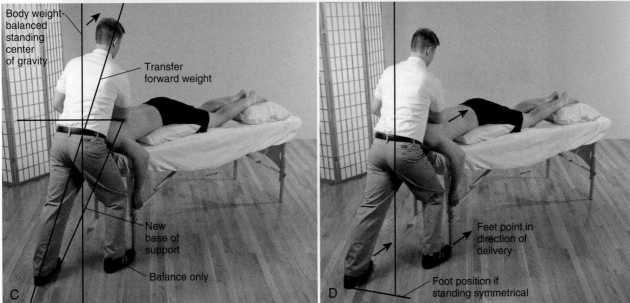

FIGURE 8-4 **A,** Using the principles of body mechanics in a weight shift. **B,** During a weight shift, the center of gravity moves between the legs to between the contact point and the original balanced center of gravity, allowing leaning to achieve a 90-degree contact on the body with the massage therapist's shoulder stabilized at approximately 45 degrees and the client's body sloped at 45 degrees. **C,** As the therapist moves from a standing center of gravity, the front leg moves forward for balance while the back leg weight-bears into the floor, transferring weight forward to apply compression. **D,** Keep the feet shoulder width apart and in an asymmetric stance.

Continued

if the hand were moved off the client. The practitioner's center of gravity moves forward between the hand or forearm contact, rather than dropping between the feet, as occurs in martial arts or similar systems.

The center of gravity is moved by "leaning" on the client, just as someone would comfortably lean against a wall or on a table. During massage application, you lean forward from the ankle as body weight is transferred to the client in the direction in which you will apply pressure, and your back leg is used for leverage (Figure 8-4) (Proficiency Exercise 8-1).

The practitioner seldom "pushes" against the client. Pushing requires a tense body and the use of muscle contraction to exert pressure. It is important that the practitioner use body weight. Although muscle strength is not a big factor, leverage is essential (Magee and Zachazewski, 2007). By leaning to transfer weight, the practitioner can substantially reduce muscle tension in the shoulders, neck, wrists, thumbs, elbows, and lower back and efficiently apply mechanical forces during the massage (Box 8-6).

When the hand is used to apply pressure during massage, the most correct position of the arm is with the elbow joint straight so that the forces produced flow directly along the bones and through the joints. This means that the elbow must be in extension (but not hyperextension) to reduce the amount

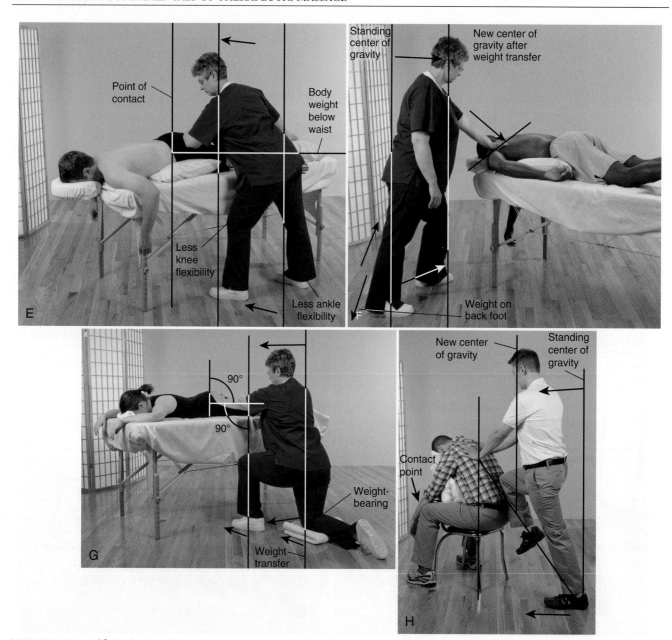

FIGURE 8-4, cont'd E, Gender differences—female example: The body weight is below the waist; less knee and ankle flexibility requires a higher massage table than for a male. **F,** The ground reaction force from weight on the back leg during a weight shift results in the application of forces at the client contact. **G,** Weight transfer while kneeling. **H,** Using the knee to apply pressure during a weight shift.

💡 PROFICIENCY EXERCISE 8-1

1. Practice leaning on a wall the correct way and the incorrect way. Feel the difference.
2. Record yourself giving a massage. Do you look graceful and relaxed, or are you working too hard?
3. Experiment with different positions with the client so that you can effectively "lean."
4. Tie one end of a short rope around your waist and the other end around your wrist. The length of the rope should allow you to reach out at a 45- to 60-degree angle. Perform a massage. The rope will prevent you from reaching too far with the stroke and will tug at your waist when it is time to shift the body by taking a step forward.

5. Practice with a standing partner. Lean on your partner as you would lean on a wall. Pay attention to how you feel as your "wall" slightly changes position by moving forward, backward, or twisting. If your partner cannot easily move you with subtle body shifts, you are stabilizing your body and pushing.
6. Have your partner lie on the table and repeat the exercise in step 5.
7. Practice using your hand as a unit and grasping objects with the palm of your hand. Make sure not to pinch during the grasping movement.

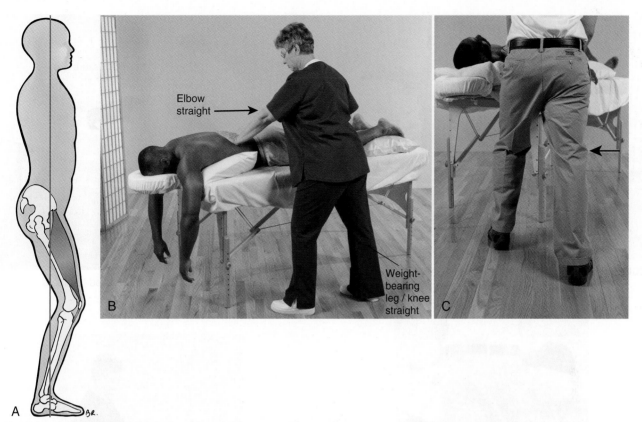

FIGURE 8-5 A, Improper leg position, which puts excessive strain on the joints and requires muscle activity to maintain balance. The gravitational line improperly falls behind the knees. **B,** Stability for a weight transfer relies on an extended (but not hyperextended) knee and elbow. **C,** Correct asymmetric standing. The right knee is extended correctly to support weight bearing.

Box 8-6 Force

Force is a push or pull on an object, which then causes an acceleration, a deceleration, or a change in shape if the object is stable. Massage application applies mechanical forces. The body can move in response to the force (joint movement), or it can change shape, as happens when the soft tissue is massaged.

Forces always occur in pairs. You cannot apply a force to the client's body without the body applying a force back out. This is the reason we can lean on something (a wall, a desk, a client's body) and not fall.

---

of muscular effort required by the massage therapist. The knee of the weight-bearing leg also must be in full extension to transmit force from the foot pushing into the floor. Muscles fatigue; bones do not. Therefore, we should develop massage techniques that rely on the maximum use of weight transfer through our bones with stable joints and the minimum use of our muscles to reduce fatigue and maintain control (Figure 8-5).

Friction and Traction: The Importance of the Feet

Body mechanics for massage begin at the feet. Ground reaction forces at the foot and floor are one of the most important—yet often the most overlooked—aspects of massage application. For our purposes, we can say that ground reaction forces occur when the body pushes into the floor and

the floor pushes back, so long as no slipping occurs. **Friction** is the force that prevents slipping. Traction is required to prevent slipping. **Traction** is the maximum frictional force that can be produced between surfaces without slipping; this applies, during massage, between the foot and the floor, or in the contact with the client's body.

Friction that allows ground reaction forces works for the massage therapist by enabling the pressure exerted during massage to move toward the client's body. Massage should not be performed in bare or stocking feet, because this hinders the ability to perform massage and also is unsanitary. The only way to ensure adequate friction (and therefore the ability to generate force) is to wear shoes that have a rubber-type sole and that can be tied or strapped around the arch (e.g., athletic shoes) (Figure 8-6).

The massage therapist can generate the greatest force when the feet are positioned shoulder width apart and with one foot being weight-bearing and the other placed approximately halfway between the point of contact with the client and the weight-bearing foot in front of the other (Figure 8-7). In this posture, the rear foot, and sometimes also the front foot, may be behind the body's center of gravity.

According to Newton's law, for every force on a body, an equal and opposite reaction force occurs. Therefore, whatever force is applied to the client's body by the hands/forearms elicits a reaction by an equal force at the foot/floor interface. For example, if you apply 15 pounds of force (moderate pressure) during massage, the friction force at your feet must be

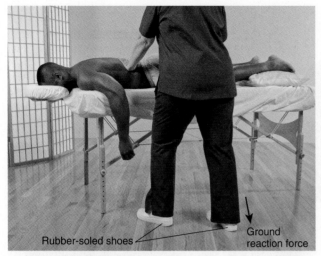

FIGURE 8-6 Ground reaction forces require nonslip surfaces.

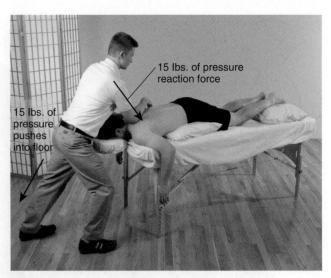

FIGURE 8-8 Ground reaction forces are used to create compressive force during massage.

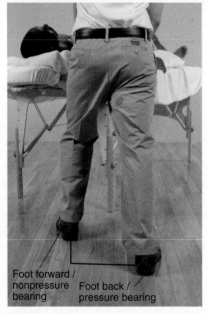

FIGURE 8-7 Feet stay shoulder width apart as non–weight-bearing leg moves forward.

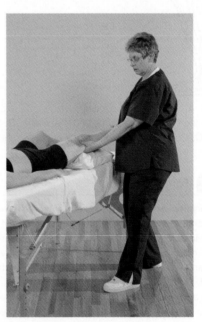

FIGURE 8-9 Pulling requires foot traction.

equal to 15 pounds. If the foot slips easily on the floor or in a sock, or even in ill-fitting shoes, the amount of force you can apply during massage is limited to the amount of friction force or traction at the feet. To get more pressure you must push with your muscles, which is inefficient (Figure 8-8).

Furthermore, with limited traction at the feet, you cannot safely lean into the client's body or away (as in a pulling stretch), because the feet will begin to slip. Researchers have shown that a person pushing with good traction can generate as much as 50% more force than can be obtained when pushing with poor traction. Applying a downward-forward push force during massage with the proper foot traction allows massage therapists to use their body weight to their advantage (Figure 8-9).

The same principles apply when sitting on a chair or stool to perform massage. The chair or stool must not slip back when the practitioner leans forward to apply pressure. The massage table, stool, or chair must not slip or have wheels or rollers unless they have a locking mechanism. Otherwise, the massage therapist must both hold the stool in place and attempt to apply pressure, which is not efficient. If therapists kneel during massage application (i.e., work on a floor mat), their knees become the contact instead of the feet (Figure 8-10).

When using the feet to perform a massage while the client is on a mat, massage therapists must make sure they are standing on a nonslip surface. A stable, nonskid cane (available at medical supply retailers) can be used to support balance in these cases (Figure 8-11).

Massage therapists also must keep in mind that although they use lubricant to reduce friction on the client's skin, this also reduces traction. If too much lubricant is used, pressure is difficult to apply.

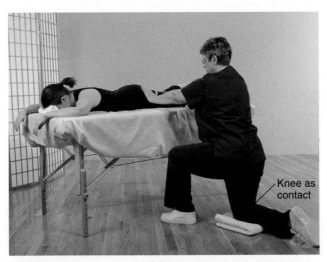

FIGURE 8-10 When the practitioner kneels to provide massage, the back knee becomes weight bearing; a folded towel can be used as a cushion.

Knee as contact

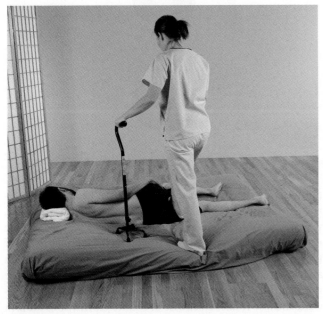

FIGURE 8-11 A cane provides support when the foot is used to apply massage.

Basic Concepts of Body Mechanics

Four basic concepts of body mechanics are common to all techniques used to apply compressive force to the body tissues during massage:

- Keeping the back straight and maintaining core stability
- Weight transfer
- Perpendicularity
- Stacking the joints

A straight back and a pressure-bearing leg are essential components of body mechanics. If the back is not straight, the practitioner often ends up pushing with the upper body instead of using the more effortless feeling of transferred weight. The practitioner's weight should be held on the back leg and flat foot, concentrated toward the heel. At first this may feel uncomfortable; however, some of the biggest muscles in

| Box 8-7 | Weight Transfer: Practical Application |

The following exercise demonstrates the concept of transferring weight by shifting the center of gravity to apply compressive force.

1. Stand facing a wall and put both hands on the wall, shoulder width apart and at shoulder height.
2. Step back with both feet so that your body is at a 45-degree angle and you are leaning into the wall. Your feet should be shoulder-width apart. Bring your hips forward and under you so that your shoulders, back, and feet are aligned. Hold your abdomen in while exhaling to stabilize the core. Hold the abdomen in but continue to breathe. Do not suck in your belly; pull it in by contracting the muscles. Notice that all your weight is on your feet and your hands.
3. Bring one leg forward and bend it. Make sure your foot is forward enough so that your toes are in front of your knee. The other leg stays back and straight. Keep your hips aligned with your shoulders and your back foot. Maintain core stability.
4. Drop the arm on the same side as your back foot. Keep the arm that remains on the wall straight and relax your shoulders. If you have range-of-motion limitations in your wrist, adjust the hand that is on the wall so that you are comfortable. Sometimes slightly curling your fingers is enough. Another option is using your fist with a straight wrist.
5. Try to hold your weight on your front leg so that your hand is not supporting you at all. Begin by slowly transferring the weight of your body from your front leg (slowly lift it from the floor) to the heel of your hand on the wall. Keep the arm that is against the wall straight and your hips aligned. Your hips do not need to move at all. Maintain core stability. As you feel the weight transfer to the heel of your hand, you will notice that weight also is moving to the heel of your back foot.

the body are in the legs. If you use the muscles of your upper body, fatigue sets in more quickly, and eventually the pain can become debilitating. The muscles of the torso, especially the abdomen, make up the body's core. Core stability is necessary for back stability (Neumann, 2010) (Figure 8-12).

With weight transfer, massage practitioners transfer their body weight by shifting the center of gravity forward to achieve a pressure that is comfortable to the client. To transfer weight, the practitioner stands (or kneels) with one foot forward and the other foot (or knee) back in an asymmetric stance. In the standing position, the front leg is in a relaxed knee flexion with the foot forward enough to be in front of the knee. The back leg is straight, and the hips and shoulders are aligned so that the back is straight. The transfer is made by taking the weight off the front leg and moving it to whichever part of the arm and hand is used to apply pressure (Figure 8-13). Pressure is increased or decreased by moving the back leg farther away from or closer to the client. The massage therapist's body weight is distributed to the flat foot of the weight-bearing leg, and the weight should be directed more toward the heel (Figure 8-14). Practitioners should not stand on their toes (Box 8-7).

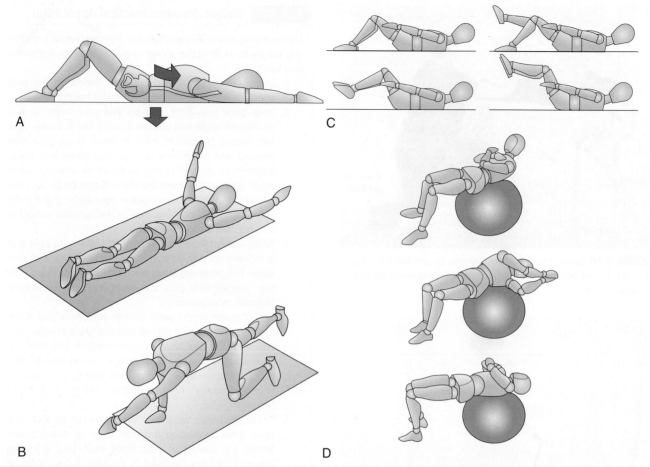

FIGURE 8-12 A, Draw-in maneuver. **B,** Prone core exercises. **C,** Supine core exercises. **D,** Ball stabilization exercises.

Perpendicularity ensures that the pressure exerted by the massage therapist sinks straight into the client's tissues. Massage primarily uses a force generated forward and downward with a 90-degree contact against the body (Figure 8-15). The combination of a 45-degree slant from the contours of the client's body plus the 45-degree angle of force used during appropriate body mechanics results in the 90-degree contact (Figure 8-16).

Stacking the joints one on top of another is essential to the concepts of perpendicularity and weight transfer. The practitioner's body must be a straight line from the feet and then through the shoulder to the forearm, or through the elbow acting as an extension of the shoulder, to the heels of the hands (Figure 8-17). The ankle, knee, hip of the back leg, and spine are stacked. The shoulder is stacked over the elbow, which in turn is stacked over the wrist. Stacking the joints in this way allows the pressure to move straight into the client's body effortlessly as the center of gravity moves forward (Figure 8-18). Stability of the shoulder girdle and elbow also is essential. Even with the best body mechanics, stabilizing the shoulder is difficult. It is important to keep the scapula fixed in place against the rib cage. The normal biomechanical position of the shoulder blade should always be resting flat against the rib cage, regardless of the position of the arm.

The two common stability problems for massage therapists are the core and the shoulder complex. The primary muscle that stabilizes the scapula to the rib cage is the serratus anterior. Other muscles that offer support in that role are the middle and lower trapezius and rhomboids. The serratus anterior fibers contract when the arm is pushing against resistance, which is what happens in giving a massage. The client is the point of resistance. In such a situation, the middle fibers of the trapezius (an adductor) and the serratus (acting as an abductor) contract simultaneously to stabilize the scapula. The shoulder blade slides upward, downward, forward, and backward and also rotates clockwise or counterclockwise as the arm moves; however, it should not come away from the rib cage.

If the muscles that hold the shoulder blade against the rib cage do not work properly and scapular winging occurs, inappropriate activation of other muscle groups will compensate, resulting in overuse and pain in these muscles (Proficiency Exercise 8-2).

Pressure, Drag, and Duration

Describing various pressures and drag intensities is difficult, because they are affected by a number of factors, including (1) the client's body size, tissue quality, and treatment preferences; (2) the massage therapist's strength, expertise, and technique preference, and (3) the location of the pressure and the desired outcome for the massage. The perception of the application depends extensively on the client. Pressure perceived as deep by one client may be perceived as lighter pressure by another. Massage students learn to gauge the most beneficial and safest pressure and drag intensity.

Pressure has been defined as compressive force; force application depth; light, medium, and deep pressure; and so on. For

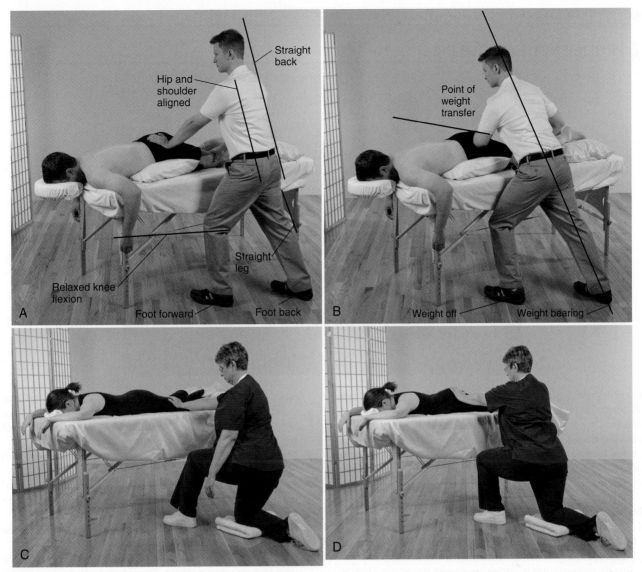

FIGURE 8-13 A, Maintaining alignment of the shoulder and pelvic girdle is part of stacking of the joints. **B,** During a weight transfer, the point of contact on the client and the therapist's back foot are weight bearing. The front foot is used only for balance. **C** and **D,** Weight transfer while kneeling.

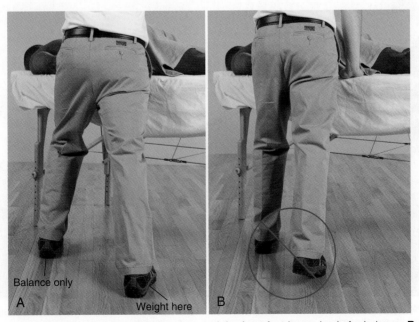

FIGURE 8-14 A, Correct stance. The back foot is weight bearing, and the front foot is used only for balance. **B,** Avoid standing on the toes, which shifts weight bearing to the front foot.

💡 PROFICIENCY EXERCISE 8-2

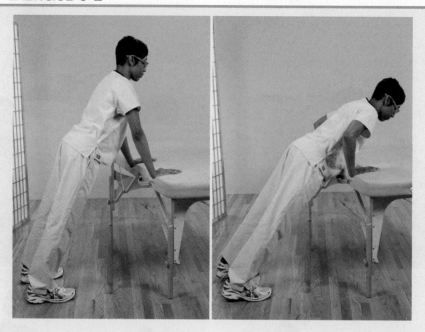

Counter push-ups are a good way to train the serratus anterior muscles. The idea is to push your chest away from a surface, and then lower it toward the surface, by using your shoulders, not your elbows. Massage therapists should perform this exercise by leaning against a counter, rather than prone on the floor, because the angle of the arms is similar to that used during massage.

Counter Push-Ups

1. Contract your abdomen to engage your core muscles. If you have difficulty maintaining core stability, use a belt or rope as an aid. First, maintain core stability while exhaling and then inhale normally (your abdomen should move out slightly).

Next, hold your breath and wrap the belt or rope around your waist and fasten it. The belt or rope should be snug but not tight or binding. If you lose core stability, the pressure against the belt will remind you to re-engage your core.

2. Stand upright about 2 or 3 feet from the counter and facing it.
3. Extend both arms and rest your palms on the edge of the counter, keeping your elbows straight. If the edge of the counter is uncomfortable, you can pad it with a towel.
4. Slowly flex your elbows and lower your chest toward the counter. Keep your feet flat on the floor.
5. Focus on using your shoulder muscles to raise yourself back up into a standing position. Repeat up to 10 times.

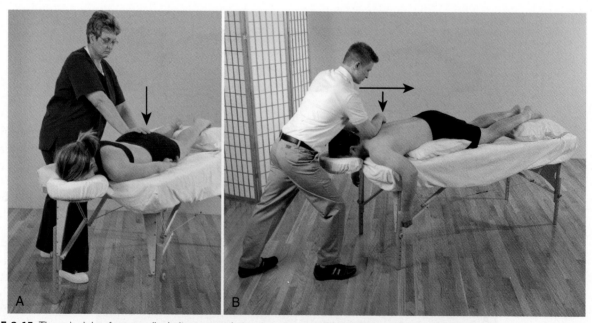

FIGURE 8-15 The principle of perpendicularity means that pressure exerted by the massage therapist sinks straight into the client's tissues when the hand **(A)** and forearm **(B)** are used.

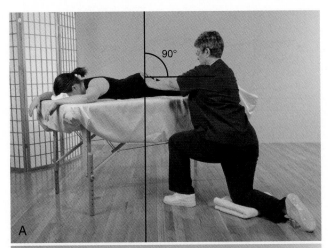

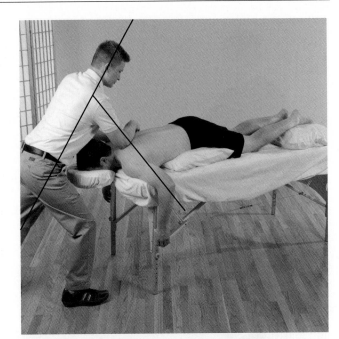

FIGURE 8-17 Position of the shoulder to achieve forearm pressure.

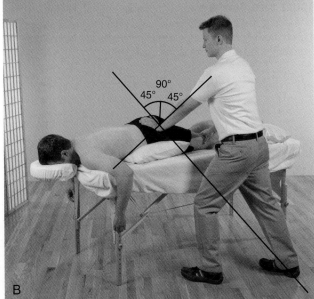

FIGURE 8-16 A, Kneeling position with transfer forward creates a 90-degree contact. **B,** In standing position, leaning by weight shift and shoulder angle about 45 degrees plus the approximate 45-degree angle at the client contact results in a 90-degree contact.

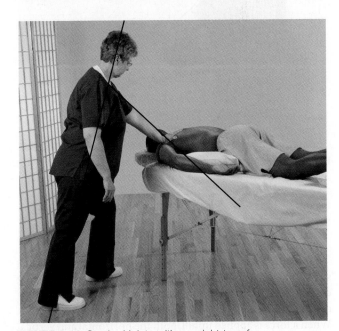

FIGURE 8-18 Stacked joints with a weight transfer.

the purposes of this text, **pressure** means compressive force exerted downward into the tissue through a 90-degree contact.

Drag is the resistance to glide. *Glide* moves horizontal to the tissues. Drag applies tension force to tissues to stretch them. The angle of force is directed away from the point of contact and can range from just less than 90 degrees to 180 degrees. Pressure combined with drag, therefore, can produce a broad range of intensities. For example, light pressure with extensive drag significantly stretches the skin. If the pressure is increased slightly and significant drag is maintained, the superficial fascia is stretched (tension force is applied).

Duration can modify intensity. In general, long duration is more intense and short duration is less intense.

Another factor that influences the application of pressure is the size of the point of contact. Clients appreciate a firm, even pressure that is distributed over a wide area. Pressure over a large contact area is less intense than that applied through a small contact point. More pressure can be applied safely with

a broad base of contact, such as the forearm or full hand, than through a small point of contact, such as the thumb. For example, firm pressure applied to the back with the forearm is pleasant. However, the same pressure applied with the point of the elbow or the thumb would be painful, because the pressure is concentrated in a small space instead of dispersed over a broad area. The tissue feels as if it is being poked, and the potential for tissue damage arises. When the practitioner's weight is maintained on the back foot and core stabilization is maintained, the pressure levels are more even; however, when the weight shifts to the front foot and core stabilization is lost, the pressure becomes more concentrated and uneven and may be uncomfortable to the client (Figure 8-19).

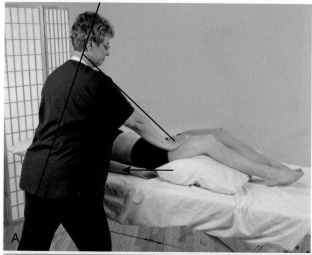

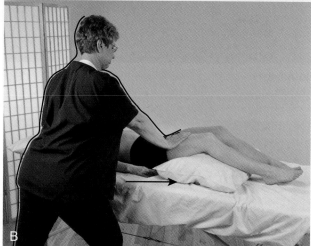

FIGURE 8-19 A, Stable core, stacked joints, and an efficient weight transfer create an even pressure delivery. **B,** An unstable core results in increased lordosis, pelvic and shoulder girdle rotation and tilt, a forward head position, and shoulder instability. A narrow contact point "pokes" the client.

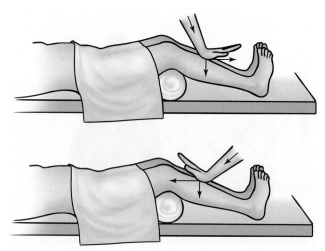

FIGURE 8-20 When a downhill stoke is applied, only the vertical component penetrates the tissue (top). When an uphill stroke is applied, both horizontal and vertical penetrate the tissue (bottom). Therefore, the uphill stroke is more efficient.

To apply pressure to a client, especially during a gliding stroke, moving uphill is always more efficient than moving downhill. When a force vector is applied at an angle, the force can be broken down into horizontal and vertical components. When a force is applied uphill, both the horizontal and vertical components are directed into the client's tissue. However, when a force is applied downhill, only the vertical component is directed into the tissue; the horizontal component is dissipated and thus wasted (Figure 8-20).

To recap, the factors that determine the intensity of a massage application are compressive force determining depth of pressure, drag, duration, and the size of the contact point. In addition, a fast, rhythmic application is more intense than a slow, rhythmic application. Obviously, determining the right pressure is more difficult than it appears (Figure 8-21).

Pressure

When compressive force is used, increasing force is needed to affect various layers of soft tissue. Hypothetically speaking, the tissues in the fleshy areas of the body (i.e., between the

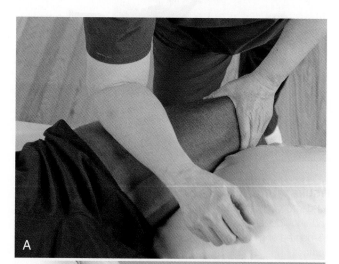

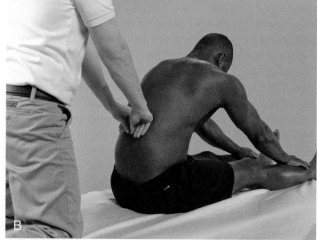

FIGURE 8-21 Using compression and the base of contact to determine the pressure level. **A,** Compression with a broad-based forearm contact. **B,** Compression applied with a loose fist on a smaller contact base.

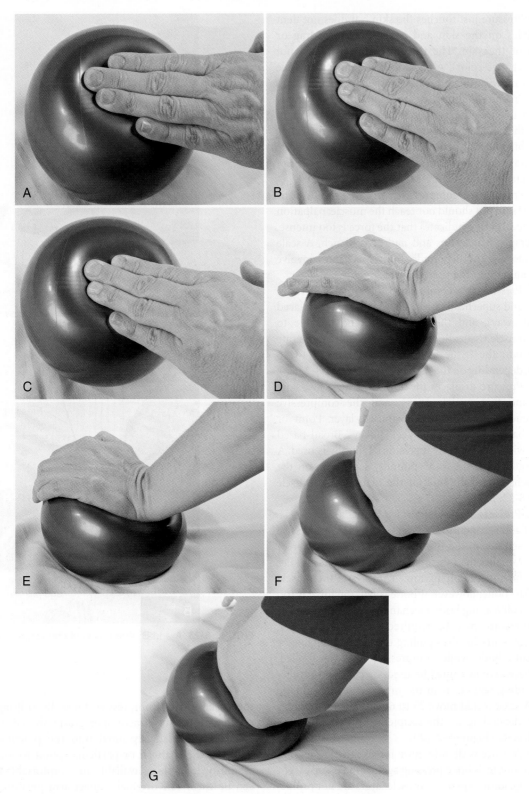

FIGURE 8-22 Pressure levels. A, Level 1, light. The therapist's fingertips do not blanch. **B,** Level 2. **C,** Level 3. **D,** Level 4. **E,** Level 5. **F,** Level 6. **G,** Level 7.

joints) can be divided into seven layers, which require seven levels of compressive force. The seven tissue layers, surface to deep, are:

Level 1—Skin surface
Level 2—Skin
Level 3—Superficial fascia

Level 4—First muscle layer
Level 5—Second muscle layer
Level 6—Third muscle layer
Level 7—Bone

The corresponding levels of pressure required to reach each of these layers are as follows (Figure 8-22):

- *Level 1:* Pressure just touches the skin but does not dent it. It slides on the skin and cannot produce drag or tension of the skin. The therapist's fingertips do not blanch (change color). A bathroom scale or other scale does not move at this pressure (Figure 8-22, *A*).
- *Level 2:* Pressure slightly dents the skin. It moves (drags) the skin to bind but cannot apply a tension force to stretch the skin past bind. The therapist's fingertips blanch, but the nail bed does not change color. A scale would move just 0 to 5 pounds, depending on the density of the person's skin (Figure 8-22, *B*).
- *Level 3:* Pressure is a compressive force that should penetrate the skin but should not reach the muscle; palpation of muscle structure indicates that the force is too intense. The therapist's fingertips and nail beds blanch. A scale would move 3 to 10 pounds. Body mechanics involve slight leaning into the tissue (Figure 8-22, *C*).
- *Level 4:* Pressure is a compressive force that penetrates the skin and superficial fascia. The skin layer is displaced (pressed away), and the therapist should be able to palpate muscle tissue. Body mechanics require moderate leaning into the tissue. A scale would move 7 to 16 pounds, depending on the tissue density (Figure 8-22, *D*).
- *Level 5:* Pressure displaces the surface tissues (i.e., skin, fascia, and first muscle layer), and the compressive force penetrates to the middle muscle layer. Point or narrow-based contact would feel "pokey." Broad-based contact with leaning body mechanics typically is used. A scale would move 12 to 35 pounds, depending on the tissue density and the bulk of the first layer of muscle (Figure 8-22, *E*).
- *Level 6:* Pressure displaces surface tissues (skin, fascia, and first and second muscle layers), and the compressive force penetrates to the third muscle layer. This layer of muscle is smaller than the first and second layers and lies next to the bone. Applying force compresses the muscle against the bone; however, if bone is felt, the force is too intense. Full leaning body mechanics with simultaneous counterpressure may be required to reach this layer. Counterpressure involves pulling up against the table or the client's body while compressive force is applied. Broad-based contact must be used, or pain and protective guarding will occur in the first and second muscle layers. A scale would move 25 to 60 pounds (sometimes higher), depending on the recipient's muscle bulk and tissue density (Figure 8-22, *F*).
- *Level 7:* Pressure is slightly more intense than at level 6. The therapist feels bone pressing against the tissue except around the joints where the muscle layers are not prominent and the bone is beneath the skin and superficial fascia (Figure 8-22, *G*).

Counterpressure

The practitioner should not push, even if intense pressure is required. Instead, the practitioner should lean on the area of the client's body that requires the intense pressure and then, using the nonworking hand, lift the body area back into

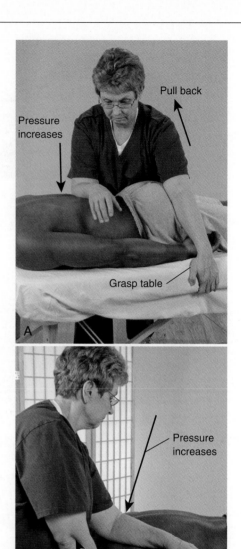

FIGURE 8-23 **A** and **B**, Application of counterpressure.

the practitioner's compressive force. By shifting the weight on the feet as the practitioner grasps the client's body, the client is automatically lifted into the practitioner (Figure 8-23). No set pattern or particular point to grasp has been established; anything available and comfortable for the client can be used. The original contact arm pressure increases as the body area is pulled into it, squeezing the pressure forces together. As the pulling arm leans back, the contact arm moves forward into the client. This technique must be monitored by the client for pressure levels. The practitioner can use the table as a source of counterpressure by pulling up on the table edge and leaning into the client's body, squeezing the forces together to increase the intensity of the pressure delivered. Contact must remain broad and must not narrow and poke the client.

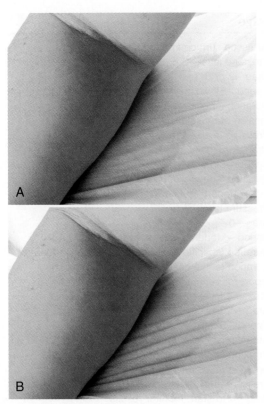

FIGURE 8-24 A, Minimal drag. **B,** Maximum drag.

Drag

The following is a suggested scale for determining drag:
0—Minimal drag (Figure 8-24, *A*)
1—Moves tissue but not to bind
2—Moves tissue to bind
3—Maximum drag: Moves tissue past bind (Figure 8-24, *B*)

Duration

Duration can modify intensity. Guidelines for duration include the following:
- For a specific application, a short duration is 10 seconds, a moderate duration is 30 seconds, and a long duration is 60 seconds.
- For a whole massage session, a short duration is 5 to 15 minutes, a moderate duration is 15 to 30 minutes, and a long duration is 45 to 60 minutes.

Speed

The speed of the massage application also can influence the intensity of the massage and the outcomes. Typically, the slower the speed, the more relaxing the massage. The faster the speed, the more stimulating the massage. Speed can be considered as follows:
- Slow—10 seconds from beginning to end of stroke
- Moderate—5 seconds from beginning to end of stroke
- Fast—2 seconds from beginning to end of stroke

Client Rhythm

It is important that massage practitioners allow their bodies to rock and sway with the massage movements. Slow rocking keeps the massage manipulations slow; this is crucial for

efficient adaptation or change in the client's muscle tissue or in the consistency of the connective tissue. The resulting rhythmic movement keeps the practitioner's body relaxed and is comforting to the client. Practitioners should remember to work with smooth, even movements, shifting position often.

The general guidelines presented in Box 8-8 can be used to combine the elements of pressure, drag, speed, and duration to achieve various massage outcomes.

GENDER DIFFERENCES

SECTION OBJECTIVES

Chapter objectives covered in this section:
5. The student will be able to alter ergonomic and biomechanical principles based on gender.
Using the information presented in this section, the student will be able to perform the following:
- Explain the necessary changes in body mechanics based on research findings in gender differences

The differences between the male body and the female body affect proper body mechanics. Most massage therapists are women (AMTA, 2011). Generally, women have more elastic tissues than do men. Also, women tend to have a slightly broader range of joint movement. Regardless of the massage therapist's gender, she or he must use the best body mechanics possible.

Center of Gravity

A woman's center of gravity is lower and farther back than that of a man. Women also carry more weight below the waist. Men are broader in the chest and shoulders and carry their weight above the waist (Figure 8-25).

Think of a man as a pear or an eggplant standing on its head and a woman as a pear or an eggplant sitting on its bottom. When a man flexes forward, his center of gravity is over his toes. When a woman flexes forward, her center of gravity is over her heels (Figure 8-26).

Pelvis and Knee

A woman's pelvis is wider than a man's pelvis, which means that a woman's femur approaches the knee at a wider angle, called the *Q angle*. A greater Q angle can result in a knock-kneed stance, which stresses the knee. The structural supports of the knee, the ligaments and tendons, are stretched on the insides and pinched on the outsides. The knee is more mobile in women because of their wider hips and the resulting tendency to knock-knees, coupled with women's greater flexibility (Figure 8-27).

Ankles

Women cannot bend at the ankles and knees as far forward as men can. They also have less total ankle strength. Because women do not have much movement at the ankle, they require a taller massage table (Figure 8-28).

Evolve Activity 8-3 Evolve Activity 8-4

Box 8-8 Guidelines for Pressure, Drag, and Duration of Massage

- Fragile patient outcomes: Comforting and soothing
  - Pressure level—1 or 2/7
  - Drag—0
- Palliative, pleasure-based massage (nonfragile)
  - Pressure level—2 or 3/7
  - Drag—1 to 2/3
  - Speed—Slow
  - Duration (full session)—Short to moderate or moderate to long
- Lymphatic drainage, surface tissues
  - Pressure level—2 or 3/7
  - Drag—2/3
  - Speed—Slow
  - Duration—Varies; moderate to long
- Lymphatic drainage, deep tissues
  - Pressure level—4 or 5/7
  - Drag—2/3
  - Speed—Slow
  - Duration—Short
- Myofascial release, superficial fascia
  - Pressure level—3/7
  - Drag—3/3
  - Speed—Slow
  - Duration (specific application)—Moderate to long
- General relaxation (inhibition of sympathetic arousal)
  - Pressure level—4 or 5/7
  - Drag—2/3
  - Speed—Slow
  - Duration—Long
- Trigger point therapy
  - Pressure level—4 to 6/7 (depending on location)
  - Drag—0
  - Speed—Not a factor
  - Duration (specific application)—Moderate

- Scar tissue surface (mature scar)
  - Pressure level—2 or 3/7
  - Drag—2 or 3/3
  - Speed—Slow
  - Duration (specific application)—Moderate
- Adhesion of muscle layers
  - Pressure level—4 to 6/7
  - Drag—3/3
  - Speed—Slow
  - Duration (specific application)—Short to moderate
- Arterial support
  - Pressure level—4 or 5/7
  - Drag—0
  - Speed—Moderate to fast over arteries
  - Duration (specific application)—Short to moderate
  - Duration (entire session)—Short to moderate
- Support for venous return
  - Pressure level—3 or 4/7
  - Drag—1/3
  - Speed—Slow
  - Duration (specific application)—Moderate
  - Duration (entire session)—Short to moderate
- Client who takes anticoagulants
  - Pressure level—1 or 2/7
  - Drag—0 to start; monitor results
- Fragile bone (osteoporosis)
  - Pressure level—1 to 3/7
  - Drag—0 to 3/3—monitor results
- Stimulation of sympathetic autonomic nervous system tone
  - Pressure level—2 to 5/7
  - Drag—0 to 1/3
  - Speed—Moderate to fast
  - Duration—Short to moderate

Pressure scale: 0–7; 0 = no pressure, 7-deep pressure.
Drag scale: 0–3; 0 = no drag, 3 = maximum drag.

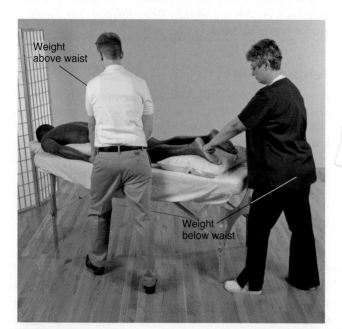

FIGURE 8-25 Comparison of male and female weight distribution.

Weight above waist

Weight below waist

Spine

In women, the spine as a whole and individual vertebrae in certain regions of a normal spine are more backwardly inclined than in men. These spinal regions are subjected to different biomechanical loading conditions. Women have less rotational stability than do men. Therefore, women must maintain alignment of the shoulder girdle and pelvic girdle during massage to prevent torsion forces (twisting) on the spine while doing massage (Janssen et al., 2009).

Physical Strength

Women generally are not as powerful as men. The average woman, because of her smaller size, works at a higher proportion of her maximum strength than does the average man. Women have only 55% to 58% of the upper body strength of men; on average, a woman is only 80% as strong as a man of identical weight. Women must leverage by leaning their body weight to apply pressure during massage application.

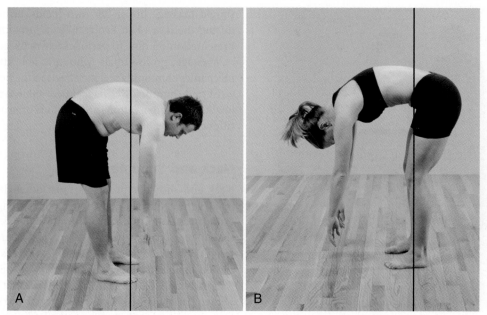

FIGURE 8-26 A, In men, weight and the center of gravity are over the toes. **B,** In women, weight and the center of gravity are over the heels.

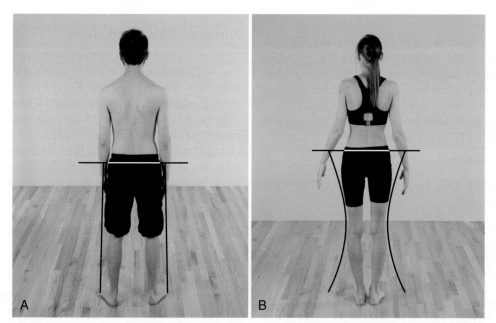

FIGURE 8-27 A, In men, the narrow pelvis keeps the hip, knee, and foot in alignment. **B,** In women, the wider pelvis places the knee and foot medial to the hip.

Male massage therapists may be able to use a shorter table without as much strain for two reasons: when they lean forward, their center of gravity also moves forward; also, they have more upper body strength. However, just because the typical man can "get away with it" does not mean that men should perform massage in any way that has the potential for harm.

So what do all these male-female differences mean with regard to massage therapy? In short, women should not attempt to perform massage in the exact same way as men.

Key Points

- Women massage practitioners generally need a higher massage table to compensate for their lower center of gravity as it shifts to the back when the torso is flexed forward.
- Women have more joint movement in general, but movement at the ankles is reduced; this also indicates the need for a higher massage table.
- Women need to curtail the tendency to flex the torso, because this moves the center of gravity behind them, and more muscle force is required to apply pressure.

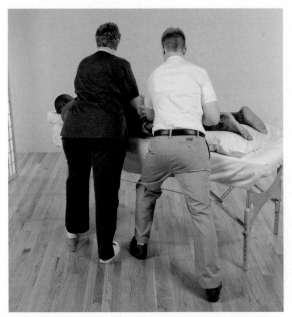

FIGURE 8-28 Men and women have different stances due to differences in ankle and knee flexibility. Stance is a factor in determining the height at which the massage table is set.

- Women need to make sure the pelvis does not tilt back during massage, causing the bottom to stick out.
- Women have more difficulty with joint stability, so they need to maintain a tighter body position and not reach or overextend the body when doing massage.
- Women need to pay specific attention to core strength and stability to stabilize the spine and scapulae.

SELF-CARE AND THE EFFECTS OF IMPROPER BODY MECHANICS

SECTION OBJECTIVES

Chapter objectives covered in this section:

6. The student will be able to identify and correct nonoptimal massage application that causes pain and discomfort for the massage therapist.

Using the information presented in this section, the student will be able to perform the following:

- Identify common dysfunctions related to poor body mechanics
- Evaluate and correct one's own body mechanics if discomfort occurs

Attention to body mechanics begins before the massage even takes place. The practitioner's body should be warmed up with general aerobic activity and gentle stretching. Massage professionals need to be comfortable and should dress in loose, unrestrictive clothing that does not interfere with movement. A short break should be taken after each massage. The massage therapist should use the time not only to set up for the next client, but also to stretch all the muscles involved in giving a massage, rehydrate, and eat a healthy snack if needed. Besides getting a professional massage regularly, the practitioner

should massage his or her own hands, arms, and shoulders during the day. (The Evolve website provides a PowerPoint presentation on how to perform self-massage.)

Massage professionals who are not attentive to body mechanics commonly feel the effects in the neck and shoulder, wrist and thumb, lower back, knee, ankle, and foot. The following recommendations are methods of protecting the practitioner's body.

Neck and Shoulder

Neck and shoulder problems most often develop when the massage practitioner uses upper body strength to push and exert pressure for massage. These problems can be avoided if the student learns to use leverage and leans with the body weight to provide pressure. The practitioner's arms and hands should be relaxed while giving a massage, because tension in the arms and hands translates to the shoulders and neck. Remember, the joints need to be stacked and stable so that the force is easily distributed from the body weight through the joint structure to create compressive force. If the core is not stable, the scapula will be unstable, making maintaining shoulder stability difficult (Figure 8-29).

Forearm, Wrist, and Hand

Massage professionals need to protect their wrists by preventing the development of excessive compressive forces from the delivery of massage methods. Using a proper wrist angle and staying behind the massage stroke protect the wrist. Tense wrists and hands also contribute to shoulder problems. It is important always to maintain a relaxed hand and wrist while giving a massage. Avoid using the thumb when applying pressure. The design of the joints in the thumb does not allow adequate stability to protect the joint. Whenever possible, use the forearm to apply massage to spare the hands and wrists (Figure 8-30).

Low Back

Some reasons for low back problems include core instability, inappropriate bending, bent static positions, twisting, improper knee position, improper foot position, bending of the elbows, and reaching for an area with the arm while giving a massage instead of moving the feet to the area. Massage professionals must learn to keep the lower back straight and avoid bending or curling at the waist while working. Maintaining a stable spinal line and a strong core helps prevent this problem. Frequent posture shifting of the massage practitioner's body also helps protect the lower back, as does learning to lift by leaning back during stretching. Using an asymmetric stance, normal knee-lock position in the weight-bearing leg provides protection for the back. The lower back is further supported by avoiding twisting and reaching (Birnbaum, 1982). The joints of the arm must be kept effectively stacked, with the elbow straight. If the elbow is bent, the body has a tendency to curl at the waist and slouch in the lower back (Figure 8-31).

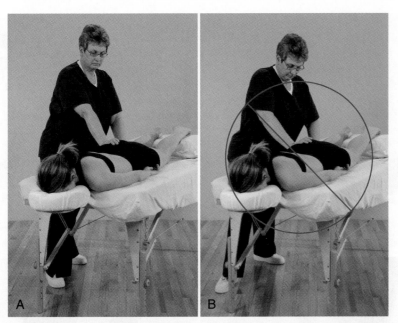

FIGURE 8-29 **A,** When core stability is functional, scapula and shoulder stability is supported. **B,** Incorrect body mechanics. An unstable core can affect the foot position, causing rotation and tilt at the pelvis and strain on the knee. The bent elbow interferes with weight transfer in the muscular effort to apply pressure. The shoulder becomes displaced and unstable, and the head moves into a forward position.

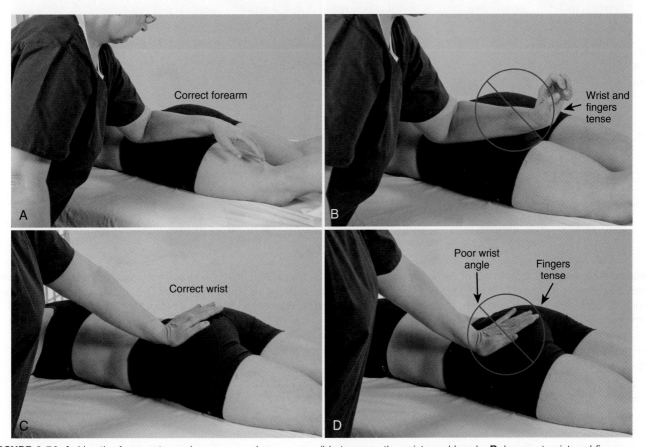

FIGURE 8-30 **A,** Use the forearm to apply massage whenever possible to spare the wrists and hands. **B,** Incorrect wrist and finger position during use of forearm for massage. **C,** Correct wrist and hand position: note the relaxed fingers and the wrist angle greater than 90 degrees. **D,** Incorrect wrist and hand position: the wrist angle is close to 90 degrees, and the fingers are tense.

Continued

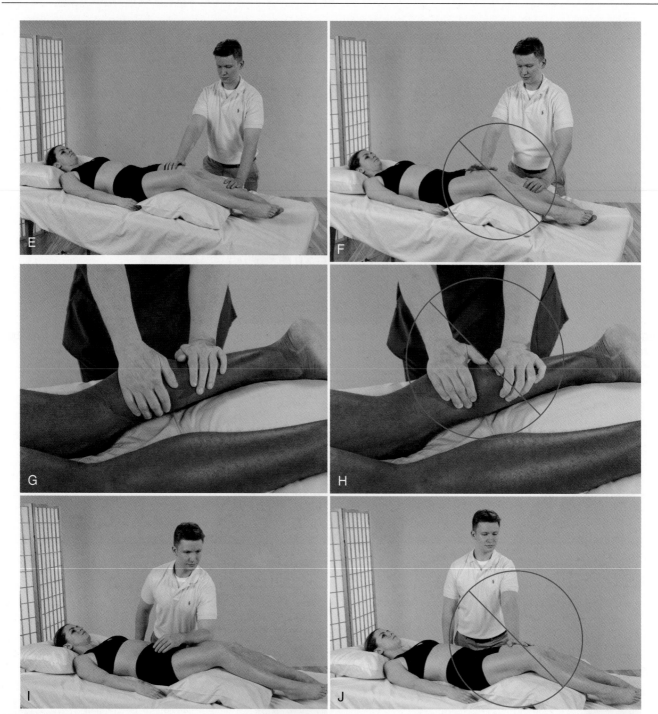

FIGURE 8-30, cont'd **E,** Correct use of the hand during massage: note the position of the elbow and shoulder. **F,** Incorrect arm, forearm, and hand position: the shoulder is rolled forward, the elbow is bent, the angle of the wrist joint is close to 90 degrees, and the fingers are tense. **G,** Correct positioning and use of the hands during kneading. **H,** Incorrect hand position for kneading: the fingers are tense and performing most of the work. **I,** Correct arm position when using the forearm for massage. **J,** Incorrect arm position: the arm is across the body toward the midline, straining the elbow and shoulder, and the body is not lined up with the direction of the weight transfer.

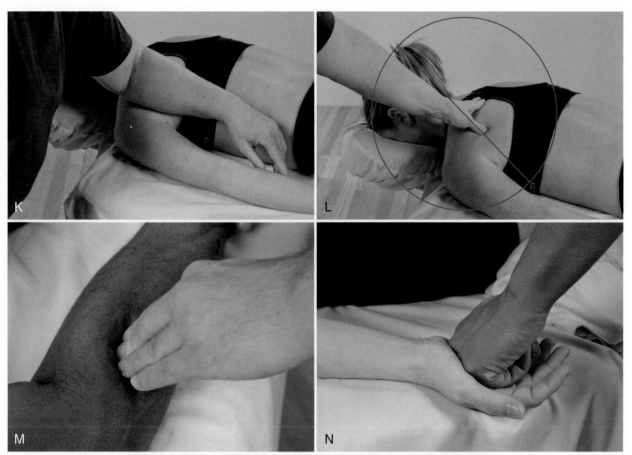

FIGURE 8-30, cont'd K, Use the forearm whenever possible to apply pressure. **L,** Incorrect: do not use the thumb to apply pressure. **M,** Correct use of braced fingers to apply pressure. **N,** Correct use of fist to apply pressure.

Knee

Knee problems can be prevented by respecting the basic stability design of the knee and frequently shifting the weight from foot to foot. The most efficient standing position involves the normal screw-home (or knee-lock) position in the last 15 degrees of extension on the back weight-bearing leg. This position provides the least compressive force on the knee capsule and the least muscular action for stability. As the knee is flexed, compressive forces increase in the joint capsule, and muscular action for stability increases. Knee hyperextension should be avoided (Figure 8-32).

Confusion and disagreement exist about the proper position of the knee while giving a massage. Some advise a slightly flexed knee, rather than the locked knee recommended by this text. Others express some concern with the locked-knee position, opposing the blocking of body energy flow and interference with concepts of grounding and centering. These concerns tend to arise from information founded on movement principles, such as tai chi, forms of dance, and martial arts. Although a flexed knee is appropriate for these systems, massage requires the application of sustained pressure from a stable position with the least amount of effort, muscular activity, and compressive force to the joint.

The knee needs to be in a slightly flexed position as the massage practitioner changes position and moves around the table (Figure 8-33). However, when pressure is applied, the anatomic design of the knee provides stability in the knee-lock position in the last 15 degrees of extension. Practitioners must honor their own bodies in terms of the individualized approach to body position. The body mechanics presented in this chapter have been developed to support the knee (Smith et al., 1996; Norkin and Levangie, 2005).

Ankle and Foot

Asymmetric standing (i.e., standing with one foot in front of the other) is the most efficient standing position. The weight is shifted from one foot to the other in an energy conservation mechanism. Symmetric standing, in which the weight is equally distributed on the two feet, is fatiguing, interferes with circulation, and should be avoided (Smith et al., 1996). The ankle and foot are protected by the asymmetric stance and frequent position changes. The body mechanics presented in this chapter are based on the asymmetric stance so as to best use the massage professional's energy and prevent fatigue (Figure 8-34) (Greene and Roberts, 2004).

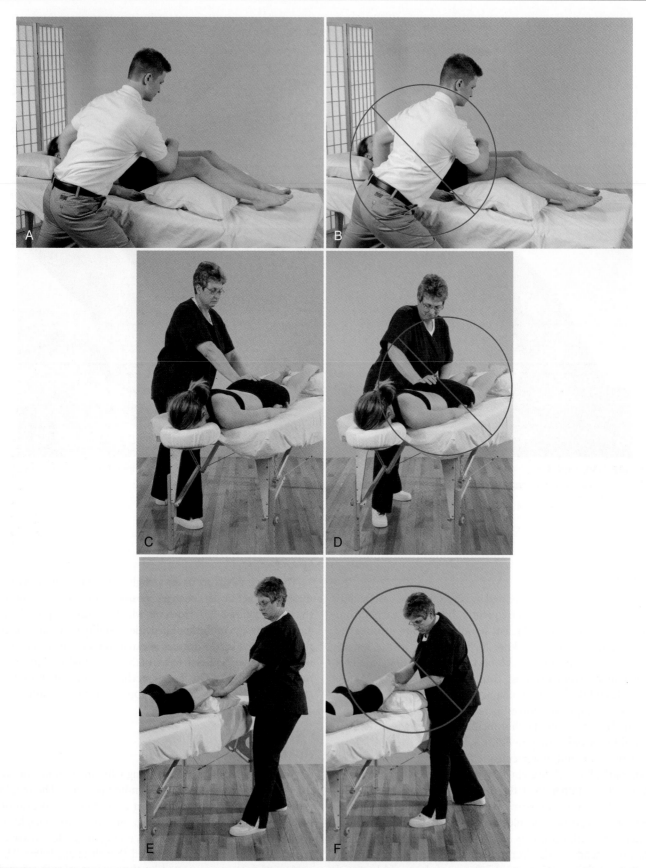

FIGURE 8-31 A, Demonstration of a stable lower back. **B,** Incorrect. The table is too short and the therapist's core is unstable, as is the scapula. The arm is medially across the body, which is not lined up with the direction of the weight transfer. All of this contributes to low back strain while giving a massage. **C,** Using an asymmetric stance and normal knee-lock position in the weight-bearing leg protects the back. **D,** Incorrect. The therapist has the weight on the front foot and is standing on the toes. The elbow is bent, and the table too high. Muscle is used to apply pressure. **E,** Stack the joints and lean back when applying a pull to stretch an area. **F,** Incorrect. Pulling using muscle strength instead of leaning back to stretch or traction the area.

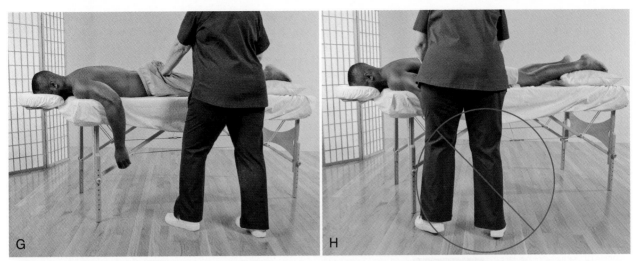

FIGURE 8-31, cont'd **G,** Correct foot position. **H,** Incorrect. Foot position is on the toes, too close to the table.

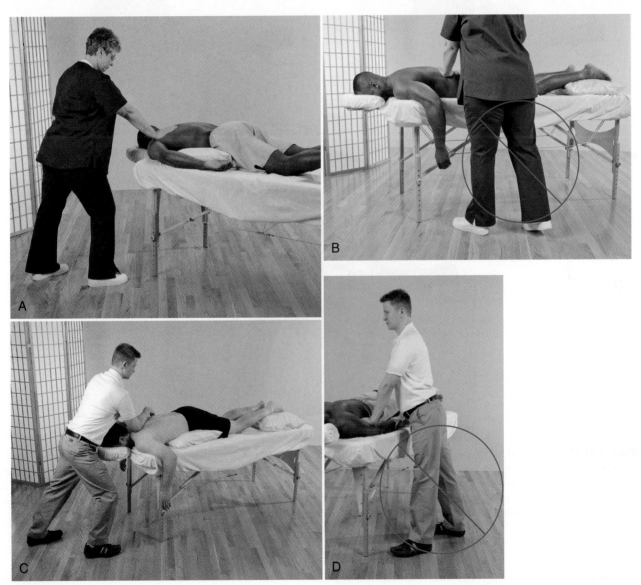

FIGURE 8-32 **A,** Proper knee position: The weight-bearing leg and knee are in extension and stable. The knee of the front balance leg is flexed to allow forward movement during weight transfer. **B,** Incorrect. The weight is on the front leg, which is straight, and the back leg is on the toes; this increases the strain on the knees. **C,** Correct knee and foot position. **D,** Incorrect. The feet are too far apart, in a symmetric stance, with both knees extended.

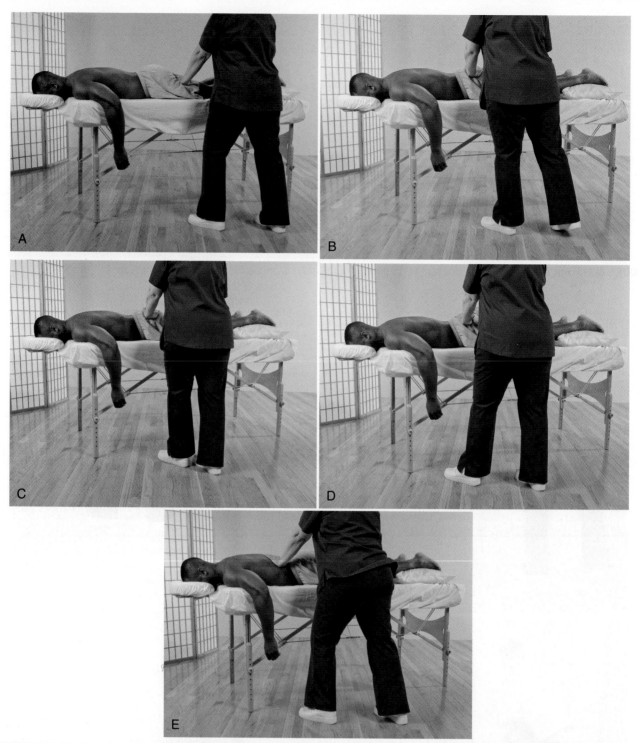

FIGURE 8-33 Moving around the massage table. **A,** Start with the correct knee position (normal knee-lock position) for stability. The moving process remains parallel to the massage table. Avoid moving closer to or farther from the table. **B,** Begin the move. Both knees are flexed; the weight is on the front foot; and the back leg is on the toes, ready to transfer the full weight to the front as the back leg is lifted off the floor. **C,** The back foot moves close to but is still behind the front foot. **D,** The weight is again shifted to the back foot, and the front foot moves to the asymmetric stance; the feet are shoulder width apart. **E,** Correct body mechanics is resumed.

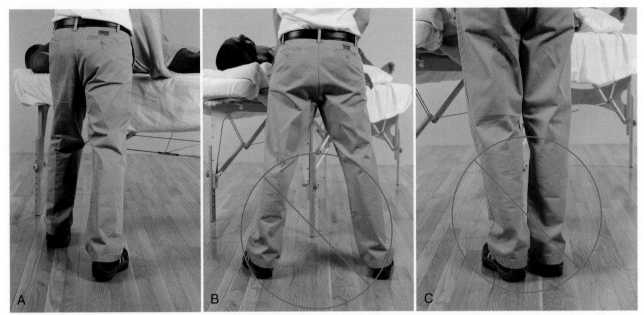

FIGURE 8-34 A, Correct asymmetric stance with the feet shoulder width apart. **B,** Incorrect. The feet are too far apart, the stance is symmetric, and both knees are flexed. **C,** Incorrect. The feet are too close together, the stance is symmetric, and both knees are flexed.

FOOT IN THE DOOR

Body mechanics begins at the feet. The ability to perform five or six excellent massage sessions a day without hurting yourself will get your foot in the door and keep you on the path to career success. If you can confidently demonstrate body mechanics that are efficient and effective, an employer (and your clients) will be impressed.

You also need an environment that supports your ability to provide massage. The massage area needs to be large enough to allow you to move around the table and change position comfortably. You need equipment that is adaptable. To be at your best, you need fresh air and a pleasant environment. When you evaluate a potential place of employment, imagine yourself in that massage area for 8 hours. Does it feel like a place you'd want your feet?

SUMMARY

Massage therapists take care of others. To sustain a massage therapy career, we must also take care of ourselves.

The massage professional's body is a vital, irreplaceable tool. It is crucial that massage professionals take care to use proper body mechanics when giving a massage. Effective ergonomics and body mechanics prevent injury. If the practitioner is uncomfortable, the client will become uncomfortable. If the practitioner can give a massage in a relaxed, efficient, and energy-conserving manner, the client will be able to relax and more easily accept the touch. Students should practice over and over until they develop graceful, efficient body mechanics.

ⓔvolve

http://evolve.elsevier.com/Fritz/fundamentals/
8-1 Review the tissue layers with this sequencing activity.
8-2 Put the seven pressure levels in correct order.
8-3 Review body mechanics terminology with a word game.
8-4 Answer multiple choice questions on time duration and tissue pressure levels.
8-5 Take a true or false quiz on proper and improper body mechanics.
8-6 Identify correct and incorrect body mechanics.
Don't forget to study for your certification and licensure exams! Review questions, along with weblinks, can be found on the Evolve website.

References

AMTA 2011 Massage Therapy Industry Fact Sheet. 2011 massage therapy industry fact sheet, February 17, 2011 http://www.amtamassage.org/articles/2/PressRelease/detail/2320 Accessed August 24, 2011.

Albert WJ, Duncan C, Currie-Jackson N, et al: Biomechanical assessment of massage therapists, *Occupational Ergonomics* 6:1, 2006.

Albert WJ, Currie-Jackson N, Duncan CA: A survey of musculoskeletal injuries amongst Canadian massage therapists, *J Bodyw Mov Ther* 12:86, 2008.

Barnett RL, Liber T: Human push capability, *Ergonomics* 49:293, 2006.

Birnbaum JS: *The musculoskeletal manual*, ed 3, Philadelphia, 1982, Academic Press.

Buck FA, Kuruganti U, Albert WJ, et al: Muscular and postural demands of using a massage chair and massage table, *J Manip Physiol Ther* 30(5):357–364, 2007.

Buckingham G, Das R, Trott P: Position of undergraduate students' thumbs during mobilisation is poor: an observational study, *Aust J Physiother* 53:55, 2007.

Evolve Activity 8-5

Evolve Activity 8-6

Campo M, Weiser S, Koenig KL, Nordin M: Work-related musculo-skeletal disorders in physical therapists: a prospective cohort study with 1-year follow-up, *Phys Ther* 88:608, 2008.

Cromie JE, Robertson VJ, Best MO: Work-related musculoskeletal disorders in physical therapists: prevalence, severity, risks, and responses, *Phys Ther* 80:336, 2000.

Greene D, Roberts S: *Kinesiology: movement in the context of activity*, ed 2, St Louis, 2004, Mosby.

Hu MT, Hsu AT, Lin SW, Su FC: Effect of general flexibility on thumb-tip force generation: implication for mobilization and manipulation, *Man Ther* 14:490, 2009.

Jang Y, Chi CF, Tsauo JY, Wang JD: Prevalence and risk factors of work-related musculoskeletal disorders in massage practitioners, *J Occup Rehabil* 16:425, 2006.

Janssen MM, Drevelle X, Humbert L, et al: Differences in male and female spino-pelvic alignment in asymptomatic young adults: a three-dimensional analysis using upright low-dose digital biplanar x-rays, *Spine* 34:E826, 2009.

Magee DJ, Zachazewski JE: *Scientific foundations and principles of practice in musculoskeletal rehabilitation*, St Louis, 2007, Mosby.

Mohr EG: Proper body mechanics from an engineering perspective, *J Bodyw Mov Ther* 14:139, 2010.

Neumann DA: *Kinesiology of the musculoskeletal system*, ed 2, St Louis, 2010, Mosby.

Norkin CC, Levangie PK: *Joint structure and function: a comprehensive analysis*, ed 2, Philadelphia, 2005, FA Davis.

Punnett L, Fine LJ, Keyserling M, et al: Back disorders and nonneutral trunk postures of automobile assembly workers, *Scan J Work Environ Health* 17:337, 1991.

Smith LK, Weiss E, Lemkuhl LD: *Brunnstrom's clinical kinesiology*, ed 5, Philadelphia, 1996, FA Davis.

Snodgrass SJ, Rivett DA, Chiarelli P, et al: Factors related to thumb pain in physiotherapists, *Aust J Physiother* 49:243, 2003.

Takahashi, I, Kikuchi S, Sato K, Sato N: Mechanical load of the lumbar spine during forward bending motion of the trunk—a biomechanical study, *Spine* 31(1):18–23, 2006.

Survey of musculoskeletal injuries among massage therapists in Australia Terra Rosa. www.terrarosa.com.au/articles/survey.pdf. Accessed August 24, 2011.

Workbook Section

All Workbook activities can be done electronically online as well as here in the book. Answers are located on ⊖volve

Short Answer

1. How do practitioners maintain good body mechanics?

2. How can massage professionals protect their necks and shoulders?

3. How can massage professionals protect their wrists?

4. How can massage professionals protect their thumbs and fingers?

5. How can massage professionals protect their lower backs?

6. How can massage professionals protect their knees?

7. How can massage professionals protect their ankles and feet while giving a massage?

8. What is asymmetric standing and why should it be used instead of symmetric standing?

9. What are the basic principles of body mechanics?

10. Where is the balance point during a massage?

11. What preparations before massage are important to support good body mechanics?

12. What are the general rules for body mechanics?

13. How do the general principles of body mechanics apply to stretching?

14. In the current research, what are the consistent findings about body mechanics with regard to massage application?

Assess Your Competencies

Now that you have studied this chapter, you should be able to:

- Interpret biomechanical research related to massage application
- Create an ergonomically effective massage environment
- Use the body, especially the hands and forearms, in an efficient and biomechanically correct manner when giving a massage.
- Alter the position of both the client and the practitioner to maximize body mechanics

On a separate sheet of paper or on the computer, write a short summary of the content of this chapter based on the preceding list of competencies. Use a conversational tone, as if you were explaining to someone (e.g., a client, prospective employer, coworker, or other interested person) the importance of the information and skills to the development of the massage profession.

Next, in small discussion groups, share your summary with your classmates and compare the ways the information was presented. (You can also post your summaries on the discussion board on the Evolve website.) In discussing the content, look for similarities, differences, possibilities for misunderstanding of the information, and clear, concise methods of description.

Problem-Solving Scenarios

1. A female massage practitioner has been doing massage for 4 years. She tends to provide deep pressure with her forearms and the point of her elbow and works very hard to sustain the pressure throughout the massage. Over the past 6 months she has developed shoulder pain with numbness and tingling. What might be the problem with her body mechanics and what corrective action could she take?

2. A male massage professional is experiencing tenderness in his wrist on the ulnar side. He has long arms and prefers a tall table. He tends to use the palms of his hands for most of his work because of concern about applying too much pressure with his forearm. What might be the problem with his body mechanics and what corrective action could he take?

3. A female massage practitioner with 10 years of experience has been aware of right knee pain over the past 2 years. She learned to keep her knees flexed as part of her initial training. She tends to rotate her right leg externally, so she often does not line up her body so that her right foot is directed toward her application of pressure. What might be the problem with her body mechanics and what corrective action could she take?

4. A female massage professional has recently developed low back pain. She tends to keep her weight on the front foot or evenly distributed between both feet in a symmetric stance. She has long legs, a short torso, and very short arms. A year ago she was advised to work at a taller table, but she never made this adjustment. What might be the problem with her body mechanics and what corrective action could she take?

5. A male massage practitioner with 2 years of experience is exhausted after giving five 1-hour massage sessions. He needs to be able to increase his client base by one massage per day, but he doesn't know whether his energy can hold out. He feels that he has good body mechanics. He usually stands and provides a variety of massages, but his specialty is a vigorous massage with a lot of pétrissage and frictioning methods. He tends to adjust his position instead of altering the client's position to his advantage. What might be the problem with his body mechanics and what corrective action could he take?

Preparation for Massage: Equipment, Professional Environment, Positioning, and Draping

CHAPTER OBJECTIVES

After completing this chapter, the student will be able to perform the following:

1. List the equipment and setup procedures required to prepare for a massage session
2. Create a massage setting in different types of environments
3. Explain massage procedures to a client
4. Identify gender issues that may influence the client's expectations and respond appropriately
5. Obtain and give relevant feedback during the massage
6. Perform premassage procedures to prepare the client and himself or herself for the massage session
7. Perform postmassage procedures to close the massage session and prepare for the next client
8. Effectively drape and position a client

CHAPTER OUTLINE

KEY TERMS

Body supports	Lubricants
Draping	Massage chair
Draping material	Massage mat
Feedback	Massage table
Focus/centering	Positioning

The massage practitioner must make certain preparations before beginning the massage. All necessary supplies must be gathered, and the room must be set up. The type of lubricant used and the way it is dispensed, the temperature of the massage room, and the warmth of the practitioner's hands are all additional considerations. The practitioner uses history-taking and assessment procedures to identify client outcomes and to formulate the approach for the massage. The plan is discussed with the client, and informed consent is obtained.

Another technique is just as important as performing the actual treatment. Massage professionals benefit from developing a method, referred to as *centering*, to help them focus on the client and the session to come.

Other considerations include client positioning and modest, appropriate draping procedures. This chapter is designed to help students develop these important premassage procedures, which support the massage relationship and the professional environment first discussed in Chapter 2.

EQUIPMENT

SECTION OBJECTIVES

Chapter objective covered in this section:

1. The student will be able to list the equipment and setup procedures required to prepare for a massage session.

Using the information presented in this section, the student will be able to perform the following:

- Care for and protect his or her hands, arms, and general health
- Make informed decisions about the purchase of a massage table, chair, mat, body supports, draping materials, and lubricants
- Make the most effective use of massage equipment

Care of the Massage Practitioner's Hands and Body

Massage professionals' most important equipment is their hands, arms, and body. They should make sure to protect their hands from abrasion and damage by wearing gloves when

| Box 9-1 | Features of a Portable Massage Table |

A portable massage table is the most versatile type of massage table. At minimum, it should have the following features:
- Sturdy construction, including cable support on the legs
- Manual height adjustment
- A face cradle
- A washable covering (usually vinyl) that also can be cleaned with disinfectant
- Adequate padding to ensure comfort and firm support
- A width of 24 to 28 inches; tables narrower than 24 inches are too narrow for the client's comfort. A width of 28 inches appears to be best suited to most situations. Tables wider than 30 inches are difficult to carry and ergonomically inefficient. Note that most tables are about 6 feet long, which can accommodate most clients.

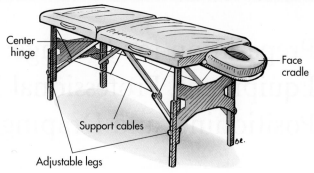

FIGURE 9-1 Portable massage table with center hinge, support cables, and face cradle.

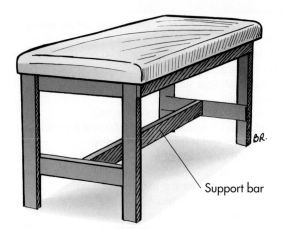

FIGURE 9-2 Stationary massage table.

doing outdoor chores or other work in which the hands may be injured. Using the forearms during a massage protects the hands and limits their use. In some circumstances, such as when working on a floor mat, the knees and feet are used for certain massage techniques. The massage practitioner has a professional responsibility always to be attentive to efficient and proper body mechanics (see Chapter 8) and the maintenance of personal health.

Massage Table

Another important piece of massage equipment is the surface on which the client may sit or lie while receiving the massage. The first choice of most practitioners for this purpose is a massage table. The table must be sturdy and properly assembled so that there is no chance of it collapsing while a client is lying on it. The two primary types of massage tables are the portable table, which folds into a smaller unit and can be carried easily from place to place (Box 9-1), and the stationary table, which remains in one location.

Most manufacturers offer a basic model, and many have tables with all sorts of features, such as automatic height and tilt adjustments, arm supports, and face cradles. The more features, the more expensive the table.

Massage tables should be purchased from an experienced manufacturer. Buying a product that has been tested for safety is worth the investment. All massage tables must be checked daily for structural stability. It is important to perform a complete maintenance check on all connectors, bolts, cables, and hinges every week and to repair any defects immediately.

Portable Tables

Almost all portable tables are built with a hinge in the middle that allows them to fold in half for ease of carrying (Figure 9-1). This hinged area is a weak spot in the table, and cable supports on the legs counterbalance the weakness. Most tables are strong and can hold about 300 pounds (136.077 kg) if the weight is distributed evenly over the entire surface of the table. Problems occur when the client sits in the middle of the table when lying down or sitting up, which focuses all the weight in

one spot. With cumulative use, the hinge weakens. It is important to check the cable tension regularly to ensure that no sag develops. Otherwise, the table may buckle, injuring the client and damaging the table. Adjustable legs allow the massage table to be lowered or raised to accommodate clients of various sizes while allowing the practitioner to use proper body mechanics.

Many clients may be concerned about the sturdiness of the table. The lightweight, portable tables may look weak, but a quality table is well built and strong. Before the massage, demonstrate the stability of the table to the client or offer alternatives, such as a chair or massage mat.

Stationary Tables

Stationary tables do not have the instability problem, because the table is heavier, and cross-bracing and leg supports make the table even safer. However, the lack of portability is a major drawback if the massage practice involves any on-site work (Figure 9-2).

Lift Tables

Two basic types of adjustable lift tables are available, hydraulic and electric. Hydraulic tables do not need electricity. With the client on the table, height adjustments are made using a hand crank or foot pump. Electric lift tables provide an electric lift mechanism with push-button controls. A lift massage table is the most ergonomically supportive massage equipment. At minimum, it should have the same features as a portable

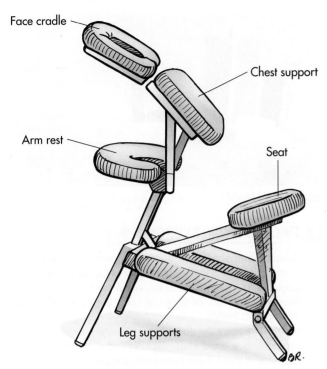

FIGURE 9-3 Massage chair.

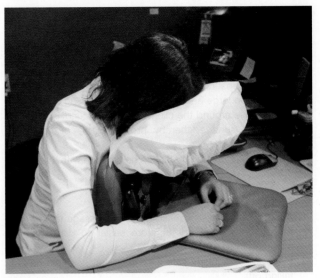

FIGURE 9-4 Massage support device for working at a desk. (From Holland P, Anderson S: *Chair massage*, St. Louis, 2010, Mosby.)

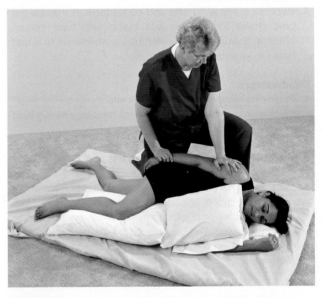

FIGURE 9-5 A generic massage mat covered with a sheet.

massage table (see Box 9-1) and a hydraulic or an electrical mechanism that allows height adjustment to at least 45 inches.

The only disadvantage of both types of lift tables is that they are not usually portable. Also, they are expensive, but they can be considered an important investment in supporting proper body mechanics.

Massage Chair

A special **massage chair** can be purchased for seated massage. These chairs are a worthwhile investment to provide options for clients (Figure 9-3). The sit-down massage, often referred to as an *on-site* or *corporate massage,* usually is provided in a public setting (e.g., business location) and is done over clothing. Massage chairs also are excellent for working with clients who are more comfortable sitting upright, such as a woman in the last trimester of pregnancy or a person who has difficulty getting on and off a massage table (Box 9-2).

A straight-backed chair with no arms also can be used. The client sits facing the back of the chair and leans on the chair back, supported by pillows. A stool or chair pushed up to a table or desk is another option. The client leans forward on a supporting pillow placed on the table. Special triangular or block-shaped foam forms can be purchased to provide support. A professionally manufactured desktop support, which could replace the pillows, is available (Figure 9-4).

Massage Mat

A mat on the floor is used for some methods of massage (Box 9-3). The **massage mat** can be a futon or an exercise mat, but it must be protected by a sanitary covering (Figure 9-5).

Box 9-2	Advantages and Disadvantages of a Massage Chair

Advantages
1. Massage chairs, which are specially designed for that purpose, usually are very comfortable and easy to use.
2. Professionally manufactured equipment adds to the professional atmosphere of the massage setting and ensures safety through quality workmanship in construction and design.
3. Professionally manufactured massage chairs are lightweight and portable.
4. Clients with certain respiratory, vascular, and cardiac conditions are best given a massage in a seated position.

Disadvantages
1. Some people have difficulty getting into and out of the semikneeling position required to use the massage chair.
2. Access to certain body areas is limited.

Box 9-3 Key Features, Advantages, and Disadvantages of a Massage Mat

Key Features
1. The mat should be soft enough and provide sufficient support to ensure the client's comfort.
2. It should be large enough to allow the massage practitioner to move around the client's body while staying on the cushioned surface, thereby protecting his or her own knees and body.
3. It should be made so that it can be covered with a sanitary covering.

Advantages
1. A mat often is less expensive than a massage table.
2. It may be lighter and therefore easier to carry than a massage table.
3. Mats are particularly safe (i.e., the client has little risk of falling off).
4. A mat is a popular choice when working with infants and children.
5. Mats are portable.
6. Because a mat is so safe and comfortable, it may be the best choice for working with clients who have certain physical disabilities; a transfer from a wheelchair to a mat may be accomplished more easily.

Disadvantages
1. Proper training is needed to work effectively on the floor; many massage practitioners are not familiar with this kind of work.
2. The floor may be drafty or cold for the client.
3. Physically challenged or elderly clients may have difficulty getting down on or up from the floor.
4. Mats do not have face cradles to maintain alignment of the neck in the prone position. However, face cradles from massage tables or bolstering systems can be adapted to use on the floor. They are placed on the floor at the end of the mat or on the mat itself, depending on the client's preference.

Body Supports

Body supports are used to bolster the body during the massage and give contour to the flat working surface (Figure 9-6).

Commercial body support products, consisting of various shapes and sizes of pillows and foam forms, can be purchased. As an alternative, the practitioner can buy assorted shapes and densities of hypoallergenic foam and make covers for them. A wedge, a round tube, and two or three square or oblong pieces will be needed, each with a different depth and density. Additional supports are needed for working with pregnant women (Proficiency Exercise 9-1).

Draping Materials

Opaque **draping material** is used to provide the client with privacy and warmth. Standard bed linens are the coverings most commonly used, because they are large enough to cover the entire body and are easily used for most draping procedures. Both full and twin-size sheets fit nicely on most massage

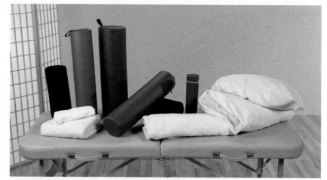

FIGURE 9-6 Different types of body supports.

⚡ PROFICIENCY EXERCISE 9-1

1. Collect information from at least three manufacturers of massage tables and massage chairs. Compare the cost, quality, and construction of the equipment.
2. Research a variety of styles of body supports for clients with specific needs.
3. Locate a source for foam (an upholstery or a mattress company is a good start). See how many different body supports you can build from foam scraps.

tables. The practitioner can either buy these linens and launder them in a sanitary fashion or use a linen service. Sheets made of cotton or cotton blends are the best choice, because they do not slip on the client. Cotton flannel sheets are a consideration for the winter months, because they feel warm to the skin. Whatever linen is used, it must be able to withstand washing with bleach or other disinfecting solution (Figure 9-7).

Large towels may be used for draping, because they are both warm and opaque. They must be at least the size of a beach towel and must have a soft texture. Be sensitive to the client's comfort and provide a choice of towels or sheets. Because towels are smaller, a client may feel more exposed and may prefer the security offered by a sheet. As an alternative, both sheets and towels can be used, with a bath-size towel used as a chest covering.

Disposable linen also is available. Some higher quality disposable products may look and feel like a cotton fabric, but they do not provide the same warmth. Disposable linens are convenient and sanitary, but they cannot be washed or recycled.

Draping Material Recommendations

Either a twin fitted sheet or a flat sheet should be put over the vinyl table top to protect the table. Laundering this additional sheet is much less expensive than replacing the covering on the table. A full or twin flat sheet then is placed over the protective covering. The top sheet can be either a full or a twin sheet. Both sheet sizes have advantages and disadvantages. Twin sheets fit a bit better on the table but sometimes can be inadequate for draping. Full sheets provide more material, which facilitates draping, but can be cumbersome. Also, for sanitary purposes, care must be taken that sheets do not drag on the floor. Face cradles should be draped with a hand towel, a pillowcase, or an additional piece of fabric sewn just to fit

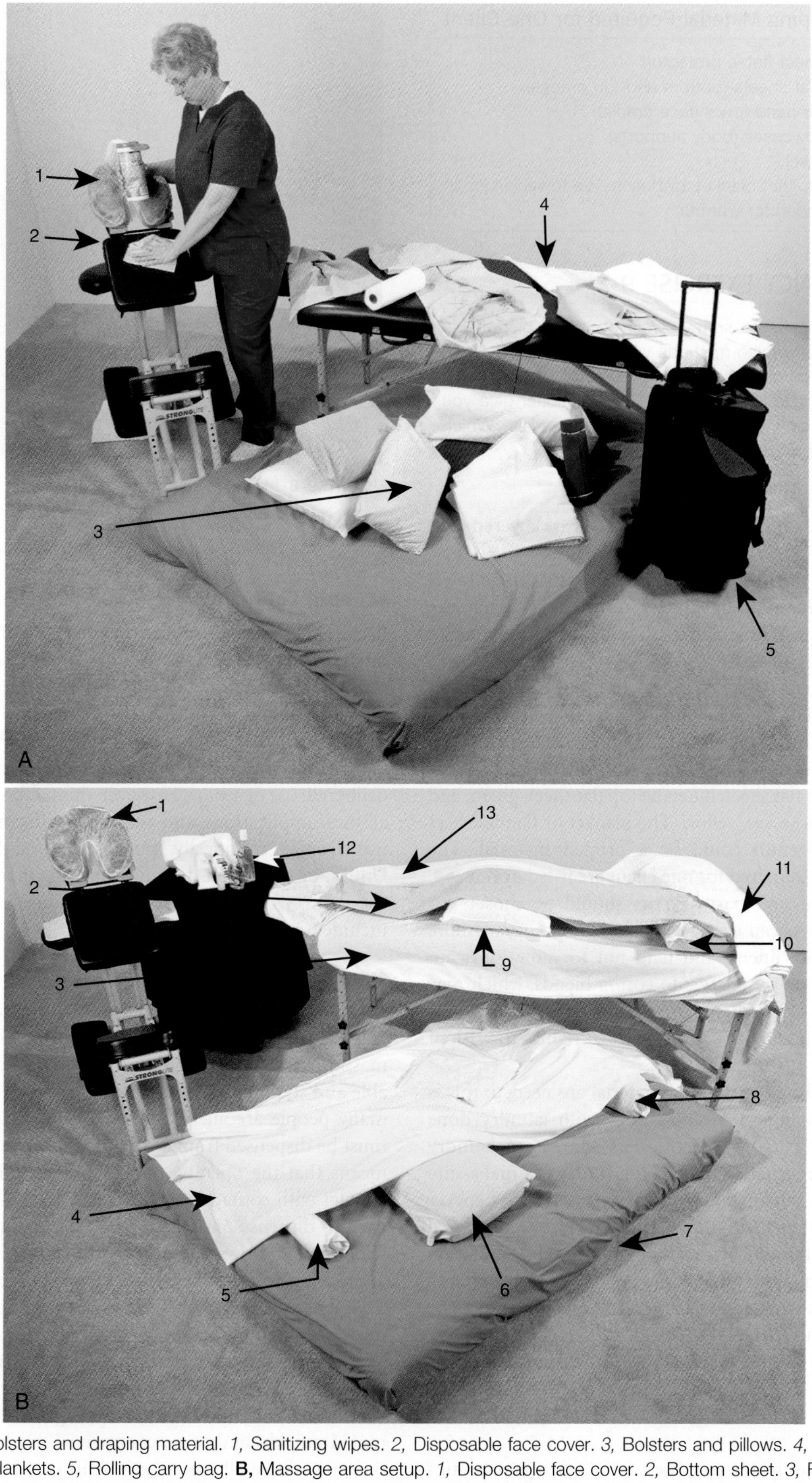

FIGURE 9-7 A, Bolsters and draping material. *1,* Sanitizing wipes. *2,* Disposable face cover. *3,* Bolsters and pillows. *4,* Sheets, pillowcases, and blankets. *5,* Rolling carry bag. **B,** Massage area setup. *1,* Disposable face cover. *2,* Bottom sheet. *3,* Fitted sheet. *4,* Top sheet. *5,* Neck roll (rolled towel). *6,* Pillow for placement beneath abdomen or knees. *7,* Mat sheet. *8,* Ankle support. *9,* Bolster (knee or abdomen). *10,* Ankle bolster. *11,* Blanket. *12,* Various lubricants and hand sanitizers. *13,* Top sheet.

Box 9-4 Draping Material Required for One Client

- 1 twin fitted sheet (table protector)
- 2 full or twin flat sheets (bottom and top drapes)
- 1 pillowcase or hand towel (face cradle)
- Additional pillowcases (body supports)
- 1 bath-size towel
- 1 flannel sheet, light blanket, or beach-size towel (which is easiest to launder) for warmth

---

PROFICIENCY EXERCISE 9-2

1. Obtain a set of sheets, some towels, and some disposable linen. Practice draping methods with them. Which type of material did you prefer to use?
2. Have another student or a massage practitioner give you a massage using the different draping materials. Which type did you prefer to have used on you?

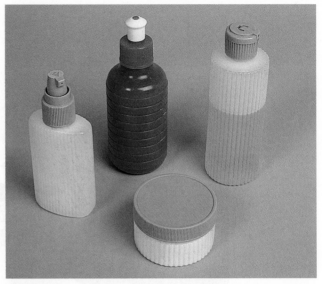

FIGURE 9-8 Massage lubricant containers.

the face cradle. All body supports and pillows are covered with pillowcases.

In addition to the sheets and pillowcases, a bath-size towel is used for various draping procedures. A large beach-size towel, a flannel sheet, or a blanket should be available in case the client becomes chilled.

Keeping different colors of sheets and towels for each set of drapery material can be helpful, because if all are the same color, distinguishing between the top and bottom sheets can be difficult. For example, the protective fitted sheet may be white; the bottom flat sheet, blue; the top flat sheet, green; and the towel and pillowcase, yellow. The blanket or flannel sheet for additional warmth could be a printed material. The draping materials required for one client are listed in Box 9-4.

When possible, soft pastel colors should be chosen for draping materials, because they withstand bleaching, are more opaque than white linens, and tend not to show lubricant stains. Some people are allergic to cotton blends, which may irritate their skin. If the client has sensitive skin, the practitioner should use white, pure cotton sheets to reduce the risk of a reaction.

At least 10 full sets of draping material are needed; this is sufficient for 2 standard business days, with laundry done every other day. Massage practitioners who use a laundry service should order enough linen for 10 days to make sure they do not run out of linens if delivery is late. Whenever linens come in contact with the client, they must be laundered in an approved fashion before they are reused. (Sanitation procedures for any linens that come in contact with a client's bodily fluids are discussed in Chapter 7.) Most linens must be replaced every 1 to 2 years if used often. Lubricants build up, and bleach wears out the fabric (Proficiency Exercise 9-2).

Lubricants

Lubricants serve only one purpose for the massage practitioner: they reduce drag on the skin during gliding-type massage strokes. Medicinal and cosmetic use of lubricants is out of the scope of practice for therapeutic massage.

Scented Lubricants

Because headaches and other allergic responses to lubricants often are caused by the volatile oils in scented products, scented lubricants should not be used. This recommendation does not discount the therapeutic benefit of aromatherapy; the sense of smell is a very powerful sensory mechanism, and many emotional and physiologic processes can be triggered by deliberate use of aroma. However, this textbook does not cover all these applications, and additional education is required to use aromas specifically, purposefully, and therapeutically. Until they receive this training, massage therapists should not use them. (A short discussion of the use of essential oils is included in Chapter 12.)

Types of Lubricants

Oils and creams can be vegetable, mineral, or petroleum based, and powders can be talc or cornstarch based. If possible, massage therapists should use the most natural products available and should avoid using petrochemicals and talc, because many people are allergic to these substances. All lubricants must be dispensed from a contamination-free container. This means that the opening of the container does not come in contact with contaminants. For example, if a squeeze tube is used to dispense massage lotion, the practitioner should not wipe the hand over the opening to stop the flow. A hygienic approach is to use small sterile containers that are filled from a larger container to hold the lubricant for an individual massage (Figure 9-8).

The lubricant traditionally used for massage is oil. It is easy to dispense from a squeeze bottle and can be kept free of contamination. However, natural vegetable oils can become rancid quickly, and some commercial products use additives that may cause allergic reactions in clients. In addition, oils are messy, they can spill and drip, and they stain linens (although specialized laundry products are available for removing oil stains).

Another popular lubricant is massage cream. Various processing methods have produced many natural vegetable oil–based massage creams and lotions that do not feel greasy. Some products are water based, and these wash out of linens without leaving stains. Massage creams must also be dispensed in a contamination-proof manner. Some creams are thin enough to be kept in a squeeze bottle. Others are thick, and the amount to be used must be removed in a sanitary fashion before the massage. Typically a single-use or sanitized spoon is used to remove the amount of cream needed for the massage.

Powders are used when creams and oils are undesirable, usually because of skin conditions (e.g., acne) or excessive body hair. The practitioner must take care not to inhale the dust from powders, which may cause respiratory problems. Powders with a cornstarch base are preferable, because they pose less of a risk of respiratory irritation. If the client and practitioner are in agreement, disposable masks can be used to reduce the risk of respiratory irritation even further.

Using Massage Lubricants

Only a small amount of lubricant is needed for a massage. Remember that the reason for using lubricant is to reduce drag on the skin from the massage movements. More lubricant is required to work over body hair. In some cases powder may be a better choice. Sometimes the use of any type of lubricant is contraindicated; therefore, it is important to be able to perform massage without a lubricant.

In Chapter 10 you will learn about different massage manipulations. The long, gliding methods are best for applying lubricant. Keep the application even and very thin. Applying more is easy, but removing excess is difficult. Keep a clean towel available in case removal is necessary.

Do not pour the lubricant directly onto the client. Warm the lubricant in your palms first by rubbing your hands together. Apply the lubricant to one area at a time rather than to the entire body. Do not use lubricant on the face or hair, because it disturbs makeup and hairstyles. For sanitary reasons, wash and dry your hands before working in the area of the face. Some practitioners begin the massage with the face and head, before using any lubricant.

Some clients may appreciate having the lubricant removed after the massage. An alcohol-based product can do this, but alcohol is drying to the skin. Rubbing the skin with an absorbent towel removes most of the lubricant.

Additional Equipment

Music

Music often is used to distract the client from or to block out surrounding noise. A less recognized use is to achieve interaction and modulation of the autonomic nervous system through entrainment. Simple, soft music with a base beat under 60 beats per minute tends to activate a parasympathetic response, which produces a soothing, relaxing effect. Music faster than 60 beats per minute encourages sympathetic responses, producing a stimulating, invigorating effect.

When using music, the practitioner must consider the effect to be created and whether both the client and the

massage practitioner enjoy the music. The best recommendation is that the massage practitioner have available a variety of music from which the client is allowed to choose. An assortment of styles, rhythms, and instruments, in addition to equipment to play music, should be available. The volume should be kept low but loud enough so that the music can be heard without straining.

The music itself can be very helpful in pacing the massage, because the massage practitioner can gain a sense of the passing of time without having to look at the clock (Proficiency Exercise 9-3).

MASSAGE ENVIRONMENT

SECTION OBJECTIVES

Chapter objective covered in this section:
2. The student will be able to create a massage setting in different types of environments.
Using the information presented in this section, the student will be able to perform the following:
- Design an efficient therapeutic massage environment
- Organize an office and massage room

Clients return for another massage because they appreciate the quality of the service and a professional personality and environment. Thoroughly plan the image you want your massage environment to convey to the public. To maintain the integrity of the professional relationship, the environment created for the massage setting, including decorations and the reading material provided for clients, should reflect the scope of practice of massage.

When most people think of massage, they picture a quiet, private room with low lighting and soft music. However, therapeutic massage can be provided almost anywhere and under almost any conditions. Successful massage practices have been developed in noisy public locations, such as airports, in a client's home, in the workplace, and outdoors at sporting events or retreats. Whatever the physical location of the massage environment, the most important aspect is to

Evolve Activity 9-1

present and deliver the highest standard of professional care to the public.

General Conditions

General conditions for massage areas that must be considered are the room temperature, the fresh air supply, privacy, and accessibility.

Room Temperature

The air temperature in the massage room should be kept at 72° to 75° F (22° to 24° C). Massage produces a vasodilative effect, which brings the blood closer to the surface of the body and allows internal heat to escape, cooling the client. Clients cannot relax if they are cold. The massage practitioner is active and fully dressed and can become warm while doing the massage. Some practitioners put an electric blanket on the table to keep clients warm. A piece of lamb's wool may be used, because it traps and retains body heat. Placing a hot water bottle or other form of heating device at the client's feet and another at the neck or wherever comfortable may increase body temperature.

The most comfortable massage practitioner's uniform is cotton or a cotton blend to wick away moisture and perspiration from the skin. It should have short sleeves and be loose fitting to help prevent the practitioner from becoming too warm.

Fresh Air and Ventilation

The room should have access to fresh air, but a window that opens to the outside is not always available. Ventilation of some sort is important. A small fan in the room pointed at the ceiling or the wall keeps the air moving without causing a draft on the client.

Privacy

Clients need privacy for removing their clothes in preparation for the massage treatment. If the massage room is separate from other public areas, the client can be left alone to get ready for the massage. Sometimes a screen or curtained area can be used to divide one large room into two distinct areas.

Accessibility

Locating the massage practice so that it is easily accessible to clients with mobility impairments is important. Barrier-free access and restrooms are required.

Lighting

The massage area must be lit well enough to meet the standards for proper cleaning and safety (see Chapter 7). Bright overhead lighting often is too harsh and glaring for the client. Indirect or natural light from a window is much better. If the massage area has overhead lights, turn them off and use a lamp in the corner of the room instead. A dimmer switch is excellent, because it allows adjustment of the lighting. Never work in a dark room, to prevent accidents caused by tripping, and never work by candlelight, because an open flame is a safety hazard.

Scents, Incense, Flowers, and Plants

Massage practitioners work with a variety of people during a day, each one with different ideas about what is pleasant and what is offensive. Many clients are also environmentally sensitive and react to scents, incense, and flowers. The best recommendation is to avoid using such items, because the fragrance lingers and can cause problems for a client.

Nonflowering (foliage) plants usually are less of a problem. However, if the practitioner serves an allergic population, the best course may be not to use them. If their use is not a problem, foliage plants are a wonderful natural air purifier that can supply oxygen to the massage areas.

Hygiene, Chemicals, Perfume, and Warm Hands

Recall from Chapter 7 that it is important for the massage professional to attend to personal hygiene and to prevent body odors, because people are sensitive to these smells. Avoid heavy use of aftershave, perfume, scented cosmetics, hair spray, or other scented products. Clients usually do not comment on offensive breath or body odors; they may simply not return for further sessions. Because recognizing odors on ourselves can be difficult, ask a family member or friend who will answer truthfully if you have such a problem.

If the massage practitioner is a smoker, the smell of smoke can linger in fabric, carpeting, and furniture and on the practitioner. This can be very distasteful to a nonsmoking client. Because removing the odor is difficult, the massage environment should be located in a nonsmoking area. Refraining from smoking during professional hours may help prevent the smell from clinging to the hands, clothes, hair, and breath.

If massage practitioners have cold hands, the hands should be heated with warm water, on a hot water bottle or other warming device, or by rubbing them together before touching the client.

Typical Massage Room, Home Office, or Clinical Setting

Business and Massage Areas

A massage area separate from the business area in the massage setting is desirable. People associate behavior with locations and expect certain activities at those locations. It is important that these two activities remain separate in the client's mind. The interaction that takes place when appointments are made and money is taken is very different from the one that takes place during a massage.

The business or reception area should be near the entrance. An appointment book, calendar, forms, receipts, pencils, and telephone, as well as a chair and a small table, should be set up in the business area. Appropriate reading material should be available for clients. The massage area should be located farther from the door or in an adjacent room (Figure 9-9).

In the massage area or room, make sure clients have a place to sit and to hang or place their clothes. Use an enclosed cabinet to store linens and lubricants and designate a place to keep the body supports. A covered hamper, located away from the massage table, is needed for used linens.

Hand-washing and restroom facilities must be easily accessible. If the massage room has no sink, a liquid hand cleanser must be available. If no direct access exists between the massage room and the restroom, make sure the client uses the facilities before the massage session begins. You should also have a plan for getting the client to the restroom during the massage session if necessary. This can get tricky if the only way to the facilities is down a public hall, past offices that share the restroom facilities. Having a robe in the room the client can put on and being willing to escort the client to the bathroom are options. When considering the location of the massage area, be mindful of the restroom location and ease of access.

Room Size

The reception and business area can be small, about 8 × 8 feet (64 square feet). A room for massage should be at least 10 × 10 feet (100 square feet), which is the minimum amount of space that allows practitioners to move comfortably around the client on the table and enables them to use proper body mechanics.

If the two areas are in the same room, a space at least 12 × 12 feet (144 square feet) is needed to provide the necessary working area (Figure 9-10).

Office at the Practitioner's Home

Designating a professional area in your home is a business option if zoning regulations allow home office businesses (see Chapter 3). Establishing a professional office in the home involves special considerations. If at all possible, the massage area should have a private entrance (zoning regulations usually require this). Barrier-free access and restrooms are a major consideration in planning a home office. Most homes are not designed with these accommodations.

If pets are in the home, potential clients must be informed in case of allergy or fear of animals. Pets should not be allowed in the business or massage areas. Family members must understand the privacy issue of the massage environment, and massage clients must understand the boundaries of the private home area. This more personal environment requires very careful attention to professional boundaries.

Public Environment: Event Sports Massage, Demonstration Massage, On-Site or Corporate Massage

In the public setting, the massage practitioner goes to the location rather than having the client come to the practitioner's office. These public massage sessions normally last less

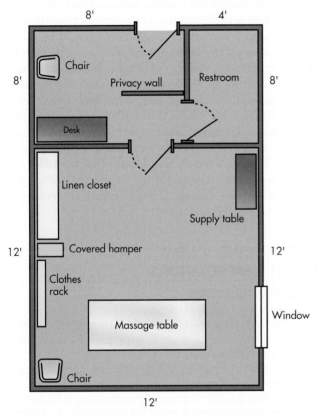

FIGURE 9-9 A sample layout of a massage office with separate business office and massage area.

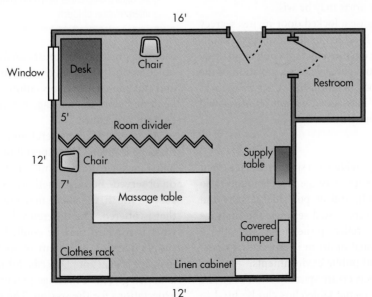

FIGURE 9-10 A sample layout of a massage office with the business office and massage area in one room.

than 30 minutes and the client remains fully clothed. As the practitioner, you usually have little control over noise, lighting, and other conditions. Clear enough space to set up the massage table or chair. If indoors, try to locate this area in a corner, which gives two walls to provide some privacy.

Regardless of the massage location, creating both a business area and a massage area is always important. Find a flat surface and use it to set up a portable office from a briefcase or similar carrying case that contains receipts, an appointment book, and handouts such as cards and brochures. Set up the massage area a few steps away.

Although the use of linens and lubricants usually is limited in these circumstances, having them available is important. They should be carried in a closed bag to maintain sanitation. Make provision for hand-washing or hand-cleaning products to maintain hygiene and sanitation.

Client's Residence (On-Site Massage)

On-site massage can be provided in the home for many reasons, including service and convenience for the client, especially if the person is housebound. A 60- or 90-minute massage usually is given in these situations. Because the massage takes place in the client's residence, this is the most difficult environment in which to maintain professionalism and professional boundaries. Therefore, a professional uniform is especially important in this environment. A portable table most often is used, but a massage chair or mat also is acceptable.

Find a private location for the massage, but avoid the bedroom; opt for a family room or den. If the only room available is a bedroom, try to use the guest room or a child's room rather than the client's bedroom. Make sure it is near an area where hands can be washed. Set up a business area using a briefcase as the office and maintain the professional atmosphere. Do not sit at the kitchen table or in the living room, because the professional role of the massage practitioner may be obscured in these traditional conversation locations.

Linens, body supports, and lubricants are needed. Also, bringing along a small fan to keep the air moving and to drown out noise from other areas may be wise.

Never lock the door, because a locked door invites secrecy and creates an environment in which maintaining professionalism is difficult. Under rare circumstances it could constitute entrapment, or the client could perceive it as a violation of the boundaries of the therapeutic relationship. Carry a sign to hang on the door that says, "Massage in session." If music will be used, bring portable equipment.

Outdoors

Outdoor massage usually is provided at a sports massage event or promotional activity. Some massage professionals also work on ships, on the beach, and at poolside at spas and resorts. Although these are very casual settings, the massage practitioner's behavior must reflect professional and ethical standards. Again, a professional uniform is especially important in these more casual and public environments.

Wind, sun, rain, and insects create special conditions. The wind blows the drapes, but picnic table clips can be used to prevent this. Instructing clients to wear a swimsuit or loose

⚙ PROFICIENCY EXERCISE 9-4

1. Arrange to give a massage in each of the four basic environments. What was different about each experience?
2. Put together a briefcase office.
3. On separate pieces of paper, design three different setups for a clinical massage environment. Indicate the business and massage areas.

clothing for an over-the-clothing massage also helps. A firm, level location is needed for the table, because tables that sink into the sand are unsafe. This can be prevented by putting sample carpet squares on the ground and placing the table legs in large empty cans such as coffee cans. The massage should be performed in the shade to prevent sunburn. A roof or canopy is helpful in case of rain. If the area is screened in, technically it is not outdoors. True outdoor massage will likely involve insects landing or crawling on the client; just blend the brushing away of insects into your massage techniques as best you can. If an area for washing hands is not available, use a disinfectant hand cleanser. Set up the portable office in an area away from the massage setting (Figure 9-11) (Proficiency Exercise 9-4).

DETERMINING A NEW CLIENT'S EXPECTATIONS

SECTION OBJECTIVES

Chapter objectives covered in this section:

3. The student will be able to explain massage procedures to a client.
4. The student will be able to identify gender issues that may influence the client's expectations and respond appropriately.

Using the information presented in this section, the student will be able to perform the following:

- Interview a new client to gain a better understanding of the client's expectations of massage in general and of the outcome for a particular massage session
- Recognize differences based on gender in clients' expectations and interpretation of touch

Massage practitioners must carefully help the client define the outcome for the massage, explain the limitations of massage, and put the client's expectations into perspective. This must be done before the massage is started as part of the informed consent procedure.

An important consideration is how the new client thinks a massage is given. The expectations of clients who have never had a massage are determined by what they have heard, read, or observed. Because methods and applications of massage vary so much, the client may not expect the style of massage that is offered. The difference between what is expected and what is received may be confusing. The client's answer to a simple question or statement such as, "What do you think a massage is like?" or "Describe for me how you think a massage is done," gives the massage practitioner an idea of the client's expectations for the session. The massage practitioner should explain the different approaches used so that the client is not

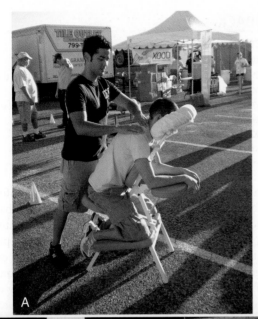

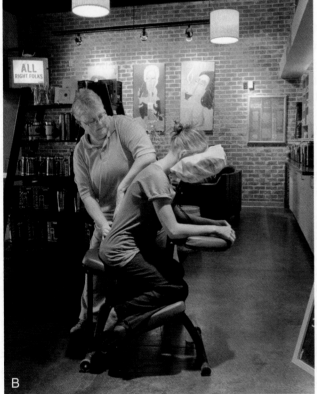

FIGURE 9-11 A, Outdoor sports massage setting involving use of a massage chair. **B,** On-site massage in a public setting. (From Holland P, Anderson S: *Chair massage*, St. Louis, 2010, Mosby.)

approach and say that your way is better; this is unethical behavior. The only exception is if the previous massage violated professional ethics, scope of practice, and standards of practice. Explain to the client that massage practitioners do not conduct themselves in a manner that violates professional codes of ethics. The code of ethics example in this textbook or one from a professional organization can be used as a framework for the discussion (see Chapter 2).

The outcome for massage is what the client can anticipate in response to the benefits of the proposed massage plan. Each massage manipulation has an anticipated response (discussed in Chapters 5 and 10). A client can be made aware of these responses and any risks inherent in the proposed massage interventions (see Chapter 6).

Do not confuse expectations with outcome. Consider this example: A new client has never had a massage, but a friend of hers in another city regularly receives therapeutic massage. The client explains that the massage her friend receives is for a chronic headache that seems to be related to daily stress and that the massage helps a lot (expectation). When you ask your client why she came for a massage (the outcome), she says that she has no real problems, although sometimes she has headaches just as her friend does. Your client thinks a massage would feel good, and her outcome is a general massage that feels good, not the more specific approach to address headaches.

The client's expectations were based on information from her friend. A first-time client naturally considers this type of information, but the outcome may be very different. If the massage practitioner is not careful to differentiate the two, the massage provided for the client may not meet the client's expectations.

The practitioner can ask a number of questions to help determine a new client's expectations, such as the following:
- How do you want to feel after the massage?
- What do you think massage will do for you?
- What results do you want from the massage?

After determining the client's expectations and the outcome, the practitioner should carefully go over all the client policies and procedures discussed in Chapter 2. Never assume that a client understands the complexities of massage practice. Explain everything in detail in terms the client can understand.

For example, when the massage therapist explains patient/client boundaries, the client may not understand the meaning of boundaries in terms of the professional relationship. Many people understand a boundary as a border, the official line that divides one area of land from another. If the massage therapist instead uses a term such as "limit," which means a restriction on what can be done, the client may better understood the concept:
- "Certain boundaries define the professional relationship between the massage therapist and the client."
- "Certain limits define the professional relationship between the massage therapist and the client."

Another example is the term "draped," which may make a client think of heavy curtains. "Covered" may be a better word:

on the table wondering why this massage is so different from what he or she expected.

If a new client has had a massage before from someone else, it is natural to compare the different styles. The massage practitioner must explain the procedures and methods used so that the client understands that massage can be done in many ways. Never discount another massage professional's methods or

- "While you receive a massage, you will be draped."
- "While you receive a massage, you will be covered."

Gender and Age Concerns

Male and female practitioners may experience some difference in a client's expectations and interpretation of touch. With first-time clients, it is important to establish clear boundaries concerning the inappropriateness of sexual interaction and to create a safe, nonsexual professional environment. These boundaries may need to be reinforced as the professional relationship evolves.

Without passing judgment on the correctness of the behavior, it is safe to say that both men and women frequently seem, at least initially, to be more comfortable with a middle-aged (30 or older) woman practitioner. This appears to be based on several factors:

- Body image on the part of women clients (they are more comfortable having another woman see their bodies)
- The discomfort of women's male partners (e.g., husbands) at having a male massage professional interact with their wives or significant others
- Women's concern about safe touch from men
- Men's discomfort with being touched in a pleasurable way by another man
- Men's social conditioning to accept comfort and touch in a caring manner from women
- Cultural influences

Men who are massage professionals must be aware of the possibility of encountering these preconceived ideas. They must present themselves in such a way as to alleviate concerns (with education when possible) and to respect the feelings of the individual client through referral to a woman massage professional if necessary. As public awareness of massage grows, this gender difference probably will begin to dissipate.

Age is also a concern. Both men and women massage practitioners under age 25 may experience bias, because older clients may see them as lacking in experience. In addition, younger practitioners may be subjected to peer stress from clients their own age.

Regardless of whether gender or age is the issue, it is essential that young massage professionals and massage professionals who are men present themselves as neutral, competent, and ethical. Acknowledging the situation also can be effective. For example, a male therapist may greet a new client as follows: "Hello, my name is John. I know it may seem unusual to have a man for a massage therapist, because currently most massage therapists are women. However, just as is happening in nursing, more and more men are entering the massage profession. I'm a fully qualified health care professional, and you can be assured of competent care."

A young (man or woman) massage practitioner might greet a client as follows: "Hello, my name is Mary (or Stephen). I know I look young, but I'm fully qualified, and I can assure you that I practice my professional responsibilities with a mature focus."

FEEDBACK

SECTION OBJECTIVES

Chapter objective covered in this section:

5. The student will be able to obtain and give relevant feedback during the massage.

Using the information presented in this section, the student will be able to perform the following:

- Elicit feedback from the client
- Provide the client with appropriate feedback

Feedback is a noninvasive, continual exchange of information between the client and the professional. Feedback is not social conversation. It is common for a client to talk during the massage and appropriate for a massage professional to listen to the client while remaining focused on the massage. *Note:* It is inappropriate for the professional to engage in social conversation with clients, particularly about their personal lives.

Client Feedback

Whether working with a new client or providing regular massage services to an existing client, encouraging feedback from the client is important. Explain the importance of feedback concerning comfort levels (e.g., warmth, positioning, restroom needs) and the quality of any pain sensations (i.e., "good pain," such as is often experienced with deeper massage methods, and "undesirable pain," which the client may feel if the methods are too aggressive). DVD 1 at the back of this book shows video case studies with premassage interviews.

The practitioner benefits from feedback about the effectiveness or ineffectiveness of the various massage methods. Session-to-session reports of progress, postmassage sensations and experiences, and the duration of effects help the practitioner adjust the application of the massage. Feedback from the client about professionalism and the quality of the professional relationship also is valuable.

Some clients may find giving feedback difficult. They may not have enough body awareness to give an accurate report on sensations during the massage or the effectiveness of the methods used. With education from the practitioner, this communication can improve.

Clients commonly find what they perceive as negative feedback difficult to communicate, such as what they did not enjoy about the massage, methods that were uncomfortable or ineffective, and inappropriate behavior by the practitioner. People generally tend to avoid confrontational situations, or they try not to hurt another's feelings. Both of these behaviors interfere with the client's ability to provide effective feedback to the practitioner. The massage professional is responsible for developing a professional trust relationship that allows the client to feel safe in giving positive, constructive feedback.

Clients should be told during premassage procedures about the importance of feedback. Explain to the client that all feedback is taken as constructive, that it is not personal, and that

---

Box 9-5 **Questions and Reminder Statements to Use with Clients**

Questions and reminder statements that could be used before the massage include the following:
- Is there a position in which you are most comfortable?
- Does the temperature of the room feel comfortable?
- I am going to place my forearm on the massage table; you apply pressure to it at a level you think you would like and explain how you want the massage to feel.
- Remember to tell me if a method is painful or the pressure is too deep.
- I would appreciate it if you would indicate when a method seems particularly beneficial or enjoyable.

Questions and reminder statements that might be used during the massage include the following:
- I'll use three different pressure levels on your back; please tell me which you prefer.
- Might there be a more comfortable position for you?
- Are you comfortable with massage in this area?
- Remember that it's okay to tell me if you are uncomfortable.
- Remember to turn over slowly.

Questions and reminder statements to use after the massage include the following:
- What methods were most effective for you today?
- What might I improve on during the next session?
- Remember to evaluate the aftereffects of the massage, and we'll discuss them at the next session.

---

it enhances the service of massage therapy. It is important to ease the client's concerns about the practitioner's possible reaction to "negative feedback." Gentle, open-ended questions before, during, and after the massage encourage feedback (Box 9-5). Reminder statements also are helpful.

Instilling the idea of "client as a teacher" is one way to encourage feedback from the client. The client teaches the massage professional about himself or herself and guides the practitioner in providing the best massage for them both. This knowledge and experience accumulate, adding depth to the knowledge base of the massage professional.

Practitioner Feedback

Massage practitioners also provide feedback to their clients. Practitioners must develop effective communication skills (see Chapter 2) to ensure that the feedback they give is not taken personally by the client, but rather as valuable information to be used. Examples of feedback the practitioner can give the client include the following:
- Do you notice that your breathing is beginning to slow a bit as you relax?
- Are you aware that you have a bruise on the back of your calf?
- The muscle tension in your shoulder appears greater than before. Can you think of a logical reason?
- You seem to tense up when I apply pressure to this area.
- I noticed that your skin color improved after the massage.

Client Conversation

New clients often talk quite a bit during the first massage, usually the result of nervousness. In future sessions, particularly those for relaxation and stress reduction outcomes, the talking usually diminishes.

Clients commonly talk more during the first 15 minutes of massage as they acclimate to the environment and begin to relax. Some talk during the entire massage; this is appropriate and should be accepted. Many people seek massage not only for the therapeutic physical benefit but also, unconsciously, for the social interaction. The professional respectfully listens to the client and limits conversation to appropriate feedback and necessary verbal exchanges to indicate understanding of what the client is saying.

The following is an example of an appropriate dialog:

Client: "My, it has been a very busy week. My son was in two band competitions. I was only able to attend one. It disturbs me when I miss these events. He placed second and third. I'm very proud of him. Do you remember that last week I told you he might get a scholarship to college for music?"

Practitioner: "Yes, I do remember you speaking of that possibility. If I remember correctly, it was to Mott College, right?"

Client: "Yes. You know, it's hard being a single parent. My work interferes with my ability to be with my son as much as I think is important."

Practitioner (replying with feedback): "Were you aware that your shoulders became more tense just now?"

Client: "Yes, it felt as if you were applying more pressure all of a sudden. Were you?"

Practitioner: "No, I didn't increase the pressure, but your muscles did tense while you were speaking about your lack of time with your son."

Client: "What would you do about this if you were me?"

Practitioner: "I appreciate your feelings about your time availability with your son. I hesitate to give you my personal opinions, and this area is outside my professional expertise. However, I can use some methods to relax your shoulders and teach you some methods to keep them relaxed throughout the week."

Here is the same dialog presented in an inappropriate way:

Client: "My, it has been a very busy week. My son was in two band competitions. I was only able to attend one. It disturbs me when I miss these events. He placed second and third. I am very proud of him. Do you remember that last week I told you he might get a scholarship to college for music?"

Practitioner: "Yes, I do remember you speaking of that possibility. If I remember correctly, it was to Mott College, right? My daughter went to Mott College. She had difficulty with the registration procedure, and it took forever to work out the snag. Make sure your son doesn't work with Mrs. Jones. She was very rude." (inappropriate because the response was personalized to therapist's experience)

Client: "Yes, Mott College is correct, but now I wonder if he'll be OK. You know, it's hard being a single parent. My work interferes with my ability to be with my son as much as I think is important."

Practitioner: "I sure do understand, because my sister is a single parent, and she just read a real good book about it. I told her she needs a day away once a month, and so do you. By the way, were you aware that your shoulders became more tense just now?" (inappropriate because the response was personalized and the advice given does not directly relate to massage).

Client: "Yes, it felt as if you were applying more pressure all of a sudden. Were you?"

Practitioner: "No, I didn't increase the pressure, but your muscles did tense while you were speaking about the guilt feelings about your lack of time with your son." (named emotions—guilt)

Client: "What would you do about this if you were me?"

Practitioner: "Well, a social group or even a support group might help. I think I would talk with my son and see if the situation really bothers him. But you know teenage boys, he probably won't tell you anything. My daughter was so hard to get any information from when she was that age. I can use some methods to relax your shoulders and teach you some methods to keep them relaxed throughout the week, since you seem to get more upset when you think about these issues, and I'm sure this entire situation is a big reason for this muscle tension." (personalized advice) (Proficiency Exercise 9-5)

💡 PROFICIENCY EXERCISE 9-5

Compare the two dialogs presented above and list three differences between them.

Example: In the first dialog, the client did most of the talking.

Your Turn
1.
2.
3.

PREMASSAGE AND POSTMASSAGE PROCEDURES

SECTION OBJECTIVES

Chapter objectives covered in this section:

6. The student will be able to perform premassage procedures to prepare the client and himself or herself for the massage session.
7. The student will be able to perform postmassage procedures to close the massage session and prepare for the next client.

Using the information presented in this section, the student will be able to perform the following:

- Set up an orientation process for a new client
- Develop a personal method of focus/centering

Premassage Procedures

Orientation Process

After the intake process, a new client is ready to learn about the massage process. The orientation proceeds in the following manner:

1. Take the client to the massage area.
2. Show her where she may hang or place her clothes and explain that she needs to remove only the clothing that is necessary and with which she is comfortable. For example, you could say "You can remove all your clothes except your underpants if that is comfortable for you (you will be covered modestly with a sheet at all times), or you may leave on your bra, shirt, pants, and so on if you would prefer to be more covered during your massage." Then explain what happens if the clothing is not removed. Most clients, especially new ones, are more comfortable leaving the underclothes on to cover the genital area. If you have any other special requirements about clothing, now is the time to explain them.
3. Demonstrate the massage table, how it is draped, and how the draping works. Explain the requested starting position on the table (prone, supine, or side-lying).
4. If you are using a massage chair or mat, show the client how to use the chair or mat for proper positioning.
5. Ask about the use of music and offer a few selections.
6. Show the client where the restroom is and how to get there if it is not next to the massage area.
7. Briefly explain any charts you may have on the walls.
8. Ask about a lubricant. Show the client what you have and offer a choice. It is important for clients to choose the type of lubricant or to have the option of no lubricant to avoid any misrepresentation by the massage practitioner of diagnosing or prescribing.
9. Explain that you will leave the room to allow the client privacy while she undresses. The exception to this is if a client is very elderly or a woman in an advanced stage of pregnancy who requests assistance, or any other special situation in which the client requires the practitioner's assistance. If you will be staying in the room, explain how you will help the client and maintain modesty. This usually is done by holding up a sheet in front of the client or by using a screen. If direct assistance is necessary for disrobing, present yourself in a professional and matter-of-fact way while providing the help needed.
10. Explain all sanitary precautions.
11. Show the client the sign on the door stating that a massage is in session and explain why the door is not locked.
12. Give a general idea of the massage flow. For example, that the massage will start on the back and take about 10 minutes, and then the legs and feet will be done for 15 minutes. Explain the effect of any change in a basic pattern; for example, that spending more time on the neck means that less time will be available for the back.
13. Instruct the client to get on the table by sitting between the end of the table and the hinged area (if the table is a portable one) or in the middle of the table (if it is a free-standing table). Next, the client should lean on one side to position herself side-lying or roll to the supine or prone position. To get off the table, the client reverses the procedure; she rolls to one side, pushes up to a seated position, and sits for a minute to prevent

dizziness. She then gets off the table. If any chance exists that the client may fall or may need assistance getting on or off the table, stay in the room to help. Demonstrate the procedures, if necessary, but do not use any draping materials on the table. It is unsanitary for anything or anyone to touch the drapes before the client uses them.

14. Ask the client if she has any questions.

15. Explain that you will be washing your hands and forearms and preparing for the massage while the client gets ready.

16. Tell the client how long you will be gone and that you will knock and announce yourself before entering the room.

Any modifications that need to be made because of the location and environment of the massage should be taken into consideration. People can become anxious if they do not know how to do what they are supposed to do. Do not assume that a client remembers the instructions or knows what is expected. Explain all steps in detail.

Reminding repeat clients of the previously mentioned procedures is important. Just as the information gathered during the intake procedure is updated each week and reassessment continues as the massage sessions progress, clients must be kept updated on any changes in procedures, new equipment, and so forth.

Focus/Centering

While waiting for the client to prepare for the massage, the practitioner should do the same through focus/centering. This can be done in many ways. Slow, deep breathing combined with stretching slows the mind and focuses the attention into the body. Looking at a nature scene or a painting is another way. Listening to music or performing some sort of repetitive behavior, such as washing your hands under warm water while visualizing the water carrying away all concerns for the next hour, can become a trigger for focus. The goal is to be present in the moment for the client and not focused on lists of things that need to be done. Developing a routine sequence for focusing enables the practitioner to become calm and centered much faster (Proficiency Exercise 9-6). During the focusing moments, the massage professional solidifies a clear intention for the massage based on the client outcomes. A very important aspect of professional behavior is to be

💡 PROFICIENCY EXERCISE 9-6

1. Develop a checklist of everything the client needs to know before preparing for the massage.

2. Role play with two other students. One student is the first-time client, another is the massage practitioner, and the third evaluates the performance. Practice using the checklist and explaining procedures to the client. Switch roles so that each student plays all three parts.

3. Develop three different ways to focus your attention before beginning a massage. Make note of your ideas for future reference.

4. Work with three students and teach each other ways to focus. Discuss what works and what does not work.

clearly focused on the client and delivering the massage with intentionally based outcomes.

Postmassage Procedures

Helping the Client Off the Massage Table

When the massage is finished, the client should be left alone for 5 to 10 minutes to rest. If necessary, re-enter the massage area to help the client off the table. Use the following procedure when helping a client off the table.

1. Reach under the client's shoulders and knees.

2. Support the sheet loosely around the client's shoulders and hold it so that it does not slip when the client is lifted.

3. Lift the client's torso off the table while swinging the knees around to the edge of the table. Make sure the client's arm is over your shoulder and not around your neck.

4. In case of dizziness, stabilize the client for a moment after he is in the seated position.

5. Still holding the sheet, help the client to a standing position.

6. Shift the position of the sheet so that the client can hold it securely.

In rare instances the client may need help dressing. Let the client do as much as possible. Be matter of fact and deliberate with any assistance.

If a client will be left to get off the table alone, remind him of the following:

1. Roll to one side.

2. Use your arms to push up to a seated position.

3. Sit for a minute before getting up.

4. Leave the sheets on the table.

5. Get dressed and return to the business area.

Closing the Session

Making the Next Appointment and Collecting the Fee

When the client is dressed and ready to leave, make the next appointment or provide a written reminder if it already has been made. If the fee was not collected in advance, the client should pay at this time.

Saying Good-Bye

After the massage is finished, do not linger in conversation. The attitude in the business area is one of courteous completion. Sometimes getting a client to leave can be difficult. After spending time in a comfortable, caring environment, many people want to talk. Breaking this pattern when business picks up can be a problem, so the best course is to establish a short, consistent departure routine in the beginning. People respond well to sameness. A client will get used to leaving and making the break from the massage practitioner in a reasonable period more easily if the sequence is always the same.

For example, the client approaches the desk, and the massage practitioner takes the money, writes a receipt, and confirms the next appointment. The massage practitioner gets up from the desk and says, "I really enjoyed working with you today. I am glad that you continue to feel that the massage is beneficial. It will be nice to see you again in 2 weeks. I hope the stretches we talked about are helpful. Keep track of any changes, and we'll discuss them next time I see you."

The massage practitioner then extends a hand for a warm handshake. In some situations, a quick, friendly hug is appropriate, but only if it is initiated by the client and the practitioner is comfortable with the interaction. Professionally and respectfully accept hugs or physical contact initiated by the client. Then say good-bye while gesturing or looking toward the door. At this point it is important for the massage practitioner to make a move to leave the area, or the client may initiate additional conversation.

After the Client Has Left

Once the client has gone, the practitioner should update all records (see Chapter 4), prepare the room for the next client, and attend to personal hygiene and self-care (Proficiency Exercise 9-7).

💡 PROFICIENCY EXERCISE 9-7

1. Practice helping people off the massage table. Find 10 different body shapes and sizes to work with and note the difference in leverage needed for each client.
2. Write down your departure routine and practice it with other students. What will you do to end a massage session successfully with a client who does not want to leave? Have one of the students in your practice group role-play this situation so that you can gauge the success of your routine.

POSITIONING AND DRAPING THE CLIENT

SECTION OBJECTIVES

Chapter objective covered in this section:
8. The student will be able to effectively drape and position a client.
Using the information presented in this section, the student will be able to perform the following:
- Position and drape a client and perform a massage using the four basic positions
- Drape effectively with two basic styles

Positioning

Positioning is placing a client into the position that best enhances the benefits of the massage. The four basic massage positions are supine (face up), prone (face down), side-lying, and seated (Figure 9-12). This section explains the use of body supports and proper draping for these basic positions.

A client may be placed in all four positions during a massage session, because remaining in one position longer than 15 minutes may become uncomfortable. The exception is a painful situation that limits the client's ability to be comfortable in a certain position.

As mentioned earlier in the chapter, pillows or other supports (e.g., folded towels, blankets, or specially designed pieces of foam) are used to make the client comfortable. The supports fill any gaps in contour when the client is positioned and provide soft areas against which the client can lean. Supports generally are used under the knees, ankles, and neck.

After the first trimester, a pregnant woman probably will be most comfortable in a side-lying position. If a client has a

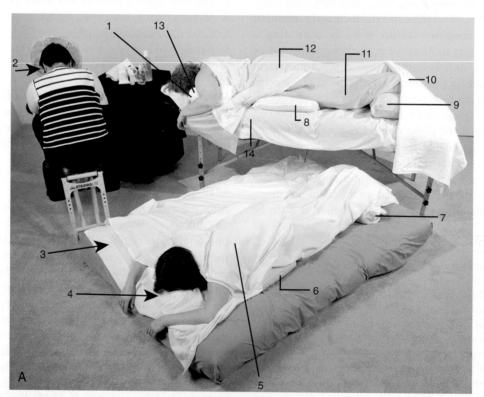

FIGURE 9-12 Positioning the client in the seated, prone, side-lying, and supine positions. **A,** Prone. *1,* Rolled towel. *2,* Face cover. *3,* Bottom sheet. *4,* Rolled towel at forehead. *5,* Top sheet. *6,* Support for abdomen or chest. *7,* Ankle support. *8,* Support for abdomen or chest. *9,* Ankle support. *10,* Blanket. *11,* Bottom sheet. *12,* Top sheet. *13,* Shoulder support. *14,* Fitted sheet.

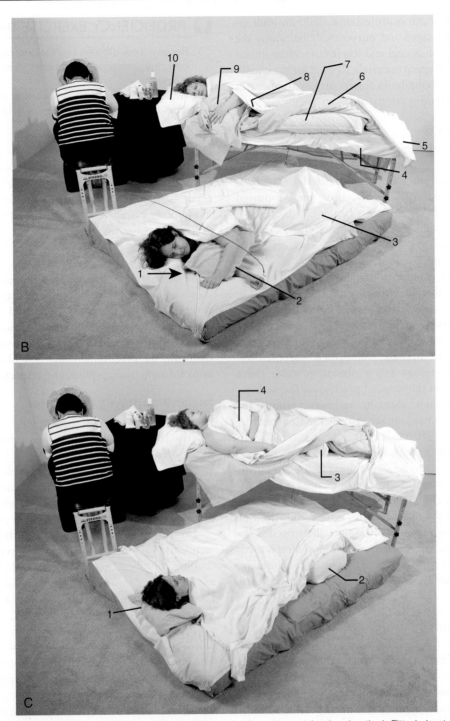

FIGURE 9-12, cont'd B, Side-lying. *1,* Towel roll or pillow. *2,* Pillow. *3,* Knee support (under sheet). *4,* Fitted sheet. *5,* Blanket. *6,* Bottom sheet. *7,* Knee/leg bolster. *8,* Top sheet. *9,* Pillow for arm and shoulder. *10,* Pillow. **C,** Supine. *1,* Pillow. *2,* Knee support. *3,* Knee support. *4,* Chest towel.

large abdomen, supports should be used to lift the chest and support the abdomen. This can be done by using a foam form with an area cut out for the abdomen. Women with large breasts may need a chest pillow.

Side-lying positions require pillows or supports for the arms and a small support between the knees. Clients with lower back pain may be more comfortable with a support under the abdomen when lying prone.

Changing the client's position requires shifting of the body supports. All supports must be under the sanitary drape or protected with sanitary coverings that are changed after each client. If the supports are located under the sheets, simply fold the bottom sheet over the top to expose the supports and move them.

Draping

Draping has two purposes: to maintain the client's privacy and sense of security and to provide warmth. The drape becomes the boundary between the practitioner and the client.

It is a way to establish touch as professional. Skillfully undraping an area to be massaged and purposefully redraping the area is much more professional and less invasive than sliding the hands under the draping materials. Respect for the client's personal privacy and boundaries fosters an environment in which the client's welfare is safeguarded.

Principles of Draping

Draping can be done in many ways, although certain primary principles apply.

- All reusable (multiple use) draping material must have been freshly laundered with bleach or other approved solution for each client (see Chapter 7). Disposable (single use) linens must be fresh for each client and then disposed of properly.
- Only the area being massaged is undraped.
- The genital area is never undraped. The breast area of women is not undraped during routine wellness massage. Specific massage targeting the breast under the supervision of a licensed medical professional may require special draping procedures for the breast area of women. In Canada, breast massage for medical purposes has a specific methodology and a consent process. These methods are out of the scope of practice for the wellness massage practitioner. (Specific recommendations for therapeutic breast massage are provided in Chapter 13.)
- Draping methods should keep the client covered in all positions, including the seated position.
- Draping materials can be a bit clumsy to use at first. To ensure the modesty of the first few practice clients, have them leave their clothing on. If the client uses a dressing area away from the massage table, a robe, top sheet, or wrap large enough to cover the body will be needed for the walk to the massage area. If a wrap or top sheet is used, it can become the top drape once the client is on the table.

The two basic types of draping are flat draping and contoured draping.

Flat Draping Methods

With flat draping, the top sheet is placed over the client in the same manner that a bed is made, with a bottom sheet and a top sheet. Instruct the client to lie supine, prone, or side-lying between the drapes on the massage table. The entire body is then covered. The top drape (and sometimes the bottom drape) is moved in various ways to cover and uncover the area to be massaged.

Note: To ensure the privacy of men, the massage practitioner should avoid smooth, flat draping over the genitals while the client is supine. The penis may become partly erect as a result of parasympathetic activation or a reflexive response to the massage. This response is purely physiologic and does not necessarily suggest sexual arousal. Loose draping that does not lie flat against the body provides for a visual shield and reduces the client's embarrassment.

Contoured Draping

Contoured draping can be done with two towels or with a sheet and a towel. The drapes are wrapped and shaped around

💡 PROFICIENCY EXERCISE 9-8

1. Receive three different professional massages and observe how the massage practitioner drapes and uses body supports.
2. With a fellow student or practice client, practice each draping method shown in Figure 9-13.

the client. This type of draping is very effective for securely covering and shielding the genital and buttock areas. Positioning of the drape may feel invasive to the client, but having the client assist in placement of the drapes preserves a sense of modesty. For women, a separate chest towel can be used to drape the breast area.

Alternative to Draping

As an alternative to draping, the client can wear a swimsuit or shorts and a loose shirt. The table or mat must have a sanitary covering, such as a bottom drape, and a top drape must be available because the client may become chilled even if partly clothed. When working with a client wearing clothing or a swimsuit, the practitioner must still observe all the precautions for sanitation, privacy, and respect.

Suggested Draping Procedures

Figure 9-13 shows the sequence for draping procedures. Practice these procedures and then combine the methods to fit the client's particular needs.

Notice how the draping material is placed so that the practitioner's clothing does not come in contact with the client. This maintains sanitation and appropriate professional distance between the practitioner and the client.

These draping procedures are a starting point for modest, secure use of towels and sheets for proper and appropriate draping. Modification is encouraged. Many other methods are available and can be used instead of or combined with the procedures presented here (Proficiency Exercise 9-8).

SUMMARY

The information discussed in this chapter is just as important as any other aspect of professional therapeutic massage. The different locations and environments for massage set the mood and reflect the personality of the massage practitioner.

Careful consideration of the type of equipment (e.g., massage tables, body supports), supplies (e.g., oils, linens), music, and other amenities that you will use in your practice results in a professional yet personalized approach.

Taking time to explain massage procedures to a client, taking a basic history, and learning and understanding the client's expectations and desired outcome for each massage help create an approach that meets the client's needs. Providing safe, respectful touch by using careful, modest draping and positioning is very important.

This chapter has described professional skills that create the confidence, respect, and trust important to successful application of therapeutic massage. Professional massage practice requires attention to these details.

Evolve Activity 9-4

Evolve Activity 9-5

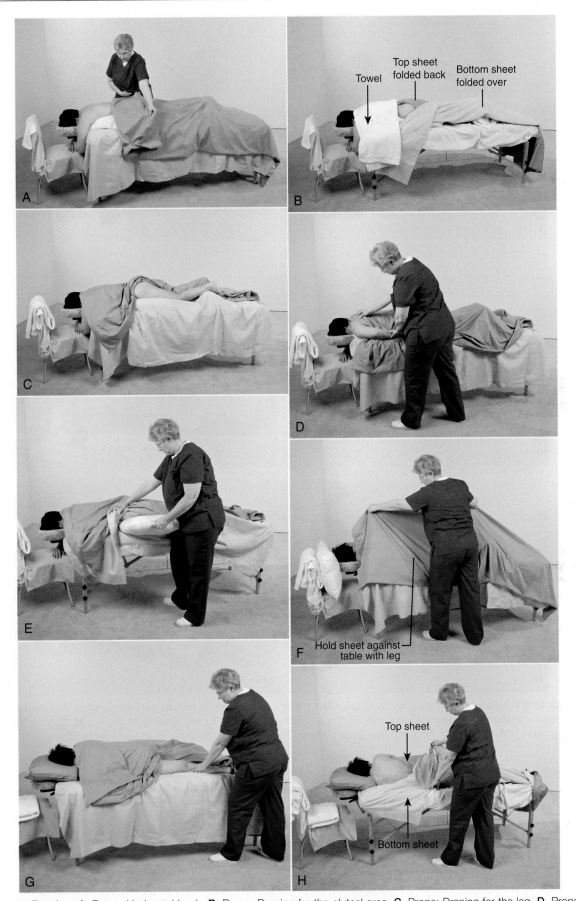

FIGURE 9-13 Draping. **A,** Prone: Undraped back. **B,** Prone: Draping for the gluteal area. **C,** Prone: Draping for the leg. **D,** Prone: Draping for the arm. **E,** Preparing to place the client in the side-lying position: remove the bolster. **F,** Lift the top sheet in the middle to allow the client to roll. **G,** Side-lying: Draping for the leg. **H,** Side-lying: Draping for the back. Use the bottom sheet to fold over the leg and glutes.

Continued

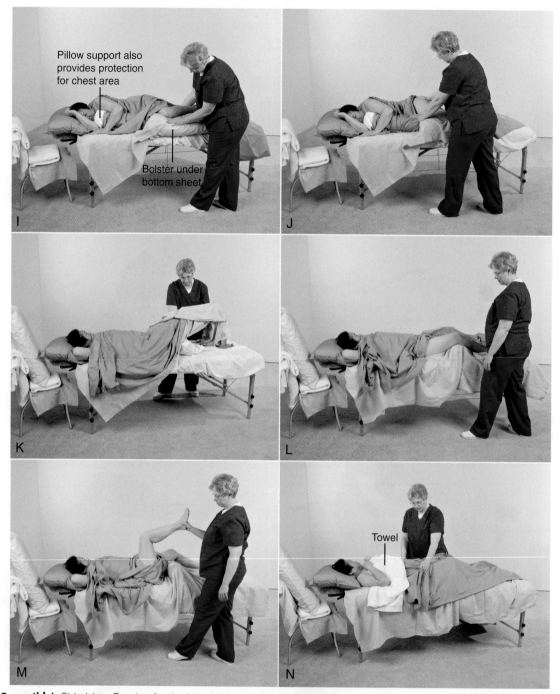

FIGURE 9-13, cont'd I, Side-lying: Draping for the leg. **J,** Move the drape to provide access to the upper thigh and gluteal area. **K,** Supine: Fold the bottom sheet over the top sheet. Lift to position the bolster. **L,** Supine: Draping for the leg. **M,** Contour the drape to prevent exposure of the groin area. **N,** Towel over the top sheet: The client holds the towel while the sheet is moved.

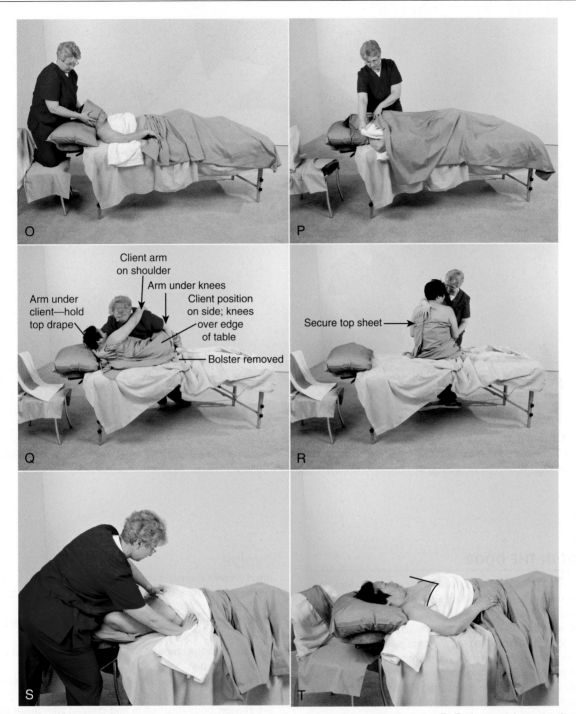

FIGURE 9-13, cont'd O, Draping for the abdomen. Optional use of a pillowcase to cover the eyes. P, Redrape and remove the towel. Q, Help the client from the table. R, Lift by standing; secure the drape. S, Working around the female breast. Use the towel to move the breast tissue. T, Contour the drape around the breast.

Continued

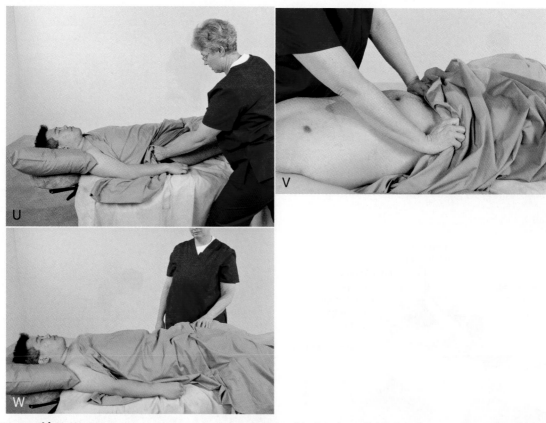

FIGURE 9-13, cont'd **U,** Working in the groin area. Use a top sheet to slide the drape tightly into the area. For males, this moves the genitals out of the massage area. **V,** Use the drape to slide to the top of the pubic bone. For males, this moves the genitals away from the massage area. **W,** Avoid flat draping on males in the supine position. Bunched sheets disguise the genital area.

FOOT IN THE DOOR

In some work environments, you will be considered the massage therapy expert. That means you may be asked for your recommendations on setting up and managing the massage environment. Certainly this is your responsibility if you plan to be self-employed. All the details, added together, create the massage experience you want to provide for your clients. If you can adapt to providing massage on either a table or a mat, you can serve more clients. Seated massage is a great promotional tool and an excellent way to get your foot in the door of many businesses. It is an effective marketing tool, once you are established in business, if you set up the massage chair in a public area such as the lobby or reception area and provide sample massages. Draping makes clients feel warm, safe, secure, and respected. The way you introduce clients to the massage environment, procedures, and methods helps them acclimate once they put their foot in your door.

evolve

http://evolve.elsevier.com/Fritz/fundamentals
9-1 Review massage equipment with this fill-in-the-blank activity.
9-2 Categorize items as appropriate or inappropriate for a massage office.
9-3 Recall all the steps of the massage process and put them in order.
9-4 Review draping and positioning with this multiple choice exercise.
9-5 Review body mechanics and draping with these videos.
Don't forget to study for your certification and licensure exams! Review questions, along with weblinks, can be found on the Evolve website.

Workbook Section

Short Answer

1. What factors must be considered before the massage actually begins?

2. What is the most important piece of massage equipment?

3. How do massage practitioners protect their hands?

4. What types of massage equipment provide a surface that supports the client while the massage is given?

5. What features should be considered when looking for a massage table?

6. What must be checked on the massage table to ensure the client's safety?

7. What are body supports?

8. What are drapes?

9. What types of draping materials are available?

10. What accommodation should be made for clients with sensitive skin?

11. What sanitary measures must be taken with draping materials?

12. What is the purpose of lubricants?

13. What types of lubricants are used?

14. What are some important things to remember about lubricants?

15. What are some general considerations for creating a professional massage environment?

16. What are the main types of massage environments?

17. What special considerations are important for the use of music?

18. What considerations are important for lighting in the massage room?

19. Why is a scentless environment so important?

20. What other considerations are necessary to ensure the client's comfort?

21. Why must the massage practitioner educate the client about appropriate expectations for the massage session?

22. Why should the massage practitioner carefully explain all procedures to the client before the massage?

23. What are the basic massage positions for a client, and how are body supports used in these positions?

24. What are the specific guidelines for draping?

25. In what way is the drape a type of boundary?

26. What are the two basic types of draping procedures?

27. How is a chest towel used?

28. How do you assist a client into a seated position?

29. What is the massage practitioner's attitude at the conclusion of the session?

30. After the client leaves, the massage practitioner should attend to what activities?

Problem-Solving Scenarios

1. A client indicates on the client information form that he does not want an oil-based lubricant used on his back, face, or chest. What are your options? List them on a separate piece of paper.

2. You booked an appointment to do a massage in a client's home. When you arrive, you realize that the house has no private location large enough to accommodate the massage table. What are some of your options? List them on a separate piece of paper.

Assess Your Competencies

Now that you have studied this chapter, you should be able to:
- List the equipment and setup procedures required to prepare for a massage session
- Create a massage setting in different types of environments
- Explain massage procedures to a client
- Identify gender issues that may influence the client's expectations and respond appropriately
- Obtain and give relevant feedback during the massage
- Perform premassage procedures to prepare the client and himself or herself for the massage session
- Perform postmassage procedures to close the massage session and prepare for the next client
- Effectively drape and position a client

On a separate sheet of paper or on the computer, write a short summary of the content of this chapter based on the preceding list of competencies. Use a conversational tone, as if you were explaining to someone (e.g., a client, prospective employer, co-worker, or other interested person) the importance of the information and skills to the development of the massage profession.

Next, in small discussion groups, share your summary with your classmates and compare the ways the information was presented. (You can also post your summaries on the discussion board on the Evolve website.) In discussing the content, look for similarities, differences, possibilities for misunderstanding of the information, and clear, concise methods of description.

Professional Application

You have signed a contract to provide on-site chair massage in a business office. Before you begin, you will have a chance to visit the location. On a piece of paper or the computer, list the specifics you will look for in locating the massage area, what supplies you need to include in the traveling office, and what materials you will need.

Research for Further Study

Check nursing texts and study the positioning and draping procedures; record any procedures that are applicable to massage.

Massage Manipulations and Techniques

http://evolve.elsevier.com/Fritz/fundamentals/

CHAPTER OBJECTIVES

After completing this chapter, the student will be able to perform the following:

1. Evaluate massage manipulations based on seven criteria
2. Use massage manipulations to apply mechanical force to the soft tissue
3. Incorporate movement of the joints as an aspect of massage application
4. Incorporate muscle energy techniques into the massage application
5. Incorporate stretching into the massage application when appropriate
6. Perform a full-body massage using the methods and techniques presented in the chapter

CHAPTER OUTLINE

KEY TERMS

Active assisted movement
Active joint movement
Active range of motion
Active resistive movement
Anatomic barriers
Approximation
Arthrokinematic movements
Comfort barrier
Compression
Concentric isotonic contraction
Depth of pressure
Direction
Direction of ease
Drag
Duration
Eccentric isotonic action
Frequency
Friction
Gliding (effleurage)
Isometric contraction
Isotonic contraction
Joint end-feel
Joint movement
Joint play
Kneading (pétrissage)
Lengthening
Multiple isotonic contractions
Muscle energy techniques
Oscillation
Osteokinematic movements
Passive joint movement
Passive range of motion
Pathologic barrier
Percussion (tapotement)
Physiologic barriers
Positional release technique (PRT)
Postisometric relaxation (PIR)
Proprioceptive neuromuscular facilitation (PNF)
Pulsed muscle energy procedures
Reciprocal inhibition (RI)
Resting position
Rhythm
Rocking
Shaking
Skin rolling
Speed
Strain/counterstrain
Stretching
Target muscle
Vibration

STUDENT NOTE: Most models in this chapter are pictured in sportswear to enhance and clarify the various body positions. A properly groomed massage professional, of course, wears a uniform. See Chapter 9 for draping procedures.

The massage profession is in the process of clarifying its terminology, and anatomic terminology also is changing. Therefore, varying terms are presented together in this chapter so that the reader can identify multiple terms for the same concept. The Massage Therapy Body of Knowledge project described in Chapter 1 began the process of standardizing terminology. At this point, the terms *technique*, *method*, and *manipulation* can be used interchangeably.

This chapter is a core technical chapter. It contains definitions, descriptions, and directions for the application and use of the most common massage techniques. As a student of therapeutic massage, you must learn to problem-solve by using clinical reasoning to devise variations of the applications of massage techniques. Because massage routines offer limited benefits, each treatment session must be designed specifically for the individual client (see Chapter 11).

It is important to understand both why and where massage methods and techniques are used and how to organize a process that uses the various therapeutic approaches efficiently. In the application of therapeutic massage, practitioners use their fingers, thumbs, hands, forearms, and sometimes their knees and feet. Although this chapter focuses on methods that use the hands and forearms, applications that use the legs and feet also are presented. Remember always to stay mindful of how best to use your body when applying massage manipulations and techniques (see Chapter 8).

Ling called the massage methods "passive movements." In 1879 the terms *effleurage*, *pétrissage*, *friction*, and *tapotement* first appeared in the *VonMosegeil* (Proceedings of the German Society for Surgery) to describe Mezger's methods (see Chapter 1). Since then, almost every textbook on massage has included these terms.

Kellogg described the resting position in terms of passive touch (Kellogg, 2010). Most historical textbooks did not distinguish between superficial stroking and effleurage, and many described compression by classifying it as part of pétrissage or pressure. Current trends divide the methods of compression into distinct categories. Most references agree that *tapotement* and *percussion* are synonymous, yet resources seem evenly split between classifying *vibration* and *shaking* separately or together. *Friction* is classified many different ways, but the definitions usually are similar.

This textbook refers to passive movements by the names developed through Ling's and Mezger's works in combination with current usage, which is moving away from the historical terminology. The current trend is to describe a method based on the way it is applied (e.g., *gliding* describes effleurage; see the massage manipulations section later in the chapter). Active movements (or gymnastics, as defined by Ling, Taylor, and others) are described under Massage Techniques Using Joint Movement using current terminology. Although the approach presented in this text is comparable to the method currently called *classical* or *Swedish* massage, it is much more expansive and should not be limited by a label. The more appropriate term is *therapeutic massage*.

All massage applications introduce mechanical forces into the soft tissues, stimulating various physiologic responses.

Mosby's Medical, Nursing, and Allied Health Dictionary defines *manipulation* as "the skillful use of the hands in therapeutic or diagnostic procedures . . . see also *massage*" (Anderson et al., 2005). This dictionary defines *massage* as "the manipulation of the soft tissue of the body through stroking, rubbing, kneading, or tapping." The term *manipulation* is used in this chapter to indicate each of these methods.

The massage methods in this textbook are explained and organized in a manner that consolidates and simplifies application. The infinite variations of massage application do not come from many different methods but from skilled use of the fundamental application and variation of the quality of touch in terms of depth of pressure, drag, direction, speed, rhythm, frequency, and duration (Box 10-1).

Box 10-1   Physiologic Effects of Massage

Assigning a wholly mechanical, reflexive, or chemical effect to massage methods is not always possible. Often the combination of the effects of massage, coupled with the client's physiologic state and receptivity to the massage, produces the response. Simply stated, imbalances fall into two categories: conditions of the body that are "too much" or "not enough." Massage methods help the body restore balance by inhibiting "too much" conditions and by stimulating "not enough" conditions. All massage methods apply forms of external mechanical force processed as sensory information that can stimulate or inhibit body processes.

When addressing muscle responses, consider imbalance reflected as a muscle that is either too short or too strong, or too long or too weak.

Connective tissue methods deal with tissue that is too hard, too soft, too thick, or too thin.

Circulation may be marked by a rushing fluid flow or a sluggish fluid flow.

With nervous system activity, think of overactivity or underactivity.

Consider these general guidelines:
- Methods that move through the skin to the underlying tissue tend to be more mechanical and stimulate localized chemical responses and arterial circulation.
- Painless, deep, broad-based compression encourages parasympathetic dominance.
- Methods that target the skin and superficial fascial layer tend to have a more direct reflexive effect on the nervous system, because many sensory nerves are located in the skin. These methods also tend to stimulate the release of hormonal and other body chemicals that provide for a general systemic (whole body) effect. The venous and lymphatic circulations are influenced. These approaches, especially if delivered briskly, stimulate sympathetic dominance.
- Methods that move the body by causing muscles to contract and relax and joint positions to change deliver sensory input to the proprioceptors and are more reflexive in nature.
- Methods that stretch or knead the tissue are more mechanical and affect the connective tissues.

QUALITY OF TOUCH

SECTION OBJECTIVES

Chapter objective covered in this section:

1. The student will be able to evaluate massage manipulations based on seven criteria.

Using the information presented in this section, the student will be able to perform the following:

- Adapt massage methods based on seven criteria called *qualities of touch*
- Effectively establish and adjust the physical contact with the client

---

Gertrude Beard (2007), a highly respected educator in massage therapy who emphasized massage as an integral part of physical therapy, described the components of massage as follows:

The factors that must be considered as components in the application of massage techniques are the direction of the movement, the amount of pressure, the rate and rhythm of the movements, the medium used, the frequency and duration of the treatment, and the position of the patient and of the physical massage practitioner.*

Variations in Touch

Individual massage methods vary in depth of pressure, drag, direction, speed, rhythm, frequency, and duration. These components of the quality of touch, compiled from Beard's work and other sources, are discussed in this textbook.

- **Depth of pressure** (compressive force) can be light, moderate, deep, or variable. Depth of pressure is extremely important. Most soft tissue areas of the body consist of three to five layers of tissue, including the skin; the superficial fascia; the superficial, middle, and deep layers of muscle; and the various fascial sheaths and connective tissue structures. Pressure must be delivered through each successive layer, displacing the tissue to reach the deeper layers without damage to the tissues or discomfort for the client. The deeper the pressure, the broader the base of contact with the surface of the body. More pressure is required to address thick, dense tissue than delicate tissue. Pressure delivers compressive force to the tissue (Figure 10-1).
- **Drag** is the amount of pull (stretch) on the tissue (tensile force). In this context the term *drag* refers to the effort required to overcome resistance. Dry skin has a high resistance to slip. Lubricant is used during massage to increase slip and thus reduce drag. When a tensile force is used during assessment or to bring about a physiologic change during the massage application, the amount of drag on the tissue increases or decreases in relationship to the degree of slipperiness of the skin.
- **Direction** means that the massage may proceed from the center of the body outward (centrifugal) or from the extremities inward to the center of the body (centripetal). It can proceed from proximal to distal attachments of the muscle (or vice versa) following the muscle fibers, transverse to the tissue fibers, or in circular motions.
- **Speed** of techniques can be fast, slow, or variable.
- **Rhythm** refers to the regularity of application of the technique. A method that is applied at regular intervals is considered even, or rhythmic. A method that is disjointed, or irregular, is considered uneven, or nonrhythmic.
- **Frequency** is the rate at which the method repeats itself within a given time frame. In general, each method is repeated about three times before the practitioner moves or switches to a different approach.
- **Duration** is the length of time the method is applied or that the technique remains in one location.

Through these variations in touch, simple massage methods are adapted to produce the client's desired outcomes. These qualities of touch provide the therapeutic benefit. The *mode of application* (e.g., gliding or kneading) provides the most efficient application. Each method can be varied, depending on the desired outcome, by adjusting depth, drag, direction, speed, rhythm, frequency, and duration. As you strive to perfect your practice of massage application, remember that the quality of touch is more important than the method.

Note that quality of touch is altered when a contraindication or caution for massage exists. For example, when a person is fatigued, the duration of application often is shortened; if a client has a fragile bone structure, the depth of pressure is altered.

---

*Beard's definition of *medium* referred to the application of lubricants or other instruments used. Her definition of *frequency* reflected how often per day or week the massage was given.

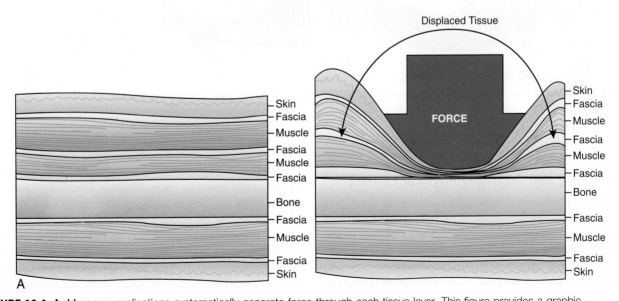

FIGURE 10-1 A, Massage applications systematically generate force through each tissue layer. This figure provides a graphic representation of the application of force. It begins with light, superficial application and progresses with increased pressure to the deepest layer.

Continued

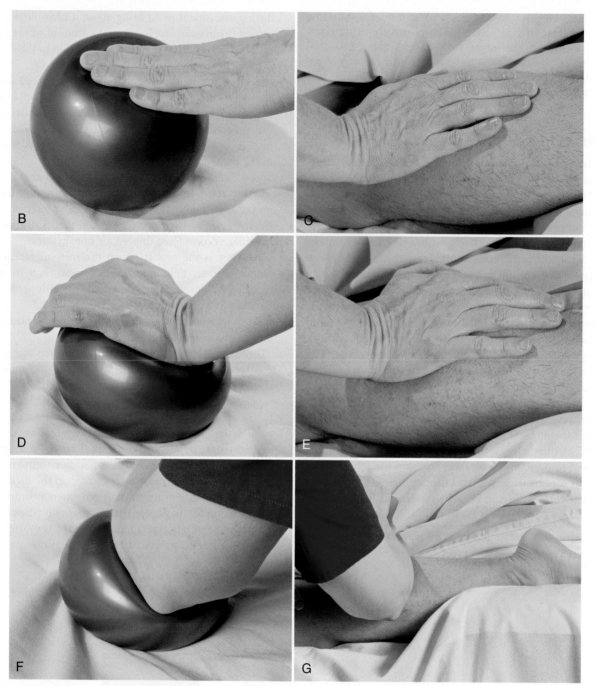

FIGURE 10-1, cont'd The varying degrees of pressure are: **B,** Light. **C,** Light. **D,** Medium. **E,** Medium. **F,** Deep. **G,** Deep.

Establishing and Adjusting Physical Contact

The massage professional must make contact with the client's body in a secure, confident way. An unsure touch is difficult to interpret and unsettling to the client. Make sure your hands are warm and then tell the client you are about to touch him or her. Your touch should be steady, not abrupt.

After touch contact has been made with the client and the massage has begun, the intention of the contact should not be broken. This means that the massage practitioner remains focused on the client for the entire session. Maintaining

contact does not mean that the practitioner never removes his or her hands from the client. Draping effectively, having the client change position, or applying lubricant to a different area is nearly impossible without removing your hands from the client's body. When removing your hands, simply establish verbal contact by telling the client you will be removing your hands for a moment, shifting the draping, or altering position. Before re-establishing touch, again tell the client you will be touching him or her and where so that the person does not startle. Centering facilitates this process of remaining focused on the client.

Positioning the Client

The four types of client positioning are prone, supine, side-lying, and seated. All four are commonly used in combination during a massage. Making sure the client is comfortable is important when positioning, and supports can be used for this purpose (see Chapter 9). The client may appreciate a positional shift during the massage to maintain general comfort. Let the client know before the massage begins that he should tell you if he is uncomfortable in any way and that you will make adjustments. If the client does not say anything during the treatment, check in about every 15 minutes to see whether he is comfortable.

TYPES OF MECHANICAL FORCE AND MASSAGE MANIPULATIONS

SECTION OBJECTIVES

Chapter objective covered in this section:
2. The student will be able to use massage manipulations to apply mechanical force to the soft tissue.
Using the information presented in this section, the student will be able to perform the following:
• Explain the five kinds of force that can affect body tissues
• Perform six basic massage manipulations and techniques: gliding, kneading, compression, oscillation (vibration, shaking, rocking), percussion/tapotement, and friction
• Combine the six basic massage manipulations into a basic full-body massage

Massage must be simple.
Albert Baumgartner (quoting Plato), *Massage in Athletics,* 1947

Many endeavor to introduce improvements into the science of massage but fail to gain adherents to their preventive methods. It would be well to advise these witty inventors of the new sub-methods to keep their improvements to themselves.
Albert Baumgartner, *Massage in Athletics,* 1947

Types of Force

Force may be perceived as mechanical or as field forces, such as gravity or magnetism. Actions that involve pushing, pulling, friction, or sudden loading (e.g., a direct blow) are examples of mechanical force, the type of force presented in this text. Mechanical forces can act on the body in a variety of ways. The different types of mechanical force and the ways they are applied therapeutically are important aspects of massage.

The five kinds of force that can affect body tissues are *compression, tension, bending, shear,* and *torsion.* Not all tissue is affected the same way by each type of force. We will look at each of the five types of force, the different ways they can cause tissue injuries, and the ways they produce important therapeutic benefits when applied by a skilled massage practitioner.

Compression

Compressive forces occur when two structures are pressed together. Compressive force is a component of massage

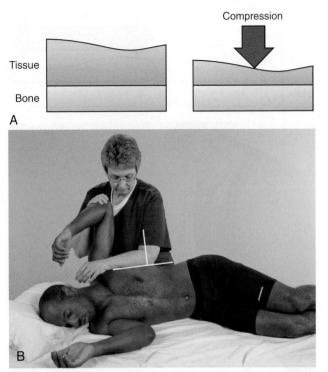

FIGURE 10-2 Illustration **(A)** and example **(B)** of compression.

application and is described as depth of pressure. This kind of force may be sudden and strong, as with a direct blow (percussion), or it may be slow and gradual, as with gliding strokes. The magnitude and duration of the force are important in determining the outcome of the application of compression (Figure 10-2).

Some tissues are quite resilient to compressive forces, and others are more susceptible. Nerve tissue is an interesting example. Nerve tissue can withstand a moderately strong compressive force if the force does not last long (e.g., a sudden blow to the back of your elbow that hits your "funny bone"). However, even slight force applied for a long time, as occurs with carpal tunnel syndrome, can cause severe nerve damage. The practitioner must take this into account when determining the duration of a massage application that involves compression over nerves. Compressive force should not be maintained on a specific area for extended periods during massage. Generally, a compressive force need not be sustained for longer than 15 seconds to achieve results.

Ligaments and tendons are quite sturdy and resistant to strong compressive loads. Muscle tissue, on the other hand, with its extensive vascular structure, is not as resistant to compressive forces. Excess compressive force can rupture or tear muscle tissue, causing bruising and connective tissue damage. This is a concern when pressure is applied to deeper layers of tissue. To prevent tissue damage, the practitioner must distribute the compressive force of massage over a broad contact area on the body; the more compressive force used, the broader the base of contact with the tissue.

Compressive force is used therapeutically to affect circulation, sensory and autonomic nerve stimulation, nerve chemicals, and connective tissue pliability.

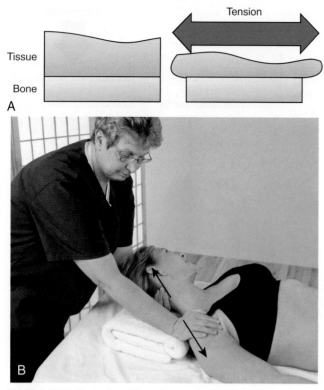

FIGURE 10-3 Illustration **(A)** and example **(B)** of tension.

Tension

Tension forces (also called *tensile forces*) occur when two ends of a structure are pulled in opposite directions. This is different from muscle tension. Muscle tension is created by excess muscular contraction, which results from an increase in motor tone or an increase in tissue density caused by fluid accumulation and connective tissue changes (muscle tone). Muscles that are long as a result of being pulled apart are affected by tensile force. Certain tissues, such as bone, are highly resistant to tensile forces. An extreme amount of force is required to break or damage a bone by pulling its two ends apart. Soft tissues, on the other hand, are very susceptible to tension injuries. In fact, tensile stress injuries are the most common soft tissue injuries. Such injuries include muscle strains, ligament sprains, tendinitis, fascial pulling or tearing, and nerve traction injuries (i.e., sudden stretching of nerves, such as occurs in whiplash).

Tension force is used during massage with applications that drag, glide, lengthen, and stretch tissue to elongate connective tissues and lengthen short muscles (Figure 10-3).

Bending

Bending forces are a combination of compression and tension. One side of a structure is exposed to compressive forces as the other side is exposed to tensile forces. Bending occurs during many massage applications. Force is applied across the fiber or across the direction of the muscles, tendons or ligaments, and fascial sheaths. Bending forces rarely damage soft tissues; however, they are a common cause of bone fractures. Bending force is very effective in increasing connective tissue pliability and affecting proprioceptors in the tendons and belly of muscles (Figure 10-4).

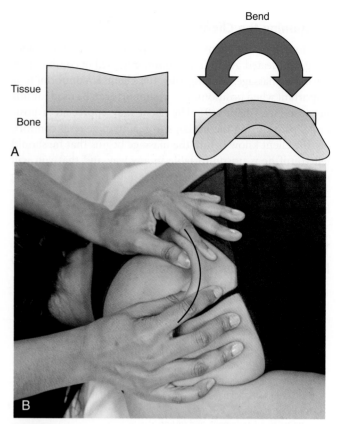

FIGURE 10-4 Illustration **(A)** and example **(B)** of bending.

Shear

Shear is a sliding force, and significant friction often is created between the structures that slide against each other. The massage method of friction uses shear forces to generate physiologic change by increasing connective tissue pliability and creating therapeutic inflammation. However, excess friction (shearing force) may produce an inflammatory irritation that causes many soft tissue problems (Figure 10-5).

Torsion

Torsion forces are best understood as twisting forces. Massage methods that use kneading introduce torsion forces and target connective tissue changes and fluid movement.

Application of torsion force to a single soft tissue structure is not very common and is rarely the cause of significant tissue injury. Torsion force applied to a group of structures (e.g., a joint) is much more likely to be the cause of significant injury. For example, when the foot is on the floor and the individual turns the body, the knee as a whole is exposed to significant torsion force (Figure 10-6).

Massage Manipulations and Techniques (Mode of Application)

The methods of massage described in the following sections introduce one or a combination of the five types of mechanical force into the body to achieve a therapeutic benefit (Figure 10-7). This process is influenced by the quality of touch, depth of pressure, drag, duration, speed, rhythm, and frequency. Appropriate use of mechanical force is necessary. If

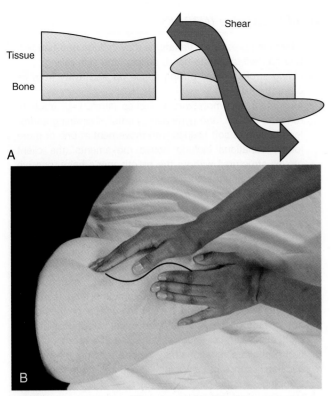

FIGURE 10-5 Illustration **(A)** and example **(B)** of shear.

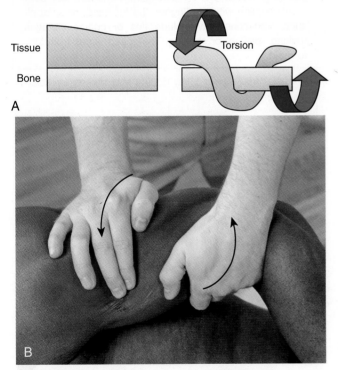

FIGURE 10-6 Illustration **(A)** and example **(B)** of torsion.

insufficient force or the wrong type of mechanical force is used, the application will not be effective; conversely, excessive or inappropriate use of force can damage tissues.

The variety of massage and bodywork modalities in the profession (see Chapter 2) can be clarified by describing what is done during the application, using qualities of touch, mechanical forces, and mode of application. For example, the modality called *deep tissue massage* is not a unique form of

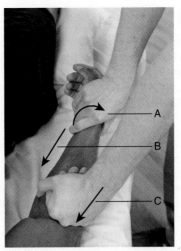

FIGURE 10-7 Example of combined loading: torsion loading *(A)* + tension loading *(B)* + compression loading *(C)*.

massage but appears to be a compressive force application at a "deeper" tissue level.

Those studying this textbook should be able to modify the massage application from surface to deep, fast to slow, and long to short, as appropriate, based on the client's individual needs. The intention and outcome of the massage application appropriately influence fluid movement, nervous system function, musculoskeletal function, and connective tissue pliability in both acute and chronic conditions. Our attention to the client is based on an intent to serve our clients in a focused and compassionate manner. The following massage manipulations, which are modes of application, are used to apply mechanical force during massage in an appropriate way to achieve the determined outcome for the massage (Box 10-2).

Resting Position (Holding)

The act of placing your hands on another person seems so simple; yet this initial contact must be made with respect and a client-centered focus with the intention of meeting the client's goals. With the resting position (holding), we enter the client's personal boundary space, as defined by sensitivity to changes in air movement and heat picked up by the sensory receptors in the skin. The root hair plexus is one of the most sensitive receptors to the movement of air. Activation of the heat sensors indicates that something is close enough to cause physical harm. Because of these sensors, the fight-or-flight responses of the sympathetic autonomic nervous system often are activated with the initial contact.

The instinctive survival and protective mechanisms designed to protect human beings from hand-to-hand combat dictate that the physiologic safety zone generally is an arm's length. If another person is at this distance, the sensory mechanisms of sympathetic arousal are less sensitive than if the person is close enough to touch. For this reason, the first approach to touch by the massage professional is very important.

Holding provides time for the client to become acclimated to the proximity of another human being. It gives the client time to evaluate, on a subconscious level, whether this touch

Box 10-2 Terminology Used in the *Massage Therapy Body of Knowledge (MTBOK)*

Discipline An area of study with shared concepts, vocabulary, and so on (e.g., Swedish massage, sports massage, myofascial release).

Modality A method of application or the employment of any physical agents and devices. The term is commonly misused to describe forms of massage (e.g., NMT, myofascial, Swedish).

Technique A procedure or skill used in massage therapy, including but not limited to the following:

- *Compression* involves use of compressive force without slip, commonly applied at a 90-degree angle to the tissue, followed by a lift or release of force. Force varies in depth and pressure.
- *Friction* strokes involve rubbing one surface over another, with little or no surface glide, providing both compressive and shearing forces. Pressure may be superficial (light) to deep, providing friction effects between various tissue levels. Examples of friction include warming, rolling, wringing, linear, stripping, cross-fiber, chucking, and circular friction. Most friction strokes are administered with little or no lubricant.
- *Gliding/stroking (effleurage)* involves gliding movements that contour to the body. The pressure may be either superficial (light) or deep. Variations may include one-handed, two-handed, alternate hand, forearm, and nerve stroking.
- *Holding* involves holding tissue without movement and with little or no force or weight in the contact.
- *Kneading (pétrissage)* strokes involve lifting, rolling, squeezing, and releasing tissue, most commonly using rhythmic alternating pressures. Variations may include one-handed, two-handed, alternate hand, pulling, and skin rolling.
- *Lifting* strokes entail pulling tissue up and away from its current position.
- *Movement and mobilization* strokes (stretching, traction, range of motion, and gymnastics) entail shortening and/or lengthening of soft tissues with movement at one or more joints. Variations include active movements (the client moves structures without the practitioner's help), passive movements (the therapist moves the structures without the client's help), resistive movement (the client moves structures against resistance provided by the therapist), and active assisted movement (the client moves structures with support and assistance from the therapist).
- *Percussion (tapotement)* strokes involve alternating or simultaneous rhythmic striking movement of the hands against the body, allowing the hand to spring back after contact, controlling the impact. Hand surfaces commonly used include the ulnar surface of the hand, tips or flats of the fingers, open palm, cupped palm and back ulnar surface, knuckles, or sides of a loosely closed fist. Technique variations may include tapping, pincement, hacking, cupping, slapping, beating, pounding, and clapping.
- *Vibration* strokes involve shaking, quivering, trembling, swinging, oscillation, or rocking movements most commonly applied with the fingers, the full hand, or an appliance. Variations may include fine or coarse vibration, rocking, jostling, or shaking. The speed varies from slow to rapid.

Modified from Massage Therapy Body of Knowledge (MTBOK) steward: *Massage therapy body of knowledge (MTBOK)*, version 1, May 15, 2010. www.mtbok.org/downloads/MTBOK_Version_1.pdf. Accessed April 1, 2011.

is safe. This first application of touch sets the stage for the first 15 to 30 minutes of the massage, because it takes that long for the sympathetic arousal fight-or-flight response, which causes the release of adrenaline into the blood, to reverse itself.

Holding also allows stillness when intermixed with the other movements of massage. The body needs time to process all the sensory information it receives during massage. Stopping the motions and simply resting the hands on the body provides this moment of stillness.

Holding is an excellent way to call attention to an area through stimulation of the cutaneous (skin) sensory receptors. Simple, sustained touch over an area of imbalance often is enough stimulation to cause a reflexive response. This technique also adds body heat from the massage practitioner's hand to an area of the client's body. In addition, it is an excellent way to re-establish contact with the client if the flow of the massage is interrupted or if physical contact is broken.

Applying the Holding Technique

An open, soft, relaxed, warm, dry hand is best for the application of holding (Figure 10-8). This signals to the physiologic survival mechanism that no weapon is nearby nor is there any intent to strike. A cool, clammy hand suggests sympathetic activation in the practitioner. Subconscious survival

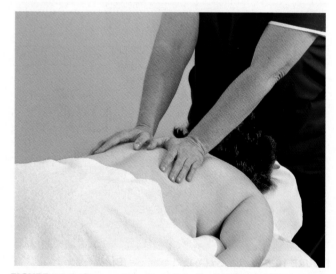

FIGURE 10-8 Open, relaxed hands in the holding position.

mechanisms in the client can recognize this and will respond to perceived danger by tensing for protection.

Practice extending an open, relaxed hand. Rub your hands together to warm them and then towel-dry them to remove any perspiration before touching the client.

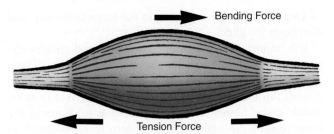

FIGURE 10-9 The focus of gliding is horizontal strokes.

PROFICIENCY EXERCISE 10-1

1. Purposeful touch may be simple, but it is not easy. Diligent practice is required. If you enjoy animals, practice your approach with them. They do not hide responses as people do. Practice using holding to touch a dog, cat, or other animal while the animal is asleep and see if you can do it without waking the animal.
2. Babies and young children also are good for practice. Practice the holding techniques with a baby or child. Acceptance of the touch is indicated if the child does not startle or move away.

In most circumstances a slow, steady approach by the practitioner, with deliberate hesitation at the arm's length boundary, accompanied by a verbal announcement that you will begin touching, is the best way to prevent excessive sympathetic arousal. Most of the time, the massage practitioner seeks to activate the restorative parasympathetic state for the client. Yet even when the massage is designed to stimulate sympathetic activation, the first touch should be slow, gradual, and deliberate, using pressure level 1 or 2 (see Chapter 8).

Apply the holding technique slowly and gradually, in a confident, secure manner. As part of the survival mechanism, the body innately responds to a hesitant touch by withdrawing. Mastering the application of the holding technique makes flowing into the other methods easy (Proficiency Exercise 10-1).

Gliding/Stroking (Effleurage)

The historical term for gliding strokes is *effleurage*. The term *effleurage* originates from the French verb meaning "to skim" and "to touch lightly on." The most superficial applications of gliding (effleurage) do this, but the full spectrum is determined by pressure, drag, speed, direction, and rhythm, making this one of the most versatile massage manipulations. The most common forces introduced by gliding are tension force, bending force, and compression force.

After application of the initial touch, gliding often is next in the sequence, especially if a lubricant is used. The long, broad movements of this method are excellent for spreading the lubricant on the skin surface. The ease of application makes this an effective manipulation to use repetitively while gradually increasing the depth of pressure. This is one of the preferred manipulations to warm or prepare the tissue for more specific bodywork. Because of the horizontal nature of the manipulation, the flow pattern of the massage can progress smoothly from one body area to another. Gliding also is a good method to use to evaluate for hard and soft tissue, hot and cold areas, or areas that seem "stuck" (i.e., areas of binding). It is the preferred method for abdominal massage and for massage to facilitate circulation.

The more superficial the stroke, the more reflexive the effect. Slow superficial strokes (pressure level 2 or 3) are very soothing, whereas fast superficial strokes (pressure level 1 or 2) are stimulating. If a deeper stroke pressure (levels 3 to 5) is applied at a slower rate, the effect is more mechanical and stimulates parasympathetic dominance (see Chapter 8).

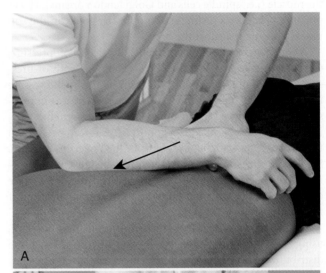

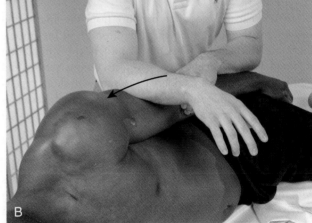

FIGURE 10-10 Two examples of gliding.

Applying Gliding Strokes

The distinguishing characteristic of gliding strokes is their horizontal application in relation to the tissue fibers, which generates a tensile force (Figure 10-9). Gliding also can be applied across fibers to create a bending force. The intensity and result of the mechanical force application are influenced by drag and depth of pressure. For example, when gliding is used to influence superficial fascia, significant drag occurs on the tissue. During a palliative (relaxation) massage approach, lubricant typically is used to reduce the drag. Compressive force (compression) is used to determine the layer of tissue affected by the tension force created by the gliding technique. Gliding on the skin surface involves little or no compression. Otherwise, all gliding techniques actually begin first with compression. Compress down into the target tissue first and then begin the glide.

It is important to use compressive force to determine the depth of pressure desired for the massage. During gliding, light pressure remains on the skin, and moderate pressure extends through the subcutaneous layer of the skin to reach muscle tissue; however, it is not so deep as to compress the tissue against the underlying bony structure. Moderate to heavy pressure that exerts sufficient drag on the tissue mechanically affects the connective tissue and the proprioceptors in the muscle (i.e., spindle cells and Golgi tendon organs). Heavy pressure produces a distinctive compressive force on the soft tissue, pressing it against the bone.

Always begin gliding by establishing depth of pressure. Compress tissue first and then begin gliding. Depth of pressure is a result of leverage and of leaning on the body. Pressure increases as the angle of the lean increases. Increases in pressure are *not* achieved by pushing with muscle strength.

Increasing pressure adds a compressive force and drag to the stroke. Light stroking is done with the fingertips or palm. Small body areas, such as the fingers, can be grasped and surrounded as gliding is applied to the entire area. The surface contact increases with full hand and forearm application of the manipulations.

Gliding that proceeds from the trunk of the body outward, using superficial pressure, usually follows the dermatome distribution and is more reflexive in its effects (Proficiency Exercise 10-2).

Strokes that use moderate pressure from the fingers and toes toward the heart, following the direction of the muscle fibers, are excellent for mechanical and reflexive stimulation of blood flow, particularly as it affects venous return and lymphatic flow. Light to moderate pressure with short, repetitive gliding that follows the patterns for the lymph vessels is the basis for manual lymphatic drainage (see Chapter 12) (Figure 10-10).

Kneading (Pétrissage)

The historical term for kneading is *pétrissage*, which comes from the French verb *petrir*, meaning "to knead." In **kneading (pétrissage)**, the soft tissue is lifted, rolled, and squeezed (Figure 10-11).

Just as gliding is focused horizontally on the body, kneading is focused vertically and involves twisting. The main purpose of this manipulation is to lift tissue, applying bend, shear, and torsion forces. After the tissues have been lifted, the full hand is used to squeeze the tissue as it rolls out of the hand while the other hand prepares to lift additional tissue and repeat the process (Figure 10-12).

Because skin and the underlying muscles cannot be lifted without first pressing into them, compression is a component of kneading and is done first. Kneading is very good for reducing motor tone. The lifting, rolling, and squeezing action affects the spindle cell proprioceptors in the muscle belly. As the belly of the muscle is squeezed, which squeezes the spindle cells, muscle tension decreases. The tendons, when lifted, are stretched, which increases tension in both the tendons and the Golgi tendon receptors. The result of this sensory input is

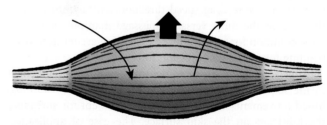

FIGURE 10-11 The focus of kneading is vertical lifting and twisting.

reflexive relaxation of the muscle to protect it from harm, restoring a more normal resting length of the muscle.

Kneading also mechanically softens the superficial fascia, making it less dense and more pliable. This type of connective tissue, located under the skin, is similar to gelatin. It is made up of a glycol (sugar) protein that binds with water. If gelatin is mixed with water and allowed to sit, it becomes thick and solidifies, resulting in reduced pliability and increased density. If the gelatin is pressed into smaller pieces and stirred, it softens. This is similar to the effect of kneading on connective tissue with the bend, shear, and tension forces exerted on the tissue. The difference in feeling in the muscles before and after kneading can be compared to the difference between the

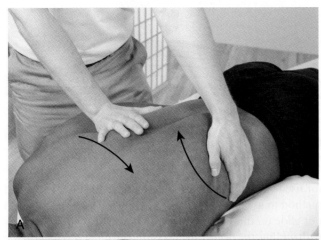

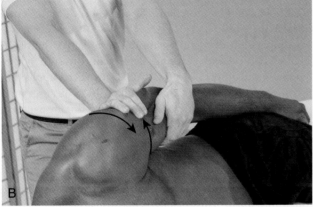

FIGURE 10-12 Two examples of kneading.

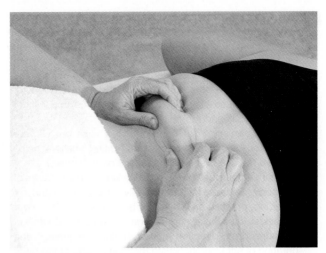

FIGURE 10-13 Skin rolling.

stiffness of a brand new pair of shoes or jeans and the comfort of an old pair of jeans or a broken-in pair of shoes.

The fascia also forms a major part of each muscle. Kneading has the mechanical effect of softening and creating space around the muscle fibers, making the tendons more pliable. The tension on the tendon as it is pulled during kneading deforms the connective tissue and mechanically warms it in a manner similar to that by which a piece of metal bent back and forth becomes warm. Instead of metal fibers, collagen fibers are bent and warmed. When something is warm, its molecules are moving faster and are farther apart. The space, which is created at the molecular level, translates into a softer, more pliable structure.

Kneading may incorporate a wringing or twisting component (torsion) after the tissue has been lifted. Changes in depth of pressure and drag determine whether the client perceives the manipulation as superficial or deep. By the nature of the manipulation, the pressure and pull peak when the tissue is lifted to its maximum and are less at the beginning and end of the manipulation.

Kneading methods are effective for supporting circulation, because they squeeze the capillary beds in the tissues and support fluid exchange.

Skin Rolling

Skin rolling is a variation of the lifting technique. Deep kneading attempts to lift the muscular component away from the bone; skin rolling, however, only lifts the skin from the

underlying muscle layer. It has a warming and softening effect on the superficial fascia, causes reflexive stimulation of the spinal nerves, and is an excellent assessment method. Areas of stuck skin (bind) often suggest underlying problems. Skin rolling is one of the very few massage methods that can safely be used directly over the spine. Only the skin is accessed, and the direction of pull on the skin is up and away from the underlying bones; therefore, no risk of injury is posed to the spine, unlike with methods that involve any type of downward pressure (Figure 10-13).

Sometimes the tissue will not lift. This may be a result of excessive edema (swollen tissue), a heavy fat layer, scarring that extends into the deeper body layers, or thickened areas of connective tissue, especially over aponeuroses (flat sheets of superficial connective tissue). If these conditions are present, kneading or skin rolling applications are uncomfortable for the client. Shifting to gliding and compression may soften the tissue enough that kneading can be used more effectively later in the session.

Excessive body hair may hamper the use of kneading or skin rolling. The massage practitioner must be careful not to pull the client's hair when using these massage manipulations.

Applying Kneading

Kneading must be rhythmic to feel correct. The speed of the technique is limited. The speed and frequency of the application are determined by how much tissue can be lifted and how long it takes to roll and squeeze the tissue through the hand. Lifting the tissue quickly or squeezing it too fast is uncomfortable for the client. Although the concept is difficult to explain, it is much like kneading bread dough; the consistency of the material determines how it is to be kneaded.

Kneading begins with palmar compression on a 45-degree angle to move the tissue forward and up. The massage practitioner produces the compression pressure by leaning into the body—not by using muscle strength to push downward. As the tissue bunches in front of the hand, the fingers, used as a unit with the palm, close over the mound of tissue. The tissue then is lifted, rolled, and squeezed through the hand as the practitioner rocks his or her entire body away from the

💡 PROFICIENCY EXERCISE 10-3

1. Knead a variety of sizes of bread dough. Small pieces can be used to practice the delicate applications used on the face and anterior neck; larger pieces can mimic big muscles, such as the gluteals. Bread dough is good for practice because it is resilient (like body tissue) and will not allow you to knead too fast.
2. Knead a partially inflated balloon. If it slips out of your grasp, you just pinched your "client." Using a balloon helps develop the use of the palm in place of the fingers.
3. For learning purposes only, practice kneading each area of the body. Because of the repetitive use of the hand for kneading, practice on a different body area each day over a week's time. Make sure to practice different depths of pressure, drag, direction, speed, rhythm, frequency, and duration of application. Notice that some parts of the body are more easily kneaded.

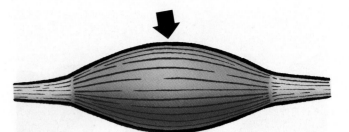

FIGURE 10-14 The focus of compression is a vertical downward pressure.

direction used to produce the compressive force and initiates the lifting action. As the practitioner's body sways back, the tissues lift and roll through the grasping hands. The massage practitioner again rocks forward and leans into the body to apply compression, and the movements are repeated to create a rhythmic pattern of kneading.

Except in very delicate areas, such as the face, the fingers and thumbs should not be used to lift the tissue because of a tendency to pinch and cause the client discomfort.

To get a feel for the method, practice with some clay. Keep your fingers pressed together, using them as a single unit pressed against the thenar eminence (the pad at the base of the thumb). Do not use the thumb itself. It is important to use as large a part of the palmar surface as possible. Slowly extend the upward pull until you feel the end of the elastic give of the tissue; this is where a sense of resistance (bind) is felt. This type of kneading works on both the skin and the tendons. In most cases only one hand at a time is used to lift, squeeze, and twist the tissue. Kneading becomes continuous when a hand-over-hand rhythm is established. Two hands also can be used against each other on larger areas, such as the hamstring muscle.

In skin rolling, the entire hand is used to lift the skin, and the thumbs then are used to feed the skin to the fingers in a rolling motion.

Note: Although kneading is very effective for softening and relaxing tissue, it is energy-consuming for the massage practitioner. As mentioned earlier, the fingers should be used as a unit with the thenar eminence of the thumb. The massage practitioner should take care not to use this manipulation excessively. A better practice is to use kneading intermittently with gliding and compression, which do not require such labor-intensive use of the hands. Constant attention must be paid to body mechanics (Proficiency Exercise 10-3).

Compression

Compression uses a press-lift method that is applied at a 90-degree angle to the tissue. Compressive force is an aspect of gliding and kneading. Compression is particularly suited for use when a lubricant is undesirable. It also is a very good method to use on hairy bodies, because the manipulations do not glide on the skin, pull the tissue, or require lubricant. As with gliding, the deeper the pressure, the more mechanical the effect. Likewise, the more superficial the pressure, the more reflexive the effect.

Compression directs pressure downward into the tissues (Figure 10-14), with varying depths of pressure adding bending and compressive forces. The superficial application of compression resembles the resting position but uses more pressure. The manipulations of compression usually penetrate the subcutaneous layer, whereas in the resting position, they remain on the skin surface. Much of the effect of compression results from pressing tissue against the underlying bone, causing it to spread and be squeezed from two sides, similar to flattening out a tortilla or a ball of clay or pressing pizza dough into a pan. This is called *tissue displacement.*

Compression can disconnect from the body with each lift and reconnect with each press in a piston-like fashion. Pressing tissue against the underlying hard bone spreads the tissue mechanically, enhancing the softening effect on the connective tissue component of the muscle. Compression is applied at 90 degree angle and adds depth of pressure to take all the slack out of the tissue (the barrier) to produce bind (a sense of resistance). Then the angle changes to push or pull at a 45-degree angle without slipping to produce a drag (tension force) on the tissue that affects the connective tissue.

Compression applied to the belly of a muscle spreads the spindle cells, causing the muscle to sense that it is stretching. To protect the muscle from overstretching, the spindle cells signal the muscle to contract. The press-lift application stimulates the muscle and nerve tissues. The combination of these two effects makes compression a good method for stimulating muscles and the nervous system. Because of this stimulation, compression is a little less desirable for a relaxation or soothing massage. If the client wants to be alert and energized, a stimulating massage using compression can be done.

A muscle must contract or at least have the nerve "fire" (as occurs in a contraction) before it can relax. This is due to the threshold stimulation pattern of the nerve and its effects on muscle tone. Nerves build up the energy needed to stimulate the nerve impulse. The automatic response of muscle fibers to contraction is a period of relaxation called the *refractory period.* Sometimes the signals are enough to get everything ready to fire, but they are not strong enough to actually cause the contraction of the muscle fibers or discharge of the nerve. If stimulation of the nerves can be increased just enough to prompt the nerve to discharge, the muscle contracts and can reset to a normal resting length. Applying compression to the belly of the muscle, and the resultant effect on the spindle cells, elicits this response. Any sustained, repetitive use of a stimulation method that causes muscle fibers to maintain a contraction or to contract repeatedly eventually fatigues the muscle fibers. Compression used in this manner initiates a relaxation response in muscles.

Compression is an excellent method for enhancing circulation. The pressure against the capillary beds changes the pressure inside the vessels and encourages fluid exchange. Compression appropriately applied to arteries allows back pressure to build, and release of the compression encourages increased arterial flow. This manipulation can be done over the clothing or without lubricant.

Very specific, pinpoint compression is called *direct pressure* or *ischemic compression* and is used on acupressure points and trigger points.

Applying Compression

Compression can be applied with stabilized fingers, the palm and heel of the hand, the fist, the knuckles, the forearm and, in some systems, the knee and heel of the foot (Figure 10-15). *Do not use the thumb to apply compression.* Compression is applied perpendicular to the tissue (i.e., 90 degrees). Usually it is applied against the contours (hills) of the body that are oriented at around 45 degrees.

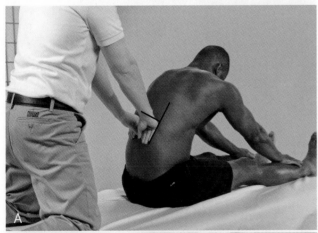
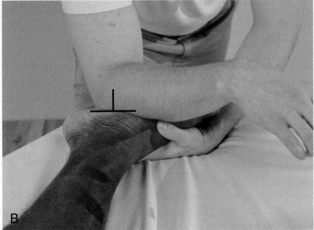

FIGURE 10-15 Two examples of compression.

When using your palm to apply compression, avoid hyperextending or hyperflexing your wrist by keeping the application hand in front of rather than directly under your shoulder. Even though the compressive pressure is perpendicular to the tissue, the position of the forearm in relation to the wrist is about 120 to 130 degrees. Application against a 45-degree angle of the body plus the 45-degree angle of the practitioner's hand and forearm results in the 90-degree contact on the tissue (remember from Chapter 8 to lean uphill). If you are using your knuckles or fist, make sure the forearm is in a direct line with the wrist. Remember: do not use your thumb to apply compression, because the thumb structures can be damaged on large muscle masses.

The tip and the radioulnar side of the elbow should not be used to apply compression. Because the ulnar nerve passes just under the skin and damage can result from extensive compression, use the forearm near the elbow for compression. The massage professional's arm and hand must be relaxed, or neck and shoulder tension develop. Leverage applied through appropriate body mechanics does the work, not muscle strength. Compression also can be applied with the practitioner's leg and foot.

The depth of compression is determined by what is to be accomplished, where compression is to be applied, and how broad or specific the contact is with the client's body. Deep compression presses tissue against the underlying bone. Because of the diagonal pattern of the muscles, the massage practitioner should stay perpendicular to the bone, with actual compression somewhere between a 60- and 90-degree angle to the body. Beyond those angles, the stroke may slip and turn into a glide.

Compression can replace gliding if gliding strokes cannot or should not be used, such as in areas of excessive body hair, areas where a person is ticklish, and areas where the skin is sensitive to lubricant. Compression bypasses the tickle response by activating deep touch receptors. Also, compression does not slip or roll on the tissue (Proficiency Exercise 10-4).

PROFICIENCY EXERCISE 10-4

1. Inflate a series of balloons with different internal pressures. Fill some with water and others with gelatin and use these to represent the density and pliability of different tissue types. Balloons are great for practicing the angle and pressure of the manipulation. The best angle allows good, firm compression into the balloon without it slipping out from under you.
2. Use pieces of foam of various densities and place them over objects of different sizes and shapes. Determine how much pressure it takes to feel each object. Pay attention to the difference between the low-density foam and the high-density foam.
3. Design a complete massage using only compression. Pay very close attention to ways in which you can use compression techniques to access the client's body successfully. Adjust depth of pressure, speed, rhythm, frequency, and duration and observe the different physiologic effects. Have a client lie on a mat and experiment with using your leg and foot to apply compression.

Oscillation

Attempts to clarify massage terminology cluster vibration, shaking, and rocking under the umbrella term *oscillation*. Oscillation is any effect that varies in a back-and-forth, or reciprocating, manner. The term *vibration* sometimes is used more narrowly to mean a mechanical oscillation.

Very simply, oscillation involves action in the form of springs and swings. In terms of springs, it is logical to include massage methods that bounce off the tissue (later called *percussion*), just as beating a drum creates oscillation. The concept of swings can be related to any massage method that moves the body. Vibration is an action of moving back and forth very rapidly; shaking is moving back and forth but is much bigger than vibration; and rocking is a rhythmic, swinging motion.

Vibration

Edgar Cyriax (1938), one of the foremost authorities on massage and manual techniques, describes vibration as follows:

Almost every author who attempts to describe the modus operandi for generating these vibrations prefaces his remarks by stating that they are extremely tiring to produce. Vibration is generated by means of the operator tensing all the muscles of his or her arm (some even include the muscles of the shoulder) into a state of powerful complete tetanus. This method is very fatiguing; no one can sustain such a contraction evenly for more than a minute or so. The correct technique for production of manual vibrations is to set up a small amount of alternating contraction and relaxation in some of the muscles of the forearm, those of the upper arm and the shoulder being kept quite passive (unless required for fixation purposes).

Vibration is very powerful if it can be done long enough and at an intensity sufficient to produce reflexive physiologic effects. The massage practitioner can use manual vibration to stimulate muscles by applying the technique at the muscle tendons for up to 30 seconds. When this is complete, the antagonist muscle pattern relaxes through neurologic reciprocal inhibition.

Vibration also can be used to break up the monotony of the massage. If the same methods are used repeatedly, the body adapts and does not respond as well to the sensation or stimulation. Because vibration is used to "wake up" nerves, it is a good method for stimulating nerve activity. The nerves of the muscles around a joint also innervate the joint itself. Muscle pain often is interpreted by the client as joint pain and vice versa. Used specifically and purposefully, vibration is a great massage manipulation to confuse and shift the muscle-joint pain perception.

Applying Vibration

All vibration begins with compression. After the depth of pressure has been achieved, the hand needs to tremble and transmit the action to the surrounding tissues. As described by Cyriax, the muscles above the elbow should be relaxed; the action comes only from the alternating contraction and relaxation of the forearm muscles (Figure 10-16) (Cyriax, 1938).

To start with coarse vibration, place one hand on the client and compress lightly. Begin moving the hand back and forth

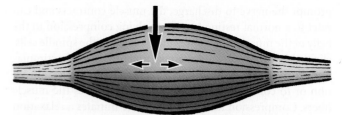

FIGURE 10-16 The focus of vibration is downward and back and forth in a fast, oscillating manner.

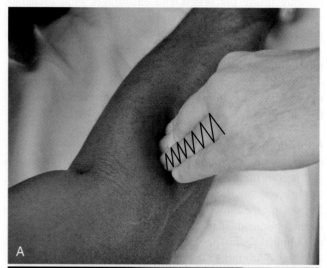

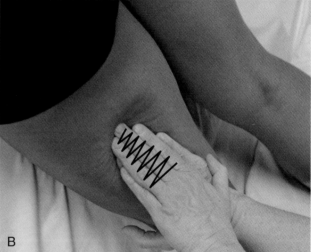

FIGURE 10-17 Two examples of vibration.

using only the forearm muscles and limiting the motion to about 2 inches of space. Gradually quicken the back-and-forth movement, checking to make sure your upper arm stays relaxed. Next, make the back-and-forth movement smaller until the hand does not move at all on the tissue but is trembling at a high intensity. This is vibration.

Because considerable energy is needed to perform this manipulation, it should be used sparingly and only for short periods. A forearm gliding method should be used after vibration, because the gliding action essentially massages and relaxes the practitioner's arm, protecting it from repetitive use problems (Figure 10-17).

💡 PROFICIENCY EXERCISE 10-5

The first two exercises to teach vibration were developed by a professional magician who is also a massage practitioner and instructor. Many sleight-of-hand movements required for his illusions use the same movements as vibration. Perfecting these two balloon exercises will enhance your vibration skills.

1. Get a clear, 5-inch balloon. Put a penny inside it and then inflate and tie the balloon. Grasp the tied end of the balloon, cupping it in the palm of your hand. Using wrist action only, circle the balloon until the penny begins to roll inside. Once you can do this, make the wrist circles smaller and smaller while continuing to roll the penny in the balloon. Eventually the action will be the movement required for vibration.

2. Use the same balloon and put the fattest part in the palm of your hand. Place your other hand on top of the balloon. Using just the bottom hand, use a coarse vibration to get the penny to jump and dance in the balloon. Once you can do this, make the movements smaller and smaller until you can make the penny dance with fine vibration movements.

3. Combine all the methods presented so far into a massage. Incorporate vibration at each tendon, paying attention to the results as the muscles contract or tense slightly in response to the stimulation.

Some professionals use mechanical vibrators to replace manual vibration. This is acceptable as long as the practice is allowed by licensing regulations, the equipment is safe, and the client approves its use (Proficiency Exercise 10-5).

Shaking

Shaking is effective for relaxing muscle groups or an entire limb. Shaking manipulations confuse the positional proprioceptors, because the sensory input is too disorganized for the brain's integrating systems to interpret; muscle relaxation is the natural response in such situations.

Shaking warms and prepares the body for deeper body-work and addresses the joints in a nonspecific manner. It is effective when the muscles seem extremely tight. Shaking has a reflexive effect, but a small mechanical influence also may be exerted on the connective tissue because of the lift-and-pull component of the method.

Shaking sometimes is classified as a form of vibration; however, the application is very different, because vibration begins with compression and shaking begins with lifting.

Applying Shaking

Shaking begins with a lift-and-pull technique. Either a muscle group or a limb is grasped, lifted, and shaken. To begin to understand shaking, think of a dog shaking water from its coat, a person shaking out a rug or blanket, a dog or cat tugging on a toy, or a horse swishing its tail.

For massage purposes, the focus of shaking is more specific and less intense than shaking a rug, but the idea is the same. It involves a lift and then a fairly abrupt downward or side-to-side movement that ends suddenly, as if something is being thrown off. Even the most subtle shaking movements deliberately move the joint or muscle tissue with the intention of a "snap" at the end of the movement.

Shaking should not be used on the skin or superficial fascia, nor is it effective for use on the entire body. Rather, it is best applied to any large muscle groups that can be grasped and to the synovial joints of the limbs. Good areas for shaking are the upper trapezius and shoulder area, biceps and triceps groups, hamstrings, quadriceps, gastrocnemius and, in some instances, the abdominals and the pectoralis muscles close to the axilla. The joints of the shoulders, hips, and extremities also respond well to shaking.

The larger the muscle or joint, the more intense the method. If the movements are performed with all the slack out of the tissue, the focal point of the shaking is very small and the technique is extremely effective. The more purposeful the approach, the smaller the focus of the shaking. The practitioner should always stay within the limits of both joint range of motion and the elastic give of the tissue. The goal is to see how small the shaking action can be and still achieve the desired physiologic effect. To accomplish this, first lift the tissue or limb, grasp it, and then lean back gently until the tissue becomes taut. Begin the shaking movement from this position (Figure 10-18).

Rocking

Rocking is a soothing, rhythmic method used to calm people. It has both reflexive and chemical effects (Figure 10-19).

Rocking also works through the vestibular system of the inner ear and feeds sensory input directly into the cerebellum. Other reflex mechanisms probably are also affected. For these reasons, rocking is one of the most productive massage methods for achieving entrainment. For rocking to be most effective, the client's body must move so that the fluid in the semicircular canals of the inner ear is affected, initiating parasympathetic mechanisms.

Applying Rocking

Rocking is rhythmic and should be applied with a deliberate, full-body movement. Rocking involves the up-and-down and side-to-side movement of shaking, but no flick or throw-off snap occurs at the end of the movement. The action moves the body as far as it will go, then allows it to return to the original position.

After two or three rocks, the practitioner can sense the client's rhythm. This attunement to the client's rhythm is a powerful point of interface point for synchronizing entrainment. The massage practitioner works within the rhythm to maintain and amplify it by attempting to gently extend the limits of movement or by slowing the rhythm. Incorporation of a rocking movement that supports this entrainment process into all massage applications effectively individualizes the application and speed of the method. The client seems to relax more easily when a subtle rocking movement, matching his or her innate rhythm pattern, is incorporated as part of the generalized massage approach, along with such techniques as gliding, kneading, compression, and joint movement, especially passive movements. The body mechanics described in this text tend to produce a rocking motion.

With a tense, anxious client who initially may resist rocking, begin the process with slightly bigger and more abrupt shaking

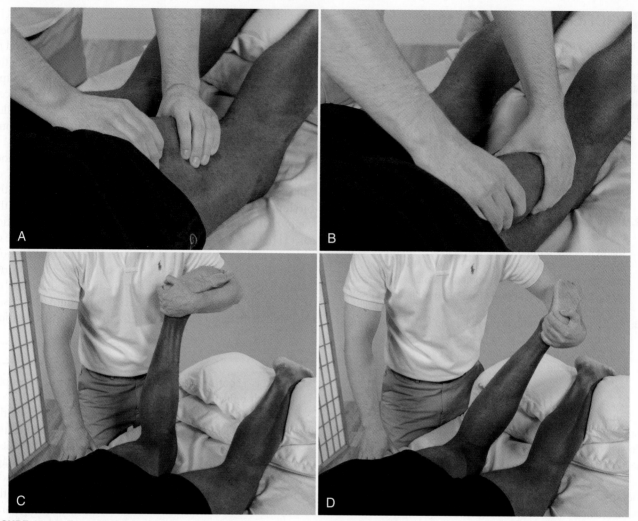

FIGURE 10-18 Examples of shaking. **A** and **B,** Shaking tissue. **C** and **D,** Shaking a limb.

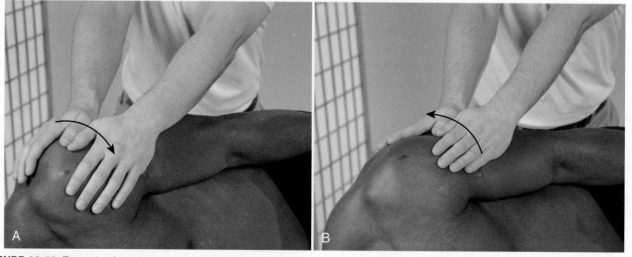

FIGURE 10-19 Example of rocking.

manipulations. As the muscles begin to relax, switch to rocking methods.

During rocking, nothing is abrupt; the methods have an even ebb and flow. All movement is flowing, like a wind chime in a gentle breeze or a porch swing on a hot summer night. Rocking is one of the most effective relaxation techniques the massage practitioner can use. Many parasympathetic responses are elicited by the rocking of the body during gliding, kneading, and compression (Proficiency Exercise 10-6).

💡 PROFICIENCY EXERCISE 10-6

1. Lay a sheet on your massage table or other flat surface. Lift one end and practice shaking the sheet to achieve a wavelike motion from one end of the sheet to the other. Practice directing the ripple to various locations on the table.
2. Swing in a playground swing, using your legs to pump yourself. This exercise gives the full-body effect of the shake. Pay close attention to the feeling as you reach the top of the swing and begin to head back.
3. Using your own body for practice, systematically shake each joint, lying down to do the legs. See how small you can make the movement and still feel the effects. Grab the muscles of your arm and leg. Lift and shake the tissue, paying attention to the sensations.
4. Sit in an old-fashioned rocking chair and let the chair rock you. See what happens when you rock the chair. Vary the speed to go faster and slower than the chair's movement. Put the chair on different surfaces, such as carpet, hard floor, sand, and grass. Again, let the chair rock you and notice the difference. Remember, each person has an individual rhythm that needs to be identified, supported, and respected.
5. Play a variety of relaxing music. Pick up the sway of the music and rock with it. Repeat the exercise with different beats of music.
6. Design an entire massage using a combination of shaking and rocking. Be aware of all the qualities of touch during the application.

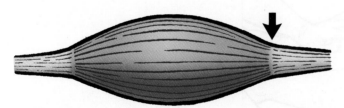

FIGURE 10-20 The focus of percussion (tapotement) is a vertical, abrupt downward snapping.

Percussion (Tapotement)

Percussion (tapotement) moves up and down on the tissue. The term *tapotement* comes from the French verb *tapoter,* which means "to rap, smack, drum, or pat." In percussion techniques, the hands or parts of the hand administer springy blows to the body at a fast rate. The blows are directed downward, creating rhythmic compression of the tissue (Figure 10-20).

Percussion is characterized as light or heavy. In light percussion, the compressive force of the blows penetrates only to the superficial tissue of the skin and subcutaneous layers; in heavy percussion, the force penetrates deeper into the muscles, tendons, and visceral (organ) structures, such as the pleura in the chest cavity.

Percussion is a stimulating technique that operates through the response of the nerves. Because of its intense stimulating effect on the nervous system, it initiates or enhances sympathetic activity of the autonomic nervous system. The effects of the manipulations are reflexive. However, percussion also can have mechanical results, which involve loosening and moving mucus in the chest. People with cystic fibrosis are treated with percussion, but massage therapy of this type is beyond the beginning skill levels of the massage practitioner.

The most noticeable effect of percussion results from the response of the tendon reflexes. A quick blow to the tendon stretches it. In response, protective muscle contraction occurs. To obtain the best result, stretch the tendon first. The most common example of this reflexive mechanism is the knee-jerk (or patellar) reflex, but this response happens in all tendons to some degree. This is very helpful when the massage practitioner is preparing the muscles for lengthening, such as when a client indicates that the hamstrings are tight and need to be lengthened. With the client supine, the hip flexed to 90 degrees, and the knee flexed to 90 degrees, percussion on the stretched quadriceps tendon causes the quadriceps to contract. As a result, the hamstrings are inhibited, which makes them easier to lengthen to a more normal resting length.

When applied to the joints, percussion affects the joint kinesthetic receptors responsible for determining the position and movement of the body. The quick blows confuse the system, similar to the effect of joint-focused rocking and shaking, but the body muscles are stimulated rather than inhibited. This method is useful for stimulating weak muscles. The force used must move the joint but should not be strong enough to damage it. For example, a single finger may be used to administer percussion over the carpal joints, whereas the fist may be used over the sacroiliac joint.

Percussion is very effective when used at motor points that usually are located in the same area as the traditional acupuncture points. The repetitive stimulation causes the nerve to fire repeatedly, stimulating the nerve tract.

Percussion focused primarily on the skin affects the superficial blood vessels of the skin, initially causing them to contract. Heavy percussion or prolonged lighter application dilates the vessels by causing the release of histamine, a vasodilator.

Applying Percussion

Two hands usually are used alternately to do percussion. One or two fingers can be used to tap a motor point located at the center of the muscle mass where the motor nerve enters the muscle (this sometimes is called *neurotapping*). The forearm muscles contract and relax in rapid succession to move the elbow joint into flexion and then allow it to release quickly. This action travels down to the relaxed wrist, extending it; the wrist then moves back and forth to provide the action of the percussion. Percussion is a controlled flailing of the arms as the wrists snap back and forth. Remember that the wrist must always stay relaxed. Beginning students usually want to use the wrists to provide the snap action. This is especially tempting when using small movements of the fingers; however, it will damage the wrist (Figure 10-21).

Heavy percussion should not be done in the kidney area or anywhere pain or discomfort is present. The following are methods of percussion.

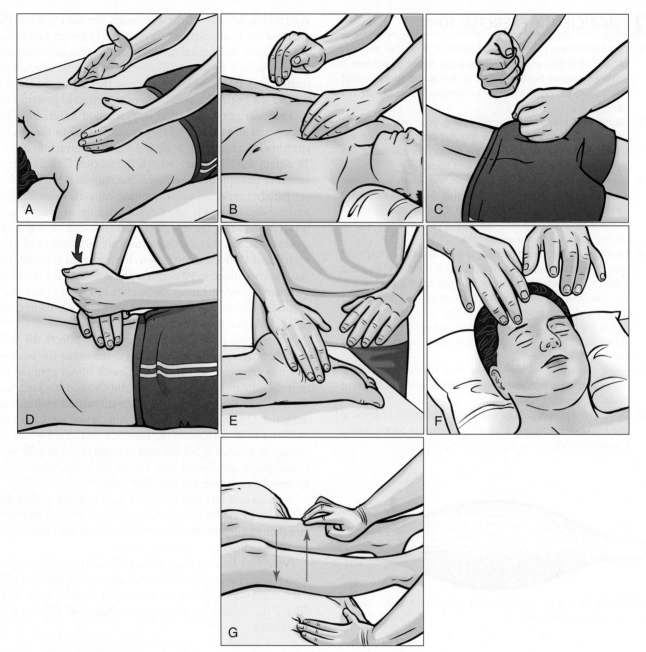

FIGURE 10-21 Examples of percussion. **A,** Hacking. **B,** Cupping. **C,** Fist beating. **D,** Beating over the palm. **E,** Slapping. **F,** Finger tapping. **G,** Finger tapping to stimulate acupuncture point.

- *Hacking.* Hacking is applied with both wrists relaxed and the fingers spread, with only the little finger or the ulnar side of the hand striking the skin surface. The other fingers hit each other with a springy touch. Point hacking can be done by using the fingertips in the same way. Hacking is done with the whole hand on the larger soft tissue areas, such as the upper back and shoulders. Point hacking is used on smaller areas, such as the individual tendons of the toes, or over motor points (Figure 10-21, *A*).
- *Cupping.* To perform cupping, the fingers and thumbs are positioned as if making a cup. The hands are turned over, and the same action used in hacking is performed. When done on the anterior and posterior thorax, cupping is

good for stimulating the respiratory system and for loosening mucus. If the client exhales and makes a monotone noise during cupping, enough pressure is used so that the tone begins to break up, changing from "AAAAAAAAAAAAHHHHHH" to "AH AH AH AH AH AH" (Figure 10-21, *B*).
- *Beating* and *pounding.* These moves can be performed with a soft fist with the knuckles down or with the fist held vertically and the action performed with the ulnar side of the palm. This technique is used over large muscles, such as the buttocks and heavy leg muscles (Figure 10-21, *C* and *D*).
- *Slapping (splatting).* For this technique, the whole palm of a flattened hand makes contact with the body. This is

a good method for causing the release of histamine, thereby increasing vasodilation and its effects on the skin. It also is a good method to use on the bottoms of the feet. The broad contact of the whole hand disperses the force laterally instead of downward, and the effects remain in the superficial tissue. Kellogg (2010) called this movement *splatting* (Figure 10-21, *E*).

- *Tapping.* For this technique, the palmar surface of the fingers alternately taps the body area with light to medium pressure. This is a good method to use around the joints, on the tendons, on the face and head, and along the spine (Figure 10-21, *F,G*) (Proficiency Exercise 10-7).

Friction

One method of friction, formalized by James Cyriax, consists of small, deep movements performed on a local area; this provides shear force to the tissue. This method uses deep transverse friction massage without the application of lubricant. The skin moves with the fingers (Figure 10-22). Friction burns may occur on the client if the fingers are allowed to slide back and forth over the client's skin or if friction is used excessively.

Friction manipulation prevents and breaks up local adhesions in connective tissue, especially over tendons, ligaments, and scars, by creating therapeutic inflammation. This method is not used over an acute injury or fresh scars. Modified use of friction, after the scar has stabilized or the acute phase has passed, may prevent adhesions and can promote a more normal healing process.

💡 PROFICIENCY EXERCISE 10-7

1. Play a drum or watch a drummer. Pay attention to the action of the arms and wrists and the grasp of the drumsticks. Notice that the drummer holds the drumsticks loosely.
2. Get a paddleball or yo-yo and see what actions it takes to make these toys work. Play with a rattle or tambourine.
3. Use the foam from the compression exercises and practice the different methods and intensity of percussion (light to deep, slow to fast).
4. While shaking your hands very quickly, use hacking to strike the foam or a practice client. Without stopping, change hand positions so that all the methods are used.
5. Design a stimulating massage with various applications of percussion. Notice which qualities of touch are most reflected with these methods.

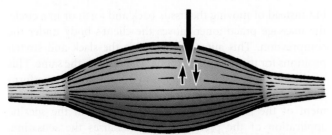

FIGURE 10-22 The focus of friction is a vertical downward pressure that is applied with a back-and-forth movement to underlying tissues.

The Cyriax application also reduces pain through the mechanisms of counterirritation and hyperstimulation analgesia. In many older textbooks, friction is explained as a back-and-forth, brisk movement focused on the skin and subcutaneous tissue to promote dilation of the vessels in the skin. Historical literature on massage indicates that friction burns were created deliberately to produce long-term stimulation of the nerve. This method of counterirritation is seldom used today.

Connective tissue has a high water content. To remain pliable, it must remain hydrated. Friction techniques may increase the water-binding capacity of the connective tissue ground substance.

The movement in friction usually is transverse to the fiber direction. Friction generally is performed for 30 seconds to 10 minutes (although some authorities have suggested a duration of 20 minutes). This type of friction initiates therapeutic inflammation. The chemicals released during inflammation result in activation of tissue repair mechanisms, with reorganization of the connective tissue. This type of work can be coupled with other proper rehabilitation techniques to aid injury healing. Because of its specific nature and direct focus on rehabilitation, deep transverse friction is not suitable for the entry-level massage practitioner. (The method is discussed in greater detail in Chapter 12.)

A modified application of friction that is used to keep high-concentration areas of connective tissue soft and pliable is appropriate for the beginner. The modified application is essentially the same as deep transverse friction in that the focus is transverse to the muscle fiber direction and moves the tissue beneath the skin; however, the duration and specificity are reduced. The direction can be transverse or circular, pinpointed or more generalized, but the tissue under the skin is still affected.

Friction is a mechanical approach best applied to areas of high concentrations of connective tissue, such as the musculotendinous junction. Microtrauma from repetitive movement and overstretching are common in this area. Microtrauma predisposes the musculotendinous junction to inflammatory problems, connective tissue changes, and adhesions. Friction is a good way to keep this tissue healthy. Experts disagree on the need to stretch an area that is to receive friction. Because both the stretching and not stretching approaches have merit, both should be included when frictioning.

Friction also can be combined with compression, a combination that adds a small stretch component. The movement includes no slide. This application has mechanical, chemical, and reflexive effects and is the most common approach used today for applying friction.

Applying Friction

When friction is used, the main focus is to move tissue under the skin. No lubricant is used, because the tissues must not slide. The area to be frictioned should be placed in a soft or slack position. The movement is produced by beginning with a specific and moderate to deep compression using the fingers, palm, or flat part of the forearm near the elbow. After the pressure required to contact the tissue has been reached, the

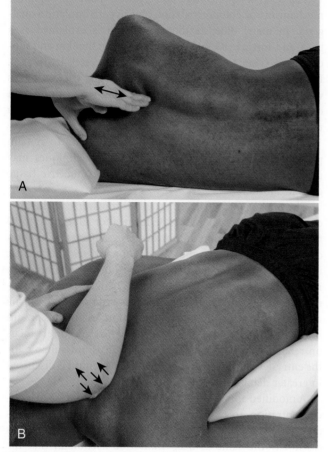

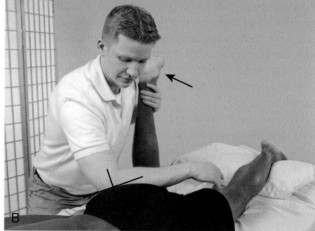

FIGURE 10-23 Two examples of friction.

FIGURE 10-24 Compression + Movement = Friction.

upper tissue is moved back and forth across the grain or fiber of the undertissue for transverse or cross-fiber friction or around in a circle for circular friction (Figure 10-23).

As the tissue responds to the friction, gradually begin to stretch the area and increase the pressure. The feeling may be intense for the client; if it is painful, the application should be modified to a tolerable level so that the client reports the sensation as a "good hurt." The recommended way to work within the client's comfort zone is to use the level of pressure at which the person feels the specific area but does not complain of pain. Friction should be continued until the sensation diminishes. Gradually increase the pressure until the client again feels the specific area. Begin friction again and repeat the sequence for up to 10 minutes.

The area being frictioned may be tender to the touch for 48 hours after use of the technique. The sensation should be similar to a mild postexercise soreness. Because the focus of friction is the controlled application of a small inflammatory response, heat and redness are caused by the release of histamine. Also, increased circulation results in a small amount of puffiness as more water binds with the connective tissue. The area should not bruise.

Another effective way to produce friction is a combination of compression and passive joint movement, with the bone under the compression used to perform the friction (Figure 10-24). The process begins with compression as just described,

but instead of moving the tissue back and forth or in a circle, the massage practitioner moves the client's body under the compression. This automatically adds the slack and stretch positions for the friction methods. The result is the same. This method is much easier for the massage professional to perform and also may be more comfortable for the client. The movement of the joint provides a distraction from the specific application of the pressure and generalizes the sensation. Broad general methods can be used with a higher degree of intensity than a pinpointed specific focus (Box 10-3) (Proficiency Exercise 10-8).

| Box 10-3 | Sequence of a Basic Massage |

Four initial methods are used on each part of the body:
1. Gliding
2. Kneading
3. Compression
4. Oscillation or percussion, depending on the body area

These four methods form the basis of therapeutic massage. Once mastered, they become the foundation for palpation assessment. Each method, whether used alone or in combination with therapeutic intervention methods, can be adjusted to create reflexive or mechanical change in the body.

Basic Sequence

The following basic sequence is performed on each body area.
1. Gliding: Use four strokes to cover the area. The first stroke is light and superficial. The second stroke is slower and deeper and moves the skin. The third stroke is progressively slower and deeper to access muscle layers. The fourth stroke is superficial again.
2. Kneading: Cover the area three times, with each application becoming slower and lifting more tissue. Make sure to use a broad base and do not pinch. Identify areas where compression plus movement is better than kneading.
3. Compression: Cover the area three times, with each application becoming slower and deeper. Use a broad base of the whole hand, double hand, forearm, or leg. To replace kneading, compress tissue away from bone and have the client move the joint below (distal to) the pressure. Move the joint back and forth or in small circles.
4. Oscillation or percussion: Apply the appropriate method to the area for about 30 to 60 seconds.
5. Repeat gliding (step 1).

Appropriate sanitation, draping, and body mechanics are used consistently.

The following example protocol is one way to approach a massage sequence. The protocol is a combination of the positioning and applications described in the chapter text. Address each area using the glide—knead—compression—oscillation or percussion—glide sequence, unless an alteration is noted. Use this written protocol along with the photographic illustrations and the example on the DVD that accompanies this book. Additional examples of massage application are available on the Evolve website.

Example Protocol

Client lies on stomach (prone).
- Use bolster under ankles (possibly also under abdomen)
- Right side back from top of gluteus to top of shoulder blade
- Left side back from top of gluteus to top of shoulder blade
- Left and right side glutes with the applications

Turn client on left side.
- Use bolster as needed
- Right upper arm
- Right lower arm
- Hand
- Left upper arm
- Left lower arm
- Hand
- Right upper shoulder
- Right side of the neck
- Right side of the head

Move to legs.
- Left inner thigh
- Left calf
- Left foot
- Right outer thigh
- Right calf
- Right foot

Turn client on right side.
- Use bolster as needed
- Left upper arm
- Left lower arm
- Hand
- Right upper arm
- Right lower arm
- Hand
- Left upper shoulder
- Left side of the neck
- Left side of the head

Move to legs.
- Right inner thigh
- Right calf
- Right foot
- Left outer thigh
- Left calf
- Left foot

Turn client on back (supine).
- Use bolster under knees and head.
- Left upper thigh
- Right upper thigh
- Abdomen
- Left chest
- Right chest

Wash or sanitize hands.
- Face
- Have client move to a seated position (you may have to assist some clients).
- Bilateral upper shoulders

Also see the General Protocol on p. 357.

MASSAGE TECHNIQUES USING JOINT MOVEMENT

SECTION OBJECTIVES

Chapter objective covered in this section:
3. The student will be able to incorporate movement of the joints as an aspect of massage application.

Using the information presented in this section, the student will be able to perform the following:

- Use movement in a purposeful way to create a specific physiologic response
- Explain the proprioceptive mechanisms and their importance in the physiologic effects of massage techniques
- Move the synovial joints through the client's physiologic range of motion using both active and passive joint movement

The purpose of an active movement is to convey to and concentrate upon a selected point, the nutrition and energies of the system. Such a movement may accomplish a twofold purpose, that of supplying a part and of relieving another part more or less distant.

The mode of effecting this purpose is as follows: the person to receive the application is placed in an easy, unconstrained position, sitting, lying, half lying, kneeling, or in a convenient position that will suitably adjust all parts of the body to the purpose. The body is fixed either by the hands of an assistant or by means of an apparatus so as to prevent as much as possible any motion of all parts of the body, except the acting part. The patient is in some cases directed to move the free part in a particular direction, the effort to do so is resisted by the operator, with a force proportionate to the exertion made very nicely graduated to the particular condition of the part and of the system at large. The resistance is not uniform, but varies according to the varying action of muscles, as perceived by the operator. In other cases the operator acts while the patient resists. The action is the same, but in one case the patient's acting muscles are shortened and in the other lengthened. The operation is a wrestle, in which a very limited portion of the organism is engaged. The motion must be much slower than the natural movement of the part engaged, which fact strongly fixes the attention and concentrates the will. The act is repeated two or three times with all the care and precision the operator can command, being cautious not to induce fatigue.

George H. Taylor, *An Illustrated Sketch of the Movement Cure*, 1866

The use of movement as described in the next section follows Taylor's guidelines and recommendations, which were his interpretations of Ling's gymnastics, or active movements (Box 10-4). The principles of massage today are built on the principles described in the historical literature. The names may be different and the physiologic explanations more precise, but the methods are the same.

The efficient use of movement techniques reduces the need for repetitive massage manipulations. If these techniques are used well, the neuromuscular mechanism can be activated and influenced quickly, with less physical effort by the massage professional.

It is important to distinguish between the soft tissue manipulations of the massage professional and the joint manipulations of the chiropractor, osteopath, or physical therapist. The massage professional does not perform specific, direct joint manipulations. The massage techniques presented in this text incorporate passive and active joint movement, as well as lengthening and stretching methods, within the comfortable limits of the joint. These methods may indirectly affect the range of motion of a joint through changes in the soft tissue. The particular focus of the massage professional is the soft tissue, not the osseous structure of the joint.

Often a combination of soft tissue work and specific joint manipulation is required to achieve the functional goals of the client. In these instances the massage practitioner, with appropriate training, becomes part of the multidisciplinary team under the supervision of the health care professional. This team approach provides the skills and expertise of multiple professionals to best serve the client.

Physiologic Influences

The passive and active joint movement and muscle energy techniques presented in this chapter work with the neuromuscular reflex system to lengthen short muscles. In contrast, stretching has both a reflexive and a mechanical aspect. The reflexive component of stretching is an initial neuromuscular lengthening phase used to prepare the area for the more mechanical stretching effect of elongating connective tissue. (Stretching is discussed in greater detail on p. 345)

A working knowledge of the proprioceptive interaction between the prime mover (muscle shortening) and the antagonist (muscle elongating), as well as body-wide reflex patterns, is necessary to understand and implement massage techniques. With this knowledge, the massage practitioner can choose methods that encourage a reset to a more normal or neutral muscular function state, which allows the optimum range of functioning. The neuromuscular mechanism (nerve muscle unit) makes adjustments based on the information it receives. If the information is clear and accurate, the muscles operate as designed; if the information is unclear, incorrect, or inconsistent, imbalances can occur.

For example, if a client spends the day talking on the phone by holding the phone with the shoulder, the lateral neck flexors and shoulder elevators are in constant contraction (tight, short, concentric contraction), whereas the other side of the neck is in constant extension (taut, long, eccentric). An adaptation takes place, and when the neck muscles are used, painful resistance occurs to any use other than that allowed by the new reset position. This type of interaction is responsible for most muscle discomfort or reduced functioning.

Muscle imbalances result because the body adapts to a different muscle spindle set point and a new muscle resting length (usually shortened). Massage techniques can provide clearer neurologic information so that the body can restore optimum function or as close to optimum as possible. This

---

Box 10-4	Taylor's Principles for the Application of Movement and Techniques

1. Be specific.
2. Be mindful of patterns of "too much" and "not enough."
3. Position the client purposefully.
4. Stabilize the body so that only the focused target area is affected.
5. You may move the area (client passive) or may cooperate in the effort with the client (client active).
6. Make sure the force and exertion are gradual and vary with the demand.
7. Remember that the purpose is to lengthen shortened tissue and stimulate weakened muscles.
8. You enable the lengthening or stimulation process by assisting the client.
9. Make sure the application is slow and purposeful.
10. Repeat the movement two or three times but not to fatigue.

allows the body's homeostatic mechanism to restore neutral muscle positions.

All the massage manipulations described previously affect proprioception reflexively but usually have a general, nonspecific effect. In this section you will learn ways to deliver accurate, specific information to the neuromuscular system that supports normal functioning. The difference is similar to providing a general announcement to a group of people (massage techniques) and calling out individuals' names and delivering a message (movement techniques).

Joint Movement and Range of Motion

Range of motion (ROM) is the angle through which a joint moves from the anatomic position to the ends of its motion in a particular direction. It is measured in degrees. Each joint has a normal range of motion. Assessment methods that move a joint can determine whether a joint is able to move within a normal range of motion. If the joint moves less than the normal range or more than the normal range, a problem may exist.

The range or amount of movement at a joint is determined by a number of factors: (1) the shape of the bones that form the joint, (2) the tautness or laxity of the ligament and capsule structure of the joint, (3) the length of the soft tissue structure that supports and moves the joint, and (4) whether the joint moves independently of other joints (open chain) or is linked to other joints in a combined movement (closed chain). Technically, ROM is a function or finding. Joint movement is an action and therefore can be a method.

To understand **joint movement,** you must first understand the structure and function of joints. A simplified review is presented here; anatomy and physiology resources can provide further clarification and descriptions of individual joints and are a valuable learning aid.

How Joints Work

Joints allow us to move. Joint position and velocity (movement) receptors inform the central nervous system where and how the body is positioned in gravity and how fast it is moving. These sensory data are the major determining factors for muscle motor tone patterns.

Joint movement techniques focus on the *synovial,* or freely movable, joints in the body (see Chapter 4). To a lesser extent the joints of the vertebral column, hand, and foot also are considered, as are other joints, such as the facet joints of the ribs, the sacroiliac joint, and the sternoclavicular joint. These joints are not directly influenced by muscles, but rather move through indirect muscle action.

We can control some joint movements voluntarily; we can move our limbs through various motions, such as flexion, extension, abduction, adduction, and rotation. These are referred to as *physiologic movements,* or **osteokinematic movements.** For normal physiologic movement, other types of movements (*accessory movements,* or **arthrokinematic movements**) must occur as a result of the inherent laxity, or **joint play,** that exists in each joint. This laxity allows the ends of the bones to slide, roll, or spin smoothly on each other

inside the joint capsule. These essential movements occur during movement of the joint and are not under voluntary control.

Comparing a Joint to a Door Hinge

A good example of joint motion is found on a door. The hinge holds the door both to the casing and away from the casing. For the door to open and close efficiently (*osteokinematic movement),* the space between the door and the door casing must be maintained and the fit must be correct. If the fit of the door in the door casing is incorrect or if the space is not maintained, the door will not open and close correctly. In the body, ligaments act as the hinges.

The door hinge must be oiled. In the joint, the synovial membrane secretes synovial fluid, produced on demand by joint movement. If a joint does not move or is not moved, it will lock up like a rusty door hinge, and movement will be restricted or lost.

If you look closely at a door hinge, you will notice the space around the pin in the hinge. If you move the hinge back and forth (not swing the door), the hinge and pin mechanism moves a little (*arthrokinematic movement).* This little movement can be likened to joint play. If the ligaments and connective tissue that make up the joint capsule are not firm enough to maintain joint space, the joint play is lost. If the capsule is too tight, joint play also is lost. Muscles around a joint can shorten, pulling the bone ends together and affecting joint play.

If the ligaments and joint capsule are not pliable, flexibility is lost. If the ligaments and joint capsule do not support the joint, the fit is disrupted. Muscle contraction may pull the joint out of alignment. Muscle groups that flex and adduct the joints are about 30% stronger and have more mass than the extensors and abductors. If the body uses muscle contraction to stabilize a joint, the uneven pull between flexors and extensors and adductors and abductors disturbs the fit of the bones at the joint.

Limitations on the Ability to Move a Joint

Joints have various degrees of range of motion. Anatomic, physiologic, and pathologic barriers to motion exist. A barrier is a point of resistance and can feel hard, such as when bone contacts bone or during binding, when soft tissue is short.

Anatomic barriers are determined by the shape and fit of the bones at the joint. The anatomic barrier is seldom reached, because the possibility of injury is greatest in this position. Instead, the body protects the joint by establishing physiologic barriers. **Physiologic barriers** are the result of the limits in range of motion imposed by protective nerve and sensory function to support optimum function. The sensation at the barrier is soft and pliable. An adaptation in a physiologic barrier that causes the protective function to limit instead of support optimum functioning is called a **pathologic barrier.** Pathologic barriers often are manifested as stiffness, pain, or a "catch."

When massage therapists use joint movement techniques, they must remain within the physiologic barriers. If a pathologic barrier exists that limits motion, techniques are used to gently and slowly encourage the joint structures to increase the limits of the range of motion to the physiologic barrier.

Joint End-Feel

When a normal joint is taken to its physiologic limit, usually still a bit more movement is possible, a sort of springiness in the joint. This type of joint end-feel is called a *soft end-feel*. When a joint movement is restricted or a muscle shortened by a pathologic barrier, resulting in reduction of the range of motion, movement is always limited in some direction. As the limit is reached and exceeded, comfortable movement is no longer possible. In the case of abnormal restriction, the limit does not have any spring, as is found at a physiologic barrier. Rather, similar to a jammed door or drawer, the joint is fixed at the barrier, and any attempt to take it farther causes discomfort and is a distinctly "binding" or leathery feel. A distinct jamming rather than springy sensation is called a *hard end-feel*.

Effects of Joint Movement Methods

Joint movement is effective because it provides a means of controlled stimulation to the joint mechanoreceptors. Movement initiates muscle tension readjustment through the reflex center of the spinal cord and lower brain centers. As positions change, the supported movement gives the nervous system an entirely different set of signals to process. The joint sensory receptors can learn not to be so hypersensitive. As a result, the protective spasm and movement restriction may lessen.

Joint movement also encourages lubrication of the enhanced joint and contributes an important addition to the lymphatic and venous circulations. Much of the pumping action that moves these fluids in the vessels results from compression against the lymph and blood vessels during joint movement and muscle contraction. The tendons, ligaments, and joint capsule are warmed from the movement. This mechanical effect helps keep these tissues pliable.

Normal joint movements often are indicated by the degree of movement available, with the anatomic, or neutral, position labeled 0 degrees. For example, the elbow is said to be able to flex 106 degrees and extend 180 degrees from neutral. Wrist flexion is 90 degrees and wrist extension 70 degrees from neutral, The "normal" range of motion for each joint should be identified for each individual. Box 10-5 presents some examples of normal range of motion for common joints addressed during massage. For additional study, consult a comprehensive anatomy and physiology book for the degrees of movement for joints.

Remember that each person is unique, and many factors influence the available range of motion. Just because a joint does not have the textbook range of motion does not mean that what is displayed is abnormal. Abnormality is indicated by nonoptimum function. This can be either a limit or an exaggeration in the "textbook normal" range of motion. Study Box 10-5 carefully. When working with clients, use it as a guide for moving each joint through its full range of motion, always remembering to go slowly and stay within the client's comfort limits. (A video of a joint movement sequence is presented on the DVD.)

Types of Joint Movement Methods

Joint movement involves moving the jointed areas within the client's physiologic limits of range of motion.

The two types of joint movement are active joint movement and passive joint movement. In active joint movement, the client moves the joint by active contraction of muscle groups. The two variations of active joint movement are active assisted movement, which occurs when both the client and the massage practitioner move the area, and active resistive movement, which occurs when the client actively moves the joint against resistance provided by the massage practitioner.

In passive joint movement, the client's muscles remain relaxed and the massage practitioner moves the joint with no assistance from the client. When doing passive joint movement, the massage practitioner should feel for the soft or hard end-feel of the joint range of motion. This is an important evaluation for determining the state of the joint and associated tissues.

Evolve Activity 10-3

2
10-4

Box 10-5 · Normal Range of Motion for Each Joint

Available range of motion is measured from the neutral anatomic position (0). If 0 appears first, the movement begins in the anatomic position. If numbers appear first, the movement begins out of the anatomic position and returns to the neutral (0) position.

Normal Values (in degrees)

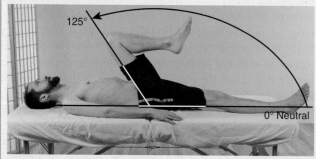

Hip flexion (0 to 125 degrees).

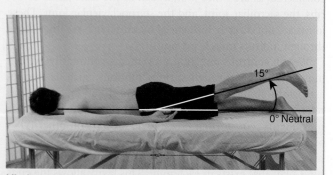

Hip hyperextension (0 to 15 degrees).

Box 10-5 Normal Range of Motion for Each Joint—cont'd

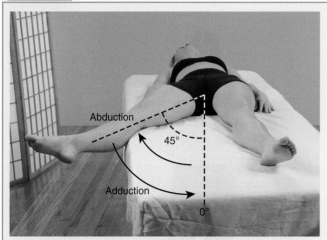

Hip abduction (0 to 45 degrees) and hip adduction (45-0 degrees).

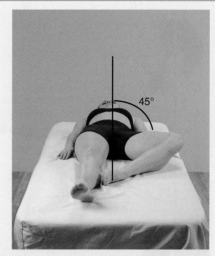

Hip lateral (extended rotator 0 to 45 degrees).

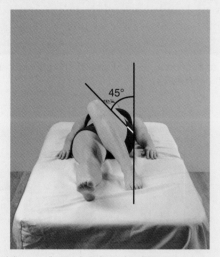

Hip medial (internal) rotation 0 to 45 degrees.

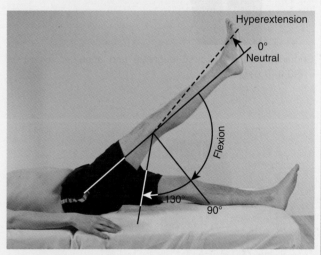

Knee flexion (0 to 130 degrees) and knee extension (120 to 0 degrees).

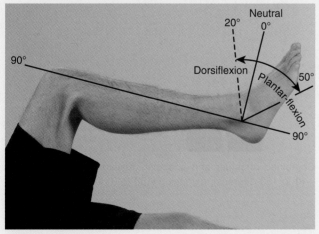

Ankle plantar flexion (0 to 50 degrees) and ankle dorsiflexion (0 to 20 degrees).

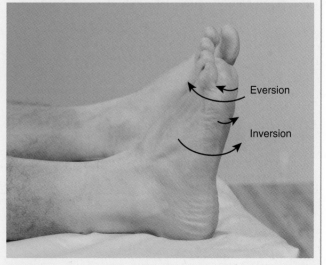

Foot inversion (0 to 35 degrees) and foot eversion (0 to 25 degrees).

Continued

Box 10-5 Normal Range of Motion for Each Joint—cont'd

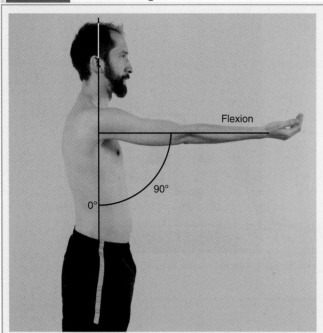

Shoulder flexion (0 to 90 degrees) and shoulder extension (90 to 0 degrees).

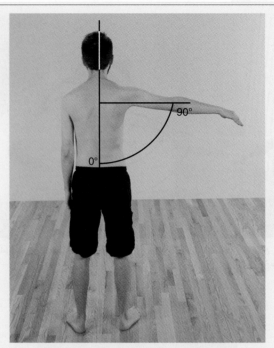

Shoulder abduction (0 to 90 degrees) and shoulder adduction (90 to 0 degrees).

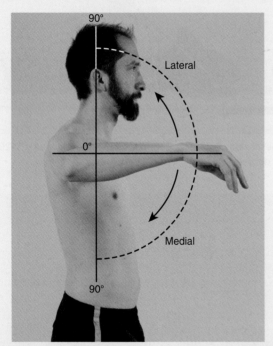

Shoulder lateral (medial) rotation (0 to 90 degrees) and shoulder medial (internal) rotation (0 to 90 degrees).

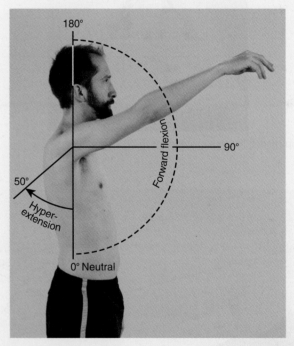

Combined shoulder and scapular movement forward flexion (0 to 180 degrees); extension (180 to 0 degrees).

Box 10-5 Normal Range of Motion for Each Joint—cont'd

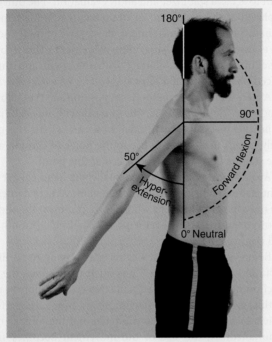

Combined shoulder and scapular movement hyperextension (0 to 50 degrees).

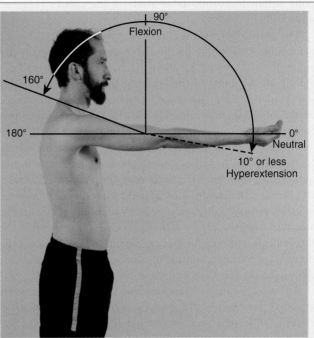

Elbow flexion (0 to 160 degrees); elbow extension (160 to 0 degrees); elbow hyperextension (0 to 10 degrees).

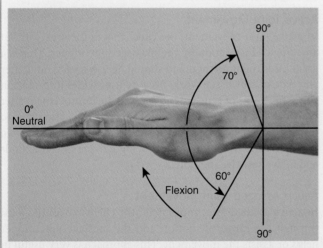

Wrist flexion (0 to 60 degrees); wrist extension (0 to 70 degrees).

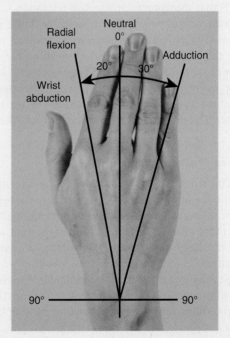

Wrist abduction (0 to 20 degrees); wrist adduction (0 to 30 degrees).

Whether active or passive, joint movements are always done within the comfortable limits of the client's range of motion.

The client's body must always be stabilized; only the joint being addressed should be allowed to move. Occasionally the entire limb is moved to allow for coordinated interaction among all the joints of the area, but the rest of the body is stabilized. It is essential to move slowly, because quick changes or abrupt moves may cause the muscles to initiate protective contractions.

Nerves stimulate muscles to contract, moving the joints. Nerves respond to sensory stimulation. If the signal is not quite strong enough, the muscle may tense but not contract; this is called *facilitation*. A facilitated area responds to a lower intensity sensory stimulation. Sensory stimulation must reach a certain intensity before activation occurs; this is called the *threshold*. If a threshold sensory signal does not occur, the nerve stays activated, waiting to contract the muscle and discharge the tension.

All massage professionals have had to deal with a leg or an arm that is extremely stiff, even though the client thinks it is relaxed. Most practitioners instruct the client to relax the muscles, or they use some other ineffective statement, such as, "Now, just let me do it." It is important to recognize that the client cannot let go of the tension in the muscles because of the facilitation of the nerves and lack of threshold stimulus.

Systems that incorporate progressive relaxation recognize that a muscle relaxes best if it contracts first. Active resistive range of motion provides a mechanism to contract muscles, discharge the nervous system, and then allow the normal relaxation phase to take over. A good approach is to have the client use active joint movement, pressing the area to be moved against stabilizing pressure provided by the massage practitioner. The practitioner then shakes or rocks the area to relax it.

Caution in Working with Joints

Joint-specific work, including any type of high-velocity thrust manipulation, is beyond the scope of practice of the beginning massage professional. Because of the interplay among the joint proprioceptors, muscle tone, innervation of the joint, and surrounding muscles by the same nerve pattern, any damage to a joint can cause long-term problems. Working within the physiologic ranges of motion for the particular client is within the scope of practice of the massage professional. Specific corrective procedures for pathologic range of motion are best applied in a supervised health care setting.

Relationship of Joint Movement to Lengthening and Stretching Methods

Joint movement is the way we position an area for the application of muscle energy techniques to lengthen muscles and stretching methods to elongate connective tissues. For this reason, the massage professional should concentrate on developing the ability to use joint movement efficiently and effectively.

Hand placement with joint movement is very important. Make sure the area is not squeezed, pinched, or restricted in its movement pattern. One hand should be placed close to the joint to act as a stabilizer and allow evaluation. The other hand is placed at the distal end of the bone; this is the hand that actually provides the movement. Proper use of body mechanics is essential when using joint movement. The stabilizing hand must remain in contact with the client and must be placed near the affected joint.

As an alternative method of positioning the stabilizing hand, the jointed area can be moved without stabilization while the massage practitioner observes where the client's body moves most in response to the range of motion action. The stabilizing hand then is placed at this point.

Avoid working cross-body. Usually, the hand closest to the joint is the stabilizing hand. The actual movement comes from the massage practitioner's whole body, not from the shoulder, elbow, or wrist. The movements are rhythmic, smooth, slow, and controlled.

Before joint movement begins, the moving hand lifts the area, and the practitioner leans back to produce the slight traction necessary to put a small stretch on the joint capsule. If this is not done, the technique is much less effective. When tractioning has been mastered and the joint is moved simultaneously, the size of the movement becomes smaller and the effectiveness increases. It is neither necessary nor desirable to have the client's limbs flailing about in the air (Figure 10-25).

Active Joint Movement

In active joint movement, the client moves the area without any type of interaction by the massage practitioner. This is a good assessment method and should be used before and after any type of soft tissue work, because it provides information about the limits of range of motion and the improvement after the work is complete. Active joint movement is also great to teach as a self-help tool. As mentioned previously, the two variations of active joint movement are active assisted methods and active resistive methods.

Active Assisted Joint Movement

In active assisted joint movement, the client moves the joint through the range of motion and the massage practitioner helps or assists the movement. This approach is very useful in cases of weakness or pain with movement. The action remains within the comfortable limits of movement for the client. The focus is to create movement within the joint capsule, encouraging the synovial fluid lubricant to warm and soften connective tissue and support muscle function.

Active Resistive Joint Movement

In active resistive joint movement, the massage practitioner firmly grasps and holds the end of the bone just distal to the affected joint. The massage practitioner leans back slightly to place a slight traction on the limb to take up the slack in the tissue. The practitioner then instructs the client to push slowly against a stabilizing hand or arm while the practitioner moves the joint through its entire range of motion. A tap or light push against the limb to begin the movement works well to focus the client's attention.

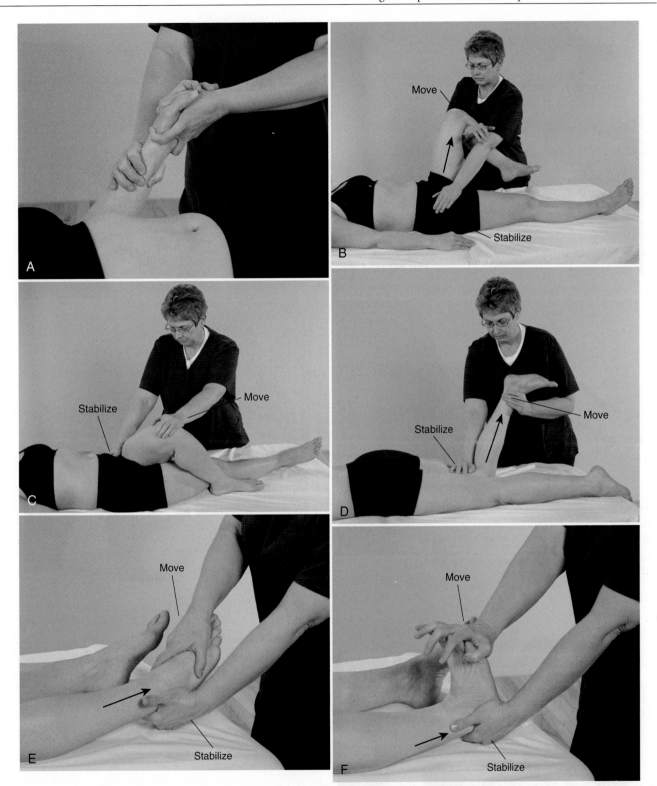

FIGURE 10-25 Examples of joint movement. **A,** Wrist joints. The stabilizing hand holds below the wrist while the moving hand produces a slight traction and moves the joint through circumduction. (*Circumduction* is a circular movement of a jointed area.) **B,** Hip joint. The stabilizing hand holds above the anterosuperior iliac spine while the moving hand and arm produce a slight traction and move the joint through circumduction. **C,** Hip joint (alternate position). The stabilizing hand holds at the hip while the moving hand moves the hip through internal and external rotation. No traction is produced in this position. **D,** Knee. The stabilizing hand holds above the knee while the moving hand produces a slight traction and moves the joint through flexion and extension. **E** and **F,** Ankle. The stabilizing hand holds above the ankle. The moving hand produces a slight traction and moves the joint through circumduction.

Continued

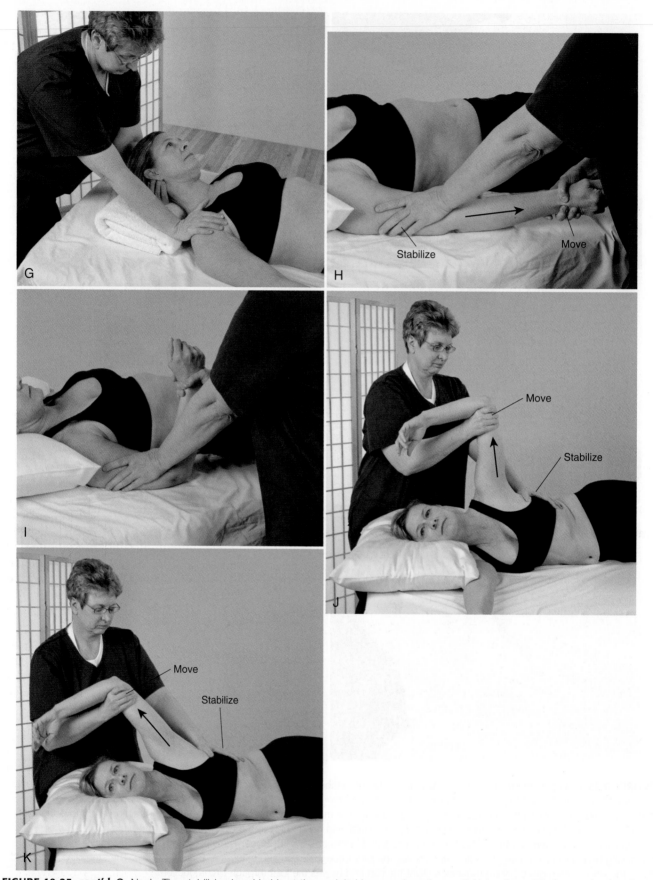

FIGURE 10-25, cont'd G, Neck. The stabilizing hand holds at the occipital base and produces slight traction while the moving hand moves the shoulder toward the feet. **H** and **I,** Elbow joint. The stabilizing hand holds above the elbow while the moving hand produces a slight traction and moves the joint through flexion and extension. Supination and pronation can also be achieved. **J** and **K,** Shoulder joint. One hand stabilizes at the shoulder joint. The other hand produces a slight traction to the shoulder joint and moves the shoulder through circumduction range of motion.

💡 PROFICIENCY EXERCISE 10-9

Using the basic massage sequence in Box 10-3, incorporate joint movement into the general sequence. At each body area use joint movement to assess for range of motion before using glide, knead, compress, oscillate, and rhythmic movement. Then use active and passive joint movement as each area is finished to assess for changes.

Another method is to stabilize the entire circumference of the limb and instruct the client to pull gently or move the area. The massage practitioner's job is to maintain a gentle traction to prevent slack in the tissue, keep the movement slow, and give the client something to push or pull against, discharging the nervous system so that the area can relax.

The counterforce applied by the massage practitioner does not exceed the pushing or pulling action of the client, but rather matches it and then allows movement.

Passive Joint Movement

If a client is paralyzed or very ill, only passive joint movement may be possible. Some clients do not wish to participate in active joint movement and prefer to take a very passive role during the massage. Client participation is not necessary.

Because the protective system of the joints does not like to be out of control, it takes time to prepare the body for passive joint movement. Shaking, rocking, and the active joint movement sequence previously described work well for this purpose.

To perform passive joint movement methods, instruct the client to relax the area by letting it lie heavy in your hands. Slowly and rhythmically move the joint through a comfortable range of motion for the jointed area. Repeat the action three or more times, increasing the limits of the range of motion as the muscles relax (Proficiency Exercise 10-9).

Suggested Sequence for Joint Movement Methods

When incorporating joint movement into the massage, follow these basic suggestions:
- If possible, perform active joint movement first. Assess range of motion by having the client move the area without participation by the practitioner.
- Have the client move the area against a stabilizing force supplied by the practitioner to increase the intensity of the signals from the contracting muscles, which discharges the nervous system.
- Incorporate any or all of the previously discussed massage methods.
- After the tissue is warm and the nervous system relaxed, do the passive joint movement.
- During a massage session, strive to move every joint approximately three times. Each time, take up any slack in the tissues and gently encourage an increase in the range of motion.
- Joint movement should be incorporated into every massage when possible (Proficiency Exercise 10-10).

💡 PROFICIENCY EXERCISE 10-10

1. Using Box 10-5 for reference, move each of your joints, using a variety of speeds, one at a time, through the normal range of motion. Notice the difference when you move slowly.
2. Pretend that a piece of plastic wrap is a joint. Hold one end tightly in your "stabilizing" hand. Now move the plastic wrap around but do not stretch it or put drag on the "tissue." Use your "moving hand" to traction the plastic wrap. Pull on it as far as it will go without stretching the tissue. Pretend to assess range of motion from this point and feel the difference. Last, pull the plastic wrap just a little more. Feel the pliability and do the joint movement from this position. Feel for the difference in effect.
3. Design and perform a massage incorporating joint movement. As always, remain aware of the variation in depth of pressure, drag, direction, speed, rhythm, frequency, and duration.

MUSCLE ENERGY METHODS

SECTION OBJECTIVES

Chapter objective covered in this section:
4. The student will be able to incorporate muscle energy techniques into the massage application.
Using the information presented in this section, the student will be able to perform the following:
- Identify the types of muscle energy methods

Muscle energy methods (MET) emerged from the osteopathic profession (Box 10-6). They fall within the scope of practice of therapeutic massage when they are used for general body normalization. The proprioceptive neuromuscular facilitation system, which was formalized as a rehabilitation method for spinal cord injury and stroke, involved the use of maximum contraction and rotary diagonal movement patterns to re-educate the nervous system. In recent years, massage professionals have begun to use pieces of the system to enhance muscle lengthening and stretching.

The diagonal movement patterns of **proprioceptive neuromuscular facilitation (PNF)** incorporate cross-body movement, which is used in repatterning for children born with various types of damage to the motor areas of the brain.

Box 10-6	Pioneers in Muscle Energy Techniques

Dr. T. J. Ruddy: Developed resistive induction technique.
Dr. Fred K. Mitchell: The father of muscle energy technique. He built on Dr. Ruddy's method, turning it into a whole body approach (Greenman, 2010).
Dr. Karel Lewit: Described the importance of methods that use postisometric relaxation (Lewit, 1998).
Dr. Leon Chaitow: Synthesized the methods of Ruddy, Mitchell, and Lewit.
Margaret Knott and Dorothy Voss: Wrote the first book on proprioceptive neuromuscular facilitation techniques, which grew out of physical therapy approaches during the 1950s (Knott and Voss, 1985).

Popularized as *cross crawl*, the technique causes the left and right brain hemispheres to function simultaneously by moving one leg and the opposite arm into flexion and adduction to cross the midline of the body. This stimulates the contralateral reflexes. The same movement is repeated with the other leg and arm. These types of movements reflexively stimulate the gait or walking pattern and are a valuable addition to any massage system. Other names for approaches based on muscle energy techniques include *manual resistance techniques, contract-relax-antagonist-contract (CRAC)*, and *active isolated stretching.*

The main differences among common methods are the origin of the approach, the intensity of the muscle contraction, and the specificity of the approach. Massage techniques as described in this text are incorporated as nonspecific aspects of a general massage. However, adaptive methods are used if massage outcomes are based on condition management or therapeutic change (see Chapter 6). Just as friction is an adaptive method used only if changes in the tissue are desired, muscle energy methods are used specifically to address shortened muscles and associated soft tissues and support optimum muscle, soft tissue, or joint function (Burns and Wells, 2006).

Additional training at more advanced levels in muscle energy techniques is available in continuing education courses. A good text to study is *Muscle Energy Techniques,* by Leon Chaitow (Churchill Livingstone, 2006). Most of the information in the following section has been adapted from Dr. Chaitow's books and workshop notes.

Muscle Energy Techniques

Muscle energy techniques involve a voluntary contraction of the client's muscles in a specific and controlled direction, at varying levels of intensity, against a specific counterforce applied by the massage practitioner. Muscle energy procedures have a variety of applications and are considered active techniques in which the client contributes the corrective force. The amount of effort may vary from a small muscle twitch to the maximum muscle contraction. The duration may be a fraction of a second to several seconds. All contractions begin and end slowly, gradually building to the desired intensity. No jerking is done in the movement.

The focus of muscle energy techniques is to stimulate the nervous system to allow a more normal muscle resting length. The **direction of ease** is the way the body allows for postural changes and muscle shortening or weakening compensation patterns, depending on its balance in gravity. Although compensation patterns may be inefficient, the patterns developed serve a purpose and need to be respected. It may seem logical to locate a shortened muscle group or a rotated movement pattern and use direct methods to reverse the pattern. However, this may not be the best approach. Protective sensory receptors prevent any forced stretch out of a compensation pattern. Instead, the pattern of compensation is respected, and the body position is exaggerated and coaxed into a more efficient position.

The term **lengthening** is used to describe this process, because lengthening is a neurologic response that allows the muscles to stop contracting and relax. **Stretching** is more

correctly defined as a mechanical force applied to elongate connective tissue. However, the terms are sometimes used interchangeably, which can be confusing.

Muscle energy techniques focus on specific muscles or muscle groups. Muscles should be positioned so that the proximal muscle attachment (origin) and the distal attachment (insertion) are either close together or in a lengthening phase with the attachments separated. Study muscle charts until you understand the configuration of the muscle structures and practice isolating as many muscles as possible, keeping in mind that proper positioning is very important. When practicing, make sure the muscles can be isolated whether the client is supine, prone, or in a side-lying or seated position (Figure 10-26).

Counterpressure is the force applied to an area that is designed to match the effort or force exactly or partially. The person providing the resistance (the massage practitioner) can apply this holding force with one or both hands, or it can be applied against an immovable object or against gravity where appropriate. The response to the method is specific to a certain muscle or muscle group, referred to as the **target muscle** (or muscles).

Types of Muscle Contractions

The massage practitioner uses three types of muscle contraction to activate muscle energy techniques: *isometric contraction, isotonic contraction,* and *multiple isotonic contractions.*

In an **isometric contraction,** the distance between the proximal and distal attachments (origin and insertion) of the target muscle is maintained at a constant length. A fixed tension develops in the target muscle as the client contracts the muscle against an equal counterforce applied by the massage practitioner; this prevents shortening of the muscle. In this contraction the effort of the muscle or group of muscles is exactly matched by a counterpressure so that no movement occurs, only effort.

In an **isotonic contraction,** the effort of the target muscle or muscles is not quite matched by the counterpressure, which allows a degree of resisted movement. With a **concentric isotonic contraction,** the massage practitioner applies a counterforce but allows the client to move the proximal and distal attachments of the target muscle together against the pressure. In an eccentric isotonic contraction (more accurately described as an **eccentric isotonic action,** because the term *contraction* specifically describes a shortening, and eccentric action results in lengthening), the massage practitioner applies a counterforce but allows the client to move the jointed area so that the proximal and distal attachments of the target muscle separate as the muscle lengthens against the pressure.

Multiple isotonic contractions require the client to move the joint through a full range of motion against partial resistance applied by the massage practitioner.

Strength of Contraction

Muscle energy techniques usually do not use the client's full contraction strength. With most isometric work, the contraction should start at about 25% of the strength of the muscle. Subsequent contractions can involve progressively greater

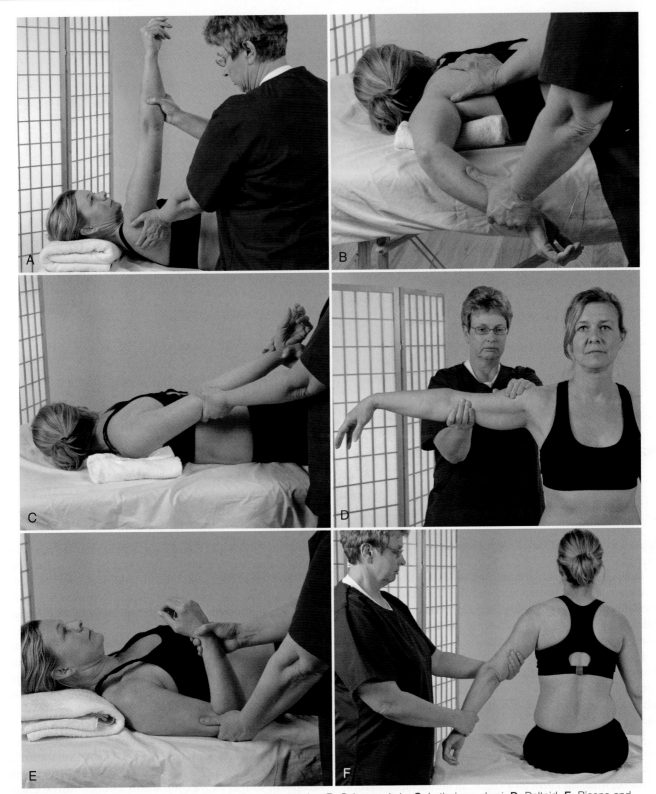

FIGURE 10-26 Positions for muscle isolation. **A,** Serratus anterior. **B,** Subscapularis. **C,** Latissimus dorsi. **D,** Deltoid. **E,** Biceps and brachialis. **F,** Triceps.

Continued

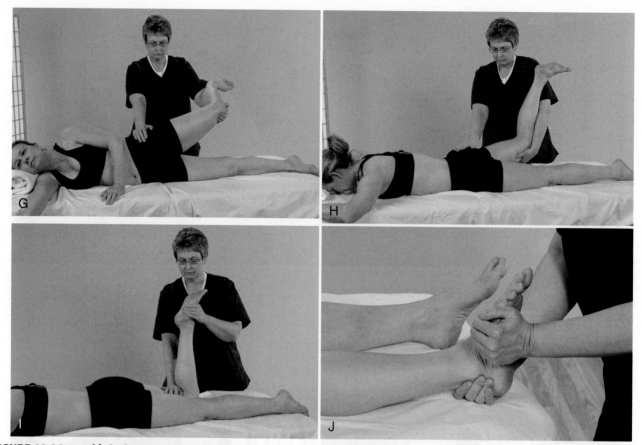

FIGURE 10-26, cont'd G, Gluteus medius. **H,** Gluteus maximus and hamstrings. **I,** Gastrocnemius and soleus. **J,** Fibularis.

degrees of effort but never more than 50% of the available strength.

Many experts use only about 10% of the available strength in muscles treated in this way, and they find that they can increase effectiveness by using longer periods of contraction. Pulsed contractions (a rapid series of repetitions) using minimal strength also are effective.

Coordinated breathing can be used to enhance particular directions of muscular effort. During muscle energy applications, all muscular effort is enhanced by having the client inhale as the effort is made and exhale during the lengthening phase.

Eye positions also can be used (Figure 10-27). Looking down activates flexors, and looking up activates extensors; when the client looks left, all muscles used to turn left are activated; when the client looks right, all muscles used to turn right are activated.

Neurophysiologic Principles

Two neurophysiologic principles have been used to explain the effect of muscle energy techniques as a result of physiologic laws, not of mechanical force, as in stretching. These principles are **postisometric relaxation (PIR)** and **reciprocal inhibition (RI)**. However, recent research indicates that the physiologic mechanism for benefit may not be directly related to PIR or RI. Rather, any type of muscle activation seems to increase tolerance to stretching by altering perceived pain and stretching sensation. In addition, some evidence indicates that the connective tissue component of the muscle is influenced, allowing for changes in tissue length (Chaitow, 2006).

Even though the scientific rationale for benefit is changing, the process of performing muscle energy applications remains basically the same; these are described in the following pages. At the end of the sections, recommendations for applications based on research findings are provided.

Postisometric Relaxation

Postisometric relaxation, occurs after isometric contraction of a muscle and is an aspect of methods called *contract/relax (CR)* and *hold/relax (HR)*. In the brief latent period of 10 seconds or so after such a contraction, a muscle can be lengthened, farther than it could before the contraction due to an increased tolerance to the stretch sensation. After the contraction, the target muscle can be lengthened passively to its comfort barrier. The **comfort barrier** is the first point of resistance before the client perceives any discomfort at either the physiologic or pathologic barrier. The isometric contraction involves minimal effort lasting 7 to 10 seconds. Repetitions continue until no further gain is noted. The procedure for PIR is as follows (Figure 10-28):

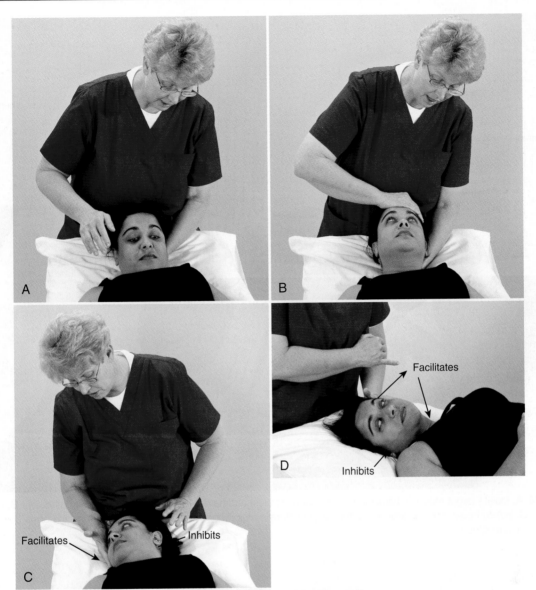

FIGURE 10-27 Eye positions. **A,** Eyes down facilitates flexors. **B,** Eyes up facilitates extension and inhibits flexors. **C,** Eyes to the right facilitates muscles that move to the right and inhibits opposing muscles. **D,** Eyes to the left inhibits previously facilitated muscle and facilitates those previously inhibited.

1. Lengthen the target muscle to the comfort barrier. Then back off slightly.
2. Tense the target muscle for 7 to 10 seconds.
3. Stop the contraction and lengthen the target muscle.
4. Repeat steps 1 through 3 until the normal full resting length is obtained.

Reciprocal Inhibition

RI takes place when a muscle contracts, causing its antagonist to relax to allow for more normal movement. While this response is no longer considered the mechanism of action, using the antagonist of the target muscle is MET variation. Such contractions usually begin in the midrange rather than near the barrier of resistance and last 7 to 10 seconds. The procedure for RI is as follows (Figure 10-29):

1. Isolate the target muscles by putting them in passive contraction (the massage practitioner moves the proximal and distal attachments of the muscles together using joint positioning).
2. Contract the antagonist muscle group (the muscle in extension).
3. Stop the contraction and slowly bring the target muscle into a lengthened state, stopping at resistance.
4. Place the target muscle slightly into passive contraction again.
5. Repeat steps 2 through 4 until the normal full resting length is obtained.

Combined Methods: Contract-Relax-Antagonist-Contract

CRAC, or contract and relax and antagonist contract, can be used to enhance the lengthening effects. The procedure for CRAC is as follows (Figure 10-30):

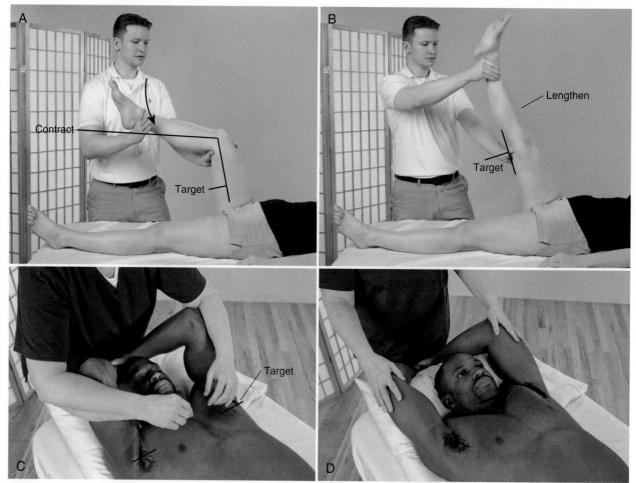

FIGURE 10-28 A, Isolate target muscles (hamstrings and gastrocnemius) and have client contract by pushing calf down. **B,** Lengthen target muscle. **C,** Isolate target muscles (latissimus dorsi and pectoralis major) and have client contract by pushing arms down toward chest. **D,** Relax and lengthen.

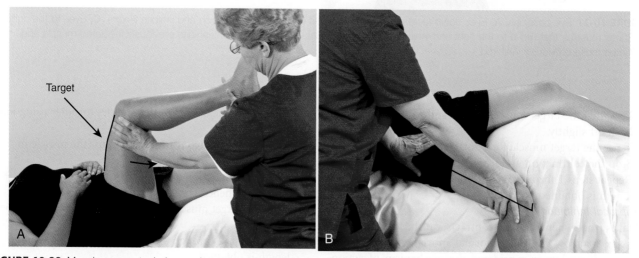

FIGURE 10-29 Muscle energy technique using antagonist contraction. **A,** Antagonist contraction (hamstrings)—target quadriceps. **B,** Lengthen quadriceps.

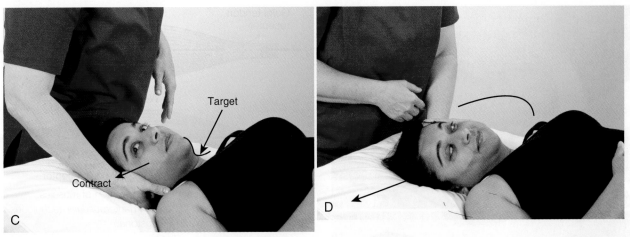

FIGURE 10-29, cont'd **C,** Identify antagonist muscles (lateral neck flexors) and contract antagonist. **D,** Lengthen target muscles.

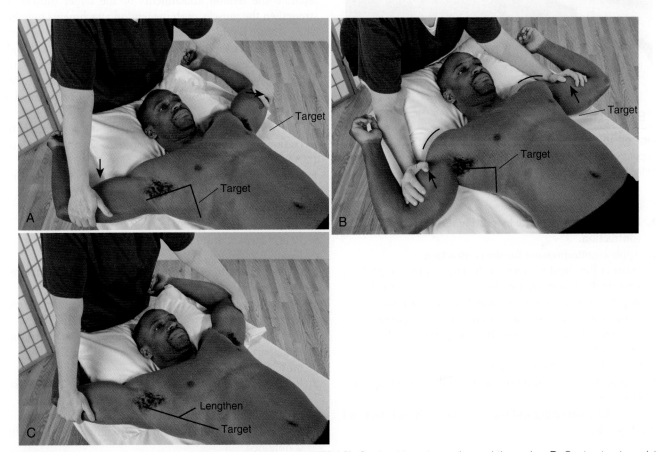

FIGURE 10-30 **A,** Example of contract–relax–antagonist-contract (CRAC). Contract target muscles and then relax. **B,** Contract antagonist muscles. **C,** Relax and lengthen target muscles.

1. Position the target muscles as in contract and relax procedures.
2. Lengthen the target muscle to the barrier. Then back off slightly.
3. Contract the target muscle for 7 to 10 seconds and then relax.
4. Contract the antagonist (reciprocal inhibition).
5. Stop the contraction of the antagonist.
6. Lengthen the target muscle to a more normal resting length.

Pulsed Muscle Energy Procedures

Pulsed muscle energy procedures involve engaging the comfort barrier and using small, resisted contractions (usually 20 in 10 seconds). The procedure for pulsed muscle energy is as follows (Figure 10-31):

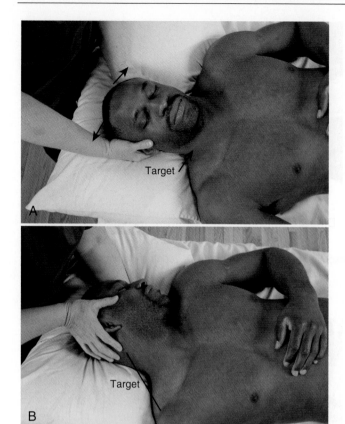

FIGURE 10-31 Pulsed muscle energy. A, Target muscle at upper trapezius. Hold area firmly and have client move back and forth. **B,** Lengthen target muscle.

1. Isolate the target muscle by putting it into a passive contraction.
2. Apply counterpressure for the contraction.
3. Instruct the client to contract the target muscle rapidly in very small movements for about 20 repetitions. Go to step 4 or use this variation: maintain the position, but switch the counterpressure location to the opposite side and have the client contract the antagonist muscles for 20 repetitions.
4. Slowly lengthen the target muscle.
5. Repeat steps 2 to 4 until the normal full resting length is obtained.

   Note: All contracting and resisting efforts should start and finish gently.

Direct Applications

In some circumstances the client does not want to participate actively in the massage or cannot. The principles of muscle energy techniques can still be used through direct manipulation of the muscle tissue. Pushing muscle fibers together in the direction of the fibers in the belly of a muscle may reduce tone. Pushing muscle fibers together in the belly of the muscle is a way to relieve a muscle cramp. This is sometimes called **approximation.**

Separating the muscle fibers in the belly of the muscle in the direction of the fibers is thought to strengthen the muscle. Manipulation of the muscle or at the ends of the muscle where

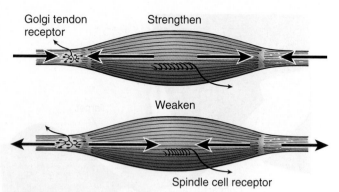

FIGURE 10-32 Proprioceptive manipulation of muscles. (Modified from Chaitow L: *Modern neuromuscular techniques,* Edinburgh, 1996, Churchill Livingstone.)

it joins the tendons is also an option. To inhibit the muscle, separate the tendon attachments of the target muscle. To strengthen the muscle, push the tendon attachments together. The pressure levels used to elicit the response must be sufficient to contact the muscle fibers. Pressure that is too light does not access the proprioceptors, and excessive pressure negates the response by activating protective reflexes. Moderate pressure, which allows the muscle itself to be palpated, is most effective.

The procedure for direct manipulation to initiate the relaxation and lengthening response is as follows (Figure 10-32):

1. Place the target muscle in comfortable passive extension.
2. Press the tissues together on the target muscle.
3. Pull the tissues apart on the antagonist muscle.
4. Lengthen the target muscle.
5. Repeat steps 2 through 4 until the normal full resting length is obtained.

Direct Manipulation of the Golgi Tendon Organs to Initiate the PIR Response

The procedure for direct manipulation of the tendon to initiate the PIR response is as follows (Figure 10-33):

1. Place the target muscle in comfortable passive extension.
2. Pull apart on the tendon attachments of the target muscle.
3. Push the tendon attachments together on the antagonist muscle.
4. Lengthen the target muscle.
5. Repeat steps 2 through 4 until normal full resting length is obtained.

Positional Release/Strain-Counterstrain

Strain/counterstrain, a technique formalized by Dr. Lawrence Jones, involves the use of tender points to guide the positioning of the body into a space where the muscle tension can release on its own.

According to Dr. Chaitow, during a **positional release technique (PRT),** a muscle's spindles are influenced by methods that take them into an ease state and that theoretically allow them an opportunity to reset and reduce hypertonicity. Strain/counterstrain and other positional release methods use the slow, controlled return of distressed tissues to the position of

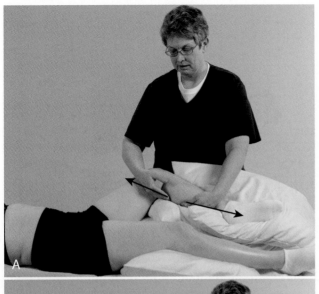

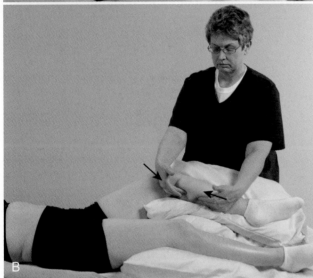

FIGURE 10-33 Direct manipulation of proprioceptive muscle. **A,** Strengthen. **B,** Weaken.

strain as a means of offering the spindles a chance to reset and thus normalize function. This is particularly effective if the spindles have inappropriately held an area in protective splinting, such as occurs around a sprain or strain to hold the injured area to avoid tissue damage.

Positional release is a more generic term used to describe these methods. Positional release methods are used on painful areas, especially recent strains, before, after, or instead of muscle energy methods. The tender points often are located in the antagonist of the tight muscle because of the diagonal balancing process the body uses to maintain an upright posture in gravity.

Repositioning of the body into the original strain, often the position of a prior injury, allows proprioceptors to reset and stop firing protective signals. By moving the body into the direction of ease (i.e., the way the body wants to go and out of the position that causes the pain), the proprioception is taken into a state of safety. Remaining in this state for a time

allows the neuromuscular mechanism to reset itself. The massage practitioner then gently and slowly repositions the area into neutral.

Positional release techniques gently allow the body to reposition and restore balance. They also are highly effective ways of dealing with tender areas regardless of the pathologic condition. Sometimes the reason the point is tender to the touch cannot be determined. However, if tenderness is present, a protective muscle spasm surrounds it. Positional release is an excellent way to release these small areas of muscle spasm without causing additional pain.

The positioning used during positional release is a full-body process. Remember, an injury or loss of balance is a full-body experience. For this reason, areas distant to the tender point must be considered during the positioning process. For example, the position of the feet very likely will have an effect on a tender point in the neck.

The procedure for positional release is as follows (Figure 10-34):

1. Locate the tender point.
2. Gently initiate the pain response with direct pressure. Remember, the sensation of pain is a guide.
3. Slowly position the body until the pain subsides.
4. Wait at least 30 seconds or longer until the client feels the release, lightly monitoring the tender point.
5. Slowly lengthen the muscle.
6. Repeat steps 1 through 5 until the normal full resting length is obtained.

Integrated Approach

Muscle energy methods can be used together or in sequence to enhance their effects. Recall that muscle tension in one area of the body often indicates imbalance and compensation patterns in other areas of the body. Tension patterns can be self-perpetuating. Often, using an integrated approach introduces the type of information the nervous system needs to self-correct. The procedure outlined here relies on the body's innate knowledge of what is out of balance and how to restore a more normal functioning pattern.

The following procedure is an integrated approach. Use the position from either option A, steps 1 and 2, or option B, steps 1 and 2, as the starting point for the rest of the process, which begins at step 3.

Option A
1. Identify the most obvious of the postural distortion symptoms.
2. Exaggerate the pattern by increasing the distortion, moving the body into ease. This position becomes the pattern of isolation of various muscles that will be addressed in the next part of the procedure (e.g., if the left shoulder is elevated and rotated forward, exaggerate and increase the elevation and rotation pattern). Continue with step 3.

Option B
1. Identify a painful point.
2. Use positional release to move the body into ease until the point is substantially less tender to pressure. The position of ease found becomes the pattern of isolation

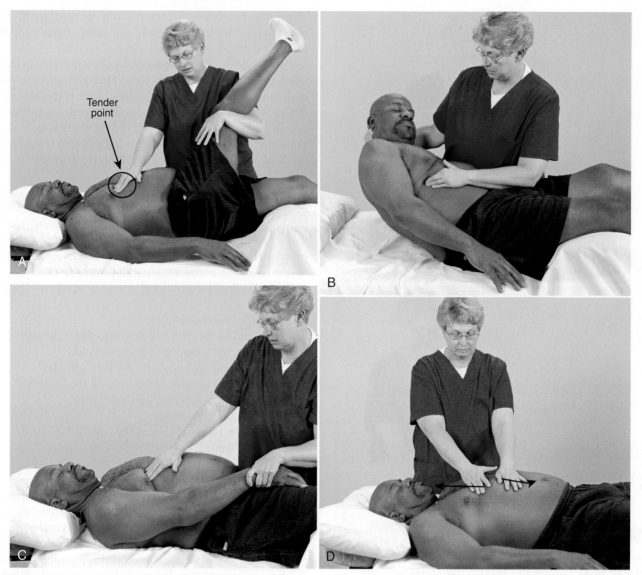

FIGURE 10-34 Generalized positional release. **A,** Identify tender points in **B** and **C** and begin to move the client into pain-relieving positions. **D,** Direct lengthening of tender area.

of various muscles that will be addressed in the next part of the procedure. Continue with step 3.

After choosing from option A or option B, continue the procedure as follows:

3. Stabilize the client in as many different directions as possible.
4. Instruct the client to move out of the pattern. Be as vague as possible and do not guide the client, because it is important for the client to identify the resistance pattern.
5. Provide resistance for the client to push or pull against.
6. Modify the resistance angle as necessary to achieve the most solid resistance pattern for the client.
7. Spend a few moments noticing when the client's breathing changes; then, while still providing modified resistance, allow the client to move through the pattern slowly.
8. When the client has achieved as much extension as she can on her own, recognize that she has achieved the lengthening pattern.

9. Gently increase the lengthening. If additional elongation in this position is desired, connective tissue stretching can be achieved.
10. Pay attention to the body areas that become involved in addition to the one addressed. This is your guide to the next position (Figure 10-35).

Making It Simple

As mentioned, some current research indicates that PIR and RI mechanisms may not be as responsible for the benefit achieved using muscle energy methods as previously believed. The approaches thus can be simplified. The act of contracting the muscles appears to be involved in a movement pattern to facilitate lengthening of the short muscles. Movement patterns occur at each jointed area and involve groups of muscles all neurologically linked—prime mover, agonist and synergist, and antagonist (eccentric control function). The eye position also influences the neurologic signaling to the muscles.

The following is a combined simplified approach (Figure 10-36):

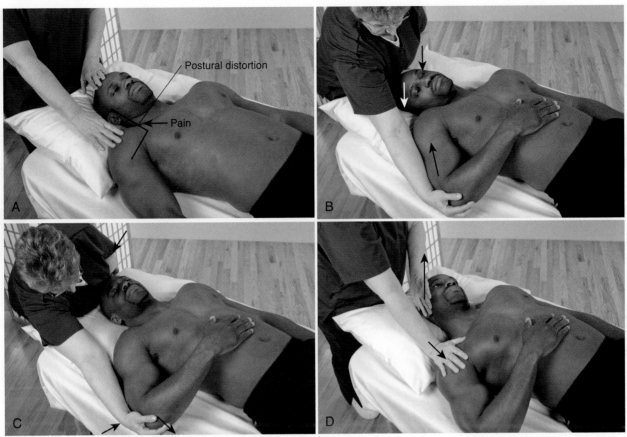

FIGURE 10-35 A, Identify area of pain and/or postural distortion. **B,** Position of release and/or increased postural distortion. **C,** Instruct client to move out of distortion pattern while providing resistance. **D,** Lengthen.

1. Assess movement patterns with passive and active joint movement and identify short tissue (the target).
2. Position short tissue in increased passively shortened position and hold it in that position.
3. Stabilize in all directions at the distal end of the area (e.g., for the elbow, stabilize just above the wrist; for the hip, just above the knee; and for the ankle, at the toes).
4. Instruct the client to push and pull back and forth for hinge joints (fingers/toes, elbows, knees) or move the area in a circle (wrist, ankle, shoulder/hip, neck, spine) while at the same time moving the eyes in a circle. The movement should be rhythmic and of moderate strength. This back and forth or circular movement against applied resistance activates all muscles in the movement pattern.
5. Slowly lengthen the target area (short tissue) to the bind (resistance barrier) and hold for a few seconds.
6. Repeat steps 3 to 5 two or three more times.
7. Massage the target tissue, primarily using gliding, compression, and kneading, both with and against the muscle fiber direction; this manually stimulates receptors, connective tissue, and fluid. Then shake or rock the area and lengthen again.

This sequence basically uses all the muscle energy methods described. See Proficiency Exercise 10-11.

💡 PROFICIENCY EXERCISE 10-11

1. Design a progressive relaxation sequence for yourself using the concept of PIR.
2. Design a lengthening sequence for yourself using pulsed muscle contraction.
3. Design a complete massage using kneading and compression on "soft muscles."
4. Experiment with positional release concepts to relax sore spots on your body.
5. Design a complete massage incorporating all the muscle energy methods presented.
6. Repeat the massage sequence from step 5 using the "making it simple" pattern. Compare the results.

STRETCHING

SECTION OBJECTIVES

Chapter objective covered in this section:

5. The student will be able to incorporate stretching into the massage application when appropriate.

Using the information presented in this section, the student will be able to perform the following:

• Describe and use two types of stretching
• Determine when stretching is appropriate and when it is not appropriate
• Use muscle energy methods to support stretching

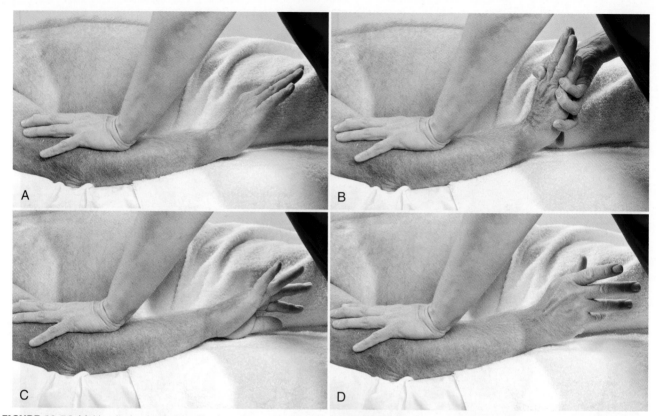

FIGURE 10-36 Making it simple. **A,** Identify short tissue. **B,** Increase passive shortening of tissue. **C** and **D,** Move distal joints in circle.

Stretching is a mechanical method of introducing various forces into connective tissue to elongate shortened areas. Research is shifting our understanding of the structure of connective tissue and its function in the body. However, for practical application purposes, the description that follows is sufficient.

Stretching introduces forces of bend, torsion, and tension that mechanically affect connective tissue. The connective tissue fibers are elongated past their normal give so that they can enter the plastic range, past the existing bind. This creates either a freeing and unraveling of fibers or a small therapeutic inflammatory response that signals for change in the fibers. Stretching also affects the ground substance, warming and softening it, thereby increasing its pliability.

Because fascial sheaths provide structural support, it is important to work with a sense of three-dimensional awareness, realizing that shifts in structure have more than a localized effect. Because the body supports stability before mobility and compensation patterns are bodywide, changes in structure must be balanced with either lengthening or strengthening activities that allow the body to maintain a sense of perpendicular orientation in gravity.

If stability and mobility are not taken into account, the body's method of reacting to changes in structure is to increase muscle spasm and acute pain. This results in a decreased ability to adapt effectively to the changes introduced, and it reduces the effectiveness of the methods.

Applying Stretching

As explained previously, stretching and lengthening are different. Before stretching, the muscles usually must be lengthened or those in the area may develop protective spasms; this occurs because stretching often moves into pathologic barriers formed by connective tissue changes. The connective tissue component cannot be accessed until the muscle has been lengthened. Without stretching, any neuromuscular lengthening may be restricted by shortened connective tissue. Although lengthening without stretching is possible and often desirable, lengthening must always be done before stretching. During stretching the two methods work together. Muscle energy techniques are used to prepare muscles to stretch by activating lengthening responses.

Longitudinal stretching pulls connective tissue in the direction of the fiber configuration. Cross-directional stretching pulls the connective tissue against the fiber direction. The two approaches accomplish the same thing, but longitudinal stretching is done in conjunction with movement at the joint and gliding manipulations applied with drag in the direction of the force. If longitudinal stretching is not advisable, if it is ineffective in situations of hypermobility of a joint, or if the area to be stretched is not effectively stretched longitudinally, cross-directional stretching is a better choice. Cross-directional stretching focuses on the tissue itself and does not depend on joint movement (Figure 10-37).

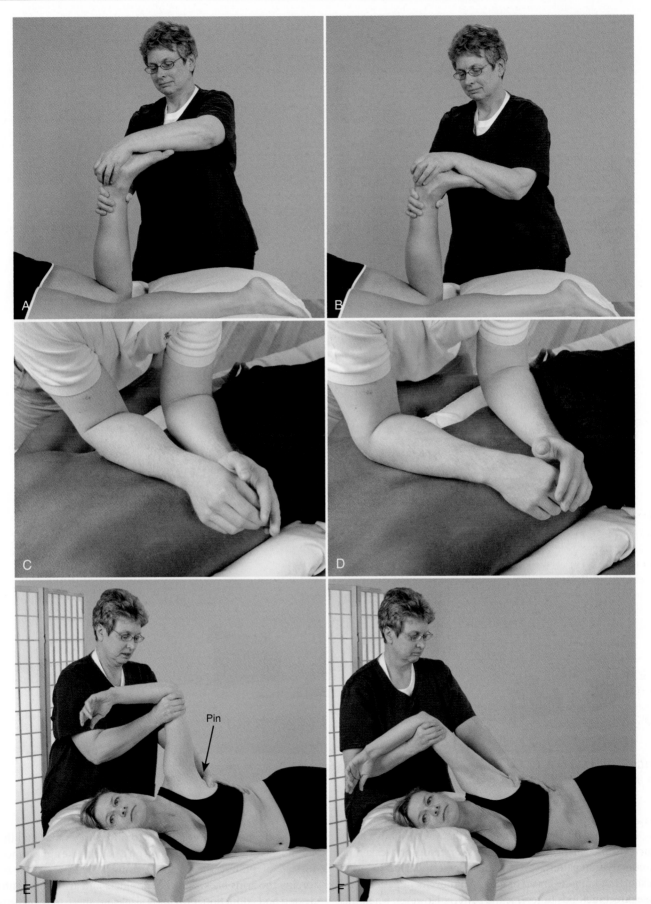

FIGURE 10-37 Beginning of **(A)** and end of **(B)** passive longitudinal stretch. Beginning of **(C)** and end of **(D)** direct tissue stretch. **E** and **F,** Pin and stretch.

Continued

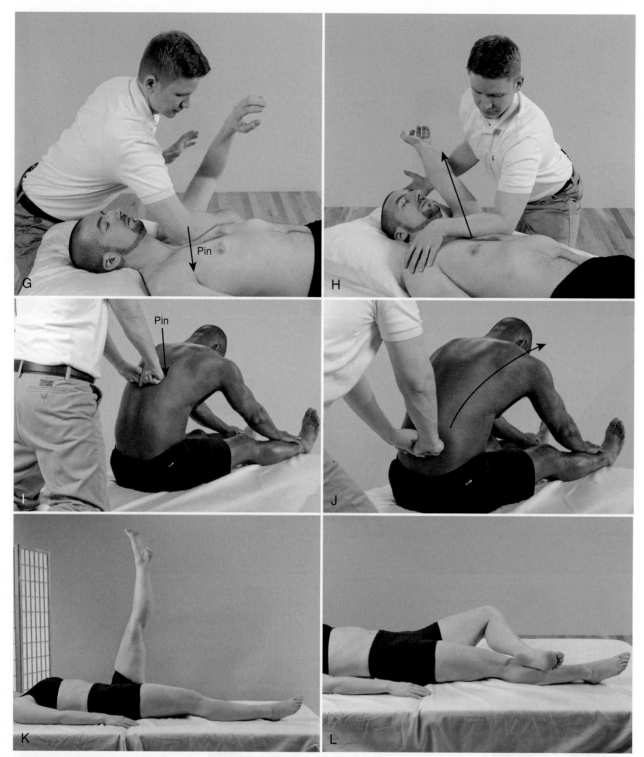

FIGURE 10-37, cont'd G, Active release, pin, and H, client moves to stretch. I, Active release, pin, and J, client moves to stretch. K and L, Examples of active self-stretching.

Recall that the direction of ease is the way the body allows for postural changes and muscle shortening or weakening compensation patterns. As stated, it may seem logical to locate a shortened muscle group or a rotated movement pattern and use direct methods to reverse the pattern. However, when this is done, protective sensory receptors tend to prevent any forced stretch out of a compensation pattern. Take the example

of a client who has shortened pectoralis muscles that pull the shoulders forward, giving the person a gorilla-like appearance. Instead of pulling the pectoralis muscles into a stretch by forcing the arms back, curl the shoulders and arms more into flexion and adduction, providing slack and space to the receptors in the pectoralis muscles. Begin corrective action from this point.

The procedure for longitudinal stretching is as follows:

1. Position the target muscle in the direction of ease. Stabilize and isolate a muscle group.
2. Choose a method to prepare the target muscle to stretch (e.g., gliding, compression, kneading).
3. After the target muscle has been prepared, stretch the muscle to its physiologic or pathologic barrier or to wherever protective contraction is engaged; this is the point of bind. Back off slightly to prevent muscle spasm. Stay in line with the muscle fibers. Exert effort or movement as the client inhales. Stretch as the client exhales.

The following two approaches are used for the actual stretch phase:

1. Hold the position just off the physiologic or pathologic barrier for at least 10 seconds to allow for the neurologic reset; this is the lengthening phase. Feel for secondary response (a small give in the muscle).
2. Take up slack by further lengthening the muscle for up to 20 seconds to create longitudinal pull (tension force) on the connective tissue. You must hold the muscle stretch as instructed to allow for changes in the connective tissue component of the muscle.

Alternate Procedures for Longitudinal Stretching

If only a small section of muscle needs to be stretched, if the muscle does not lend itself to stretching with joint movement, or if the joints are so flexible that not enough pull is put on the muscles to achieve an effective stretch to the tissues, the following alternate procedure for longitudinal stretching should be used:

1. Locate the fibers or muscle to be stretched.
2. Place the hands, fingers, or forearms in the belly of the muscle or directly over the area to be stretched.
3. Contact the muscle with sufficient pressure to reset the neuromuscular mechanism.
4. Separate the fingers, hands, or forearms (tension force) or lift the tissue with pressure sufficient to stretch the muscle (bending or torsion force). Take up all slack from lengthening, then increase the intensity slightly and wait for the connective tissue component to respond (this may take as long as 30 seconds).

Note: All requirements for preparation of the muscle and direction of stretch are the same as those described for the previous longitudinal stretching procedure.

The following procedure is used for active assisted longitudinal stretching:

1. Identify and isolate the muscle, making sure it is not working against gravity in this position. Remind the client to exhale during the stretching phase of this technique.
2. Lengthen the muscle to its physiologic or pathologic barrier, move slightly beyond this point, and stretch gently for 1 to 2 seconds.
3. Return the muscle to its starting position. Repeat this action in a rhythmic, pulselike fashion for 5 to 20 repetitions.

4. The client can benefit from contracting the antagonist while the target muscle is lengthened and stretched. As in all proper lengthening and stretching movements, attention must be paid to the stretch reflex; bouncing is never done because it initiates this reflex.

Other effective methods involve the application of compression into the short binding tissue to hold it, followed by either active or passive movement:

1. Locate the area to be stretched.
2. Apply compression into the short tissue and hold it in a fixed position.
3. The client moves the adjacent joints and lengthens the tissue (sometimes called *active release*), or the massage practitioner uses the other hand to move the tissue or joint into a stretched position (sometimes called *pin and stretch*).

Cross-directional tissue stretching uses a pull and twist component, introducing torsion and bend forces. The procedure for cross-directional stretching is as follows:

1. Access the area to be stretched by moving against the fiber direction using compression.
2. Lift or deform the area slightly and hold for 30 to 60 seconds until the area gets warm or seems to soften.

Use the following procedure for skin and superficial connective tissue:

1. Locate the area of restriction.
2. Lift and pull (like taffy), first moving into the restriction and then pulling and twisting out of it, keeping a constant tension on the tissue (remember the plastic wrap exercise). Go slowly. Take up slack until the area warms and softens.

Use of Cold Applications and Stretching

Dr. Janet Travell popularized the cold spray and stretch technique (Travell and Simons, 1999). The cold spray stimulates cold receptors, blocking other sensory signals; the proprioceptors thus are inhibited momentarily, allowing the muscle to relax.

Ice application can be used to create the same effect as cold spray. Make an ice pop by filling a paper cup with water, inserting a wooden stick, and freezing. Remove the paper cup and then move the ice pop on the skin from the proximal to the distal attachment along the path of the target muscle. Move the ice pop about 1 inch per second while stretching the muscle.

Use of Percussion with Stretching

Using forms of percussion on the skin over the muscle along the same pathway as the ice pop massage facilitates stretching. The skin is snapped quickly with a move that is like flicking lint off a coat. If a tendon is tapped quickly, the muscle contracts. To assist stretching, apply the tap to the antagonist muscles so that they contract reflexively. The target muscle thus is inhibited reciprocally, allowing for a relaxation response and the ability to stretch with reduced protective muscle spasm.

💡 PROFICIENCY EXERCISE 10-12

1. Knead extra flour into bread dough so that the consistency is quite firm. Practice stretching the dough. Feel for the give of the dough as opposed to the dough breaking.
2. Design a lengthening and stretching sequence for yourself that accesses the major muscle groups and connective tissue areas. Pay attention to the difference in the feel of neuromuscular lengthening, with its quick release, and connective tissue stretching, with its softer, slower give.
3. Have a fellow student assume various stretch positions. Tell him or her to stretch as far as is comfortable and hold. Take the area and stretch it $\frac{1}{8}$-inch farther and hold it. Pay attention to the feeling and talk with the student to get feedback.
4. Practice tapping antagonist tendons and using ice massage on a client as you position the body for various stretches.
5. Working with a partner, see how many massage manipulations and techniques you can combine and perform at one time (e.g., joint movement combined with compression, gliding combined with a stretch, percussion combined with a stretch, kneading combined with muscle energy methods).
6. Design a massage incorporating at least two massage or movement techniques for every body area.

Stretching Deep Fascial Planes

Accessing deep fascial planes requires an understanding of the deep structures involved. Specific soft tissue systems, such as myofascial release and soft tissue manipulation, provide instruction in these very valuable methods. Chapter 12 expands on this information.

It is important to realize that the human body is made up of interconnecting parts; consequently, all stretching affects deep connective tissue structures. The body cannot be divided into separate layers; the only difference is the access point. A house may have three or four doors, each of which will let you inside. Where you enter may be different, but once you are inside, you are able to have an effect on all the areas. Therefore, effective stretching of the more superficial connective tissues, as presented in this chapter, also indirectly affects the deeper connective tissue structures (Proficiency Exercise 10-12).

SEQUENCE AND FLOW: THE BASIC FULL-BODY MASSAGE

SECTION OBJECTIVES

Chapter objective covered in this section:
6. The student will be able to perform a full-body massage using the methods and techniques presented in the chapter.

Using the information presented in this section, the student will be able to perform the following:
- Understand how to deal with difficult or unusual situations regarding body hair, skin problems, and avoidance of tickling
- Make thoughtful decisions about the application of massage techniques by body region
- Adapt massage application based on the needs of individual clients
- Design a basic full-body massage

The previous section presented massage and movement techniques. The next concern is how to combine the methods into a focused massage session. A massage can be given in many ways. The choices massage therapists make each time they give a massage need to come from an understanding of the principles and practice of therapeutic massage. Each massage is different, because the client is different each time, even if that client has been seen for many massage sessions. The illustrations in the protocol and the DVD included with this text show body placement. Any methods and techniques can be used in any combination in a particular body area. Some students will find these simple guidelines helpful, whereas others will find it easier to develop a structure themselves. For learning purposes, beginning with the suggestions provided and then modifying them as needed is a good way to start. Remember, the examples in the book and on the DVD are only a place to begin as you work to understand the organization of massage application. (A sample protocol is presented on p. 357.)

The different approaches can be combined in many different ways to create different massage patterns. You may find it helpful to study the illustrations and incorporate the suggestions into your practice massage sessions. Use the illustrations while generating your own ideas and be open to experimentation, creation, and modification of massage applications based on individual clients according to body shape, style of massage, and equipment available.

The focus of the session depends on the outcomes the client is seeking. To understand those outcomes, the massage practitioner must be able to take a general history and do a basic assessment of the client (see Chapter 4). Based on the information gathered in the history and assessment process, the therapeutic massage professional designs the best massage for that particular client by choosing the appropriate methods, pressure, rhythm, pacing, intensity, duration, and amenities (e.g., music). (Refinement of the assessment process and the criteria for decision making are addressed in Chapter 11 and in the case studies in Chapter 16.)

When doing a massage, the massage practitioner uses a variety of techniques in a manner that allows easy transition from one method to another as a particular part of the body is addressed. Once students learn the technical aspects of performing methods, they learn to perfect the massage sequence; that is, to combine the methods in a logical way to address specific body areas and eventually to generate specific outcomes, such as relaxation, pain control, mobility, and improved circulation.

General sequencing principles guide the massage application. These principles describe the direction and progression of manipulations. They are:

General → Specific → General
Superficial → Deep → Superficial

General to specific to general and *superficial to deep to superficial* refer to the ways in which methods are applied to an area of the body. The first application of a method is done generally and superficially; this is followed by applications that are more specific and deeper. The methods then return to more general and superficial techniques before the practitioner moves to another area.

This sequencing has many effects. It accustoms the client to the touch, and it allows the practitioner to palpate through layers of tissue in a systematic manner for assessment or application for therapeutic change. Without this approach, especially after deep work, the client may experience postmassage soreness for hours or days after the session.

Another important concept is that compressive force is always applied first. After that a secondary force is added, such as tension produced by gliding or torsion produced by kneading.

A good rule to remember is "down first, then out or around." Compression (down) is used to determine the tissue layer being targeted. For example, holding methods typically are skin level, so very light compressive force is applied. The superficial fascia is below the skin; therefore, the compressive force (pressure) moves your hand, forearm, or foot through the skin and into the superficial fascia. Once the tissue layer has been reached, the next force is added (out or around), such as tension force with gliding methods, torsion force with kneading, local stretching with bending force, or shear force with frictioning.

Basic Full-Body Massage

The basic full-body massage is a common approach in massage. The session lasts about 1 hour. The full-body general massage stimulates all the sensory nerve receptors, contacts all the layers and types of tissues, and moves all the major joints of the body. The general protocol is shown on p. 357 and also on the DVD that accompanies this textbook.

The purpose of the massage is to affect the whole body using primarily gliding, compression, oscillation, and movement of the joints, along with limited use of kneading, shaking, and general friction methods. The other manipulations and techniques are chosen as needed to address specific problem areas.

Regardless of the type of massage approach, the first and perhaps most important massage technique is holding, or the first touch. The next massage techniques are used for general, broad applications and to connect all the other methods during the massage session. Methods most commonly used for general broad applications are gliding strokes, compression, rhythmic rocking and shaking, and joint movement (Box 10-7).

The full-body general massage has a sense of wholeness, with a beginning point and an ending point. The massage should have a general sense of continuity. It needs to flow, to feel connected, like one continuous experience made up of all the applications of the massage methods chosen to achieve the individual client's outcomes.

The general sequence of contact is gliding, kneading, oscillation (rocking, shaking), and movement (usually passive joint movement). Remember, a compressive force is used to determine the depth of pressure for gliding and kneading.

Each body area is addressed. Each method usually is applied three or four times (frequency), becoming slower and deeper with each application. The rhythm, duration, and direction vary, depending on the goal of the massage. A basic sequence

| Box 10-7 | When to Use What Massage Method |

Gliding strokes are effective in the following situations:
- A lubricant will be used.
- A large surface area must be covered efficiently.
- Changes are made between techniques.
- The practitioner moves from one area to another.
- The client prefers a soothing massage with generalized body responses.

Compression is effective in the following situations:
- A lubricant will not be used.
- The client is hairy or ticklish.
- The client prefers a more stimulating massage.

Rhythmic rocking and *shaking* are effective in the following situations:
- A lubricant will not be used.
- Excessive rubbing or pressing on the skin or underlying tissue is not desirable.
- The client wants a soothing massage with generalized body responses.

Joint movement is effective in the following situations:
- A lubricant will not be used.
- The client is hairy or ticklish.
- Excessive rubbing or pressing on the skin or underlying tissue is not desirable.
- The client wants a general increase in mobility.

Blending these four methods to provide the general base of the massage is beneficial. The other massage techniques provide uniqueness to the massage.

can be developed (e.g., glide, glide, glide—knead, knead, knead—compress, compress, compress—rock or shake or move a joint as appropriate). The practitioner then can move to a different body area and repeat the sequence.

General Massage Suggestions

Body Hair

Excessive body hair requires an alteration in the massage procedure. Gliding and kneading methods can pull the hair. A lubricant may feel uncomfortable. Compression and oscillation (vibration, rocking, and shaking), coupled with lengthening and stretching procedures, can be an effective alternative.

Skin Problems

Massage procedures must be altered for people with rashes, acne, psoriasis, and other skin problems. The integrity of healthy skin prevents the transmission of pathogens. Physician referral and approval may be required. Massage usually can be provided by placing a clean, white bath towel or triple-folded sheet over the affected area and using compression methods over the fabric. Be very careful to avoid contact with any body fluids.

Working over a clean towel or sheet can be helpful for clients who have sensitive skin and find the movement of massage irritating. Any method that does not glide on the skin can be used over a towel, sheet, or loose, nonrestrictive clothing. Using a towel to lift tissue, especially the tissue of the abdomen, is helpful for gaining an effective grip and is more comfortable.

Avoidance of Tickling

Tickling usually can be avoided by reducing the speed and increasing the pressure of the stroke. Also, because tickling oneself is difficult, the problem often can be solved by placing the client's hand on the area you want to massage and massaging with it. Tickling frequently can be avoided by working over a towel or sheet.

Considerations and Suggestions for Massage Applications by Body Region

Head and Face Massage

Because of the extensive motor/sensory sensitivity of the face, massage can stimulate considerable nervous system activity, which may be beneficial for relaxation and pain control. Also, the facial muscles create the expressions that reflect our moods and emotions. Changes in expression are processed in the emotional centers of the brain. Careful massage of the face may gently interact with the way the client feels emotionally.

Key Points

- To avoid disturbing the client's hairstyle and makeup, always ask before massaging the head and face.
- Use lubricants carefully, keeping in mind the sensitivity of the facial skin. Avoid using lubricant on the face if possible.
- Remember that the delicate nature of the facial skin and muscles requires a confident yet moderate approach.
- Always clean your hands before massaging the face. Pathogens can easily be spread through the mucous membranes of the eyes, nose, and mouth. Avoid direct contact with these areas.

Neck Massage

The neck is a crowded, complex area. It can be affected by responses to stress and by chest and shoulder breathing, which can cause the neck muscles to become rigid and hypertonic. Effective massage of the neck is necessary to provide for relaxed breathing and reduced perception of stress.

Careful study of the anatomy of the neck shows that the direct soft tissue influence extends from the forehead to the second and third ribs, the middle thoracic vertebrae, and the middle of the humerus. Because the neck area balances the head against gravity, postural distortion anywhere in the body is reflected in the neck. Massage to this area, in conjunction with an entire body approach, is most beneficial.

The brachial nerve plexus exits from the neck. It is helpful to think of most arm, wrist, and hand problems as beginning at the neck. Problems result either from direct dysfunction of the neck or from difficulties in the arm and hand, which often indirectly cause a neck problem.

Key Points

- Although the neck can be massaged effectively with the client lying supine or prone, side-lying is also an effective position for massage of the neck. The head is stabilized against the table, and the neck area is opened up for easy access.
- Always provide lengthening and stretching for the neck from the shoulder with the head held still. Injury may result if the neck is lengthened or stretched by moving the head.
- Avoid deep pressure into the anterior triangle of the neck (the general area between the sternocleidomastoid muscle and the trachea). Such pressure can damage blood vessels and nerves in this area.
- When massaging the neck, use broad, generalized methods of massage applied with the forearm or the whole hand; this feels less invasive than using the fingers and thumbs.

Shoulder Massage

The shoulder complex (scapula, clavicle, humerus, and associated muscles, ligaments, and tendons) floats on the trunk. It is constructed with a loose fit at the shoulder (glenohumeral) joint to provide for a wide range of motion. Soft tissue (muscles, tendons, ligaments, and fascia) connects the shoulder to the trunk, with multidirectional forces coming from the back, chest, and neck. The practitioner should consider all these areas when massaging the shoulder.

The joint design reflects the fact that flexor muscles (which narrow a joint angle) and adductor muscles (which pull toward the midline of the body) exert more pull and are stronger than the extensors (which increase the joint angle) and abductors (which pull away from the midline). Joint fit may be compromised by an imbalance in the tone pattern of these muscles. The practitioner should keep this in mind when working with the shoulder.

The brachial nerve plexus, which supplies the arm, may be affected by soft tissue dysfunction in the shoulder area. This is a very important consideration for clients who have arm pain and discomfort, often resulting from repetitive use injury. Massaging the shoulder may help reduce muscle tension and soften connective tissue in the area, which may alleviate discomfort in the shoulder and arm.

Key Points

- Although the shoulders can be massaged with the client lying supine or prone, side-lying is quite an effective position for massage, range of motion, and lengthening and stretching of the shoulder.
- The shoulder is stabilized at the iliac crest and sacrum by the latissimus dorsi muscle and the lumbar dorsal fascia. With any shoulder massage, the practitioner should consider massage of the low back area.

Arm Massage

The nerves of the brachial nerve plexus run the entire length of the arm. Nerve impingement from soft tissue at the neck, shoulder, and elsewhere in the entire length of the arm needs to be considered if pain is radiating into the area.

When massaging the arm, it is useful to remember that the fingers actually begin at the elbow, and the shoulder mechanism extends to the elbow.

The elbow joint area is more complex than a hinge joint because of the pronation (palm down)/supination (palm up) action at the elbow. Flexion, extension, pronation, and supination movement patterns need to be considered when massaging the arm.

Key Points

- Positioning and stabilization of the arm for massage can be aided by massaging the arm in all the basic positions: supine, prone, and side-lying. Each offers advantages.
- Massage only the areas of the arm that are easily accessible in each position. Return to the arm as the client changes position.
- Massage the arm with the forearm stabilized against the massage table in the prone or supine position or against the body in the side-lying position.
- The arm often is small enough in circumference to grasp with the hands, surrounding a bulk of the tissue. This approach provides a compressive glide to facilitate fluid movement.

Hand and Wrist Massage

Because of the extensive motor/sensory sensitivity of the hand, massage can provide intense neurologic stimulation. The hand is an effective area for massage to initiate relaxation and pain control. The hand and wrist have an intricate, complex joint and soft tissue structure. Thorough attention to massage of these structures and range of motion of the hand and wrist requires time and a focus on detail.

Massage of the hand can be a time of increased connection between the client and the massage practitioner. This is a result of the hand-in-hand position. The sense of intimacy created by the act of holding hands may shift the therapeutic focus from the client to the massage practitioner. Extra care is suggested to prevent transference/countertransference and professional boundary issues without disturbing the closeness created at this time.

Slow circumduction (moving in a circle) of the wrists, both passive and active against resistance, accesses the joint movement patterns of the wrist. The carpal and metacarpal (palm) joints of the hand can be addressed with a scissoring action. The phalangeal (finger) joints are hinge joints that respond well to active movement against resistance and passive range of motion.

Key Points

- Because the hand usually is in a flexed position, opening and spreading the tissue of the palm is very beneficial.
- Using compression to provide a pumping action on the palm stimulates the lymphatic plexus in the palm, which in turn encourages lymphatic flow. This can be very helpful for clients whose hands swell.

Chest Massage

The pectoralis muscles and associated connective tissue are involved in arm and shoulder movement. This large soft tissue area often is shortened, not only affecting arm action, but also causing breathing difficulties. Effective massage, lengthening, and stretching are beneficial.

The intercostal muscles (those between the ribs) are very important in respiratory function. Slow, deliberate work between the ribs with the client in the side-lying position can be valuable for restoring mobility and breathing function.

Key Points

- On women, the breast area can pose difficulties in accessing the chest. The side-lying position is effective for massage of the chest area, because the breast tissue falls toward the table, allowing access to the side of the chest and the axilla. Using the client's hand as a "buffer" between the practitioner's hand and the client (e.g., as when avoiding tickling) can be helpful when working around the clavicles and ribs.
- Broad compressive applications to the rib area in the side-lying position are effective in providing general range of motion to the ribs.
- Avoid the breast tissue and nipple area on both men and women. No reason exists to massage this area during general massage, and the tissue often is very sensitive to touch and can be easily irritated.
- Be extra attentive to changes in the tissue in the chest area. Without any alarm reaction, refer clients to their physician if you notice any lumps or tissue changes.

Abdominal Massage

Many times the abdomen is given only superficial attention during massage—avoid this tendency. This is an important area that deserves effective massage application. The abdomen has an expansive fascial system. Lifting methods to stretch this connective tissue can be beneficial. Using a towel to lift the abdominal tissue provides grip and protects against pinching.

Be careful of pressure down into the abdomen. Always move slowly, allowing the tissue to soften under the touch. If you feel a pulse or throbbing, immediately reduce the pressure.

Not all researchers agree that massage has a substantial effect on peristalsis or even that mechanical emptying of the colon is possible. Nonetheless, with abdominal massage, it seems prudent to approach the area as though massage does have an effect. Theoretically, to support peristalsis and mechanical emptying of the colon, all massage manipulations are directed in a clockwise fashion. To prevent any chance of impaction of fecal material, the manipulations begin in the lower left quadrant at the sigmoid colon. The methods progressively contact the large intestine and eventually end up encompassing the entire colon area. The abdomen often is ticklish; this is a protective mechanism. Follow the instructions given earlier for avoiding tickling.

Key Points

- The abdomen can be massaged with the client in the supine or side-lying position. Side-lying on the left is the most effective position. During abdominal massage the knees

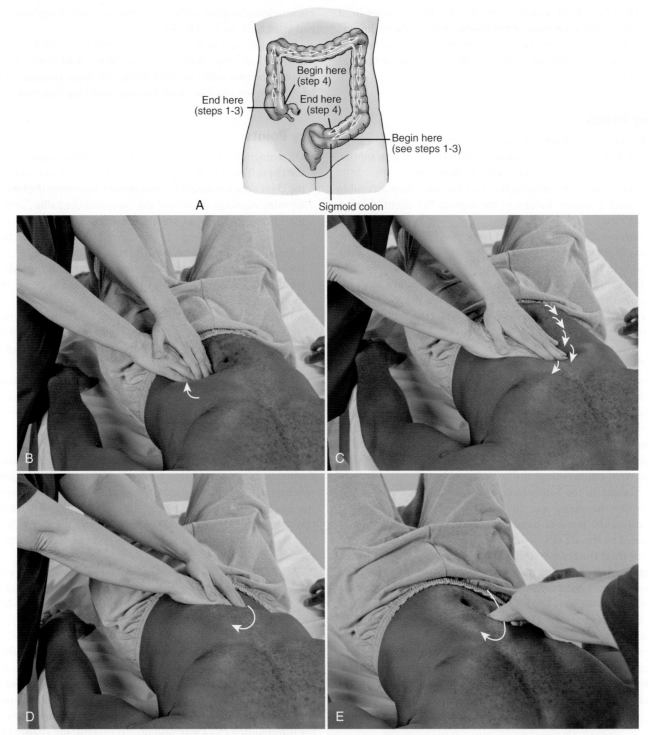

FIGURE 10-38 A, Colon (arrows indicate the flow pattern). All massage manipulations are directed in a clockwise fashion. The manipulations begin in the lower left quadrant (on the right side as you view the illustration [**A**]) at the sigmoid colon. The methods progressively contact all of the large intestine and eventually cover the entire colon area. **B,** Abdominal sequence. The direction of flow for emptying of the large intestine and colon. Make the change as suggested. Massage down the left side of the descending colon using short strokes directed toward the sigmoid colon. **C,** Massage across the transverse colon to the left side using short strokes directed toward the sigmoid colon. **D,** Massage up the ascending colon on the right side of the body using short strokes directed toward the sigmoid colon. End at the right-side ileocecal valve, which is located in the lower right quadrant of the abdomen. **E,** Massage the entire flow pattern of the abdominal sequence, using long, light to moderate strokes, from the ileocecal valve to the sigmoid colon. Then repeat the sequence.

usually are bent about 90 degrees to the trunk to tilt the pelvis and allow for more relaxed abdominal muscles.

- Because the abdomen contains no bony structure against which to apply pressure, much abdominal work is done with lateral pressure. The tissue is pushed against pressure from the massage practitioner's opposing hand or with kneading that lifts the tissue.

Abdominal Sequence

Standing on the left side of the body when the client is in the supine position facilitates the body mechanics of the practitioner (Figure 10-38). The body mechanics for the massage practitioner and elimination patterns are most efficient when the client is lying on his or her left side.

The direction of flow for emptying the large intestine and colon is as follows:

1. Massage down the left side of the descending colon, using short strokes directed to the sigmoid colon.
2. Massage across the transverse colon to the left side, using short strokes directed to the sigmoid colon.
3. Massage up the ascending colon on the right side of the body, using short strokes directed to the sigmoid colon.
4. End at the right ileocecal valve, located in the lower right quadrant of the abdomen.
5. Massage the entire flow pattern, using long, light to moderate strokes, from the ileocecal valve to the sigmoid colon. Repeat the sequence.

Back Massage

The back often is the starting place for the massage because for many clients, the back does not feel as vulnerable an area as the abdomen. Even though shortening of the anterior tissues is causing the client's backache, beginning massage on the back directly addresses the client's experience of discomfort. Nerve roots are located all along the spine. Massage close to but not on the spine is beneficial. The low back, including the deep quadratus lumborum muscle, is easily massaged in the side-lying position with the client's arm raised over the head to lift the rib cage away from the iliac crest. Deep, even pressure with the forearm often feels best to the client.

Gentle range of motion to provide for rotation of the spinal column is most effectively done in the side-lying position.

Key Points

- Avoid spending excessive time on massage of the back. Often the reason for back pain or stiffness is shortening and weakness of muscles in the chest and abdomen. The resulting change in posture is responsible for the back tension.
- The back is effectively massaged in the prone, side-lying, and seated positions.
- Use of the forearm is very effective for back massage. The lumbar dorsal fascia responds well to skin rolling (tissue lifting) and connective tissue stretching methods. Pressure directly over the spine is not appropriate. However, skin rolling techniques that lift the skin over the spine are effective.

Gluteal and Hip Massage

The lumbar and sacral plexuses both innervate the gluteal and hip region. Nerve distribution patterns include the entire lower body, and the largest nerve is the sciatic nerve. When using heavy pressure to address the soft tissue, avoid sustained deep pressure on the nerve tracts.

The sacroiliac joints are large joints that are not directly moved by muscular action. Range-of-motion actions are indirectly achieved through movement of the leg through a range-of-motion sequence.

The coxal articulations (hip joints) are massive joints with an extensive ligament structure. The joint provides considerable range of motion, second only to the shoulder joint. When doing range-of-motion methods, include as many variations of flexion, extension, abduction, adduction, and internal and external rotation as possible to involve all the soft tissue elements.

Key Points

- Massage of the gluteals and hips is most effective when the client is in the side-lying or prone position. Lengthening and stretching methods are most easily done in the side-lying or supine position. This area is heavily muscled and reinforced with extensive ligament and tendon structures. The bones and joints in this area are large compared with those in other body areas. Deeper pressure, with increased duration, often is required to relax these tissues.
- Methods need to work slowly into the tissue. Avoid work with the hands and make extensive use of the forearm, knee, or foot; these are less intimate, which may be an important consideration when working with the gluteals and hips.

Leg Massage

The lumbosacral plexus nerves supply the leg, with the sciatic nerve running the entire length of the leg. Impingement can occur anywhere along the nerve pathways. The distribution of leg pain can indicate the nerve portion affected. When located, the entire nerve tract needs to be searched above and below the impingement site for soft tissue restriction to provide soft tissue normalization around the nerves. Light stroking along the nerve tracts is very soothing.

The knee is a complex joint influenced by muscles from above and below the joint. Knee instability often is compensated for by increased motor tone in the leg muscles and thickening and shortening of the iliotibial tract (a large connective tissue structure on the outside of the leg). This is resourceful compensation, and the protective nature of the muscle and connective tissue tension must be considered. The gluteus maximus and tensor fascia lata muscle exert a pull at the iliotibial crest. Relax these muscle structures to reduce tension on the iliotibial tract and knee. If the client has a hypermobile knee, you can use the proper methods to reduce excessive motor tone and connective tissue shortening, but you should not try to remove the splinting action entirely. To do so may result in increased knee pain.

Key Points

- Supine, prone, and side-lying are all effective positions for massage of the leg and are best used in combination to access all parts of the leg easily. For the most efficient use of time in the massage session, make sure each area of the leg is massaged only once. For instance, if you massage the back of the leg in the prone position, it is not necessary to repeat the back of the leg again in the supine position unless a specific reason exists for doing so.
- The side-lying position offers the easiest access to the medial and lateral aspects of the leg. The supine position provides access to all aspects of the leg, whereas the prone position is the most limited.
- The soft tissue mass of the leg lends itself to massage with the forearm, leg, and foot. Kneading often is uncomfortable on the leg because of body hair and the tight adherence of the skin and superficial fascia to the underlying tissue. Gliding and compression are effective methods to use instead.
- Varicose veins most often occur in the leg, particularly in the saphenous veins. Thromboembolism and thrombophlebitis are serious conditions involving a blood clot in a vein. If the clot moves, it can lodge in the heart, lung, kidney, or brain, with serious consequences. Symptoms of deep vein thrombophlebitis in the legs are aching and cramping that can be mistaken for muscle pain. Massage of any type is contraindicated, and immediate referral is indicated for varicose veins, thromboembolism, and thrombophlebitis. Diagnosis is beyond the scope of practice for therapeutic massage; therefore, massage practitioners should remain cautious of any leg pain and refer the client to the appropriate health care professional.
- Range of motion for the leg above the knee is hip range of motion. Make sure to stabilize effectively at the pelvis. Stabilizing pressure in this area can be uncomfortable. A small pillow or folded towel can be used over the stabilizing point to ensure comfort.

Foot and Ankle Massage

The foot and ankle mechanism is a highly complex structure. It has many joints, muscles, and nerves that provide stability and neurologic positional information during walking and standing. An extensive connective tissue network provides stability. Any disruption of normal foot and ankle action often results in a compensatory pattern through the entire musculoskeletal system.

Massage of the foot is one of the best ways to provide a high degree of nervous system input for relaxation and pain control. Many beneficial effects are obtained with foot massage because of the stimulation of parasympathetic activity, which results in the relaxation or quieting response.

The sole of the foot contains a vast lymphatic plexus that acts as a pump to move lymphatic fluid in the foot and legs. Compression used in a rhythmic pumping action is effective in stimulating the lymphatic system.

The tibial nerve, off the sciatic nerve, branches into the medial and lateral plantar nerve, which in turn branches to provide extensive nerve distribution in the foot. Sciatic nerve impingement can be felt into the foot. Nerve pain in the foot can indicate impingement anywhere along the nerve tract from the lumbosacral plexus to the foot. Nerve pain in the foot needs to be addressed with massage of the entire leg, and the practitioner should notice which areas of restriction refer pain to the foot.

Key Points

- For a client who is nervous or in pain, the feet often are a safe place to begin a massage.
- Because of the number of joints in the foot and ankle, careful and deliberate range-of-motion work is beneficial in this area. Slow circumduction (circular movements), both passive and active against resistance, accesses the ankle movement patterns. The tarsal and metatarsal (main foot) joints can be accessed with a scissoring or bending movement of the foot. Phalangeal (toe) joints are hinge joints that benefit from both **active range of motion** against resistance and **passive range of motion**.

Designing a Massage

The following series of photographs provides one example of how a massage can be designed. Examples of massage applications are provided, incorporating the various methods and techniques described in this chapter. It is assumed that the student would perform the techniques on both sides of the body where appropriate. Variations also are shown, providing options for massage of a particular area. This series of photographs is complemented by the demonstration provided on the DVD. By studying these examples, you should be able to modify and adapt applications to make each massage unique (Proficiency Exercise 10-13).

The series of photographs that follow is organized as an example of a full-body massage in three positions: prone, side-lying, and supine. Draping is shown, but not in such a way as to obstruct the view of the application. Ideally, the massage is applied using all of the best positioning. Most areas of the body can be massaged in the three positions; however, some positions related to body areas support optimum body mechanics, and circumstances may require that variations be used.

🔋 PROFICIENCY EXERCISE 10-13

Design a 1-hour massage sequence on paper using a variety of methods and techniques from this chapter. Trade papers with another student and perform the other person's massage sequence on him or her. When you are finished, list what you learned from the experience and share the list with your partner in this exercise. Have your partner critique his or her massage design.

GENERAL MASSAGE PROTOCOL

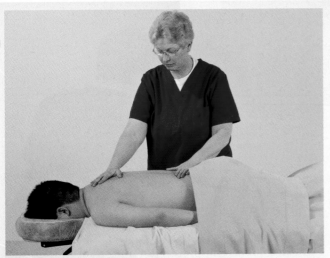

1. Calmly and with compassion approach client with intention focused on massage outcomes. Center. Then apply holding stroke.

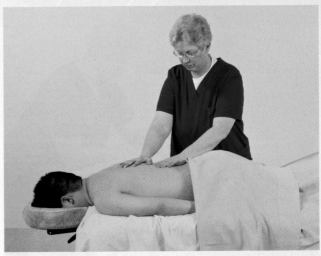

2. Palpation. Wet/dry skin drag, ease/bind, hot/cold, rough/smooth.

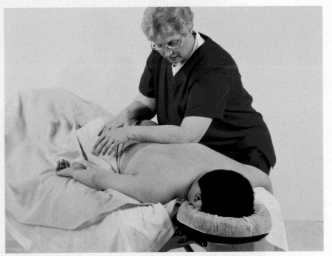

3. Glide on back. Vary speed, drag, and depth of pressure.

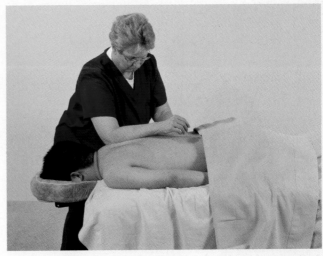

4. Shift position. Glide/compress.

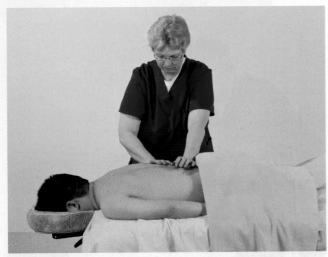

5. Knead.

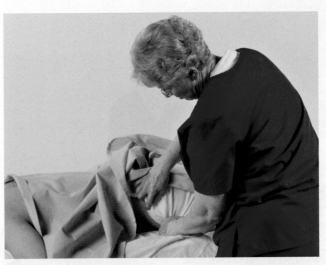

6. Move underwear.

Continued

GENERAL MASSAGE PROTOCOL—cont'd

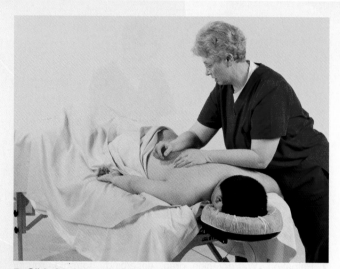

7. Glide lumbar and gluteal region.

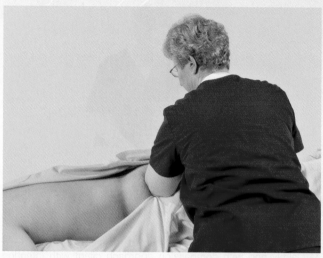

8. Compression to gluteal area.

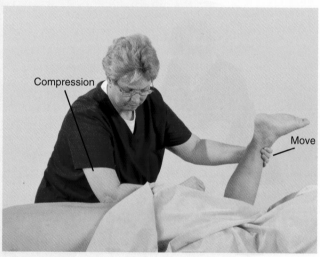

9. Combined loading. Compression and move.

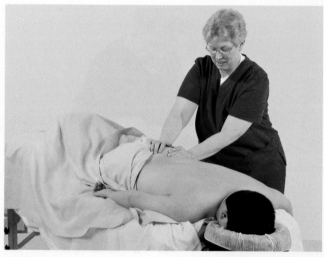

10. Knead.

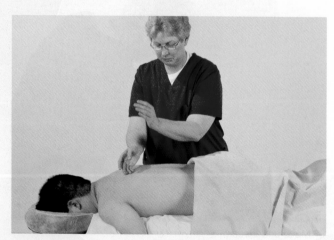

11. Percussion. Repeat opposite side.

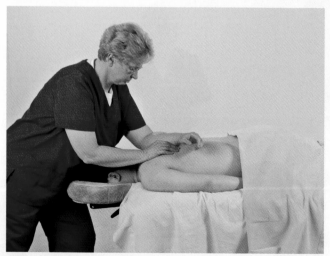

12. Shift position. Compression/glide upper back/shoulder.

GENERAL MASSAGE PROTOCOL—cont'd

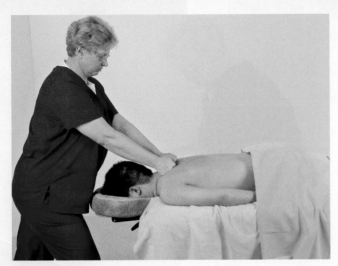

13. Compression.

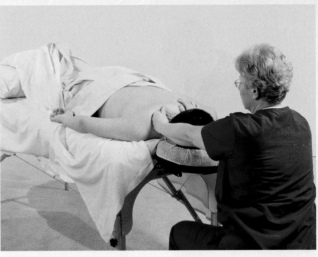

14. Compression with therapist kneeling.

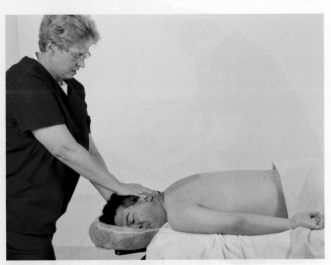

15. Turn head, massage scalp.

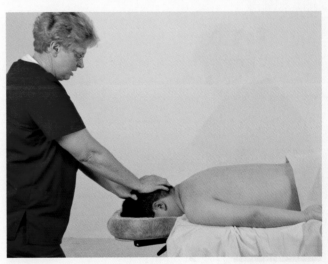

16. Reposition head. Compress muscles of the head.

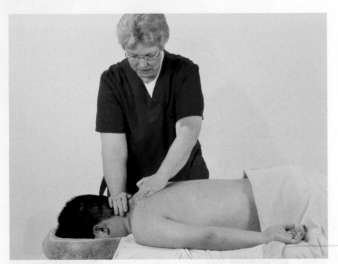

17. Knead neck.

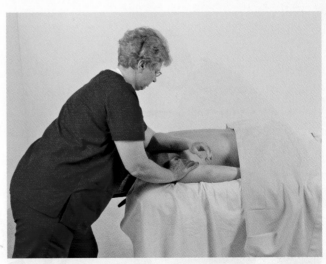

18. Compression/glide on shoulder.

Continued

GENERAL MASSAGE PROTOCOL—cont'd

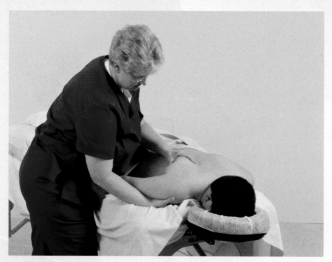

19. Oscillation. Shaking and move scapula.

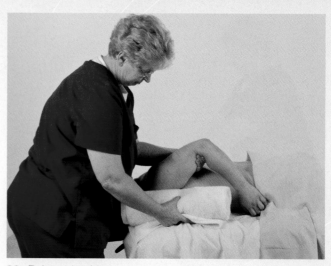

20. Bolster shoulder.

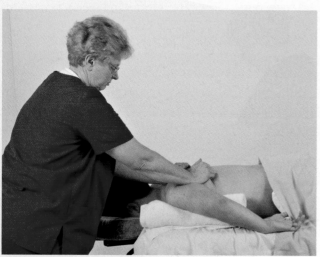

21. Knead and glide around scapula.

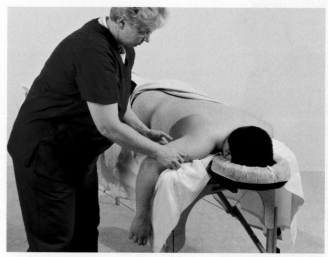

22. Position arm, rock and shake, then assess.

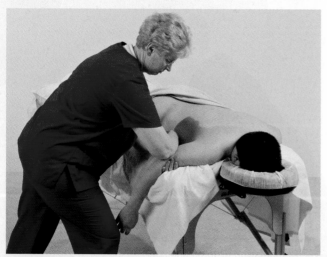

23. Glide arm using forearm.

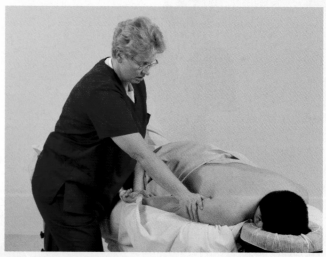

24. Glide using palm.

GENERAL MASSAGE PROTOCOL—cont'd

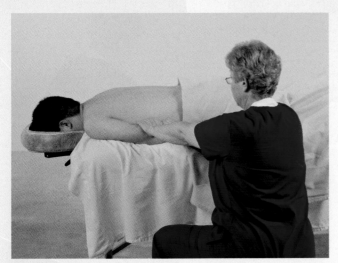

25. Knead arm and forearm.

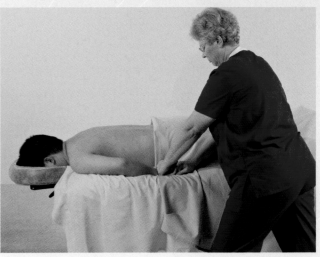

26. Compress forearm and hand. Repeat opposite side.

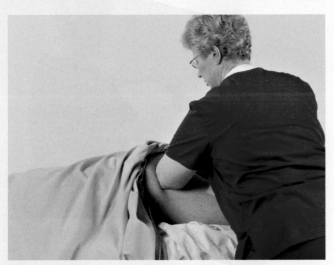

27. Move to hip and thigh. Compression/glide with forearm.

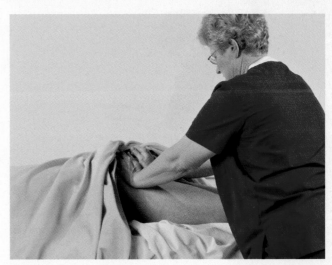

28. Palm compression.

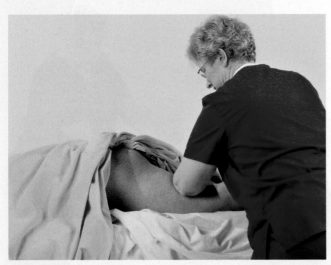

29. Repeat gliding—slower and deeper.

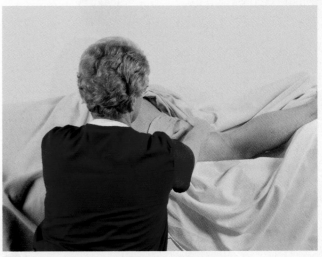

30. Knead posterior thigh while kneeling.

Continued

GENERAL MASSAGE PROTOCOL—cont'd

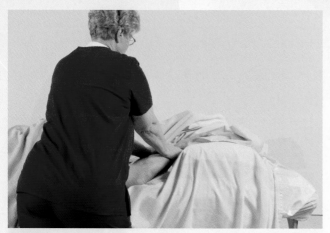

31. Glide on calf.

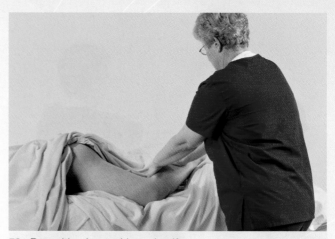

32. Reposition leg and knead calf.

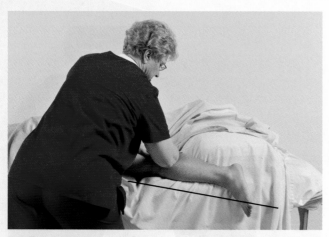

33. Reposition leg, straighten knee, compress, glide, and knead.

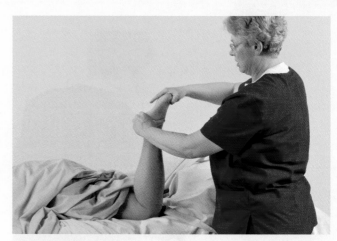

34. Joint movement of knee, ankle, foot.

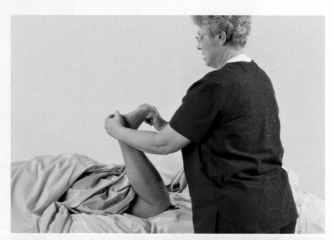

35. Stretch and move. Position leg for foot massage.

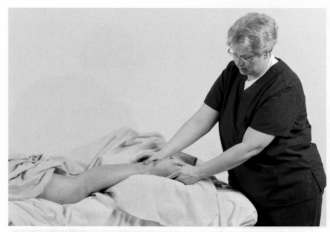

36. Compression of lateral foot using palm. Reposition leg.

GENERAL MASSAGE PROTOCOL—cont'd

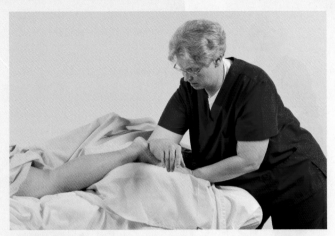

37. Compression of sole of foot using forearm.

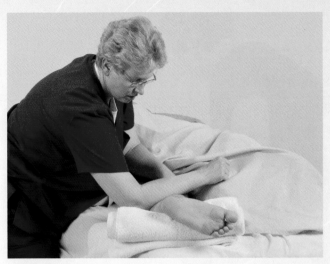

38. Reposition client side-lying with glide/compression of calf and foot.

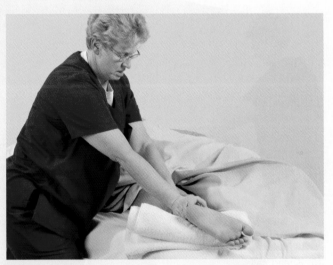

39. Compression/glide of ankle and heel, medial side.

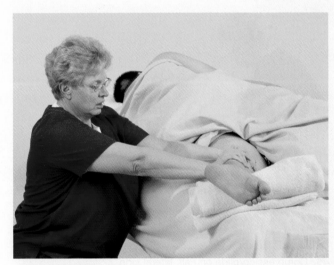

40. Knead calf.

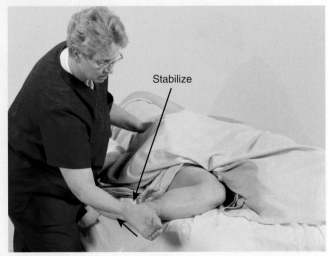

Stabilize

41. Muscle energy techniques using antagonist contraction.

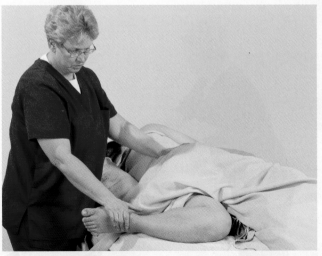

42. Stretch anterior thigh.

Continued

GENERAL MASSAGE PROTOCOL—cont'd

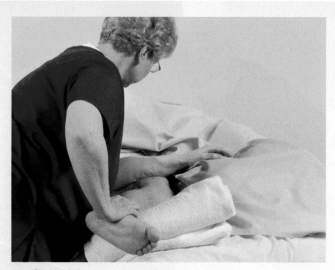

43. Glide of the inner (medial) thigh.

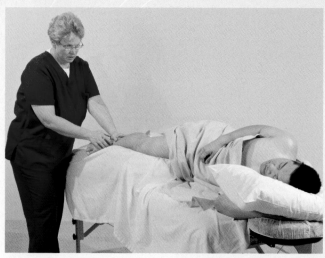

44. Client remains side-lying. Switch to opposite leg.

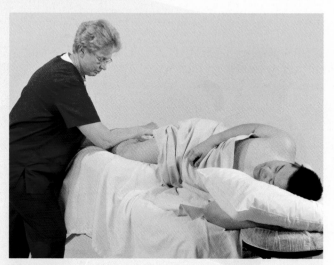

45. Compression/glide on calf, lateral side.

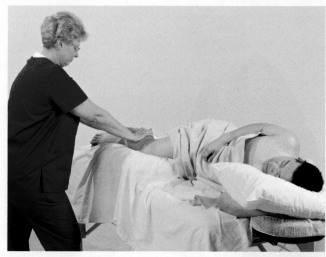

46. Knead calf.

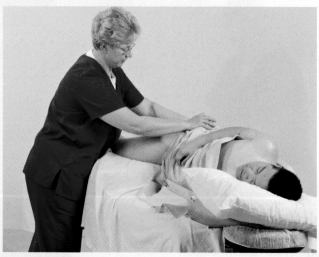

47. Move drape to provide access to thigh and hip.

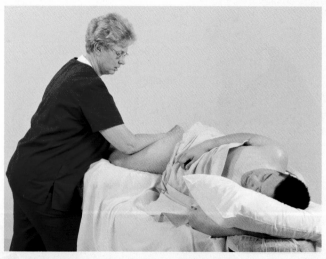

48. Glide, lateral thigh. Caution: do not compress tissue into underlying bone.

GENERAL MASSAGE PROTOCOL—cont'd

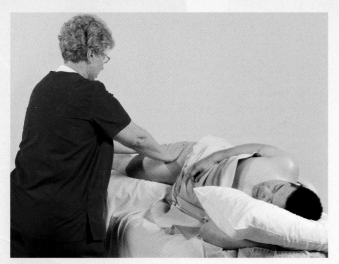

49. Knead lateral thigh.

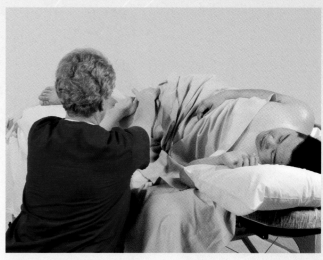

50. Knead while kneeling.

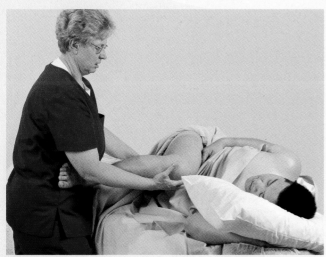

51. Joint movement.

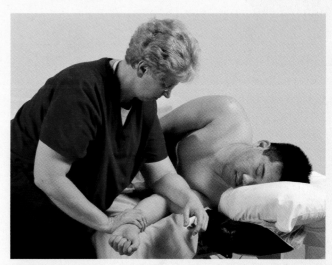

52. Arm. Compression/glide using forearm.

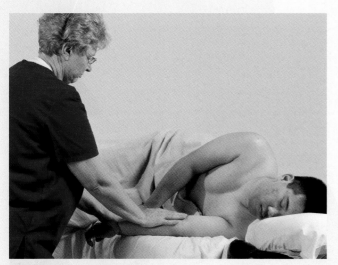

53. Glide using palm.

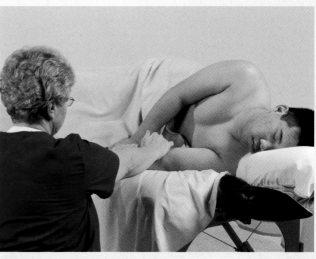

54. Knead while kneeling.

Continued

GENERAL MASSAGE PROTOCOL—cont'd

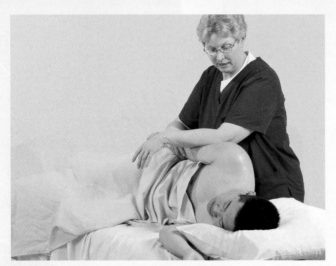

55. Move to opposite arm. Compression/glide.

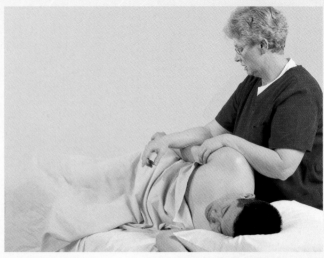

56. Change position to access forearm. Compression/glide using forearm.

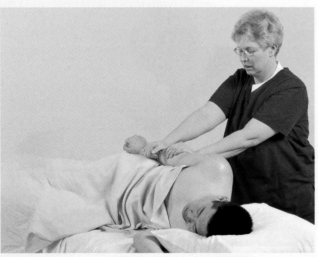

57. Knead arm.

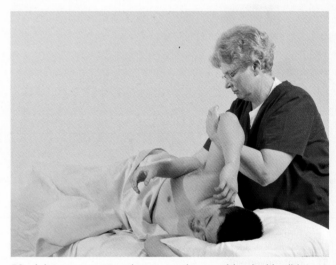

58. Joint movement and compression combined with glide.

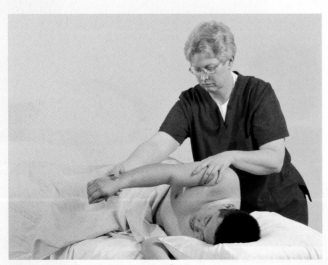

59. Joint movement and position arm.

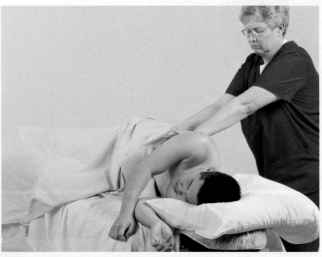

60. Knead lateral chest and back.

GENERAL MASSAGE PROTOCOL—cont'd

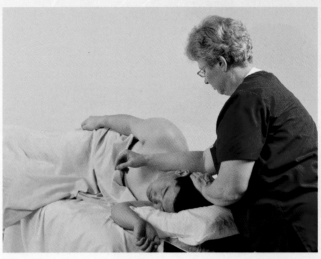

61. Compression of neck—stay behind the sternocleidomastoid muscle.

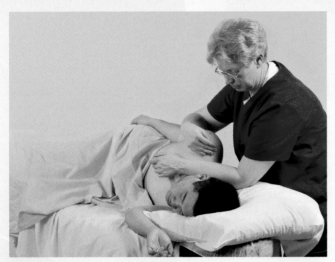

62. Compression of shoulder.

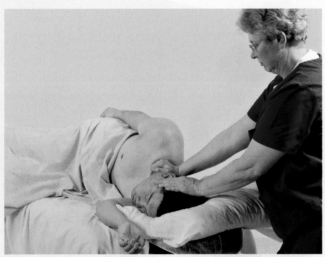

63. Knead neck.

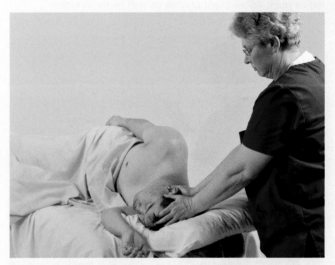

64. Massage the head. Repeat opposite side.

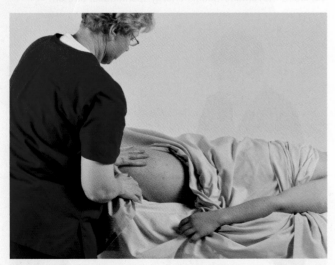

65. Turn client supine—begin with leg. Assess and palpate.

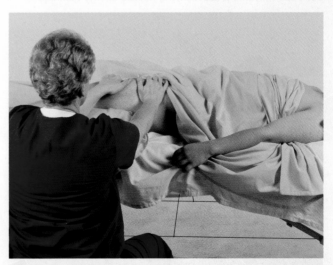

66. Knead anterior thigh.

Continued

GENERAL MASSAGE PROTOCOL—cont'd

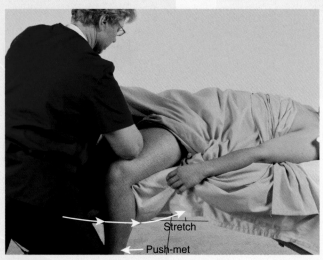

67. Position leg. Glide anterior thigh combined with muscle energy technique and lengthen and stretch using the therapist's leg as point where client pushes as well as for stretch.

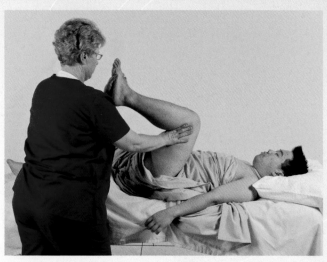

68. Joint movement of hip/assessment.

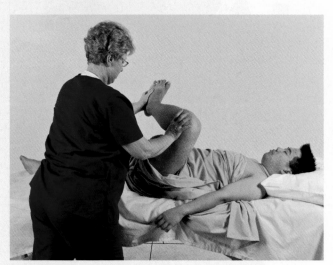

69. Joint movement/assessment, muscle energy techniques.

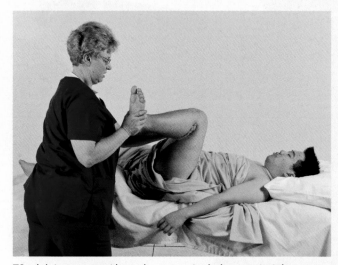

70. Joint movement/muscle energy techniques, stretch.

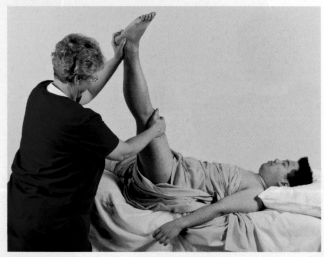

71. Assessment/joint movement, stretch (hip and knee).

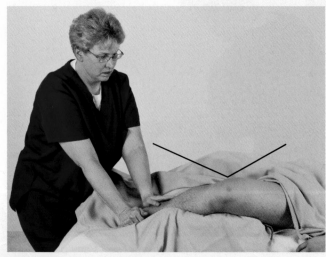

72. Position leg to massage foot, medial leg.

GENERAL MASSAGE PROTOCOL—cont'd

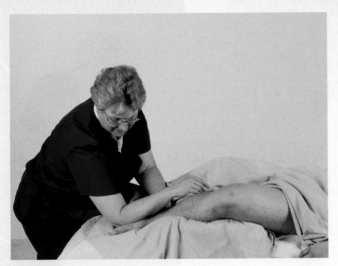

73. Compression of foot.

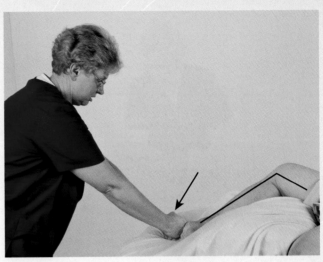

74. Compression of foot. Note: leg position.

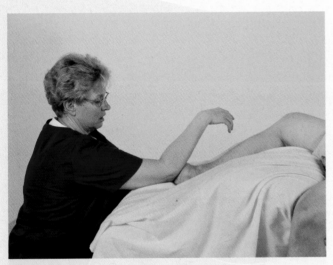

75. Compression of foot while therapist kneels.

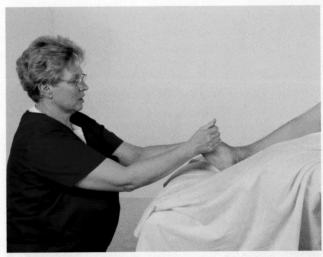

76. Stretch toes. Repeat other side.

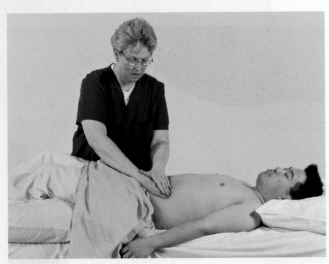

77. Massage abdomen.

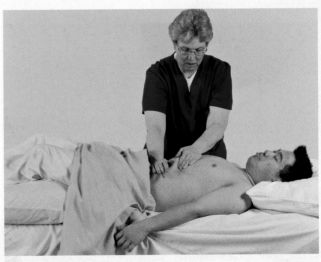

78. Knead abdomen.

Continued

GENERAL MASSAGE PROTOCOL—cont'd

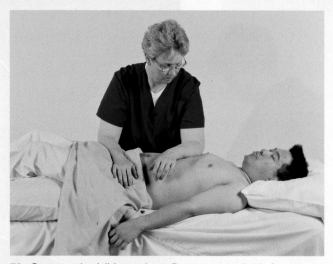

79. Compression/glide on chest. Drape appropriately for women.

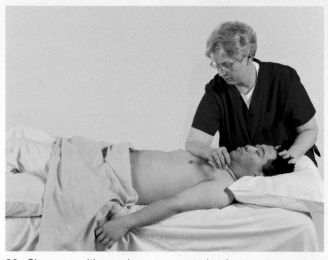

80. Change position and massage anterior thorax.

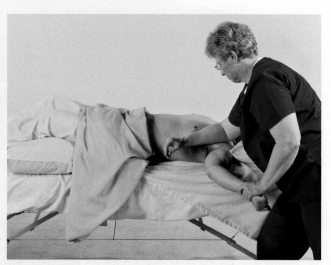

81. Move arm. Compression/glide on pectoralis muscle.

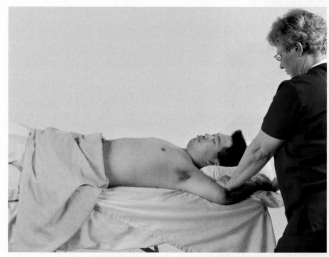

82. Position arm. Compression and kneading.

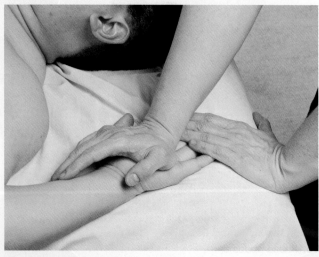

83. Compression of hand.

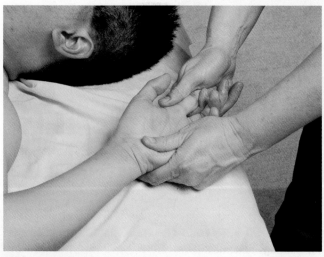

84. Massage fingers.

GENERAL MASSAGE PROTOCOL—cont'd

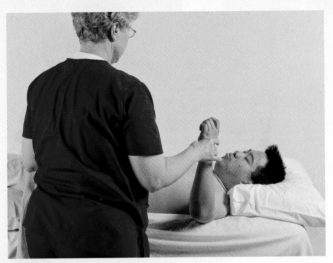

85. Joint movement of shoulder and elbow.

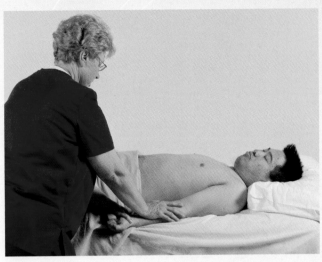

86. Position arm. Compress/glide forearm and arm.

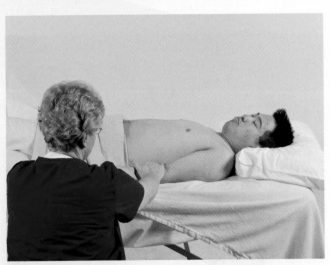

87. Kneading of forearm and arm, therapist kneeling.

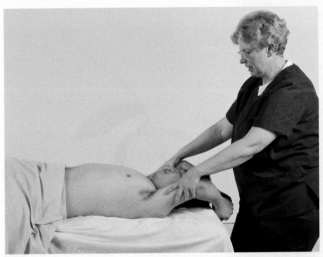

88. Bring arms up. Joint movement and muscle energy techniques.

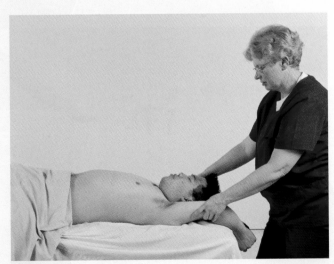

89. Lengthen and stretch.

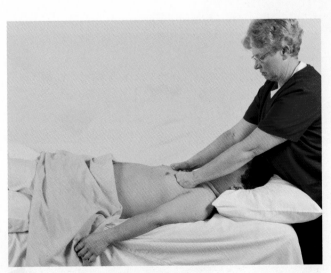

90. Compression of upper anterior thorax.

Continued

GENERAL MASSAGE PROTOCOL—cont'd

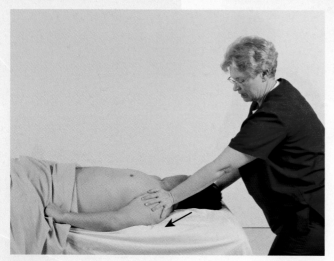

91. Joint movement of neck. Stretch is applied at shoulder.

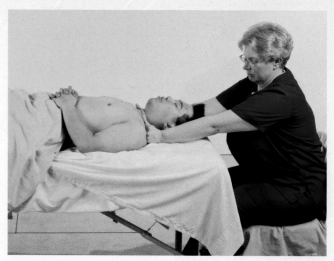

92. Compression of shoulder and neck massage, therapist seated.

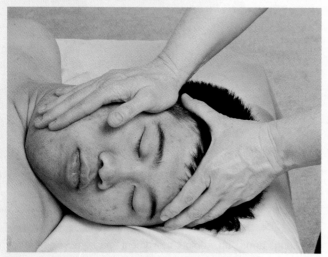

93. Compression/glide muscles of mastication.

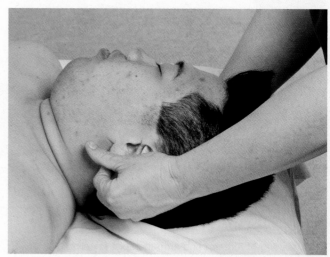

94. Ears.

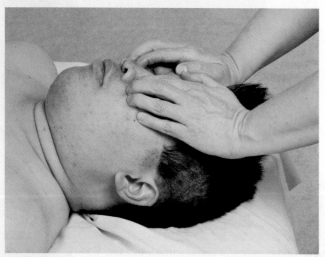

95. Face/compression of sinus points.

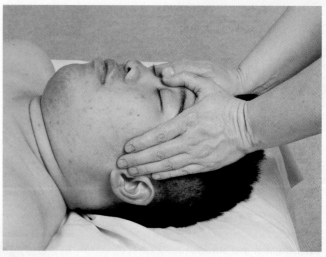

96. Finish.

GENERAL SEATED MASSAGE PROTOCOL

Massage methods can be adapted to the seated position. The accompanying photographs demonstrate how to apply massage to the various body regions using primarily compression and movement, because clothing typically is left on during a seated massage. (See the DVD for a complete demonstration of the general seated massage protocol.)

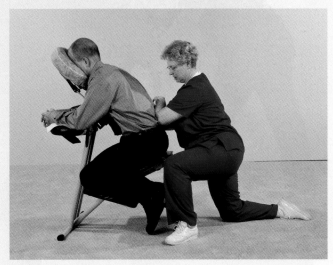

1. Forearm compression, standing.

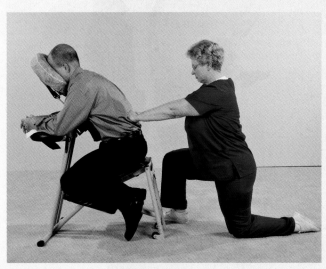

2. Fist compression, kneeling.

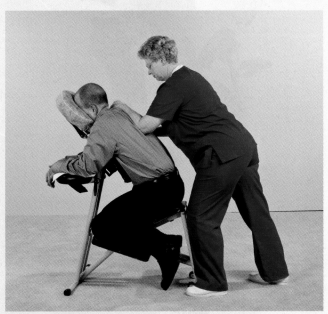

3. Forearm position, kneeling.

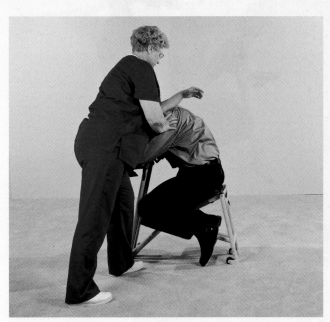

4. Forearm compression, shoulder.

Continued

GENERAL SEATED MASSAGE PROTOCOL—cont'd

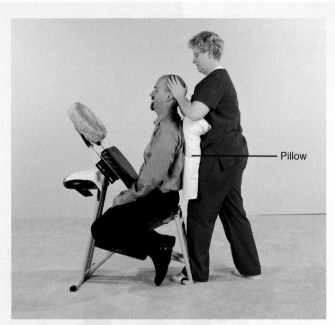

5. Position client against pillow.

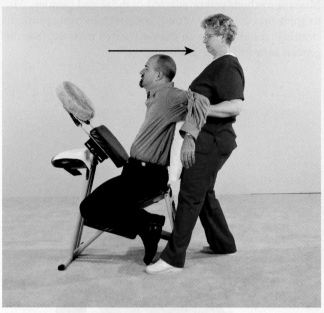

6. Stretch, lean back.

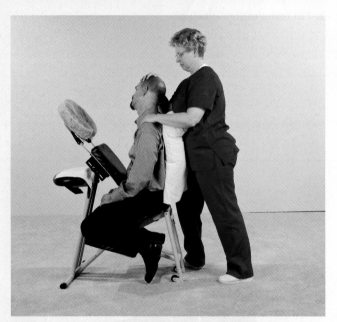

7. Movement of the neck.

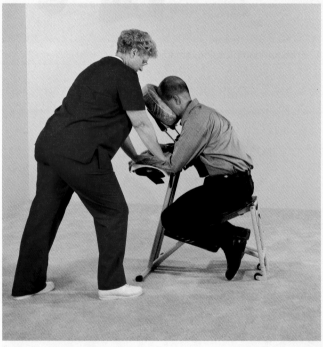

8. Palm compression, forearm.

GENERAL SEATED MASSAGE PROTOCOL—cont'd

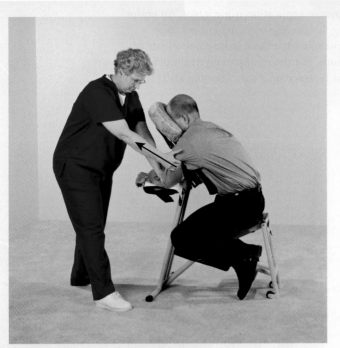

9. Pull back to massage upper arm.

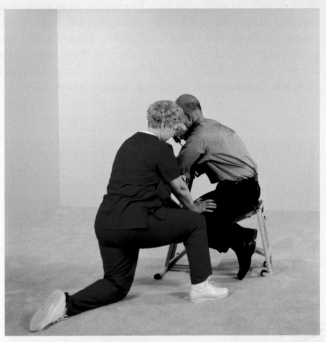

10. Kneel to compress thigh.

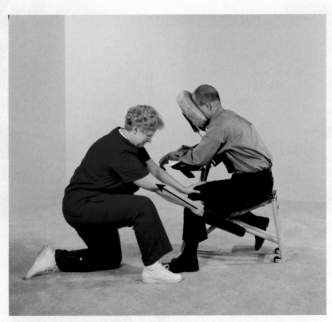

11. Pull and lean back to massage calf.

MAT MASSAGE PROTOCOL

1
10-3
The following series of photographs provides an example of massage application using a mat. An entire sequence is not provided, but the photographs show positioning, bolstering, sequencing, and body mechanics, along with examples of gliding, kneading, and compression, the three basic components of general massage. It is impossible to show all the massage variations, but the examples given should provide enough structure to allow you to begin to perfect techniques for massage on a mat. (See the DVD for a complete demonstration of the mat massage protocol.)

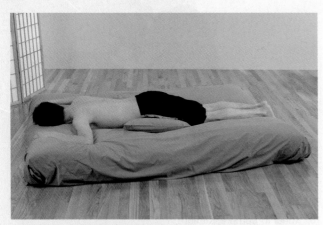

1. Client positioned prone on mat.

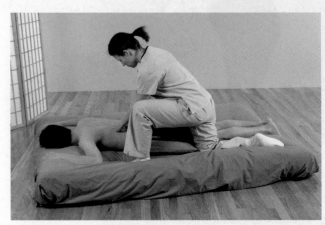

2. Kneeling body mechanics.

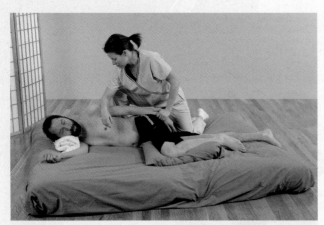

3. Side-lying using forearm compression/glide.

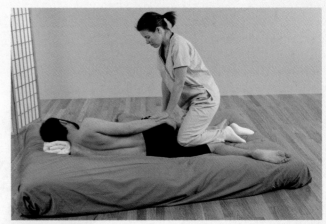

4. Using leg to apply compression.

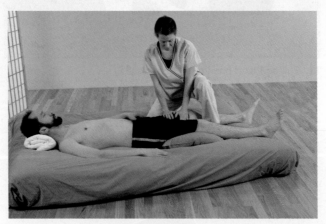

5. Working on legs in supine position.

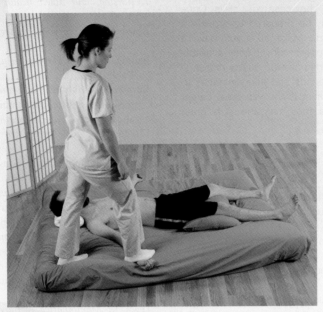

6. Using foot to perform massage.

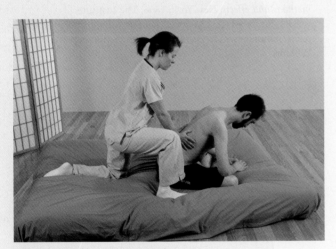

7. Back massage, client seated.

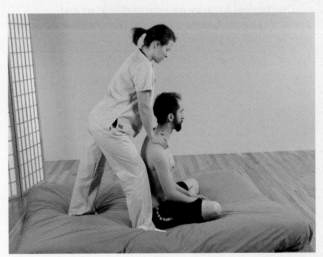

8. Shoulder and neck compression.

SUMMARY

Now that you have all the individual skills to give a great massage, your job is to practice using them in combination. It is common to be clumsy with massage applications at first. Skills evolve with experience and practice. Very few people, if any, do something perfectly on their first attempt. Expertise is a never-ending process of learning, modification, and change. If you work with a client-centered focus, allow the client's needs to direct the massage, and do not try to force a particular response; the client should experience beneficial results.

Massage manipulations and techniques can be combined to produce an infinite number of therapeutic massage applications. Give yourself permission to practice and improvise. As you practice, ask the client for feedback on how a particular application of a technique or massage manipulation feels and what its effects are. Always be open to innovation, and do not be afraid to experiment with new techniques.

ⓘ FOOT IN THE DOOR

Offering to provide a massage to the person interviewing you for a job is an excellent way to showcase your skills. Once you have your foot in the door, be prepared to provide a massage to potential employers. Make sure you have a uniform, massage table, and supplies conveniently available (i.e., in your car). If you consistently provide quality massage to clients, they will refer their friends and acquaintances to you. Referral from a satisfied client is the very best career builder there is. Incidentally, a foot massage is a great "massage sample."

ⓔvolve

http://evolve.elsevier.com/Fritz/fundamentals/
10-1 Review the variations of touch with a matching exercise.
10-2 Practice new vocabulary on types of force and techniques.
10-3 Practice identifying the direction and range of motion for the joints.
10-4 Review the suggested sequence for joint movement methods.
10-5 Check out the Evolve website for additional massage protocol video.

Don't forget to study for your certification and licensure exams! Review questions, along with weblinks, can be found on the Evolve website.

References

Anderson KE, Anderson LE, Glanze D, editors: *Mosby's medical, nursing, and allied health dictionary*, ed 6, St Louis, 2005, Mosby.

Beard G: *A history of massage technique*, ed 5, St Louis, 2007, Saunders.

Baumgartner AJ: *Massage in athletics*, Minneapolis, 1947, Brugess Publishing.

Burns DK, Wells MR: Gross range of motion in the cervical spine: the effects of osteopathic muscle energy technique in asymptomatic subjects, *J Am Osteopath Assoc* 106:137, 2006.

Chaitow L: *Muscle energy techniques*, Edinburgh, 2006, Churchill Livingstone.

Cyriax E: Some misconceptions concerning mechano-therapy, *Br J Physical Med* October 1938.

Greenman PE: *Principles of manual medicine*, ed 4, Baltimore, 2010, Lippincott Williams & Wilkins.

Kellogg JH: *The art of massage: a practical manual for the nurse, the student and the practitioner*, Kila, Mont, 2010, Kessinger Publishing.

Knott M, Voss D: *Proprioceptive neuromuscular facilitation: patterns and techniques*, ed 3, Baltimore, 1985, Lippincott Williams & Wilkins.

Lewit K: *Manipulative therapy in rehabilitation of the locomotor system*, ed 3, Oxford, 1998, Butterworth-Heinemann.

Taylor GH: *An illustrated sketch of the movement cure: its principal methods and effects*, New York, 1866, The Institute.

Travell JG, Simons DG: *Myofascial pain and dysfunction: the trigger point manual*, vol 2, Baltimore, 1999, Lippincott Williams & Wilkins.

Workbook Section

All Workbook activities can be done electronically online as well as here in the book. Answers are located on ⊖volve

Short Answer

1. What are the three effects massage techniques have on the body? Explain each one.

2. Which massage methods seem more mechanical?

3. Which methods seem more reflexive?

4. What are the seven aspects of quality of touch?

5. What is the importance of varying the quality of touch with regard to speed, rate, rhythm, and duration?

6. Why do you think that similar trends, applications, and methods continue to make up the body of knowledge of therapeutic massage?

7. What are the major differences between massage manipulations and massage techniques using joint motion?

8. What are the main uses for the holding position?

9. How does the massage practitioner first approach the client?

10. What is the distinguishing characteristic of gliding?

11. Why should deeper applications of gliding always move slowly?

12. What are some specific uses of the gliding massage manipulation?

13. What are the distinguishing qualities of kneading?

14. Why should the massage professional use kneading sparingly?

15. What conditions interfere with the use of kneading?

16. What are the physiologic effects of compression?

17. What are some things massage practitioners should remember to protect their hands and arms while doing compression?

18. Where are the best anatomic locations to do vibration? Why?

19. How is rocking different from shaking?

20. What is the strongest physiologic effect of percussion (tapotement)?

21. From where does the movement for percussion come?

22. What are the distinguishing characteristics of friction?

23. How long does friction need to be done to accomplish the desired results?

24. Describe two methods for applying friction.

25. Why does the use of joint movement and muscle energy techniques make massage manipulations more effective?

26. What are the three types of proprioceptors affected by movement techniques? What do they detect?

27. What are the two different types of joint movement described in this text?

28. What is the pathologic range-of-motion barrier?

29. Explain hand placement for joint movement.

30. What are the major uses of muscle energy techniques?

31. Describe the concept of lengthening.

32. What is the importance of positioning?

33. What types of muscle contraction are used for muscle energy techniques? Explain each one.

34. What is postisometric relaxation (PIR)?

35. What is reciprocal inhibition (RI)?

36. How do pulsed muscle energy methods differ from the other methods described?

37. What is the target muscle?

38. How much strength is required during the contraction for the muscle energy method to work?

39. When is direct manipulation of the muscle used?

40. When is positional release/strain-counterstrain used?

41. Define stretching.

42. Why should lengthening methods be used before stretching?

43. When might stretching be an inappropriate method to use?

44. What are the two basic types of stretch?

45. What is direction of ease and why is it important?

46. Explain the concept of massage as a mixture of techniques.

47. What is the goal of the general massage?

Matching I

Match the massage manipulation or technique with its description.

_____ 1. Active joint movement
_____ 2. Beating
_____ 3. Compression
_____ 4. Cross-directional stretching
_____ 5. Cupping
_____ 6. Gliding stroke
_____ 7. Friction
_____ 8. Hacking
_____ 9. Joint movement
_____ 10. Kneading
_____ 11. Lengthening
_____ 12. Longitudinal stretching
_____ 13. Manipulation
_____ 14. Muscle energy techniques
_____ 15. Passive joint movement
_____ 16. Positional release
_____ 17. Postisometric relaxation (PIR)
_____ 18. Proprioceptive neuromuscular facilitation (PNF)
_____ 19. Pulsed muscle energy
_____ 20. Reciprocal inhibition (RI)
_____ 21. Resting stroke
_____ 22. Rocking
_____ 23. Shaking
_____ 24. Skin rolling
_____ 25. Slapping
_____ 26. Stretching
_____ 27. Tapotement
_____ 28. Tapping
_____ 29. Techniques
_____ 30. Vibration

a. A type of alternating tapotement in which the massage therapist strikes the surface of the body with quick snapping movements

b. The movement of the joint through its normal range of motion

c. Assumption of a normal resting length by a muscle through the neuromuscular mechanism

d. A stretch applied along the fiber direction of the connective tissues and muscles

e. Tissue stretching that pulls and twists connective tissue against its fiber direction

f. Moving the body out of a position causing discomfort and into the direction it wants to go, thereby taking proprioception into a state of safety, which may allow it to stop signaling for protective spasm

g. Occurs after isometric contraction of a muscle, resulting from the activity of minute neural reporting stations called the *Golgi tendon bodies*

h. Application of muscle energy techniques that combine muscle contractions with stretching and muscular pattern retraining

i. Rhythmic movement of the body

j. Grasping and shaking a body area in a quick, loose movement; sometimes classified as rhythmic mobilization

k. A form of pétrissage that lifts skin

l. Movement of a joint through its range of motion by the client

m. Methods of therapeutic massage that provide sensory stimulation or mechanical alteration of the soft tissues of the body

n. Pressure exerted into the body to spread tissue against underlying structures; a massage manipulation sometimes classified with pétrissage/kneading

o. A fine or coarse tremulous movement that creates reflexive responses

p. A type of tapotement that uses a cupped hand; it is often used over the thorax

q. Horizontal strokes, applied with the fingers, hand, or forearm, that follow the fiber direction of the underlying muscle or fascial planes or a dermatome pattern

r. Circular or transverse movements that are focused on the underlying tissue and do not glide on the skin

s. Procedures that involve engaging the barrier and using minute, resisted contractions (usually 20 in 10 seconds), which introduces mechanical pumping and PIR or RI (depending on the muscles used)

t. Takes place when a muscle contracts, obliging its antagonist to relax to allow normal movement

u. The first stroke of the massage; the simple laying on of hands

v. A form of tapotement that uses a flat hand

w. Mechanical tension applied to lengthen the myofascial unit (muscles and fascia); the two types are longitudinal and cross-directional

x. A form of heavy tapotement that uses the fist

y. Springy, fast blows to the body to create rhythmic compression to the tissue; also called *percussion*

z. A type of tapotement done with the fingertips

aa. Skillful use of the hands in a therapeutic manner; massage manipulations focus on the soft tissues of the body and are not to be confused with joint manipulation using a high-velocity thrust

bb. Specific use of active contraction in individual muscles or groups of muscles to initiate a relaxation response;

activation of the proprioceptors to facilitate muscle tone, relaxation, and stretching

cc. Movement of jointed areas by the massage practitioner without the client's assistance

dd. Rhythmic rolling, lifting, squeezing, and wringing of soft tissue

Matching II

Match the movement activity with its proper description.

_____ 1. Arthrokinematic movement
_____ 2. Concentric isotonic contraction
_____ 3. Counterpressure
_____ 4. Eccentric isotonic contraction
_____ 5. Isometric contraction
_____ 6. Osteokinematic movements

a. Accessory movements that occur because of inherent laxity or joint play that exists in each joint; these essential movements occur passively with movement of the joint and are not under voluntary control

b. During the contraction of a muscle, the massage practitioner applies a counterforce but allows the client to move, bringing the origin and insertion of the target muscle together against the pressure

c. Flexion, extension, abduction, adduction, and rotation; also referred to as *physiologic movements*

d. A contraction in which the effort of the muscle, or group of muscles, is exactly matched by a counterpressure so that no movement occurs, only effort

e. During the extension of a muscle, the massage practitioner applies a counterforce but allows the client to move the muscle, enabling the origin and insertion to separate

f. The force produced by the muscles of a specific area, designed to match the effort exactly (isometric contraction) or partially (isotonic contraction)

Problem-Solving Scenarios

1. A client has achy legs. She also has a history of varicose veins. This contraindicates direct massage of the area. What methods can be used to relax the legs?

2. A client has very sensitive skin that cannot tolerate any type of lubricant. What massage methods can you use that do not involve lubricant?

3. A client's nose becomes stuffy and he gets a sinus headache when he lies on his stomach. How will you give him a massage?

Assess Your Competencies

Now that you have studied this chapter, you should be able to:

- Evaluate massage manipulations based on seven criteria
- Use massage manipulations to apply mechanical force to the soft tissue
- Incorporate movement of the joints as an aspect of massage application
- Incorporate muscle energy techniques into the massage application
- Incorporate stretching into the massage application when appropriate
- Perform a full-body massage using the methods and techniques presented in the chapter
- Organize massage methods and techniques for application in four positions
- Explain the basic theories of the physiologic effects of massage methods and techniques

Now, write a short summary of the content of this chapter based on the preceding list of competencies. Use a conversational tone, as if you were explaining to someone (e.g., a client, prospective employer, co-worker, or other interested person). Write the paper as if you were having a conversation and explaining the importance of the information and skills to the development of the massage profession.

Next, in small student discussion groups, share your thoughts with your classmates and compare and contrast how you presented the information. In discussing the content, look for similarities, differences, and potential possibilities for misunderstanding the information as well as examples of clear, concise description.

Professional Application

A massage professional finds that he becomes fatigued with the style of massage he tends to provide, which consists mostly of gliding, kneading, and percussion. He would like to be able to perform massage more effectively. What recommendations would you make?

Assessment Procedures for Developing a Care/Treatment Plan

 http://evolve.elsevier.com/Fritz/fundamentals/

KEY TERMS

Applied kinesiology	Palpation
Assessment	Phasic muscles
End-feel	Postural muscles
Kinesiology	Rapport
Neurologic muscle testing	Resourceful compensation
Orthopedic tests	Strength testing

As you begin your education in massage therapy, it is important that you understand the value of the sequence and general flow of the massage application. Modeling precise massage routines is a valuable learning exercise; however, after you grasp the concepts, the routine must evolve to meet the unique needs of the individual client. Massage practitioners who have the ability to modify and alter the application of therapeutic massage are better able to serve their clients. People do not fit neatly into a routine sequence of massage techniques. To achieve the best results, the student must use the concepts learned from performing the routines to design an application based on physiologic outcomes, rather than trying to make the client fit the routine.

Instead of providing the structure of a precise, step-by-step routine, this chapter teaches you to perform an assessment to evaluate current function and ways to determine short- and long-term outcome goals for the client. Because most of the physiologic changes and benefits of massage result from the most basic technical skills, expertise comes from the decisions made in applying those skills. The practitioner's ability to make those decisions depends on his or her ability to gather the client's history data, perform assessment and analysis, and interpret the information collected during assessment. Then, with the information gathered and the client outcomes determined, the massage methods and variations (depth of pressure, drag, frequency, direction, speed, and rhythm) are identified to develop an individualized treatment plan.

The assessment process can be as simple as ruling out contraindications for a one-time session in a personal service environment (e.g., day spa, cruise ship, resort) or as comprehensive as determining a client's needs for therapeutic massage provided as a health care component (e.g., as part of a rehabilitation or pain management program or in the development of coping strategies for addressing the physical effects of anxiety disorder). The care/treatment plan also can be simple (e.g., providing a 1-hour vacation from daily stress, a present for Mother's Day or Father's Day, or a session of pleasure and pampering for a client) or complex (e.g., using massage to aid the management of asthma, depression, stroke rehabilitation, side effects caused by chemotherapy, and sports training protocols).

This chapter also presents the assessment skills a practitioner needs to function effectively with supervision in a health care setting, providing massage as part of a comprehensive treatment plan developed by health care professionals. The massage professional should be able to participate in this process by providing reliable information to be considered in the development of the treatment plan. These skills exceed those usually required in the personal service massage setting; however, as more employment opportunities open in the health care setting, it is important to be able to function as part of a multidisciplinary health care team. The ability to reason clinically at this level supports the effectiveness of all massage interactions, be it for relaxation and pleasure outcomes or for the management of complex health conditions.

To understand the results of the massage session, the student must learn to separate assessment information obtained before, during, and after the massage from methods of intervention. To support the learning process, this chapter is divided into two distinct areas:

- Assessment procedures
- Interpretation of assessment information with general suggestions for massage intervention

Always begin each massage session with this question, "What information do I need to develop a safe, effective massage therapy treatment plan for this client?"

ASSESSMENT

SECTION OBJECTIVES

Chapter objective covered in this section:

1. Conduct an effective client interview.

Using the information presented in this section, the student will be able to perform the following:

- Explain the importance of assessment
- Identify resourceful compensation

- Define rapport and establish rapport with a client
- Interview a client effectively
- Use effective listening skills
- Use a sample script for the assessment interview process

Assessment is a learned skill. The ability to incorporate this skill into massage sessions enhances the quality of treatment given by the massage professional. **Assessment** is the collection and interpretation of information provided by the client, the client's consent advocates (parent or guardian), and the referring medical professionals, in addition to information gathered by the massage practitioner. In a growing number of clinical health care settings, the massage professional's assessment is considered in the treatment plan developed by the multidisciplinary health care team. Therefore, being able to perform standard assessment and charting procedures is crucial. Chapter 4 introduced these concepts; this chapter refines and integrates them. Although the massage professional observes, interprets, and makes decisions based on information gathered during assessment procedures, it is important to remember that the massage professional is not equipped to diagnose any specific medical condition or to treat one except under the direct supervision of a licensed medical professional.

Components of the Assessment

For the massage practitioner, the information gathered during a premassage assessment has four purposes:

- To determine whether the client should be referred to a medical professional
- To discover any cautions that would modify the massage application
- To obtain input from the client that is used to help develop the massage care/treatment plan
- To design the best massage for the client; specifically, the types of methods used and the mechanical forces generated by those methods, in addition to the proper application of depth of pressure, drag, direction, speed, rhythm, frequency, and duration of each method, to achieve the desired physiologic outcome (Figure 11-1)

In reality, the assessment and the application of massage techniques are almost the same thing. Often massage manipulations and techniques are used during a massage first to evaluate the tissue; then, altered slightly in intensity, to support tissue-appropriate change; and finally to reassess for tissue changes. To aid student learning, the two approaches have been separated.

Without assessment, treatment focuses on only certain areas of the client's body; this may prevent the massage practitioner from noting a larger pattern of dysfunction and its consequences. Therefore, massage professionals must keep in mind that:

- Assessment does not change a condition; rather, it is an attempt to understand it.
- Interventions (e.g., massage applications) change the abnormal findings revealed by the assessment.

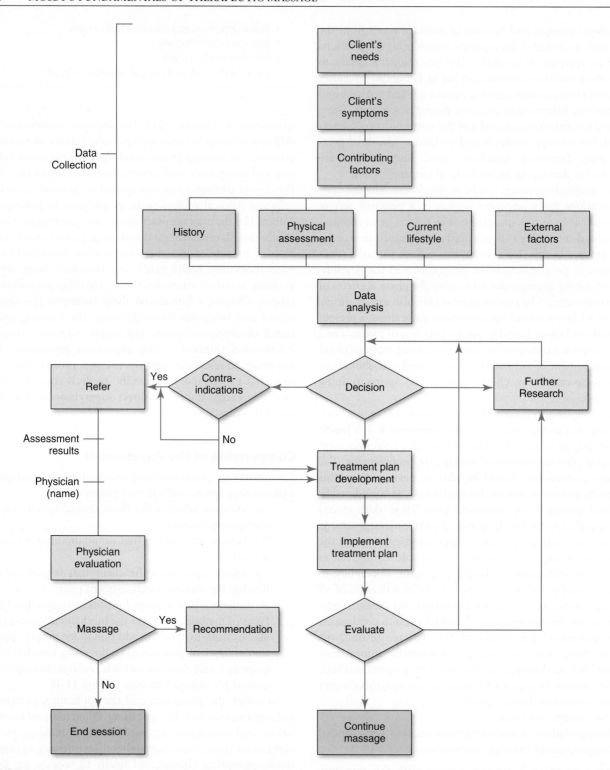

FIGURE 11-1 Algorithm for the development of a care/treatment plan.

Compensation Patterns

Compensation patterns are the result of the body's adjustment to some sort of dysfunction. Years of clinical experience have taught many therapists that most symptoms are compensatory patterns. Some problems are recent, and some qualify for archeologic exploration, having developed in early life and been compounded over time. Compensatory patterns often are complex, but the client's body frequently can show us the way if we will listen to the story it tells. The importance of compensation must be considered in an assessment.

Resourceful Compensation

Assessment identifies what is functioning normally, what is abnormal, and whether the abnormal condition is problematic (maladaptive), requiring attention, or is a resourceful and successful adaptive compensation.

Patterns of resourceful compensation develop when the body has been required to adapt to some sort of trauma or repetitive use pattern. Permanent resourceful adaptive changes, although not as efficient as optimum functioning, are the best pattern the body can develop in response to an irreversible change in the system. Resourceful compensation must be supported, not eliminated, because determining whether the changes in the body are helpful or harmful can be difficult.

The main reason for physical change in the body is adaptive demand. Recall that anatomy is form and physiology is function.

Form and function influence each other. If a person breaks a bone, the healing process changes the shape of the bone to some extent; the bone typically becomes thicker at the point of the healed fracture. This can be both a help and a hindrance to the body. For example, the healed bone may be strong, but the changes in the bone's shape caused by the thickening process may result in impingement on another tissue or interference with range of motion.

This situation often arises when the clavicle is broken. It usually heals well, but because of the clavicle's proximity to the ribs, the change in shape might cause pinching or rubbing of structures between the clavicle and the ribs, resulting in nerve impingement, inflammation, and pain. Massage cannot change the shape of bone. However, it can be used to maintain as much tissue pliability as possible, which may reduce symptoms.

Another example of resourceful compensation is swelling and muscle tension around a joint sprain. The increased stiffness of the area prevents movement during the early stages of healing, almost in the same way that a cast does. This type of compensation should not be altered. However, if these tissue changes persist into the later stages of healing, they will interfere with a return to normal function. Massage may be used to reduce unproductive tissue changes and support a full return to function.

In massage, a general guideline for detecting resourceful compensation is that the body resists the changes introduced by massage. This resistance to change may occur as follows:

- During massage, the client stiffens or flinches away from the application. This also may be caused by inappropriate application of a technique. However, if the application style is altered and the tissues continue to resist change, a beneficial reason likely exists for the adaptation in the body. Do not force tissue changes. Massage the area in general and manage symptoms.
- Immediately after the massage, the client indicates that he feels good and really loose. Then 24 to 48 hours after the massage, the client is sore and his symptoms have increased. This occurs when the massage destabilizes a resourceful pattern.

During assessment procedures, if you are unable to come up with a logical reason for the tissue and movement changes, the best course is to use general methods in the area and to avoid aggressive specific procedures during the massage. When resourceful compensation is present, therapeutic massage methods are used to support the altered pattern and prevent any greater increase in postural distortion than is necessary to support the body change (compensation).

Some compensatory patterns develop to accommodate short-term conditions that do not require permanent adaptation. Having a leg in a cast and walking on crutches for a time is a classic example. The body catching itself during an "almost" fall is another classic setup pattern. Unfortunately, the body often habituates these patterns and maintains them well beyond their usefulness. Over time, the body begins to show symptoms of pain or inefficient function or both.

A simple means of differentiating resourceful from unresourceful compensation is as follows:

1. If the client reports improvement immediately after the massage and at least 50% of the improvement remains 24 to 48 hours later, the compensation pattern likely is reversible. Massage application is therapeutic change (see Chapter 6).
2. If the client reports improvement immediately after massage, but 24 to 48 hours later the symptoms return at the same or greater intensity, the compensation pattern likely is resourceful and cannot be reversed at this time. Massage application becomes condition management.
3. If the client has no significant reduction in symptoms immediately after massage (adaptive capacity is exhausted), only palliative care is appropriate.

Dysfunction as a Solution

No education on assessment is complete without a discussion of whether the pattern discovered is a problem or a solution. The previous section defined resourceful compensation as the best that can be expected under the circumstances. The concept of dysfunction as a solution is similar to the patterns of resourceful compensation. If all the information gathered during assessment can be viewed as an attempt at a solution, this broadens the practitioner's perspective in the decision making required for effective massage care plans. As discussed in Chapter 6, it is important to consider the client's whole situation in determining whether a condition is a dysfunction or a solution. For example:

- A workaholic client has continual tension headaches. When the client has a headache, she tends to slow her pace and work fewer hours. Is the headache a problem or a solution?
- A massage therapist who regularly provides massage sessions for 30 to 40 clients a week develops a low back condition that prevents her from working with more than 10 clients a week. Management of the low back condition requires the massage professional to receive regular massages, exercise regularly, and manage stress. She has to cut her workload, which opens time for teaching and community service. Is the low back dysfunction a problem or a solution?

Understanding the bigger picture when analyzing assessment information adds a very important dimension to the development of essential and appropriate massage care plans. View each pattern as a solution and realize that problems are solutions that no longer provide benefit. Solutions are to be supported. Problems must be understood and other possibilities offered for a solution. Massage effectively provides both for the body.

Establishing Rapport

The client is the most important resource involved in the assessment process. The four primary skills a massage professional needs for the process of gathering information from a client are:

- The ability to establish rapport
- Keen observation
- Successful interviewing methods
- Active listening

Rapport is the development of a relationship based on mutual trust and harmony. It is the massage professional's responsibility to establish a sense of rapport with clients. The best way to begin establishing rapport is to learn and use the client's name. The massage practitioner needs to show a genuine interest in the person that goes beyond the problems and goals the person presents. What happens to a person affects the whole being.

Rapport is enhanced if the massage professional uses words, a tone of voice, and body language similar to those of the client. The process of rapport involves neurons in the brain, called *mirror neurons,* that coordinate the process of looking and acting like the person with whom we are communicating. This process is a very instinctual survival mechanism. If the body language and tone of voice are similar (like a dance), the client and massage therapist connect. If the mirroring is not established for some reason, the people communicating will feel odd and may avoid contact. This is an overlooked issue in client retention. Unless the client feels rapport, he or she will not be able to relax during the massage and likely will avoid further contact.

Some practitioners may have difficulty mirroring their mannerisms or tone of voice to their potential clients, which may result in difficulty establishing rapport. Social conditioning or some sort of physical issue may be the cause of this disconnect. For example, if a person has suffered a closed head injury, he may not be able to modulate eye contact or body language. If the reason for the disconnect is not evident, the potential client will not understand why he or she feels uncomfortable.

Medication also can interfere with rapport mechanisms, as do almost all substances of abuse. Massage professionals who have a physical condition that makes "mirroring" difficult for them should briefly explain the situation to clients and coworkers. Massage professionals who find that they have clients with whom they are out of sync must learn more effective rapport skills. This may require taking communication classes or seeking help to understand the nature of their own behavior and that of the client.

How to Observe

Attention to detail and the client's needs provide a sensitive, well-trained massage therapist with essential information.

Clients notice the difference between a massage professional who takes the time to honor the client's space and adjust to it and one who tries to make the client fit into a routine method of massage application. During the initial conversation, it is important to pay very close attention to the client visually. If the practitioner has a visual impairment, information gathered from the interview and physical assessment replaces visual assessment. An effective therapist uses all the senses—hearing, sight, smell, touch, and intuition—in the assessment of the client.

At the beginning of each session, the massage therapist should get a sense of the client's general presence. How well does the client move and breathe? Does the client's presence suggest sympathetic or parasympathetic dominance? Sympathetic dominance is the display of restlessness, anxiety, fear, anger, agitation, elation, or exuberance. Parasympathetic dominance is indicated by a generally relaxed appearance, contentment, slowness or, in the extreme, depression. Because therapeutic massage can either stimulate or relax, this needs to be considered in the massage design.

If a client is active and exuberant (sympathetic dominance), the initial massage approach and the massage practitioner's energy level need to match the client's energy level. If the focus of the session is to calm the client, the therapist begins to slow down as the massage progresses and may introduce appropriate rhythmic entrainment approaches to provide a calming effect.

If the client is tired or moderately depressed, the therapist should proceed slowly in the initial pace of the massage. During the session, the energy and activity level of the massage practitioner and the methods used can be increased as the client's energy increases. In general, excessive sympathetic activation would be balanced by a relaxing, full-body rhythmic massage with a general nonspecific approach. Excessive parasympathetic activation would be balanced by a stimulating massage with a specific focus. If the client seems "out of sorts," operating more as a collection of parts than the sum of the parts, entrainment processes may be off. The centered, coordinated presence of the professional providing a harmonized, rhythmic approach to the massage is beneficial.

Gestures

People tend to be consistent with their gestures and word phrases within their internal body language system. However, body language is as individual as the person. Particular gestures or styles of body language cannot be generalized to mean one specific thing. The professional is responsible for learning what a gesture means for a particular individual.

Because of nervous system patterns and the basic universal body language connected with survival emotions such as fear, anger, distress, and happiness, some body language is fairly consistent from person to person. However, the massage practitioner cannot assume that a certain gesture means the same thing with every person. Time and careful observation are required to decipher an individual's body language code. This is done by watching for repetitive body language and connecting the particular gesture or posture to the client's mood and state and the content of the conversation. Eventually the client

🔍 PROFICIENCY EXERCISE 11-1

1. Watch people in a public place, such as a mall or an airport. Is the general presence of each person you observe sympathetic or parasympathetic in nature?

2. Ask 10 people to explain a physical ache or pain to you. Watch their gestures carefully. What similarities do you notice in their explanations?

3. Walk into your own treatment space or that of a fellow student. Look at it the way a client would see it. Are the sheets wrinkle free; the lotion dispensed from a closed, single-use container; the counters clean; the doorknobs free of a greasy feeling; and the lighting adequate but not glaring? Also, do you see a therapist who is calm and welcoming, not nervous, rushed, or unengaged?

repeats the body language patterns often enough that the individual pattern is evident.

The skilled massage practitioner pays attention to where and how a client indicates a problem on the body. These gestures often reveal whether a client has a muscle, joint, or visceral problem. It also is important for the therapist to observe the client's body language and nonverbal responses while discussing various topics. Everything the person does is important. Everyone's behavior has a pattern, and all the bits of information combine to reveal that pattern (Proficiency Exercise 11-1).

The following are common gestures and indications.

- A finger pointed to a specific area suggests hyperactivity of an acupressure or a motor point or possibly a joint problem. The meaning of the pointing depends on the area indicated.
- If a finger is pointed to a specific area but the hand then swipes in a certain direction, a trigger point problem may be the issue.
- Grabbing, pulling, or holding and moving an area as if to stretch it often indicates muscle or fascial shortening.
- If movement is needed to show the area of tightness, the area may need muscle lengthening combined with muscle energy work to prepare for stretching and for resetting of neuromuscular patterns.
- If the client moves into a position and then acts as if stuck, the area may need connective tissue stretching.
- Drawing lines on the body may indicate nerve entrapment in the fascial planes or grooves.

Interviewing and Listening: Subjective Aspect of Assessment

Communication skills first were presented in Chapter 2. These skills are used during interviewing sessions and throughout client-practitioner interactions.

The point of the interview is to help the client communicate his or her health history and to reveal the goal for the massage. During an interview information is only gathered, not interpreted—resist the urge to try to understand what all the information means. Interpretation comes after all

the information has been gathered, which may take several sessions. Any massage provided at this initial stage is a form of assessment. Although the client experiences generalized benefits from the assessment-focused massage, only when sufficient information has been gathered can the client's expected outcomes be specifically addressed.

When you speak to a client, it is important to use words the client can understand. Although professionalism is important, medical terminology need not be used if it will confuse the client. If the client uses a word that is unclear, the therapist should ask what the person means. Asking for clarification enhances knowledge and understanding of the information obtained from the client. Do not use slang or jargon when speaking in the professional setting to either coworkers or clients.

Certain specific information must be obtained from the client. The massage professional can easily forget to ask the important questions. A client information form provides a framework for obtaining necessary and important information during the interview.

Open-ended questions encourage conversation. Questions that can be answered with only one word should be avoided.

EXAMPLE

The question, "Have you ever had a professional massage before?" requires the client to answer only "Yes" or "No." A better question would be, "What is your experience with therapeutic massage?" This question requires the client to give more detail when answering.

When listening, the massage practitioner must do nothing but listen. You cannot listen while thinking about what is going to be said or while writing or interpreting information. An active listener nods or shows other signs of interest to encourage the person to continue speaking.

Many people need time to sort out their thoughts and feelings and develop their statements. The conversation should proceed slowly, and the client should never be rushed. Some people rehearse what they say internally before speaking. They speak with pauses between statements, and you must wait for the client to complete thoughts before speaking. If interrupted, the client often forgets what she was going to tell you. Other clients talk quite a bit. They may need to sort through their information by saying it aloud. Practitioners who give the person their full attention and observe what makes the client most comfortable find it easier to resist the urge to treat everyone in the same manner.

When the client provides information, the practitioner should restate what the client has said. The client then has the opportunity to correct any information and is reassured that the therapist was listening and understands what has been said. It is amazing how often information is misinterpreted (Proficiency Exercise 11-2).

In addition, a competent professional is careful about having preconceived ideas and keeps an open mind while the assessment is in progress (Box 11-1).

Box 11-1 **Sample Script for the Assessment Interview**

1. **Greet the client. Smile, introduce yourself, extend your hand, and give a firm handshake.**
   Example:
   • Hi, my name is Bailey, and I will be your massage therapist.

2. **Initiate conversation. Ask how the client would like to be addressed: Mr., Mrs., Ms., or by first name. Explain the assessment process and the forms used. Include information on confidentiality.**
   Example:
   • Your name is Jane Smith, correct? Do you prefer to be called Ms. Smith or Mrs. Smith, or by your first name?
   • Because this is your first massage session, we will be doing an information gathering process.
   • Together we will gather information about your health history relevant to massage so that I will be able to plan the safest and most beneficial massage for you.
   • I will use two forms. One is a history form, on which I will record the information you give me. The other is a physical assessment form, on which I will record the results of various physical assessment procedures. Examples of these procedures include a postural symmetry assessment, in which I will compare the left and right and front and back of your body for evenness; muscle assessments to identify how the muscles are functioning; and joint assessments for stability and ease of movement.
   • I will analyze this information, and we will discuss it to determine whether there may be any reason for you to be evaluated by another health professional (referral) and also to determine the goals for the massage outcome. Finally, we will agree on a massage care plan.
   • This process is always more extensive for the first visit.
   • When you return for future massage sessions, we recap what was done in the last session and update the records for anything new.
   • At least once a year we will again do a comprehensive reassessment and review of the outcomes of previous massage sessions.
   • I want to assure you that all the information gathered will be maintained in a secure system to protect your privacy.
   • You may have a copy of your records at anytime.
   • If I ask a question and you do not wish to answer, feel free to tell me.
   • At all times, if you are uncomfortable with any conversation, questions, or massage assessment or method, please tell me right away.
   • Please feel free at anytime to ask questions or give me feedback and please do not be concerned about hurting my feelings. I depend on you to make sure that what I am doing during the assessment and massage is safe and beneficial.
   • Do you have any questions or comments?

3. **Give the client time to respond.**

4. **Begin the health history.**
   Example:
   • Let's start with your reasons for wanting a massage.
   • What results do you want from the massage? For example, is your goal better sleep, reduced neck stiffness, decreased knee pain, more energy, a minivacation from life?

   • Another way to think about your goals for massage would be to tell me how you want to feel or what you want to be able to do more easily after the massage.

5. **Give the client the history form.**
   Example:
   • I am going to use the history form to help me ask questions so that I stay on track and do not forget something.
   • Would you like to fill out this form first and then we can discuss it, or would you prefer that I ask the questions and fill in the responses you give?

6. **Follow the sequence on the form to gather the information. Any areas indicating some sort of past illness, injury, experience with massage, and so forth should be explored in more detail.**
   Example:
   • I noticed that you indicated that you are taking some vitamins and herbs.
   • Would you please tell me what you are taking and the reason for it. Sometimes I have to alter the massage because of an unwanted effect that massage could cause.
   • For example, if you are taking fish oil and aspirin, both of which are anticoagulants and can thin the blood, I would want to make sure that the depth of pressure and the type of application did not cause any bruising.
   Example:
   • Based on the information you provided on the history form, am I correct that you have a family history of cardiac disease?
   • You indicate that your mother and grandmother both had heart disease.
   • Have you been monitored by your physician for these types of conditions?
   • What is your current health status with regard to cardiovascular disease?

7. **After completing the history form, summarize the information.**
   Example:
   • Let's see if I understand all this data.
   • Your primary reasons for receiving massage are relieving shoulder stiffness to see whether that reduces the frequency of tension headaches, and you would like relaxation, and pleasure and pampering. Correct?
   • These are all reasonable goals and within my scope of practice.
   • Since your doctor suggested massage for the headaches, we know she is aware of your condition and has made a diagnosis.
   • If she likes, I can forward her the summaries of the results of the massage sessions.
   • You will need to sign a release of information form for me to be able to do this.
   • It may be enough for you to keep her updated.
   • You indicated that you will take over-the-counter pain medication for the tension headache, so please tell me before each massage session if you have taken any medication, when you took it, and what you took so I can alter the massage application if necessary.

Box 11-1   Sample Script for the Assessment Interview—Cont'd

- I will also observe the condition of your skin, because you indicated that you work out in the sun and you have had some areas of possible skin cancer treated.
- When I do massage, I see parts of your body that you usually do not, such as your back or your neck.
- If I find any areas that look as if the doctor should see them, I will let you know, and then please follow up with your physician. Okay?
- Is there anything you would like to add or do you have any questions?

8. **Respectfully wait for a moment, then move to the physical assessment process.**
    Example:
    - Now we will begin the physical assessment.
    - Actually, the entire time I am giving you a massage, I am performing assessment.
    - When I move your tissues by gliding and kneading, for example, I am performing palpation assessment.
    - It is kind of like listening to your tissues with my hand or forearm.
    - Your skin, fascia, muscles, and joints give me information, such as hot, cold, wet, dry, rough, smooth, stiff, short, long, and so forth.
    - I will also move your joints during the massage to assess for range of motion.
    - Sometimes I might ask you to maintain a position I place you in or to push or pull against me.
    - These are all forms of muscle testing assessment.
    - I will ask for feedback; for example, "Is this painful?" or "Does this feel stiff to you?"
    - Even if I don't ask the question and you have those types of sensations, tell me, okay?
    - If the way your tissues feel or your joints move seems to be somewhat less than optimum, I may do a more specific assessment.
    - When I do these assessments, I am checking to see whether there might be something I need to be particularly cautious about or whether I think I should refer you to your doctor.
    - For example, if I think your leg feels swollen, I might press into it to identify whether the swelling is pitting edema or simple edema.
    - I may ask a couple of questions to see whether the situation has a logical explanation; for example, "Have you been sitting a long time?" or "Is it near your menstrual cycle?"
    - If the condition does not appear to have a logical explanation, I may suggest that you see your physician.
    - Before the massage I will do postural and walking assessments and some simple assessments to check for efficient breathing function.
    - I may do some specific assessment procedures based on something you tell me.
    - For example, if you tell me your low back is aching, I might have you bend forward, sideways, and backward.
    - After the massage we will redo some of the assessments to see whether any change has occurred, either for the better or for the worse.

- This is called postassessment, and the information collected helps me plan the next massage session.
- I also will explain things during the massage.
- These assessment procedures will be performed in a relaxing way so that you are also pampered and feel relaxed at the end of the massage.
- Any questions or comments?

9. **Hand the client the physical assessment form and explain it briefly.**
    Example:
    - This is the form I will use so that I stay organized.
    - I will show you how to do the things I ask you to do.
    - For example, if I want you to move your shoulder a certain way, I will demonstrate first.
    - If anything I ask you to do is uncomfortable or painful, stop doing it and tell me.
    - If any of the assessments reproduce the symptoms you are experiencing, such as recreate headache pain, tell me right away.
    - I really appreciate your participation, so let's get started.

10. **Use the physical assessment form to perform the assessments. Do as many as possible as part of the massage. All of the passive and active joint movement assessments and palpation assessments can be incorporated into the massage session.**

11. **Summarize your findings.**
    Example:
    - Because your physician indicates that the pain in your knee is likely osteoarthrosis, I performed various assessments to help me determine the safest and most beneficial approach to massage. Because there is joint pathology, massage will be best targeted to managing symptoms and supporting movement.
    - There appears to be some fascia binding in the area of the surgical scar that could be contributing to the stiffness in your shoulder. Massage should be able to loosen that up somewhat. We will re-evaluate in five or six sessions to see whether the connective tissue methods have been beneficial.
    - Your left ankle moves beyond the normal range of motion. This is called hypermobility, and often the joint is unstable. You told me you had sprained it a couple of times and that could be the cause. You also said that it does not bother you, so unless you ask or I think it may be contributing to some other situation, such as knee pain, I will include the area in the general massage application but not specifically target it for intervention.

12. **In writing up the history and the physical assessment, follow these rules:**
    - Record all pertinent data
    - Avoid extraneous data
    - Use common terms
    - Avoid abbreviations
    - Be objective
    - Use diagrams when indicated

💡 PROFICIENCY EXERCISE 11-2

1. With a partner, practice asking three open-ended questions that you might use during an interview.
2. Hold conversations with 10 different people. Practice restating information you are given in response to a question you had asked.
3. Practice using and modifying the script example provided in Box 11-1.

Table 11-1 Forces and Resulting Injuries

Force	Injury
Tension force	Soft tissue stretching: tears, strains
Compression force	Contusions, tearing, direct blows
Bending force	Ligament tears, fractures
Shearing force (forces occur perpendicular to tissue fibers)	Ligament tears, blisters, abrasions
Rotational/torsion force (combined tension and shearing forces)	Ligament tears, spiral fractures

PHYSICAL ASSESSMENT: OBJECTIVE ASPECT OF ASSESSMENT

SECTION OBJECTIVES

Chapter objective covered in this section:

2. Explain and implement subjective and objective instruments into the assessment process.

Using the information presented in this section, the student will be able to perform the following:

- Define biomechanics and kinesiology
- Use standardized documentation instruments to measure and record assessment findings

After the subjective assessment has been completed, the massage therapist may choose to do a physical assessment before beginning the massage. For a single-session general massage, the physical assessment usually is limited to having the client show the massage therapist any movements that feel restricted or may be causing pain. It is important to ask the client to point out any bruises, varicose veins, or areas of inflammation so that they can be avoided or the methods used over them can be altered. The massage practitioner should ask, "Are there any areas you feel I should avoid?" Be sure the information is indicated on the client information form and then take care to avoid those areas.

The assessment for basic therapeutic massage, including the development of a care/treatment plan and agreed-on outcomes over a series of massage sessions, includes a general evaluation of the client's posture gait (walking pattern) and biomechanical function. To understand posture and gait function, we must learn a bit about biomechanics and kinesiology.

Biomechanics and Kinesiology

Biomechanics is the science of the action of forces, internal or external, on the living body. *Kinetics* is a branch of the study of biomechanics that describes the effect of forces on the body. The topic of kinetics is introduced here as it applies to the musculoskeletal system.

A force can be considered a push or a pull that can produce, stop, or modify movement. Force application is what a massage professional does when giving a massage. In Chapter 10 each massage method was explained in terms of the force applied and the expected outcome as the tissues responded to the force. These same forces also can cause injury (Table 11-1). When we perform various assessments, these forces are applied to identify whether the area is injured.

Kinesiology is the science of the study of movement and the active and passive structures involved, including bones, joints, muscle tissues and all associated connective tissues. The following are elements of kinesiology.

- *Stability* is required o provide a stable base for functioning. Stability concerns usually focus on the proximal musculature in the trunk, shoulders, and hips, which allow for movement of the extremities. Stability is required before balance can exist.
- *Balance* is the ability to execute complex patterns of movement with the right timing and sequence. Balance is essential to motor function, as is the ability to maintain the center of gravity over the available base of support.
- *Coordination* is the efficient execution of a movement. Coordination usually involves motor learning and practice.
- *Endurance* (lasting power) is based on efficiency and stamina.

An important development in biomechanics research is the concept of the kinetic chain (also known as the *kinetic link*). The concept gained prominence in mechanical engineering in the 1970s and was applied to biomechanics. The kinetic chain describes the body as a linked system of interdependent segments. Just as there is no such thing as an individual muscle, body segments do not exist in isolation. By understanding the relationship of the body segments to each other, we can maximize the effectiveness of massage application, because we understand the importance of whole body massage rather than isolated spot work. The diagram in Figure 11-2 shows the common areas of interrelated kinetic chain function. Follow the colored lines to locate the interconnections.

The components of biomechanics and kinesiology appear throughout this chapter each time a specific type of assessment is presented.

Outcome Documentation Instruments

Because health care intervention is based on evidence of benefit, the massage therapist must be able to show that beneficial changes occur in the client's status as a result of massage. Both the value and quality of evidence-based interventions can be assessed using standardized assessment tools, or instruments.

Two important aspects of the development of a care/treatment plan and effective documentation (charting) are preassessment and postassessment. When the preassessment and postassessment data are compared, the benefits of massage can be identified, as can parts of the care/treatment plan that may need to be adjusted in future massage sessions. To assess outcomes accurately, massage therapists must use the same instruments for follow-up evaluations that they used for the baseline (beginning) evaluation.

Instruments for evaluating outcomes can be divided into two categories: those that use subjective measurements, which focus on data provided by the client, and those that use objective measurements, which focus on data provide by the practitioner's assessment.

Subjective Measurements

Pain Evaluation

The evaluation of pain classically has been a subjective measurement. Pain assessment tools help patients describe their pain. Three examples of assessment instruments that focus on subjective outcomes are:

- Pain scales (measure the intensity of pain)
- Pain drawing (measures the location and quality of pain)
- McGill Pain Questionnaire (measures the sensory and cognitive experience of pain)

Pain scales are commonly used to describe the intensity of the pain or how much pain the patient feels. Types of pain scales include the numeric rating scale, the visual analog scale, the categorical scale, and the pain faces scale.

- On the numeric rating scale, individuals are asked to identify how much pain they are having by choosing a number from 0 (no pain) to 10 (the worst pain imaginable).
- The visual analog scale is a straight line on which the left end represents no pain and the right end represents the worst pain. Individuals are asked to mark the line at the point they think represents their level of pain.
- The categorical pain scale has four categories: none, mild, moderate, and severe. Individuals are asked to select the category that best describes their pain.
- The pain faces scale uses six faces with different expressions on each face. Each face represents a person who feels happy because he or she has no pain or who feels sad because he or she has some or a lot of pain. Individuals are asked to choose the face that best shows how they are feeling. This rating scale can be used by people age 3 years or older (Figure 11-3).

Pain drawing involves providing documentation with generic human body forms representing the anterior, posterior, and lateral views of the body. Clients use colored pencils or pens to draw their symptoms on the body forms. It is possible to identify intensity and distribution of the pain or other symptom based on the quality of the drawing. Those areas that are heavily marked indicate intense pain. Large or small symptom distribution can be determined by when and what shape the client has drawn. Colors such as orange and red can be used to indicate intense pain. See Figure 11-31, the

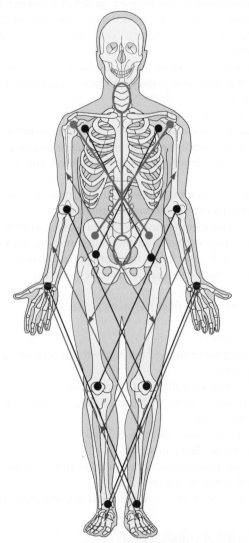

FIGURE 11-2 Interrelated kinetic chain function. Arm—Thigh; Forearm—Leg; Hand—Foot; Shoulder—Hip; Elbow—Knee; Wrist—Ankle; Cervical—Sacrum; Shoulder Girdle—Pelvic Girdle. (From Fritz S: *Sports and exercise massage,* St Louis, 2005, Mosby.)

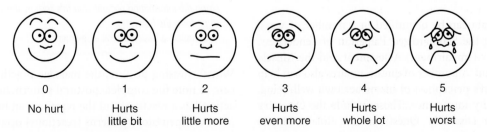

0	1	2	3	4	5
No hurt	Hurts little bit	Hurts little more	Hurts even more	Hurts whole lot	Hurts worst

FIGURE 11-3 Categorical/numeric pain scale.
(Modified from Whaley L, Wong D: *Nursing care of infants and children,* ed 3, St Louis, 1987, Mosby.)

physical assessment form, for an example of figures that can be used for pain drawing.

On the McGill Pain Questionnaire (MPQ), individuals use sensory, affective, and evaluative word descriptors to specify their subjective pain experience. The three primary measures are (1) the pain rating index, which is based on two types of numeric values that can be assigned to each word descriptor; (2) the number of words chosen; and (3) the present pain intensity, which is rated on a 1 to 5 intensity scale (Melzack, 1983).

The short form of the McGill Pain Questionnaire (SF-MPQ) has 11 questions related to the sensory dimension of the pain experience and four related to the affective dimension (Melzack, 1987). Each descriptor is ranked on a four-point intensity scale (0 = none, 1 = mild, 2 = moderate, 3 = severe). The pain rating index of the standard MPQ is included, as is a visual analog scale. You may encounter these types of pain measurement documents in various work environments, especially medical settings.

Objective Measurements

Physical Evaluation

Physical assessment procedures typically are classified as objective. The main considerations are body balance, efficient function, and basic symmetry. These assessment procedures cover isolated function of muscles or joints (or both), range of motion, strength, and endurance. These functions are measured and compared to what is considered normal function, and the differences (deviations from the norm) are recorded.

People are not perfectly symmetric, but the right and left halves of the body should be similar in shape, range of motion, and ability to function. For example, the ear, shoulder, hip, and ankle should be in a vertical line. The greater the discrepancy in symmetry, the greater the potential for soft tissue and joint dysfunction.

Functional capacity, or whole body movement capabilities, also can be measured. Functional assessment considers posture, gait, and range of motion. Disruption of the gait (walking) reflexes creates the potential for many problems. Common gait problems include a functional short leg caused by soft tissue shortening, short neck and shoulder muscles, aching feet, and fatigue. The massage therapist must understand basic biomechanics, including posture, interaction of joint functions, and gait.

Examples of functional capacity tests include lifting, carrying, walking, sitting, standing, balancing, and hand function. These types of assessment procedures are especially helpful for measuring qualitative goals, such as improvement in performing activities of daily living and occupation-related rehabilitation.

Assessment data can be quantified in a number of ways, such as by using the Standardized Palpation of Tenderness, Physical Capacity (Impairment) Assessment and the Muscle Testing Assessment. A number of questionnaires also can help identify the client's perception of his or her own well-being, distress, or activity intolerance. These include the Oswestry Low Back Pain Disability Questionnaire, Roland-Morris Questionnaire, and Functional Assessment Screening Questionnaire (FASQ).

Standardized Palpation of Tenderness

The American College of Rheumatology has developed a quantifiable method of assessing tissue tenderness (Wolfe et al., 1990). The examiner observes the response to palpatory stimulus by noting pain behaviors, such as facial grimacing and signs of withdrawal. By comparing the painful sites to uninvolved body areas, the examiner can determine whether the response is due to increased physiologic activity; this same assessment process can be used to detect a change in pain perception at the same pressure. Instruments for gauging pressure, called *algometers,* can further objectify the assessment.

A baseline of 4 kg of pressure is used (enough to blanch the tip of a thumbnail pressed on a table), and results are rated as follows:

Grade 0—No tenderness
Grade I—Tenderness with no physical or verbal response
Grade II—Tenderness with grimacing or flinching or both
Grade III—Tenderness with withdrawal (positive jump sign)
Grade IV—Withdrawal from non-noxious stimuli

Physical Capacity (Impairment) Assessment

Physical capacity tests measure functions such as joint mobility and muscle strength and endurance, such as cervical rotation mobility, hip range of motion, and trunk extensor endurance. Such tests may include the following:

- Walking 1 mile
- Climbing two flights of stairs (16 steps)
- Squatting
- Kneeling
- Sitting for prolonged periods with the knees bent in one position
- Climbing four flights of stairs (32 steps)
- Running a short distance (100 yards, the length of a football field)
- Walking a short distance (1 block)

Muscle Testing Assessment

Various instruments have been developed to measure muscle and joint function (Figure 11-4).

Box 11-2 presents a quick physical assessment procedure.

POSTURE ASSESSMENT: STANDING POSITION

SECTION OBJECTIVES

Chapter objective covered in this section:

3. Identify and address during massage elements relating to function and dysfunction of posture.

Using the information presented in this section, the student will be able to perform the following:

- Complete a basic postural assessment

When assessing posture, the massage practitioner must take care to note the complete postural pattern, head to toe. Every action has a reaction, and the reaction can be compensation. Most compensatory patterns (reactions) occur in response to external forces imposed on the body. The body makes countless compensatory changes daily. This is normal, and if other

Box 11-2 Abbreviated Physical Assessment Protocol

In some cases, only a simple physical assessment is necessary, or it is all that time allows. Begin by viewing the client from three standing positions: front, back, and side. Note any areas of asymmetry. Then proceed according to the following outline.

Back

Instruct the client to reach for the toes, keeping the knees straight.

Observe for:

- Scoliosis
- Kyphosis
- Asymmetry

Instruct the client to side-bend by sliding the hand down the side of the leg; compare the two sides.

Instruct the client to twist the torso left and right; compare the two sides.

Cervical Spine Range of Motion

Instruct the client to do the following:

- Look at ceiling (extension)
- Look at floor (flexion)
- Look over each shoulder (rotation)
- Bend the ear to each shoulder (abduction/lateral flexion)

Shoulder Range of Motion

Instruct the client to do the following:

- Scratch the back with each hand from over the shoulder (external rotation and abduction)
- Scratch the back with each hand from under the shoulder (internal rotation and adduction)

Muscle Tests—Instruct the client to do the following:

- Shrug the shoulders
- Flex the shoulders to 90 degrees
- Abduct the shoulders to 90 degrees
- Rotate each shoulder internally and externally

Upper Extremity Range of Motion

Instruct the client to do the following:

- Flex and extend the elbows

- Pronate and supinate the wrists with the arms at the sides and the elbows flexed to 90 degrees
- Spread the fingers
- Make a fist

Muscle Tests—Instruct the client to do the following:

- Flex and extend the elbows
- Pronate and supinate the wrists with the arms at the sides and the elbows flexed to 90 degrees
- Spread the fingers
- Make a fist

Lower Extremity—Hip Motion

Instruct the client to bend forward at the hip joints to touch the toes.

- Observe for hamstring shortening at the hip and the knee.

Instruct the client to do the following:

- Contract and relax the quadriceps; observe for symmetry
- Contract and relax the quadriceps; observe for patellar tracking

Next:

- Observe for knee effusion
- Observe for ankle effusion

Instruct the client to do the following:

- Rise up on toes; observe for calf strength
- Rise up on heels; observe for leg strength

Instruct the client to perform the one leg standing balance test:

- Have the client stand first on one foot and then on the other; compare the two sides and observe for balance and coordination

Instruct the client to perform the squat test:

- Have the client raise the arms over the head and then squat by pretending to sit down in a chair; observe for symmetry and reduced or excessive movement, core strength, hip, knee ankle flexion, hip adduction, shoulder abduction, and latissimus shortening

pathologic conditions are not present, they seldom become problematic. However, if the client has had an injury, maintains a certain position for a prolonged period, or overuses a body area, the body may not be able to return to a normal dynamic balance efficiently. The balance of the body against the force of gravity is the fundamental determining factor in a person's posture, or upright position. Even subtle shifts in posture demand a whole body compensatory pattern (Figure 11-5 and Box 11-3).

The cervical, thoracic, lumbar, and sacral curves (Figure 11-6) develop because of the body's need to maintain an upright position against gravity. In adults, the cervical vertebrae, when viewed laterally, form a symmetric anterior convex curve. The thoracic vertebrae curve posteriorly, and the lumbar vertebrae reverse and curve in the anterior direction, with a posterior curve of the sacrum. The sharp angulation above C1, the atlas, which allows the head to maintain a level,

horizontal plane, also has been considered a curve. Changes in the normal spinal curves result in scoliosis, lordosis, and kyphosis.

Mechanical Balance

A mechanically balanced, weight-bearing joint is in the gravitational line of the mass it supports and is located exactly through the axis of rotation. The axis of rotation is the center around which something rotates. Placement of the feet influences the stability of the standing position by providing a base of support. The most common position is one leg in front of the other, with mild external rotation of the forward leg. People commonly have a functionally long and short leg. When a person is standing, the long leg often is the front one. When the person is seated with the legs crossed, the long leg often is on top.

Muscle Strength Grading Scale (Oxford Scale)
Medical Research Council [MRC] grading scale

Grade	Value	Muscle Strength
5	Normal	Complete range of motion (ROM) against gravity with full resistance
4	Good	• Complete ROM against gravity with some resistance: Full range of motion with decreased strength • (Sometimes this category is subdivided further into 4^-/5, 4/5, and 4^+/5)
3	Fair	Complete ROM against gravity with no resistance; active ROM
2	Poor	Complete ROM with some assistance and gravity eliminated
1	Trace	Evidence of slight muscular contraction, no joint motion evident
0	Zero	No evidence of muscle contraction NT: Not testable

FIGURE 11-4 Muscle strength grading scale (Oxford Scale). (From Medical Research Council: *Aids to the examination of the peripheral nervous system,* London, 1976, Her Majesty's Stationary Office.)

  Box 11-3 Habitual Factors Leading to Posture Distortion

Three major factors influence posture: heredity, disease, and habit. These factors must be considered in the evaluation of posture. The easiest factor to adjust is habit.

- Occupational habits (e.g., a shoulder raised from talking on the phone) and recreational habits (e.g., a forward-shoulder position in a bike rider) can have an effect on posture.
- Clothing and shoes can affect the way a person uses the body. Tight collars or ties restrict breathing and contribute to neck and shoulder problems. Restrictive belts, control-top undergarments, and tight pants also limit breathing and affect the neck, shoulders, and midback. Shoes with high heels or those that do not fit the feet comfortably interfere with postural muscles. Shoes with worn soles imprint the old postural pattern, and the client's body assumes the dysfunctional pattern if she puts them back on after the massage. To maintain postural changes, the client must change to shoes that do not have a worn sole.
- Sleep positions can contribute to a wide range of problems such as neck strain when sleeping on one's stomach or sleeping on one's side, which can affect the shoulders.
- Furniture that does not support the back or that is too high or too low perpetuates muscular dysfunction.

By normalizing the soft tissue and teaching balancing exercises, the massage therapist can play a beneficial role in helping clients overcome habitual postural distortion.

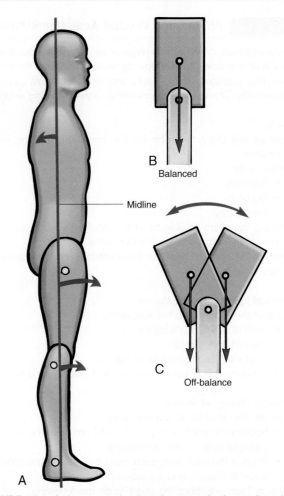

FIGURE 11-5 A, In a normal, relaxed stance, the leg and trunk tend to rotate slightly off the midline of the body but maintain a counterbalance force. Balance is achieved in **B** but not in **C.** Anytime the trunk moves off this midline balance point, the body must compensate.

The standing posture requires various segments of the body to cooperate mechanically as a whole. Passive tension of ligaments, fascia, and the connective tissue elements of the muscles supports the skeleton. Muscle activity plays a small but important role. Postural muscles maintain small amounts of contraction that stabilize the body upright in gravity by continually repositioning the body weight over the mechanical balance point.

In relaxed symmetric standing, both the hip and the knee joints assume a position of full extension to provide for the most efficient weight-bearing position. The knee joint has an additional stabilizing element in its screw-home mechanism. The femur rides backward on the medial condyle and rotates medially about its vertical axis to lock the joint for weight bearing; this happens only in the final phase of extension. The normal screw-home extension pattern of the knee is not hyperextension, which puts a strain on the knee. The hamstrings are the major muscles that resist the force of gravity at the knee (Smith et al., 1996; Norkin and Levangie, 2005).

At the ankle joint, bones and ligaments do little to limit motion. Passive tension of the two-joint gastrocnemius muscle (i.e., the muscle crosses two joints) becomes an important factor. This stabilizing force is diminished if high-heeled shoes are worn. The heel of the shoe puts the gastrocnemius on a slack. If these heels are worn constantly, the muscle and the Achilles tendon shorten.

During prolonged standing, the average person shifts position frequently. The two basic positions used are the symmetric stance, with the weight distributed equally on both feet, and the asymmetric stance, in which nearly all the weight rests on one foot (Figure 11-7). The asymmetric stance is the most common, with the weight shifted back and forth between the two feet. This allows for rest periods and shifting of the gravitational forces. Body sway is limited by the intermittent action of appropriate antigravitational postural muscles.

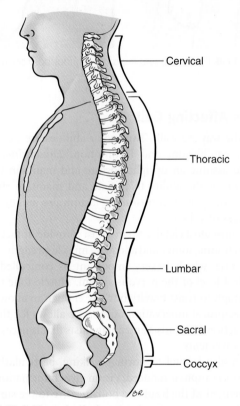

FIGURE 11-6 Normal spinal curves.

Cervical

Thoracic

Lumbar

Sacral

Coccyx

Asymmetry usually results when short muscles (increased motor tone) or shortened connective tissue, or both, pulls the body out of alignment. Direct trauma pushes joints out of alignment. Weak stabilizing mechanisms, such as overstretched ligaments or inhibited antagonist muscles, contribute to the problem. A chiropractor, an osteopath, or another trained medical professional skilled in skeletal manipulation is needed for these conditions. Often a multidisciplinary approach to client care is required.

Postural Assessment: Procedure for the Standing Position

1. To assess posture in the standing position, have the client use the symmetric stance.
2. The feet are about shoulder-width apart, and the eyes are closed.
3. With the eyes closed, most of the client's postural patterns are exaggerated, because the client is unable to orient the body visually.
4. Often the client tips the head or rotates it slightly to feel balanced; this indicates muscular imbalance and internal postural imbalance information relayed by positional receptors.

Box 11-4 presents a list of indicators of lack of symmetry. The physical assessment form in Chapter 4 is a helpful tool for performing the physical assessment.

Intervention Guidelines

Misalignment of body areas can be caused by muscles that pull or that do not stabilize, by connective tissue shortening or laxity or, more likely, by a combination of these. The best course is to follow the lead provided by the client's body.

When performing massage, the practitioner should honor what the body is doing. This can be done by creating an exaggeration of the asymmetric pattern found and then slowly encouraging the body to shift to a more symmetric pattern. The integrated muscle energy approach explained in Chapter 10 is effective in these situations.

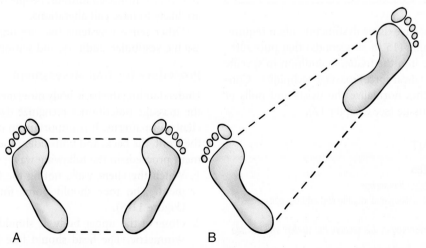

A   B

FIGURE 11-7 A, Symmetric stance. **B,** Asymmetric stance. The asymmetric stance, with the weight shifted from foot to foot, is the most efficient standing position.

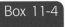

Box 11-4 Landmarks That Help Identify Lack of Symmetry

The following landmarks can be used to compare the symmetry of the body in different aspects. Be sure to observe the client from the back, the front, and the left and right sides.

- The middle of the chin should sit directly under the tip of the nose. Check the chin alignment with the sternal notch. These two landmarks should be in a direct line.
- The shoulders and clavicles should be level with each other. The shoulders should not roll forward or backward or be rotated with one forward and one backward.
- The arms should hang freely and at the same rotation out of the glenohumeral (shoulder) joint.
- The elbows, wrists, and fingertips should be in the same plane.
- The skin of the thorax (chest and back) should be even and should not look as if it pulls or is puffy.
- The navel, located on the same line as the nose, chin, and sternal notch, should not look pulled.
- The ribs should be even and springy.
- The abdomen should be firm but relaxed and slightly rounded.
- The curves at the waist should be even on both sides.
- The spine should be in a direct line from the base of the skull and on the same plane as the line connecting the nose and the navel. The curves of the spine should not be exaggerated.
- The scapulae should appear even and should move freely. You should be able to draw an imaginary straight line between the tips of the scapulae.
- The gluteal muscle mass should be even.
- The tops of the iliac crests should be even.
- The greater trochanter, knees, and ankles should be level.
- The circumferences of the thigh and calf should be similar on the left and right sides.
- The legs should rotate out of the acetabulum (hip joint) evenly in a slight external rotation.
- The knees should be locked in the standing position but should not be hyperextended. The patellae (kneecaps) should be level and pointed slightly laterally.
- A line dropped from the nose should fall through the sternum and the navel and should be spaced evenly between.

Working with connective tissue dysfunction often requires slow, sustained stretching (15 to 30 seconds) that puts sufficient mechanical force into the tissue, in addition to specific application of friction (shear force) massage techniques. Connective tissue approaches normalize the twists and pulls of shortened connective tissue (see Chapter 12).

GAIT ASSESSMENT

2
11-2

SECTION OBJECTIVES

Chapter objective covered in this section:
4. Explain the process of walking and identify and address gait dysfunction.
Using the information presented in this section, the student will be able to perform the following:
- Complete a basic gait assessment

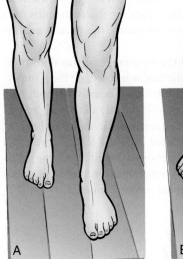
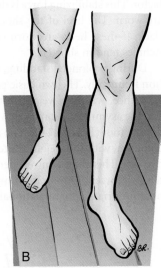

FIGURE 11-8 Proper **(A)** and improper **(B)** foot position in walking.

Factors Affecting Gait

Gait is the way we walk. Two major abilities are essential to walking: equilibrium and locomotion. *Equilibrium* is the ability to assume an upright posture and maintain balance. *Locomotion* is the ability to initiate and maintain rhythmic stepping. Many other contributing factors also are involved in the process of walking.

The musculoskeletal system must provide intact bones, well-functioning joints, and adequate muscle strength. Normal muscle tone, which is very important, is controlled at the subcortical level of the nervous system. Muscle tone must be high enough to resist gravity but low enough to allow movement. Reciprocal innervation of muscles allows for the coordinated action of agonists and antagonists that is necessary for skilled movements.

Vision also is vital to normal walking, particularly when other sensory input is reduced. Vision gives information about the movement of the head and body relative to the surroundings and is important for the automatic balance responses to changes in surface conditions. People with visual impairments are likely to have gait alterations.

Other sensory systems that are important in this process are the vestibular, auditory, and sensory motor systems.

Procedure for Gait Assessment

Understanding the basic body movements of walking can help the massage practitioner recognize dysfunctional and inefficient gait patterns. It is important to observe the client from the front, the back, and both sides. The process of gait assessment proceeds in the following way.

1. Watch the client walk, noting the heel-to-toe foot placement. The toes should point forward with each step (Figure 11-8).
2. Observe the upper body. It should be relaxed and fairly symmetric. The head should face forward with the eyes level with the horizontal plane. A natural arm swing should occur opposite the leg swing. The arm swing begins at the

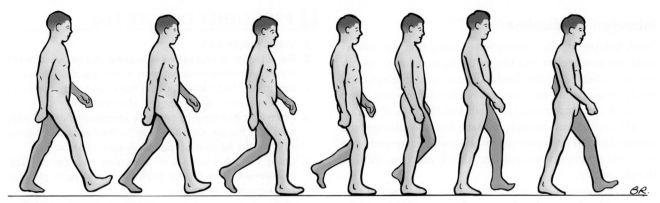

FIGURE 11-9 Efficient gait position.

shoulder joint. On each step, the left arm moves forward as the right leg moves forward and vice versa. This pattern provides balance. The rhythm and pace of the arm and leg swing should be similar. Increasing the walking speed should increase the speed of the arm swing. The length of the stride determines the arc of the arm swing (Figure 11-9).

3. Observe the client walking and note the person's general appearance. The optimum walking pattern is as follows:

   a. The head and trunk are vertical, with the eyes easily maintaining forward position and level with the horizontal plane; the shoulders are level and perpendicular to the vertical line.

   b. The arms swing freely opposite the leg swing, allowing the shoulder girdle to rotate opposite the pelvic girdle.

   c. The step length and timing are even.

   d. The body oscillates vertically with each step.

   e. The entire body moves rhythmically with each step.

   f. At the heel strike, the foot is approximately at a right angle to the leg.

   g. The knee is extended, not locked, in slight flexion.

   h. The body weight is shifted forward into the stance phase.

   i. At push-off, the foot is strongly plantar flexed, with defined hyperextension of the metatarsophalangeal joints of the toes.

   j. During the leg swing, the foot easily clears the floor with good alignment, and the rhythm of movement remains unchanged.

   k. The heel contacts the floor first.

   l. The weight then rolls to the outside of the arch.

   m. The arch flattens slightly in response to the weight load.

   n. The weight then is shifted to the ball of the foot in preparation for the spring-off from the toes and the shifting of the weight to the other foot.

4. During walking the pelvis moves slightly in a side-lying, figure-eight pattern. The movements that make up this sequence are transverse, medial, and lateral rotation. The stability and mobility of the sacroiliac (SI) joints play very important roles in this alternating side, figure-eight movement. If these joints are not functioning properly, the entire gait is disrupted. The SI joint is one of the few joints in the body that is not directly affected by muscles that cross the joint. It is a large joint, and the bony contact between

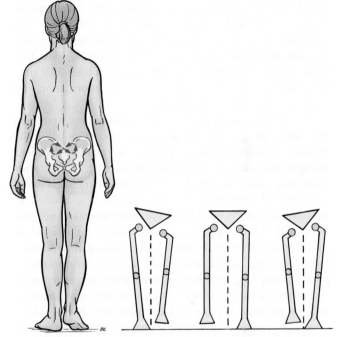

FIGURE 11-10 Mechanism of the slight rocking movement of the sacroiliac joint.

the sacrum and the ilium is broad. The rocking of this joint often is disrupted (Figure 11-10).

5. The hips rotate in a slightly oval pattern, beginning with a medial rotation during the leg swing and heel strike, followed by a lateral rotation through the push-off.

6. The knees move in a flexion and extension pattern opposite each other. The extension phase never reaches enough extension to initiate the normal knee-lock pattern that is used in standing.

7. The ankles rotate in an arc around the heel at heel strike and around a center in the forefoot at push-off.

8. Maximum dorsiflexion at the end of the stance phase and maximum plantar flexion at the end of push-off are necessary.

Common Findings from Gait Assessment

Any disruption of the gait demands that the body compensate by shifting movement patterns and posture. Observing areas of the body that do not move efficiently during walking is a good means of detecting dysfunctional areas.

Intervention Guidelines

When interpreting the information gathered from gait assessment, the massage practitioner should focus on areas that do not move easily when the client walks and areas that move too much. Areas that do not move are restricted; areas that move too much are compensating for inefficient function. By releasing the restrictions through massage and re-educating the reflexes through neuromuscular work, such as correcting gait reflex and exercise, the practitioner can help the client improve the gait pattern.

The techniques used are similar to those for postural corrections. The shortened and restricted areas are softened with massage, then the neuromuscular mechanism is reset with muscle energy techniques, muscle lengthening, and stretches. During visual and palpation assessment, shortened and restricted areas form concavities or metaphorical caves. Accompanying the adaptation of short tissues, long taut tissues form into convexities or metaphorical hills. This simplification can quickly provide assessment information and guide massage intervention plans.

The client should be taught slow lengthening and stretching procedures for the short areas (caves). After stimulating the muscles in weakened areas, the practitioner can teach the client strengthening exercises for the long areas (hills). The therapist must make sure to incorporate the adaptation methods into a complete, full-body massage rather than doing spot work on isolated parts of the body to support adaptation and integration. Suggestions could be made to the client to evaluate factors that may contribute to identified dysfunctions, such as posture, footwear, chairs, tables, beds, clothing, shoes, work stations, physical tasks (e.g., shoveling), and repetitive exercise patterns.

Proper functioning of the SI joint is an important factor in walking patterns. Because SI joint movement has no direct muscular component, it is difficult to use any kind of muscle energy lengthening when working with this joint. The joint is embedded deep in supporting ligaments. To keep the surrounding ligaments pliable, direct and specific connective tissue techniques are indicated unless the joint is hypermobile. If that is the case, external bracing combined with rehabilitative movement may be indicated. Sometimes the ligaments restabilize the area. Stabilization of the jointed area should be interspersed with massage and gentle stretching to ensure that the ligaments remain pliable and do not adhere to each other. This process takes time.

The diagnosis of specific joint problems and fitting for external bracing are outside the scope of practice for therapeutic massage, and the client must be referred to the appropriate professional.

Recall that all dysfunctional patterns are whole body phenomena. Working only on the symptomatic area is ineffective and offers limited relief. Therapeutic massage with a whole body focus is extremely valuable for dealing with gait dysfunction (Proficiency Exercise 11-3). Additional muscle testing assessments for gait function are found in Proficiency Exercises 11-5 and 11-6 later in this chapter. (For further information on gait, see Chapter 10 of *Mosby's Essential Sciences for Therapeutic Massage*, Mosby, 2013.)

💡 PROFICIENCY EXERCISE 11-3

1. Watch people walk.
2. Pay attention to yourself when walking. Put on two different shoes and notice what happens when you walk. Bind one arm to your torso to restrict the movement of that arm and pay attention to what happens when you walk.
3. Place your thumbs on a person's sacroiliac joints and walk behind as the person walks. Feel for the movement. Notice whether the figure-eight pattern is even or lopsided.
4. Using the information just presented and the physical assessment form on the Evolve website, do a physical assessment of 10 people.

Key Points

- Pain causes the body to tighten and alters the normal relaxed flow of walking.
- Muscle weakness and shortening interfere with the neurologic control of the agonist (prime mover) and antagonist muscle action.
- Limitation of joint movement and joint hypermobility result in protective muscle contraction. If the situation becomes chronic, shortening of both muscle groups (agonist and antagonist) and muscle weakness result.
- Changes in the soft tissue, including all the connective tissue elements of the tendons, ligaments, and fascial sheaths, restrict the normal action of muscles and joints. Connective tissue usually shortens and becomes less pliable.
- Amputation disrupts the body's normal diagonal counterbalance function. Obviously, amputation of any part of the leg disturbs the walking pattern; what is not so obvious is that amputation of any part of the arm affects the counterbalance movement of the arm swing during walking. The rest of the body must compensate for the loss. Loss of any of the toes greatly affects the postural information sent to the brain from the feet. These details may be overlooked when in fact they could be major contributing factors in posture and gait problems.
- Soft tissue dysfunction can exist without joint involvement.
- Any change in the tissue around a joint has a direct effect on the joint function. Changes in joint function eventually cause problems with the joint. Any dysfunction with the joint immediately involves the surrounding muscles and other soft tissue.

ASSESSMENT OF JOINT RANGE OF MOTION

SECTION OBJECTIVES

Chapter objective covered in this section:
5. Integrate joint movement into the massage for assessment purposes.
Using the information presented in this section, the student will be able to perform the following:
- Complete a range-of-motion assessment

Recall from Chapter 10 that active and passive joint movement can assess the range of motion of a joint. Active joint movement is performed when the client moves the joint through the planes of motion that are normal for that joint. Any pain, crepitus, or limitation that manifests during the action is reported. This assessment identifies what the client is willing or able to do.

Passive joint movement to assess range of motion is performed when the massage therapist moves the joint passively through the planes of motion that are normal for the joint. The assessment identifies limitation (hypomobility) or excess movement (hypermobility) of the joint. Passive movement is performed carefully and gently to allow the client to fully relax the muscles during the assessment. The client reports the point at which pain or bind, if present, occurs. The massage therapist stops the motion at the point of pain or bind. Passive joint movement provides information about the joint capsule and ligaments and other restricting mechanisms, such as muscles (Figure 11-11).

Measuring Joint Range of Motion

The range of motion of joints is measured in degrees, starting at the neutral line of anatomic position, which is considered 0. Movement of a joint in the sagittal, frontal, or transverse plane is described as the number of degrees of flexion, extension, adduction, abduction, and internal and external rotation (Figure 11-12). For example, the elbow has approximately 150 degrees of flexion at the end range. Anything less than this is hypomobility, and anything more is considered hypermobility. The degrees of movement are recorded as 0 to X° if the motion began in the anatomic position and as X°to 0 if the motion began out of the anatomic position.

Overpressure and End-Feel

The stretch on the soft tissues (i.e., muscles, tendons, fascia, and ligaments) and the arrangement of the joint surfaces

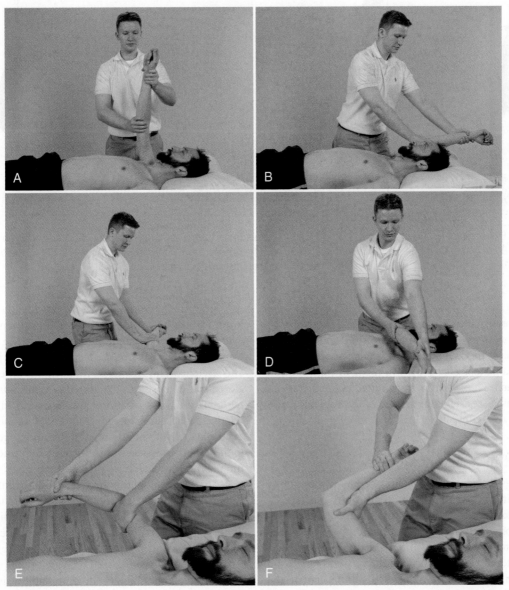

FIGURE 11-11 Assessment of shoulder using passive joint motion. **A,** Flexion glenohumeral joint only. **B,** Full flexion shoulder complex including glenohumeral joint and scapular movement. **C,** Horizontal abduction. **D,** Horizontal adduction. **E,** Internal/medial rotation. **F,** External/lateral rotation.

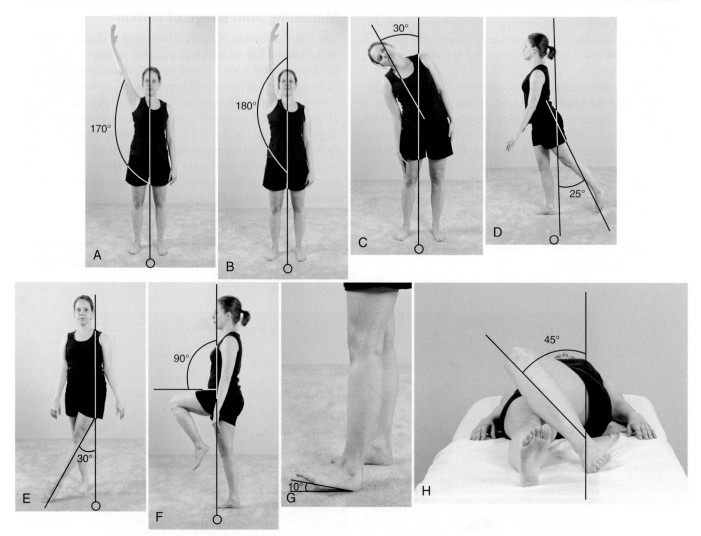

FIGURE 11-12 Examples of visual assessment of active joint movements and degrees of range of motion. **A,** 170 degrees shoulder abduction. **B,** 180 degrees. **C,** 30 degrees, lateral trunk flexion. **D,** 25 degrees, leg extension. **E,** 30 degrees, hip adductor. **F,** 90 degrees, hip flexion. **G,** 10 degrees, dorsiflexion. **H,** 40 to 45 degrees, internal hip rotation.

determine the range of motion of the joint and therefore the joint's normal **end-feel** (see Chapter 10). In using overpressure, the massage therapist gradually applies more pressure when the end of the available passive range of joint motion has been reached. The sensation transmitted to the therapist's hands by the tissue resistance at the end of the available range is the end-feel of a joint (Box 11-5).

Assessment of Range of Motion

Active and passive joint movement can identify limits of movement. Joint movement determines the joint position. In the closed packed position, the articular surfaces of the bones within most joints are closest together and the shapes of the bones best fit together. This position is the most stable position for a joint and usually in or near the very end range of a motion. In this position, most ligaments and parts of the capsule are pulled taut, providing an element of natural stability to the joint. For many joints in the lower extremity, the closed packed position is essential to normal function. At the

knee, for example, the closed packed position, which is full extension, provides stability to the knee in the standing position through the combined effect of maximum joint congruity and stretched/taut ligaments. All positions other than a joint's closed packed position are referred to as the joint's *loose packed positions.* In these positions, the ligaments and capsule are relatively slackened, allowing increased mobility. The joint generally is least congruent near its midrange. Therefore, a joint in the loose packed position, especially midrange, is most mobile but least stable.

If an empty capsular or hard end-feel is identified, the joint is damaged. Referral is needed for acute conditions. Range of motion limited by muscle contraction may indicate an underlying problem with joint laxity or injury, and caution is indicated before muscle guarding is reduced. Proceed slowly until a balance is achieved between increased range of motion and maintaining joint stability. If joint stability is reduced, the client usually experiences pain in the joint for a day or two after the massage; also, increased stiffness in the area may be noted as stability is restored.

Box 11-5 Types of End-Feel	
Normal End-Feel	**Abnormal End-Feel**
• Soft tissue approximation end-feel occurs when the full range of the joint is restricted by the normal muscle bulk; it is painless and has a feeling of soft compression. • Muscular (tissue stretch) end-feel occurs at the extremes of muscle stretch, such as in the hamstrings during a straight leg raise; it has a feeling of increasing tension, springiness, or elasticity. • Capsular stretch (leathery) end-feel occurs when the joint capsule is stretched at the end of its normal range, such as with external rotation of the glenohumeral joint; it is painless and has the sensation of stretching a piece of leather. • Bony (hard) end-feel occurs when bone contacts bone at the end of normal range, as in extension of the elbow; it is abrupt and hard.	• Empty end-feel occurs when no physical restriction to movement exists except the pain expressed by the client. Muscle spasm end-feel occurs when passive movement stops abruptly because of pain; a springy rebound may occur as a result of reflexive muscle spasm. • Boggy end-feel occurs when edema is present; it has a mushy, soft quality. • Springy block (internal derangement) end-feel is a springy or rebounding sensation and indicates loose cartilage or meniscal tissue within the joint. • Capsular stretch (leathery) end-feel that occurs before normal range indicates capsular fibrosis with no inflammation. • Bony (hard) end-feel that occurs before normal range indicates bony changes or degenerative joint disease or malunion of a joint after a fracture.

Intervention Guidelines

Simple edema around a joint is managed with lymphatic drainage (see Chapter 12). If any unexplained edema develops, the client should be referred for diagnosis. In general, if a joint range is reduced (hypomobile), massage should target the short soft tissues to increase length and pliability, which would allow for more joint range of motion. Muscle energy methods and stretching methods can also be used to improve joint movement. Do not stretch a joint beyond the typical physiological barriers. Never force an increase in range of motion; instead, allow it to occur as a natural outcome of effective massage application to the soft tissues of the body. Range of motion should improve as the client's tissues normalize with general massage.

BASIC ORTHOPEDIC TESTS

SECTION OBJECTIVES

Chapter objective covered in this section:
6. Define and use simple orthopedic tests during the assessment process.
Using the information presented in this section, the student will be able to perform the following:
• Perform basic orthopedic tests to assess for the need for referral

Orthopedic tests are performed primarily to assess for bone, joint, ligament, and tendon injury. They also identify areas of impingement. The most common structures in which impingement is seen are nerves, blood vessels, tendons, and occasionally muscles. Orthopedic tests also can help determine whether a referral is necessary. Even if you do not perform them as part of your massage assessment, clients are likely to inform you of the findings of any such tests that may have been done by another health professional, such as an athletic trainer, physical therapist, chiropractic physician, or medical or osteopathic doctor.

Most orthopedic tests assess stress areas to evaluate pain, joint play, and muscle extensibility. Because of the strain involved during some orthopedic tests, care must be taken to avoid further injury. Before any orthopedic tests can be done, the massage practitioner must make sure the area is free of fractures or neoplasms (abnormal growths). Furthermore, any client with severe spasms, pain of unknown origin, or pain that awakens the person at night should not undergo orthopedic tests until a full medical evaluation has been done to address these symptoms.

Reproduction of the client's symptoms is a positive test result. If the client does not want a test performed, this is called an *apprehension sign*. Additional positive signs are a change in the stability of the joint and changes in pulses. Many types of orthopedic tests can be performed. Box 11-6 presents those that are most relevant to therapeutic massage practice.

Sequence for Joint Assessment

Learning any new process, such as joint assessment, is easier with a procedure to follow, such as this example of a sequence for assessing joint function.

History

1. Have you been injured? If yes, how and when did the injury happen?
2. Do you have any pain, impaired mobility or stiffness? If yes, where is it located? Can you show me?
3. Do your joints feel and move evenly on both sides of your body? If no, please explain. Can you show me?
   If an injury or symptoms such as stiffness are present, continue with the following questions.
4. Does it hurt all the time or only when you bump or press on it or when you move?
5. Did you hear or feel a "pop" or "snap"?
6. Have you had a similar injury? If yes, please explain.

Observation

1. Is there any obvious deformity that suggests a fracture or dislocation?
2. Is the area swollen, including edema and effusion?
3. Is there any discoloration?

Box 11-6   Orthopedic Assessment Tests

This box contains a few common orthopedic tests.

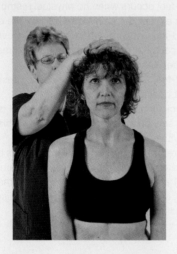

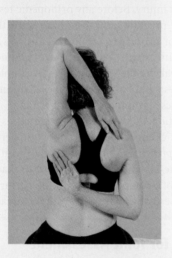

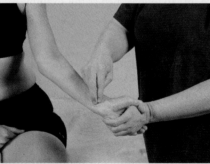

Axial Compression Test

- The client is either sitting or lying and you press down on the top of the client's head causing narrowing of the neural foramen and pressure on the facet joints, or muscle spasm.
- A positive test causes increased pain and indicates that there is some type of pressure on a nerve. *Refer client.*

Apley's Scratch Test

- The client is seated or standing. Ask the client reach over their head with one hand to scratch their back while keeping the other hand behind the back.
- Or, tell the client to touch the opposite scapula to test range of motion of the shoulder.
- Reaching over the head allows you to assess abduction and external rotation.
- Reaching behind the back allows you to assess adduction and internal rotation.
- Compare both sides for symmetry.
- If pain or limited range of motion there may be a rotator cuff tear or shoulder impingement (there may also be a potential for adhesive capsulitis or glenohumeral osteoarthritis). *Refer client.*

Tinel's Test

- Assesses for unlar nerve irritability.
- Assessment is performed at elbow and wrist.
- Place elbow flexion and wrist in extension.
- Tap at the cubital and/or carpal tunnel.
- A positive test produces paresthesias (numbing) or tingling along the distal course of the ulnar indicating irritability and or impingement of the ulnar nerve. *Refer client.*

Box 11-6   Orthopedic Assessment Tests—Cont'd

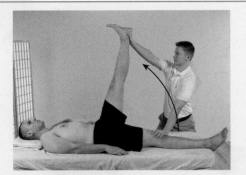

Straight Leg Raising Test
- With the knee extended and the client supine, the hip is flexed (with the leg straight).
- A positive test results in pain in the sciatic nerve pathway down the leg and suggests a disc herniation. *Refer client.*

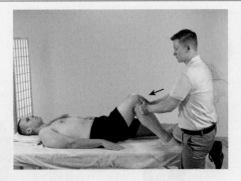

Posterior Drawer Test
- With the knee flexed approximately 90 degrees, push the proximal tibia posteriorly.
- Excessive movement indicates a tear of the posterior cruciate ligament. *Refer client.*

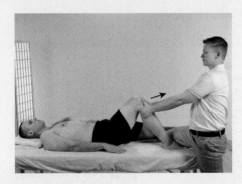

Anterior Drawer Test
- The client reclines with the knee flexed to 90 degrees.
- Grasp the proximal tibia and pull forward.
- If the tibia displaces anteriorly, the anterior cruciate ligament may be injured. *Refer client.*

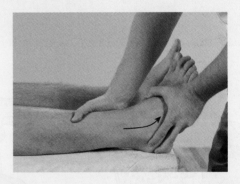

Talar Tilt Test
- The distal tibia is stabilized while the other hand "tilts" the talus to test the integrity of the lateral ligament complex.
- A positive sign would indicate injury such as a sprain. *Refer client.*

Continued

4. Compare injured and uninjured areas and identify changes.

Note: When performing the following assessments, remember that pain is the indication of a pathologic condition—do not cause an increase in pain; only locate the source of the pain.

Palpation

1. Perform palpation on the uninvolved side first. The uninvolved area is "normal."
2. Palpate all bony landmarks.
3. Briskly tap the bone and ask the client whether an increased pain sensation was felt. If so, this may indicate a stress fracture. Avoid the area during the massage and refer the client.
4. Palpate all ligament and tendon attachments.

5. Palpate all muscles that act on the area.
6. Palpate for edema and effusion.

Range of Motion

1. Perform active joint movement assessments to evaluate for changes in range of motion.
2. Perform a passive joint movement assessment and compare the range of motion to that seen with active movement assessment.

Manual Muscle Testing

1. Perform strength and neurologic testing on the normal side.
2. Perform strength and neurologic testing on the affected area. Do not cause additional pain or strain the injured area.

Box 11-6 Orthopedic Assessment Tests—Cont'd

→ Compression
→ Tension

Trunk Extension—an anterior herniation in which the gel-like nucleus has pushed forward.

→ Compression
→ Tension

Trunk Flexion—a posterior herniation in which the gel-like nucleus has pushed backward.

→ Compression
→ Tension

Trunk Lateral Flexion—a lateral herniation in which the gel-like nucleus has pushed to the side.

Specific Orthopedic Tests

1. Carefully perform appropriate orthopedic tests.

Intervention Guidelines

If the practitioner notes no pain, stiffness, mobility issues, or other concerns during the assessment, the joint can be considered normal. General massage for the jointed area is indicated to support normal function.

If the practitioner notes pain with movement or on palpation, discoloration, indications of inflammation, unusual stiffness, exaggerated hypermobility or hypomobility, weakness, or some other positive orthopedic test result, caution is indicated. If no logical cause exists for the finding (e.g., recent unusual activity or a fall) or if the client does not have pertinent information or is being treated by a physician, referral

may be necessary to determine the cause. Once the cause has been identified, massage treatment plans can be developed.

ASSESSMENT BY PALPATION

SECTION OBJECTIVES

Chapter objective covered in this section:

7. Use massage application as palpation assessment.

Using the information presented in this section, the student will be able to perform the following:

• Complete a 14-level palpation assessment

Palpation is the use of touch to examine the body. Our hands are our most versatile and refined assessment tool. Technology does not come close to the sensitivity and accuracy of a trained assessing hand. Our hands need to be trained to interpret what they perceive accurately. Palpation is more than touching and information gathered by sensory receptors in the hands and joints of the upper limb. Sometimes the foot and leg are used during massage and can be effective for palpation assessment. For the therapeutic massage professional, palpation is an essential and continuous process, and the hands as well as other parts of the body used to perform massage become skilled with experience.

With palpation assessment, the main considerations for basic massage are:

- The ability to differentiate between different types of tissue
- The ability to distinguish differences of tissue texture in the same tissue types
- The ability to palpate through the various tissue layers from superficial to deep

The tissues the massage therapist should be able to distinguish are the skin, superficial fascia, fascial sheaths, tendons, ligaments, blood vessels, muscle layers, and bone.

Palpation also includes assessment for hot and cold, and various body rhythms, including breathing patterns and pulses. During palpation of the skin, it is prudent to observe general skin condition and color.

Mechanisms of Palpation

Before actual palpation skills are discussed, it helps to understand the mechanism that makes palpation an effective assessment tool. The proprioceptors and mechanoreceptors of the shoulder, arm, and hand (or hip, leg, and foot) receive stimulation from the tissue being palpated. This is the reception phase. These impulses are transmitted through the peripheral and central nervous systems to the brain, where they are interpreted.

The somatosensory region of the brain that interprets this sensory information devotes a massive area to the hand. The refined discriminatory sense of the hand can perceive very subtle shifts and changes. The ability to interpret usually is a sense of comparison; that is, this tissue is softer than that tissue, or this feels rougher than that. Because comparison is a necessity, you must be careful to compare apples with apples; for example, the skin on the back cannot be compared with the skin on the feet.

This same mechanism makes self-massage less effective. The brain has difficulty deciding which signals to pay attention to when the hand is doing the massage and trying to send sensory information, and the body area being massaged is also trying to decide what is happening. Because the hand sensory and motor areas in the brain are so large, the information from the hand may supersede the information from the part of the body being self-massaged. The body seems to respond to the strongest set of signals. Consequently, the brain pays attention to the hand and does not focus enough motor response to the area being massaged. If the same area is massaged by another person, it can respond without conflicting sensory input.

It is essential that the massage therapist's entire self become sensitive to subtle differences in the client's body. With palpation, what is going on must be felt and not thought about. Too much thinking shifts awareness away from kinesthetic input.

How to Palpate

Palpation can begin in many different ways. After you have learned the skills, you need not follow the particular protocol presented in this text. The best course is to begin with the lightest palpation and move to the deepest levels, because after the hands have been used for deep compression, the sensitivity of the light touch sensors is momentarily diminished.

During palpation, varying depths of pressure must be used to reach all the tissue types and layers. Do not stay in one area too long or concentrate on a particular spot. The receptors in the practitioner's hands, forearms, or other body areas adapt quickly, and what is subsequently felt or perceived is then lost. The practitioner's first impression should be trusted; if the area feels hot, it probably is. The differences often are small. For practice, put your thumb and first finger together. Close your eyes and then just move the finger on the thumb only enough so that you feel the movement. Open your eyes and notice that the observable difference is tiny. Palpation assessment occurs at this level of awareness.

Palpation assessment becomes part of the massage. In any massage, about 90% of the touching can be considered assesssment as part of gliding, kneading, compression, shaking and rocking, and joint movement. Palpation assessment contacts the tissue but does not override it or encourage it to change. This type of work generally relaxes or stimulates the client, depending on the type of strokes used and the rhythm, duration, and speed of application.

Near-Touch Palpation

The first application of palpation does not involve touching the body; rather, the intent is to detect hot and cold areas. This is best done just off the skin using the back of the hand, which is very sensitive to heat. The general temperature of the area and any variations should be noted. It is important to move fairly quickly in a sweeping motion over the areas assessed because heat receptors adapt quickly.

Very sensitive cutaneous (skin) sensory receptors also detect changes in air pressure and currents and the movement of the air. This is one reason we can feel someone come up behind us when we cannot see the person. The movement and change in the surrounding air pressure alert us; this is a protective survival mechanism. Being able to consciously detect subtle sensations is an invaluable assessment tool. It is important to realize where the information comes from and why it can be sensed, to dispel the notion that this is an extrasensory ability. We are subconsciously aware of all the sensory stimulation that we have receptor mechanisms to detect. With practice, we can become consciously aware of these more subtle sensory experiences. Sensitivity, or intuition, is the ability to work with this information on a conscious level.

Intervention Guidelines

Near-touch assessment just above the skin feels somewhat similar to putting two poles of a magnet together; a very subtle resistance occurs. Areas that seem thick, dense, or bumpy or that tend to push the therapist away are hyperactive. Deeper palpation often reveals muscular hyperactivity or hot spots.

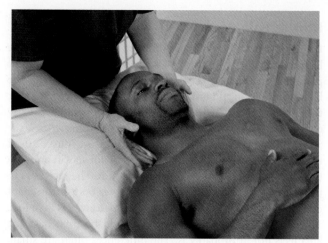

FIGURE 11-13 Near-touch palpation to determine hot-cold temperature differences and potential bioenergy fields.

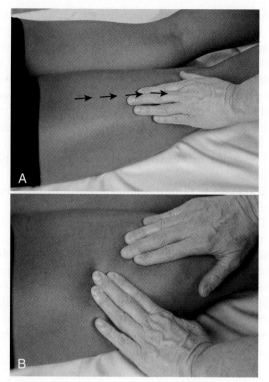

FIGURE 11-14 A, Skin drag assesses for hot/cold, wet/dry, rough/smooth. **B,** Skin stretch palpation assesses for local areas of ease and bind.

Areas that seem thin or feel as though holes are present usually are underactive. Impaired circulation, fibrotic tissue, and inhibited muscle activity often develop in underactive areas. Hot areas may be caused by inflammation, muscle spasm, or increased surface circulation. When the focus of intervention is to cool the hot areas, a method such as application of ice can be used (see the section on hydrotherapy in Chapter 12). A hot area can also be cooled by reducing the muscle spasms and encouraging more efficient blood flow in the surrounding areas.

Cold areas often are areas of diminished blood flow, increased connective tissue formation, or muscle flaccidity. Heat can be applied to cold areas. Stimulation massage techniques increase muscle activity, heating up the area. Connective tissue approaches soften connective tissue, help restore space around the capillaries, and release histamine, a vasodilator, to increase circulation. These approaches can warm a cold area (Figure 11-13).

Palpation of the Skin

The second application of palpation is very light surface stroking of the skin. First, determine whether the skin is dry or damp. Damp areas feel a little sticky, or the fingers drag. This light stroking also causes the root hair plexus that senses light touch to respond. It is important to notice whether a particular area gets more goose bumps (i.e., the pilomotor reflex) than other areas. This is a good time to observe for color, especially blue or yellow coloration. In addition, the practitioner should note and keep track of all moles and surface skin growths, pay attention to the quality and texture of the hair, and observe the shape and condition of the nails.

In palpation, the examiner uses gentle, small stretching of the skin in all directions and compares the elasticity of these areas (Figure 11-14). The skin also can be palpated for surface texture. Roughness or smoothness can be felt by applying light pressure to the skin surface.

The skin should move evenly and glide on the underlying superficial fascial tissues. Areas that are stuck, restricted, or too loose should be noted, as should any areas of the skin that become redder than surrounding areas.

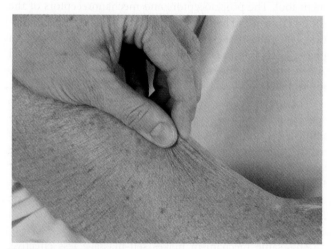

FIGURE 11-15 Dehydration test.

Intervention Guidelines

Skin should be contained, hydrated, resilient, elastic, and even and have rich coloring. If the skin does not spring back into its original position after a slight pinch, this may be a sign of dehydration (Figure 11-15). The skin should have no blue, yellow, or red tinges. Blue coloration suggests lack of oxygen; yellow indicates liver problems, such as jaundice; and redness suggests fever, alcohol intake, trauma, or inflammation. Color changes are most noticeable in the lips, around the eyes, and under the nails.

Bruises must be noted and avoided during massage except for simple lymphatic drainage (see Chapter 12). A client whose body shows any hot redness or red streaking should be referred to a physician immediately. This is especially important with the lower leg because of the possibility of deep vein thrombosis (blood clot).

The skin should be watched carefully for changes in any moles or lumps. As massage professionals, we often spend more time touching and observing a person's skin than anyone else, including the person. If we keep a keen eye for changes and refer clients to physicians early, many skin problems can be treated before they become serious.

Depending on the area, the skin may be thick or thin. The skin of the face is thinner than the skin of the lower back. The skin in each particular area, however, should be similar. The skin loses its resilience and elasticity over areas of dysfunction. It is important to know the visceral referred pain areas on the skin. If changes occur in the skin in these areas, the client should be referred to a physician.

The superficial skin is a blood reservoir. At any particular time, it can hold 10% of the available blood in the body. The connective tissue must be pliable to allow the capillary system to expand to hold the blood. Histamine, which is released from mast cells found in the connective tissue of the superficial fascial layer, dilates the blood vessels. Histamine also is responsible for the client's reported sense of "warming and itching" in an area that has been massaged.

Damp areas on the skin are indications that the nervous system has been activated in that area. This small amount of perspiration is part of a sympathetic activation called a *facilitated segment*. Surface stroking with enough pressure to drag over the skin will identify these slightly damp areas because there is a tiny sensation of stickiness. In addition, repeated stroking over the sticky area elicits a red response over the area of a hyperactive muscle. Deeper palpation of the area usually elicits a tender response. The small erector pili muscles attached to each hair also are under the control of the sympathetic autonomic nervous system. Light fingertip stroking produces goose bumps over areas of nerve hyperactivity. All of these responses can indicate potential activity, such as trigger points in the layers of muscle under the indicated area.

Hair and Nails

The hair and nails are part of the integumentary system and can reflect health conditions. The hair should be resilient and secure; hair loss should not be excessive when the scalp is massaged.

The nails should be smooth. Vertical ridges can indicate nutritional difficulties, and horizontal ridges can be signs of stress caused by changes in circulation that affect nail growth. Clubbed nails may indicate circulation problems. The skin around the nails should be soft and free of hangnails.

During times of stress, the epithelial tissues are affected first. Hangnails; split skin around the lips and nails; mouth sores; hair loss; dry, scaly skin; and excessively oily skin are all signs of prolonged stress, medication side effects, or other pathologic conditions. Only a physician can diagnose the cause of the condition (refer to the contraindications in Appendix A for more information).

Palpation of the Superficial Connective Tissue

The third application of palpation is the superficial connective tissue, which separates and connects the skin and muscle

tissue. It allows the skin to glide over the muscles during movement. This layer of tissue is found by using compression until the fibers of the underlying muscle are felt. The pressure then should be lightened so that the muscle cannot be felt, but if the hand is moved, the skin also moves. The tissue should feel resilient and springy, as if you were touching gelatin. The superficial fascia holds fluid and fat. If surface edema is present, it is in the superficial fascia. This water-binding quality gives this area the feel of a water balloon, but it should not feel boggy or soggy or show pitting edema (i.e., the dent from the pressure stays in the skin). Fat is stored in the superficial fascia; the method known as skin rolling should really be called superficial fascia rolling. By lifting and rolling the tissue folds, the massage practitioner can compare binding and density (Figure 11-16).

The sensation of bind comes from tissue being restrained from motion. To experience the sensation, hold one end of a rubber band or a piece of cloth, tissue, paper with one hand; hold the other end and the material in between with the other hand. Then, keeping one hand still, slowly begin to pull the

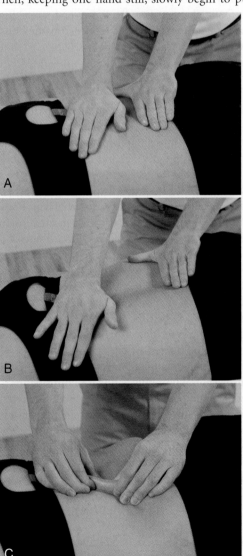

FIGURE 11-16 Beginning (**A**) and end (**B**) for palpation assessment of superficial fascia for ease and bind mobility. **C,** Skin roll palpation assesses for ease, bind, mobility, and pliability in the superficial fascia.

material with the other hand. When you feel a tiny tug on the hand that is still, you have reach bind. The sensation of something dense can be understood as a thick consistency and firmness with a greater depth than typical. To experience the sensation of dense tissue, squeeze an orange or grapefruit and then a kiwi or strawberry; also try this with a couch or chair cushion compared to a bed pillow and a sponge compared to a cotton ball.

Methods of palpation that lift the skin, such as kneading and skin rolling, provide much information. Depending on the area of the body and the concentration of underlying connective tissue, the superficial fascia should lift and roll easily.

Intervention Guidelines

Loosening and increasing the pliability of the superficial connective tissue are very beneficial. This can be done by applying the assessment methods more slowly and deliberately, allowing for softening in the tissues.

Any areas that become redder than the surrounding tissue or that stay red longer than other areas are suspect for connective tissue changes. Usually, lifting and stretching (bend, shear, and torsion forces) of the reddened tissue or use of the myofascial approaches presented in Chapter 12 normalizes these areas.

Palpation of Vessels and Lymph Nodes

The fourth application of palpation involves the circulatory vessels and lymph nodes. The more superficial blood vessels lie just above the muscle and in the superficial connective tissue. The vessels are distinct and feel like soft tubes. Pulses can be palpated, but the feel of the pulse is lost if the pressure is too intense. Feeling for pulses helps detect this layer of tissue.

In this same area are the more superficial lymph vessels and lymph nodes. Lymph nodes usually are located in joint areas and feel like small, soft gel caps. The compression of the joint action assists in lymphatic flow. A client with enlarged lymph nodes should be referred to a medical professional for diagnosis. Very light, gentle palpation of lymph nodes and vessels is indicated in this circumstance (Figure 11-17).

Vessels should feel firm but pliable and supported. If any areas of bulging, mushiness, or constriction are noted, the practitioner should refer the client to a physician.

The practitioner should compare the pulses by feeling for a strong, even, full pumping action on both sides of the body. If differences are perceived, the client should be referred to a physician. Sometimes the differences in the pulses can be attributed to soft tissue restriction of the artery or a more serious condition that can be diagnosed by the physician. To assess for capillary function of the circulatory system, press each nail in the fingers and toes firmly, but not painfully, until the nail bed blanches (whitens). Then release and observe how long it takes for the nail to return to normal color. Refill of capillaries in the nail beds should take approximately 3 to 5 seconds and should be equal in all fingers.

Intervention Guidelines

Enlarged lymph nodes may indicate local or systemic infection or more serious conditions. The client should be referred to a

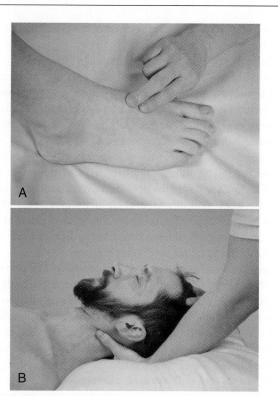

FIGURE 11-17 A, Palpation assessment of vessels for circulation. **B,** Assessment of lymph nodes.

physician immediately if these are noted. Tissue should not be boggy and taut from water retention. It is important to refer the client to a physician if the person has unexplained and persistent edema. General massage appears to support fluid movement, at least at a local level. (Specific applications that affect blood and lymph circulation are presented in Chapter 12.)

Palpation of Muscles

The fifth application of palpation is skeletal muscle. Muscle has a distinct fiber direction that can be felt. This texture feels somewhat like corded fabric or fine rope. Muscle is made up of contractile fibers embedded in connective tissue. Individual muscles are contained in layers of deep fascia. The area of the muscle that becomes the largest when the muscle is concentrically contracted is in the belly of the muscle. The tendon develops where the muscle fibers end and the connective tissue continues; this is called the *musculotendinous junction.* A good practice activity involves locating both of these areas for all surface muscles and as many underlying ones as possible. Almost all muscular dysfunctions, such as trigger points or microscarring from minute muscle tears, occur at the musculotendinous junction or in the belly of the muscle. Most acupressure points and motor points are also located in these areas.

Often three or more layers of muscle are present in an area. These layers are separated by deep fascia, and each muscle layer should slide over the one beneath it (Figure 11-18). It is important to compress systematically through each layer until the bone is felt. Pressure used to reach and palpate the deeper layers of muscle must travel from the superficial layers down to the deeper layers. To accomplish this, the compressive force

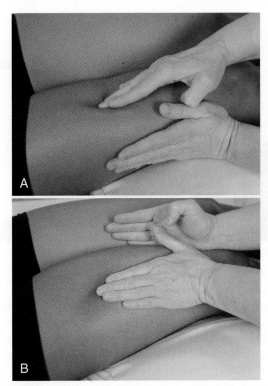

FIGURE 11-18 Palpation of muscle and sliding assessment for mobility.

must be even, broad based, and slow. The touch should not have a "poking" quality, and abrupt pressure should not be used to push through muscle layers, because the surface layers of muscle will tense up and guard, preventing access to the deeper layers.

Muscle tends to push up against palpating pressure when it is concentrically contracting. Having the client slowly move the joint that the muscle moves can help the practitioner identify the proper location of muscles being assessed (Figure 11-19).

Make sure to slide each layer of muscle back and forth over the underlying layer to detect any adherence between the muscle layers. The layers usually run cross-grain to each other. The best example of this is the abdominal muscle group. Even in the arm and leg, where all the muscles seem to run in the same direction, a diagonal crossing and spiraling of the muscle groups is evident. If a muscle layer becomes adherent to (stuck to) the one beneath it, movement is limited to the available movement of the tissue to which the muscle layer is attached.

Muscles can feel tense and ropy in both concentric (short) and eccentric (long) patterns. Therefore, think of muscle functioning as short and tight and long and taut.

Skeletal muscle is assessed for both texture and function. It should be firm and pliable. Soft, spongy muscle or hard, dense muscle indicates connective tissue and fluid dysfunction (muscle tone problems). Muscle atrophy results in a muscle that feels smaller than normal. Hypertrophy results in a muscle that feels larger than normal.

Intervention Guidelines

Application of the appropriate techniques can normalize the connective tissue component of the muscle, and circulation

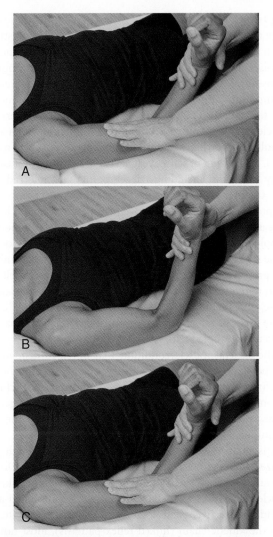

FIGURE 11-19 Palpation of muscle. **A,** Contact the area. **B,** Have the client contract the muscles. **C,** Palpate the muscles as they contract.

methods can address fluid movement. Excessively strong or weak muscles can result from problems with neuromuscular control or imbalanced work or exercise demand. Weak muscles can be a result of wasting (atrophy) of the muscle fibers or a result of neurologic inhibition (reciprocal inhibition). Tension/tightness can be felt in muscles that are either concentrically short or eccentrically long. Tension/tightness that manifests in short muscles that are concentrically contracted results in tissue that feels hard and bunched (caves). When muscles are tense/tight from being pulled into an extension pattern, they feel like long, taut bundles with some contraction and shortened muscle fiber groups (hills). Usually, flexors, adductors, and internal rotators become short, whereas extensors, abductors, and external rotators palpate tight but are really taut because they long and have eccentric dysfunctional patterns.

Massage addresses the short concentrically contracted muscles (caves) to lengthen them, rather than the long muscles (hills), because massage methods usually result in longer tissues. Remember, massage is effective at making tissues longer and more pliable; it is not very effective at making long tissues shorter. Therapeutic exercise is necessary to restore normal tone to the "long" muscles. Massage is applied to the long tissue areas, but the focus is on relieving discomfort by using massage as a form of counterirritation and hyperstimulation analgesia. The massage application does not include invasive intervention (e.g., frictioning or trigger points) intense stretching, or pressure into the deep muscle layers.

Important target areas are the musculotendinous junction and the muscle belly, where the nerve usually enters the muscle. Motor points cause a muscle contraction with a small stimulus, somewhat like a pilot light for a gas stove (motor tone). Disruption of sensory signals at the motor point causes many problems, including trigger points and referred pain (see Chapter 12), hypersensitive acupressure points (see Chapter 12), and restricted movement patterns caused by the increase in the physiologic barrier and the development of pathologic barriers. Typically, when these tissues are located in the short "cave" areas, compression is used to create inhibitory pressure at the muscle attachment or the muscle belly (or both) to reduce motor tone and restore normal resting length. These same methods are not used in the long, taut "hill" areas. These areas benefit from a more superficial general massage application coupled with exercise.

The skeletal muscle condition that develops depends on the person's heredity, activity level, and general health. Careful assessment of the entire pattern, use of clinical reasoning and problem-solving skills, and good general massage that addresses all tissue components are the best recommendations.

It is amazing what sorts itself out during a thorough generalized massage when the entire body is addressed. Do not discount the effectiveness of this type of massage when skeletal muscle imbalances are detected. Spot work on isolated areas is seldom effective. Neurologic muscle imbalances interfere with the kinetic chain (linked reflex patterns), most notably the gait reflexes and the interaction between postural and phasic muscles. The best intervention is a general full-body approach that is modified based on qualities of touch (e.g., depth, drag, and so on).

Palpation of Tendons

The sixth application of palpation is the tendons. Tendons have a higher concentration of collagen fibers and feel more pliable and less ribbed than muscle. Tendons feel like duct tape. Tendons attach muscles to bones. These attachments can be directly on the bone, but just as often tendons attach to ligaments, other tendons, and deep fascia for indirect attachment to the bone. The important point to remember is that these attachment areas are made up of various types of connective tissue. The difference in the connective tissue is the ratio of collagen, elastin, and water. Beneath many tendons is a fluid-filled bursa, or cushion, that assists the movement of the bone under the tendon. Bursae feel like small water balloons or bubbles.

Intervention Guidelines

Tendons should feel elastic and mobile. If a tendon has been torn (sprain), it may adhere to the underlying bone during the healing process. Some tendons, such as those of the fingers and toes, are enclosed in a sheath and must be able to glide

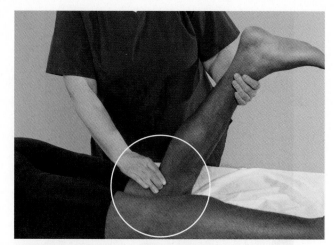

FIGURE 11-20 Palpation of tendons assesses for stability, mobility, and pain.

within the sheath. If they cannot glide, inflammation occurs, and the result is tendinitis. Overuse also can cause inflammation. Inflammation signals tissue healing with the formation of connective tissue, which can interfere with movement and cause the tendons to adhere to surrounding tissue. Frictioning techniques may help these conditions. Usually, tight tendon structures normalize when the muscle's resting length is normalized (Figure 11-20).

Palpation of the Deep Fasciae

The seventh application of palpation is the deep fasciae. The deep fasciae feel like sheets of plastic wrap and duct tape. Unlike the superficial fascia, which is thick and spongy, the deep fasciae are thin but very fibrous. Deep fasciae separate muscles and expand the connective tissue area of bone for muscular attachment. Some deep fasciae, such as the lumbodorsal fascia, the abdominal fascia, and the iliotibial band, run on the surface of the body and are thick, like a tarp. Other types of deep fasciae, such as the linea alba and the nuchal ligament, run perpendicular to the surface of the body and the bone, like a rope. Still others run horizontally through the body. The horizontal pattern occurs at joints, the diaphragm muscle (which is mostly connective tissue), and the pelvic floor. Deep fasciae separate muscle groups and provide a continuous, interconnected framework for the body that follows the principles of tensegrity. The shapes and sheets of deep fasciae are kept taut by the design of the cross-pattern and the action of muscles that lie between sheaths, such as the gluteus maximus, which lies between the iliotibial band and the lumbodorsal fascia.

The larger nerves and blood vessels lie in grooves created by the fascial separations. Careful comparison reveals that the location of the traditional acupuncture meridians corresponds to these nerve and blood vessel tracts. The fascial separations can be felt by palpating with the fingers. With sufficient pressure, the fingers tend to fall into these grooves, which can then be followed. These areas need to be resilient but distinct, because they serve as both stabilizers and separators (Figure 11-21). Deep fascial sheaths should be pliable, but because they are stabilizers, they may be more dense than tendons in

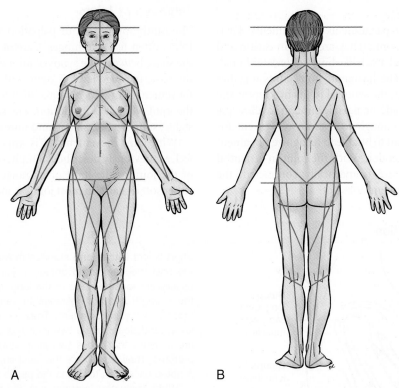

FIGURE 11-21 Fascial sheaths. **A,** Anterior view. **B,** Posterior view.

some areas. Problems arise if the tissues that are separated or stabilized by these sheaths become stuck to the sheath. Chronic health conditions almost always show dysfunction with the connective tissue. Any techniques discussed as connective tissue approaches are effective as long as the practitioner proceeds slowly and follows the tissue pattern. The massage therapist should not override the tissue or force the tissue into a corrective pattern. Instead, the tissue must be untangled or unwound gradually.

Intervention Guidelines

Fascial separations between muscles create pathways for the nerves and blood vessels. When palpated, these pathways feel like grooves running between muscles. If these areas become narrow or restricted, blood vessels may be constricted and nerves impinged. A slow, specific, but careful stripping/gliding along these pathways can be beneficial. If the application is too aggressive, vessels and nerves can be damaged. As a general guide, the client should not grimace, flinch or protectively tense up during the application. The nerves run in these fascial pathways, and the nerve trunks correlate with the traditional meridian system. Therefore most meridian and acupressure work takes place along these fascial grooves.

Muscle layers are also separated by deep fascia, and because muscles must be able to slide over each other, the practitioner must make sure there is no restrictive adherence between muscle layers. This situation often occurs in the legs. If assessment indicates that the muscles are stuck to each other, kneading and gliding can be used to slide one muscle layer over the other (Figure 11-22).

Myofascial approaches are best suited to dealing with the deep fascia (see Chapter 12). Mechanical work, such as slow,

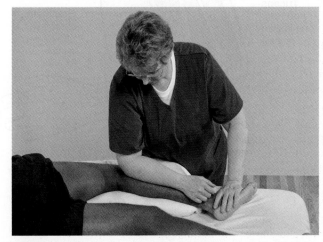

FIGURE 11-22 Palpation of fascial sheaths assesses for bind and mobility. Here we see an example of the sheath between the lateral and posterior compartment of the leg.

sustained stretching, and methods that pull and drag on the tissue are used to soften deep fascia. Because this work often is uncomfortable, it should not be undertaken unless the client is willing to commit to regular appointments until the area has been normalized. This may take 6 months to 1 year.

Highly developed assessment and palpation skills are a must for working specifically with connective tissue dysfunction. General massage methods that are applied slowly and that generate a drag to introduce bend, shear, and torsion forces on tissues that are short and stuck should be used until more specific training is obtained.

Because water is an important element of connective tissue, optimum fluid intake should be recommended to clients.

Palpation of Ligaments

The eighth application of palpation is the ligaments. Ligaments are found around joints. They are high in elastin and somewhat stretchy; they feel much like bungee cords, although some ligaments are flat. The ligaments hold joints together and maintain joint space in the synovial joints by keeping the joint apart. Ligaments should be flexible enough to allow the joint to move, yet stable enough to restrain movement for joint stability. It is important to be able to recognize a ligament and not mistake it for a tendon. With the joint in a neutral position, if the muscles are isometrically contracted, the tendon moves but the ligament does not.

Palpation of Joints

The ninth application of palpation is the joints (Box 11-7). Joints often feel like hinges. Careful palpation should reveal the space between the synovial joint ends. Most assessment, at the basic massage level, is done with active and passive joint movements. An added source of information is palpation of the joint while it is in motion. The sense should be that of a stable, supported, resilient, and unrestricted range of motion.

With joint movements, it is important to assess for end-feel, as previously described. Simply, end-feel is the perception of the joint at the limit of its range of motion, and it feels either soft or hard. In most joints it should feel soft; this means

---

Box 11-7 Joint Function

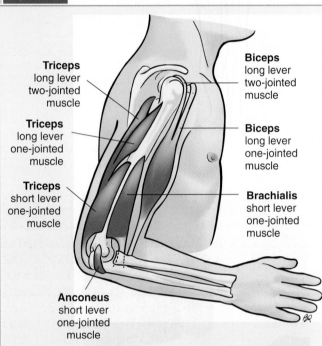

Triceps
long lever
two-jointed
muscle

Triceps
long lever
one-jointed
muscle

Triceps
short lever
one-jointed
muscle

Biceps
long lever
two-jointed
muscle

Biceps
long lever
one-jointed
muscle

Brachialis
short lever
one-jointed
muscle

Anconeus
short lever
one-jointed
muscle

One- and two-joint muscles; functional short- and long-lever muscles.

For the most part, massage practitioners work with synovial (freely movable) joints. These joints are the focus of this text. The amount of joint movement depends on the bone structure, supportive elements of the ligaments, and arrangement of the muscles. Joints are designed to fit together in a specific way. For a joint to move, there must be a space between the bone ends. The bone ends must be smooth and lubricated to prevent friction. Also, the muscular elements must function properly, and the joint structure, including the cartilage, must be functional. Anything that interferes with these key elements interferes with joint function.

Balance is another key element in joint function. If the positional receptors in a joint relay information to the central nervous system indicating that damage to the joint may occur, motor activity (i.e., muscular action) is affected.

Joints are characterized as having one-joint muscles or two-joint muscles, depending on the basic configuration of the muscles around the joint. One-joint muscles are muscles that cross a single joint; they consist of short levers and long levers.

Short levers initiate and stabilize movement. They often have the best mechanical advantage in joint movement, and they usually are located deep to the long levers. Long levers have the strength and pulling range to carry out the full range of motion of the joint pattern. They are superficial to the short levers and deep to the two-joint muscles. Two-joint muscles are muscles that cross two joints and coordinate movement patterns. They usually are the most superficial of the muscles. A noted exception to this is the psoas muscle.

When evaluating joint function, the massage professional is most concerned with pain-free, symmetric range of motion. Determining whether pain on movement is a muscle or tendon problem or a ligament or joint problem can be difficult. Because therapeutic massage deals with nonspecific soft tissue dysfunction, joint dysfunction is out of the scope of practice for massage professionals unless they are specifically supervised by a chiropractor, physician, or physical therapist.

It is important to be able to distinguish between the muscle and tendon components and the ligament and joint components in a restricted movement pattern. When in doubt, always refer suspected joint problems to a medical professional.

Muscle and tendon problems can be differentiated from ligament and joint problems in two ways:

- Pain on gentle traction usually indicates a soft tissue problem, such as a muscle or tendon condition; pain with gentle compression usually indicates a ligament or joint problem.
- If active range of motion produces pain and passive range of motion does not, the cause usually is a muscle or tendon problem. If both passive and active range of motion produce pain, the cause usually is a ligament or joint problem.

When massage practitioners work with joints, it is important that they distinguish between the *anatomic barrier* and the *physiologic barrier*. The anatomic barrier is the bone contour and the soft tissue (especially the ligaments) that serve as the final limit to motion in a joint. Beyond this motion limit, tissue damage occurs. The physiologic barrier is more of a nervous system protective barrier that prevents access to the anatomic barrier when damage to the joint could occur. A pathologic barrier exists when the movement is limited by some sort of injury, dysfunction, or inappropriate compensation pattern. The massage therapist must stay within the limits of the physiologic barrier to avoid possible hypermovement of a joint. Therapeutic massage may increase the range of motion of a jointed area by resetting the confines of the pathologic barrier.

that the body is unable to move any more through muscular contraction, but a small additional move by the therapist still produces some give. A hard end-feel is what the bony stabilization of the elbow feels like on extension. No more active movement is possible, and passive movement is restricted by bone.

It is important to assess for fluid changes around joints. Tissues around the joint can swell because of edema or excess fluid, which can build up inside the joint capsule. Edema is caused by extra water in the system and typically occurs around the joint. Swelling caused by extra water inside the joint capsule is called *effusion*. A small amount of fluid exists in normal joints. This fluid acts as a lubricant for the bones moving against each other and maintains the space in the joint between the bones. Effusion can be a protective mechanism for arthritic joints, because a small amount of excess fluid keeps the bone ends apart. Excessive effusion can be an indication of serious injury or a pathologic condition. Edema feels spongy, and pressure leaves an indentation. Effusion feels more like a water balloon. Movement of the joints through comfortable ranges of motion can be used as an evaluation method. Comparison of the symmetry of range of motion (e.g., comparing the circumduction pattern of one arm against that of the other) is effective for detecting limitations of a particular movement.

Intervention Guidelines

Muscle energy methods, in addition to all massage manipulations, can be used to support symmetric range-of-motion functions. All these tissues and structures are supported by general massage applications, which result in increased circulation, increased pliability of soft tissue, and normalized neuromuscular patterns.

Massage can positively affect the normal limits of the physiologic barrier. When joints are traumatized, the surrounding tissue becomes "scared," almost as if saying, "This joint will never get in that position again." When this happens, all the proprioceptive mechanisms reset to limit the range of motion, setting up a pathologic barrier. Massage and appropriate muscle lengthening and general stretching, combined with muscle energy techniques and self-help, can have a beneficial effect on ligaments, joint function, and bone health. Ligaments are relatively slow to regenerate, and sustained improvement takes time.

Application of various mechanical forces (e.g., kneading) to the soft tissue around joints can increase tissue pliability; however, the most common soft tissue dysfunction around joints is laxity, not shortening. Lax (loose) joint structures should not be massaged directly; instead, the muscles around the joint should be the main target.

Palpation of Bones

The tenth application of palpation is the bones. Those who have developed their palpation skills find a firm but detectable pliability to bone. Bones feel like young sapling tree trunks and branches.

For the massage practitioner, it is important to be able to palpate the bony landmarks that indicate the tendinous

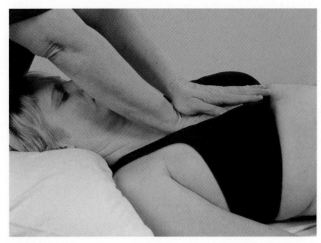

FIGURE 11-23 Palpation of bone (e.g., the sternum).

attachment points for the muscles and to trace the bone's shape (Figure 11-23).

Palpation of Abdominal Viscera

The eleventh application of palpation is the viscera, which are the internal organs of the body. The abdomen contains the viscera. It is important for the massage professional to be able to locate the organs in the abdominal cavity and to know their positioning.

The massage therapist should be able to palpate the distinct firmness of the liver and the large intestine. Although deep massage to the abdomen is not suggested for those trained in basic massage, light to moderate stroking of the abdomen is beneficial for the large intestine. The massage therapist should be able to locate and palpate this organ. Refer the client to a physician if any hard, rigid, stiff, or tense areas are noted in the abdomen. Close attention must be paid to the visceral referred pain areas (see Chapter 6). If tissue changes are noted, the practitioner must refer the client to a physician.

Intervention Guidelines

The skin often is tighter in areas of visceral referred pain. As a result of cutaneous and visceral reflexes, benefit may be obtained by stretching the skin in these areas. There is some indication that normalizing the pliability of the skin over these areas has a positive effect on the functioning of the organ. If nothing else, circulation may be increased and peristalsis (intestinal movement) may be stimulated.

In accordance with the recommendations for colon massage (see Chapter 10), repetitive stroking in the proper directions may stimulate smooth muscle contraction and can improve elimination problems and excessive intestinal gas. A professional practitioner is prepared for the results and will inquire as to whether the client wants to visit the restroom (Figure 11-24).

Palpation of Body Rhythms

The twelfth application of palpation is the body rhythms, which are felt as tiny, swaying undulations and pulsations. Body rhythms are designed to operate in a coordinated, balanced, and synchronized manner. In the body the rhythms all

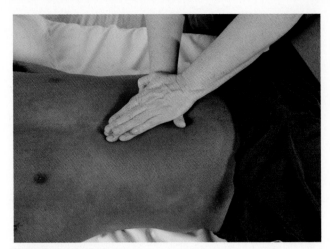

FIGURE 11-24 Palpation of viscera assesses for pliability, mobility, and pain.

entrain (synchronize). When palpating body rhythms, the practitioner should get a sense of this harmony. Although the trained hand can pick out some of the individual rhythms, just as one can hear individual notes in a song, it is the whole connected effect that is important. When a person feels "off" or "out of sync," he or she often is speaking of disruption in the entrainment process of body rhythms.

The three basic rhythms assessed are the respiration, blood circulation, and lymph circulation. Some bodywork systems also concentrate on craniosacral rhythms. More subtle energetic rhythms may be present in the body that can be identified with increased palpation sensitivity. However, the three basic rhythms are supported by the most scientific understanding.

- *Respiration.* The breath is easy to feel. It should be even and should follow good principles of inhalation and exhalation (see Chapter 15). Palpation of the breath is done by placing the hands over the ribs and allowing the body to go through three or more cycles as the practitioner evaluates the evenness and fullness of the breath. Relaxed breathing should result in a slight rounding of the upper abdomen and lateral movement of the lower ribs during inhalation. Movement in the shoulders or upper chest indicates potential difficulties with the breathing mechanism.

- *Blood circulation.* The rhythmic beating of the heart moves the blood in the body. The movement of the blood is felt at the major pulse points. The pulses should be balanced on both sides of the body. Basic palpation of the movement of the blood is done by placing the fingertips over pulse points on both sides of the body and comparing for evenness. The vascular refill rate is another means of assessing the efficiency and rhythm of the circulation. To assess this rate, press the nail beds until they blanch (push blood out), then let go and count the seconds until color returns. The nail bed color should return within a few seconds.

- *Lymph circulation.* Lymph vessels have an undulating, peristalsis type of rhythm. The movement is very subtle and wavelike. The sensation is full body and not limited to vessels, as with the blood circulation.

Craniosacral Rhythm

The craniosacral rhythm is somewhat controversial. It is said to be experienced as a subtle but detectable widening and narrowing movement of the cranial bones. A to-and-fro (back and forth) oscillation of the sacrum should be felt (DeStefano, 2010). Specific training for craniosacral therapy focuses on this mechanism. Basic palpation of the craniosacral rhythm is done by lightly placing the hands on either side of the head and sensing for the widening and narrowing of the skull. The same undulation can be sensed in any symmetrically placed hand position on the body, such as on both shoulders, the two sides of the back, the two sides of the rib cage, the iliac crests, the knees, and the feet. Also, place a hand over the sacrum and feel for the to-and-fro movement. These sensations normally occur at a rate of 10 to 14 times per minute (DeStefano, 2010). The movement should feel coordinated and even. This sensation may be the rhythmic lymphatic undulation instead of a specific focus on the craniosacral system or some other combined low-frequency oscillations in the human body, such as blood pressure, blood flow velocity, heart rate variability, and intracranial fluid oscillations (Nelson et al, 2006; Perrin, 2007).

Intervention Guidelines

The body rhythms are assessed before and after the massage. An improvement in rate and evenness should be noticed after the massage. Massage offered by a centered practitioner with a focused, rhythmic intent provides patterns for the client's body to use to entrain its own rhythms. The massage practitioner must remain focused on the natural rhythm of the client. Although the entrainment pattern of the practitioner and the massage provides a pattern for the client, it should not superimpose an unnatural rhythm on the client. Any foreign patterns ultimately will be rejected by the client's body. Instead, the practitioner should support the client in re-establishing her innate entrainment rhythm. Supported by rocking methods and a rhythmic approach to the massage and the appropriate use of music, the body can re-establish synchronized rhythmic function.

Breathing

Improved breathing function helps the entire body. Recall from Chapter 5 that the muscular mechanism for inhalation and exhalation depends on unrestricted movement of the musculoskeletal components of the thorax. The muscles of respiration include the scalenes, intercostals, anterior serratus, diaphragm, abdominals, and pelvic floor muscles. If a breathing pattern disorder (see Chapter 5) is a factor and the person is prone to anxiety, massage intervention can help normalize the upper body and support the breathing mechanism.

Because of the whole body interplay between muscle groups in all actions, tight lower leg and foot muscles often are found to interfere with breathing. By contracting the lower legs and feet and taking a deep breath, a person can discover for himself that breathing is a whole body function (Figure 11-25).

Disruption of function in any of these muscle groups inhibits full and easy breathing. (For additional information on breathing, see Chapter 15.)

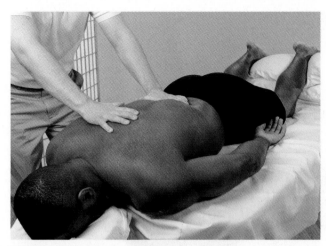

FIGURE 11-25 Palpation assessment of breathing and body rhythm.

General relaxation massage and stress reduction methods seem to help breathing the most. The client can be taught slow lengthening and stretching methods and the breathing retraining pattern found in Chapter 15. The client also can be advised to avoid wearing restrictive clothing.

Proficiency Exercise 11-4 provides a palpation exercise; follow Figure 11-26 for the palpation of arterial pulses.

ASSESSMENT PROCEDURES FOR MUSCLE TESTING

SECTION OBJECTIVES

Chapter objective covered in this section:

8. Adapt joint movement methods to perform muscle testing assessment.

Using the information presented in this section, the student will be able to perform the following:

• Complete a basic muscle testing assessment

Traditional anatomy involves learning about individual muscles in the body as they have been dissected and named by anatomists. However, the most current research indicates that this is a very artificial way of understanding the body. No such structure as an individual muscle actually exists. Instead, the body functions in movement patterns, and all of the elements involved in the movement are connected. The contractile structures that we call *muscles* are concentrated within connective tissue networks that also hold nerves and blood vessels. The *tendons,* as we call them, are not separate but consist of this same material, although with fewer contractile fibers; as they approach the jointed areas, they become part of the material that makes up the ligaments, joint capsule, and bone. As these structures cross over the joints, they again begin to increase in contractile fibers and start to look like muscles.

If the body were dissected in a way to identify function, these long chains would appear. The connective tissue sheaths bundle up functional units such as the structures that flex the knee or stabilize the back. These units collectively would be called by the function performed, such as elbow flexors or cervical extensors. Even this level of separation is not quite correct. The functional relationships of the muscles

💡 PROFICIENCY EXERCISE 11-4

1. Palpate several objects with different textures. Then palpate the same objects through a sheet, a towel, a blanket, and foam. See how many you can identify.
2. Have people walk up to you while you are blindfolded. Pay attention to when you sense the person's presence.
3. Feel for heat radiating off various objects. How far away can you get from the object before you cannot feel the heat?
4. Feel appliances or machinery as the motor runs. Pay attention to the vibrations. How far away can you get and still feel the vibrations?
5. Put a dime in a phone book under two pages. Locate the dime. Keep increasing the number of pages over the dime until you cannot feel it.
6. Get two magnets and play with them. Feel for the "force field."
7. Palpate and/or observe all of the following on five clients.
   • Heat and cold
   • Air pressure and current shifts
   • Damp or dry skin
   • Goose bumps
   • Color
   • Hair
   • Nails
   • Skin texture
   • Skin roughness or smoothness
   • Superficial connective tissue and superficial fascia
   • Blood vessels
   • Pulses
   • Lymph nodes
   • Direction of skeletal muscle fiber
   • Musculotendinous junction
   • Motor points
   • Muscle layers
   • Tendons
   • Fascial sheaths
   • Ligaments
   • Bursae
   • Joints
   • Joint space
   • Joint movement
   • Joint movement end-feel
   • Bone
   • Bony landmarks
   • Bone shape
   • Viscera
   • Craniosacral rhythms or lymphatic undulation
   • Breathing

surrounding a jointed area cannot be separated. For example, knee flexion occurs when what we call the hamstring muscles shorten. However, all of the structures that act on the knee are active and communicating during this specific movement. One segment is shortening, another is controlling the speed and direction of the movement, and yet another is providing stability, and so forth.

Actually, the concept of function lines of tissue, as conceptualized in traditional Chinese meridians, is more accurate (see Chapter 12). These meridians follow pathways around the

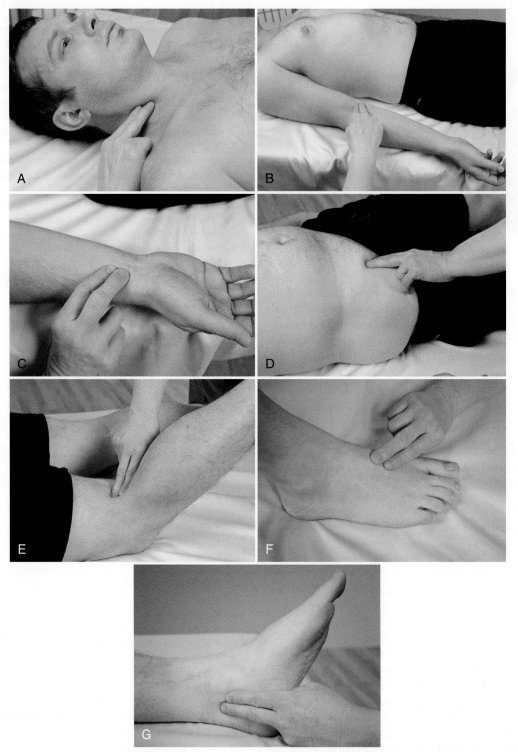

FIGURE 11-26 Palpation of the arterial pulses. **A,** Carotid pulse. **B,** Brachial pulse. **C,** Radial pulse. **D,** Femoral pulse. **E,** Popliteal pulse. **F,** Dorsalis pulse. **G,** Posterior tibial pulse.

body that are similar to what anatomists now are attempting to describe as functional units. If the massage practitioner understands the interconnectedness of the body, the muscle testing assessment makes more sense.

Types of Muscle Testing

Muscle testing procedures are used for different purposes. The purpose of strength testing is to discover whether the muscle responds with sufficient strength to perform the required body functions. The purpose of neurologic muscle testing is to discover whether the neurologic interaction of the muscles is working smoothly. The third type of muscle testing, which is used in applied kinesiology, relies on muscle strength or weakness as an indicator of body function. It is somewhat like a body biofeedback mechanism. The system itself is controversial and too complex to cover in this book, but it is important to identify applied kinesiologic muscle testing procedures as a method of assessment and evaluation so that students are aware of the system (Haas et al., 2007; Hall et al., 2008).

Strength Testing

In general, the purpose of strength testing is to determine whether the muscle or muscle groups are able to respond with adequate force to a demand without excessive recruitment of other muscles and whether the muscle strength patterns are similar on both sides of the body. Strength testing determines a muscle's force of concentric contraction.

Procedure for Strength Testing

1. The preferred method is to isolate the muscle or muscle group by positioning the joint that the muscle acts on in the middle of the available range of motion.
2. The muscle or muscle group being tested should be isolated as specifically as possible.
3. The client holds or maintains the contracted position of the muscle isolation while the therapist slowly and evenly applies a counterpressure to pull or press the muscle out of its isolated position.
4. The massage therapist must use sufficient force to recruit a full response by the muscles being tested but not enough to recruit other muscles in the body.

If strength testing is done this way, there is little chance the therapist will injure the client. As with palpation, the muscle test must be compared with a similar area, usually the same muscle group on the opposite side (see Chapter 10 of *Mosby's Essential Sciences for Therapeutic Massage*).

Various assessment scales are used to describe the findings from strength testing. The most common is a numeric scale. Grades for a manual muscle test are recorded as numeric scores ranging from 1, which represents no activity, to 5, which represents a "normal" or best-possible response to the test or as great a response as can be evaluated by a manual muscle test. The grades are as follows:

5—Normal strength
4—Movement against gravity and resistance
3—Movement against gravity (resistance eliminated)
2—Movement with gravity eliminated
1—Only a flicker of movement

Because this text is based on tests of motions rather than tests of individual muscles, the grade represents the performance of all muscles in that motion.

Procedures for Muscle Testing

Muscle strength is assessed by making the muscles hold against an imposed force. The term "resistance" is used to describe a force that acts in opposition to a contracting muscle. Manual resistance should always be applied in the direction of the "line of pull" of the participating muscle or muscles. Resistance is applied at a 90-degree angle to the primary axis of the body part tested.

1. To ensure correct positioning and stabilization for the test, place the muscle group to be tested in the test position rather than have the client actively move it there.

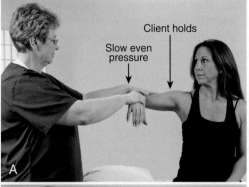
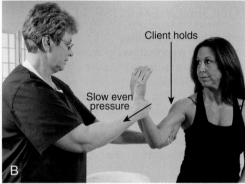

FIGURE 11-27 A, Muscle test for medial deltoid. **B,** Muscle test for biceps.

2. Stabilize the rest of the body so that only the joint targeted for assessment will move in response to the muscle contraction.
3. Apply resistance near the distal end of the segment to which the muscle attaches.
4. Make sure the application of manual resistance to a part is never sudden or uneven (jerky). Apply resistance slowly and gradually, allowing it to build to the maximum tolerable intensity.

A tested muscle or muscle group may be unable to hold against applied force for many reasons, including atrophy, joint dysfunction, and neurologic inhibition (Figure 11-27).

Assessing the Coordination of the Agonist-Antagonist Interaction

Another muscle testing method used for assessment is to compare a muscle group's strength with its antagonist muscle group pattern. The body is designed so that the flexor, internal rotator, and adductor muscles are about 25% to 30% larger and therefore stronger than the extensor, external rotator, and abductor muscles. It also is designed so that flexors and adductors usually work against gravity to move a joint. The main purposes of extensors and abductors are to restrain and control the flexor and adductor movement and to return the joint to a neutral position. Less strength is required, because gravity is assisting the function.

Strength testing should reveal a difference in the pattern between the flexors, internal rotators, and adductors, and the extensors, external rotators, and abductors in an agonist/antagonist pattern. These groups should not be equally strong (i.e., able to hold against the same applied force). Flexors, internal rotators, and adductors should show more muscle strength than extensors, external rotators, and abductors.

Muscle Testing of Gait Patterns

It also is important to consider the pattern of muscle interactions that occurs with walking. Remember that gait has a certain pattern for efficient movement. For example, if the left leg is extended for the heel strike, the right arm also is extended. This results in activation of the flexors of both the arm and leg and inhibition of the extensors. Strength imbalances are common in this gait pattern. One muscle out of sequence with the others can set up increased motor tone (too strong) or inhibited (unable to hold) muscle imbalances. Whenever a muscle contracts with too much force, it overpowers the antagonist group, resulting in inhibited muscle function. The imbalances can occur anywhere in the pattern (Proficiency Exercise 11-5).

💡 PROFICIENCY EXERCISE 11-5

Protocol for Gait Muscle Testing
This procedure is demonstrated in detail on the DVD.

To perform this exercise successfully, you must understand two important definitions:
- *Control group:* For this particular purpose, the control group is the group of muscles that initiates the reflex response.
- *Test group:* Also in this case, the test group is the muscle group that responds to the stimulus from the control group.

The body has many gait-related kinetic chain patterns. This exercise concentrates on the main patterns involved in flexion, extension, abduction, and adduction at the shoulder and pelvic girdle. For testing of the arm flexors and extensors, the humerus should be stabilized superior to the elbow joint, and the femur should be stabilized above the knee.

The control group is activated first, the test group is next, and the contractions in the two groups are held simultaneously. Both groups should hold strong and steady during the test. Chart the data to show any inhibitions.

The antagonist pattern should be inhibited during the test; that is, the antagonists should let go. If they do not, the contraction maintained is concentric rather than eccentric. Be sure to chart the data.

I. Contralateral Flexors
A. Left Arm Flexor Test (Figures A1 to A4)
1. Isolate and stabilize the left arm and the right leg in supine flexion.
2. Control group: Use the right leg as the control and have the client hold the right leg position against inferior/caudal pressure provided by you.

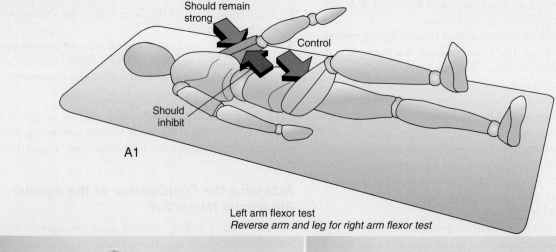

Left arm flexor test
Reverse arm and leg for right arm flexor test

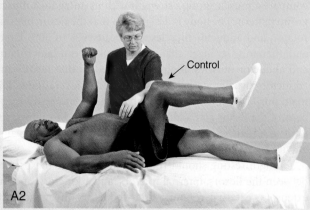

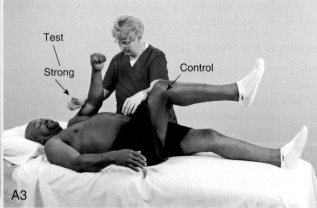

💡 PROFICIENCY EXERCISE 11-5—Cont'd

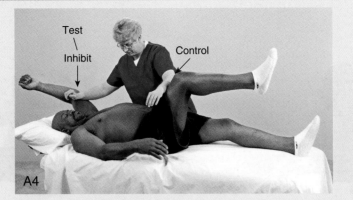

A4

3. Test group: Test the left arm flexors by having the client hold the left arm position against inferior/caudal pressure provided by you.
4. The two groups should be equally strong and steady. If the test group is inhibited (i.e., lets go), chart the data.

Antagonist test: Test the left arm extensors by having the client hold against superior/cranial pressure provided by you. These muscles should inhibit (let go). If the test group remains concentrically contracted and holds, chart the data.

B. Right Arm Flexor Test

1. Isolate and stabilize the left leg and the right arm in supine flexion.
2. Control group: Use the left leg as the control and have the client hold the left leg position against inferior/caudal pressure provided by you.
3. Test group: Test the right arm flexors by having the client hold the right arm position against inferior/caudal pressure provided by you.
4. The two groups should be equally strong and steady. If the test group is inhibited, chart the data.

Antagonist test: Test the right arm extensors by having the client hold the right arm position against superior/cranial pressure provided by you. These muscles should inhibit. If the test group remains concentrically contracted and holds, chart the data.

C. Left Leg Flexor Test

1. Isolate and stabilize the left leg and the right arm in supine flexion.

2. Control group: Use the right arm as the control and have the client hold the right arm position against inferior/caudal pressure provided by you.
3. Test group: Test the left leg flexors by having the client hold the left leg position against inferior/caudal pressure provided by you.
4. The two groups should be equally strong and steady. If the test group is inhibited, chart the data.

Antagonist test: Test the left leg extensors by having the client hold against superior/cranial pressure provided by you. These muscles should inhibit. If the test group remains concentrically contracted and holds, chart the data.

D. Right Leg Flexor Test (Figures B1 to B4)

1. Isolate and stabilize the left arm and the right leg in supine flexion.
2. Control group: Use the left arm as the control and have the client hold the left arm position against inferior/caudal pressure provided by you.
3. Test group: Test the right leg flexors by having the client hold the right leg position against inferior/caudal pressure provided by you.
4. The two groups should be equally strong and steady. If the test group is inhibited, chart the data.

Antagonist test: Test the right leg extensors by having the client hold the right leg position against superior/cranial pressure provided by you. These muscles should inhibit. If the test group remains concentrically contracted and holds, chart the data.

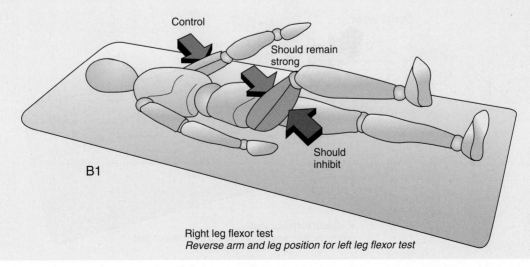

B1

Right leg flexor test
Reverse arm and leg position for left leg flexor test

Continued

💡 PROFICIENCY EXERCISE 11-5—Cont'd

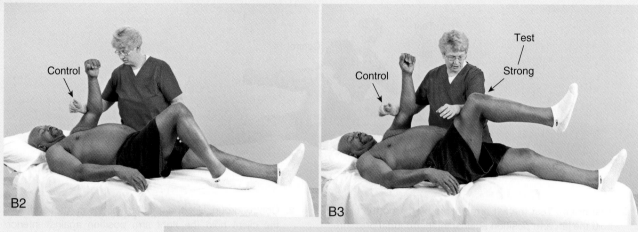

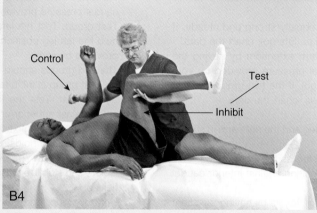

II. Contralateral Extensors

A. Left Arm Extensor Test (Figures C1 to C6)

1. Isolate and stabilize the left arm and the right leg in supine flexion.
2. Control group: Use the right leg as the control and have the client hold the leg position against superior/cephalad pressure provided by you.
3. Test group: Test the left arm extensors by having the client hold the arm position against superior/cephalad pressure provided by you.

4. The two groups should be equally strong and steady. If the test group is inhibited, chart the data.

Antagonist test: Test the left arm flexors by having the client hold the left arm position against inferior/caudal pressure provided by you. These muscles should inhibit. If the test group remains concentrically contracted and holds, chart the data.

B. Right Arm Extensor Test

1. Isolate and stabilize the left leg and the right arm in supine flexion.

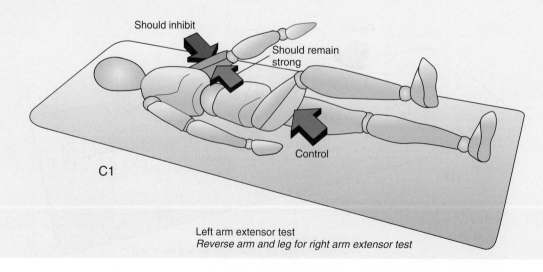

Left arm extensor test
Reverse arm and leg for right arm extensor test

💡 PROFICIENCY EXERCISE 11-5—Cont'd

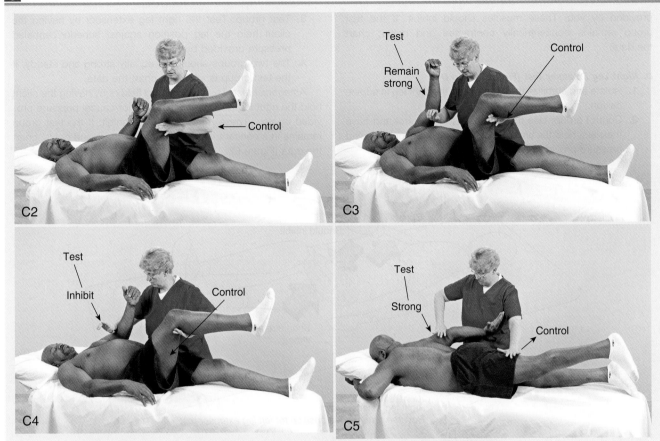

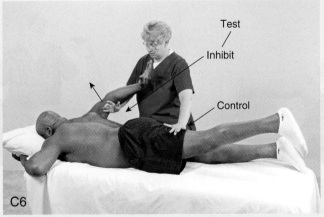

2. Control group: Use the left leg as the control and have the client hold the leg position against superior/cephalad pressure provided by you.

3. Test group: Test the right arm extensors by having the client hold the arm position against superior/cephalad pressure provided by you.

4. The two groups should be equally strong and steady. If the test group is inhibited, chart the data.

Antagonist test: Test the right arm flexors by having the client hold the right arm position against inferior/caudal pressure provided by you. These muscles should inhibit. If the test group remains concentrically contracted and holds, chart the data.

C. Left Leg Extensor Test

1. Isolate and stabilize the left leg and the right arm in supine flexion.

2. Control group: Use the right arm as the control and have the client hold the arm position against superior/cephalad pressure provided by you.

3. Test group: Test the left leg extensors by having the client hold the leg position against superior/cephalad pressure provided by you.

4. The two groups should be equally strong and steady. If the test group is inhibited, chart the data.

Antagonist test: Test the left leg flexors by having the client hold the left leg position against inferior/caudal pressure

Continued

💡 PROFICIENCY EXERCISE 11-5—Cont'd

provided by you. These muscles should inhibit. If the test group remains concentrically contracted and holds, chart the data.

D. Right Leg Extensor Test (Figures D1 to D4)

1. Isolate and stabilize the left arm and the right leg in supine flexion.
2. Control group: Use the left arm as the control and have the client hold the arm position against superior/cephalad pressure provided by you.

3. Test group: Test the right leg extensors by having the client hold the leg position against superior/cephalad pressure provided by you.
4. The two groups should be equally strong and steady. If the test group is inhibited, chart the data.

Antagonist test: Test the right leg flexors by having the client hold the right leg position against inferior/caudal pressure provided by you. These muscles should inhibit. If the test group remains in a concentrically contracted pattern and holds, chart the data (Figure E).

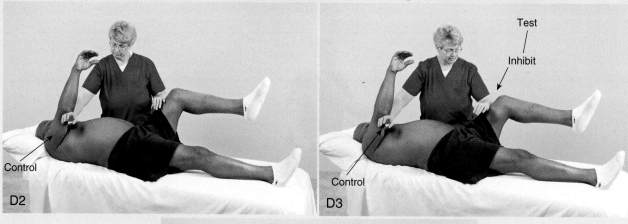

D1

Right leg extensor test
Reverse arm and leg position for left leg extensor test

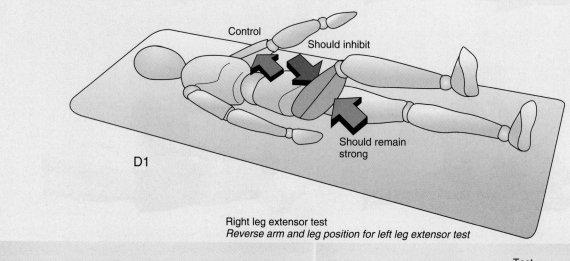

D2 — Control

D3 — Test, Inhibit, Control

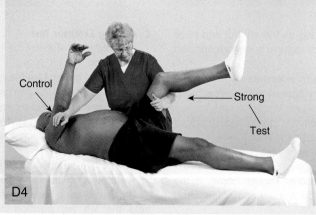

D4 — Control, Strong, Test

PROFICIENCY EXERCISE 11-5—Cont'd

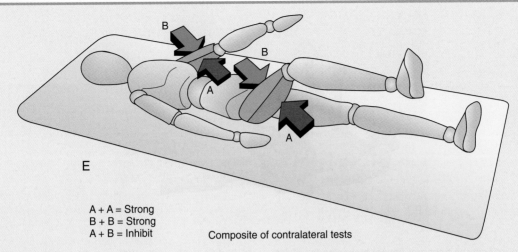

A + A = Strong
B + B = Strong
A + B = Inhibit

Composite of contralateral tests

III. Unilateral Flexors

A. *Left Arm Flexor Test (Figures F1 to F4)*

1. Isolate and stabilize the left arm and the left leg in supine flexion.
2. Control group: Use the left leg as the control and have the client hold the leg position against superior/cephalad pressure (contracting extensors) provided by you.
3. Test group: Test the left arm flexors by having the client hold the arm position against inferior/caudal pressure (testing flexors) provided by you.
4. The two groups should be equally strong and steady. If the test group is inhibited, chart the data.

Antagonist test: Test the left arm extensors by having the client hold the left arm position against superior/cranial pressure provided by you. These muscles should inhibit. If the test group remains concentrically contracted and holds, chart the data.

B. *Right Arm Flexor Test*

1. Isolate and stabilize the right arm and the right leg in supine flexion.
2. Control group: Use the right leg as the control and have the client hold the leg position against superior/cephalad pressure (contracting extensors) provided by you.

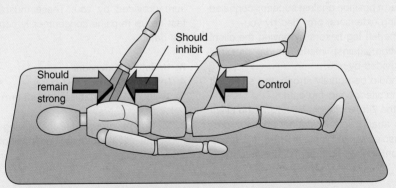

Should inhibit

Should remain strong

Control

F1 Left arm flexor test
Reverse arm and leg position for right arm flexor test

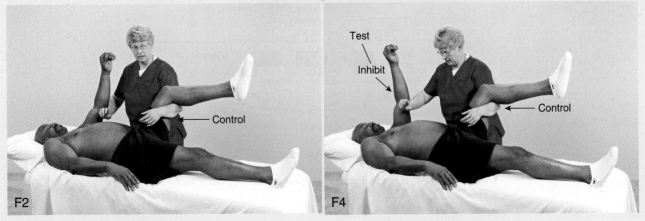

F2 Control

F4 Test Inhibit Control

Continued

💡 PROFICIENCY EXERCISE 11-5—Cont'd

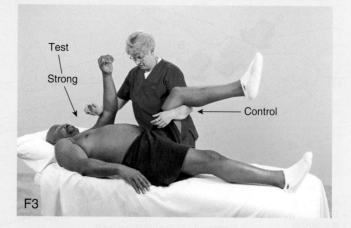

F3

3. Test group: Test the right arm flexors by having the client hold the arm position against inferior/caudal pressure (testing flexors) provided by you.

4. The two groups should be equally strong and steady. If the test group is inhibited, chart the data.

Antagonist test: Test the right arm extensors by having the client hold the right arm position against superior/cranial pressure provided by you. These muscles should inhibit. If the test group remains concentrically contracted and holds, chart the data.

C. Left Leg Flexor Test

1. Isolate and stabilize the left arm and the left leg in supine flexion.

2. Control group: Use the left arm as the control and have the client hold the arm position against superior/cephalad pressure (contracting extensors) provided by you.

3. Test group: Test the left leg flexors by having the client hold the leg position against inferior/caudal pressure (testing flexors) provided by you.

4. The two groups should be equally strong and steady. If the test group is inhibited, chart the data.

Antagonist test: Test the left leg flexors by having the client hold the left leg position against inferior/caudal pressure provided by you. These muscles should inhibit. If the test group remains concentrically contracted and holds, chart the data.

D. Right Leg Flexor Test (Figures G1 to G4)

1. Isolate and stabilize the right arm and the right leg in supine flexion.

2. Control group: Use the right arm as the control and have the client hold the arm position against superior/cephalad pressure (contracting extensors) provided by you.

3. Test group: Test the right leg flexors by having the client hold the leg position against inferior/caudal pressure (testing flexors) provided by you.

4. The two groups should be equally strong and steady. If the test group is inhibited, chart the data.

Antagonist test: Test the right leg extensors by having the client hold the leg position against superior/cranial pressure provided by you. These muscles should inhibit. If the test group remains concentrically contracted and holds, chart the data.

IV. Unilateral Extensors

A. Left Arm Extensor Test

1. Isolate and stabilize the left arm and the left leg in supine flexion.

2. Control group: Use the left leg as the control and have the client hold the leg position against inferior/caudal pressure (contracting flexors) provided by you.

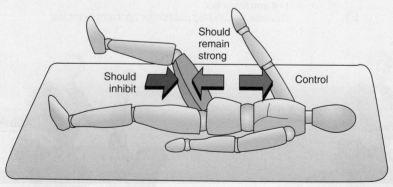

G1

Right leg flexor test
Reverse arm and leg position for left leg flexor test

💡 PROFICIENCY EXERCISE 11-5—Cont'd

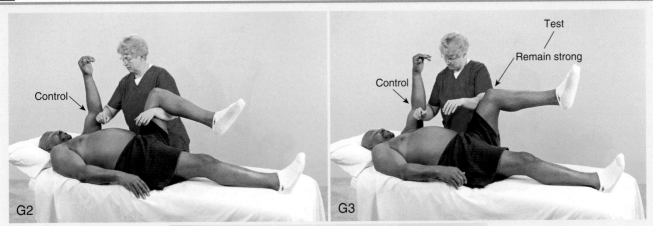

G2   Control

G3   Test   Remain strong   Control

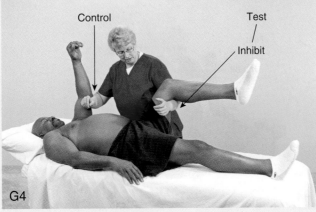

G4   Control   Test   Inhibit

3. Test group: Test the left arm extensors by having the client hold the arm position against superior/cephalad pressure (testing extensors) provided by you.

4. The two groups should be equally strong and steady. If the test group is inhibited, chart the data.

Antagonist test: Test the left arm flexors by applying inferior/caudal pressure. These muscles should inhibit. If the test group remains concentrically contracted and holds, chart the data.

B. Right Arm Extensor Test (Figures H1 to H4)

1. Isolate and stabilize the right arm and the right leg in supine flexion.

2. Control group: Use the right leg as the control and have the client hold the leg position against inferior/caudal pressure (contracting flexors) provided by you.

3. Test group: Test the right arm extensors by having the client hold the arm position against superior/cephalad pressure (testing extensors) provided by you.

4. The two groups should be equally strong and steady. If the test group is inhibited, chart the data.

Antagonist test: Test the right arm flexors by applying inferior/caudal pressure. These muscles should inhibit. If the

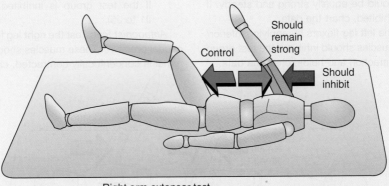

Control   Should remain strong   Should inhibit

H1   Right arm extensor test
Reverse arm and leg position for left arm extensor test

Continued

💡 PROFICIENCY EXERCISE 11-5—Cont'd

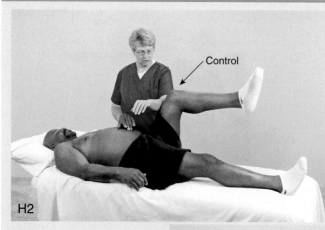

H2

Control

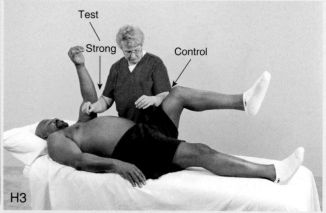

H3

Test
Strong
Control

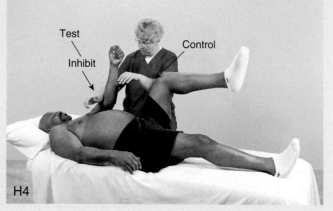

H4

Test
Inhibit
Control

test group remains concentrically contractor and holds, chart the data.

C. Left Leg Extensor Test
1. Isolate and stabilize the left arm and the left leg in supine flexion.
2. Control group: Use the left arm as the control and have the client hold the arm position against inferior/caudal pressure (contracting flexors) provided by you.
3. Test group: Test the left leg extensors by having the client hold the leg position against superior/cephalad pressure (testing extensors) provided by you.
4. The two groups should be equally strong and steady. If the test group is inhibited, chart the data.

Antagonist test: Test the left leg flexors by applying inferior/caudal pressure. These muscles should inhibit. If the test group remains in concentric contraction and holds, chart the data.

D. Right Leg Extensor Test (Figures I1 to I4)
1. Isolate and stabilize the right arm and the right leg in supine flexion.
2. Control group: Use the right arm as the control and have the client hold the arm position against inferior/caudal pressure (contracting flexors) provided by you.
3. Test group: Test the right leg extensors by having the client hold the leg position against superior/cephalad pressure (testing extensors) provided by you.
4. The two groups should be equally strong and steady. If the test group is inhibited, chart the data (Figures J1 to J5).

Antagonist test: Test the right leg flexors by applying inferior/caudal pressure. These muscles should inhibit. If the test group remains concentrically contracted, chart the data.

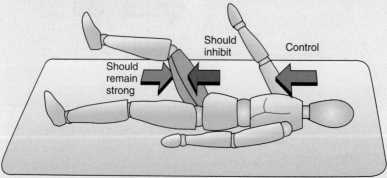

Should inhibit
Control
Should remain strong

I1

Right leg extensor test
Reverse arm and leg position for left leg extensor test

💡 PROFICIENCY EXERCISE 11-5—Cont'd

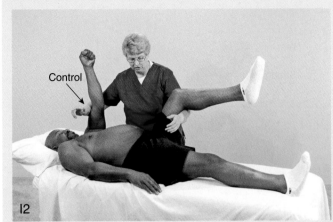

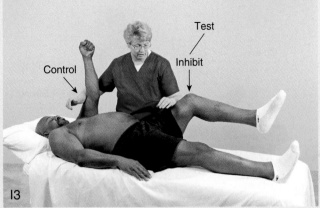

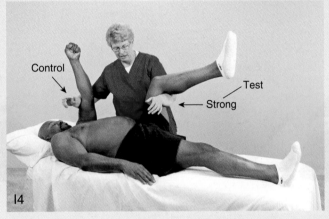

V. Medial/Lateral Symmetry

A. Bilateral Arm Adductor Test (Figures J1 to J5)

1. Isolate and stabilize the arms bilaterally in supine 90% flexion and the legs bilaterally in flexion.

2. Control group: Use the bilateral legs as the control and have the client either hold position against lateral pressure provided by you or squeeze a ball (contracting adductors).

3. Test group: Test the bilateral arm adductors by having the client hold the arm position against lateral pressure (testing adductors) provided by you.

4. The two groups should be equally strong and steady. If the test group is inhibited, chart the data.

Antagonist test: Test bilateral arm abduction by having the client hold position against medial pressure provided by you. These muscles should inhibit. If the test group remains concentrically contracted, chart the data.

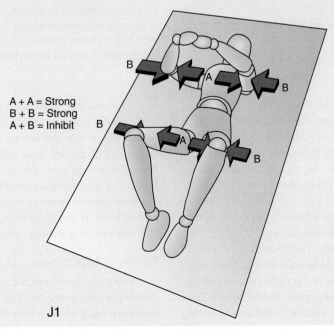

A + A = Strong
B + B = Strong
A + B = Inhibit

J1

Continued

💡 PROFICIENCY EXERCISE 11-5—Cont'd

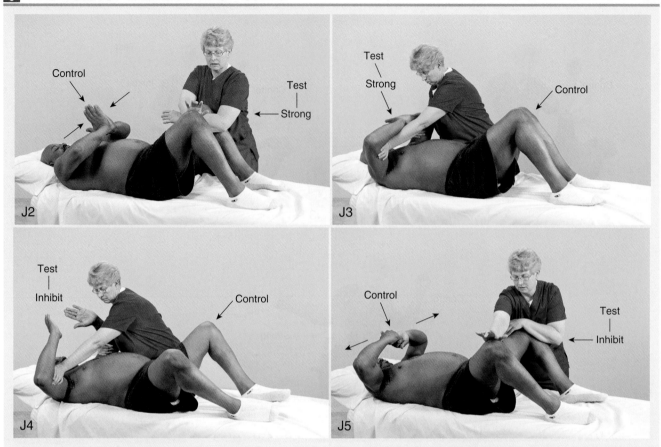

B. Bilateral Leg Adductor Test

1. Isolate and stabilize the arms bilaterally in supine 90% flexion and the legs bilaterally in flexion.
2. Control group: Use the bilateral arms as the control and have the client hold position against lateral pressure provided by you or have the client press the palms together (contracting adductors).
3. Test group: Test the bilateral leg adductors by having the client hold position against pressure provided by you (testing adductors).
4. The two groups should be equally strong and steady. If the test group is inhibited, chart the data.

Antagonist test: Test the bilateral leg abductors by having the client hold position against medial pressure provided by you. These muscles should inhibit. If the test group remains concentrically contracted, chart the data.

Intervention

Use massage methods to inhibit muscles that test as too strong by remaining in concentric contraction patterns when they should inhibit. Appropriate methods are slow compression, kneading, gliding, and shaking. Strengthen muscles that inhibit when they should hold strong. Appropriate methods are percussion and rhythmic contraction of inhibited muscles. Then retest the pattern; it should be normal.

Strength muscle testing should reveal that the flexor and adductor muscles of the right arm should activate, facilitate, and coordinate with the flexors and adductors of the left leg. The opposite also is true: left arm flexors and adductors activate and facilitate with the right leg flexors and adductors. Extensors and abductors in the limbs coordinate in a similar fashion.

If the flexors of the left leg are activated, as occurs during strength testing, the flexors and adductors of the right arm should be facilitated and test strong. The flexors and adductors of the right leg and left arm should be inhibited and test weak. Also, the extensors and abductors in the right arm and left leg should be inhibited. All associated patterns follow suit (i.e., activation of the right arm flexor pattern facilitates the left leg flexor pattern and inhibits left arm and right leg flexor muscles while facilitating extensors and abductors). In a similar way, activation of the adductors of the right leg facilitates the adductors of the left arm and inhibits the abductors of the left leg and right arm. The other adductor/abductor patterns follow the same interaction pattern.

All of these patterns are associated with gait mechanisms and reflexes. If any pattern is out of sync, gait, posture, and efficient function are disrupted.

Practical Application

It is helpful to break apart the gait cycle and look at the relationship of the arms and legs (see Figure 11-9). You can use your own body to learn how the muscles of the shoulders and arms and hips and legs work in sequence. Begin to take a step and then stop and notice the position of the body. Notice what part of the body is moving forward and what is behind the body. Now continue the step and freeze. Observe again. Continue this process until you complete an entire gait cycle.

An understanding of gait provides the foundation for assessment and information for intervention. For example, a person trips and strains the left leg extensor muscles. Gait muscle testing reveals the imbalanced pattern by showing that the left leg extensor muscles are weak, whereas the flexors in the left leg and right arm are overly tense. The leg is sore and cannot be used for work, but the arm muscles are fine. By activating the extensors in the right arm, the left leg extensor muscles can be facilitated. By activating the flexors of the left arm, the flexors of the left leg are inhibited. This process may restore balance in the gait pattern. Many combinations are possible based on the gait pattern and reflexes. Gait muscle testing provides the means of identifying these interactions.

Careful study of this interaction is important for work with individuals such as athletes or dancers. An understanding of this interaction also is helpful in working with people who have various forms of spastic paralysis and spastic muscle conditions. For example, a child with a head injury that causes flexor spasms in the right arm may be helped temporarily by a reduction in the spasm pattern through activation of left leg extensor patterns, especially if the child has more coordination in that area. All other possible interactions follow suit. If voluntary activation of the muscles is not possible, percussion at the tendons of the muscle required to contract usually provides the appropriate neurologic signal.

Neurologic Muscle Testing

Neurologic muscle testing focuses more on the patterns of muscle communication. A small force is used for testing, because only the nervous system is assessed. An efficient pattern is one in which the muscles contract evenly, without jerking and without a lot of synergistic (helper muscle) activity. The same isolation of muscle groups is used as in strength testing. The client holds the contraction, and the massage therapist provides moderately light pressure against the muscle. Different neurologic interactions can be assessed, including muscle group interactions, muscle activation sequences and firing patterns, and postural (stabilizer) and phasic (mover) muscle interactions.

As always, the goal is to locate the muscle interaction pattern, not only for the muscle directly tested but also for all other muscles linked through functional units and gait and postural reflexes. In tests of neuromuscular activity, it is important that the massage practitioner notice what the rest of the body does when the isolated muscle group is tested. For example, if testing of the neck flexor muscles causes the left leg to roll in, a pattern of interaction has shown itself. These patterns may be natural, such as the gait reflexes, but they often are a mixed-up set of signals that cause the body to respond inappropriately. Inefficient patterns cause some muscles to contract with more force than is necessary. After contraction, muscles may not be able to resume a normal resting length; they may remain short and thus maintain tension patterns. Whenever a pattern of overly short muscles exists, a pattern of inhibited and weak muscles also is present. When the prime mover for a particular function does not respond appropriately, the synergist attempts to compensate, altering optimum movement. Synergistic dominance is a common form of neuromuscular dysfunction. These imbalances use energy and contribute to fatigue and pain.

Muscle Group Interactions

Remember that most joints in the body are moved by muscles that cross a single joint or muscles that cross two joints. Muscles are tested in groups because isolating a single muscle is almost impossible; the brain does not process movement of individual muscles. It is more important to work with muscles in patterns of flexion and extension, adduction and abduction, or elevation and depression than to be concerned with the function of individual muscles. The movement pattern of each synovial joint is based on the flexion and extension principle. To move in gravity, each joint must be stabilized by some sort of diagonal pattern that functions as a counterbalance. Therefore, the entire body is involved in all movement patterns.

Muscle Activation Sequences and Muscle Firing Patterns

Muscles contract, or fire, in a neurologic sequence to produce coordinated movement. If the optimum muscle activation sequence is disrupted and muscles fire out of sequence or do not contract when they should, labored movement and postural strain result. Firing patterns can be assessed by initiating a particular sequence of joint movements and palpating for muscle activity to determine which muscle is responding first, second, or third to the movement.

The central nervous system recruits the appropriate muscles in specific activation sequences to generate the appropriate muscle function of acceleration, deceleration, or stability. If these firing patterns are abnormal and the synergist becomes dominant, efficient movement is compromised and the joint position is strained. The general firing pattern is prime movers, then stabilizers, then synergists. If the stabilizer must also move the area (acceleration) or control movement (deceleration), it typically becomes short. If the synergist fires before the prime mover, the movement is awkward and labored.

If one muscle is short and has increased motor tone, reciprocal inhibition typically occurs. Reciprocal inhibition exists when a short, tight muscle decreases nervous stimulation to its functional antagonist, causing it to reduce activity (i.e., inhibition). For example, a short psoas reduces the function of the gluteus maximus. The activation and force production of the prime mover (the gluteus maximus) are decreased, leading to compensation and substitution by the synergists (hamstrings) and stabilizers (erector spinae), creating an altered firing pattern. The most common firing pattern dysfunction is synergistic dominance, in which a synergist compensates for a prime mover to produce the movement. For example, if a client has an inhibited gluteus medius, synergists (the tensor fasciae latae, adductor complex, and quadratus

| Box 11-8 | Major Postural and Phasic Muscles |

Major Postural Muscles
Gastrocnemius
Soleus
Adductors
Medial hamstrings
Psoas
Abdominals
Rectus femoris
Tensor fascia lata
Piriformis
Quadratus lumborum
Erector spinae group
Pectorals
Latissimus dorsi
Neck extensors
Trapezius
Scalenes
Sternocleidomastoid
Levator scapulae

Major Phasic Muscles
Neck flexors
Deltoid
Biceps
Triceps
Brachioradialis
Quadriceps
Hamstrings
Gluteus maximus
Anterior tibialis

lumborum) become dominant to compensate for the weakness. This alters normal joint alignment, which further alters the normal length-tension relationships of the muscles around the joint. (The most commonly used assessment procedures and the intervention for altered firing patterns are presented in Proficiency Exercise 11-6.)

Postural (Stabilizer) and Phasic (Mover) Muscle Interactions

The two basic types of muscles are those that support the body in gravity (postural muscles) and those that move it through gravity (phasic muscles) (Chaitow, 1988). Muscles can perform both functions (Box 11-8).

These two types of muscle are made up of different kinds of muscle fibers. Postural muscles have a higher percentage of slow-twitch red fibers, which can hold a contraction for a long time before fatiguing. Phasic muscles have a higher percentage of fast-twitch white fibers, which contract quickly but tire easily. These two types of muscle are tested differently and develop different types of dysfunction.

Postural Muscles

Postural (stabilizer) muscles are relatively slow to respond compared with phasic (mover) muscles. They do not produce bursts of strength if asked to respond quickly, and they may cramp. They are the deliberate, slow, steady muscles that require time to respond. Using the analogy of the tortoise and

the hare, these muscles are the tortoise. Inefficient neurologic patterns, muscle tension, reorganization of connective tissue with fibrotic changes, and trigger points are common in postural muscles (Chaitow, 1988).

If posture is not balanced, postural muscles must function more like ligaments and bones to provide stability. When this happens, trigger points and additional connective tissue can develop in the muscle to provide the ability to stabilize the body in gravity. The problem is that the connective tissue freezes the body in the dysfunctional position, because unlike muscle, which can actively contract and lengthen, connective tissue is a more static tissue.

Postural muscles tend to shorten and have increased motor tone when under strain. This is an important consideration when massage practitioners attempt to assess which muscles are short, apt to develop trigger points and connective tissue changes, and require lengthening and stretching (see Chapter 12). Connective tissue shortening is dealt with mechanically through forms of stretch. Trigger points usually respond to muscle energy methods and inhibitory pressure. Short concentric contraction muscles are dealt with through muscle energy methods and lengthening procedures (see Chapter 10).

Phasic Muscles

Phasic (mover) muscles jump into action quickly and tire quickly. Musculotendinous junction problems are more common in phasic muscles. The four most common problems are microtearing of the muscle fibers at the tendon, inflamed tendons (tendinitis), adherence of muscles and tendons to underlying tissue, and bursitis.

Phasic muscles usually are inhibited (weaker) in response to postural muscle shortening. Sometimes the inhibited muscles also shorten as a form of compensation, which allows the weak muscle the same contraction power on the joint. It is important not to confuse this condition with hypertense muscles. These muscles are inhibited and weak.

Phasic muscles occasionally become short. This almost always results from some sort of repetitive behavior Phasic muscles also become short in response to a sudden posture change that causes the muscles to assist the postural muscles in maintaining balance. These common, inappropriate muscle patterns often result from an unexpected fall or near fall, an automobile accident, or some other trauma. Often the only intervention needed is using the general full-body massage methods discussed in this text. This general, nonspecific massage seems to act as a reset button for out-of-sync muscles. If a more specific intervention is needed, the gait muscle assessment and corrections and the assessment for muscle activation sequences and firing patterns with appropriate correction can be used (Proficiency Exercise 11-7).

The muscular and skeletal systems coordinate function through the nervous system. Movement occurs through a series of patterns that are both inherent (e.g., reflexes) and learned (e.g., tying shoelaces). The patterns most relevant to the massage therapist are related to posture and gait. No set system exists for figuring out neuromuscular patterns. These patterns are activated in response to a disruption of balance in gravity, such as a fall or repetitive movement. Usually the

PROFICIENCY EXERCISE 11-6

Protocol for Assessing Common Muscle Activation Sequences and Muscle Firing Patterns

Trunk Flexion (Figures A1, A2)

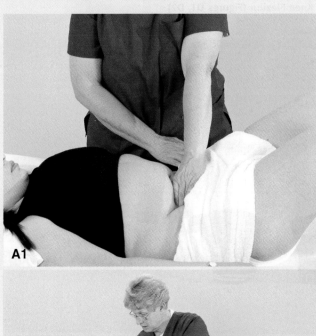

A1

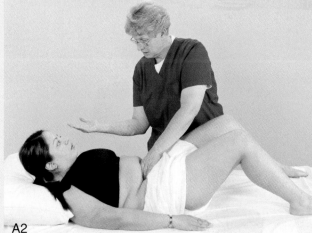

A2

Palpate either side of the rectus abdominis to assess contraction of the obliques and the transverse abdominis abdomen.

1. Normal firing pattern
   a. Transverse abdominis
   b. Abdominal obliques
   c. Rectus abdominis
2. Assessment
   a. Position the client supine with the knees and hips in approximately 90 degrees of flexion.
   b. Instruct the client to perform a normal curl up.
   c. Assess the abdominal muscles' ability to functionally stabilize the lumbar-pelvic-hip complex by having the client draw the abdominal muscle in (as when bringing the umbilicus toward the back) and then do a curl just lifting the scapula off the table while keeping both feet flat. Inability to maintain the drawing-in position and/or to activate the rectus abdominis during the assessment demonstrates an altered firing pattern of the abdominal stabilization mechanism.

3. Altered firing pattern
   a. Weak agonist—abdominal complex
   b. Overactive antagonist—erector spinae
   c. Overactive synergist—psoas, rectus abdominis
4. Symptoms
   a. Low back pain
   b. Buttock pain
   c. Hamstring shortening

Hip Extension (Figures B1, B2)

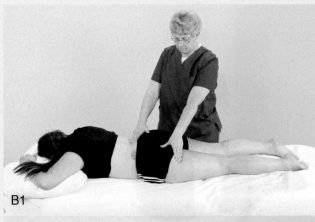

B1

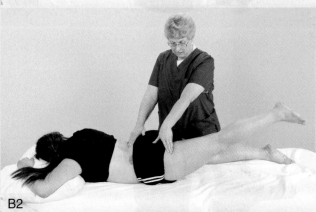

B2

1. Normal firing pattern
   a. Gluteus maximus
   b. Opposite erector spinae
   c. Same-side erector spinae and hamstring
   or
   a. Gluteus maximus
   b. Hamstring
   c. Opposite erector spinae
   d. Same-side erector spinae
2. Assessment
   a. Place the client in the prone position.
   b. Palpate the erector spinae with the fingers of one hand while palpating the muscle belly of the opposite gluteus maximus and hamstring with the little finger and thumb of the other hand.
   c. Instruct the client to raise the hip more than 15 degrees off the table.

Continued

💡 PROFICIENCY EXERCISE 11-6—Cont'd

3. Altered firing pattern
   a. Weak agonist—gluteus maximus
   b. Overactive antagonist—psoas
   c. Overactive stabilizer—erector spinae
   d. Overactive synergist—hamstring
4. Symptoms
   a. Low back pain
   b. Buttock pain
   c. Recurrent hamstring strains

Hip Abduction (Figures C1, C2)

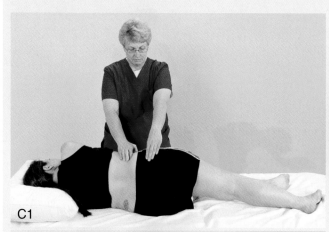

C1

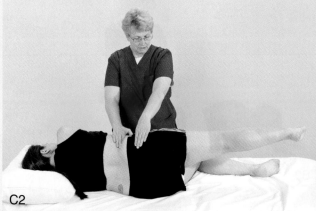

C2

1. Normal firing pattern
   a. Gluteus medius
   b. Tensor fasciae latae
   c. Quadratus lumborum
2. Assessment
   a. Place the client in the side-lying position.
   b. Stand next to the client and palpate the quadratus lumborum with one hand and the tensor fasciae latae and gluteus medius with the other hand.
   c. Instruct the client to abduct the leg from the table.
3. Altered firing pattern
   a. Weak agonist—gluteus medius
   b. Overactive antagonist—adductors
   c. Overactive synergist—tensor fasciae latae
   d. Overactive stabilizer—quadratus lumborum
4. Symptoms
   a. Low back pain
   b. Sacroiliac joint pain

c. Buttock pain
d. Lateral knee pain
e. Anterior knee pain

Knee Flexion (Figures D1, D2)

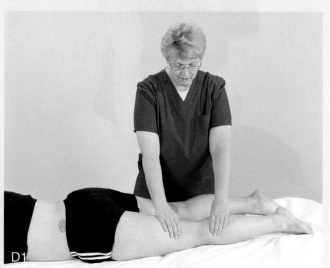

D1

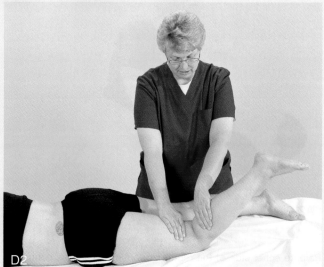

D2

1. Normal firing pattern
   a. Hamstrings
   b. Gastrocnemius
2. Assessment
   a. Place the client in the prone position.
   b. Place your fingers on the hamstring and the gastrocnemius.
   c. Instruct the client to flex the knee.
3. Altered firing pattern
   a. Weak agonist—hamstrings
   b. Overactive synergist—gastrocnemius
4. Symptoms
   a. Pain behind the knee
   b. Achilles tendinitis

💡 PROFICIENCY EXERCISE **11-6**—Cont'd

Knee Extension (Figures E1, E2)

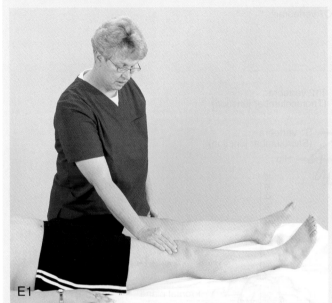

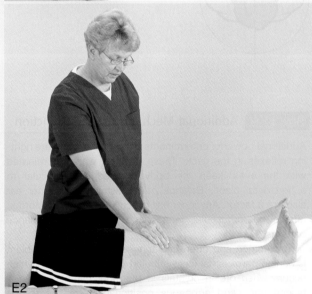

1. Normal firing pattern
   a. Vastus medialis
   b. Vastus intermedius and vastus lateralis
   c. Rectus femoris
2. Assessment
   a. Place the client in the supine position with the leg flat.
   b. Instruct the client to pull the patella cranially (toward the head).
   c. Place your fingers on the vastus medialis oblique portion, vastus lateralis, and rectus femoris.
3. Altered firing pattern
   a. Weak agonist—vastus medius, primarily oblique portion
   b. Overactive synergist—vastus lateralis
4. Symptoms
   a. Knee pain under the patella
   b. Patellar tendinitis

Shoulder Flexion (Figures F1, F2)

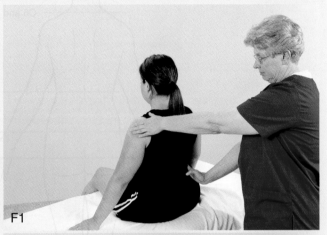

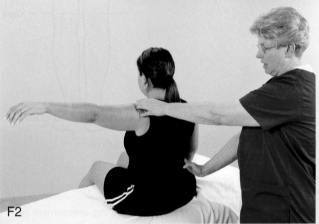

1. Normal firing pattern
   a. Supraspinatus
   b. Deltoid
   c. Infraspinatus
   d. Middle and lower trapezius
   e. Contralateral quadratus lumborum
2. Assessment
   a. Place the client in the seated position. Stand behind the client and put one hand on the client's shoulder and the other on the contralateral quadratus area.
   b. Instruct the client to abduct the shoulder to 90 degrees.
3. Altered firing pattern
   a. Weak agonist—levator scapulae
   b. Overactive agonist—upper trapezius
   c. Overactive stabilizer—ipsilateral quadratus lumborum
4. Symptoms
   a. Shoulder tension
   b. Headache at the base of the skull
   c. Upper chest breathing
   d. Low back pain

Intervention for Altered Firing Patterns
Use appropriate massage applications to inhibit the dominant muscle, then strengthen the weak muscles.

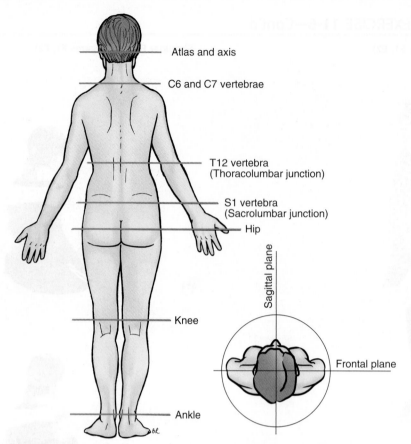

FIGURE 11-28 Quadrants and movement segments.

body's response is to correct the disruption and then return to normal. Sometimes the body does not resume normal function, and dysfunction occurs. A general pattern of dysfunction can be detected during the assessment, and modification methods can be initiated during the massage intervention (Box 11-9).

Kinetic Chain

The postural and movement functions of the body are organized into interconnected segments called the *kinetic chain.* When all segments function well, posture and movement are good. However, if a problem arises in any part of a segment, the entire segment is affected.

Kinetic Chain and Posture

The body is a circular form divided into four quadrants: a front, a back, a right side, and a left side. With divisions on the sagittal and frontal planes (Figure 11-28), the body must be

| Box 11-9 | Additional Mechanisms of Dysfunction |

Additional powerful determinants of normal function are righting reflexes in the neck. These reflexes, when coordinated with the eyes, keep the body oriented perpendicular to a horizontal plane. Balance mechanisms of the inner ear also are a factor. Any inner ear difficulties or visual distortion affects neuromuscular interactions and postural balance patterns.

A common and often undiagnosed eye and ear problem is benign paroxysmal (or vestibular) positional vertigo, which occurs when otolith crystals in the inner ear become displaced and send erroneous positional information to the balance and muscle coordination centers in the lower brain. The eyes are linked through the righting reflex mechanism. Various muscle tension patterns can be linked to this and other, similar conditions. Referral to the appropriate health care professional is important for proper diagnosis.

balanced in three dimensions to withstand the forces of gravity and maintain normal function.

The body moves and is balanced in gravity in the following skeletal areas through the atlas; the C6 and C7 vertebrae; the T12 and L1 vertebrae (the thoracolumbar junction); the L4, L5, and S1 vertebrae (the sacrolumbar junction); and at the hips, knees, and ankles (see Figure 11-28), with stabilization at the shoulder. If a postural distortion exists in any of the four quadrants or within one of the jointed areas (e.g., the tissue

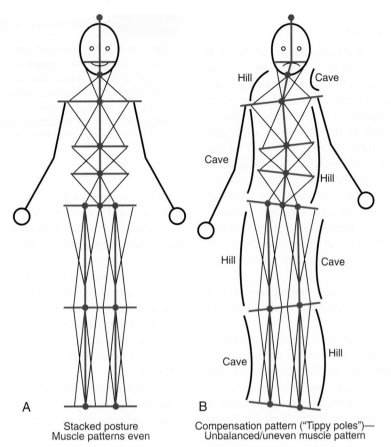

A
Stacked posture
Muscle patterns even

B
Compensation pattern ("Tippy poles")—
Unbalanced/uneven muscle pattern

FIGURE 11-29 Stacked pole **(A)** versus tippy pole **(B)** postural influences on the body.

between the atlas and the axis or the hip and the knee), the entire balance mechanism must be adjusted to maintain upright posture and keep the eyes horizontal. This occurs as a pinball-like effect that jumps front to back and side to side in the soft tissue between the movement lines at the joints.

For example, if one segment, such as the area between L1 and L4-5 and S1 (lumbar, low back area) is altered (e.g., tipped or rotated), the segments above and below must tip or twist in the opposite direction to provide counterbalance and maintain the eye position and center of gravity. As expected, the next segments up and down also adjust, and the eventual result is distortion from head to toe.

The following demonstration can help you gain an understanding of postural balance:

1. Get a pole of some type (a broom handle without the broom portion will work).
2. Tie a string around the pole.
3. Try to balance the pole on its end with the string.
4. Note that in trying to counter the fall pattern of the pole, you work opposite that fall pattern.
5. If the pole tends to fall forward and to the left, you apply a counterforce back and to the right.

This concept can be explained in another way. That is, the body is made up of many different poles stacked on top of one another. The poles stack at each of the jointed areas previously mentioned. Muscles and other soft tissue between the joints form movement segments that must be three-dimensionally balanced in all four quadrants to support the pole in that area.

Each area must be balanced. If one pole area tips a bit to the right, the body compensates by tipping the adjacent pole areas (above or below or both) to the left. If a pole area is tipped forward, adjacent poles are tipped back. A chain reaction occurs, such that when compensating poles tip back, their adjacent areas must counterbalance the action by tipping forward. As explained previously, this is how the body-wide compensation pattern is set up.

Whether the pole areas sit nicely on top of each other with evenly distributed muscle and other soft tissue action or whether they are tipped in various positions and counterbalanced by compensatory muscle and fascial actions, the body remains balanced in gravity. However, the "tippy pole" pattern is much more inefficient than the balanced pole pattern (Figure 11-29). Tippy poles create caves (concave areas) and hills (convex areas); caves have short tissue, and hills have long tissue. Because massage affects short tissue most and supports elongation and relaxation, most massage intervention occurs in the concave areas; tissues that are long need to be exercised.

Interventions focus on normalizing the balance process by lengthening short, tight areas and strengthening muscles in corresponding long, taut, but weak areas, allowing the poles to straighten out. If a pole is permanently tippy, such as with scoliosis or kyphosis, intervention plans attempt to support the appropriate compensation patterns and prevent them from increasing beyond what is necessary for postural balance.

Kinetic Chain and Movement

Movement can occur either in an *open kinetic chain* or in a *closed kinetic chain*. For example, if you move an arm (or a leg) and your hand (or foot) also is free to move, an open kinetic chain exists. Waving your hand is an open kinetic chain movement. However, if your arm (or leg) is fixed against a surface, such as the floor or a desk, and you push, this is closed kinetic chain movement. Closed kinetic chain movements provide simultaneous movements of the interconnected segments. As in our example, if you place your hands against a wall and push, the joints of the wrist, elbow, and shoulder all work together. Problems arise when the joints are not mobile enough to function independently during open kinetic chain movement or when they cannot remain stable in closed kinetic chain movements.

Intervention involves increasing soft tissue pliability in a joint with limited mobility and supporting exercise for a joint that is unstable.

Each jointed area has an ideal movement activation sequence (firing pattern). The movement is a product of the entire mechanism, including bones; joints; ligaments; capsular components tendons; muscle shapes and fiber types; interlinked fascial networks; nerve distribution; myotactic units of prime movers, antagonists, synergists, and fixators; neurologic kinetic chain interactions; the body-wide influence of reflexes, including the positional and righting reflexes of vision and the inner ear; circulatory distribution; general systemic balance; and nutritional influences. Assessment of a movement pattern as normal indicates that all parts are functioning in a well-orchestrated manner. When a dysfunction is identified, the causal factors may arise from any one or a combination of these elements. Often a multidisciplinary diagnosis is necessary to identify clearly the interconnected nature of the pathologic condition.

Intervention Guidelines

Muscle dysfunction, discovered through muscle testing procedures, often indicates how the body is compensating for postural and movement imbalances. Muscle testing also can locate the main muscle problems. When the primary dysfunctional group of muscles is tested, the main compensatory patterns are activated, and other body compensation patterns activate and exaggerate. The massage professional must become a detective, looking for clues to unwind the pattern. By concentrating on methods that restore symmetry of function, the practitioner can help the client's body work out the details.

An example of a major muscle problem is short muscles with increased motor tone. If these muscles can be relaxed, lengthened and, if necessary, stretched to support connective tissue changes, the rest of the dysfunctional pattern often resolves (Box 11-10).

If the extensors and abductors are stronger than the flexors and adductors, major postural imbalance and postural distortion result. Similarly, if the extensors and abductors are too

---

Box 11-10 Muscle Tone and Motor Tone

The term *muscle tone* describes the density and length of a muscle structure with regard to connective tissues and the amount of fluid present (blood, interstitial fluid, lymph). The term *motor tone* describes how long or short a muscle is based on nervous system functions, such as agonist-antagonist interplay and other relationships.

---

weak to balance the other movement patterns, the body curls into itself, and nothing works properly.

If gait and kinetic chain postural patterns are inefficient, more energy is required for movement, and fatigue and pain can result.

Shortened postural (stabilizer) muscles must be lengthened and then stretched. This takes time and uses all the massage practitioner's technical skills. The fiber configuration of the muscle tissue (slow-twitch red fibers or fast-twitch white fibers) dictates that techniques must be sufficiently intense and must be applied long enough to allow the muscle to respond.

Shortened and weak phasic (mover) muscles first must be lengthened and stretched. Eventually, strengthening techniques and exercises are needed.

If the hypertense phasic muscle pattern is caused by repetitive use, the muscles can be normalized with muscle energy techniques and then lengthened. Overworked muscles often increase in size (hypertrophy). The client must reduce the activity of that muscle group until balance is restored, which usually takes about 4 weeks. Muscle tissue that has undergone hypertrophy begins to return to normal if it is not used for the excessive activity during that time. Athletes often have this pattern and very likely will resist complete inactivity. A reduced activity level and a more balanced exercise program, combined with flexibility training, can be beneficial for them. Refer these individuals to appropriate training and coaching professionals if indicated.

Inappropriate muscle activation sequences (firing patterns) can be addressed by inhibiting the muscles that are contracting out of sequence and stimulating the appropriate muscles to fire. Using compression at the attachment and in the muscle belly inhibits motor tone. Tapotement is a good technique for stimulating muscles. If the problem does not normalize easily, referral to an exercise professional may be indicated.

The range of motion of a joint is measured in degrees. A full circle is 360 degrees. A flat horizontal line is 180 degrees. Two perpendicular lines (as in the shape of a capital L) create a 90-degree angle. Various ranges of motion are possible. For example, when the range of motion of a joint allows 0 to 90 degrees of flexion, anything less is hypomobile and anything more is hypermobile. A great degree of variability exists among individuals as to the actual normal range of motion; the degrees provided are general guidelines. Range of motion is measured from the anatomic position. Whether the client is standing, supine, or side-lying, anatomic position is considered 0 degrees of motion.

PUTTING IT ALL TOGETHER: FUNCTIONAL BIOMECHANICAL ASSESSMENT

SECTION OBJECTIVES

Chapter objective covered in this section:
9. Interpret and categorize assessment information.
Using the information presented in this section, the student will be able to perform the following:
• Organize assessment information into categories of distortion and stages to develop a massage care/treatment plan

Functional biomechanical assessment defines mobility based on active and passive movements of the body, through the use of palpation and observation to detect distortion in these movements. Muscle testing and identification of the functional relationships of muscles also are performed.

Typical dysfunction includes the following:
• Local joint hypermobility or hypomobility
• Gait dysfunction
• Altered firing patterns (activation sequences)
• Postural imbalance (tippy pole)

Any one or combination of these conditions can lead to changes in motor function and can be accompanied by temporary or chronic joint, muscular, and nervous system disorders.

Performing a Functional Assessment

The assessment skills presented so far in this chapter are the tools used to perform a functional assessment of the client. Remember that each individual joint movement pattern is part of an interconnected aspect of the neurologic coordination pattern of muscle movement (the kinetic chain) and of the tensegrity of the body's design. Both posture and movement dysfunctions identified in an individual joint pattern must be assessed and treated in broader terms of kinetic chain interactions, muscle length relationships, and the effects of stress and strain on the entire system and the person's ability to adapt and respond to intervention.

When a movement pattern is evaluated, multiple types of information are obtained in one functional assessment.

When a jointed area moves into flexion and the joint angle is decreased, the prime mover and synergists concentrically contract, antagonists eccentrically function with controlled lengthening, and the fixators isometrically contract and stabilize. Body-wide stabilization patterns also come into play to assist in allowing the motion.

During assessment, resistance applied to load the prime mover groups and synergists is used to assess for neurologic function of strength and, to a lesser degree, endurance as the contraction is held. At the same time, the antagonist pattern or the tissues that are lengthened when positioning for the functional assessment can be assessed for increased muscle or connective tissue shortening.

Dysfunction shows itself in limited range of motion by restricting the movement pattern. Therefore, when placing a jointed area into flexion, the examiner assesses the extensors for increased motor tone and muscle tone, which can cause

shortening that would limit movement. When the jointed area moves into extension, the opposite becomes the case. The same is true for adduction and abduction, internal and external rotation, plantar and dorsal flexion, and so on.

Each movement pattern (e.g., flexion and extension of the elbow and knee, circumduction and rotation of the shoulder and hip, movement of the trunk and neck) is assessed by sequence positioning in each area in all available movement patterns and by testing for strength, range, and ease of movement.

Resistance (pressure against) applied to the muscles is focused at the end of the lever system. For example:
• When the function of the shoulder is assessed, resistance is focused at the distal end of the humerus, not at the wrist.
• Elbow function is assessed with resistance at the wrist, not the hand.
• When extension of the hip is assessed, resistance is applied at the end of the femur.
• When flexion of the knee is assessed, resistance is applied at the distal end of the tibia.

Resistance is applied slowly, smoothly, and firmly at an appropriate intensity, as determined by the size of the muscle mass.

Stabilization is essential for accurate assessment of movement patterns. Only the area assessed is allowed to move. Movement in any other part of the body must be stabilized. The massage therapist usually applies a stabilizing force. As one hand applies resistance, the other provides the stabilization. Sometimes the client can provide the stabilization. Some methods use straps to provide stabilization.

The easiest way to identify the area to be stabilized is as follows:
1. Move the area to be assessed through the range of motion.
2. At the end of the range, some other part of the body begins to move; this is the area where stabilization is applied.
4. Return the body to a neutral position.
5. Provide the appropriate stabilization to the area identified and begin the assessment procedure.

During assessments, muscles should be able to hold against appropriate resistance without strain or pain from the pressure and without recruiting or using other muscles. Appropriate resistance is applied slowly and steadily and with just enough force to induce the muscles to respond to the stimulus. Large muscle groups require more force than small ones. The position should be easy to assume and comfortable to maintain for 10 to 30 seconds. Contraindications to this type of assessment include joint and disk dysfunction, acute pain, recent trauma, and inflammation.

Distortion Categories

Distortions in functioning often are measured and categorized in the following way.
• *First-degree distortion:* Shortening or weakening of some muscles or the formation of local changes in muscle and motor tone. The person must use additional muscles

from different parts of the body for usual and simple movements. As a result, movement becomes uneconomical and labored.

- *Second-degree distortion:* Moderately expressed shortening of postural muscles and inhibition and weakening of antagonist muscles. Moderately peculiar postures and movements of some parts of the body are present. Postural and movement distortion, such as altered firing patterns, begin to occur.
- *Third-degree distortion:* Clearly expressed shortening of postural muscles and weakening of antagonist muscles occur, and specific, nonoptimum movement develops. Significantly expressed peculiarity in postures and movement occurs. Increased postural and movement distortions result in defined changes in muscle and motor tone and related connective tissues.

It is very important to determine which muscles are shortened and which are inhibited to choose the appropriate therapeutic intervention.

Based on the three levels of distorted function, the development of postural and movement pathologic conditions is divided into three stages:

- Stage 1: *Functional tension.* In stage 1, the person tires more quickly than normal. This fatigue is accompanied by first- or second-degree limitation of mobility, painless local myodystonia (changes in the muscle length-tension relationship), postural imbalance in the first or second degree, and nonoptimum motor function of the first degree.

As a result: The person can do what he or she wants, but it takes more energy.

- Stage 2: *Functional stress.* Stage 2 is characterized by fatigue with moderate activity, discomfort, slight pain, and the appearance of singular or multiple degrees of limited mobility that is painless or that results in first-degree pain. It may be accompanied by local hypermobility or hypomobility. Functional stress also is characterized by reflex vertebral-sensory dysfunction, fascial and connective tissue changes, and regional postural imbalance. It is also accompanied by distortion of motor function in the first or second degree and firing pattern alterations.

As a result: The person can still do most things but perhaps not as easily. The individual eventually begins to avoid certain activities and uses more energy to achieve reduced function.

- Stage 3: *Connective tissue changes in the musculoskeletal system.* The reasons for connective tissue changes are overloading, disturbances of tissue nutrition, microtrauma, microhemorrhage, unresolved edema, and other factors, both endogenous (inside the body) and exogenous (outside the body). Hereditary predisposition also is a consideration. In stage 3, changes in the spine and weight-bearing joints may appear, with areas of local hypermobility and instability of several vertebral motion segments, hypomobility, widespread painful muscle tension, fascial and connective tissue changes in the muscles, regional postural imbalance in the second or third degree in many joints, and temporary nonoptimum motor function with second- or third-degree distortion. Visceral disturbances may be present. Individuals in stage 3 have significantly reduced function.

As a result: The person is no longer able to perform many common occupational and daily life activities. He or she avoids most activities, and when the person does participate, extreme fatigue occurs.

Distortion Management

Stage 1 (functional tension) often can be managed effectively by massage methods and by massage practitioners who are competent in the skills presented in this text. It is important that the client have all symptoms evaluated by the appropriate health care professional, because the early phases of many serious conditions present the same symptoms as those seen in stage 1 postural conditions. Working with stage 2 and stage 3 conditions (functional stress and connective tissue changes) usually requires more training and proper supervision within a multidisciplinary approach.

Assessment Results

The results of the assessment identify either appropriate function of each area or dysfunction, which is rated as first, second, or third degree. When all assessments have been completed, the overall result is described as normal or as stage 1, stage 2, or stage 3 dysfunction, as described previously. First-degree and stage 1 dysfunction usually can be managed by general massage application. (Remember to make sure the client has no underlying serious conditions.) Clients with stage 2 or stage 3 dysfunction should be referred to the appropriate health care professional, and cooperative multidisciplinary treatment plans should be developed (Figure 11-30).

Intervention Guidelines

Guidelines for analyzing problems found through the functional biomechanical assessment include the following:

- If an area is hypomobile, consider increased motor or muscle tone or shortening in the antagonist pattern as a possible cause.
- If an area is hypermobile, consider instability of the joint structure or muscle weakness in the fixation pattern or problems with antagonist/agonist co-contraction function as possible causes.
- If an area cannot hold against resistance, consider weakness from reciprocal inhibition of the muscles of the prime mover and synergist pattern and tension in the antagonist pattern as possible causes.
- If pain occurs on passive movement, consider joint capsule dysfunction and nerve entrapment syndromes as possible causes.
- If pain occurs on active movement, consider muscle firing patterns and fascial involvement as a possible cause.
- Always consider body-wide reflexive patterns, as discussed in the section on posture and gait and kinetic chain, as possible causes.

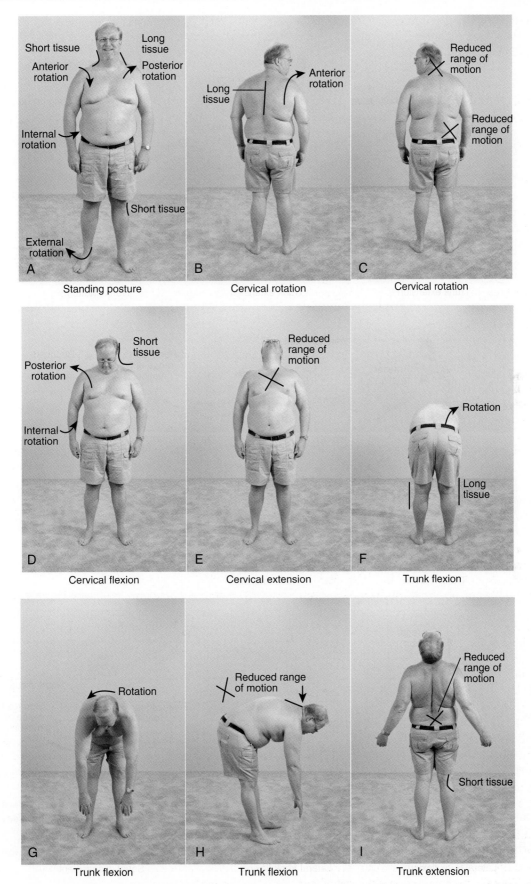

FIGURE 11-30 Postural and functional movement assessment. Examples of dysfunction patterns.

Continued

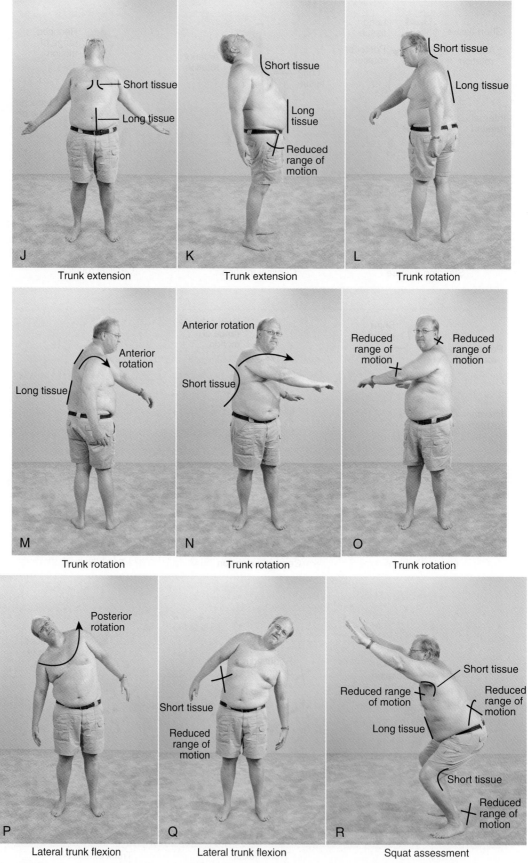

FIGURE 11-30, cont'd

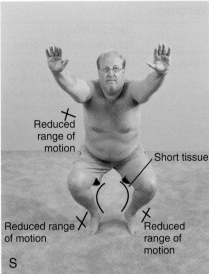
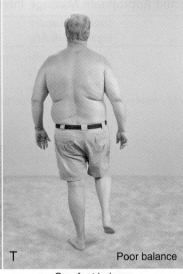
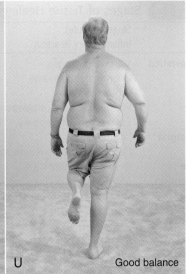

Reduced range of motion

Short tissue

Reduced range of motion

Reduced range of motion

S Squat assessment

T Poor balance One-foot balance

U Good balance One-foot balance

FIGURE 11-30, cont'd

The following guidelines also are important:

- The ability to easily resist the applied force should be the same or very similar bilaterally.
- Opposite movement patterns should be easy to assume.
- Bilateral asymmetry, pain, weakness, inability to assume the isolation position or to move into the opposite position, fatigue, or a heavy sensation may indicate dysfunction.
- Intervention or referral depends on the severity of the condition (stage 1, 2, or 3) and whether the dysfunction is related to joint, neuromuscular, or myofascial problems.

A plan based on efficient biomechanical movement focuses on re-establishing or supporting effective movement patterns. Biomechanically efficient movement is smooth, bilaterally symmetric, and coordinated, with an easy, effortless use of the body. Functional assessment measures the efficiency of coordinated movement. During assessment, noticeable variations need to be considered.

CLINICAL REASONING AND PROBLEM SOLVING

SECTION OBJECTIVES

Chapter objective covered in this section:

10. Use clinical reasoning skills to apply assessment data to treatment plan development.

Using the information presented in this section, the student will be able to perform the following:

- Use the clinical reasoning model as a decision-making tool in the development of massage care/treatment plans

Once the assessment information has been gathered, it is time to connect all the pieces in an interpretation and analysis process to develop the best massage treatment plan for the individual client. The massage does not depend on a modality or protocol; rather, it is an individualized approach based on care/treatment plans. To provide an outcome-based massage,

the practitioner must use clinical reasoning and problem-solving skills (Tables 11-2 and 11-3).

The main purpose of intervention is to help the body regain homeostasis, symmetry, ease of movement, and optimum function. Therefore, when observing gait or posture, the practitioner should note areas that seem pulled, twisted, low, or high. The massage therapist's job is to use massage methods to lengthen shortened areas, untwist twisted areas, raise low areas, lower high areas, soften hard areas, firm up soft areas, warm cold areas, and cool hot areas.

After rapport has been established, clients are comfortable and begin to trust the massage therapist. They will communicate a variety of information during the discussion or the massage session. The practitioner should listen for repeated phrases, such as "It's a real pain in the neck" or "I can hardly stand up to it." The massage therapist should not counsel or explain the ramifications of the information, only notice the pattern and keep general clinical notes.

Careful attention should be paid to the order of priority in which the client relays the information. If the headache is mentioned first, the knee ache second, and the tight elbow last, the areas should be dealt with in that order, if possible, in the massage flow. A client typically says, "It's tight there," if a motor tone problem is the trouble. "Stiff" can apply either to a connective tissue problem or a fluid retention problem (muscle tone), and "stuck" often indicates a joint problem.

The importance of listening to understand is paramount. Many experienced professionals have learned that if we listen to our clients, they will tell us what is wrong and how to help them restore balance. The best way to do this is not to jump to conclusions, to pay attention, and to let the information unfold. Realize that each client is the expert about himself or herself. Clients are your teachers about themselves, and in teaching you they often begin to understand themselves better. In every session, approach each client with fascination about what you will learn from him. No textbook, class, or instructor can equal the teaching provided by careful attention to the client.

Table 11-2   Stages of Tissue Healing and Appropriate Massage Interventions

	Stage 1 (Acute): Inflammatory Reaction	Stage 2 (Subacute): Repair and Healing	Stage 3 (Chronic): Maturation and Remodeling
Characteristics	Vascular changes Inflammatory exudate Clot formation Phagocytosis, neutralization of irritants Early fibroblastic activity	Growth of capillary beds into area Collagen formation Granulation tissue Fragile, easily injured tissue	Maturation and remodeling of scar Contracture of scar tissue Alignment of collagen along lines of stress forces (tensegrity)
Clinical signs	Inflammation Pain before tissue resistance	Decreased inflammation Pain during tissue resistance	Absence of inflammation Pain after tissue resistance
Massage intervention	(3 to 7 days after injury) *Main goal:* Protection • Control and support effects of inflammation • PRICE treatment (protection, rest, ice, compression, and elevation) • Promote healing and prevent compensation patterns • Passive movement midrange • General massage and lymphatic drainage with caution • Support for rest with full-body massage	(14 to 21 days after injury) *Main goal:* Controlled motion • Promote development of mobile scar • Cautious, controlled soft tissue mobilization of scar tissue along fiber direction toward injury • Active and passive, open and closed-chain range of motion (midrange) • Support for healing with full-body massage	(3 to 12 months after injury) *Main goal:* Return to function • Increase strength and alignment of scar tissue • Cross-fiber friction of scar tissue coupled with directional stroking along lines of tension away from injury • Progressive stretching and active and resisted range of motion (full range) • Support for rehabilitation activities with full-body massage

Table 11-3   Massage Approach During Healing

Acute Phase
• Manage pain
• Support

Subacute Phase (Early)
• Manage pain
• Support sleep
• Manage edema
• Manage compensation patterns

Subacute Phase (Later)
• Manage pain
• Support sleep
• Manage edema
• Manage compensation patters
• Support rehabilitative activity
• Support mobile scar development
• Support tissue regeneration process

Remodeling Phase
• Support rehabilitation activity
• Encourage appropriate scar tissue development
• Manage adhesions
• Restore firing patterns, gait reflexes, and neuromuscular responses
• Eliminate reversible compensation patterns
• Manage irreversible compensation patterns
• Restore tissue pliability

From Fritz S: *Sports and exercise massage: comprehensive care in fitness, athletics, and rehabilitation,* St Louis, 2006, Mosby.

As previously stated, specific protocols (recipes) or modalities for therapeutic intervention seldom work without modification, because each person is different. Protocols provide a model of how to begin a therapeutic process, but the massage professional must modify applications of methods based on the client's individual needs and circumstances. The ability to process information effectively in the development of a therapeutic plan is based on a clinical reasoning approach rather than protocols.

The ability to apply what is learned comes from a clinical reasoning/problem-solving process. Effective work with clients becomes a continual learning process of performing a premassage assessment, determining intervention procedures, analyzing their effectiveness through postmassage assessment, and recognizing progress made from session to session. Even in the most basic sessions with a client, when the goals are pleasure and relaxation, decisions must be made about the best way to encourage the body to respond to meet the particular client's goals.

After a history has been completed and an assessment performed, the information gathered is analyzed and interpreted. The next step is to make decisions about what to do and how to develop the process into a coordinated, effective plan for achieving the client's goals. This information was first presented in Chapter 4; now we put it all together.

As noted in Chapter 4, sessions with massage professionals are goal oriented. Goals describe desired outcomes. A primary reason for developing care/treatment plans is to set achievable goals and outline a general plan for reaching them. It is important to develop measurable, activity-based (functional) goals that are meaningful to the client. Goals must be *quantifiable* (measurable) and *qualifiable* (experiential; that is, what they can achieve for the client).

EXAMPLE

• Goal for massage is to increase pliability in burn-related scar tissue to allow increase in range of motion of the shoulder from 80 degrees of abduction to 100 degrees of abduction. *(Quantifiable)*
• The client will be able to reach above shoulder height. *(Qualifiable)*

The database developed in history taking and assessment procedures, combined with any health care treatment orders from other professionals, provides the foundation for clinical reasoning and decision making. Decisions are based on an analysis of the database information. The following four-part analysis process has been presented in many ways throughout this text.

1. **Review the facts and information collected.**

   Questions that can help with this process include the following:
   - What are the facts?
   - What is considered normal or balanced function?
   - What has happened? (Spell out events.)
   - What caused the imbalance? (Can it be identified?)
   - What was done or is being done?
   - What has worked or not worked?

2. **Brainstorm the possibilities.**

   Questions that can help with this process include the following:
   - What are the possibilities? (What could it all mean?)
   - What does my intuition suggest?
   - What are the possible patterns of dysfunction?
   - What are the possible contributing factors?
   - What are possible interventions?
   - What might work?
   - What are other ways to look at the situation?

3. **Consider the logical outcome of each possibility.**

   Questions that can help with this process include the following:
   - What is the logical progression of the symptom pattern, contributing factors, and current behaviors?
   - What is the logical cause and effect of each intervention identified during brainstorming?
   - What are the pros and cons of each intervention suggested? (Remember to look at both sides of the issue.)
   - What are the consequences of not acting?
   - What are the consequences of acting?

4. **Consider how the people involved would be affected by each possibility.**

   Questions that can help with this process include the following:
   - For each intervention considered, what is the impact on the people involved: client, practitioner, and other professionals working with the client?
   - How does each person involved feel about the possible interventions?
   - Is the practitioner within his or her scope of practice to work with such situations?
   - Does the practitioner feel qualified to work with such situations?
   - Does a feeling of cooperation and agreement exist among all parties involved?

5. **Results of the process.**

   Based on your analysis, answer the following questions:
   1. Does the client need referral? If so, to which professionals?
   2. What are the measurable function goals for the care/treatment plan?
   3. What interventions would you choose to achieve those goals?
   4. How would you use them to address the various imbalances?
   5. What results do you expect?
   6. How long do you think it will take to achieve the goals?

Creating the Care/Treatment Plan

The development of a care/treatment plan is based on the five-part analysis just described. After completing the analysis, the practitioner can decide what will be involved in the care/treatment plan. Methods are chosen to achieve the agreed-on goals for the session. The plan is not an exact protocol set in stone; rather, it is a guideline. The care/treatment plan may evolve over the first three or four sessions and may be altered if a change occurs in the therapeutic goals or the client's status.

Decision making becomes a part of each session. As the care/treatment plan unfolds with each successive session, an update on effects, progress, and setbacks is discussed with the client before the massage begins. An updated targeted assessment based on goals is performed, and clinical reasoning and problem solving are used to choose the most effective methods for achieving the best results for the current session. As the plan is implemented, it is recorded sequentially, session by session, in some form of charting or documentation process (e.g., SOAP notes [see Chapter 4]).

The effectiveness or ineffectiveness of intervention procedures is analyzed and compared with the results of previous sessions. Review of the charting notes from previous sessions becomes the foundation for this analysis. The plan is refined, re-evaluated, and adjusted as necessary as the sessions progress (Proficiency Exercise 11-8).

During the massage, assessment and intervention intermingle. Differentiating the two is difficult, except through careful observation. For the experienced massage therapist, assessment and intervention interact in the context of the massage session. An area of imbalance is discovered through various methods of palpation and passive and active range of motion. Assessment leads into intervention, often simply by gently increasing the intensity or duration of the original evaluation method and repeating the methods three or four times.

Reassessment

After the massage is complete, a reassessment must be done to determine what changes the body has made. This can be done efficiently by targeting a few major areas that were the core focus of the massage. The reassessment process helps the client integrate the body changes. The before-and-after awareness also is a reinforcing factor for the client regarding the benefits of massage.

The entire process of massage is an assessment, an intervention for adaptation, and then a reassessment to see whether the approach was beneficial. This takes practice. During

💡 PROFICIENCY EXERCISE 11-8

These case studies can help you practice making decisions about the meaning of the information you gather during the assessment process. They also can teach you how to make decisions about methods for achieving the client's goals. Remember, decision making is always a process. There are no right answers for this activity; effective applications are those that benefit the client.

This decision-making process should feel familiar by now. It was introduced in Chapter 2 to help you learn ethical decision making, and it is a thread that winds throughout the text. The same process is used to make decisions on interventions and ways to apply the best approach for a massage session. (For additional case studies, see Chapter 16.)

Case Study 1

A 54-year-old man has decided to try massage to deal with a nagging catch in his low back. No medical reason for the problem has been identified, and the physician states that age, an old injury, and flat feet are the probable culprits. The client was fitted with orthopedic shoes, and massage was suggested as an adjunct strategy.

The client's history reveals that the problem has been worsening over the past 2 years. The client played many high school and college sports, particularly football, and had many injuries that he did not allow to heal before playing again. He was an Air Force jet pilot for many years, which required long periods of sitting in confined areas and body positioning to accommodate the gravitational forces of aerial combat maneuvers.

The client's current profession requires long hours of sitting and being attentive to people. Because of a change in physical activity, he had gained 40 pounds over the past 4 years and had practically eliminated any physical exercise program. However, in the past 6 months he has lost the weight and begun exercising regularly.

The client broke his foot 6 years ago, and 4 years ago it was rebroken and pinned to correct difficulties with the original healing process.

He has been under increased emotional stress for both professional and personal reasons. His sleep has been disrupted off and on for the past 2 years.

The client shows symptoms of adult attention deficit disorder but chooses not to use medication to treat it. He has no other health concerns. His last physical examination indicated normal functioning.

During the assessment interview, the client poked at his low back on the right, pulled at his neck, moved his left shoulder around, and pointed to the glenohumeral joint numerous times. He seemed edgy and spoke rapidly. He also seemed impatient with the pain in his back. He kept saying that he was too busy to deal with this and that he wished he could ignore it.

The physical assessment showed the following:

- The head is held in a forward position, with the chin elevated and the posterior neck area shortened.
- The shoulders are rolled forward, more so on the left.
- A slight lordosis is present.
- The most notable deviation is flat feet and a rolling to the outside of the heel of the foot, more so on the left.

Gait assessment indicated reduced arm and leg movement on the left side. The entire right side of the body seemed to lunge forward during walking. This assessment also revealed the following:

- The sacroiliac joint was more fixed on the right side.
- The weight is carried mostly on the heels and to the outside of the foot.
- The shoes show an uneven wear pattern.

Palpation indicated areas of cold on the back of the neck and a thickened skin texture, in addition to the following:

- The right lumbar area was warmer than surrounding tissue, with a damp area and exaggerated reddening just below the last rib.
- The superficial connective tissue all seemed short and thick, and lifting the skin in any area was difficult.
- The muscle mass in the legs seemed overdeveloped in relation to the muscle mass of the upper body.
- The left shoulder had restricted range of motion and a hard end-feel in all directions.
- The left foot and ankle were restricted and had limited range of motion compared with the right foot and ankle.
- The breath was even but seemed out of sync with the rest of the rhythms.

Muscle testing indicated body-wide imbalance in adduction/abduction patterns, with the adductors short and the abductors weak, taut, and long. The quadratus lumborum fired first during abduction.

Using the information just given, complete the clinical reasoning process and develop a series of massage interventions and referrals to help this client. It can be helpful to puzzle through the information individually and then work in groups to compare analysis processes and decisions.

1. **Review the facts and information collected.**
   Questions that can help with this process include the following:
   - What are the facts?
   - What is considered normal or balanced function?
   - What has happened? (Spell out events.)
   - What caused the imbalance? (Can it be identified?)
   - What was done or is being done?
   - What has worked or not worked?

2. **Brainstorm the possibilities.**
   Questions that can help with this process include the following:
   - What are the possibilities? (What could it all mean?)
   - What does my intuition suggest?
   - What are the possible patterns of dysfunction?
   - What are the possible contributing factors?
   - What are possible interventions?
   - What might work?
   - What are other ways to look at the situation?
   - What do the data suggest?

3. **Consider the logical outcome of each possibility.**
   Questions that can help with this process include the following:
   - What is the logical progression of the symptom pattern, contributing factors, and current behaviors?
   - What is the logical cause and effect of each intervention identified?
   - What are the pros and cons of each intervention suggested? (Remember to look at both sides of the issue.)
   - What are the consequences of not acting?
   - What are the consequences of acting?

💡 PROFICIENCY EXERCISE 11-8—Cont'd

4. **Consider how the people involved would be affected by each possibility.**

   Questions that can help with this process include the following:

   - For each intervention considered, what would be the impact on the people involved: client, practitioner, and other professionals working with the client?
   - How does each person involved feel about the possible interventions?
   - Is the practitioner within his or her scope of practice to work with such situations?
   - Is the practitioner qualified to work with such situations?
   - Does the practitioner feel qualified to work with such situations?
   - Does a feeling of cooperation and agreement exist among all parties involved?

5. **Results of the process.**

   Based on your analysis, answer the following questions:

   1. Does the client need referral? If so, to which professionals?
   2. What are the measurable functional goals for the care/treatment plan?
   3. What interventions would you choose to achieve those goals?
   4. How would you use them to address the various imbalances?
   5. What results do you expect?
   6. How long do you think it will take to achieve the goals?

Case Study 2

The client, a 16-year-old young woman, shows atypical seizure patterns daily; however, neurologic tests have not found any abnormality. The neurologist referred the patient to a mental health professional, suggesting stress as the causal factor. Physiologic evaluation indicates several emotional stressors, including the life-threatening illness of a family member, the recent relocation of a special friend, relationship problems, learning difficulties, and a tendency for obsessive-compulsive behavior. A breathing pattern disorder is evident. The client's self-esteem is low.

In the past 2 years the client has had two car accidents. She is taking several medications to try to control the seizure activity. Her diet is low in vitamins and minerals, and medications and counseling have had minimal benefit. A mental health professional referred the client for massage as part of a comprehensive treatment plan monitored by the neurologist.

The physical assessment indicated restricted breathing, with primarily an upper chest pattern, shortened muscles, and an elevated scapula on the left with trigger points that generate the suspected seizure activity when palpated. No other indications were evident on the physical and gait assessments.

During the assessment process, the client seemed cooperative but distant and distracted. Her mother was supportive but overwhelmed. Both seemed somewhat desperate for an answer to what is happening.

Using the information just given, complete the clinical reasoning process and develop a series of massage interventions and referrals to help this client. It can be helpful to puzzle through the information individually and then work in groups to compare analysis processes and decisions.

1. **Review the facts and information collected.**

   Questions that can help with this process include the following:

   - What are the facts?
   - What is considered normal or balanced function?
   - What has happened? (Spell out events.)
   - What caused the imbalance? (Can it be identified?)
   - What was done or is being done?
   - What has worked or not worked?

2. **Brainstorm the possibilities.**

   Questions that can help with this process include the following:

   - What are the possibilities? (What could it all mean?)
   - What does my intuition suggest?
   - What are the possible patterns of dysfunction?
   - What are the possible contributing factors?
   - What are possible interventions?
   - What might work?
   - What are other ways to look at the situation?
   - What do the data suggest?

3. **Consider the logical outcome of each possibility.**

   Questions that can help with this process include the following:

   - What is the logical progression of the symptom pattern, contributing factors, and current behaviors?
   - What is the logical cause and effect of each intervention identified?
   - What are the pros and cons of each intervention suggested? (Remember to look at both sides of the issue.)
   - What are the consequences of not acting?
   - What are the consequences of acting?

4. **Consider how the people involved would be affected by each possibility.**

   Questions that can help with this process include the following:

   - For each intervention considered, what would be the impact on the people involved: client, practitioner, and other professionals working with the client?
   - How does each person involved feel about the possible interventions?
   - Is the practitioner within his or her scope of practice to work with such situations?
   - Is the practitioner qualified to work with such situations?
   - Does the practitioner feel qualified to work with such situations?
   - Does a feeling of cooperation and agreement exist among all parties involved?

5. **Results of the process.**

   Based on your analysis, answer the following questions:

   1. Does the client need referral? If so, to which professionals?
   2. What are the measurable functional goals for the care/treatment plan?
   3. What interventions would you choose to achieve those goals?
   4. How would you use them to address the various imbalances?
   5. What results do you expect?
   6. How long do you think it will take to achieve the goals?

Continued

💡 PROFICIENCY EXERCISE 11-8—Cont'd

Case Study 3
The client is a 40-year-old woman. Today is her birthday, and she received a gift certificate for a massage from her daughter. Her history does not indicate any contraindications. The client has no particular goals for the session and is not sure whether she will have any other massage sessions. The physical assessment does not reveal any major deviations of symmetry.

Using the information just given, complete the clinical reasoning process and develop a series of massage interventions and referrals to help this client. It can be helpful to puzzle through the information individually and then work in groups to compare analysis processes and decisions.

1. **Review the facts and information collected.**
   Questions that can help with this process include the following:
   • What are the facts?
   • What is considered normal or balanced function?
   • What has happened? (Spell out events.)
   • What caused the imbalance? (Can it be identified?)
   • What was done or is being done?
   • What has worked or not worked?

2. **Brainstorm the possibilities.**
   Questions that can help with this process include the following:
   • What are the possibilities? (What could it all mean?)
   • What does my intuition suggest?
   • What are the possible patterns of dysfunction?
   • What are the possible contributing factors?
   • What are possible interventions?
   • What might work?
   • What are other ways to look at the situation?
   • What do the data suggest?

3. **Consider the logical outcome of each possibility.**
   Questions that can help with this process include the following:

   • What is the logical progression of the symptom pattern, contributing factors, and current behaviors?
   • What is the logical cause and effect of each intervention identified?
   • What are the pros and cons of each intervention suggested? (Remember to look at both sides of the issue.)
   • What are the consequences of not acting?
   • What are the consequences of acting?

4. **Consider how the people involved would be affected by each possibility.**
   Questions that can help with this process include the following:
   • For each intervention considered, what would be the impact on the people involved: client, practitioner, and other professionals working with the client?
   • How does each person involved feel about the possible interventions?
   • Is the practitioner within his or her scope of practice to work with such situations?
   • Is the practitioner qualified to work with such situations?
   • Does the practitioner feel qualified to work with such situations?
   • Does a feeling of cooperation and agreement exist among all parties involved?

5. **Results of the process.**
   Based on your analysis, answer the following questions:
   1. Does the client need referral? If so, to which professionals?
   2. What are the measurable functional goals for the care/treatment plan?
   3. What interventions would you choose to achieve those goals?
   4. How would you use them to address the various imbalances?
   5. What results do you expect?
   6. How long do you think it will take to achieve the goals?

💡 PROFICIENCY EXERCISE 11-9

Design and conduct five massage sessions, following the assessment guidelines provided in this chapter.

the learning process, assessment and reassessment can feel choppy. The skilled massage therapist learns through practice to flow between the three steps of assessment, intervention/adaptation, and reassessment during the massage, providing a sense of continuity and fluidity to the session (Proficiency Exercise 11-9).

SUMMARY

Massage is a whole body discipline. Assessment skills are the basis for developing intuition; this is done by learning to pay closer attention and becoming more skilled in the interpretation of the assessment information. With practice and experience, these skills become almost second nature.

Trained massage professionals who consider themselves therapists modify methods to best address the client's needs.

Massage therapists not only perform massage "routines," as does the massage technician, they also adjust and adapt massage applications in an outcome-based approach. Massage methods are simple; however, when they are applied with the right intensity and in the right location, the body recognizes the stimulation and can respond resourcefully. This is the approach used by a competent massage therapist. This learning is continuous; the client never stops teaching the therapist.

The more reliable the assessment information, the more likely it is to be accurately interpreted. The more accurate the interpretation, the more specific the application of massage methods. Massage and bodywork techniques are relatively basic. Soft tissue can be pushed, pulled, shaken, stretched, and pounded, regardless of the bodywork system. Forces applied to accentuate change are tension, bend, shear, compression, and torsion. The only variables are the location of the application; the intensity, including drag, depth of pressure, and rhythm; the direction; the frequency; and the duration. The detective work and skills required to assist the client in figuring out each individual pattern prevents the massage therapist

▣ FOOT IN THE DOOR

If you want a successful career as a massage therapist, designing and adapting massage application to each individual is absolutely essential. If you want to get your foot in the door where health care insurance may pay for massage, you need to perfect your assessment skills and be able to justify the benefits of the massage treatment plan. You can get your foot in the door of health care practices such as chiropractors, hospitals, clinics, and so forth by demonstrating the ability to fine-tune massage application with assessment skills and treatment planning.

from becoming bored, which can occur if the same protocol is administered over and over.

A master of massage has learned to respect the client and follow the client's lead. This takes years of practice.

The bottom line is, the client knows his or her body best. The practitioner's job is to understand what the client says verbally, visually, through body language, and in the tissues and movement patterns. Each person's body language is unique. It takes time to learn it. Only through listening, observing, touching, and then using effective clinical reasoning skills can massage therapists begin to recognize the patterns, which ultimately allows them to find solutions for the individual.

The massage therapist should not hesitate to ask for help and should refer a client when the problem is beyond the professional skills determined by the scope of practice for massage therapy and the professional's individual training. By joining in the team approach with other health professionals, the massage practitioner can become an important part of the complex client treatment process.

Practice enables the massage professional's skills to grow. After completing 1,000 massage sessions, the massage professional begins to own the information learned in school. After 5,000 massage sessions, the massage professional has enough experience to begin to trust the process of massage. After 10,000 massages, the massage therapist allows the massage to happen.

Robert Fulghum (1991) tells a story about hiccups that epitomizes massage:

> The reason most cures work, at some time on some people, is that hiccups usually last from between seven and 63 hicks before stopping of their own accord. Whatever you do to pass the time while the episode runs its course seems to qualify as a cure, so the more entertaining the cure is, the better. The hiccuper will be treated with great solicitation while in the throes of these miniconvulsions, and the shaman who has come up with the winning cure will be looked upon with respect.

Applications of therapeutic massage certainly are "entertaining" for the body, and conditions often do improve with therapeutic massage. When a massage intervention allows more efficient functioning for a client, massage professionals should focus on educating the client about the body's responses so that the client begins to experience personal empowerment and recognizes the body's own healing potential.

⊖volve

http://evolve.elsevier.com/Fritz/fundamentals/

11-1 Answer true or false questions on the components of assessment.

11-2 Review physical assessment terms with a crossword puzzle.

11-3 Read an additional case study on posture assessment and answer a few questions.

11-4 Watch an additional video clip on gait assessment.

Don't forget to study for your certification and licensure exams! Review questions, along with weblinks, can be found on the Evolve website.

References

Chaitow L: *Soft-tissue manipulation: a practitioner's guide to the diagnosis and treatment of soft-tissue dysfunction and reflex activity,* ed 4, Rochester, Vt, 1988, Healing Arts Press.

DeStefano L: *Greenman's principles of manual medicine,* ed 4, Baltimore, 2010, Williams & Wilkins.

Fulghum R: *Uh-oh,* New York, 1991, Villard Books.

Haas M, Cooperstein R, Peterson D: Disentangling manual muscle testing and applied kinesiology: critique and reinterpretation of a literature review, *Chiropr Osteopat* 15:11, 2007.

Hall S, Lewith G, Brien S, Little P: A review of the literature in applied and specialized kinesiology, *Forsch Komplementmed* 15:40, 2008.

Melzack R: The McGill Pain Questionnaire. In Melzack R, editor: *Pain measurement and assessment,* New York, 1983, Raven Press.

Melzack R: The short-form McGill Pain Questionnaire, *Pain* 30:191, 1987.

Nelson KE, Sergueef N, Glonek T: Recording the rate of the cranial rhythmic impulse, *J Am Osteopath Assoc* 106:337, 2006.

Norkin CC, Levangie PK: *Joint structure and function: a comprehensive analysis,* ed 4, Philadelphia, 2005, FA Davis.

Perrin RN: Lymphatic drainage of the neuraxis in chronic fatigue syndrome: a hypothetical model for the cranial rhythmic impulse, *J Am Osteopath Assoc* 107:218, 2007. Available online at www.jaoa.org/cgi/content/full/107/6/218.

Shankman GA: *Fundamental orthopedic management for the physical therapist assistant,* ed 2, St Louis, 2004, Mosby.

Smith LK, Weiss E, Lehmkuhl L: *Brunnstrom's clinical kinesiology,* ed 5, Philadelphia, 1996, FA Davis.

Wolfe F, et al: The American College of Rheumatology: 1990 criteria for classification of fibromyalgia, *Arthritis Rheum* 33:160, 1990.

Workbook Section

All Workbook activities can be done electronically online as well as here in the book. Answers are located on ⊖volve

Short Answer

1. What is an assessment?

2. Why does the massage practitioner perform an assessment?

3. What or who is the most important source of information during the assessment process?

4. What is rapport?

5. What does the massage practitioner consider when observing the general presence of the client?

6. What information can be gathered by watching a person's gestures?

7. What is the importance of open-ended questions?

8. Why is it important to repeat what the client has told you?

9. What interferes with the ability to listen?

10. What is the importance of measurement during assessment?

11. What are the three factors that influence posture and which is easiest to affect?

12. What is the essence of mechanical balance?

13. What is required to stand?

14. What is the screw-home mechanism of the knee?

15. What is the position of the client during assessment of the standing position?

16. What is the importance of bony landmarks in the assessment process?

17. Why assess for efficient gait patterns?

18. What is the importance of the sacroiliac joint during walking?

19. What are the two main factors to look for during the assessment of gait?

20. What are the most common reasons for dysfunctional walking patterns?

21. Why is full-body massage beneficial for efficient gait patterns?

22. What is palpation?

23. Why is the hand such an effective assessment tool?

24. Are palpation skills limited to the hand?

25. Why is it important to trust first impressions during palpation?

26. Why can we feel something that does not touch us?

27. What is intuition?

28. What type of information is gathered with near-touch, or palpation that does not actually touch the body?

29. What types of things are noticed when one palpates the skin?

30. What does the superficial connective tissue layer feel like?

31. Where are the superficial blood and lymph vessels located?

32. Why refer clients with enlarged lymph nodes to a physician?

33. How can you tell if you are feeling skeletal muscle?

34. What is the importance of the musculotendinous junction?

35. Do tendons attach only to bone? Why or why not?

36. What is the function of deep fascia?

37. Why is it important for the massage therapist to be able to palpate and recognize a ligament?

38. What is joint end-feel?

39. What should a normal joint feel like?

40. What is the basic configuration of muscles around a joint?

41. What would pull the alignment of a joint out of its anatomic position?

42. Why is it important to differentiate between joint and soft tissue dysfunction?

43. Explain why you palpate bone.

44. What are the important things to look for when palpating the abdomen?

45. What are body rhythms?

46. What are the three basic types of muscle testing?

47. What is the difference between strength testing and neurologic muscle testing?

48. When muscles are evaluated both for strength and neurologic function, what is the importance of the firing pattern (muscle activation sequence)?

49. What are the two basic types of muscles?

50. Typically, how do muscle imbalances set up dysfunctional patterns?

51. When is the information from the assessment interpreted?

52. What are some key elements in developing a care/treatment plan?

53. What is the purpose of the care/treatment plan?

54. How does the massage therapist decide which method to use for intervention?

55. What is the importance of reassessment?

56. How does the quote from Robert Fulghum, found in the chapter summary, pertain to massage?

Doing the Paperwork

The following is an example massage session, from initial interview to completion of the massage. Read the example carefully. Then complete the physical assessment form (Figure 11-31). It helps if you assume the different postures as indicated in the example and then assess yourself in a mirror. Next, complete the care/treatment plan form (Figure 11-31). Finally, complete the SOAP notes form (Figure 11-32) using only the information given in the example. Remember that much of this information is recorded on the client history form. Record only the information relevant for SOAP notes.

Sue Williams, who is 37 and a new client, arrives for her first massage with you. She has received bodywork before while a member of a health spa. She says the massages were light and relaxing. At work she is a middle management supervisor for a local manufacturing company. Her job requires time on the phone and many hours of meetings. The company is in the process of downsizing.

She has been experiencing tingling in her arms and also headaches (which she rates usually as 6 to 8 on a pain scale of 1 to 10), mainly at the back of her head. You notice that she squeezes the occipital area and pulls her hair in that

MASSAGE ASSESSMENT/PHYSICAL OBSERVATION/PALPATION AND GAIT

PRE
POST

Client Name:_____ Date:_____

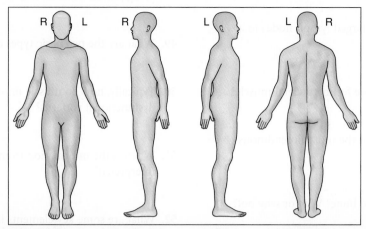

OBSERVATION & PALPATION		
ALIGNMENT	**RIBS**	**SCAPULA**
Chin in line with nose, sternal notch, navel	Even	Even
Other:	Springy	Move freely
HEAD	Other:	Other:
Tilted (L)	**ABDOMEN**	**CLAVICLES**
Tilted (R)	Firm and pliable	Level
Rotated (L)	Hard areas	Other:
Rotated (R)	Other:	**ARMS**
EYES	**WAIST**	Hang evenly (internal) (external)
Level	Level	(L) rotated ☐ medial ☐ lateral
Equally set in socket	Other:	(R) rotated ☐ medial ☐ lateral
Other:	**SPINE CURVES**	**ELBOWS**
EARS	Normal	Even
Level	Other:	Other:
Other:	**GLUTEAL MUSCLE MASS**	**WRISTS**
SHOULDERS	Even	Even
Level	Other:	Other:
(R) high / (L) low	**ILIAC CREST**	**FINGERTIPS**
(L) high / (R) low	Level	Even
(L) rounded forward	Other:	Other:
(R) rounded forward	**KNEES**	**PATELLA**
Muscle development even	Even/symmetrical	(L) ☐ movable ☐ rigid
Other:	Other:	(R) ☐ movable ☐ rigid

FIGURE 11-31 Massage assessment/physical observation/palpation and gait.

location as she explains the headaches. She has had some shortness of breath and lately has not been sleeping well. She had a full physical checkup in which nothing untoward was found. Her physician told her that she was stressed and needed to find some ways to relax. Massage and exercise were suggested as options. She is in a long-term relationship and has two children, a 16-year-old and a 9-year-old. She was in a car accident 4 years ago and suffered minor head trauma and whiplash. She broke her left ankle while cheerleading in high school and tends to walk on the outside of that foot.

You notice that she also tends to roll her shoulders while breathing and that she sighs a lot. During the physical assessment, you find that she swings her left leg farther than the right leg when walking and that her right shoulder is high. She definitely is using shoulder muscles when she breathes. Her head is tilted toward her right shoulder. She has a very mild kyphosis and is pulled forward in the chest area, more so on the right, so that a rotation is present at the thoracolumbar junction. You note limited movement in her right scapula and the right side of her rib cage. Palpation and muscle testing reveal that the upper thorax

ANKLES		TRUNK		LEGS	
Even		Remains vertical		Swing freely at hip	
Other:		Other:		Other:	
FEET		**SHOULDERS**		**KNEES**	
Mobile		Remain level		Flex and extend freely through stance and swing phase	
Other:		Rotate during walking		Other:	
ARCHES		Other:		**FEET**	
Even		**ARMS**		Heel strikes first at start of stance	
Other:		Motion is opposite leg swing		Plantar flexed at push-off	
TOES		Motion is even (L) and (R)		Foot clears floor during swing phase	
Straight		Other:		Other:	
Other:		(L) swings freely		**STEP**	
SKIN		(R) swings freely		Length is even	
Moves freely and resilient		Other:		Timing is even	
Pulls/restricted		**HIPS**		Other:	
Puffy/baggy		Remain level		**OVERALL**	
Other:		Other:		Rhythmic	
HEAD		Rotate during walking		Other:	
Remains steady/eyes forward		Other:			
Other:					

FIGURE 11-31, cont'd

is rigid. Her lower leg muscles are short, and her abdominals are weak.

You give Sue a general massage using muscle energy methods to lengthen the shoulders, lower legs, and upper posterior neck. You explain to her that she has some connective tissue shortening in the upper chest, low back, and posterior neck areas. You teach her lengthening exercises for the shoulders and lower leg. You also suggest weekly massage sessions for about 6 weeks and then a re-evaluation.

Sue agrees. She also says after the session that her headache is better (a 3 on a 0 to 10 pain scale) but not entirely gone, and she thinks she can breathe pain better. Overall she feels more relaxed and wants to go home and take a nap.

After Sue leaves, you review her chart and wonder about the pattern arising from the broken ankle, the whiplash, and the short lower legs, shoulders, chest, and neck structures. You also wonder whether the fact that she wears high heels a lot, in addition to the considerable amount of sitting in meetings and talking on the phone that she does, may have something to do with the pattern.

Problem-Solving Scenarios

1. A client is obviously stressed and tense after a traffic tie-up on the freeway. She is pacing and talking loudly and fast. How would you begin the massage?

2. A client complains of a leg problem and shows you a spot on his knee. He keeps pointing to a particular area and drilling into the spot. What kinds of problems could be present in that area?

3. A client has a damp area by her scapula that gets goose bumps when it is lightly touched. It also gets very red when massaged. What could be happening to cause these signs?

4. When comparing the pulses in a client's feet, you notice that the pulse on the right side is not as strong as the pulse on the left side. The client says his right leg has been tingling. What should you do?

5. A factory worker has very short pectoralis muscles and taut trapezius muscles on the right side. His left hip recently has begun to ache and spasm. What might be going on?

6. A regular client reports during her weekly visit that last night she almost fell when she tripped over one of her son's toy cars. She thought she had sprained her ankle, so she put ice on it and wrapped it. The ankle is sore today, but what surprises her is that her knee is really painful. She is reluctant to go to the doctor. What orthopedic tests would you perform to determine whether she should see her physician?

SESSION NOTES
SOAP CHARTING FORM

Client Name: _____ Date: _____
Practitioner Name: _____

S ubjective

CLIENT STATUS
• **Information from client, referral source, or reference books:**
1) Current conditions/changes from last session: _____
_____
_____
_____

O bjective

2) Information from <u>assessment</u> (physical, gait, palpation, muscle testing): _____
_____
_____

CONTENT OF SESSION
• **Generate goal (possibilities) from analysis of information in <u>client status</u>.**
1) Goals worked on this session. (Base information on client status this session and goals previously established in Treatment Plan): _____
_____

What was <u>done</u> this session: _____
_____
_____

A nalysis

RESULTS
• **Analyze results of session in relationship to what was done and how this relates to the session goals. (This is based on <u>cause</u> and <u>effect</u> of methods used and the effects on the persons involved).**
1) What worked/what didn't: (Based on measurable and objective Post Assessment) _____
_____
_____

P lan

PLAN: Plans for next session, what client will work on, what next massage will reassess and continue to assess: _____
_____
_____

CLIENT COMMENTS: _____
_____

Time In: _____ Time Out: _____

Therapist signature: _____

FIGURE 11-32 Session notes.

7. A client tells you that his shoulder is painful. If the Apley scratch test is positive, what does this tell you? What orthopedic test would you use if you were assessing for disc problems and nerve impingement in the lumbar area?

Assess Your Competencies

Now that you have studied this chapter, you should be able to:
• Conduct an effective client interview
• Perform a basic physical assessment
• Interpret assessment information
• Develop a care/treatment plan

On a separate sheet of paper or on the computer, write a short summary of the content of this chapter based on the preceding list of competencies. Use a conversational tone, as if you were explaining to someone (e.g., a client,

prospective employer, coworker, or other interested person) the importance of the information and skills to the development of the massage profession.

Next, in small discussion groups, share your summary with your classmates and compare the ways the information was presented. In discussing the content, look for similarities, differences, possibilities for misunderstanding of the information, and clear, concise methods of description.

Professional Application

You are being considered for a massage position with a chiropractor. The chiropractor wants to expand the wellness program currently provided by her office, and she believes that massage would be a wonderful health service to offer. A major concern of all the staff members is the ability of another person to work effectively as part of the team. How will assessment skills be an important influencing factor for this job?

Complementary Bodywork Systems

CHAPTER OBJECTIVES

After completing this chapter, the student will be able to perform the following:

1. Describe the physiologic mechanisms of complementary bodywork systems.
2. Explain and implement hydrotherapy as an adjunct to massage application.
3. Describe the use of stones and other tools used for thermotherapy.
4. Safely integrate aromatherapy into the massage process.
5. Modify massage application to support beneficial blood and lymph movement in the body.
6. Modify massage application to target the connective tissues of the body.
7. Identify and properly use massage to address trigger points.
8. Explain the fundamental concepts of Asian bodywork and incorporate simple application of acupuncture and acupressure methods into massage therapy.
9. Compare Shiatsu and Thai massage and incorporate mat methods into massage.
10. Explore the healing philosophy of Ayurveda.
11. Use the principles of polarity therapy as an energetic component of massage application.
12. Modify foot massage to incorporate the philosophy of reflexology.

CHAPTER OUTLINE

KEY TERMS

Acupressure	Neuromuscular therapy
Acupuncture	Polarity
Aromatherapy	PRICE first aid
Ayurveda	Reflexology
Deep transverse frictioning	Shiatsu
Essential oils	Systemic massage
Hydrotherapy	Thai massage
Lymphatic drainage	Thermotherapy
Meridians	Trigger point
Myofascial approaches	

This chapter presents a brief overview of bodywork systems that can be incorporated into massage, suggestions for implementing the basic concepts and techniques that overlap well with massage therapy, and guidance for the development of an integrated system.

The many different systems of bodywork cluster into six categories:

- Reflex systems (e.g., hydrotherapy)
- Fluid movement systems (e.g., lymphatic drainage)
- Structural systems (e.g., Rolfing and myofascial release)
- Neuromuscular methods (e.g., trigger point therapy)
- Eastern and Asian methods involving vital energy, chakras, meridians, and points
- Energetic systems (e.g., polarity)

The chapter is organized to take advantage of similarities among bodywork systems. The first systems discussed are hydrotherapy, thermotherapy, and aromatherapy. Hydrotherapy and thermotherapy are excellent adjuncts to massage and can be included in the massage session by using hot and cold packs or stones or footbaths in addition to the massage. Often aromatherapy is combined with hydrotherapy, such as in scented footbaths or steam inhalation during the massage. Essential oils typically are used as an additive to the massage lubricant.

The next category of methods addresses the movement of fluids in the body. The lymphatic and circulatory systems are the main focus. Hydrotherapy, thermotherapy, and aromatherapy also influence fluid movement; or in the case of aromatherapy, move through the body using blood as a means of transport.

After the fluid movement segment are the connective tissue, myofascial, and trigger point methods. When combined, these approaches form the basic techniques of neuromuscular therapy, which is similar to what has been called *deep tissue massage*. Understanding how all these approaches and their effects interact can be confusing.

Asian and Eastern bodywork systems are presented next. It is interesting that most trigger points (93% to 97%) are in the same location as traditional Chinese acupuncture points. Another interesting fact is that acupuncture points and meridian locations are closely related to the enveloping deep fascia around muscle groups. Current thought is that trigger points and acupuncture points likely describe the same physiologic phenomena.

The Asian systems described are traditional Chinese medicine (TCM) and shiatsu (Japanese). Reflexology is actually based on TCM even though it has been Westernized; therefore, it appears with this group. Also included in the Eastern system is Ayurveda from India and traditional Thai massage from Thailand, which has its roots in Ayurveda. The chakras are included in the Ayurvedic physiology. Dr. Randolf Stone combined these systems with principles of body energy flow into polarity therapy. A short segment on color therapy is included, because the Asian and Eastern systems place importance on the value of color both in assessment and treatment.

The element that all these systems have in common with therapeutic massage is the application of touch in a structured way to introduce various forms of sensory and mechanical information to the body so as to effect positive physiologic change. The language of each system is different, and the theory bases vary. The methods of assessment for each approach are distinctive and generally unique to that approach. Do not become too concerned with, or overwhelmed by, the different terminologies that describe the same elements of anatomy and physiology in each bodywork method.

This text does not attempt to describe the various systems in depth; rather, it is devoted to the professional practice of therapeutic massage. Expertise in any of the systems requires specific study. Massage students have enough to learn about therapeutic massage; they should not also be expected to develop expertise in the other styles. Nor does it seem necessary to attempt to become proficient in multiple bodywork styles, because the ultimate result of the application for all of them is essentially the same. In simple terms, pick one (maybe two) and learn it (them) well.

The information in this chapter is not sufficient training to enable the practitioner to understand and use these methods purposefully and intelligently for anything other than general enhancement of the skills already developed. However, with a commitment to further education, these methods can add efficiency, effectiveness, and enthusiasm for the benefits that therapeutic massage has to offer with regard to wellness, prevention, rehabilitation, and client-directed healing. It is important for massage practitioners to understand the basis of other methods so that they know when a client might be better served by referral to another practitioner.

As you practice the various methods presented, pay attention to areas in which you display a particular interest and talent; this can help direct you to specific avenues for continuing education.

COMPLEMENTARY BODYWORK SYSTEMS

SECTION OBJECTIVES

Chapter objective covered in this section:
1. Describe the physiologic mechanisms of complementary bodywork systems.
Using the information presented in this section, the student will be able to perform the following:
- Identify similarities in bodywork methods

In their book, *Zen Shiatsu: How to Harmonize Yin and Yang for Better Health*, Shitzuto Masunaga and Wataru Ohashi (1977) describe the interface of various bodywork methods:

Some professional therapists insist that a great difference exists among the three (Amma [Chinese], Western massage, shiatsu [Japanese]) forms of treatment. I believe that a great difference cannot exist within a general field, in this case, manually applied stimulation to the human body. Of course, there are a variety of methods and schools, but basically they are similar. It is important to note that effectiveness of any treatment depends on both the practitioner and the method working together. So the effectiveness of any treatment can vary greatly from one practitioner to another. All three methods of manipulation aim at stabilizing the functioning of the human body, the difference being whether they stimulate blood circulation and nerve interactions directly or indirectly. The effectiveness of manipulative therapy has been proven by modern scientific experiments involving cutaneous stimulation. From this point of view, no difference exists among the basic three techniques, though they were developed from different principles. The purpose of manipulative therapy is to work with a person's natural healing force to correct any internal malfunctioning particular to that person.

Many massage professionals continue their therapeutic massage learning through the comprehensive study of a single additional bodywork approach. Other practitioners study many different bodywork modalities, some in considerable depth and others more superficially. They then integrate the information into therapeutic massage, variations, concepts, and an expanded look at the body.

Basis of Bodywork

You can apply pressure, lift and stretch tissue, rock the body, stroke the skin, entrain the rhythms, move the joints, generate tissue repair by creating therapeutic inflammation, stimulate reflex responses, soothe the energy field, and provide the client with interpersonal and professional support, compassion, and acceptance. Regardless of the theoretical, historical, and cultural base, all the bodywork systems, including therapeutic massage, are built on this foundation.

Expertise in any bodywork system consists of quality assessment for the purpose of making effective decisions about the application of treatment to provide a service that benefits the client. Within these bodywork systems a unique form of assessment may exist. For example, traditional Chinese medicine includes assessment of the tongue for color, coating, and shape and of the pulse as it relates to various meridians. Information is gathered, analyzed, and a plan is made and implemented and results evaluated.

Benefits derived from receiving these various methods range from pleasure and comfort to ongoing management of chronic conditions and stress, in addition to a therapeutic change process.

Body, Mind, and Spirit

Bodywork—therapeutic massage as a complete system within the broader realm—serves the wholeness of the individual through a direct influence on the body and a respect for the mind and spirit. The concept of the body/mind/spirit connection found in many complementary systems of bodywork leads to the acceptance of the unity and integrity of the individual. Consideration must include different aspects of the person, although never separate from the whole. As discussed at the beginning of this textbook, the skin is not separate from the emotions, nor the emotions separate from the organs, nor the organs separate from the muscles. No part is separate from the spirit or the context of our influence on others, society, culture, and the larger expanse of the universe.

In many bodywork traditions, this interconnectedness is also apparent. For example, the Ayurvedic medicine of India is similar to Asian medicine. These practices are similar to the tribal medicine of Native Americans and other indigenous peoples. In Thailand, Tibet, Russia, and other parts of the world, the ancient traditions of medicine and folk health wisdom have a common difference with Western scientific thought: these systems identify body/mind/spirit lifestyle imbalance, a concept referred to in this text as dysfunction or "almost sick and not quite well." They introduce interventions to reverse this process before it cycles into body/mind/spirit

disease. Western health care is beginning to embrace this concept of wholeness through prevention, and whole personal care is now a consistent component of health care.

Therapeutic Massage, Relaxing Massage, Medical Massage, and All the Rest

Many names are attached to massage therapy, such as *wellness massage, sports massage, medical massage, prenatal massage, geriatric massage,* and so forth. This becomes very confusing to the student and the public. For example, sports massage is massage that focuses on an athlete. Prenatal massage focuses on a pregnant woman. Regardless of the population served (see Chapter 14), the most effective massage uses fundamental massage skills adapted to the client's unique circumstances (see Chapter 16). This type of massage uses now called *outcome-based massage,* yet another name to confuse students and the public.

The main purpose of this textbook is to train the massage professional to use massage methods intelligently, based on quality evidence (see Chapter 5), to promote health and well-being for anyone seeking massage. Massage is best used in the prevention of disease and the support of optimum health. Generally healthy people can benefit from the normalizing physiologic effects of hydrotherapy, massage adapted to address connective tissue, lymphatic and blood circulation, trigger points, acupressure, reflexology, and so forth. These methods can add another dimension to the effectiveness of the massage. The current trend is toward expanding the role of the massage profession in the spa industry. Typically, this setting reflects the integrated approach and offers clients many modalities in various combinations of service menus. For example, a hydrotherapy application, including the use of essential oils, mud and clay packs, and salt scrubs, may be combined with massage. (Specific information on spa applications is presented in Chapter 13.)

Sometimes the client may present the massage professional with minor problems that can be helped by the use of the techniques discussed in this chapter. These same methods can be used in various forms of health care and rehabilitative procedures or with athletes. To use the methods in a more specific way, massage professionals require additional training, especially in pathophysiology, pharmacology, and medical treatment protocols, so that they can understand the integration of massage therapy into these approaches. Even when the massage practitioner deals with medical conditions and works in the health care environment (see Chapter 13), the methods (i.e., massage manipulations and techniques as described in Chapter 10 or any of the methods described in this chapter) do not change. Some methods are more appropriate for certain conditions and others are chosen for different outcomes. The difference is the condition of the person receiving the massage. Additional education not only focuses on learning new methods, but also on learning how to choose and apply methods with clients who have various complex circumstances.

Massage professionals who work with a client in the sports and fitness or health care setting need to increase their knowledge based on the function, dysfunction, or disease addressed. For example:

- Serving the athlete requires an understanding of training protocols, common stress patterns, and injury rehabilitation of that particular sport.
- Working with stroke rehabilitation requires increased knowledge of stroke etiology, rehabilitation, and the use of massage as part of the overall rehabilitation and management process.
- Working with clients who suffer from depression is enhanced by an understanding of the manifestations of depression, mental health interventions, and psychotropic pharmacology.

The massage professional should confer with the medical team when dealing with clients who are undergoing medical intervention (e.g., medications, physical therapy, psychotherapy, or chiropractic treatment). The massage should be integrated into the entire treatment protocol. Supervision by the medical team can help ensure that methods used for a client are monitored and evaluated for effectiveness and safety.

HYDROTHERAPY

SECTION OBJECTIVES

Chapter objective covered in this section:
2. Explain and implement hydrotherapy as an adjunct to massage application.
Using the information presented in this section, the student will be able to perform the following:
- Explain the general effects of hot and cold water applications
- Incorporate simple hydrotherapy methods into a massage session
- Suggest easy, basic hydrotherapy self-help techniques for clients

Hydrotherapy is a distinct form of treatment that combines well with massage. Water can be used in many different ways, depending on the client's health needs and condition and the facilities available for therapy. Hydrotherapy is a component of the spa environment, sports treatment, and health care. Skillful use of hydrotherapy methods requires long-term study. The advanced level massage therapist should be well trained in hydrotherapy.

History of Hydrotherapy

Water therapy is as old as the human race. One of the first recorded mentions of the use of water as medicine involves the temples of the Greek god of medicine, Aesculapius. At the temples, bathing and massage were part of the treatment of the sick. Hippocrates used water as a beverage for reducing fever and treating many diseases. He also stressed the value of using various types of baths, each with a different temperature, as a therapeutic tool to combat illness. Later, the ancient Roman physicians Galen and Celsus also recommended specific baths as an integral part of their remedies. Almost every warm climate civilization has at some point in its history used baths for therapeutic purposes (Buchman, 1979).

These methods have very powerful physiologic effects and have been used for centuries as part of the healing process.

Before the development of antidepressant and stimulant medications, hot, warm, and cold applications were used to stimulate or sedate the autonomic nervous system. Cold shock was used instead of electric shock to treat depression. Warm baths of long duration were used to calm anxious individuals. For centuries, herb and mineral additives were used to enhance the effects of water treatments.

Hydrotherapy Uses and Indications

Water is a near-perfect natural body balancer and is necessary for life. It accounts for the largest percentage of our body weight. A universal solvent, it can act as a detoxifier for the body. It is available in many forms, all of which have the potential to be therapeutically beneficial. Water can relax or stimulate, anesthetize, and reduce or increase circulation. It works naturally and is nonallergenic, tissue tolerant, inexpensive, and readily available.

Water's three forms (liquid, steam, and ice) allow it to be used at a variety of temperatures and in a variety of ways, such as full or partial baths, showers, compresses, packs, hot water bottles, frozen ice bandages, wrapped ice, and as steam (Table 12-1).

Table 12-1 Therapeutic Uses of Water

Use	Application
Analgesic (relieves pain)	Hot, warm, and cold applications
Anesthetic (reduces sensation)	Cold application
Antiedemic (reduces swelling)	Cold application
Antipyretic (reduces fever)	Cool to cold application
Antiseptic (kills pathogens)	Boiling water, high-pressure steam (not for use on the body)
Antispasmodic (reduces muscle spasms)	Hot, warm, and cold applications
Astringent (causes tissues to contract)	Cold application
Burn treatment (first-degree and mild second-degree burns only)	Cool application
Diaphoretic (produces sweating)	Hot application
Diuretic (increases urine formation)	Drinking water
Emetic (produces vomiting)	Drinking warm water
Expectorant (loosens mucus)	Hot and steam applications
Immunologic enhancement (increases white cell production)	Cold application
Laxative (promotes peristalsis of the bowel)	Drinking cold water or use of an enema
Purifier (eliminates toxins)	All forms of water
Sedative (reduces sympathetic arousal and encourages sleep)	Drinking warm water
Stimulant (increases sympathetic arousal)	Short hot and cold applications
Tonic (increases muscle tone)	Cold and alternating hot and cold applications

Modified from Nikola RJ: *Creatures of water: hydrotherapy textbook,* Salt Lake City, 2005, Europa Therapeutic LLC.

The therapeutic properties of hydrotherapy are based on its mechanical or thermal effects (or both) and the body's reaction to hot and cold stimuli. Therapeutic effects also occur in response to the hydrostatic pressure exerted by the water when the body (or body part) is immersed in (surrounded by) water, and in response to the sensation of the water against the skin. The peripheral nerves are stimulated by the temperature or pressure of the water, and impulses from the sensation on the skin are carried deeper into the body, stimulating the central nervous system, the autonomic nervous system and, indirectly, all the other body systems.

In general, heat quiets and soothes the body, slowing the activity of internal organs. Cold, in contrast, stimulates and invigorates, increasing internal activity. When the body is submerged in water, such as a bath, a pool, or a whirlpool, the constant pull of gravity is reduced. Water also has a hydrostatic pressure effect; it has a massage like effect, because water in motion stimulates touch receptors on the skin.

Rest and relaxation are potential benefits of hydrotherapy; it is useful for some anxious clients because it promotes general relaxation of the nervous system. Hydrotherapy usually is one component of an overall health and wellness program. It also can offer specific relief to people with a number of conditions, such as:

- Arthritis problems
- Back and neck pain
- Sports injuries
- Work-related injuries
- Cerebral palsy
- Orthopedic injuries

Used correctly, hot and cold applications are probably the most powerful antiinflammatory treatments, and they have essentially no side effects.

Key Points

Water is effective as a therapeutic agent for several reasons:

- It can store and transmit heat.
- It is a good conductor of heat.
- It has solvent properties.
- It is nontoxic.
- It can change states within a narrow, easily obtainable temperature range.
- In its solid form (ice), it is an effective cooling agent.
- It its liquid form (water), it may be applied using many pressures and temperatures, in addition to methods ranging from total immersion to local compression.
- In its gaseous form (steam), it may be used in vapor or steam baths or for inhalation treatments.
- The density of water is near that of the human body; therefore, it supports exercise for clients with joint disease, paralysis, or atrophy.
- The hydrostatic pressure exerted on the body surface during immersion increases urine output and venous and lymphatic flow from the periphery.

Effects of Hydrotherapy

The effects of water are primarily reflexive and focus on the autonomic nervous system. The addition of heat energy or the dissipation of heat energy from tissues can be classified as a mechanical effect. In general, cold stimulates sympathetic responses, and warmth activates parasympathetic responses. Short- and long-term applications of heat or cold differ in effect. For the most part, short cold applications stimulate and vasoconstrict and have a secondary effect of increased circulation as blood is channeled to the area to warm it. Long cold applications depress and reduce circulation. Short applications of heat vasodilate vessels and depress and deplete tone, whereas long heat applications result in a combined depressant and stimulant reaction.

Visceral Reflex

Cutaneous and Somatic Effects

Stimulation of certain nerve endings in organs results in both a muscle and a skin response in a reflex loop. Usually the muscles spasm or increase in tension, and the skin becomes more taut. This reflex is responsible for visceral referred pain patterns (see Chapter 6). Theoretically the reflex is a loop; therefore, stimulation of muscle and skin can reflexively affect the corresponding organ. In general, an organ is in a reflex pattern with the muscles and skin over it. Applications of hydrotherapy seem to have either sedative or stimulating effects on the specific organ.

Mechanical Effects

Different water pressures can exert a powerful mechanical effect on the nerve and blood supplies of the skin. Techniques that are used include a friction rub with a sponge or wet mitten and pressurized streams of hot and cold water directed at various parts of the body (Box 12-1 and Table 12-2).

Osmosis is a principle of hydrotherapy by which water moves across a permeable or semipermeable membrane from a mineral salt concentration that is low to a high concentration to equalize solution consistency. In theory, if the water used for hydrotherapy application is lower in salt content than body fluids, water moves from the outside of the body to the inside through the semipermeable superficial tissue of the skin and superficial fascia. If the salt content of the water external to the skin is higher, such as when mineral salt baths are used, water from the body moves into the external soak water. When this happens, surface edema might be reduced. Unfortunately, as yet no research has either confirmed or discounted this effect.

Table 12-2	Classification of Water Temperatures Used for Treatment	
	Temperature Range	**Effect**
Very cold	32°–56° F	Painful
Cold	56°–65° F	Uncomfortable
Cool	65°–92° F	Goosebumps
Neutral	92°–98° F	Normal skin temperature
Warm to hot	98°–104° F	Comfortable
Very hot	104°–110° F*	Reddened skin

*Temperatures higher than 110° F should not be used.

Box 12-1 Effects of Hydrotherapy Using Heat, Cold, and Ice Applications

Effects of Heat
- Increases circulation
- Increases metabolism
- Increases inflammation
- Increases respiration
- Increases perspiration
- Decreases pain
- Decreases muscle spasm
- Decreases tissue stiffness
- Decreases white blood cell production

Applications of Heat Hydrotherapy

As a sedative
Water is a very efficient, nontoxic, calming substance. It soothes the body and promotes sleep.

Techniques: Use hot and warm baths to quiet and relax the entire body. Salt baths, neutral showers, or damp sheet packs can be used to relax certain areas.

For elimination
The skin is the largest organ of the body, and simple immersion in a long, hot bath or a session in a sauna or steam room can stimulate the excretion of toxins through the skin. Inducing perspiration is useful for treating acute diseases and many chronic health problems.

Techniques: Use hot baths, Epsom salt or common salt baths, hot packs, dry blanket packs, and hot herbal drinks.

As an antispasmodic
Water effectively reduces cramps and muscle spasm.

Techniques: Use hot compresses (depending on the problem), herbal teas, and abdominal compresses.

Effects of Cold and Ice

Cold
- Increases stimulation
- Increases muscle tone
- Increases tissue stiffness
- Increases white blood cell production
- Increases red blood cell production
- Decreases circulation (primary effect); increases circulation (secondary effect)
- Decreases inflammation
- Decreases pain
- Decreases respiration
- Decreases digestive processes

Ice
- Increases tissue stiffness
- Decreases circulation
- Decreases metabolism
- Decreases inflammation
- Decreases pain
- Decreases muscle spasm

Types of Applications
- Ice packs
- Ice immersion (ice water)
- Ice massage
- Cold whirlpool

- Chemical cold packs
- Cold gel packs (use with caution)

Contraindications to Use of Ice
- Vasospastic disease (spasming of blood vessels)
- Cold hypersensitivity; signs include:
  - *Skin:* Itching, sweating
  - *Respiratory:* Hoarseness, sneezing, chest pain
  - *Gastrointestinal:* Abdominal pain, diarrhea, vomiting
  - *Eyes:* Puffy eyelids
  - *General:* Headache, discomfort, uneasiness
- Cardiac disorder
- Compromised local circulation

Precautions for Use of Ice
- Do not use frozen gel packs directly on the skin.
- Do not use ice applications (cryotherapy) for longer than 30 minutes continuously.
- Do not do exercises that cause pain after cold applications.
- Do not use cryotherapy on individuals with certain rheumatoid conditions or those who are paralyzed or have coronary artery disease.

Applications of Cold Hydrotherapy
Ice is a primary therapy for strains, sprains, contusions, hematomas, and fractures. It has a numbing, anesthetic effect and helps control internal hemorrhaging by reducing circulation to and metabolic processes within the area.

For restoring and increasing muscle strength and increasing the body's resistance to disease
Cold water boosts vigor, adds energy and tone, and aids in digestion.

Techniques: Use cold water treading (standing or walking in cold water), whirlpool baths, cold sprays, alternate hot and cold contrast baths, showers and compresses, salt rubs, apple cider vinegar baths, and partial packs.

For injuries
Application of an ice pack controls the flow of blood and reduces tissue swelling.

Technique: Use an ice bag in addition to compression and elevation.

As an anesthetic
Water can dull the sense of pain or sensation.

Technique: Use ice to chill the tissue.

For minor burns
Water, particularly cold and ice water, has been rediscovered as a primary healing agent.

Technique: Use ice water immersion or saline water immersion.

To reduce fever
Water is nature's best cooling agent. Unlike medications, which usually only diminish internal heat, water both lowers temperature and removes heat by conduction.

Technique: Use ice bags at the base of the neck and on the forehead and feet; cold water sponge baths; and drinking cold water.

Physiologic Effects

Hydrotherapy techniques with heat and cold are thought to produce physiologic effects that help improve circulation, stimulate the immune system, provide relief from pain, reduce stress, and tone the body. Water itself helps to restore and rejuvenate the body.

The physiologic effects of hydrotherapy can be thermal and mechanical, Thermal effects are produced when the water temperature is higher or lower than the current body temperature. When the temperature difference is small, the effect is mild; when the temperature difference is large, the effect is strong. Mechanical effects occur from the pressure of the water on the body, such as occurs in showers or whirlpools, and hydrostatic pressure forces that occur in baths.

In hydrotherapy, heating and cooling effects occur when heat from the water is transferred to the body or vice versa.

Circulation Enhancement

Supporting circulation is an important aspect of promoting healing. Circulation can be enhanced very effectively with hydrotherapy. Massage also is very effective for moving blood in the body. The combined effects of massage and hydrotherapy can increase the rate of blood flow, decrease the rate of blood, increase blood flow to an ischemic area (an area with too little blood), and decrease blood flow in a congested area (an area with too much blood). To accomplish these changes in blood flow, three physiologic effects are necessary:

- The revulsive effect
- The derivative effect
- The collateral circulation effect

Revulsive Effect

The revulsive effect occurs when blood flow through an area increases. The most effective means of accomplishing this is to use alternating hot and cold applications. The revulsive effect depends on repeated application. A series of three hot/cold applications is typical. The cold application should last 20 to 30 seconds, which is long enough to produce vasoconstriction. The warm application typically lasts twice as long as the cold application.

The revulsive effect is most beneficial for conditions involving tissue congestion. For example, if the client is experiencing sinus congestion, alternating hot and cold compresses over the face can reduce sinus pressure.

Derivative Effect

The derivative effect is the opposite of the revulsive effect. Instead of encouraging blood flow to or through an area, the goal is to shift blood flow away from an area, thereby creating blood volume changes from one area of the body to another. An example of the derivative effect is application of heat to the feet to reduce congestion in the head. Vascular headaches, in which too much blood in the vessels causes pressure, also may respond to this type of intervention.

Cold or heat can be applied for long periods (up to 30 minutes) and at varying temperature extremes, depending on the size of the treated area and desired effect.

Collateral Circulation Effect

In the body, superficial and deep tissues receive blood through the same arteries as they branch. These branches are called *collateral arteries.* The collateral circulation effect creates change in the deep, rather than superficial, collateral branches of the same artery. Application of heat to an area causes surface vessels to dilate, increasing blood flow to the superficial tissues and also reducing blood flow to the deep tissues. Application of cold has the opposite effect. Local application of hydrotherapy techniques (generally by compress or pack) is used to produce collateral circulatory changes in a specific area of the body.

Effects of Cold Applications

In the skin, cold receptors are more numerous than heat receptors. The temperature-regulating mechanism in the hypothalamus responds to signals by attempting to prevent cooling or overheating. The primary or direct effect of cold applications is depressant. A decrease in function can occur locally if cold is applied to an area of the body or systemically if the entire body is exposed to cold. When the application of cold lasts a long time and the temperature is significantly colder than body temperature, the effects require a more adaptive response from the body. Caution is required for those who do not have sufficient adaptive capacity to respond to cold.

Cold applications typically cause shivering, goose bumps, increased pulse and respiration, dilation of blood vessels, and increased muscle tone. These effects are referred to as a *tonic,* a stimulating reaction to cold. As the body responds to the cold application, the return to normal function results in the secondary, or indirect, effect of cold, called the *reaction.* The secondary effect, or reaction, occurs only when the body has the adaptive capacity to respond to the cold by warming the area by increasing blood flow. In general, the colder the application, the greater the reaction. Many hydrotherapy techniques are directed at producing the reaction to the cold application.

Effects of Hot Applications

Hot applications stimulate the body to eliminate heat and thereby prevent tissue damage. Heat applications have different effects, depending on the temperature, duration of application, and method used. Water temperatures of 98° to 104° F (37°–40° C) generally are considered "hot." A temperature above 104° F is considered very hot. Many people can tolerate hot air, such as in a sauna, for fairly long periods, even though temperatures in a sauna may reach as high as 200° F, well above an individual's tolerance for heat in water. Often, after exposure to heat, cold is applied, such as a cold shower.

Exposure to the high temperatures of hot tubs and saunas has become popular, but it can be dangerous. Prolonged use may weaken the individual or trigger dangerous changes in respiratory and cardiac function. In pregnant women, prolonged exposure to hot temperatures may harm the fetus.

Box 12-2 lists additional risks, cautions, and contraindications for heat and cold applications of hydrotherapy. Specific indications and contraindications are discussed with each

---

Box 12-2 | **Risks, Cautions, and Contraindications for Heat and Cold Hydrotherapy**

- Clients whose ability to sense temperature changes is impaired are at risk for burns, scalding, or frostbite, because they are unable to determine whether tissue is being damaged.
- Clients with diabetes should avoid hot applications to the feet or legs and full-body heating treatments, such as hot baths and body wraps.
- Cold applications should not be used if the client has been diagnosed with Raynaud's disease.
- Elderly people and young children may not be able to adapt to long exposure to heat and should avoid long, full-body hot treatments, such as whirlpools and saunas.
- Long-duration exposure to hot treatments such as immersion baths and hot saunas are not recommended for individuals with multiple sclerosis, women who are pregnant, anyone with high or low blood pressure, or individuals with any type of heart condition.
- Temperatures higher than 104° F should never be used, because the body temperature increases very quickly and cannot adapt.

---

particular application in the Hydrotherapy Treatments and Common Techniques section.

Hydrotherapy Supplies

Hydrotherapy can be used as an adjunct to massage with the aid of a few basic supplies:

- Tubs, bowls, and other containers of various sizes to hold water
- Thermometer
- Large watering can
- Hot plate, large pot, or slow cooker, or electric roaster to heat water
- Small refrigerator to cool water and make ice
- Cotton sheets
- Wool or acrylic blankets
- Flannel material or towels and washcloths
- Some sort of waterproof sheeting (e.g., tarp, vinyl, or plastic tablecloth)
- Plastic sheeting
- Classic hot water bottle
- Elastic bandages for wrapping around an area to hold a compress or pack in place
- Rice-filled cloth bags
- Microwave oven
- Access to a tub and shower (if immersion methods will be used)

Note: The equipment required for techniques must be sanitized and maintained properly.

Hydrotherapy Treatments and Common Techniques

Hydrotherapy Baths

A *bath* is a full or partial immersion of the body into water. The water temperature and the duration of the bath depend on the desired outcome. Substances can be added to the water to produce specific results. Additives most commonly used are salts, essential oils, milk, oatmeal, and seaweed preparations. The water may be moving, as in a whirlpool, or still.

Hot Full Immersion Bath

- Water temperature range: 100° to 104° F (38°–40° C)
- Bath duration: Up to 20 minutes

Indications for a Hot Full Immersion Bath

- Muscular spasms
- Detoxification through sweating
- Relaxation and stress reduction

Note: Hot baths typically are followed by a brief cool treatment, such as a cool shower.

> **Caution:** Prolonged hot immersion baths are contraindicated for the elderly, infants, young children, immunosuppressed individuals, pregnant women, and people with cardiac or kidney disease.

Neutral Full Immersion Bath

- Average temperature of the skin: 92° to 95° F (33°–35° C)
- Bath duration: 15 minutes to 4 hours

Note: If the bath lasts longer than 20 minutes, warm water must be added to maintain the temperature.

Indications for a Neutral Full Immersion Bath

- Supporting parasympathetic dominance (considered a sedative effect)
- Creating increased urinary output (a result of the absorption of water into the body during prolonged immersion and hydrostatic pressure of the water against the body)
- Treating peripheral edema
- Reducing the surface temperature of the body (when the elevated temperature is the result of lack of the normal heat-producing stimulus of cool air on the skin)
- Anxiety and irritability
- Exhaustion from insomnia
- Chronic pain

> **Caution:** Clients commonly feel chilled after a neutral bath, and care must be taken to keep them warm.

Variations of Full Immersion Baths

Whirlpool. A whirlpool is a tub with air jets that move the water to stimulate the tissues. Generally, the water temperature is hot. Whirlpools open pores and promote sweating. They also promote psychological and mechanical muscular relaxation.

Mud Bath. In a mud bath, a combination of volcanic ash or clay, peat moss, and natural spring water is used to draw out the body's toxins and exfoliate and nourish the skin.

Herbal Bath. For a herbal bath, herbs are added to the water, producing the combined therapeutic properties of the herbs and the water. Two preparation methods are used:

Method 1: One cup of herbs is added to 2 quarts of water and simmered for 15 minutes to create an infusion. The herbs then are strained from the infusion, and the liquid is added to the bathwater.

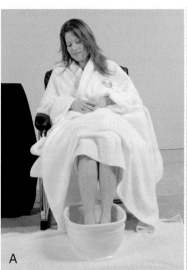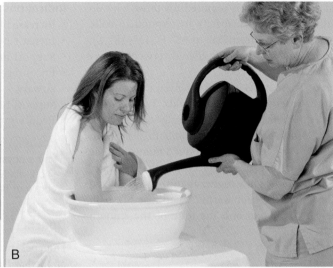

FIGURE 12-1 **A,** Foot bath. **B,** Arm bath.

Method 2: A thin cloth or mesh bag is filled with about 1 cup of herbs. It is either placed in the bathwater or tied to the spigot so that the hot water runs through it as the tub fills.

Cold Foot Bath. The feet are placed in a tub filled calf deep with cold water. The client should stop soaking the feet when the water is no longer perceived as cold.

Indications for a Cold Foot Bath

- Varicose veins
- Edema
- Vascular headaches
- Low blood pressure
- Circulatory problems
- Ankle sprain, strain, or bruise
- Sweaty feet
- Aching feet

> **Caution:** Cold foot baths are not used for clients who suffer from cold feet, very high blood pressure, diabetes, or peripheral vascular disease.

Rising Temperature or Warm Foot Bath

- *Rising temperature foot bath:* The feet are immersed in a foot bath filled with water at body temperature (Figure 12-1, *A*). Hot water is added gradually to produce a final temperature of 103° to 104° F (39°–40° C).
- *Warm foot bath:* The feet are immersed in a warm foot bath with the water at 100° to 104° F (38°–40° C). The foot bath should last 10 to 15 minutes and can be done daily.

Indications for a Rising Temperature or Warm Foot Bath

- Cold feet
- Onset of a common cold
- Relaxation

> **Caution:** Do not use a rising temperature or warm foot bath if the client has varicose veins, lymphostasis, or edema.

Cold Arm Bath

For a cold arm bath, a tub is filled with cold water until it reaches a depth several inches above the immersed elbow (Figure 12-1, *B*).

Indications for a Cold Arm Bath

- Headaches
- Shoulder, elbow, wrist, and hand pain

> **Caution:** Do not use a cold arm bath if the client has heart or circulatory problems.

Rising Temperature and Warm Arm Bath

- *Rising temperature arm bath:* The arm is immersed in a tub filled with water at body temperature. Hot water is added gradually to produce a final temperature of 103° to 104° F (39°–40° C).
- *Warm arm bath:* The arm is immersed in a warm bath with the water at 100° to 104° F (38°–40° C). The arm bath should last 10 to 15 minutes and can be done daily.

Indications for a Rising Temperature or Warm Arm Bath

- Bronchitis
- Asthma
- Respiratory infection
- Circulatory conditions

> **Caution:** Rising temperature or warm arm baths are not indicated in cases of acute inflammation.

Sitz Bath

An immersion bath of the pelvic region typically is performed using a specially constructed tub, but it also may be done in a regular bathtub. A sitz bath may be hot, neutral, cold, contrasting hot and cold, rising temperature, or warm. Before a sitz bath, the feet should be warmed with a warm foot bath.

Variations of Sitz Baths

Hot sitz bath: Water temperature generally is 105° to 110° F (40°–43° C); bath lasts 3 to 10 minutes. The primary effect is analgesic. Effects require a more adaptive response from the body *Neutral sitz bath:* Water temperature is 92° to 95° F (33°–35° C); bath lasts 15 minutes to 2 hours. To manage inflammation, the client must be kept warm during treatment.

Cold sitz bath: Water temperature is 55° to 75° F (13°–24° C); bath lasts 30 seconds to 5 minutes. Cold sitz baths are given to increase the tone of the smooth muscles of the uterus, bladder, and colon. Caution is required for those who do not have sufficient adaptive capacity to respond to cold. Cold temperatures range from 55° to 65° F (13°–18° C). Anything colder, such as ice, is considered very cold. Anything warmer is considered cool.

Contrast sitz baths: These baths usually are given in groups of three (i.e., three repetitions of hot to cold). Two separate tubs are needed. For the hot bath, the water temperature is 105° to 110° F (40°–44° C); for the cold bath, it is 55° to 85° F (13°–29° C). The client spends about 3 minutes in the hot bath and then 30 seconds in the cold bath. The water level in the hot tub is slightly higher than that in the cold tub. The client must be kept warm. A contrast sitz bath increases pelvic circulation and the tone of the smooth muscles in the area.

Indications for a Sitz Bath
- Uterine cramps
- Hemorrhoids or inflammation (cold sitz bath)
- Irritable bladder (warm or rising temperature sitz bath)

Note: All contrast hydrotherapy treatments finish with the cold application.

Caution: A warm or rising temperature sitz bath should not be used for hemorrhoids. Hot sitz baths are not indicated in cases of acute inflammation.

Saunas and Steam Baths

Saunas and steam baths have similar effects. A sauna is dry heat, and the heat acts more quickly to eliminate toxins through the skin as the body sweats. The moist air of a steam bath seems to have a greater effect on the respiratory system. The client should spend no more than 15 to 20 minutes at a time in a sauna and should wipe the face frequently with a cold cloth and drink cool water to prevent overheating.

Indications for Saunas and Steam Baths
- Increase blood flow
- Increase heart rate
- Support immune system
- Encourage secretions in the respiratory system and open the airways
- Support relaxation
- Reduce muscle aching from overexertion

Caution: Clients should not use a sauna, unless supervised by a physician, if they have rheumatoid arthritis, acute infection, acute or chronic inflammation, vascular changes in the brain or heart, circulatory problems, or cancer.

Douches

Douches are a gentle flow of water over an area and can be applied with a watering can or hose. The water should not splash, but rather gently surround and flow over the area. The water stream is directed from distal to proximal. Excess water is stroked off with the hands.

Douche Variations

Knee Douche

The water stream begins at the lateral side of the foot and moves along the outside of the lower leg to the back of the knee, then back along the inside and over the sole of the foot. The process is repeated for the other leg (Figure 12-2, *A*).

Indications for a Knee Douche
- Headaches and migraines
- Low blood pressure
- Insomnia
- Contusions
- Varicose veins
- Knee pain

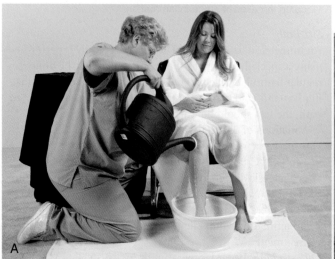
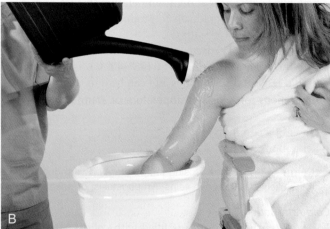

FIGURE 12-2 Examples of douches. **A,** Knee douche. **B,** Arm douche.

Thigh Douche

The procedure for a thigh douche is the same as for a knee douche but includes the upper thigh.

Lower Trunk Douche

The procedure for a lower trunk douche is the same as for a thigh douche, but the lower abdomen and gluteal area are included.

Indications for a Thigh and Lower Trunk Douche

• Poor circulation
• Varicose veins
• Muscle aches

Arm Douche

The water stream begins on the outside of the hand and moves to the shoulder, then back on the inside of the arm. The process is repeated for the other arm (Figure 12-2, *B*).

Indications for an Arm Douche

• Cold hands
• Anxiety
• Muscle ache of the arms
• Headaches

Upper Trunk, Back, and Neck Douche

An upper trunk, back, and neck douche involves the upper torso and arms. It can be used to improve blood flow to the lungs, heart, and pleura.

Indications for an Upper Trunk, Back, and Neck Douche

• Bronchitis
• Upper respiratory conditions
• Headaches
• Nervous excitability
• Toning up
• Weakened back muscles
• Back pain
• Shoulder and neck pain

Face Douche

The water stream begins at the right temple and moves downward to the chin, upward to the left temple, from right to left over the forehead, and repeatedly from the forehead to the chin, then in circles over the face. Make sure the client keeps the eyes closed.

Indications for a Face Douche

• Headaches
• Tension and migraines
• Tired eyes

Compresses and Packs

The difference between a bath and a compress or a pack can be understood in this way: with baths, the body is in the water; with a compress or pack (a material or bag that holds the water), water is layered on the body. The three basic types of compresses are hot, cold, and alternating hot and cold (Figure 12-3).

Compresses and packs are applied using cloth, or some other compress material, which is wrung out to the desired amount of moisture and then applied to any surface of the body. A single compress consists only of layers of the wet material. A double compress is a wet cloth completely covered

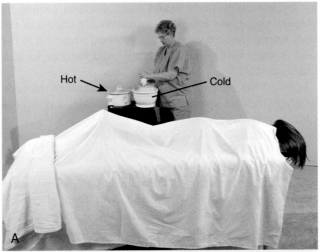

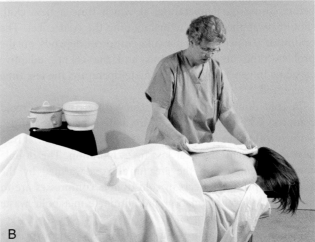

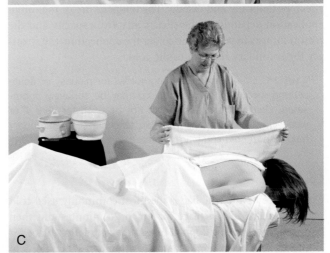

FIGURE 12-3 Applying a compress. **A,** Wet the compress with hot or cold water and wring it out. **B,** Apply it to the area. **C,** Cover the compress with a towel.

by dry material (usually wool), which prevents cooling by evaporation or heat loss. With a cold double compress, the body warms the area, producing a secondary reaction to the cold. A water bottle filled with hot or cold water or ice also can be used.

Compresses are named according to the area of the body to which they are applied (e.g., a head compress or a knee compress).

Cold Compresses

For a cold compress, a cloth is immersed in cold water (sometimes ice water), wrung out, and then placed on the body. Substances often are added to the water, such as baking soda, Epsom salts, boric acid, herbs, or cider vinegar. A cold compress can remain on the body 1 to 5 minutes before losing its temperature, at which time a new cloth should be applied, thereby maintaining the cold effect. The optimum temperature for a cold compress depends on the problem, the desired outcome, and the client's adaptive capacity. In general, the colder the temperature, the less time is required.

A cold double compress is achieved by covering a cold compress with several layers of dry material, such as flannel, wool, or other heavy fabrics. These layers of dry material trap heat and prevent any heat loss by evaporation. The double compress remains on the area until it is warmed by the body. The primary effects of cold double compresses are to increase the local circulation and eliminate metabolic waste from the area.

A cold single compress has a primarily vasoconstrictive effect, both locally and distally. The temperature of the initial application depends on the client's adaptive capacity and the reason for use. In general, the colder the application, the stronger the secondary reaction to the cold.

Caution: Do not use a cold compress for pleurisy or acute asthma, because these conditions may be seriously aggravated. Cold compresses should not be used for very ill or weak individuals, who are unable to generate a secondary response to cold and warm the area.

Cold Packs

Crushed ice in a plastic bag is the most commonly used cold pack. It can be left in place for up to 20 minutes and then removed, or it may be applied repeatedly (i.e., left in place for 1 minute and then removed for 5 minutes). Reusable cold packs that contain gel can be used. A bag of frozen peas or corn makes an effective cold pack.

Indications for a Cold Compress or Pack
- Reduce edema after injury
- Inhibit inflammation
- Relieve pain caused by congestion
- Reduce body temperature (e.g., fever), especially when applied over a large area
- Upper respiratory infections
- Sore throat
- Swollen lymph nodes

Caution: When using ice packs, place a thin cloth between the pack and the skin to prevent frostbite.

Hot Compresses

A hot compress is a prolonged application of moist heat, generally to a local area of the body, which may create an analgesic effect, especially for pain caused by muscle spasm and intestinal or uterine cramping. Fairly hot compresses may be applied directly to the skin surface, with care taken to avoid burning the client.

A *fomentation* is a special type of hot compress that provides prolonged exposure at a higher temperature. Fomentations must be applied over a bath towel placed on the affected area, because the temperature of these compresses cannot be tolerated when applied directly to the skin.

Warm Packs

A warm pack can be created by soaking wrapping cloth in a hot infusion or decoction of herbs, wringing it out, and then applying it to the client's body. Alternatively, various sizes of bags can be filled with rice and then heated in a microwave oven. The typical heating time is 1 minute per pound, not to exceed 5 minutes. This type of pack stays warm longer than a water-based pack; therefore, it is important to monitor the client to prevent burns.

Indications for Hot Compresses or Packs
- Increase blood flow to the periphery
- Decrease internal congestion
- Tissue warming and relaxation
- Insomnia
- Nervous tension
- Mild muscular spasms
- Arthrosis
- Sluggish blood flow
- Headaches (muscle tension type)

Note: Extreme caution is required when electric heating pads are used. Burns are common, because the device does not cool down as does a hot pack or hot water bottle.

Caution: Hot applications are contraindicated on the extremities of diabetic individuals. Special precautions must also be observed when treating the elderly, infants, and individuals with impaired neurologic function, edema, or decreased circulation. It is important to monitor the skin to make sure the client is not burned.

Wet Sheet Pack

Treatment with a wet sheet pack is one of the most useful hydrotherapy procedures. It requires 1 to 3 hours, depending on the client's condition (Figure 12-4).

1. Place two wool or acrylic blankets lengthwise on the table with a small pillow at the head and a small bolster under the knees for comfort. The blankets must be large enough to cover the client.
2. Have the client take a warm shower or bath before applying the treatment. Soak a clean white cotton sheet in cold water and then wring it out as dry as possible.

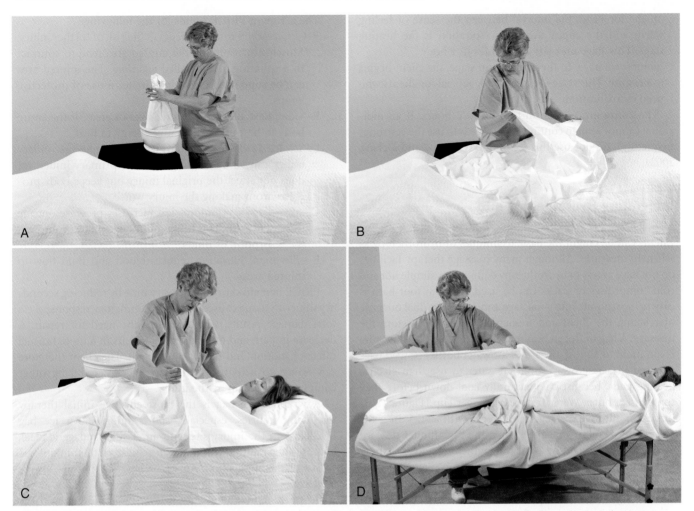

FIGURE 12-4 Using a wet sheet pack. **A,** Place two blankets on the table. Wet a sheet and wring it out. **B,** Place the wet sheet over the top blanket. **C,** Have the client lie down on the wet sheet and then wrap the sheet around the person. **D,** Wrap the surface blanket around the client and then finally wrap the second blanket for warmth.

Open the sheet and place it lengthwise along the table with equal amounts draped over each side. The sheet should be slightly smaller than the blankets.

3. Have the client remove his or her clothing (underwear can be left on) and lie down on the wet sheet. The shoulders should be 4 to 6 inches below the top of the sheet. Have the client raise both arms over the head. Wrap one side of the sheet around the client's body, tucking it in snugly on the opposite side. Below the hips, wrap the sheet around the leg on the same side.

4. Have the client lower the arms. Then, bring the opposite side of the sheet over the body, covering both arms, and wrap the opposite leg.

5. Smooth the wet sheet over the body to ensure complete contact and tuck it in around the feet.

6. Quickly pull the blankets on the table over the client's body and tuck them in firmly, making sure there are no drafts around the client's neck or feet.

7. Additional blankets may be placed over the client, and a stocking cap can be pulled over the head to increase the heating effect.

8. Supervise the client closely. If the person feels claustrophobic or anxious, first remove the sheet from the feet. If

this is unsuccessful, the procedure may need to be stopped. If the client complains of chilliness, add blankets, place a hot water bottle on the feet, or provide warm drinks.

A wet sheet pack proceeds through four stages: tonic (cooling), neutral, heating, and eliminative. Depending on the desired effect, the therapist may prolong any specific stage.

- *Tonic stage:* This stage lasts 2 to 15 minutes and is finished when the client no longer perceives the sheet as cold. The tonic stage creates an intense thermic reaction. The duration of this stage depends completely on the amount of water left in the sheet. For a shorter duration (used for those who are ill or fragile), the sheet should be wrung out as completely as possible. If the client is relatively healthy, more moisture can be left in the sheet to prolong this stage.
- *Neutral stage:* The neutral stage begins when the client is no longer cold. It may last 15 minutes to 1 hour, depending on the client's adaptive capacity. During this phase the client experiences a sense of calm similar to that experienced during a neutral bath. Very often the client falls asleep during this stage.
- *Heating stage:* Heat from the client accumulates beneath the blankets, and light perspiration eventually begins to appear

on the forehead; the interval between the sense of feeling warm and the appearance of perspiration is the heating stage. This stage may last 15 minutes to 1 hour.

• *Eliminative stage.* In the elimination stage, the client begins to perspire. This stage is especially beneficial for clients who need detoxification.

The entire procedure can take up to 3 hours. If an individual cannot remain confined (e.g., needs to use the restroom frequently), do not use this technique (Chaitow and Delany, 2002).

Integrating Hydrotherapy into Therapeutic Massage

Clients can be taught the basic techniques of hydrotherapy as self-help measures. Although many massage therapy facilities do not have access to hydrotherapy equipment, simple hot and cold compresses or packs can be used. A warm foot bath is easy to incorporate into a massage and serves the dual purpose of relaxing the client and freshening "stale" feet before the massage. A bag of frozen peas makes a great cold pack, because it can mold to almost any area. Hot water bottles or seed bags warmed in a microwave oven are safer to use than electric heating pads, because they naturally cool down before they can cause a burn. Water frozen in a paper cup (Figure 12-5) makes an effective massage tool (freeze with a stick in it for even better results), especially when the practitioner uses ice as a counterstimulant to assist in lengthening and stretching procedures. Drinking water also should be available for both the client and the therapist. Meticulous attention to sanitation is necessary when water applications are used (Box 12-3).

PRICE First Aid

Everyone should understand basic first aid. The **PRICE first aid** application includes hydrotherapy and is appropriate for most soft tissue injuries, especially sprains and strains. Serious injuries are always referred to a medical doctor.

The acronym PRICE stands for the following:

P—*Protection:* Protection reduces the risk of further injury. Muscles surrounding the injured area tend to contract in a splinting action called *guarding.* The injured area can be supported through short-term use of protective wraps.

R—*Rest:* Rest allows the injured area or areas or the entire body to best use regenerative energy to heal.

I—*Ice:* Ice slows the metabolism, resulting in less secondary injury caused by swelling from the primary injury. Ice does not affect the original injury but keeps body processes from making the injury worse.

C—*Compression:* Compression increases pressure outside the vasculature. This helps control edema by promoting the resorption of fluids.

E—*Elevation:* Elevation reduces blood and fluid flow to injured areas.

PRICE first aid shortens recovery time by reducing secondary injury to tissue caused by the inflammatory response. Less total damage results, which reduces the need for repair. A decrease in pain and muscle spasms results in a more normal range of motion and muscular strength. The client therefore can return to activity much more quickly, reducing other complications set up by the injury.

A wrapped ice bag is the most effective initial therapy for many injuries, especially sports injuries. An ice bag held close to the injury site with an elastic bandage is ideal, because the resulting compression reinforces the physiologic action of the application. An ice bath or ice massage also is effective.

To prevent frostbite, place a layer of fabric between the ice and the skin. Ice therapy varies with the injury and its severity. Most injuries respond within 24 to 48 hours. Ice bag compression should be used for 20 minutes twice a day or for shorter applications four times a day. Apply ice periodically, not continuously. Between ice applications, rub the body part briskly with the hand. When heat is ineffective for muscle spasms, use ice. Often a sciatica attack that does

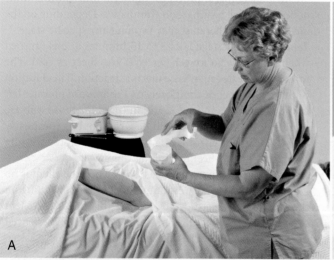
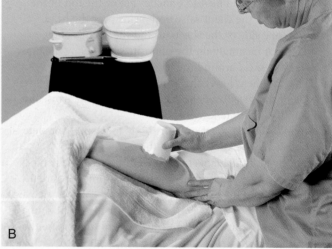

FIGURE 12-5 Ice massage. **A,** To use the ice pop, peel away the edge of the cup or freeze the ice with a stick inserted and peel away the cup. **B,** Apply ice massage to a local area. Catch dripping water with a towel.

Box 12-3 Rules of Hydrotherapy

Hydrotherapy has a powerful effect on the body. The following rules, taken from the Ontario, Canada, curriculum guidelines for massage therapy, should be followed when hydrotherapy is used in the massage setting.

1. Always take a thorough case history to check for possible contraindications. Contraindications include circulatory and kidney problems and skin conditions.
2. Always adapt the method to the individual, not vice versa. The time, temperatures, and other variables used in procedures should be considered guidelines, not absolutes.
3. Have the client go to the bathroom before treatment begins.
4. Stay with the client during treatment or have some way for the client to contact you, such as by using a bell.
5. Explain the complete treatment to the client beforehand so that he or she knows what to expect and what is expected.
6. Make sure the room is draft free, clean, and quiet. All equipment should be sanitary and in good working condition. Each client should have clean towels and sheets.
7. Keep the client from becoming chilled during or after the treatment.
8. For cold water treatments, the water should be as cold as possible, within the client's tolerance. A difference of 10° F from the client's body temperature (hydrotherapy application) is the minimum needed to produce stimulation and change in the circulation.
9. For warm water treatments, the water should be as warm as necessary, within the client's tolerance. A temperature that is too hot can be debilitating.
10. More is not better. Using greater extremes of temperature or longer durations is not always more effective. The aim is to achieve a positive change, and too much can overtax, damage, or set back the condition.
11. Ask pertinent questions during the treatment, including questions about comfort level and thirst, but keep talking to a minimum to allow the client to relax.
12. Check the client's respiratory rate and pulse before, during, and after treatments as required, especially with prolonged hot treatments. The pulse should stay fairly even.
13. Watch for discomfort or negative reactions or both to the treatment.
14. Stop the treatment if a negative reaction occurs.
15. Generally, short cold treatments are followed by active exercise. Prolonged cold and hot treatments are followed by bed rest and then exercise.
16. Apply cold compresses to the head with hot treatments and prolonged cold treatments.
17. Never give a cold treatment to a cold body. Always warm the body first. The easiest method for this is a warm foot bath.

See Table 12-2 for the classification of water temperatures for treatments.

Water Applications for Health Purposes

1. *Local heat:* Apply heat to a specific area of the body, such as a joint, the chest, throat, shoulders, or spine. Use a hot, moist compress or a hot water bottle.
2. *Local cold:* Apply cold to a specific area of the body. Use a cold compress, ice bag, ice pack, ice hat, or frozen bandage.
3. *Sponging:* Use alcohol, water, or witch hazel applied with a sponge to wash the body.
4. *Tonic friction:* Combining water sponging and washing with some form of friction, either from the hand or a rough washcloth, produces a tonic effect in the body. Use cold friction massage or a cold sponge rub.
5. *Baths:* Baths involve immersion of the body in cold, hot, or tepid water. Use foot, sitz, full, mineral, or herb baths. Any part of the body may be partly bathed, as in an arm, eye, or finger bath. A whirlpool is a bath in which the water is moving under pressure.
6. *Compresses and packs:* Compresses and packs are folded cotton, flannel, or gauze soaked in water or liquid medications or herbs. A pack covers a larger area than a compress.
7. *Showers:* Several kinds of water streams can be directed against the body. Alternate streams can also be directed against the body, or large amounts of water can be poured from a height.
8. *Shampoo:* Using soap and water together on one or all parts of the body creates a shampoo. Use shampoo to cleanse the hair or after a sauna or steam room session.
9. *Steam:* A vaporizer can cleanse the upper respiratory system, and a steam room or sauna increases body perspiration and releases many stored toxins. Cold steam, as from a humidifier, moistens dry rooms in winter and is important in preventing colds and sinus headaches.
10. *Sauna (dry heat):* A sauna is an intense but tolerably heated room. A tepid or cold shower should be taken after a sauna treatment.

not respond to moist heat responds to one or two frozen bandages.

Make sure the injury has been evaluated by a physician. Apply ice to the injured area by immersion in ice water (ice bath) and massage with ice cubes or pops, an ice bag, or ice packs.

Ice application continues through four sensations (over a 10- to 15-minute period): appreciation of cold (pain), warming, ache or throbbing, and skin anesthesia (numbness).

The effects of alternating hot and cold include constriction and dilation of vessels and decreased congestion. Techniques include hot and cold compresses, ice bags, warm or hot baths, hot packs, whirlpool baths, and alternating hot and warm or hot and cold showers. Do not use heat on a fresh injury; it increases the blood flow and inflammation and therefore causes tissue swelling (Proficiency Exercise 12-1).

💡 PROFICIENCY EXERCISE 12-1

Gather some of the recommended supplies for hydrotherapy (e.g., bowls, towels, and a watering can). Experiment with hot and cold applications that you feel are convenient to offer as part of the massage process, such as a warm foot bath and a cool eye compress.

HOT AND COLD STONES

SECTION OBJECTIVES

Chapter objective covered in this section:

3. Describe the use of stones and other tools used for thermotherapy.

Using the information presented in this section, the student will be able to perform the following:

• Describe the physiologic effects of thermotherapy (the use of stones) as an aspect of massage

• Use hot and cold stones safely

The use of stones is an ancient healing art that has been rediscovered, particularly in the spa setting. Its modern form came in the early 1990s, when massage therapist Mary Hannigan of Tucson trademarked her particular style and called it LaStone Therapy. Since then, it very quickly became a popular treatment in the spa industry in North America, and it has taken many forms. Most spas offer their own versions.

Stone therapy is a type of **thermotherapy**. It uses deep penetrating heat from smooth, heated stones and alternating cold from chilled stones. There is nothing magical about stones. The simple fact is that stones have an innate ability to hold heat well. As shown in the hydrotherapy section, the physiologic benefits of applying alternating temperatures to the body have long been scientifically investigated and validated. The weight of the stones also has value for providing a sustained compressive force against the tissue while the stone is in place.

Types of Stones Commonly Used for Massage

Basalt stones are commonly used. Basalt is an igneous rock (explained later in the chapter) and holds heat well, but many other types of stone work just fine. The size, weight, and shape of the stone are more important than the type of stone. When the stones are wet or oiled, they change color, becoming darker and acquiring a satinlike appearance.

River rock is commonly used for stone thermal applications in massage. River rocks have smooth rounded edges from movement in river and streambeds. It also is important that the river rock used have some flat surfaces. Quality is determined by the type of parent rock (e.g., sandstone, granite, basalt) and the distance the rock has traveled in the river. Some stones are smoother than others, and color varies; not all river rock is smooth and black. A stone's ability to hold heat depends on the amount of ore in the stone. Ore can appear in the rock as tints of green, grey, rust, blue, and other colors. Black stones do not necessarily hold heat better than lighter colored ones.

Another rock commonly used for stone massage is nephrite (jade). Nephrite is composed of calcium, magnesium, and iron silicate. Nephrite is unique and versatile, because it can hold heat just as well as it can hold cold.

Healing Properties of Minerals

The properties of the crystalline structures of minerals have led to a belief in the healing qualities of various stones. The rarer the stone, the greater its value, and therefore the more healing properties or mystical qualities that are attributed to the mineral.

Gemstones and crystals exhibit rather unusual electrical properties. Four types of electrical phenomena have been described for gemstones.

• *Frictional electrical charges.* Certain gemstones develop an electrical charge when rubbed by a particular material. Thales recognized this quality in amber around 600 BC; in fact, the Greek word for amber is *electron*. In essence, the outer layers of electrons are exchanged between the two materials, and the charge generated depends on the materials. For instance, glass develops a positive charge when rubbed with silk and a negative charge when rubbed with flannel. Diamond, tourmaline, and topaz can be electrically charged by friction.

• *Pyroelectricity.* Pyroelectricity is electrical forces induced by heat. Tourmaline and quartz exhibit this effect, which is the reason they attract dust in a display case if they are located near a heat source, such as a light bulb. This effect was first recognized in tourmaline by Theophrastus in 315 BC and was fully researched during the eighteenth century. The German name for tourmaline originally was *aschentrekker*, which means "ash drawer," a reference to the gem's tendency to attract dust when charged. The color of the tourmaline seems to make a difference; black is the least chargeable, and red is the most chargeable.

• *Piezoelectrical charges.* Piezoelectrical charges are created by mechanical compression of a material; that is, the electrical charge is generated by squeezing, pulling, or compressing the material. Quartz and tourmaline show this property. Even more important is the reverse effect; that is, when an electrical current is passed through the material, it thickens or lengthens. This is the process by which quartz is used to regulate a clock. An electric current causes the quartz to oscillate (vibrate) at a very consistent rate. The same principle was used in submarine detection as early as 1918 and in radio broadcasting frequency control in 1922. An intriguing and still unanswered question is whether piezoelectric forces in certain of the earth's minerals may be what animals sense, either in their systems or on the ground, when they "predict" earthquakes by exhibiting strange behavior. Strong changes in atmospheric pressure may cause this effect. Piezoelectrical forces are known to exist in the bones, cartilage, and tendons of vertebrates.

• *Electrical conduction.* Some gemstones also conduct electricity.

Use of Stones During Massage
Gliding Tool

The smoothness and shape of stones allow some to be used for gliding techniques. A little oil applied to the stone allows a smooth gliding movement as the muscle is warmed; this is similar to "ironing" a muscle. However, some body mechanics concerns for the practitioner arise with regard to gripping the stone. When the massage therapist holds the stone, the muscles in the forearm are activated, which has the potential to cause damage; therefore, the stone should be held with a very light grip. The use of stones for actual massage should be limited.

Pressure Point Tool

Stones of a certain shape can be used for compression. For example, reflexology trigger point treatments can be provided with stones. Client safety is always a concern when implements are used, and caution is necessary.

Compression Tool

The weight of the stones provides physical and mental comfort and enhances compression applications. As the stones cool, they can remain on the body while massage is applied to other areas. Care must be taken to ensure that stones are not overly hot, because they can cause burns.

Thermotherapy Tool

Because of their ability to hold heat and cold, stones make excellent thermotherapy tools. Warm stones transfer heat to the client's muscles and produce relaxation. When frozen or chilled, the stone can be used in all cases in which ice would be appropriate. Alternating application of heat and ice is a well-practiced method of increasing circulation. Stones provide a uniform element for applying the heat and cold without the drawback of cold drips, as may occur with an ice bag.

Note: Stones used as massage tools must be polished very smooth so that they do not catch or pull the client's body hair or scrape the skin.

Proper Body Mechanics While Using Stones

Some applications of stone massage include holding the stone in the hand and using it to apply gliding or compression pressure on a trigger point or acupuncture point. However, body mechanics concerns arise with this process. Gripping the stone while using it to apply pressure strains the practitioner's forearm muscles. The hand must remain relaxed during the massage application, or the muscles in the forearms are strained. Even if the stone is not gripped but rather slid around the body, just using the palm of the hand tends to activate the forearm muscles.

Another safety concern when using stones, or any object, to apply compression is that the massage practitioner's hand is not in direct contact with the client's body, monitoring feedback and pressure depth, and therefore injury might occur.

Justifying the Use of Stones with Massage

Massage therapists should avoid using gimmicks, fads, and buzz words, because these compromise the practitioner's professionalism and the validity of the treatment. Some may question whether the use of stones can be justified in the massage setting. A case can be made for using stones as an adjunct therapy, but this reasoning is based on the properties of the stones.

If you are going to use stones during massage, you should do some research about them. *Petrology* is the study of the classification and mineral and chemical composition of rocks (the term *petrology* is derived from the word *petroleum*). The terms *stones* and *rocks* can be used interchangeably. Body parts that can be treated with stones include the following:

- Forehead
- Area between the toes
- Thigh and back of the calf
- Arm (elbow joint, forearm)
- Sternum, stomach
- Back
- Shoulder
- Neck
- Lumbar area
- Gluteals
- Scapulae

Stones typically are placed on areas of the body with concentrated neurovascular activity; joints, nerve plexuses, acupuncture points, and meridians, in addition to chakras, respond to the compressive thermal influence.

Simply allowing the stones to rest on the body is beneficial. The therapeutic quality of the stone, coupled with the sustained compressive force from the weight of the stone and possibly the energy influence from the crystal structure and color, is sufficient to achieve a therapeutic effect, and the practitioner avoids the potential for repetitive strain injuries caused by using the stones to apply the massage.

Selecting Stones

Make the stone selection process unique by searching for your own or, for convenience, purchase a set from a distributor. To select stones, you can go to a quarry, the beach, a landscaper, or your garden. Many distributors sell crystals. You can find smooth or tumbled stones in many places. Make it a fun practice to search for stones that intrigue you and begin your collection.

Stones used therapeutically have to have a weight and shape that are conducive to body placement. The stones must be fairly flat so that they do not roll around on the body, and they should be fairly smooth so that they do not cause injury. Typically, a flat, oval shape lies on the body without rolling off. River rock often has shapes that fit these criteria. Different sizes of stones can be used on different areas. For example, a stone for the forehead would be flat, rectangular, approximately 3 inches by 5 inches, and $\frac{1}{2}$-inch thick. A stone used for placement on the sacrum could be flat, triangular, and about the size of your hand.

Keep in mind that stones used during massage must be able to withstand constant immersion in hot or cold water and must be sanitized by boiling them in a sanitizing agent (e.g., 10% bleach solution) after each use.

Procedure for Using Stones During Massage
(Figure 12-6)

1. Before the client arrives, sanitize the stones and heat them in water at a temperature of 120° to 150° F (49°–65° C), then cool the stones to 100° to 104° F (38°–40° C) for hot and warm application, or cool in ice water or refrigeration for cold applications. Stones can also be warmed in a slow cooker. A cooking

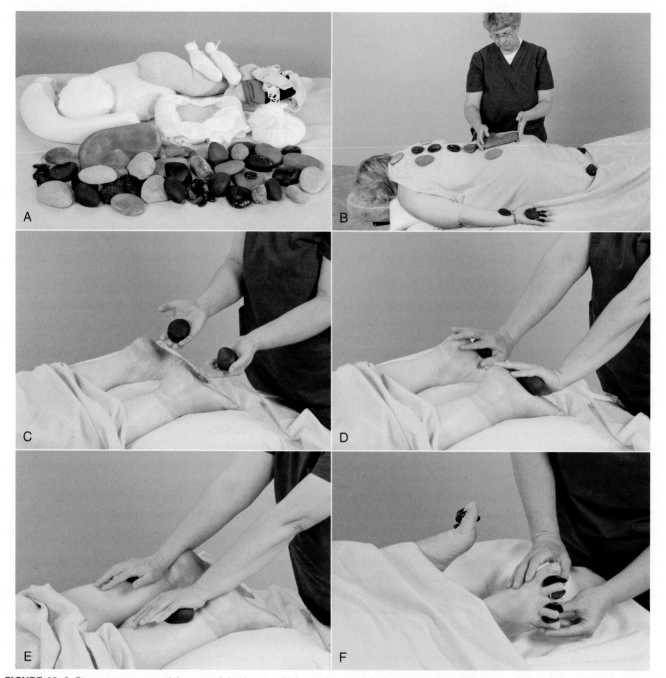

FIGURE 12-6 Stone massage and the use of rice bags, which can be used for hot and cold applications. **A,** Examples of stones and rice bags. **B,** Application of stones on the posterior of the body. **C–E,** Examples of using stones to perform massage. **F,** Example of placing stones between the toes.

thermometer is necessary to achieve a beneficial and safe temperature.

2. Use gliding strokes with the heated stone. When the stone loses heat, replace it with another. Observe precautions for body mechanics.

3. Preferably, use the warm stone to heat your hands. Then use your warm hands for massage and place the stone as described in the next step.

4. Place heated stones at specific points along the body meridians, the spine, in the palms of the hand, or between the toes (anywhere they will stay) to improve the flow of energy in the body. Instruct the client to speak up if the stones are too warm or the pressure is too intense.

5. If the client has inflammation or a muscle injury, use cold stones in those areas.

6. Cover the area with a sheet and then place the stones on the sheet rather than directly on the skin; this is the safest and most sanitary method. With direct application to the skin, the most serious concern is burning the client if the stone is too hot for the individual's skin and/or if it is left on too long. Always use warm, not hot, stones.

7. Massage practitioners are rarely the target of lawsuits; however, incorrect use of hot stones, resulting in burns to the client, has produced a number of cases of litigation. Practitioners must be especially mindful to avoid burning a client by using stones that are too hot,

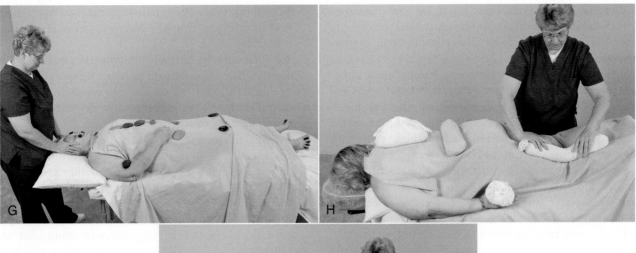

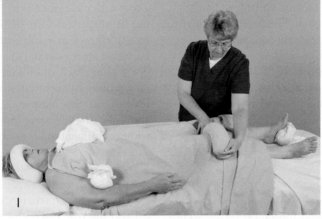

FIGURE 12-6, cont'd G, Application of stones on the anterior of the body. H–I, Examples of using rice bags for compression and thermotherapy.

especially when they are left in one place on the client's body.

8. Apply the stones with an intentional, centered approach.

9. Placement of stones can be combined with general massage. Also, it might be fun to have a selection of stones to give clients for self-help methods. However, make sure the client understands the importance of safe temperature.

10. If the therapeutic benefit of stone application depends on temperature and weight, cloth bags filled with rice or other grains can be used. A pair of socks makes a great bag for this purpose. Fill one sock with the grain (the most inexpensive rice you can buy works fine) and tie the end tightly with string. Then slip the other sock over the filled one and tie it off with a string in a bow that can be tied and untied. The top sock can easily be removed and laundered. Various sizes and shapes of bags can be made using different sizes of socks.

Different colors of socks can be used to add a color element to the process. If appropriate, an essential oil can be placed on the surface sock. These bags—rice, socks, and string—cost less than $5 to make. Sock bags can be heated in the microwave or cooled in the freezer. They also can be molded to the area where they are placed, and they tend to stay put. These grain bags provide all the same therapeutic elements as stones except possibly piezoelectric qualities.

AROMATHERAPY

SECTION OBJECTIVES

Chapter objective covered in this section:
4. Safely integrate aromatherapy into the massage process.
Using the information presented in this section, the student will be able to perform the following:
* Define aromatherapy and essential oils
* Explain the potential benefits of aromatherapy
* Use essential oils safely

Aromatherapy involves the use of essential oils, which are distilled extracts from aromatic plants. Aromatic plants and infusions prepared from them have been used in medicines and cosmetics for thousands of years, but the use of distilled oils dates back only 1,000 years. Ancient civilizations used these oils to protect against disease, to ward off evil, and to aid spiritual healing. As various societies came in contact with each other and shared these oils, knowledge spread. The term *aromatherapy* was coined in the early twentieth century and was recognized as a healing discipline (Tissarand and Balacs, 1995; Schnaubelt, 1998; Price and Price, 2006).

Modern aromatherapy is used in healing the mind, body, and spirit, and its uses range from spiritual to relaxation to therapeutic. Essential oils can be directly inhaled or absorbed through the skin to achieve therapeutic effect. Massage can be combined with aromatherapy. This combination stems from the fact that essential oils, being lipids, are easily absorbed through the skin. Topical application also allows the client to benefit through inhalation for absorption through mucous membranes.

Medical aromatherapy is common in Europe, where physicians prescribe essential oils for the treatment of diseases and conditions. In the United States, nurses and other health care providers often are trained in aromatherapy. Because essential oils have antiseptic, antibacterial, and antibiotic properties, they complement most forms of health care.

Aromatherapy training ensures that the practitioner is prepared to take a client history and can perform an assessment, recognize contraindications, and create essential oil blends designed to address the client's specific concerns. This approach would be considered a medical treatment. Essential oils can also be used for many spa applications (particularly in relation to skin care), such as cleansing and reducing pores, soothing burns, treating sensitive or cracked skin, detoxification, oil gland regulation, hair growth, and skin nourishment. These are common focuses in the spa setting.

Note: The client's consent should be obtained before essential oils are used.

Essential Oils

Essential oils are subtle, volatile chemicals distilled from plants, shrubs, flowers, trees, roots, bushes, and seeds. Essential oils are beneficial both through inhalation of the scent, which affects the limbic system, and through lipid absorption of the oil through the skin. Aromatherapy is an extensive study, and care and caution are advised in the use of essential oils. Only therapeutic grade (100% pure) essential oils should be used, and they should be diluted in a carrier oil (e.g., olive, jojoba, grapeseed, or almond oil) before they are applied to the skin. Only three or four drops of essential oil are needed in 2 ounces of carrier oil. When a drop of oil is mixed with a small amount of salt ($\frac{1}{4}$ cup), it can be dissolved in a warm water immersion, such as a bath. Essential oils in the pure state should never be applied directly to the skin.

Only oils that are generally considered safe, such as the ones listed in this text, should be used.

The following are some of the effects of essential oils:

- *Skin:* They can dissolve dead surface cells, increase cell turnover, stimulate metabolism, improve texture, add softness, give radiance, stimulate, and tone.
- *Nervous system:* They can calm, soothe nerve endings, cause a sense of euphoria, and promote relaxation.
- *Glands:* They can have a soothing and sedating effect, or a toning and stimulating effect.
- *Muscles:* They can relieve fatigue, reduce soreness and stiffness, and improve the resilience and elasticity of muscle.

Additives for an aromatherapy bath or massage oil might include the following:

- Relaxing: Lavender, clary sage, melissa, ylang ylang, bergamot, chamomile
- Stimulating: Rosemary, thyme, lavender (good for toning), pine, cypress
- Soothing: Chamomile, jasmine, geranium, rose
- Moisturizing: Orange blossom, neroli, patchouli, lavender

Essential oils have hormonelike properties and are natural antiseptics. Each oil is thought to have a unique effect on the body and mind, but the oil also can be easily classified as antiseptic, analgesic, antiinflammatory, detoxifying, regenerating, stimulating, or sedating.

Essential oils are not oily; rather, they are more like water. They generally are transparent and can be various colors. Because essential oils are lipid (fat) based, they are soluble in alcohol, oils, and fats, but not water.

Degradation can be an issue with essential oils. Store them in dark glass bottles, away from heat and sunlight. Storage in a cool dark place, such as a refrigerator, is recommended. Also, use of stoppered caps helps prevent oxidation, which can reduce efficacy or result in chemical changes in the essential oil. Never store essential oils in plastic and make sure they are not within reach of children. Most essential oils should be used within 1 year of purchase, although refrigeration can at least double this lifespan. Some oils, such as orange, lemon, and lime, degrade more quickly and may last only 6 months without refrigeration.

Fragrance Oils

Essential oils are the organic constituents of fragrant plant matter and are extracted by distillation or cold pressing. They contain the true essence of the plant. Fragrance or perfume oils are blended synthetic aroma compounds diluted with carrier oils. These artificial oils are used most often in perfumes, cosmetics, and flavoring and are not therapeutically effective.

Because use of the term *aromatherapy* is not regulated by the U.S. government, caution is required when using products. Many beauty and skin care preparations, candles, and other products are improperly labeled with the term *aromatherapy,* although the scent actually is artificial and derived from synthetic fragrance oils. As mentioned, fragrance oils do not offer the therapeutic value of pure high-grade essential oils.

Distillation is a primary determinant of therapeutic grade status. The higher the pressure used in distillation, the higher the yield of oil; however, this also causes unnecessary fractionation of the oil molecules as a result of the higher temperatures created by increasing the pressure. Flavor and fragrance companies produce their oils this way, because they are interested in the scent or flavor applications for food, soft drinks, and other beverages, at the lowest possible cost. Oils produced by high-pressure distillation work fine for flavor and fragrance; they just are not therapeutic grade. Therapeutic-grade oils are produced under lower pressure to preserve their molecular structures with the highest integrity. Lower pressure yields less essential oil, which is one reason therapeutic oils generally are more expensive than commercial-grade oils (Watt, 2011).

Carrier Oils

As mentioned, essential oils are mixed with a carrier oil. Carrier oils are high-quality, fresh vegetable oils that are used

Table 12-3 Common Carrier Oils

Oil	Uses
Apricot kernel oil (Prunus armeniaca)	Extremely moisturizing; use to help revitalize dry skin, delicate skin, mature skin, and sensitive skin and to help soothe minor skin inflammations.
Avocado oil (Persea americana)	Rich in vitamins A, B_1, and B_2; excellent for cases of extremely dry skin (e.g., calluses on the feet). Use on dry, cracked, chapped, and irritated skin and for eczema and psoriasis.
Corn oil	Soothing for all skin types.
Evening primrose oil (Oenothera biennis)	Reduces the appearance of wrinkles; also beneficial for sluggish skin, scarring, inflammation, eczema, acne, and minor skin irritations.
Grapeseed oil (Vitis vinifera)	Used in most cosmetics as a base oil; use for thin skin around the eyes and for normal to combination skin as a light moisturizer.
Hazelnut oil (Corylus avellana)	Helps to tone and tighten skin and to restore elastin to the skin; use to help promote cell regeneration; apply on oily and combination skin.
Hemp seed oil (Cannabis sativa)	Penetrates the skin to moisturize, stimulate, and repair cells damaged by the elements, sun, wind, and ultraviolet light; useful for any skin type.
Jojoba golden (Simmondsia chinensis)	Similar to sebum (the oil human skin produces). Skin absorbs it very quickly, and no oily residue is left on the surface; good for dry, chapped, and cracked skin.
Olive oil	A heavy oil used in cosmetics and soaps; for massage, it is best blended with a lighter vegetable oil.
Rose hip seed (Rosa mosqueta)	Has the highest natural vitamin C content of all the carrier oils and is a renowned cell-renewal agent. Use for scars, stretch marks, wrinkles, cracked skin, dry skin, and sunburn and to support collagen in the skin.
Sesame oil (Sesamum indicum)	Nourishes damaged skin. Use on dry, chapped, discolored, flaky, sun-damaged, and burned skin.
Soybean oil	Use on mature skin.
Sunflower oil (Helianthus annuus)	Has excellent healing properties. Use as a treatment for acne on the body and for accelerating the healing of wounds and insect bites.
Sweet almond oil (Prunus dulcis)	A favorite of massage therapists because of its nutritive and moisturizing qualities. Great for sensitive skin and high in vitamins A, B_1, B_6, and E. Use for dry skin, itchiness, and irritated and inflamed skin.
Wheat germ oil (Triticum vulgare)	Known for its high content of vitamins E and C. Use on mature skin, wrinkles, sun damage, dark spots, eczema, psoriasis, stretch marks, and skin showing signs of premature aging.

to dilute essential oils. Carrier oils also have their own therapeutic properties. The most popular carrier oils are listed in Table 12-3. Make sure all carrier oils are fresh.

Benefits of Aromatherapy

The physiologic effect of essential oils is primarily chemical. The chemistry of essential oils is very complex. Hundreds of components, such as terpenes, aldehydes, and esters, make up the oils. Lavender, for example, has antiseptic, antibacterial, antibiotic, antidepressant, analgesic, decongestant, and sedative properties. Essential oils also reach the bloodstream through inhalation. When inhaled, they pass through the tiny air sacs to the surrounding blood capillaries by the process of diffusion. Once in the bloodstream, the aromatic molecules interact with the body's chemistry.

In addition to their medicinal properties, essential oils have the ability to uplift the client's spirits through inhalation. The sense of smell is interrelated with the limbic system, an area of the brain primarily concerned with emotion and memory. This influence of aromas on the psyche has led many aromatherapists to practice a form of aromatherapy called *psychoaromatherapy*, in which essential oils are used to enhance the client's mood and emotions. The massage therapist needs to be cautious of the scope of practice and ethical boundaries when oils are used for specific treatment of physical or mental disorders.

When an essential oil is inhaled, the chemicals in it stimulate the olfactory center, which receives the odor and carries it to the limbic system. The signal passes between the pituitary and pineal glands, targeting the amygdala (memory center for fear and trauma). The olfactory system is used to bypass the blood-brain barrier. These areas of the brain influence mood, and the hippocampus and amygdala are specifically related to emotion and memory. Scent memory is longer than visual memory. The experience is one of déjà vu; that is, feeling as if the current experience is familiar and seems to be triggered by memory.

An aromatherapy massage can help a person deeply relax and let go of worries, even if only for a short time. Relaxation is powerful enough to activate the body's self-healing ability. Combining the physical and emotional effects of massage with the medicinal and therapeutic properties of essential oils can alleviate stress and improves a person's mood.

Essential oils can help with moderate anxiety and depression, insomnia, digestive disorders, headaches, and muscle aches and pains. Many essential oils are wonderful for skin care. They balance sebum (the skin's natural oil secretion) and can help tone the complexion in supporting capillary function. Essential oils can be used in hair and scalp products to improve circulation to the scalp, to prevent dandruff and promote healthy new hair growth. Essential oils can help heal many minor skin problems, such as athlete's foot, cold sores, ringworm, scabies, psoriasis, dry skin, and oily skin, when used with appropriate health care supervision. Steam or direct inhalation of essential oils can help reduce cold and flu symptoms such as coughs, tonsillitis, sore throats, sinusitis, and bronchitis.

Safety Guidelines for the Use of Essential Oils

As mentioned, essential oils are highly concentrated, volatile substances that, if used correctly, can have therapeutic benefit. Although many oils are useful, some are not safe to use at all, and proper safety guidelines must always be followed when using essential oils. Practitioners should receive advanced training in the use of essential oils before offering aromatherapy massage.

Note: The following cautions and information do not in any way replace medical and professional advice and may not include all cautionary information available.

- Always dilute essential oils in a carrier oil to prevent skin irritation and burning. Never use undiluted essential oils directly on the skin. Experienced aromatherapists may break with this rule, but without extensive training, it is important to work with these substances with caution. Some clients can tolerate some oils, such as tea tree and lavender, in an undiluted form, but again, caution is advised, because severe reactions and sensitivity are possible.
- When using a new oil on your client, it is important to patch test for sensitization and irritation. To patch test, apply a small amount of the diluted oil to the client's skin and leave for 24 to 48 hours to determine whether a reaction occurs. Even if working with an oil that does not commonly cause irritation, the patch test is important as a measure of safety.
- Be familiar with essential oils that are contraindicated during pregnancy or for clients with diseases and illnesses such as asthma and epilepsy.
- Only small amounts of essential oils are needed, and you should use the smallest amount possible for effective treatment. If an additional drop is not necessary, do not use it.
- Many essential oils are not appropriate for use in aromatherapy. Do not assume that every essential oil can be used safely. Some oils, such as wormwood, onion, bitter almond, pennyroyal, camphor, horseradish, wintergreen, rue, and sassafras, should only be used by a qualified aromatherapist. Some oils should not be used at all.
- Keep essential oils out of children's reach. These oils can be tempting, because the scents are appealing and children may think they are lotions or even candy or sweet drinks (e.g., citrus oil). Treat these oils as medicines or poisons when considering storage.
- Keep essential oils away from animals.
- Do not eat, drink, or otherwise ingest essential oils. With extreme caution, a qualified aromatherapy practitioner may prescribe internal use of an essential oil, but only after detailed consultation with the client.
- Essential oils are flammable. Store them properly and keep them away from fire hazards.

- Keep oils away from the eyes. If a drop or so of oil accidentally gets in the eye, put some vegetable oil (e.g., almond oil) in the eye; the vegetable oil will absorb the essential oil, and a tissue then can be used to remove the oil. Do not use water, which will spread the oil. If burning or itching occurs, seek medical treatment.
- Do not use the same oils for a prolonged period.
- Use photosensitizing oils cautiously (i.e., bergamot, verbena, lime, angelica root, bitter orange, lemon, and grapefruit). Advise the client to avoid sun exposure and the use of tanning beds for 12 hours after application of these oils. Photosensitization occurs when oils containing furanocoumarin compounds are applied to the skin and the skin is immediately exposed to sunlight or ultraviolet (UV) light. Furanocoumarin compounds allow the UV rays to penetrate the skin more readily, resulting in abnormal skin pigmentation or mild to severe burns. Remember, UV rays are present even on cloudy days.
- Store essential oils away from light and heat and keep the cap tightly closed. Essential oils are volatile and evaporate readily.

Some aromatherapy experts believe that certain essential oils should not be used unless administered by qualified aromatherapists, and some oils should not be used even by qualified practitioners. Box 12-4 provides a list of potentially hazardous essential oils; do not assume that an oil is safe to use if it is not included in the box. This information is for general educational purposes only and is not considered complete nor is it guaranteed to be accurate.

Aromatherapy Applications

Essential oils can be used in various ways in combination with hydrotherapy and massage.

Aromatic bath, hot tub, or sauna: Put 4 to 10 drops of essential oil in the water just before the person gets into it. Gently stir the water to disperse the oil. For a sauna, dilute the oil with 70% to 90% water and spray it on the rocks and into the air. The bottle must be shaken continually to keep the oil in suspension in the water.

Aromatic compress: Put 3 to 5 drops of oil into 1 to 2 cups of hot or cold water, depending on the need for a compress. Fold a clean cloth and submerge it in the water, then squeeze the excess water from the compress into the basin. Apply immediately to the treatment area.

Aromatic facial steam: Use 1 to 2 drops of oil per 1 cup of boiling water. Place the oil in the bowl or basin after the water has boiled. Stir the water to disperse the oil. Immediately place a towel over the head and place the face as close as possible to the aromatic steam without causing any discomfort.

Environmental and room fragrance: Electronic diffusers are an easy, effective way to fragrance a room for esthetic and therapeutic purposes. Use only pure essential oils or synergies of pure essential oils. Never use essential oils cut with carrier oils in diffusers, because this clogs the diffuser.

Aroma lamps: Aroma lamps are great for adding environmental fragrance. Add 10 drops of essential oils to 1 teaspoon

Box 12-4	Potentially Hazardous Essential Oils

Oils that should *not* be used on any client include:
- Bitter almond
- Boldo leaf
- Calamus
- Camphor (yellow)
- Horseradish
- Jaborandi leaf
- Mugwort
- Mustard
- Pennyroyal
- Rue
- Sassafras
- Savin (*Juniperus sabina*)
- Southernwood
- Tansy
- Thuja
- Western red cedar (*Thuja plicata*)
- Wintergreen
- Wormseed
- Wormwood

Oils that should *not* be used on pregnant clients include:
- Aniseed
- Basil
- Cinnamon
- Clary sage
- Cypress
- Fennel
- Hyssop
- Jasmine
- Juniper
- Marjoram
- Myrrh
- Origanum
- Peppermint
- Rose
- Rosemary
- Sage
- Thyme

Oils that should *not* be used on or by individuals with epilepsy include:
- Camphor
- Fennel
- Hyssop
- Sage
- Rosemary

of water and place in the designated receptacle on the lamp. The heat of the light disperses the fragrance.

Inhalation: An effective and simple way to inhale essential oils is to place a couple drops of an oil or blend on a handkerchief or cotton cloth and inhale throughout the day. This is a nice gift for the person who just received the massage.

Aromatic spray: Mix about 100 drops of essential oil (a single oil or a blend of oils) with 4 ounces of vodka. This creates a concentrate that can be added to water to create the aromatic spray. Add about 100 drops of the concentrate to 2 ounces of distilled water and shake well. To create a spritzer

for the face or body, use only water and essential oils. For the body, add about 40 to 50 drops of essential oil or a blend to 4 ounces of distilled water. For the face, add 8 to 10 drops to 4 ounces of water.

Massage: Use a dilution of about 1% to 2.5% of essential oil to carrier oil when preparing the massage oil. This means approximately 5 to 15 drops of essential oil per 1 ounce of carrier oil. If you are using more than one essential oil, blend them first and then add no more than 15 drops of the blend to the carrier oil. Remember, when creating a massage blend, less is more, and in fact the desired result can be achieved with very low dilutions.

Choosing Essential Oils to Complement Massage

A number of factors can affect the selection of essential oils to be used for massage. The choice can be based on the therapeutic quality of the oil or oils (Table 12-4), the client's emotional well-being (Table 12-5), or the presence of a specific condition (Table 12-6).

- Offer a selection of oils you can tolerate (no more than 10).
- Let the client sniff each oil; have the person choose one or two he or she really likes and then the one the individual least likes. Look up the characteristics of the oils with the client (see Table 12-4) and see how they relate to the client's current condition.
- Create a unique blend for the client with 2 drops of each of the preferred oils (4 drops total) and 1 drop of the least favorite oil (blend no more than three oils). Then blend the mixture into a carrier oil chosen according to the client's skin type and the qualities of the carrier oil.

LYMPH, BLOOD, AND CIRCULATION ENHANCEMENT

SECTION OBJECTIVES

Chapter objectives covered in this section:
5. Modify massage application to support beneficial blood and lymph movement in the body.

Using the information presented in this section, the student will be able to perform the following:
- Explain the general effects of lymphatic and circulation enhancement massage
- Identify indications for and contraindications to lymphatic drainage massage.
- Incorporate the principles of lymphatic and circulation massage into a general massage session

Massage targeting this area can be considered fluid movement. Stimulation of the lymphatic and circulatory systems once was considered a well-documented benefit of massage. However, current research has not supported that contention Review Chapter 5 to better understand the shift from accepting that massage altered circulation as a benefit to questioning the evidence. Nevertheless, in one study of manual lymphatic drainage, a specialized form of massage therapy, data from a rat model of obstructive lymphedema suggests

Table 12-4	Therapeutic Qualities of Individual Essential Oils
Oil	**Therapeutic Qualities**
Bergamot	Skin conditioner, soothing agent, antiseptic, phototoxic
Cajeput	Stimulating agent, mood enhancer, antiseptic
Cardamom	Muscle relaxant, skin conditioner, soothing agent
Carrot seed	Muscle relaxant, soothing agent, skin conditioner
Cedarwood	Antiseptic, skin conditioner, deodorant, soothing agent
Clary sage	Skin conditioner, astringent, soothing agent, muscle relaxant. Do not use if client is pregnant or drinks alcohol.
Eucalyptus	Antiseptic, soothing agent, skin conditioner, sinus clearing
Frankincense	Skin conditioner, soothing agent
Geranium	Skin refresher, muscle relaxant
Ginger	Astringent
Grapefruit	Soothing agent, astringent, skin conditioner
Jasmine absolute	Emollient, soothing agent, antiseptic
Juniper	Skin detoxifier, astringent, soothing agent; flammable
Lavender	Muscle relaxant, skin conditioner, soothing agent, astringent
Lemon	Soothing agent, antiseptic
Lemongrass	Skin conditioner, soothing agent, muscle relaxant, antiseptic
Lime	Soothing agent, skin conditioner, astringent
Mandarin	Soothing agent, skin conditioner, astringent
Myrrh	Antiinflammatory, emollient, antiseptic. Use in moderation if client is pregnant.
Neroli	Antiseptic, emollient
Nutmeg	Antiseptic, muscle relaxant; soothes irritated skin
Orange	Astringent, soothing agent, skin conditioner
Peppermint	Emollient, antiseptic, muscle relaxant
Pine	Antiseptic
Roman chamomile	Muscle relaxant, skin conditioner
Rose absolute	Skin conditioner
Rose otto	Astringent
Rosemary	Antiseptic, muscle relaxant, soothing agent, skin conditioner. Do not use if client is pregnant or has high blood pressure.
Rosewood	Muscle relaxant
Sandalwood	Antiseptic, emollient, soothing agent, skin conditioner
Spearmint	Emollient, astringent, soothing agent. Use sparingly.
Tea tree	Antiseptic, acne fighter, dandruff fighter
Ylang-ylang	Reduces stress and tension

Table 12-5	Oils for Emotional Well-Being
Condition	**Treatment Oils**
Anger	Bergamot, jasmine, orange, patchouli, rose, ylang-ylang
Anxiety	Clary sage, frankincense, geranium, lavender, mandarin, rose, sandalwood
Confidence	Bergamot, grapefruit, jasmine, orange, rosemary
Depression	Bergamot, clary sage, frankincense, geranium, grapefruit, jasmine, lavender, lemon, mandarin, neroli, orange, rose
Fatigue, exhaustion, and burnout	Bergamot, clary sage, frankincense, grapefruit, jasmine, lemon, peppermint, rosemary, sandalwood
Fear	Clary sage, frankincense, grapefruit, jasmine, lemon, neroli, orange
Grief	Frankincense, neroli, rose
Happiness, peace	Frankincense, geranium, grapefruit, lemon, neroli, orange, rose sandalwood, ylang-ylang
Insecurity	Frankincense, jasmine, sandalwood
Irritability	Lavender, mandarin, neroli, Roman chamomile, sandalwood
Loneliness	Bergamot, clary sage, frankincense, rose
Memory, concentration problems	Lemon, peppermint, rosemary
Stress	Bergamot, clary sage, frankincense, geranium, grapefruit, jasmine, lavender, mandarin, neroli, Roman chamomile, rose sandalwood, ylang-ylang

Data from Aromatherapy for Emotional Well-Being, Aroma Web, LLC at http://www.aroma.com/articles/emotional/wellbeing.asp.

decongestive therapy and manual lymphatic drainage in patients with breast cancer–related lymphedema are positive, (Koul et al., 2007).

Based on these studies, a case can be made for the influence of massage on the movement of lymphatic fluid, even though we do not totally understand the mechanisms and research findings are conflicting.

As informed and ethical massage therapists, we need to consider the myths that now exist concerning the effects of massage on body fluid, and re-educate clients and others about the current evidence on massage's effects on circulation. As mentioned, it is reasonable to believe that massage has some effect on body fluid movement, but it is not clear what causes the circulatory changes and whether they are significant enough to result in specific benefit. Therefore, the following section presents adaptations to the massage approach that would be most likely to affect the movement of the lymph and blood in the body.

Many variations and styles of massage have been and are used to stimulate lymphatic and blood circulation. When the massage is focused to stimulate the lymphatic or circulatory system specifically, some modifications to the massage application are necessary. Because an entire body system is being stimulated, the approach is sometimes called systemic massage. In this section we discuss the important physiology and methods of focusing the massage to enhance the lymphatic and blood circulations.

that massage alone can reduce fluid volume (Bernas et al., 2005). Typically this form of massage is combined with compression bandaging. Another study found that in a cohort of patients with mild, stable, upper-limb lymphedema, massage alone was as effective as massage combined with compression bandaging (Bernas et al., 2005). The results of combined

Table 12-6	Essential Oils for Common Physical Conditions

Condition	Oils
Abdominal cramps	Lavender, clary sage
Acne	Bergamot, chamomile, geranium, lavender, patchouli, sandalwood, tea tree
Aging skin	Carrot seed, frankincense
Arthritis	Chamomile, eucalyptus, ginger
Athlete's foot	Tea tree
Brain fog	Grapefruit, lemongrass, lime, orange
Colds, flu, bronchitis	Cajeput, eucalyptus, frankincense, ginger, lavender, peppermint, tea tree
Corns, warts	Lemon, tea tree
Bruises	Chamomile, lavender
Burns	Lavender
Children's stomach upsets	Mandarin, tangerine
Cold sores	Eucalyptus, tea tree
Coughs	Eucalyptus, ginger, tea tree
Dandruff	Lavender
Dermatitis	Chamomile, lavender
Dry skin	Geranium (especially skin with oily patches), sandalwood
Dysmenorrhea (painful periods/menstrual cramps)	Chamomile, clary sage, cypress, lavender
Edema	Carrot seed, grapefruit
Fevers	Eucalyptus, lemongrass
Flatulence	Lime
Headache	Chamomile, lavender, peppermint
Herpes	Tea tree
High blood pressure (hypertension)	Lavender, ylang-ylang
Indigestion	Chamomile, orange
Inflammation	Chamomile, lavender
Insect bites and stings	Chamomile, lavender, tea tree
Insect repellent	Lemongrass, lavender
Insomnia	Chamomile, lavender
Laryngitis, sore throat	Ginger, lavender, thyme
Muscle aches and pains	Chamomile, eucalyptus, ginger, grapefruit, lavender, rosemary
Nausea	Chamomile, lavender
Nervous exhaustion, fatigue	Peppermint, rosemary
Nervous tension, stress	Chamomile, clary sage, frankincense, lavender, sandalwood
Neuralgia	Chamomile
Poor circulation	Ginger, rosemary
Premenstrual syndrome (PMS)	Geranium, lavender
Scars	Frankincense, lavender
Sinusitis	Eucalyptus, pine
Sprains, strains	Chamomile, eucalyptus, lavender
Stretch marks	Mandarin, lavender
Vertigo	Lavender, peppermint

Lymphatic Drainage

Various styles of bodywork are used for **lymphatic drainage.** One such style is manual lymphatic drainage, which was developed by Emil Vodder. Another style, described by Eyal Lederman, an osteopathic physician, takes a somewhat different approach. Recently, a third approach was added, taught by Bruno Chikly. These three methods provide the foundation for this section.

Lymphatic drainage to address pathologic lymphedema is a therapeutic method requiring specialized training that combines specific manual techniques and compression bandaging. The following information and suggested applications may be beneficial for the lymphatic system in general and for nonpathologic simple edema that occasionally occurs. As with all methods of massage, we need to appreciate the anatomy and physiology of body functions that are the target of the massage.

Lymphatic System

The lymphatic system is a specialized component of the circulatory system that is responsible for waste disposal and immune response. The lymphatic system transports fluid from around the cells through a system of filters. Lymph and blood are very similar, except that lymph does not have red blood cells or platelets. Lymph has a slightly higher protein content than blood, and it carries large molecules, such as proteins, lipids, and bacteria, and other debris. Lymph is the interstitial fluid (i.e., the fluid that surrounds the cell). It is generated when plasma is forced out of the blood capillaries into cellular spaces to bathe and nourish the cells (Figure 12-7).

The lymphatic system permeates the entire tissue structure of the body in a one-way drainage network of vessels, ducts, nodes, lacteals, and lymphoid organs such as the spleen, tonsils, and thymus.

The spleen, the largest organ of the lymphatic system, filters the blood. It manufactures lymphocytes, stores red blood cells, releases blood to the body in cases of extreme blood loss, and removes foreign substances and dead red blood cells. The spleen contains red and white pulp. The white pulp contains white blood cells and surrounds arteries that enter the spleen, and the red pulp surrounds veins that leave the spleen. Macrophages in the red pulp remove foreign substances and worn out or dead red blood cells.

The tonsils form a ring of lymphatic tissue that surrounds the opening to the digestive and respiratory tracts, an area where harmful substances can easily enter the body. The three pairs of tonsils are the pharyngeal, palatine, and lingual tonsils.

The thymus forms antibodies in newborns and is involved in the initial development of the immune system. Lymphocytes produced in the red bone marrow migrate to the thymus, where they develop into T cells. The thymus also produces the hormone thymosin. The activity of the thymus gland declines with age.

Aggregated lymph nodules are collections of lymphatic tissue in mucous membranes that are continuous with the skin; examples of these nodules include the tonsils, the bronchi of the respiratory tract, the small intestine, and the appendix. Aggregated lymph nodules respond to antigens in those areas and create antibodies.

To get an idea of the extensive lymph network, visualize the roots on a plant. Tiny lymph vessels, known as *lymph*

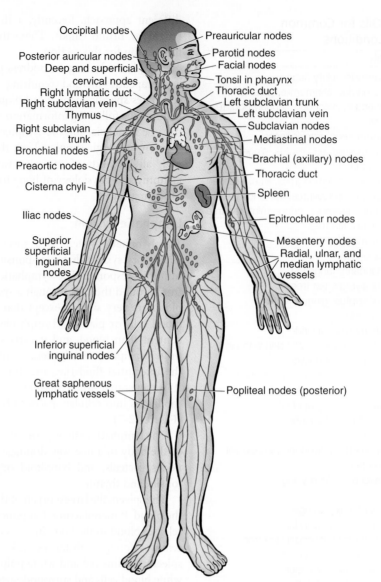

FIGURE 12-7 The lymphatic system and lymphatic drainage pathways throughout the body.

capillaries, are distributed throughout the body, except in the eyes, brain, and spinal cord. Fluid collects in the lymph capillaries in a manner somewhat similar to the way water is drawn up into a plant's roots. Segments of lymph capillaries are divided by one-way valves and a spiral set of smooth muscles called *lymphangions.* This system moves fluid against gravity in a peristalsis-type undulation.

The lymphatic tubes merge until major channels and vessels are formed. These vessels run from the distal parts of the body toward the neck, usually alongside veins and arteries. Valves in the vessels prevent the back flow of lymph.

Lymph nodes are enlarged portions of the lymph vessels that generally cluster at the joints. This arrangement assists movement of the lymph through the nodes by means of the pumping action from joint movement. These nodes filter the fluid and produce lymphocytes.

All of the body's lymph vessels converge into two main channels, the thoracic duct and the right lymphatic duct. Vessels from the entire left side of the body and from the right side of the body below the chest converge into the thoracic

duct, which in turn empties into the left subclavian vein, situated beneath the left clavicle. The right lymphatic duct collects lymph from the vessels on the right side of the head, neck, upper chest, and right arm. It empties into the right subclavian vein beneath the right clavicle. Waste products then are carried by the bloodstream to the spleen, intestines, and kidneys for detoxification.

Lymph moves along a pressure gradient from areas of high pressure to areas of low pressure. It moves from the interstitial space (high pressure) into the lymph capillaries (low pressure) through a pressure mechanism exerted by respiration, peristalsis of the large intestine, the compression of muscles, and the pull of the skin and fascia during movement. This action is especially prominent at the plexuses in the hands and feet. Major lymph plexuses are found on the soles of the feet and the palms of the hands. The rhythmic pumping of walking and grasping probably facilitates lymphatic flow. As mentioned in Chapter 5, recent research indicates the existence of a primary intrinsic pumping mechanism in the lymphatic system.

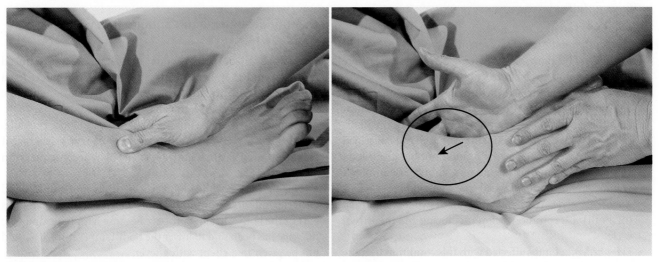

FIGURE 12-8 Assessment for edema.

Lymph circulation involves two steps:
- First, plasma is forced out of blood capillaries into the space around the cells. The fluid now located around the cells is called *interstitial fluid*. As fluid pressure increases between the cells, the cells move apart, pulling on the microfilaments that connect the endothelial cells of the lymph capillaries to tissue cells. The pull on the microfilaments causes the lymph capillaries to open like flaps, allowing interstitial fluid to enter the lymph capillaries. Once the fluid is in the lymph capillaries, it is called *lymph*.
- Next, the lymph moves through the network of contractile lymphatic vessels. The lymphatic system does not have a central pump like the heart. Various factors assist the transport of lymph through the lymphatic vessels.

The "lymphatic pump" is the spontaneous contraction of lymphatic vessels as a result of the increased pressure of lymphatic fluid. These contractions usually start in the lymphangions adjacent to the terminal end of the lymph capillaries and spread progressively from one lymphangion to the next, toward the thoracic duct or the right lymphatic duct. The contractions are similar to abdominal peristalsis and are stimulated by increases in pressure inside lymphatic vessels. Contractions of the lymphatic vessels are not coordinated with the heart or breath rate. If the pressure inside the lymphatic vessels exceeds or falls below certain levels, lymphatic contractions stop.

During inhalation, the thoracic duct is squeezed, which pushes fluid forward and creates a vacuum in the duct. During exhalation, fluid is pulled from the lymphatics into the thoracic duct to fill the partial vacuum.

Edema

Edema, which is an increase in interstitial fluid, can be caused by a variety of factors (Figure 12-8 and Box 12-5).
- *Lack of exercise.* Exercise, in which muscles alternately contract and relax, stimulates lymph circulation and cleans muscle tissue. If the muscles stay contracted or

> **Box 12-5** **Assessment for and Treatment of Fluid Imbalance**
>
> 1. Ask the client if tissue feels taut, distended, fat, or stiff. If the answer is no, palpate to confirm that edema is not present and then proceed with the general massage. If the answer is yes, ask for the history.
> 2. The history should include any injury, swelling, bruising, static position, and unusual increase in physical activity followed by extended inactivity. If the client answers yes to any of these, then observe.
> 3. Observe for a decrease in muscle definition, bruising, tissue distention, and changes in color. If any of these are found, palpate.
> 4. Palpate for increased muscle tone, specifically tissue tautness and an increase in fluid (pitting edema) or venous congestion. If these are noted, observe and palpate for signs of inflammation.
> 5. Palpate for heat and observe for redness. Ask about pain.
> 6. If the area is swollen, hot, red, and painful, refer the client to a medical professional. If inflammation is present, massage the area only after the reason for the condition has been determined.
> 7. If the area is not hot or red, determine whether the tissue is congested or swollen.
> 8. Congested tissue has increased blood in the veins and capillaries; the tissue feels dense and stiff but does not show pitting edema. Swollen tissue has increased interstitial fluid; this tissue pits when pressure is applied.
> 9. If the tissue is congested, massage methods that enhance venous return are indicated. Observe cautions for thrombosis, kidney disease, and heart disease.
> 10. If the tissue is swollen, lymphatic drainage is indicated. Observe cautions for infection, kidney disease, and heart disease.

flaccid, lymph circulation declines drastically inside the muscles, and edema can result.
- *Increase in exercise.* An increase in exercise can strain the lymph system by causing blood capillary permeability, resulting in an increase in fluid movement to the

interstitial spaces. This is one cause of the delayed onset of muscle soreness.

- *Salt consumption.* The body retains a specific ratio of salt to fluids. The more salt a person consumes, the more water is retained to balance it, resulting in edema.
- *Heart or kidney disease.* These diseases affect the blood and lymphatic circulations. Lymphatic massage stimulates the circulation of lymph. However, caution is indicated, because the increase in fluid volume could overload an already weakened heart. In addition, because blood volume is regulated by the kidneys, an increase in blood volume could overload already weakened kidneys.
- *Menstrual cycle.* Water retention or a swollen abdomen (or both) are common before or during the menstrual cycle.
- *Lymphedema.* Limbs affected with this condition become very swollen and painful, resulting in difficulty moving the affected limb and disfigurement. Lymphedema can be life threatening, because the interstitial fluid is contaminated, injuries to the skin do not heal, and even small abrasions and sores can become infected.
- *Inflammation.* Increased blood flow to an injured area and the release of vasodilators, which are part of the inflammatory response, can cause edema in the localized area.
- *Other causes.* Medications, including steroids, hormones, and chemotherapy for cancer, may cause edema as a side effect. Scar tissue and muscle tension can cause obstructive edema by restricting lymph vessels.

Indications for Lymphatic Drainage Massage

Simple edema, with screening for contraindications, appears to respond to massage focused on the lymphatic system even though the research evidence is sparse. The following conditions may benefit from massage that focuses on the movement of lymph:

- Simple edema that results from inactivity (e.g., a long car ride, sitting at computer).
- Traveler's edema, which is the result of enforced inactivity, such as sitting in an airplane or a car for several hours (the same is true for anyone who sits for extended periods). Interstitial fluid (tissue fluid) responds to gravity, causing swelling in the feet, hands, and buttocks of a person who has to sit without moving very much for a few hours. Lymphatic drainage massage can move the fluid and reduce the pain and stiffness caused by the edema. Caution is indicated because of the possibility of the formation of blood clots with prolonged activity.
- Exercise-induced, delayed-onset muscle soreness, which may be partly caused by increased fluid pressure in the soft tissues. Lymphatic drainage massage appears to be effective for reducing the pain and stiffness of this condition.
- Fluid retention caused by premenstrual hormonal changes.
- Residual edema in the later stages of the healing of strains, sprains, and other types of injuries.

Contraindications and Cautions for Lymphatic Drainage Massage

Edematous tissues have poor oxygenation and reduced function, and they heal slowly after injury. Chronic edema results in chronic inflammation and fibrosis, which makes the edematous tissue coarse, thicker, and less flexible.

Lymphatic drainage massage can lower blood pressure. If the client has low blood pressure, the danger exists that it may drop even farther, and the client may become dizzy on standing.

During a fever, white blood cells multiply more rapidly and bacteria and viruses multiply more slowly; fever, therefore, is part of the body's healing process. Because lymphatic drainage massage has been said to lower the body temperature, it should not be given to a client with a fever.

Lymphatic drainage massage may affect the circulation of fluid in the body, which may overwhelm an already compromised heart or kidneys. Do not give lymphatic drainage massage to anyone with congestive heart failure or kidney failure or anyone undergoing kidney dialysis unless it is specifically ordered by the physician.

Principles of Lymphatic Drainage Massage

If massage does indeed affect the movement of lymph in the body, then somehow massage would need to mimic the natural mechanism of lymph movement.

The pressure provided by massage mimics the drag and compressive forces of movement and respiration and can move the skin to open the lymph capillaries. The pressure gradient from high pressure to low pressure is supported by creating low-pressure areas in the vessels proximal to the area to be drained. The depth of pressure, speed and frequency, direction, rhythm, duration, and drag are adjusted to support the lymphatic system.

Depth of pressure. According to Vodder, the softer the tissue or the greater the edema, the lighter the pressure that should be used. Vodder estimated the proper pressure for lymphatic drainage to be 8 to 12 ounces per square inch, with the pressure in the peripheral lymphatics even lighter (less than 1 to 8 ounces per square inch). You can develop a sense of these levels of pressure by stroking the surface of a postage scale until you can easily keep the pressure within the recommended range. This pressure is just enough to move the skin. The lymphatics are located mostly in superficial tissues, in the outer 0.3 mm of the skin, and surface edema occurs in those superficial tissues, not in the deep tissue.

Simple muscle tension puts pressure on the lymph vessels and may block them, interfering with efficient drainage. Massage can normalize this muscle tension. As the muscles relax, the lymph vessels open, and drainage becomes more efficient. Work on the areas of muscle tension first, using appropriate massage methods and pressure, and then finish the area with lymphatic drainage.

Disagreement exists about the intensity of the pressure used. Some schools of thought recommend very light pressure, such as that described by Vodder. Other methods, such as the technique described by Lederman, use a deeper pressure. Lederman holds that the stronger the compression used, the greater the increase in the flow rate of the lymph. Light pressure is used initially, and the pressure is methodically increased as the area is drained (Lederman, 2005). Moving the skin moves the lymphatics. Stretching the lymphatics longitudinally, horizontally, and diagonally stimulates them to contract.

Speed and frequency. The greater the amount of fluid in the tissue, the slower the massage movements. Massage strokes are repeated at a rate of approximately 10 per minute in an area, the approximate rate at which the peripheral lymphatics contract.

Direction. The lymph is moved toward the closest cluster of lymph nodes, which are located in the neck, axilla, and groin for the most part. Massage near nodes first, then move fluid toward them, working proximally from the swollen area toward the nodes. Massage the unaffected side first, then the obstructed side. For instance, if the right arm is swollen because of scar tissue from a muscle tear, massage the left arm first.

Rhythm. Slow, rhythmic repetition of the massage movements stimulates a wave in the lymph fluid similar to intestinal peristalsis (e.g., a pump).

Duration. Full-body lymphatic drainage massage lasts about 45 minutes. Focus on local areas for about 5 to 15 minutes.

Drag. Drag on the tissue pulls open the terminal ends of the lymphatic capillaries (flap), allowing interstitial fluid to enter. Drag moves the superficial tissues (skin and superficial fascia) into and out of bind.

Application of Lymphatic Drainage Massage

The massage approach described next specifically targets the lymphatic system and is appropriate for clients who are generally healthy. People commonly develop a somewhat sluggish lymphatic flow. The usual culprits are inactivity, consumption of junk food and beverages, and reduced water intake. All these factors stress the lymphatic system. General massage with a focus as presented in this section, coupled with corrective action by the client (i.e., increased water intake, increased activity, and reduced junk food intake) can reverse the problem.

Additional training and medical supervision are required for professionals who intend to work with clients with lymphatic conditions. Although disagreement exists about methodology, and whether massage can even affect lymphatic movement sufficiently to provide benefit, all approaches have some validity. Therefore, the method described in this text combines the various methods to support lymphatic movement in the body (Proficiency Exercise 12-2).

Procedure for Lymphatic Drainage Targeted Massage

1. Begin the massage session with a pumping action on the thorax.
2. Place both hands on the anterior surface of the thoracic cage.

PROFICIENCY EXERCISE 12-2

1. Fill a long balloon with water. Leave an air bubble in it. Use short gliding strokes with a drag component to move the bubble. Notice the level of pressure that moves the bubble most effectively.
2. Design a lymphatic self-massage. Incorporate deep breathing movement and compression action at the joints, palms, and soles of the feet.

3. As the client exhales completely, allow your hands to passively follow the movements of the thorax.
4. When the client starts to inhale, resist the movement of the thorax with counterpressure for 5 to 7 seconds.
5. Repeat this procedure four or five times.

Pumping action on the thorax increases lymphatic drainage through the lymph ducts by additionally lowering intrapleural pressure and exaggerating the action of inhalation and exhalation.

The massage application consists of a combination of short, light, pumping, gliding strokes beginning close to the torso at the node cluster and directed toward the torso; the strokes methodically move distally. The stroke does not slip, but rather drags the tissue to bind. The phase of applying pressure and drag must be longer than the phase of pressure and drag release. The releasing phase cannot be too short, because the lymph needs time to drain from the distal segment. Therefore the optimum duration of the pressure and drag phase is 6 to 7 seconds; for the release phase, it is about 5 seconds. Traditionally, this application was described as stationary circles, which essentially produces a bind/release movement. This pattern is followed by long surface gliding strokes with a bit more pressure to influence deeper lymph vessels. The direction is toward the drainage points.

The focus of the initial pressure and finishing strokes is the dermis, just below the surface layer of skin, and the layer of tissue just beneath the skin and above the muscles. This is the superficial fascial layer, which contains 60% to 70% of the lymphatic circulation in the extremities. Not much pressure is required to contact the area. If too much pressure is applied, the capillaries are pressed closed; this nullifies any effect on the more superficial vessels. With lymphatic massage, generally light pressure is indicated initially, which increases to a moderate level (including kneading, compression, and gliding) during repeated application to the area to reach the deep lymphatic vessels; the technique then returns to lighter pressure over the area.

Drag is necessary to affect the microfilaments and to open the flaps at the ends of the capillary vessels. A pumping, rhythmic compression on the soles and palms supports lymph movement.

Rhythmic, gentle, passive and active joint movement reproduces the body's normal means of pumping lymph. The client helps the process by deep, slow breathing, which stimulates lymph flow in the deeper vessels. When possible, position the area being massaged above the heart so that gravity can assist lymph flow. This approach is very methodical and repetitious. Drinking water supports the system (see the combind fluid movement protocol on p. 482).

2
12-2

Circulatory Massage

The purpose of circulatory massage is to stimulate the efficient flow of blood through the body. As described for lymphatic drainage massage, the current research is inconclusive and sparse; therefore, caution is urged when making claims about the benefits of massage that specifically targets fluid movement. As with lymphatic massage, specific application for circulatory disease is out of the scope of practice for the massage professional unless the massage is performed under appropriate supervision. In this situation, massage may be beneficial as part of the overall treatment plan.

Clients who are not sick can benefit greatly from increased efficiency in the circulatory system. Aerobic exercise (see Chapter 15) is possibly the best way to support circulation. Massage tends to normalize blood pressure, tone the cardiovascular system, and reduce the negative effects of occasional stress. It is an excellent massage approach to use with athletes and anyone else after exercise. Circulatory massage also supports the inactive client by potentially increasing blood movement mechanically; however, it in no way replaces exercise. Both the circulatory and lymphatic types of massage would seem to be beneficial for a client who is unable to walk or exercise aerobically.

Circulatory System

The circulatory system is a closed system composed of a series of connected tubes and a pump. The heart's pumping action provides pressure to move the blood through the body via the arteries and eventually into the small capillaries, where blood gas and nutrient exchange happens. The blood returns to the heart by way of the veins. Venous blood flow is not under pressure from the heart. Rather, it relies on muscle compression against the veins to change the interior venous pressure. As in the lymphatic system, back flow of blood is prevented by a valve system.

Massage Methods for the Circulatory System

Massage to encourage blood flow to the tissues (arterial circulation) is different from massage to encourage blood flow from the tissues back to the heart (venous circulation). Because the veins and lymph vessels have a valve system, deep, narrow-based stroking over these vessels from proximal to distal (from the heart outward) is contraindicated. A small chance exists of breaking down the valves if this is done. Compression, which does not slide, as does gliding or stripping, is appropriate for stimulating arterial circulation.

FLUID MOVEMENT PROTOCOL

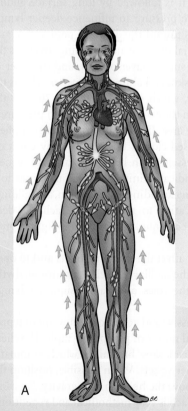

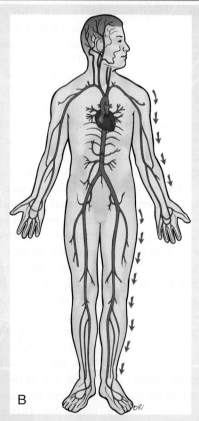

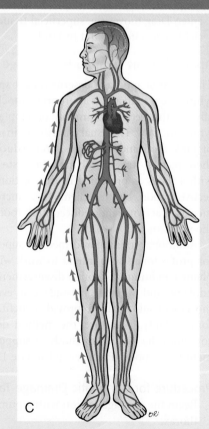

A, Direction of strokes for facilitating lymphatic flow.

B, Direction of compression over arteries to increase arterial flow.

C, Direction of gliding strokes to facilitate venous flow.

1. Compression is applied over the main arteries, beginning close to the heart (proximal) and moving systematically toward the tips of the fingers or toes (distal).
2. The manipulations are applied with a pumping action at a rhythm of approximately 60 beats per minute, or at a rhythm that matches the client's resting heart rate.
3. Compressive force changes the internal pressure in the arteries, stimulates the intrinsic contraction of arteries, and encourages the movement of blood out to the distal areas of the body.
4. Compression also begins to empty venous vessels and forms an arteriovenous pressure gradient, encouraging arterial blood flow.
5. Rhythmic, gentle contraction and relaxation of the muscles powerfully encourage arterial blood flow. Both active and passive joint movements support the transport of arterial blood.
6. The squeezing action of compression and kneading helps empty the capillary beds, allowing them to refill with arterial blood, and also supports venous return.

After compression, the next step is to assist venous return flow. This process is similar to lymphatic massage in that a combination of short and long gliding strokes is used in conjunction with movement. The difference is that lymphatic

PROFICIENCY EXERCISE 12-3

1. Hook up a hose to a faucet and barely turn on the water; this simulates the heart pump. Use compression to facilitate the movement, or "circulation," of the water in the hose.
2. Obtain a 3-foot piece of clear, soft plastic tubing. As if sucking on a straw, draw up a small amount of water into the tubing. Massage the water to the other end of the tube; this is similar to venous return massage.

massage is done over the entire body and the movements usually are passive (Proficiency Exercise 12-3).

1. With venous return flow massage, the gliding strokes move distal to proximal (from the fingers and toes to the heart) over the major veins, and the strokes actually slide somewhat like a squeegee washing a window.
2. The gliding stroke is short, only about 3 inches long; this enables the blood to move from valve to valve.
3. Long gliding strokes carry the blood through the entire vein. Both passive and active joint movements encourage venous circulation.
4. Placing the limb or other area above the heart brings gravity into assistance.

See the fluid movement protocols for a visual demonstration of these methods.

FLUID MOVEMENT PROTOCOL: LYMPHATIC DRAINAGE AND VENOUS RETURN

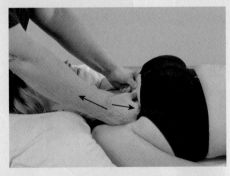

1. Pumping the thorax to support lymph drainage.

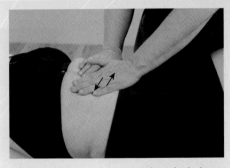

2. Pumping the abdomen to support lymph drainage.

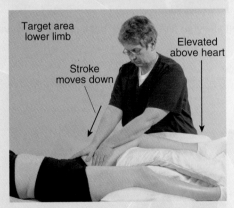

Target area lower limb

Elevated above heart

Stroke moves down

3. Elevate the area to be drained above the heart to support both lymph and venous flow. Begin close to the torso.

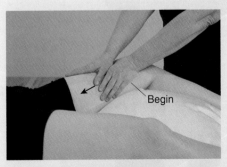

Begin

4. For specific focus on lymphatics, do not let the hands slip on the skin while moving tissue into and out of bind.

Continued

LYMPHATIC DRAINAGE AND VENOUS RETURN—cont'd

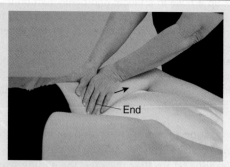

5. Do not let the hands slip on the skin as each area is moved into and out of bind.

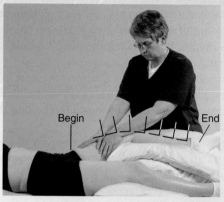

6. Move tissue into and out of bind as you travel slowly down the area.

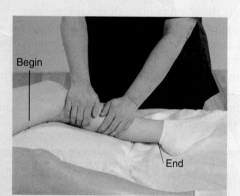

7. Knead tissue.

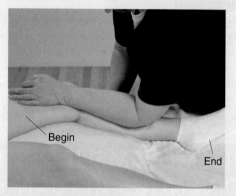

8. Compress tissue.

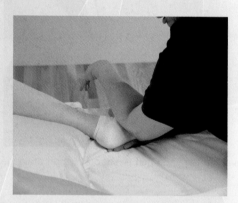

9. Compress the plexus in the foot.

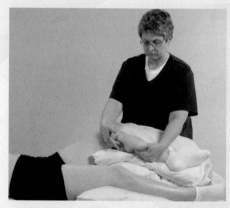

10. When shaking, flip the tissue back and forth rhythmically.

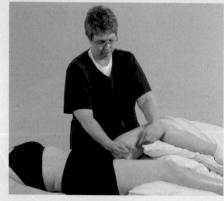

11. Move up the area being drained and flip the entire area rhythmically.

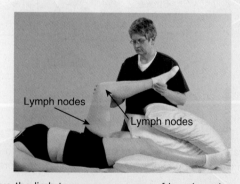

12. Move the limb to compress areas of lymph nodes.

LYMPHATIC DRAINAGE AND VENOUS RETURN—cont'd

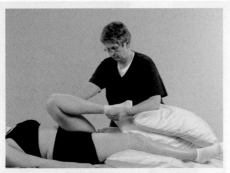

13. Move rhythmically back and forth to create a pumping action on the lymph nodes.

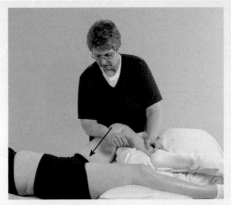

14. Reposition for venous return. Glide over veins moving distal to proximal with broad-based compression.

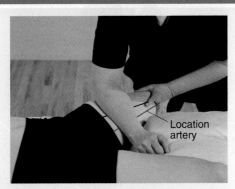

15. Repeat gliding.

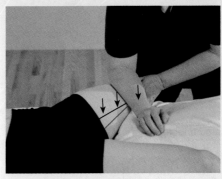

16. Repeat sequence.

FLUID MOVEMENT PROTOCOL: ARTERIAL CIRCULATION

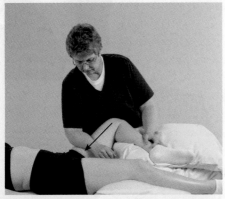

Location artery

1. To support arterial circulation begin with the area positioned below the heart. Focus compression over the arteries.

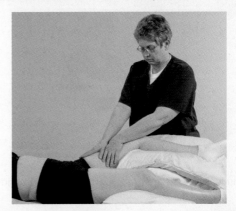

2. Move the compression down (away) from the heart at about 1 compression per second.

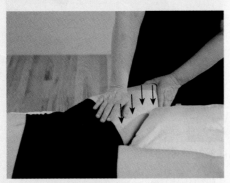

3. Repeat.

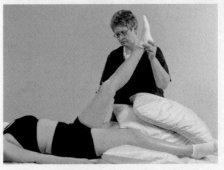

4. Move area and reposition for lymphatic drainage and venous return.

FLUID MOVEMENT PROTOCOL: INTEGRATED SEQUENCE

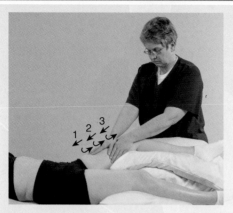

1. Begin lymphatic drainage.

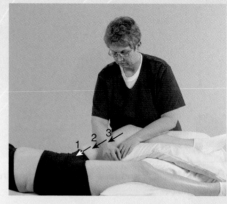

2. Switch to venous return.

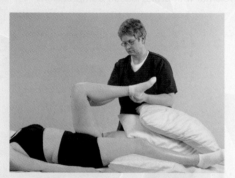

3. Rhythmically move area to support both lymph and venous flow.

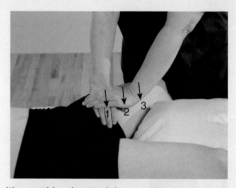

4. Reposition and begin arterial support.

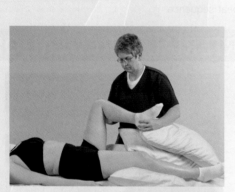

5. Move area again and reposition.

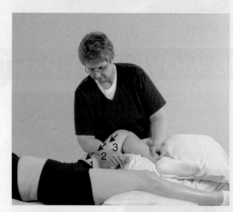

6. Target venous flow again.

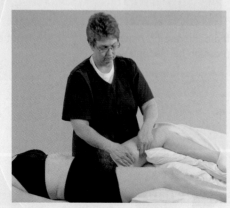

7. Shake tissue.

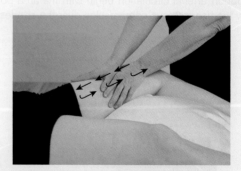

8. Resume lymphatic drainage.

12-3

CONNECTIVE TISSUE APPROACHES

SECTION OBJECTIVES

Chapter objectives covered in this section:

6. Modify massage application to target the connective tissues of the body. *Using the information presented in this section, the student will be able to perform the following:*

- Modify massage methods to address the connective tissue specifically
- Explain the principles of deep transverse friction massage

Methods that affect the connective tissue of the body have been discussed throughout the text, and research has supported the benefits of connective tissue massage. Connective tissue techniques use manually guided forces in numerous strain directions to treat injuries and somatic dysfunctions. Connective tissue bodywork systems range from the very subtle, light work of some systems of myofascial release to the very mechanical, deep transverse frictioning developed by Dr. James Cyriax.

This section provides introductory information about deep transverse friction and myofascial approaches. Refer to Chapters 5 and 6 for research information and indications and contraindications, and Chapter 10 to review the information on how mechanical forces created by massage affect connective tissue.

Review of Fascia Research

Recall from Chapter 5 that neuromuscular therapy is a combination of connective tissue methods that target the superficial and deep fascia (a type of connective tissue). The formation of myofascial trigger points is related to microtrauma and/or localized circulatory issues resulting in a localized acidic environment that irritates the nerve endings.

The basic connective tissue approach consists of influencing the tissue by introducing various mechanical forces that result in pressure, pulling, movement, and stretch on the tissues.

We would expect massage to make tissue softer or pliable, yet studies indicate otherwise. To understand this, you must understand the properties of elasticity and stiffness. *Elasticity* is the property by which an object changes shape when a force is applied but returns to its original shape when the force is removed. *Stiffness* is the degree to which an elastic material stretches when a force is applied. Think about bending a piece of wire. The stiffer it is, the harder it is to bend.

The two basic types of fiber in connective tissue are collagen and elastin. The ropelike collagen fibers give tissues and organs the rigidity needed for function. Collagen is stiff. Elastin gives elasticity to tissues and functions in partnership with collagen. Collagen provides rigidity. Elastin is the protein that allows the connective tissues to stretch and then recoil to their original positions. The elastin chain cannot be pulled too far during connective tissue work, because the companion stiff collagen fibers in the connective tissue limit the stretching of the elastin fibers (Box 12-6) (Zorn, 2007).

The fascia has contractile cells, which respond to the application of mechanical force, and smooth muscle cells, which

---

Box 12-6 Tissue Responses to Massage

When a mechanical force (e.g., massage) is applied to the body, three tissue responses can occur:

- The tissue can break. This happens in tissue injuries such as a sprain or when the intent of the massage is to separate tissue adhesions.
- The tissue can plastically deform and remain in its new shape. This happens in lax ligament syndrome, in which the ligaments have been overstretched. The massage practitioner may attempt to permanently change the shape of short tissues, such as a scar.
- The tissue can behave elastically (as does a rubber band or bungee cord), changing shape and then returning to its original shape. This is normal behavior in most fascial types, including bone, which is more elastic than it appears.

A combination of these responses also is possible.

---

are controlled by the autonomic nervous system. The fascial tonus (tone) may be influenced and regulated by the state of the autonomic nervous system. Any intervention targeting the fascia also is an intervention on the autonomic system and vice versa (Schleip, 1998). The smooth muscle cell contraction most likely is controlled by the sympathetic aspect of the autonomic nervous system, but confirming research is sparse. If the sympathetic nervous system is the regulator, then that activation would increase the overall fascial tension (Klingler et al., 2004). For example, imagine you are in clothing that is one size too small. Sympathetic activations are perceived as stressed. Might a massage that reduces the fight-or-flight response (sympathetic dominance) and supports relaxation (parasympathetic dominance) be like getting out of those too-tight clothes and getting into loose, soft pajamas?

Fascial responsiveness to massage cannot be explained by its mechanical properties alone. Earlier we discussed how myofascial trigger points and traditional acupuncture points are in the same location. Microscopic study has shown that in many places in the fascia, a vein, an artery, and a nerve perforate (poke through) it. Called *neurovascular bundles,* these points are in the same location as most of the trigger points and acupuncture points.

In addition, connective tissue may function as a whole body communication system. The loose connective tissue type (think spider web) has a language of tiny tugs and pulls that communicates mechanical messages throughout the body because of the principle of tensegrity (Langevin, 2006).

The common location of the neurovascular bundles, myofascial trigger points, and places where the fascial fibers interconnect may explain how dysfunction in these focal points can cause body-wide disturbance. Massage application that normalizes these areas may result in a normalizing body-wide response. The entire concept of myofascial release remains somewhat of a mystery (Remvig et al., 2008).

When tissue is strained unequally (think a snag in the fibers of a sweater), human fibroblasts respond with increased secretion of proinflammatory chemicals, resulting in increased cell proliferation, distinct changes in cellular structure, and a delayed inflammatory response. For example, delayed-onset muscle soreness may take up to 3 days to manifest and is associated with inflammation and cytokine induction, among other possible causes. The inflammatory response triggers abnormal collagen secretion and may lead to fibrosis, reducing the tissue's elasticity and ability to slide.

Both direct and indirect connective tissue methods have been shown to reverse the inflammatory effects in cells that have been strained repetitively. A direct technique moves the restricted tissue into the barrier caused by binding. An indirect technique moves the tissue away from the restrictive barrier to a point of ease. Changing the strain pattern in cells (indirect, away from the bind or direct, toward the bind) may result in improvement in symptoms. It may take only 60 seconds for changes to occur (Meltzer and Standley, 2007; Standley and Meltzer, 2008).

Connective Tissue Dysfunctions

People can develop several basic connective tissue dysfunctions. Connective tissue may shorten, lose fluidity, and adhere, causing binding, pulling, and restricted movement. Another common problem is overstretched connective tissue at the joint, resulting in laxity and destabilization of the joint. This sets the stage for protective muscle spasms, which reduce joint space.

Normalization of connective tissue may allow the joint to function properly; however, this process may become problematic. One important function of the connective tissue is to stabilize; stabilization may require that the joint remain out of optimum alignment. As explained by Dr. David Gurevich, a Russian physician, the pattern of degeneration usually begins with dystonia, or disruption of motor tone. (Sometimes direct trauma to a joint may cause misalignment, rather than increased or decreased muscle tension pulling joints out of alignment.) Bones are designed to fit at the joint in a specific way. When this fit is disrupted, the next step is a protective muscle spasm, followed by connective tissue reorganization to stabilize the area. Areas of disruption in joint play or joint alignment eventually include a connective tissue component in the dysfunction (Kreighbaum and Barthels, 1995).

Treatment of Dysfunctions

Gurevich taught that the treatment sequence is first massage, including connective tissue approaches; then mobilization (movement of jointed areas within a comfortable range of motion); and finally joint manipulation. Massage and mobilization are within the scope of bodywork practice, whereas joint manipulation is not. The services of a chiropractor, osteopath, or other professional trained in joint manipulation are needed for problems that require direct manipulation of the joint.

Professional experience suggests that the longer the problem has existed, the more mechanical the techniques required initially. Mechanical techniques include all gliding, kneading, skin rolling, and compression styles of bodywork, as long as the contact slowly elongates and drags or pulls on the tissue for sustained periods. The connective tissue responds relatively slowly, sometimes taking 30 seconds. Conversely, neuromuscular techniques usually elicit a response in 15 seconds.

The stretching, pulling, or pressure on the connective tissue is a little different from that of neuromuscular methods. Neuromuscular techniques usually flow in the direction of the fibers to affect the proprioceptive mechanism and create a quick response. Connective tissue approaches are slow and involve deliberate drag, usually against or across the fibers. Connective tissue stretching is elongated or telescoped at the point of the bind (Chaitow, 1988b, 1991, 1992, 1993). In chronic conditions, it is important to induce a small inflammatory response in the dysfunctional area. This process initiates the reorganization of tissue by stimulating tissue repair mechanisms (Chaitow and Delany, 2000; Lederman, 2005).

Controlled Injury Healing

Another of the body's responses to inflammation is the generation of healing potentials through controlled injury. Injured tissue produces a current known as the *current of injury*. First detected by Galvani in 1797, this current can encourage healing processes for days until the miniature wound heals (Gunn, 1992).

Studies also have shown that on the microscopic level, imperfections in acupuncture needles literally snag the filaments found in fascia, meaning that acupuncture can be considered a type of connective tissue method, at least microscopically (Langevin et al., 2004; Dorsher, 2006; Dorsher and Fleckenstein, 2008). In acupuncture the insertion of a needle into a muscle generates a burst of electrical discharges, which can cause a shortened or hypertonic muscle to relax instantly or within minutes.

Deep Transverse Frictioning

The most specific localized example of connective tissue work is Cyriax's cross-fiber frictioning method, or **deep transverse frictioning**. This method is especially effective around joints, where the tendons and ligaments become bound. Deep transverse frictioning is always a specific rehabilitation intervention; it introduces therapeutic inflammation through the creation of a specific and controlled reinjury of the tissues. Cyriax asserts that the essential component of a transverse friction massage is the application of concentrated therapeutic movement over a very small area. The key element is the use of friction to move the tissue against its grain. In Cyriax's words:

> During treatment by deep friction, great precision in seating (positioning) of the patient and of the physiotherapist's hand is essential; throughout the session the physiotherapist keeps her mind on her fingertip. This type of work involves much more concentration and care than most of the physiotherapist's other work. Nothing about it is routine; each patient and each lesion must be assessed and given expert and individual attention (Cyriax and Coldham, 1984).

Although mastery of this type of deep transverse friction is beyond the scope of the technical development of this textbook, it is a valuable form of rehabilitative massage. Any massage practitioner working in a medical or sports setting should be trained in the techniques. The additional skills

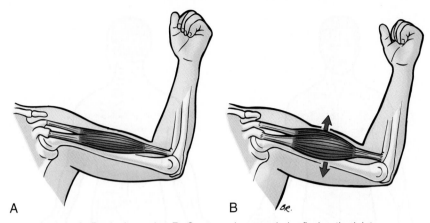

FIGURE 12-9 Broadening contraction. **A,** Beginning point. **B,** Contract the muscle by flexing the joint.

required are not so much in the delivery of the methods, which are fairly straightforward, but in the assessment of where to friction and how to incorporate it into a comprehensive rehabilitation plan. Specific anatomic knowledge is required for the precision of which Cyriax speaks.

The frictioning can last as long as 15 minutes to create the controlled reinjury of the tissue, which introduces a small amount of inflammation and traumatic hyperemia to the area. The result is the restructuring of the connective tissue, increased circulation to the area, and temporary analgesia (Cyriax and Coldham, 1984).

Proper rehabilitation after the massage is essential for the friction technique to be effective and to produce a mobile scar on rehealing of the tissue. The frictioned area must be contracted painlessly, without any strain put on the frictioned tissue. This is done by fixing the joint in a position in which the muscle is relaxed and then having the client contract the muscle as far as it will go. This is sometimes called a *broadening contraction* (Figure 12-9).

As Cyriax has said:

> Deep transverse friction restores mobility to muscle in the same way as manipulation frees a joint. Indeed, the action of deep transverse friction may be summed up as affording a mobilization that passive stretching or active exercises cannot achieve. After the friction has restored a full range of painless broadening to the muscle belly, this added mobility must be maintained. To this end, the patient should perform a series of active contractions with the joint placed in a position that fully relaxes the affected muscle, that is, the position that allows the greatest broadening. Strong resisted movement should be avoided until the scar has consolidated itself; otherwise, started too soon, [such movements] tend to strain the healing breach again (Cyriax and Coldham, 1984).

Methods of Deep Transverse Frictioning

Cyriax teaches that when massage is given to a muscle, tendon, ligament, or joint capsule, the following principles must be observed (Figure 12-10):

1. The right spot must be found.
2. The therapist's fingers and the client's skin must move as one. Care must be taken not to cause a blister. The client must understand that deep friction massage to a tender point can be painful.

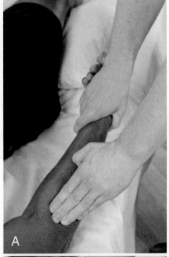
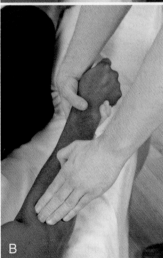

FIGURE 12-10 A and **B,** Friction/compression with movement.

3. The friction must be given across the fibers composing the affected structure.
4. The friction must be given with sufficient sweep. Pressure only accesses the tender area; it does not replace the friction. Circular friction is not recommended. Only a back-and-forth friction is effective.
5. The friction must reach deep enough. If it does not reach the lesion, it is of no value.

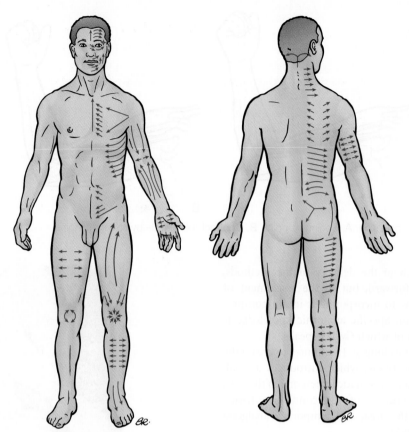

FIGURE 12-11 Application of connective tissue massage, modified from Bindegewebmassage. This system primarily introduced the mechanical forces of tension, bend, shear, and torsion into the soft tissues. The arrows indicate the direction of the massage application to most efficiently target connective tissue structures.

6. The client must be placed in a suitable position that ensures the appropriate degree of tension or relaxation of the tissues to be frictioned.

7. Muscles must be kept relaxed while being frictioned. Because the connective tissue of the muscle is affected, the massage must penetrate into the muscle and not stay on the surface.

8. Tendons with a sheath must be kept taut during friction massage.

9. Broadening contractions are used between sessions to promote circulation and mobile scar development during the healing process.

Using Cyriax's principles, this textbook introduces a modified version of these methods that can be incorporated into a general massage session for small areas of adhered tissue. The modified version of deep transverse friction does not have the same effects on an area of adhesion, but the ability to move the tissue in a transverse way may keep the development of adhesions in check when a person develops minor soft tissue tears from overstretching or minor muscle pulls.

To accommodate the lack of precise location of the anatomic structures, the friction suggested is done over a broader area for a shorter time, using the following procedure:

1. Locate the area to be frictioned.
2. Place the muscle in a relaxed position.
3. Provide friction as described in Chapter 10.

Myofascial Approaches

Other forms of connective tissue massage also can be used. *Bindegewebmassage*, developed by Elizabeth Dickie, consists of light strokes without oil that focus on the superficial fascial layer (between the skin and muscles). The method involves movement of the superficial fascial layer in a specific pattern related to the neurologic dermatome distribution. The results are both neurochemical and mechanical. The depth of pressure is sufficient to move the superficial fascia on top of the muscle layer (Figure 12-11).

Rolfing, developed by Ida Rolf, and its various offshoots, such as Hellerwork, are methods of structural integration focused to bring the physical structure of the body into an efficient relationship with the perpendicular alignment of the body in gravity. The focus is normalization and redirection of the deeper fascial components of muscles and fascial sheaths. Osteopathy and physical therapy theory and practice contribute to the body of knowledge for **myofascial approaches.**

These styles of bodywork are often called *soft tissue manipulation* or *myofascial release*. The procedures described in this textbook are only part of these systems, and additional training is required to learn these valuable methods in more detail.

Nature of the Fascia

Fascia in some form surrounds and separates almost every structure and cell in the body. It forms the *interstitial space* (the space between individual cells). Fascia is involved in structural and visceral support and in separation and protection; it therefore influences respiration, elimination, metabolism, fluid flow, and the immune system. Fascia is stress responsive; it becomes stiffer in response to real or perceived threats and any other activation of the sympathetic autonomic nervous system. This response is sometimes called *body armoring*, which is a factor in the relationship between body and emotional expression. Body armoring also is often a component of body/mind approaches.

Because the body is a tensegrity structure, an injury at any given site often begins as long-term strain in other parts of the body. The injury manifests where it does because of inherent weakness or previous injury, not purely and always because of local strain or a direct impact. Discovering these points of tension and easing chronic strain in the body become a natural part of restoring balance in the structure and tend to prevent future injuries (Myers, 2008).

Transmission of tension through a tensegrity array provides a way to distribute forces to all interconnected elements and at the same time to tune the entire system mechanically as one. Creating a balance across the bones, myofascial component and, further, across the entire fascial net could have profound implications for health, both cellular and general. The goal for massage is to support balance in the myofascial systems (Myers, 2008).

Location of the Fascia

Anatomically, fascia can be classified as superficial (subcutaneous) fascia or deep fascia; however, it really is one interconnected structure. Superficial fascia lies between the skin and the muscles. Deep fascia surrounding the muscles weaves diagonally through the body, creating fascial sheaths. Subserous fascia lies between the deep fascia and the membranes lining the body cavities. A deep level of fascia interconnects the cranium, spine, and sacrum, joining the connective tissue coverings of the central nervous system with the unity of the body. The body also has three or four transverse fascial planes. These are located in the cranial base, cervical thoracic area, diaphragm, and lumbar and pelvic floor areas. Transverse planes also exist for joints.

These classifications of fascial layering are artificial, because as previously described, the tensegrity of fascia composes one large, interconnected, three-dimensional microscopic dynamic grid structure that connects everything with everything. Through the fascial system, if you pull on the little toe, you affect the nose, and if the structure of the nose is dysfunctional, it can pull anywhere in the body, including the little toe.

Although fascia generally orients itself vertically in the body, it orients in any directional stress pattern. For example, scar tissue may redirect fascial structures, as can trauma, repetitive strain patterns, and immobility. This redirection of structural forces occurs as a result of compensation patterns. During physical assessment, the body appears "pulled" out of symmetry or stuck.

Myofascial Dysfunction

Dysfunction in the fascial network compromises the efficiency of the body, requiring an increase in energy expenditure to achieve functioning ability. Fatigue and pain often result. Fascial shortening and thickening restrict movement, and the easy undulation of the expression of body rhythms and entrainment mechanisms is disturbed. Twists and torsions of the fascia bind and restrict movement from the cellular level outward to affect joint mobility. This bind can be likened to ill-fitting clothing or, more graphically, "fascial wedgies." The dysfunctions are difficult to diagnose medically, are not apparent with standard medical testing, and are a factor in many elusive chronic pain and fatigue patterns. Adhesions result when fascia attempts to stabilize itself by attaching to surrounding tissue. Stabilizing formations can orient in any direction. Breakdown of the fascial system is a primary factor in the aging process.

Fascial dysfunction is seldom simple and almost always multidimensional, often encompassing body and emotional phenomena, because body armoring is an effective coping strategy. As explained in Chapter 6, introducing corrective intervention is a therapeutic change process akin to remodeling a house. If the person is unable to respond effectively to a change process, management approaches can be offered, but the result is more symptom management than structural change.

The methods themselves are deceptively simple in relation to the degree of change that can be experienced. Therefore a solid respect for myofascial approaches is in order. Use them wisely after considering the broader picture of the client's state of being and ability to cope with active change.

Myofascial Massage Methods

In most cases a lubricant is not used with myofascial approaches, because the drag quality on the tissue is necessary to produce results, and lubricant reduces drag.

Methods that affect primarily the ground substance require a quality of slow, sustained pressure and agitation. Most massage methods can soften the ground substance as long as the application is not abrupt. Tapotement/percussion and abrupt compression are less effective than slow gliding methods that have a drag quality. Kneading and skin rolling that incorporate a slow pulling action also are effective. The appropriate application introduces one or a combination of the mechanical forces of tension, compression, bend, shear, and torsion to achieve results.

The fiber component is affected by stretching methods that elongate the fibers past the normal give of the fiber and enter the plastic range past the bind. This creates either a freeing and unraveling of fibers or a small therapeutic (beneficial and controlled) inflammatory response that signals for change in the fibers. The important consideration for all connective tissue massage methods is that the pressure exerted vertically and horizontally must actually move the tissue to create tension, torsion, shear, or bend forces; in addition, these forces must alter the ground substance long enough for energy to

💡 PROFICIENCY EXERCISE 12-4

1. Make some gelatin using only half the specified amount of water. Let it set. Massage it into liquid form. Pay attention to the type of massage you use.
2. Twist and wad some plastic wrap into a ball. Then smooth it out. What methods did you need to use?
3. Take the same plastic wrap and pull it. Take out all the slack and telescope and elongate the tissue. What did you have to do to accomplish the stretch?

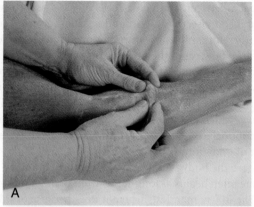

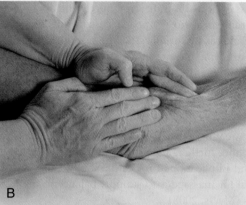

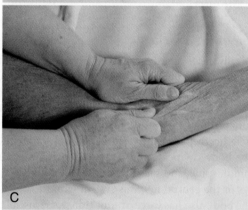

FIGURE 12-12 Using connective tissue methods to increase the pliability of scar tissue. **A,** Application of bending force to lift scar tissue. **B,** Application of shear force. **C,** Application of tension force.

build up, soften the ground substance, and influence the smooth muscle bundles. Research has shown that this process occurs in 10 to 30 seconds, and any change that will occur happens within that time frame (Findley, 2009).

The development of connective tissue patterns is highly individualized; therefore, systems that follow a precise protocol and sequence often are less effective for dealing with these complex patterns (Box 12-7 and Figure 12-12) (Proficiency Exercise 12-4).

Tissue Movement Methods Specific for the Superficial Fascia

To apply the more subtle connective tissue approaches, the practitioner must develop the skill to follow tissue movement under the skin.

1. Make firm but gentle contact with the skin.
2. Increase the downward (vertical) pressure slowly until resistance is felt (bind); this barrier is soft and subtle.
3. Maintain the downward pressure at this point; now, add horizontal pressure until the resistance barrier (bind) is felt again.
4. Sustain the horizontal pressure and wait.
5. The tissue will seem to creep, unravel, melt, slide, quiver, twist, or dip, or some other movement sensation will be apparent.
6. Follow the movement; stay at bind.
7. Slowly and gently release first the horizontal force and then the vertical force.

Following tissue movement becomes simple once the practitioner stops thinking about the process and begins to experience it. A curious result of this type of work is the development of vasomotor responses on parts of the skin not directly addressed during the fascial tissue movement method. One theory suggests that these are areas with internal fascial connections that were pulled during the method. To continue the process, introduce vertical pressure over the vasomotor reddening and begin again.

Fascial Restriction Method

Fascial restriction involves an area larger than a small, localized spot. A restricted area is palpated as a barrier or an area of immobility (bind) within the tissue. The area is worked initially using routine massage techniques; if it does not soften, the pressure must be more specific.

1. Stabilize the tissue with one hand.
2. With the fingers of the other hand, pull the tissue in the direction of the restriction.
3. Use the heel of the hand or the arm to separate the tissue.
4. Maintain the pressure until a softening occurs.

Twist-and-release kneading and compression applied in the direction of the restriction also can release these fascial barriers. See the connective tissue/myofascial protocol for a demonstration.

CONNECTIVE TISSUE PROTOCOL

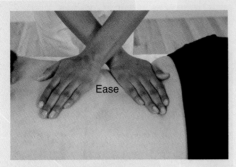

1. Place crossed hands over tissue and meld hands to the skin.

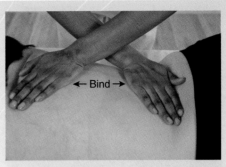

2. Separate hands moving tissue to and just into bind. Do not slip.

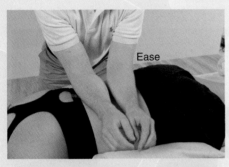

3. Forearms can be used. Place on the tissue and meld to it.

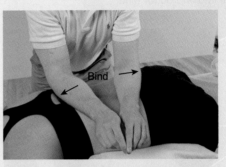

4. Separate arms moving tissue to and just into bind.

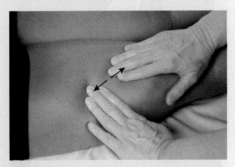

5. Small areas of tissue can be stretched by placing the short tissue between the fingers of both hands, and then without slipping separate tissues into the bind.

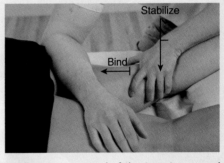

6. Stabilize tissue at one end of the target area and hold fast. Then slowly glide, with drag maintaining tension on the tissues at all times.

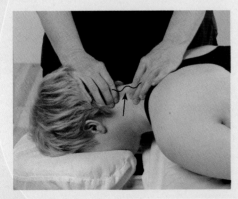

7. Use shear forces to move tissue in and out of bind.

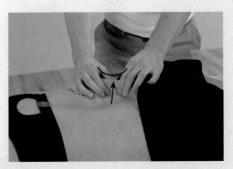

8. Use bending force to move tissue into bind (skin rolling).

Continued

CONNECTIVE TISSUE PROTOCOL—cont'd

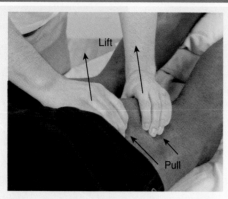

9. Grasp, lift, and pull to create combined loading to move tissue into and out of bind.

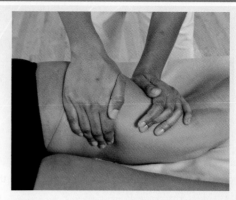

10. Use torsion force to twist tissue into and out of bind.

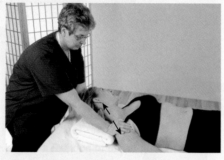

11. Stretching methods take tissue into bind. Hold at the ends of the area to be stretched and move away to create tension force.

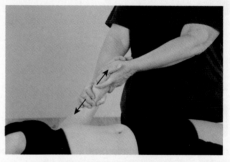

12. Traction applies tension force to the tissues surrounding a joint. Grasp firmly above and below the joint and move hands apart to create tension force into bind.

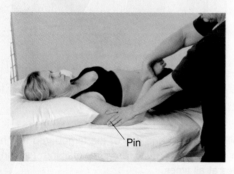

13. Pin and stretch variation. Move target tissue from ease position toward bind and hold in place.

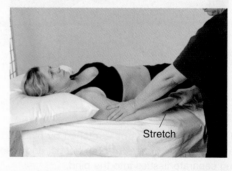

14. As the target tissue is held fixed, move the joint area to create the tension force into the bind.

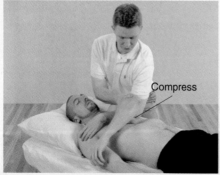

15. Active release variation. Compress target tissue while in ease and then move from ease to bind position.

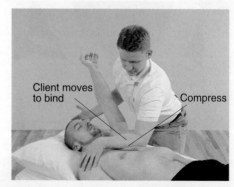

16. Client moves the jointed area away while the tissue is fixed to create the tension force to move tissues into bind.

TRIGGER POINT TREATMENT APPROACHES

SECTION OBJECTIVES

Chapter objectives covered in this section:

7. Identify and properly use massage to address trigger points.

Using the information presented in this section, the student will be able to perform the following:

- Describe a trigger point
- Locate a trigger point
- Use two methods to massage a trigger point
- Implement connective tissue approaches and trigger point treatment methods as part of a larger, neuromuscular therapy system

Some confusion exists about the synonymous use of the terms *neuromuscular therapy* and *trigger point therapy.* Neuromuscular therapy is an umbrella term that encompasses a variety of treatment approaches, many of which can be used for addressing trigger points. As with most of the methods discussed in this chapter, massage therapists require additional training to use trigger point methods specifically and efficiently. However, in general massage applications, the practitioner can deal with mild trigger point activity effectively by using the methods discussed in this section.

A trigger point is a condition, not a method. Many different methods can be used to address trigger point–related dysfunction and pain. Hydrotherapy, acupuncture, therapeutic exercise, massage, and nutrition are just a few possibilities. It is important to understand that with any altered physiology, such as the development of trigger points or connective tissue changes, these adaptive responses may constitute resourceful compensation and should *not* be changed. Knowing when to apply massage specifically and when *not* to is the hallmark of a professional. It is simple to find points on the body that are painful when pressed and then press on them. The individual may even feel better after the intervention; however, feeling better and being better are not the same thing. Assessment using the general massage approach as a sequence for palpation and joint movement is performed to identify potential tender points. Clinical reasoning skills then are used to determine what these points are and what should be done.

Myofascial pain symptoms usually involve muscle pain with specific "trigger" or "tender" points. Many experts in the field recognize the ubiquity of this condition. However, if you put all the experts on trigger points in a room and asked them if they truly know what causes trigger points, they would honestly have to say no.

Central sensitization can be defined simply as an increased sensitivity to stimulation resulting in a hypersensitive central nervous system (CNS) response. The stimulation does not need to be strong enough to cause pain, but it is processed as pain. Sometimes after an injury, a typically painless stimulation may recruit activity in these same central neurons, and the CNS thinks it is experiencing pain. This is actually a form of learned behavior, but it is not conscious behavior. The person with pain related to central sensitization is experiencing real pain, but the pain is no longer related to tissue damage. If this is one of the mechanisms of trigger point pain, then just pushing on these points actually may reinforce the pathway. On the other hand, pressure on the point may reset the abnormal sensitivity back to normal. The question you may be asking as you read is, "So do you apply compression to trigger points or not?" The answer is, "It depends. Sometimes yes and sometimes no."

Researchers have found concentrations of immune system histochemicals in the trigger point locations. These chemicals, sometimes called *proinflammatory mediators,* are related to inflammation and pain. They create an acidic fluid around the trigger point location that acts as an irritant, causing localized pain not caused by muscle tissue damage (Simons, 2008). Localized shortening of tissue in the area (taut band) seems to occur, which in turn can reduce circulation to the area, either causing the problem or perpetuating it (Dorsher, 2006, 2009; Simons, 2008; Shah et al., 2008).

All this information can become confusing. However, it is important that ethical massage professionals provide massage care from an informed position and use current evidence to support and explain their work.

Dr. Janet Travell did extensive research on myofascial pain involving trigger points and was considered the foremost authority in this area (Travell and Simons, 1999). Although some of her early research now is considered obsolete, most of her findings remain relevant. The work of Dr. Leon Chaitow has provided additional information about trigger point therapy (Chaitow 1988a, 1988b, 1991, 1992, 1993; Chaitow and Delany, 2002). These two experts are the resources for the information in this section about trigger point therapy.

Definition of a Trigger Point

A trigger point is an area of local nerve facilitation of a muscle that is aggravated by stress of any sort that affects the body or mind. The most current theory of what causes trigger points to form involves an interaction of calcium and adenosine triphosphate (ATP) on muscles that have been stressed in some way. This causes the muscles to shorten in a localized area, producing a taut band and a nodule of sorts. The taut band/nodule generates considerable localized and uncontrolled metabolic activity in the area and a localized acidic fluid environment, which makes the nerve endings hyperirritable; the result is pain. As this process persists, the ongoing inflammation in the area can cause connective tissue changes, and the tiny microfilaments in the muscles start to stick together (adhesions) (Gerwin, 2008; Shah et al., 2008).

A good, simple definition of trigger points is small areas of hyperirritability within muscles (Box 12-8). If these areas are located near motor nerve points, the person may experience referred pain caused by nerve stimulation. The area of the trigger point often is the motor point where nerve stimulation initiates a contraction in a small, sensitive bundle of muscle fibers that in turn activates the entire muscle (Travell and Simons, 1999; Chaitow and Delany, 2002).

A trigger point area often is located in a tight band of muscle fibers. Palpation across the band may elicit a twitch response, which is a slight jump in the muscle fibers. This is difficult to detect when the trigger point is in the deeper muscle layers.

Box 12-8	Theory of Trigger Point Formation

The following progression has been proposed to explain the formation of trigger points.

1. Dysfunctional endplate activity occurs, commonly associated with a strain, overuse, or direct trauma.
2. Stored calcium is released at the site as a result of overuse or of tearing of the sarcoplasmic reticulum.
3. Acetylcholine (Ach) is released excessively at the synapse because of calcium-charged gates.
4. High calcium levels at the site keep the calcium-charged gates open, and the release of Ach continues.
5. Ischemia develops in the area, resulting in an oxygen and nutrient deficit.
6. A local energy crisis develops.
7. Because adenosine triphosphate (ATP) is no longer available, the tissue is unable to remove the calcium ions, and Ach continues flowing.
8. Removal of the superfluous calcium requires more energy than sustaining a contracture; therefore, the contracture remains.
9. The contracture is sustained not by action potentials from the spinal cord but by the chemistry at the innervation site.
10. The actin/myosin filaments slide to a fully shortened position (a weakened state) in the immediate area around the motor endplate (at the center of the fiber).
11. As the sarcomeres shorten, a contracture knot forms.
12. The contracture knot is the "nodule," a palpable characteristic of a trigger point.
13. The remainder of the sarcomeres of that fiber are stretched, creating the usually palpable taut band that also is a common trigger point characteristic.
14. Attachment trigger points may develop at the attachment sites of these shortened tissues (periosteal, myotendinous) where muscular tension provokes inflammation.

Modified from Chaitow L, Delany J: *Clinical application of neuromuscular techniques,* vol 1, *The upper body,* London, 2002, Churchill Livingstone.

Box 12-9	Palpation for Trigger Points

In performing light palpation, the therapist may notice trigger points from the following responses.

Skin changes: The skin may feel tense and show resistance to gliding strokes. It may be slightly damp as a result of perspiration from sympathetic facilitation, causing the therapist's hand to stick or drag.

Temperature changes: The temperature in a local area increases with acute dysfunction but decreases with ischemia, which indicates fibrotic changes in the tissues.

Edema: Edema is an impression of fullness and congestion in the tissues. With chronic dysfunction, edema gradually is replaced by fibrotic (connective tissue) changes.

Deep palpation: During deep palpation, the therapist establishes contact with the deeper fibers of the soft tissues and explores them for any of the following:

- Immobility
- Tenderness
- Edema
- Deep muscle tension
- Fibrotic changes
- Interosseous changes

Mechanical perpetuating factors include the following:
- Standing postural distortion
- Seated postural distortion
- Gait distortion
- Immobilization
- Vocational stress
- Restrictive or ill-fitting clothing and shoes
- Furniture

Systemic perpetuating factors include the following:
- Enzyme dysfunction
- Metabolic and endocrine dysfunction
- Chronic infection
- Dietary insufficiencies
- Psychological stress

Assessment for Trigger Points

Determining whether a tender spot is really a trigger point, a point of fascial adhesion requiring friction, a motor point, or some other irritable reflex point, including any active acupuncture points, can be difficult. However, stretching of trigger point areas is essential to effective treatment; therefore, if doubt exists about the nature of the point, it should be treated as a trigger point.

The massage therapist usually finds trigger points during palpation or general massage using both light and deep palpation consisting of gliding strokes (Box 12-9). Chaitow recommends that gliding strokes cover a region of 2 to 3 inches at a time.

Travell and Chaitow agree that some pain is elicited during assessment and treatment; however, the pain elicited during treatment should be well within the client's comfort zone, so that the client is aware of the trigger point but does not initiate protective mechanisms such as guarding (tightening up), breath holding, or flinching. The muscle must be relaxed to be examined effectively. If the pressure is too great, severe local

Any of the more than 400 muscles in the body can develop trigger points. The development of trigger points is accompanied by the characteristic referred pain pattern and the restriction of motion associated with myofascial pain. With classic trigger points, the referred pain pattern can be traced to its site of origin. The distribution of the referred trigger point pain does not usually follow the entire distribution of a peripheral nerve or dermatome segment (Figure 12-13) (Travell and Simons, 1999; Chaitow and Delany, 2008).

Perpetuating Factors

The development of trigger points can be perpetuated by reflexive, mechanical, and systemic factors. Reflexive perpetuating factors include the following:

- Skin sensitivity in the area of the trigger point
- Joint dysfunction
- Visceral dysfunction in the viscerally referred pain pattern
- Vasoconstriction
- A facilitated nerve segment

pain may overwhelm the referred pain sensation, making accurate evaluation impossible. Trigger points that are so active that referred pain is already produced have no need of exaggerated pressure.

Only muscles that can actually be treated at the same visit should be examined. Palpation for trigger points can aggravate their referred pain activity; therefore, only areas intended for treatment should be palpated.

Methods of Treating Trigger Points

Trigger point therapy must not be done for extended periods. Because of the nature of the syndrome and the irritation involved, 15 minutes is sufficient time to spend on trigger points. On some occasions 30 minutes of therapy can be tolerated, but this should not become a standard practice, and it should be incorporated into a more general approach, such as full-body massage.

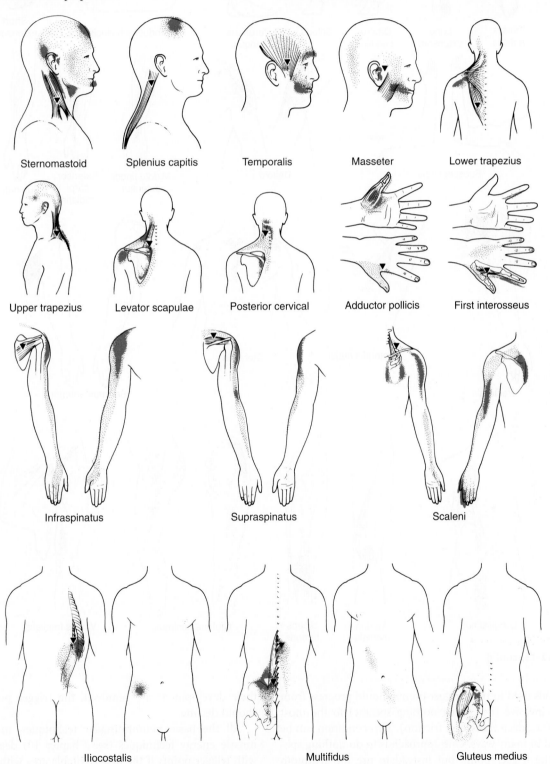

FIGURE 12-13 Common trigger points. (From Chaitow L: *Modern neuromuscular techniques,* ed 2, Edinburgh, 2003, Churchill Livingstone.)

Continued

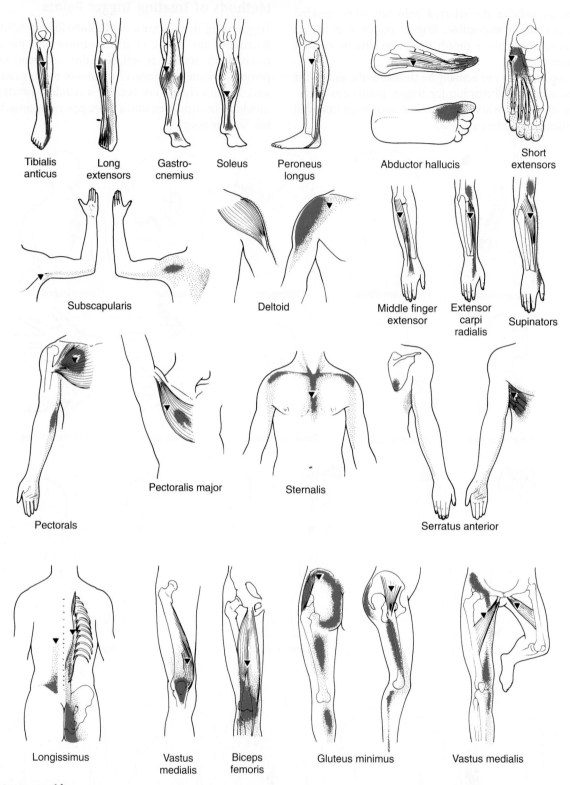

Tibialis anticus   Long extensors   Gastro-cnemius   Soleus   Peroneus longus   Abductor hallucis   Short extensors

Subscapularis   Deltoid   Middle finger extensor   Extensor carpi radialis   Supinators

Pectorals   Pectoralis major   Sternalis   Serratus anterior

Longissimus   Vastus medialis   Biceps femoris   Gluteus minimus   Vastus medialis

FIGURE 12-13, cont'd

Methods used to treat trigger points should progress from the least invasive (i.e., doing nothing specific) to the most invasive (i.e., deep transverse friction). This condition can be addressed in many ways. One approach is to do nothing specific to the trigger point, but instead to use the symptom intensity of the trigger points as preassessment and postassessment. Because trigger points are a condition, if the reasons for their development are removed, the trigger point activity should decline.

All the basic neuromuscular techniques, including the muscle energy techniques (see Chapter 10) deal effectively with trigger points if the hyperirritable area within a muscle is hyperstimulated and then lengthened, and the connective tissue in the area is softened and stretched. Travell and other professionals in the field suggest direct pressure, dry needling (acupuncture), and ice massage for trigger point areas. Direct manipulation of proprioceptors by pushing or pulling on a muscle belly or its attachments also is very effective. Positional release with the appropriate stretching is one of the most effective ways to treat trigger points.

Positional release and lengthening and direct manipulation are the least invasive and gentlest methods. The integrated muscle energy method is more aggressive than positional release or direct manipulation but less aggressive than pressure or pinching methods. These methods often are effective and are worth trying before the more intense pressure or pinching techniques.

As a reminder, positional release consists of identifying the painful point and positioning the body in the easiest position that reduces the pain at the point. Positional release is the first step in the integrated muscle energy method, which then introduces muscle contraction before lengthening (see Chapter 10).

Direct manipulation methods consist of pushing together at the belly of a muscle to affect spindle cells and pushing apart on tendons to affect tendon receptors. If the belly of the muscle is pressed together and the desired effect is not experienced, the next step should be to separate the tissue from the middle of the muscle belly toward the tendons. The local area must be lengthened. This lengthening is performed either directly on the tissues or through movement of a joint.

If the trigger point remains after the less invasive methods have been attempted, pressure techniques (i.e., inhibitory pressure) should be tried. The pressure may take the form of direct pressure, in which the trigger point is pressed by the therapist against an underlying hard structure (bone), or pinching pressure, when no bony tissue lies underneath, as in the "squeezing" of the sternocleidomastoid muscle.

Pressure techniques can end the hyperirritability by mechanical disruption of the sensory nerve endings mediating the trigger point activity. When using the direct pressure technique, the therapist must hold the compression long enough to stimulate the spindle cells.

The pressure technique must be done properly. Travell has pointed out that the client usually senses referred pain within 10 seconds of the application of pressure; therefore, the practitioner need not maintain pressure longer than 10 seconds when trying to locate the trigger.

After the trigger has been located, the time of applied pressure is different from the time used to locate the trigger. Chaitow recommends a procedure of gradually intensifying pressure, building up to 8 seconds, then repeating the process for up to 30 seconds or as long as 2 minutes. The procedure should end when the client reports that the referred pain has stopped or when the therapist feels a "release" in the trigger point tissue.

Sufficient duration is determined by the fiber construction of the muscle. Muscles are made up of red or white fibers, which can be slow twitch or fast twitch. The type of fiber that makes up a muscle is determined by whether the muscle functions as a postural (stabilizer) muscle or a phasic (mover) muscle and the demands of the client's lifestyle. Phasic muscle fibers are easier to fatigue than postural muscle fibers. After

the muscle is fatigued, a period of recovery ensues in which the fibers will not contract, and the muscle can be lengthened effectively and stretched if necessary.

Chaitow also recommends variable pressure, rather than constantly held pressure from beginning to end, to prevent further irritation of the trigger area. Students should not misinterpret this idea of variable pressure; it is not a "bouncing" in and out of the tissue, but rather a carefully changing pressure for a specific purpose. The pressure used reflects the therapist's sensitivity to what is happening as the tissue responds; the therapist applies more pressure as the tissue shows that it is relaxing and accepting more pressure. When the massage therapist senses that the tissues are becoming tense, pressure is reduced.

As an alternative, deep cross-fiber frictioning over the trigger point can be effective, followed by lengthening and stretching. This method is beneficial if the massage therapist suspects that the connective tissue around the trigger point has become immobile.

Travell recommends that after treating the trigger point with pressure methods, the practitioner again stimulate circulation to the local area with circular friction, kneading, and/or vibratory massage techniques. Localized treatment of the muscle should always end with lengthening and stretching, whether passive or active, of the affected muscle.

Travell and Chaitow agree that gradual, gentle lengthening to reset the normal resting length of the neuromuscular mechanism of a muscle and stretching to elongate shortened connective tissue of the treated (involved) muscle must follow any other interventions. Incomplete restoration of the full length of the muscle means incomplete relief of pain. Failure to lengthen and stretch the area results in the eventual return of the original symptoms. Muscle energy approaches are more effective than passive stretching in achieving the proper response. They enable the muscle to "learn" that it can now return to a fuller resting length and more complete range of motion. Trigger points in deep layers of muscle or in a muscle that is difficult to lengthen by moving the body are addressed with local bend, shear, and torsion techniques.

After treating a trigger point, the practitioner should search the target (referred) area to uncover and deal with satellite or embryonic triggers. Immediately after treatment, moist heat (a hot towel) over the region is soothing and useful. The area requires rest for a few days and avoidance of all stressful activity.

Deciding Which Trigger Points to Treat

Trigger points in the muscle belly usually are found in short, concentrically contracted muscles. Trigger points located near the attachments usually are found in eccentric patterns and in long, inhibited muscles acting as antagonists to concentrically contracted muscles. Muscle contractions may serve as a response for compensation purposes. The best course is to address the trigger point activity in the short tissues first and wait to see whether the trigger points in the long muscles and at the attachments resolve as the posture of muscle interaction normalizes. The sequence for addressing trigger points is as follows:

💡 PROFICIENCY EXERCISE 12-5

1. Place a dried pea under a ½-inch piece of foam. Locate the pea with light and deep palpation.
2. Working with a partner, use light palpation to locate an area of suspected trigger point activity. After an area has been found, use deep palpation to find the exact area of the trigger point. Then use the methods described in this section to normalize the area.

1. Those that are most painful and that reproduce familiar symptoms
2. Those most medial
3. Those in the short tissue
4. Those in the muscle belly

As seen with the previous skills, the actual application of trigger point methods is fairly basic. The trained professional's skill is required more in the assessment, in decision making about the appropriateness and intensity of treatment, and in the choice of methods. As with myofascial methods, the application of treatment protocols is deceptively simple, especially when the client's condition is multifaceted and complex. Often more than one method is required in these cases. Trigger point release is a good example of the integration of multiple methods, because effective intervention involves the use of several treatment protocols, massage manipulations, muscle energy methods, stretching methods, and hydrotherapy methods (Figure 12-14) (Proficiency Exercise 12-5).

Neuromuscular Therapy

Before ending this grouping of approaches, let's review the concept of neuromuscular therapy. A distinction must be made between the terms "neuromuscular techniques" and "neuromuscular therapy." All massage methods can be used as neuromuscular techniques, but additional training is required to achieve competence in neuromuscular therapy. Neuromuscular therapy (NMT) is a very specialized form of manual therapy. The European version continues to be practiced as originally developed. An alteration of that system now is called the American version. A therapist trained in NMT is educated in the physiology of the nervous system and its effect on the muscular and skeletal systems. The neuromuscular therapist also is educated in kinesiology and biomechanics and how to work in a clinical or medical environment.

Neuromuscular therapy enhances the function of joints, muscles, and the general arthrokinematics of the body. It covers six basic elements that cause pain:

- Postural distortion
- Biomechanical dysfunction
- Trigger points
- Nerve compression/entrapment
- Ischemia
- Postural distortion

These six areas are addressed using massage as described in this textbook, especially in Chapter 11 and also in this chapter. The distinction between a massage therapist using neuromuscular techniques and a neuromuscular therapist is that for the latter, the training is more focused on targeting dysfunction and massage is not specifically an aspect of that training.

ASIAN BODYWORK METHODS

SECTION OBJECTIVES

Chapter objectives covered in this section:

8. Explain the fundamental concepts and incorporate simple application of Asian bodywork methods into massage therapy.
9. Compare Shiatsu and Thai massage and incorporate mat methods into massage.

Using the information presented in this section, the student will be able to perform the following:

- Explain the basic physiology of acupuncture points and the effects of acupuncture
- Locate an acupuncture point
- Use simple methods to normalize acupuncture points
- Compare the theory of shiatsu to the meridian theory of traditional Chinese medicine
- Compare the application of shiatsu to the application of Thai massage
- Integrate mat methods from shiatsu and Thai massage into a massage session

The richness of Asian health theory and the unity of its body/mind/spirit connection are based on the energy of life. Life force, called *chi* (or *qi/ri*) energy, flows through the body through interconnected pathways as water flows through the streams, rivers, lakes, and oceans of the earth. When *chi* energy flows through the body like pure water, all of life's processes are balanced. However, if obstruction or stagnation in the life force develops, it becomes the basis for disease.

The Tao, or "Way," supports the balanced functioning of all the senses and teaches a lifestyle of moderation that avoids both deprivation and excess. *Chi* energy is the vital force of life, and Tao is the path or way to sustain the *chi* energy.

Some people are concerned about taking pieces from the totality of being expressed in the Tao. Western science has lifted techniques from this simultaneously simple and complex, all-encompassing system. Very often, a technique separated from its theoretical basis is less effective. Although techniques can stimulate physiologic functions, they cannot support the human experience. The small section presented in this textbook is based on a very limited part of the total Asian medicine system. As you begin to develop an understanding of these methods, be mindful and respectful of the larger body of knowledge from which they have been taken.*

Acupuncture

Acupuncture increasingly is gaining acceptance by Western science. It is a branch of Chinese medicine that has proved effective in the treatment of many diseases and dysfunctions. The exact origin of acupuncture is unknown. Although the process remains a mystery in some respects, Western science is

---

*Masunaga and Ohashi, 1977; Yao, 1984; Gunn, 1992; Ohashi, 1993; Wiseman and Feng, 1997; Yu and Rose, 1999; Veith and Rose, 2002.

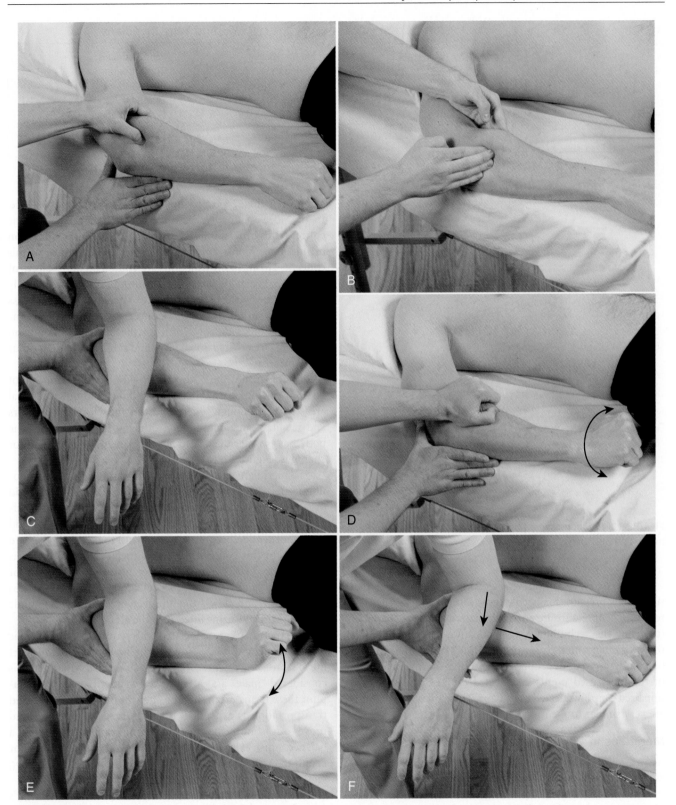

FIGURE 12-14 Treatment sequence in a trigger point. **A,** Location of a trigger point. **B,** Holding at ease. **C,** Broad-based compression to area. **D,** Pinching/squeezing compression with movement active or passive. **E,** Active release. **F,** Direct pressure, then glide.

close to validating its phenomena. Whatever physiologic factors underlie acupuncture, the beneficial changes that occur clearly provide a sound basis for acupuncture treatment.

Acupuncture can be defined as the stimulation of certain points with needles inserted along the meridians (channels) and *ah shi* (meaning "ouch") points outside the meridians. Interestingly, *ah shi* and traditional acupuncture points have a high degree of correlation with trigger points. The purpose of acupuncture is to prevent and modify the perception of pain (analgesia) or to normalize physiologic functions.

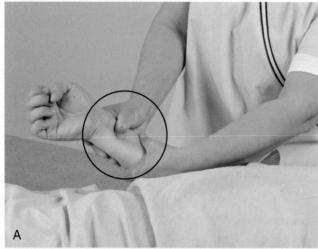

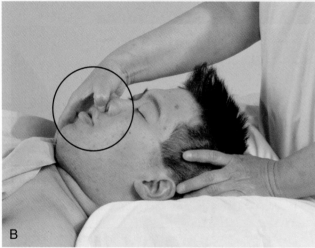

FIGURE 12-15 Acupressure points. **A,** Inside wrist. **B,** Between the lip and the nose.

Box 12-10	Yin and Yang Meridians
Yin Meridians	**Yang Meridians**
Pericardium	Triple heater
Liver	Gallbladder
Kidney	Bladder
Heart	Small intestine
Spleen	Stomach
Lung	Large intestine

stand on a circle, you can look across and see the other side. In this idea of duality, we often forget that a circle is one concept; it is broken into sections only through the limitation of our perceptions. *Yin* and *yang* are representations of this concept. *Yin* and *yang* functions are complementary pieces of the whole. When all parts of the continuum function equally and in harmony, the natural balance of health exists in all areas of the body, mind, and spirit. Conversely, if part of the continuum becomes out of sync with the rest, stress is put on the entire circle. Thus imbalances and symptoms might occur in many areas.

Physiologically, the body is a closed system. There cannot be areas of "too much" energy in the body without reciprocal areas of "not enough" energy. Just as muscles work in pairs and facilitate and inhibit each other, so do meridians. The body has *yin* meridians, or channels, and *yang* meridians, or channels (Figure 12-16).

Yin meridians are associated with parasympathetic autonomic nervous system responses and functions of the solid organs essential to life (e.g., the heart). The energy is considered "female" and a "negative" charge. (Terminology and metaphor tend to become confused with the terms *female* and *negative*. In this context, the terms mean that the functions draw energy of sustenance and nurturing in and restore or reproduce.) *Yin* meridians are located on the inside soft areas of the body and flow from the feet up (Chinese anatomic position with the arms lifted into the air).

Yang meridians are associated with sympathetic autonomic nervous system responses and with hollow organs that support life but are not essential (e.g., the stomach). The energy is considered "male" and a "positive" charge. (Again, in metaphor these terms mean that the energy of transformation and transportation is expended in short bursts as necessary and moves out from the body). Chinese philosophy teaches that a balance must exist between the forces of *yin* and *yang* for health to exist. This balance changes according to the weather, seasons, and other rhythms of nature (Box 12-10).

The patterns that acupuncture points make on the body's surface have been charted by practitioners of acupuncture for centuries. They have been grouped together in lines (called *channels* or *meridians*) and have been allocated to the organs or functions upon which they appear to act. In addition to the 12 pairs of bilateral meridians, two meridians lie on the anterior and posterior midline of the trunk and head. Various extra meridians appear to relate to the body's organs and functions. Other points in the ear surfaces, the hands, and the face have specific reflex effects.

Acupressure is a modified version of acupuncture that substitutes pressure for needle insertion (Figure 12-15). The results of acupressure are not as dramatic as those of acupuncture, but the technique is still effective, especially if it is repeated often with the pressure held long enough. The human body has hundreds of acupuncture points. Approximately 360 of the most used points are located on 12 paired and two unpaired centrally located meridians. These meridian patterns are very similar to the meridians used in shiatsu.

Meridians in Chinese Bodywork Systems

According to Chinese theory, the meridians are internally associated with organs and externally associated with the surface of the head, trunk, and extremities. **Meridians** seem to be energy flows from nerve tracts in the tissue and are located in the fascial grooves (Cunningham, 2002; Dorsher, 2009).

Yin and *Yang*

The Chinese perspective considers body functions in terms of balance between complementary forces. These complements, which often are thought of as opposites, actually are parts of a continuum. A circle is a good example; no matter where you

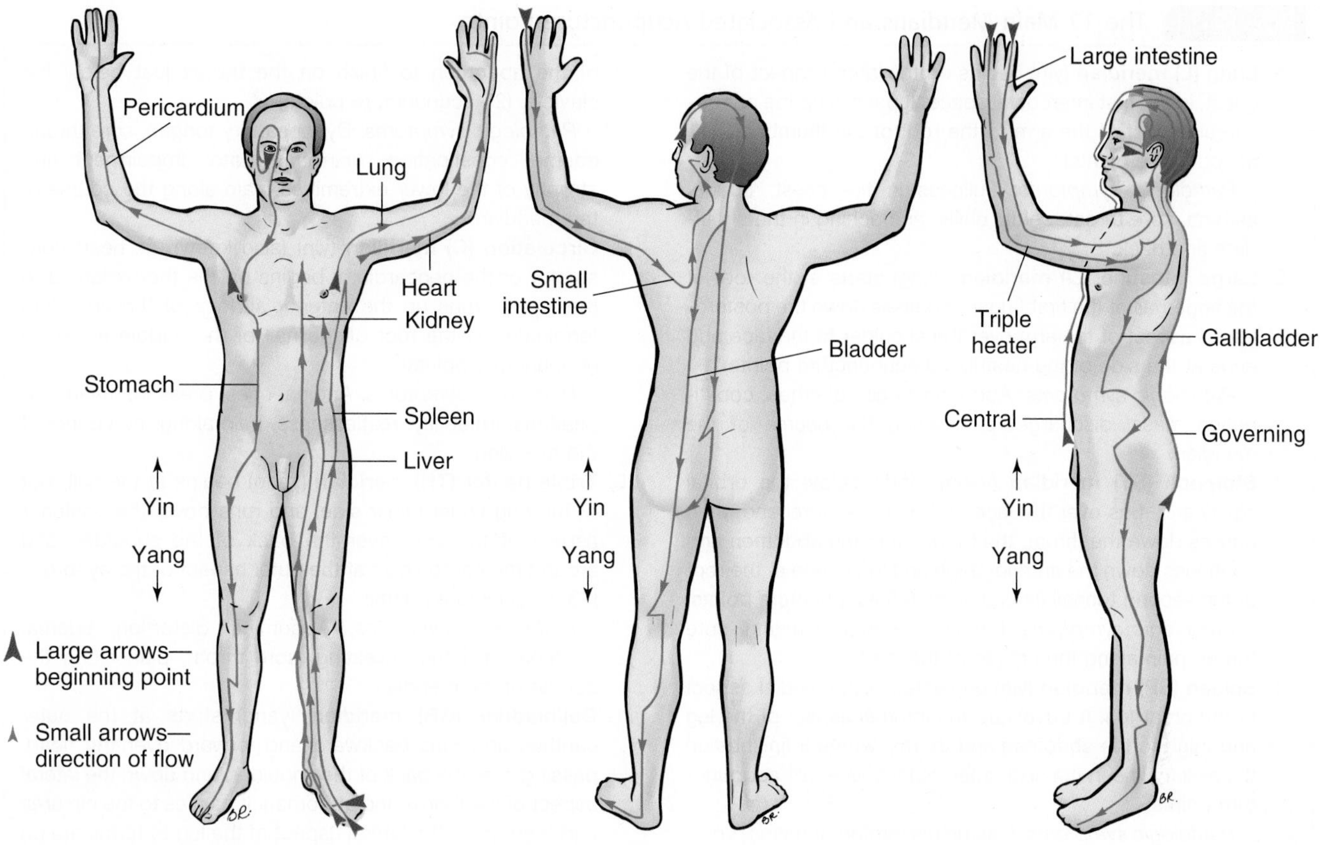

FIGURE 12-16 Typical location of meridians. Meridians tend to follow nerves.

The 12 Main Meridians

The 12 main meridians are bilateral, symmetrically distributed lines of acupuncture points with affinity for or effects upon the functions or organs for which they are named (Box 12-11).

Clinically, abundant evidence indicates the existence of reflex links between acupuncture points and specific organs and functions. In fact, no one really knows what an acupuncture point is. A body of information about acupuncture points, their nature, structure, function, interrelationships, and interactions also exists, and we have the experience derived from thousands of years of using acupuncture points to treat illness. Nevertheless, the most reliable authorities in Chinese medicine seem to agree that there is something mysterious about acupuncture points. An acupuncture point is a component of a system. Acupuncture points have a reflexive characteristic in relation to this system. They reflect information, energy, states of being, conditions of existence of the body and the mind, of the being as a whole and its component parts. The system that comprises the acupuncture points is likewise a reflexive system of information generation and conveyance. In traditional Chinese medicine, this system is known as *jing luo,* usually translated into English as either "meridians" or "channels and network vessels."

Thus the system of acupuncture points can be visualized as a matrix that passes through the body, connecting all its parts and serving as an energy and communications grid that generates, propagates, stores, and releases information and

force related to the body and its various components. Every place in the body is permeated by and connected with every other place in the body by means of the *jing luo* system, which is, in short, the fundamental infrastructure of Chinese anatomy and physiology. The similarity between this description and current research on the fascial network is exciting.

The Chinese word-concept that we translate into English as "acupuncture point" is composed of elements conveying the sense of "body transport (of communications) hole." It is written *shu xue.* Functionally, acupuncture points seem to have two most basic actions: they open, and they close. The names of the many points include words that mean gate, pass, or door. In opening, they release information and energy. In closing, they store it.

The channels contain and convey *chi* and *xue* (blood). The basic nature of *chi* is the manifestation of transformation. From the Chinese viewpoint, everything that is sensed or experienced is a form of *chi.*

Yin-yang theory is one of the oldest doctrines in Chinese culture. The words *yin* and *yang* originally were pictographic representations of the shady and sunny sides, respectively, of a mountain or a hill. They came to represent two primordial forces that were the fundamental constituents of the universe and everything in it. *Chi* is the result of the interplay between *yin* and *yang. Yin* and *yang* mix together, and *chi* issues forth; when *yin* and *yang* were separated from the singularity at the beginning of existence, the resulting potential gave rise to *chi.*

Box 12-11 The 12 Main Meridians and Associated Acupuncture Points

1. **Lung (L) meridian** (yin) begins on the lateral aspect of the chest, in the first intercostal space. It passes up the antero-lateral aspect of the arm to the root of the thumbnail. (11 acupuncture points)

   Pathologic symptoms: Fullness in the chest, cough, asthma, sore throat, colds, chills, and aching in the shoulders and back.

2. **Large intestine (LI) meridian** (yang) starts at the root of the fingernail of the first finger. It passes down the postero-lateral aspect of the arm over the shoulder to the face and ends at the side of the nostril. (20 acupuncture points)

   Pathologic symptoms: Abdominal pain, diarrhea, constipation, nasal discharge, pain along the course of the meridian.

3. **Stomach (ST) meridian** (yang) starts below the orbital cavity and runs over the face and up to the forehead, then passes down the throat, the thorax, and the abdomen and continues down the anterior thigh and leg to end at the root of the second toenail (lateral side). (45 acupuncture points)

   Pathologic symptoms: Bloating, edema, vomiting, sore throat, pain along the course of the meridian.

4. **Spleen (SP) meridian** (yin) originates at the medial aspect of the great toe. It travels up the internal aspect of the leg and thigh to the abdomen and thorax, where it finishes on the axillary line in the sixth intercostal space. (21 acupuncture points)

   Pathologic symptoms: Gastric discomfort, bloating, vomiting, weakness, heaviness of the body, pain along the course of the meridian.

5. **Heart (H) meridian** (yin) begins in the axilla and runs up the anteromedial aspect of the arm to end at the root of the little fingernail (medial aspect). (9 acupuncture points)

   Pathologic symptoms: Dry throat, thirst, cardiac area pain, pain along the course of the meridian.

6. **Small intestine (SI) meridian** (yang) starts at the root of the small fingernail (lateral aspect) and travels down the posteromedial aspect of the arm and over the shoulder to the face, where it terminates in front of the ear. (19 acupuncture points)

   Pathologic symptoms: Pain in the lower abdomen, deafness, swelling in the face, sore throat, pain along the course of the meridian.

7. **Bladder (B) meridian** (yang) starts at the inner canthus, ascends, and passes over the head and down the back and the leg to terminate at the root of the nail of the little toe (lateral aspect). (67 acupuncture points)

   Pathologic symptoms: Urinary problems, mania, headaches, eye problems, pain along the course of the meridian.

8. **Kidney (K) meridian** (yin) starts on the sole of the foot, ascends the medial aspect of the leg, and runs up the front

   of the abdomen to finish on the thorax just below the clavicle. (27 acupuncture points)

   Pathologic symptoms: Dyspnea, dry tongue, sore throat, edema, constipation, diarrhea, motor impairment and atrophy of the lower extremities, pain along the course of the meridian.

9. **Circulation (C) meridian** (yin) (also known as heart constrictor or the pericardium) begins on the thorax lateral to the nipple, runs up the anterior surface of the arm, and terminates at the root of the nail of the middle finger. (9 acupuncture points)

   Pathologic symptoms: Angina, chest pressure, heart palpitations, irritability, restlessness, pain along the course of the meridian.

10. **Triple heater (TH) meridian** (yang) begins at the nail root of the ring finger (ulnar side) and runs down the posterior aspect of the arm, over the back of the shoulder, and around the ear to finish at the outer aspect of the eyebrow. (23 acupuncture points)

    Pathologic symptoms: Abdominal distortion, edema, deafness, tinnitus, sweating, sore throat, pain along the course of the meridian.

11. **Gallbladder (GB) meridian** (yang) starts at the outer canthus and runs backward and forward over the head, passing over the back of the shoulder, and down the lateral aspect of the thorax and abdomen. It passes to the hip area and then down the lateral aspect of the leg to terminate on the fourth toe. (44 acupuncture points)

    Pathologic symptoms: Bitter taste in the mouth, dizziness, headache, ear problems, pain along the course of the meridian.

12. **Liver (LIV) meridian** (yin) begins on the great toe, runs up the medial aspect of the leg, up the abdomen, and terminates on the costal margin (vertically below the nipple). (14 acupuncture points)

    Pathologic symptoms: Lumbago, digestive problems, retention of urine, pain in the lower abdomen, pain along the course of the meridian.

Midline Meridians

The body has two midline meridians.

- The conception (or central) vessel (CV) meridian (yin) starts in the center of the perineum and runs up the midline of the anterior aspect of the body to terminate just below the lower lip (24 acupuncture points); it is responsible for all yin meridians.
- The governor vessel (GV) meridian (yang) starts at the coccyx and runs up the center of the spine and over the midline of the head, terminating on the front of the upper gum (28 acupuncture points); it is responsible for all yang meridians.

The Five Elements

Chinese medical thinking is based on the relationship of the human being with nature. The five elements of nature become a basis for examination, diagnosis, and treatment to support health and relieve disease. The concepts of health parallel natural occurrences of life force energy as represented in the five elements. The five elements are wood, fire, earth, metal,

and water. Each organ is represented by an element, and each element has qualities of colors, sounds, smells, fluid secretion, anatomy, emotions, time, seasons, numbers, flavor, foods, planets, moon phases, dreams, and more (Figure 12-17 and Table 12-7).

The human being is a reflection of the universe, and the five elements become a metaphor for the life processes of people. The qualities of the five elements become the basis for

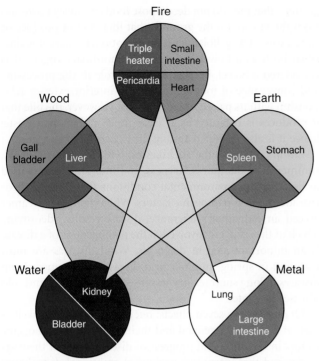

Fire

Wood

Earth

Water

Metal

Triple heater

Small intestine

Pericardia

Heart

Gall bladder

Liver

Stomach

Spleen

Kidney

Bladder

Lung

Large intestine

FIGURE 12-17 The wheel illustrates the relationships connecting the five elements and the organs of the body. The center star depicts the *ko,* or control cycle. Wood controls earth by covering it or holding it in place with roots. Earth controls water by damming it or containing it. Water controls fire by dousing or extinguishing it. Fire controls metal by melting it. Metal controls wood by cutting it. The next set of lines that form a circle depict the *sheng,* or creative cycle. Water engenders wood. Wood fuels fire. Fire creates earth (ashes). Earth engenders metal. Metal engenders water. The five circles indicate the solid *(yin)* on the inside and hollow *(yang)* organs on the outside that are associated with the elements. Movement around the wheel— Fire-> Earth-> Metal-> Water->Wood-> Fire->—is the flow or support cycle, the clockwise movement from one element to the next.

life. As mentioned previously, in Chinese medicine the five elements are the basis for examination, diagnosis, and treatment. Each element is a *yin-yang* relationship of two meridians.

- Earth—Spleen/stomach
- Metal—Lung/large intestine
- Water—Kidney/bladder
- Wood—Liver/gallbladder
- Fire—Heart/small intestine, pericardium/triple heater

The outside circle of the five-element figure represents the *sheng,* or creative cycle. The metaphor is as follows: during the birth phase of the universe, wood came to represent all that grows. As wood grows, it surges out to fire and matures as earth. As continued breakdown occurs, the metal, or inorganic, separates from the organic, with water representing death and rebirth of wood, and so the cycle continues. On the inside, a five-pointed star represents the *ko,* or control cycles. The dynamic balance between creation and control is representative of homeostatic mechanisms in Western science and is explained in the metaphor as follows:

- Wood controls earth by penetrating it with roots.
- Earth controls water by containing it (a pond or lake).
- Water controls fire by extinguishing it.
- Fire controls metal by melting it.
- Metal controls wood by chopping it.

These elegant metaphors in relation to the natural world are easy to understand and become the basis for understanding health and well-being, in addition to methods for assessment and treatment. If processes become disturbed in either the creative or the control cycle, homeostasis is disrupted.

Like *yin* and *yang,* the five elements are categories of quality and relationship. The ancient Chinese saw phenomena in the universe as the products of the movement and mutation of the five entities. These elements represent qualities that relate to each other in specific ways. They function metaphorically, providing images that ancient theorists used to

Table 12-7 Qualities of the Five Elements

	ELEMENT				
Phase	Metal	Earth	Fire	Water	Wood
Yin	Lung	Spleen	Heart	Kidney	Liver
Yang	Large intestine	Stomach	Triple heater	Bladder Small intestine	Gallbladder
Sense	Smell	Taste	Speech	Hearing	Sight
Organ	Nose	Mouth, lips	Tongue	Ears	Eyes
Liquid	Mucus	Saliva	Sweat	Urine	Tears
Color	White	Yellow	Red	Blue/black	Green
Expression	Weeping	Singing	Laughing	Groaning	Shouting
Extreme emotion	Grief, anxiety	Worry, reminiscence	Shock, overjoyed	Fear	Anger
Balanced emotion	Openness, receptivity	Sympathy, empathy	Joy, compassion	Resolution, trust	Assertion, motivation
Taste	Pungent, spicy	Sweet	Bitter, burned	Salty	Sour
Season	Fall	Indian summer	Summer	Winter	Spring
Related activity	Releasing	Thinking	Inspiration	Willpower and intimacy	Planning and decision making
Times	Lung, 3-5 AM Large intestine, 5-7 AM	Stomach, 7-9 AM Spleen, 9-11 AM	Heart, 11 AM–1 PM Small intestine, 1-3 PM	Bladder, 3-5 PM Kidney, 5-7 PM Triple heater, 9-11 PM	Gallbladder, 11 PM–1 AM Pericardium, 7-9 PM Liver, 1-3 AM

organize their thinking about the physical world (Veith and Rose, 2002).

Principles of Traditional Chinese Medicine

Si shi is the term for the four seasons—spring, summer, autumn, and winter—in which the third month of summer (the sixth month of the Chinese lunar year) is called *long summer*. The four seasons correlate with the five elements: spring/wood; summer/fire; long summer/earth; autumn/metal; winter/water.

Shen is the spirit, seen as a general term for vital activities, especially as reflected in the external appearance of the internal (physiologic and/or psychological) condition of the body. As such, it is the primary criterion for diagnosis and prognosis. The word *shen* refers to the eternal dimension of life, to the magical or heavenly aspects of being alive. It means, "god, deity, divinity or divine nature; supernatural; magical expression, look, appearance; smart, clever."

Xue is the blood, described as an essential component of the body derived from the refined foodstuff that is consumed and made capable of being assimilated through the processes of digestion and metabolism. It is the liquid substance that circulates in the blood vessels to deliver nourishment to all parts of the body. The word *xue* is used to mean the blood itself in the same sense as it is understood in modern physiology. It is also used to mean something specific to Chinese medicine: the substantial fraction of the circulatory system in a unique relationship with the circulation of *chi*.

Ying is an essential ingredient of the blood and is responsible for the production of blood and the nourishment of body tissues. The blood and the *ying* are inseparable, thus they often are referred to as *ying xue*.

Jin ye is a general term for all fluids of the body other than the blood. It is one of the basic substances that transforms into blood. It exists extensively within the human body, between organs and tissues, and serves a nutritive function. It is composed of two categorically different substances that form a single entity and that can transform one into the other.

Wu zang describes the five viscera, the so-called solid organs. This is a name given collectively to the heart, liver, spleen, lungs, and kidneys. These organs constitute one category that is distinguished from the six *fu* organs in both structure and function. The *zang* organs are thought of as solid, essence-containing organs. *Liu fu* is the word for the six bowels, the six hollow organs; it is a term given collectively to the gallbladder, stomach, large intestine, small intestine, urinary bladder, and the difficult to define "triple burner" *(san jiao)*. In contrast to the five *zang* organs, the six *fu* organs are considered to be involved in the transportation of substances rather than the storing of essential substances. The word *liu* means "six." The word *fu* means "bowel." Like *zang*, it is a special term of Chinese medicine.

Qi heng zhi fu literally means "extraordinary organs." This designation is given to a group of organs that resemble the *fu* organs in structure and the *zang* organs in function; they include the bones, blood vessels, gallbladder, and uterus. The brain and bone marrow also are in this category. These extraordinary organs are distinguished from the bowels on the grounds that they do not decompose food or convey waste and from the viscera on the grounds that they do not produce or store excess. The gallbladder is an exception, because it is classified both as a bowel and as an extraordinary organ. It is considered a bowel, because it plays a role in the processing and conveyance of food and stands in interior-exterior relationship with its paired organ, the liver. However, the bile that it produces is regarded as a "clear fluid" rather than waste; hence it is also classified among the extraordinary organs.

Liu qi comprises the six excesses, referring to wind, cold, summer heat, dampness, dryness, and fire. This term is used to describe the environmental conditions that ancient theorists identified as pathogenic factors. When changes in weather exceed an individual's tolerance, disease results. Identifying which of the six *qi* are involved in the pathogenesis of a disease is an important step in diagnosis. Wind diseases are most common in spring, summer heat diseases in summer, damp diseases in long summer, dryness diseases in autumn, and cold diseases in winter.

Qi qing, or the seven affects, refers to emotional as well as mental activities in general and their potential as pathogenic factors in the onset and progress of disease. Ancient theorists recognized that intense or prolonged emotional disturbance can act as a pathogenic factor, and they identified seven such states: anger, melancholy, anxiety, sorrow, terror, fright, and excessive joy. Each of these can act to disturb the normal function of the *chi*, blood, and viscera, resulting in disease. This notion embraced thinking itself, which is understood as having the potential to exhaust the *chi* of the spleen if one thinks (or worries) excessively. The word qi means "seven." The word *qing* means "feeling, affection, sentiment, emotional."

Xu shi means vacuity and repletion or deficiency and excess, insubstantial and substantial (particularly in the martial arts), replete and deplete, full and empty. *Xu shi* refers to two principles for estimating the condition of both the person's resistance and the pathogenic factors present. *Vacuity* generally refers to a general insufficiency of vitality, energy, and functioning of the body and is usually expressed in terms of *yin, yang, chi,* and blood. *Repletion* typically is used to refer to the hyperactivity of pathogenic factors and the resulting symptoms of conflict between the body's healthy resistance and these pathogenic factors.

Han re describes cold and heat and is considered the primary manifestation of *yin* and *yang* (i.e., symptoms that evidence predominance of cold or heat). These two signs of disease are considered of primary importance in the selection of herbal ingredients for prescriptions to treat illness. The word *han* means "cold." The word *re* means "heat."

Si zhen is the term for the *four methods of diagnosis*

Wang zhen is *diagnosis by observation*, which includes observation of the patient's complexion, skin color, physical build, development and nutrition, and observation of tongue

Wen zhen is *diagnosis by hearing and smelling*

Wen zhen is *diagnosis by interrogation*

Qie zhen is *pulse-taking and palpation*

The four examinations provide the raw data for diagnosis. It is essential that the data from all four examinations be correlated to arrive at a complete diagnosis. The four examinations are followed by pattern identification.

The first and most fundamental method of gathering diagnostic information consists of looking at the patient's physical appearance, posture, mental and emotional status (as reflected in outward signs), color, and so forth. This includes inspection of urine, stool, and other secretions and excretions. For the well-trained Chinese doctor, it includes a comprehensive inventory of all relevant data that can be gathered through observation. The word *wang* means "inspection; looking with the eyes." Special attention focuses on the complexion and tongue, which are important indicators of the bowels and viscera. Listening and smelling consists of gathering data by means of the olfactory and auditory organs. The doctor of Chinese medicine listens to the various sounds the person makes, such as voice, breathing, coughing, moaning, and notes any particular odors.

Shi wen, the 10 questions, refers to the 10 basic aspects of a patient that a doctor inquires about in gathering diagnostic information. These include feelings of heat or coldness; perspiration; the condition of the head, trunk, and limbs; urination and defecation; appetite; the condition of the chest and abdomen; hearing and sleeping; thirst; menstruation, leukorrhea, and so forth, including the growth and nourishment of children; the past history; and the cause of disease.

Wu se, or the five colors, refers to the colors associated with the five elements and the five *zang* organs. These are green (a greenish-blue associated with wood, liver); red (fire, heart); yellow (earth, spleen); white (metal, lungs); and black (water, kidneys). Observation of these colors as they appear in the body is taken together with other clinical data and forms an important aspect of diagnosis.

San yin describes a method of classifying pathogenic factors, in terms of their point of origin, as endogenous, exogenous, or neutral (literally non-external-internal). These three categories are *nei yin,* endogenous pathogenic factors, which include abnormal emotional activities; *wai yin,* exogenous pathogenic factors, including wind, cold, summer heat, damp, dry, and fire; and *bu nei wai yin,* improper diet, trauma, animal bites, insect stings, and fatigue. The word *yin* means "cause, because of, as a result of." The word *nei* means "inner, within, inside." The word *wai* means "outer, outward, outside, external."

External factors are the six excesses. Internal causes are the seven effects. Neutral causes ("non-external-internal") include eating too much or too little, falls, crushing, drowning, and animal injuries.

A thousand sufferings fall into just three categories. First, the evil invades the *jing luo* and enters the *zang fu;* this is known as *external causes.* Second, blood and vessels connect the four limbs and nine orifices. When these become congested, illness follows; these are called *internal causes.* The third category contains such aspects as sexual life, wounds from knives, bites from insects, and beasts; these are "neither internal nor external."

Si qi si xing refers to the essential synergistic characteristics of medicine or treatment. The four natures are cold, hot, cool, and warm. They are categorized according to *yin* and *yang.* Hot and warm are in the *yang* category; cold and cool are in the *yin* category. The purpose of categorizing medicinal substances in this fashion is to permit herbal practitioners to follow a basic precept of Chinese herbal medicine: "Use heat to overcome cold pathogenic factors; use cold to overcome hot pathogenic factors." Herbs with a cold nature typically are used to clear hot or warm pathogenic factors and internally generated heat. They are used to treat heat patterns and *yang* patterns. Herbs with a hot nature are used to dispel cold pathogenic factors by warming the interior, invigorating *yang,* and nourishing *chi.* They are used in the treatment of cold patterns and *yin* patterns.

Wu wei, the five flavors, refers to the tastes of herbs: acrid, sweet, sour, bitter, and salty. These flavors are understood to correspond with the five *zang* organs according to the following arrangement:

- Heart—Bitter
- Liver—Sour
- Spleen—Sweet
- Lungs—Acrid
- Kidney—Salty

The flavors can be classified as *yin* and *yang.* Acrid and sweet effusing (i.e., diaphoretic) and dissipating medicinals are *yang;* sour and bitter upwelling (i.e., emetic) and discharging (i.e., draining) medicinals are *yin;* salty upwelling and discharging medicinals are *yin;* bland percolating and discharging medicinals are *yang.*

Zhen jiu translates as "needle" and "long-lasting fire." Together, these two words form the term that is typically translated in English as "acupuncture and moxibustion" or "acumoxa therapy," commonly referred to simply as acupuncture. The term refers to two allied forms of therapy, *zhen fa* and *jiu fa. Zhen fa* refers to the therapeutic method of applying any of a variety of types of needles, including filiform needles, three-edged needles, plum-blossom needles, and intradermal needles, among others. The needles are applied to stimulate certain points that lie among channels for the treatment of disease. *Jiu fa* consists of the application of an herb, artemisia, which is prepared in various ways and then burned either near or on certain points to warm and thereby stimulate the movement of *chi.*

Shu xue, or *in bach shu,* means transport point and is a term for a category of acupoints found on the back in two lines, one approximately 11 inches lateral to the spine and the other at about 3 inches lateral to the spine. These points are related to the functioning of the internal organs and various other aspects of physiology.

Mu xue means an alarm point and refers to a group of points on the anterior surface of the body that have both diagnostic and therapeutic interrelationships. Because changes in the *chi* frequently precede any other clinical symptoms or signs, *mu xue* points can "sound an alarm" prior to the onset of disease. The word *mu* means to "collect, gather, or muster together."

Wu shu xue is the Chinese term for the five transport points, referring to a group of points on each of the 12 primary channels. These points include well points, spring points, stream points, river points, and uniting (sea) points. Here the word *shu* means "transportation or communication."

Tui na is a general name for massage. The word *tui* means "push, push forward, promote." The word *na* means to "hold, to grasp." *Tui na* thus means pushing and holding (i.e., massage).

An mo is another general term for massage. The word *an* means "press, push down, keep one's hand on (something)." The word *mo* means "to rub, scrape, touch." *An mo* is a method of preventing and treating diseases using various massage techniques and methods and of undertaking manipulation and adjustment of the joints and the extremities. More specifically, *an mo* is one of the eight manipulations used in bone setting to relax muscle tissue, dissipate blood stasis, and reduce swelling.

Health Preservation and Exercise

An important part of Chinese medicine is the discipline of preserving health and extending life. Foremost among the various methods that fall in this category are exercise and disciplines aimed at cultivating the inborn treasures of the body, mind, and spirit.

- *Qi gong. Qi gong,* or breathing exercise, refers to a variety of traditional practices consisting of physical, mental, and spiritual exercises. The regulation of the breath *(qi)* is a common feature of such exercise methods. The word *gong* means "achievement, result; skill; work; exercise." It is composed of two radicals. The radical on the left is also pronounced *gong* and means "work." The radical on the right is the word *li* and means "strength or force." *Qi gong* can be understood as exercise designed to strengthen and harmonize the *chi,* regulate the body and mind, and calm the spirit.
- *Tai ji quan. Tai ji quan (tai chi)* is both a martial and a meditative art. It therefore has complementary aspects that combine in a comprehensive discipline of physical culture and mental and spiritual discipline. The word *quan* means "fist; boxing; punch."
- *Dao yin.* This discipline involves meditation and breathing exercises that seek to develop the ability to lead and guide the *chi* throughout the body for the benefit of the spirit, mind, and body. *Dao yin* exercises have a long history in China. They consist of bending, stretching, and otherwise mobilizing the extremities and the joints to free the flow of *chi* throughout the whole body. Like *Qi gong, dao yin* emphasizes control of the breath *(chi). Dao yin* also includes self-massage techniques that relieve fatigue and prolong life by activating and harmonizing the circulation of blood and *chi.* These techniques also stress the development of strength in the muscles and bones.

The vastness of the Asian medicine model and its elegance are far beyond the scope of this textbook; therefore, no attempt is made to present scaled-down versions of these systems. The student is directed to the reference list for sources of further study. Students who are drawn to these concepts are encouraged to explore them in depth as they continue on their path of knowledge.

During the natural course of therapeutic massage, the physical aspects of meridians and points are addressed. The following section briefly investigates methods of incorporating this approach into therapeutic massage.

Methods of Treating Acupuncture Points

Acupuncture points usually lie in a fascial division between muscles and near origins and insertions. A point feels like a small hole, and pressure elicits a "nervy" feeling. Unlike a trigger point, which may be found only on one side of the body, acupuncture points are bilateral (i.e., found on both sides of the body) and are located on the central, or governing, meridian. To confirm the location of an acupuncture point, locate the point in the same place on the other side of the body.

To stimulate a hypoactive acupuncture point (one with insufficient energy), use a short vibrating or tapping action. This method is effective if the area is sluggish or if a specific body function needs to be stimulated.

To sedate a hyperactive acupuncture point (one with too much energy) to reduce pain, elicit the pain response within the point itself. Use a sustained holding pressure until the painful over energy dissipates and the body's own natural painkillers are released into the bloodstream (Tappan and Benjamin, 2004). The pressure techniques are similar to those used for trigger points; however, an acupuncture point does not need to be lengthened and stretched after treatment.

As with other reflex points, if you are unsure whether the acupuncture point is hypoactive or hyperactive, alternately apply both techniques and allow the body to adjust to the intervention.

Determining whether you are dealing with a trigger point or an acupressure point often is difficult, because the two often overlap. It may be wise to lengthen and stretch the area gently after using direct pressure methods; this does not interfere with the effect on an acupressure point, but without it a trigger point cannot be treated effectively (Chaitow, 1990) (Proficiency Exercise 12-6).

Asian methods work for sound physiologic reasons through the neuroendocrine and fascial systems. Particular effects can be demonstrated after acupuncture treatment. Some of these effects involve alteration of the function of organs or systems. An analgesic effect and an anesthetic effect also are seen. It is not necessary to hold that imbalance between *yin* and *yang* (the two equal and opposite forces of the universe, which act through *chi*) causes disease. Instead, the acupuncture benefit can be framed in terms of the body's homeostatic tendency, whereby a stable internal environment is maintained through

💡 PROFICIENCY EXERCISE 12-6

1. Working with a partner, perform a massage that incorporates running the hand down each of the meridian grooves in the body. Stop at each hole or point you feel.
2. When you locate a point while performing this massage, decide whether the point needs to be stimulated with vibration or tapping, or sedated with sustained direct pressure. How did you decide?

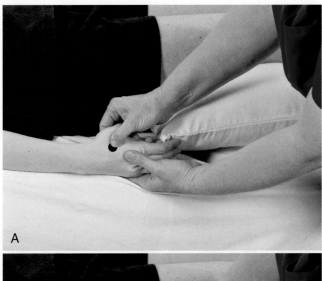

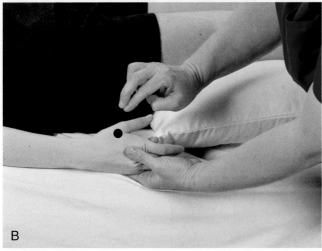

A

B

FIGURE 12-18 Treatment of acupuncture points. **A,** Press, sedate. **B,** Tap, stimulate.

the interaction of the various body processes and systems. For many years osteopaths and chiropractors have used reflex pressure techniques to assist the body in its efforts toward health. Many of the points used correspond with acupuncture points.

If one accepts that the body constantly strives for health, then one must agree that the body uses all helpful stimuli to that end. If this function can be assisted through acupuncture or manual pressure, the homeostatic interplay of organ systems will carry on the work to the extent possible at that time (Figure 12-18).

Acupuncture successfully induces the desired feeling of soreness and fullness that is a forerunner of the anesthetic effect (pain modulator). Electrophysiologic studies have shown that deep pressure applied to muscles and tendons has a definite inhibitory effect on the unit discharge of neurons in the nonspecific nucleus of the thalamus, which would support the claimed benefit of acupressure.

Pain relief might well be the result of neutrally mediated changes in the brain's receptivity to pain impulses, in addition to an effect of biochemical changes caused by the release of hormonelike substances both locally and generally.

Western research so far has produced no great breakthrough in our understanding of acupuncture, although

Melzack and Wall have proposed the gate control theory, and endogenous polypeptides that link to opiate receptors in the brain and central nervous system offer an explanation of the acupuncture phenomenon. Regardless, skillful application of the method provides benefits and can easily be integrated into therapeutic massage.

Shiatsu

Shiatsu (finger pressure), which was developed in Japan, is one of the more familiar Asian bodywork systems. Shiatsu and acupressure sometimes are considered the same method. However, shiatsu is much broader in its application of methods and diagnosis. Shiatsu was recognized in Japan as a manipulative therapy about 70 years ago. Basically, it is a form of massage in which the fingers are pressed onto particular points of the body to ease aches, pain, tension, fatigue, and symptoms of disease. These points, called *tsubo,* or acupuncture points, are located along the meridians described later in this section. One distinguishing method of shiatsu diagnosis is done through areas on the *hara* (abdomen or center) and the back. Pressure in these areas or along the meridians identifies energy flow (in Japanese, *ki*) as either *kyo* (under energy) or *jitsu* (over energy). Shiatsu restores balance by strengthening or stimulating (toning) the *kyo* and sedating the *jitsu.*

The traditional meridian system is the foundation of the shiatsu system (Figure 12-19). The following list describes each meridian function and the imbalances that manifest as *kyo* and *jitsu* symptoms (Figure 12-20) (Masunaga and Ohashi, 1977). It is interesting to compare these meridian descriptions to those most closely identified with Chinese theory (see Box 12-11).

- *Lung meridian:* Functions with the intake of *ki* energy from the air to build up strength and to eliminate unneeded gases through exhalation.
  - *Kyo* imbalances: Hypersensitivity, anxiety, breathing difficulties, antisocial demeanor, shortness of breath, coughing; also excess body weight, elimination difficulties, upper body fatigue, susceptibility to respiratory infection, shoulder pain.
  - *Jitsu* imbalances: Anxiety over small details; tendency to sigh and choke while breathing; susceptibility to nasal congestion, colds, constipation, shoulder pain, bronchitis, asthma, excess production of mucus, thumb pain, and tightness in the chest muscles.
- *Large intestine meridian:* Assists functioning of the lung; secretes and excretes from inside and outside the body; eliminates the stagnation of *ki* energy.
  - *Kyo* imbalances: Lack of determination, disappointment, overdependency, negative thinking; dry or congested nasal passage; weak bronchial tubes, constipation; prone to diarrhea when digesting coarse foods; poor circulation in the lower abdomen; tendency to shiver; malfunctioning of the large intestine; fatigue in the lower body below the hips; lack of vitality, susceptibility to inflammation.
  - *Jitsu* imbalances: Perpetual dissatisfaction; headaches, flushed complexion; runny nose, nasal congestion, nose

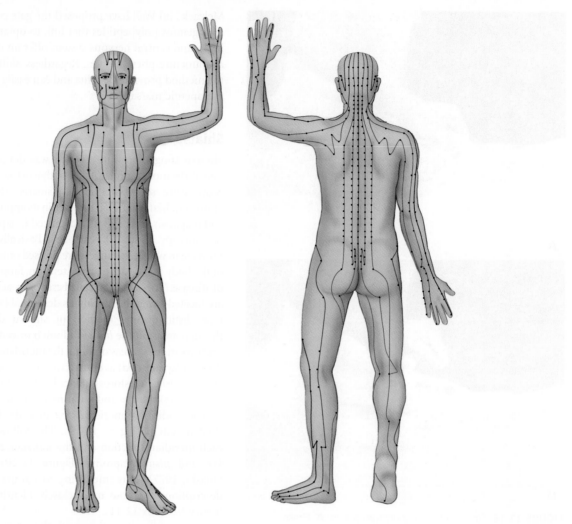

FIGURE 12-19 The main meridian pathways of shiatsu. (From Anderson SK: *The practice of shiatsu,* St Louis, 2008, Mosby.)

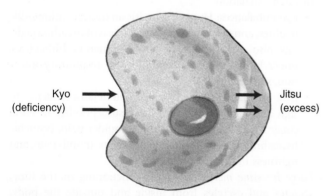

FIGURE 12-20 Cell with *kyo* and *jitsu.* Every area of *jitsu* has a resulting area of *kyo.* Every area of *kyo* has a resulting area of *jitsu.* (From Anderson SK: *The practice of shiatsu,* St. Louis, 2008, Mosby.)

bleed, prone to respiratory infection; painful sensation in the lower teeth; shoulder pain; tension in the chest and arm muscles; constipation but occasional diarrhea; tendency to overeat; itchy skin, puffiness in lower abdomen and hemorrhoids; epilepsy.

- *Spleen meridian:* In modern terms the spleen is considered to be the pancreas. It supports digestion, including the secretion of saliva and gastric bile, secretions from the small intestine, and secretion of reproductive hormones related to the breasts and ovaries. Mental fatigue adversely affects the spleen meridian, and lack of exercise causes malfunctioning digestion and hormone secretion.
  - *Kyo* imbalances: Obsession with details; restless, anxious, and dissatisfied; tendency to overeat and eat quickly; busy brain, memory loss; sleepiness; diminished gastric acid and saliva; sticky, dry taste in the mouth, thirst; inability to consume food without liquid; diminished taste sensations, poor digestion, inability to taste food; brownish cast of the face, lack of energy for exercise, poor circulation in the legs and feet.
  - *Jitsu* imbalances: Tendency to be isolated; hesitant, timid, and thinks too much; cautious and anxious; eats quickly with craving for sweets; thirsty, sticky feeling in the mouth; no appetite, no appreciation for tasting foods; gastric hyperacidity, overeating, obesity; heaviness in the legs, no strength, and stiffness in the shoulders and arms.
- *Stomach meridian:* Related to functioning of the stomach, esophagus, and duodenum, as well as functioning of the reproductive and menstrual cycles, lactation, ovaries, and appetite mechanism.

- *Kyo* imbalances: Busy brain with tendency to want to lie down; craves cold and soft food; emotional eating, lack of chewing with tendency to eat while doing something, and irregular meal intake; chronic gastric problems, eats with no appetite; shoulder pain caused by problems with ovaries; yawning; fat legs; fatigue, coldness felt in the front part of the body; lack of flexibility in the muscles.
  - *Jitsu* imbalances: Nervous about details; frustrated, lacking in affection; overeats; time urgency, neurotic; gastric hyperacidity; cold sores; thirst; stiffness in the shoulder, pain and stiffness in the solar plexus and the heart; prone to upper respiratory infections; poor circulation in the legs; rough, dry complexion; intestinal gas; yawning; redness on top of the nose; tendency to be anemic; female reproductive system problems.
- *Heart meridian:* Related to functions of compassion and emotions, as well as blood circulation. Also the mechanism that adapts external stimuli to the body's internal environment.
  - *Kyo* imbalances: Mental fatigue, shock, nervous tension, stress, neurosis, poor appetite, restlessness, memory loss; timidity, tendency to be disappointed, no will power; upper abdomen weakness, tightness in the solar plexus area; strong palpitations; heart organ problems; abdominal tension; sweaty palms; fatigue, angina, coated tongue, myocardial infarction.
  - *Jitsu* imbalances: Chronic tension and stiffness in the chest; tries to contain anxiety and restlessness; perpetual fatigue; tendency to stammer; stiffness in the solar plexus area; thirst; laughing; always clearing the throat; tightness in the heart area; stiff body; hysteria; sweaty palms, perspires easily, sensitive skin; shoulder pain; desire for cold drinks; nervous stomach; palpitations.
- *Small intestine meridian:* Exerts a total body influence through digestion of food.
  - *Kyo* imbalances: Narrow focus, oversensitivity to small details, anxiety; strong determination, decreased ability to control deep emotional sadness, emotional shock; anemia caused by poor nutrition and digestion; blood stagnation and poor circulation and heaviness in the hips and legs; fainting; dysfunction of the intestinal organs; easily fatigued in the hip area, low back problems, weak abdominal muscles; hearing difficulty; eye fatigue; abnormal menstrual cycle; pain in the ovaries; shoulder pain; migraine headaches.
  - *Jitsu* imbalances: Patient, determined, overworked; restless rapid eye movements, headaches; stiffness of the cervical vertebrae; puffiness of the eyes and ears; feeling of having a chilled body and heat in the head; redness in the cheeks; bladder and bowel urgency; poor circulation in the extremities; poor digestion, constipation; ovary malfunctioning; lower back ache; shoulder pain; pain in the upper part of the teeth; dry mouth, lack of saliva.
- *Kidney meridian:* Functions to control the spirit and energy to the body and to promote resistance against mental stress through control of hormone secretions, including cortisol; detoxifies and purifies the blood, preventing acidosis.

- *Kyo* imbalances: Anxiety, fear, restlessness, nervousness, pessimism; family stress, lack of patience and determination, mental fatigue; dry, puffy, inelastic skin; poor circulation in the hips and abdomen; bladder frequency; low back ache; malfunctioning of hormone secretions; insomnia; sexual dysfunction, reproductive organ problems; cracks in the nails; prone to bone fractures; tendency to stumble; stiffness in the abdominal and torso muscles.
  - *Jitsu* imbalances: Impatient, "workaholic," nervousness, restlessness, constant complaining, overfocuses on details, lack of determination; blackish cast to face; vomiting, blood in the saliva; prone to nose bleeds and fainting; thirst; ringing in the ears; back stiffness; tension in the torso muscles; abnormal hormone secretion; dark urine; bad breath and bitter taste in the mouth; prone to inflammation; work-related burnout.
- *Bladder meridian:* Connected to midbrain; function is to support kidney hormone system and pituitary gland; also connected to the autonomic nervous system, especially reproductive and urinary organs; eliminates urine.
  - *Kyo* imbalances: Strained nerves, stiff body; complains and is easily frightened, night sweats, anxiety; nasal congestion; heaviness and pain in the eyes; migraine headache; malfunctioning of the autonomic nervous system, poor circulation, especially in the lower back; frequent urination, bladder inflammation and pain.
  - *Jitsu* imbalances: Worry and oversensitivity; stiff neck pain, head and eye heaviness, shoulder muscle tension; tightness in the backs of the legs; nasal congestion; frequent urination; inflammation or pain in the bladder or prostate area; autonomic nervous system strain.
- *Heart constrictor meridian:* Supports and assists functioning of the heart related to the circulatory system; also controls total nutrition.
  - *Kyo* imbalances: Absent-mindedness; insomnia and vivid dreams, heart palpitations and shortness of breath, squeezing sensation around the chest; swallowing problems; heart dysfunctions, easily fatigued; low blood pressure; dropsy, poor circulation; pain in the stomach and duodenum; abnormal blood pressure; pain in the chest and rib cage.
  - *Jitsu* imbalances: Restless when asleep or awake; social anxiety; difficulty focusing on tasks; inappropriate emotions and hypersensitivity; strong heart palpitations; high blood pressure; dizziness, easily fatigued; poor circulation; headache; tightness in the abdomen, stomach pain; tingling in the fingers; hot palms; colitis; coated tongue.
- *Triple heater meridian:* Supports functioning of the small intestine; controls visceral organs circulating energy to the entire body; supports functions of the lymphatic system.
  - *Kyo* imbalances: Mental obsessions; headaches, ringing in the ears, heaviness and dizziness in the head; sensitivity to heat, cold, and dampness; weak and strained lymphatic system; nasal problems; sensitivity to humidity and temperature change, easily catches cold; tired eyes; sensitive skin, allergy; tightness in the chest and abdomen; abnormal blood pressure, pain in the back of the head and in the temples.

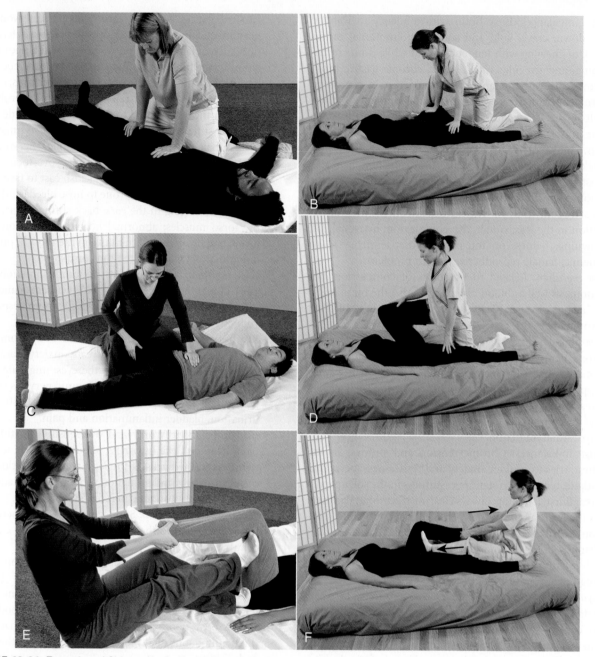

FIGURE 12-21 Examples of Shiatsu **(A, C, E)** and Thai **(B, D, F)** massage.
(A, C, and E from Anderson SK: *The practice of shiatsu,* St. Louis, 2008, Mosby.)

- *Jitsu* imbalances: Extremely cautious with tendency to be hypervigilant; nervous reaction to external changes in heat, cold, and humidity; heaviness in chest (upper heater), stomach (middle heater), and lower abdomen; sensitivity; foggy brain; eye pressure; neck, shoulder, and arm pain; lymphatic inflammation; itchy skin; poor circulation in the legs; susceptible to humidity; ticklish.
- *Liver meridian:* Stores nutrients and energy for physical activity; supports resistance against disease and maintains blood for physical energy.
  - *Kyo* imbalances: Lack of determination; easily upset, inconsistent; inability to gain weight; weak joints, easily fatigued; dizziness, tendency to stumble, tired eyes; body system easily poisoned because of poor detoxification; fever; lack of appetite; stiff muscles; sexual dysfunction.

- *Jitsu* imbalances: Stubbornness, works impatiently and impulsively until exhausted; easily affected emotionally, displays emotion and then controls it; burnout; overeating (especially sweets), excessive drinking; swollen chest and stomach; headaches; poor digestion; lack of exercise; dizziness; high fever without cause; liver organ malfunction; hemorrhoids; prostate problems; pain in the sacrum and coccyx; general bending stiffness; flatulence; prone to inflammations.
- *Gallbladder meridian:* Distributes nutrients and balances energy, supporting internal hormones and secretions such as bile, saliva, gastric acid, insulin, and intestinal hormones.
  - *Kyo* imbalances: Susceptible to emotional excitement; sudden fatigue after stress; timid, lack of determination, strained nerves, light sleeper, lack of energy; tired, weak

eyes, lack of energy caused by deficiency of nutrients, tired legs; poor digestion of fats, prone to diarrhea and constipation; neuralgia; dizziness; pale complexion; obesity despite poor appetite, accumulation of fatty tissues without consumption of greasy foods, gastric hyperacidity; improper nutritional distribution.

- *Jitsu* imbalances: Takes on too much responsibility; fatigued, impatient, time urgency; lack of sleep, causing tired eyes; bloated stomach, loss of appetite; yellowish tinge in white part of eye and skin; tendency to blink frequently; stiffness in the extremities; bitter taste in the mouth; gallstones and spasms in the gallbladder; shoulder pain; heaviness in the head; migraine headache; mucosal stagnation; coughing; excessive intake of sweets; lack of sour food consumption.

Thai Massage

Called **Thai massage** in the Western world, *nuad phaen boran*, as it is called in Thailand, translates as "ancient massage" or "traditional massage." It can be traced to Thailand more than 2,500 years ago from the Vajrayana or the Diamond Healing lineage of Tibet. It made its way to Thailand, where the Ayurvedic techniques and principles gradually became influenced by traditional Chinese medicine. For centuries, Thai massage was performed by monks as one component of Thai medicine.

It combines elements of yoga, shiatsu, and acupressure, working with the energy pathways of the body and the therapy points located along these lines. Thai massage is believed to have been developed by Jivaka Kumar Bhaccha, physician to Buddha in India. The practice is deeply influenced by Indian Ayurveda and TCM.

Thai massage incorporates elements of mindfulness, gentle rocking, deep stretching, and rhythmic compression to create a singular healing experience. It uses assisted yoga *asanas* (yoga postures) to open the joints and relieve the tension in surrounding muscles, which allows *prana, chi,* or healing energy to move more freely through the body. Thai massage is also called Thai yoga massage, because the therapist uses his or her hands, knees, legs, and feet to move the client into a series of yogalike stretches. Thai massage is performed on a mat on the floor, and the client wears light, loose-fitting clothing. The session can last 1 to 3 hours or longer. The treatment style is slow, deliberate, and gentle. Thai massage is more energizing and rigorous than more classic forms of massage (Figure 12-21).

AYURVEDA

SECTION OBJECTIVES

Chapter objectives covered in this section:

10. Explore the healing philosophy of Ayurveda.

Using the information presented in this section, the student will be able to perform the following:

- Identify and understand introductory Ayurvedic terminology
- Locate the major chakras and explain the qualities of each
- Explain and use color as a therapeutic element during massage

Ayurveda is a system of health and medicine developed in India. The foundation of its theory base is similar to that of Asian systems. As with all the complementary systems presented in this chapter, Ayurveda is a distinct and rich body of knowledge. The language of Ayurveda is being used more often in Western society, and massage professionals should be familiar with some of the terms that describe Ayurvedic principles of thought (Johari, 1996).

The word *Ayurveda* means "life knowledge" or "right living." Ayurveda is grounded as a body/mind/spirit system in the Vedic scriptures. The tridosha theory is unique to this system. A *dosha* is a body chemical pattern. When the doshas combine, they constitute the nature of every living organism. The three doshas are *vata* (wind), *pitta* (bile), and *kapha* (mucus). These three combine to form the five elements (similar to Asian theory) of ether, air, fire, water, and earth.

Bones, flesh, skin, and nerves belong to the earth element. Semen, blood, fat, urine, mucus, saliva, and lymph belong to the water element. Hunger, thirst, temperature, sleep, intelligence, anger, hate, jealousy, and radiance belong to the fire element. All movement, breathing, natural urges, sensory and motor functions, secretions, excretions, and transformation of tissues belong to the air element. Love, shyness, fear, and attachment belong to the ether element.

People display temperament based on the degree of influence or dominance of a particular dosha; this is considered an inherited genetic quality that influences a person through his or her entire life. The balance of function within the dosha system equates with health.

The points connected with this system are called *marmas*. There are about 100 marmas, which are concentrated at the junctions of muscles, vessels, ligaments, bones, and joints. These junctions form the seat of vital life force (in Hindi, *prana*). Marmas have a strong correlation with common trigger points and the location of the traditional meridians (Figure 12-22).

In Ayurveda, chakras are considered the seven centers of the *prana* (see Figure 1-4). They are located along the spinal column, interrelated with the nervous system and endocrine glands. These are subtle centers of consciousness that are the link between the universal source of intelligence and the human body. Chakras are wheels of energy, and they govern the various physical organs, in addition to etheric bodies, such as the emotional body (the feelings). Within every living body, although on the subtle rather than the gross or the physical level, there is said to be a series of energy fields or centers of consciousness, which in traditional Tantric teachings are called *chakras* (wheels) or *padmas* (lotuses). They are said to be located either along or just in front of the backbone, even though they might express themselves externally at points along the front of the body (e.g., navel, heart, throat). Associated with the chakras is a latent subtle energy, called *kundalini* in Shaktism and *tumo* in Tibetan Buddhist Tantra.

The massage methods of Ayurveda are tapping, kneading, rubbing, and squeezing. The use of specialized oil preparations is integral to the systems (Johari, 1996).

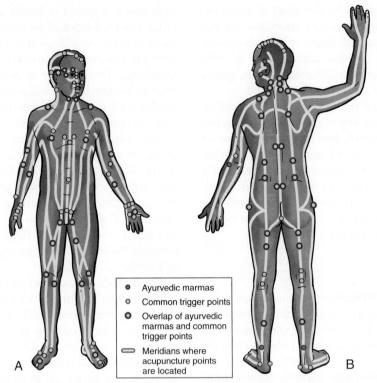

FIGURE 12-22 Comparison of ayurvedic marmas, common trigger points, and traditional meridians where acupuncture points are located. Anterior **(A)** and posterior **(B)** views of overlapping locations of various points suggest that the points have a common anatomy and physiology.

Color and Chakra Therapy

Light can be used therapeutically. When the light spectrum is spread, a rainbow appears. Each color has a specific frequency that is thought to influence the body. Color can be incorporated into massage through uniforms, linens, or tinted lighting. The traditional Chinese medicine system also relies on color. Chakra therapy often is related to color. The following is a brief, basic discussion of the individual chakras and the color relationship (Box 12-12; also see Figure 1-4).

- The chakras are numbered, beginning with the lowest vibration, which is the first chakra, or root chakra. Located at the base of the spine, the first chakra is associated with the color red. Energy is tied to the element of earth, grounding us and connecting us to the physical plane. Glandular system: gonads.
- The second chakra, or sacral chakra, sits in the area of the reproductive organs and vibrates to the color orange. The sacral chakra controls emotions and sexuality. Glandular system: adrenal.
- The third chakra, or solar plexus chakra, is tied to the color yellow and is located just below the diaphragm. This chakra deals with intellect and ego. Glandular system: pancreas.
- The fourth chakra, or heart chakra, is located in the chest and is linked to the color green. It controls love and relationships, especially agape, or divine love. Glandular system: lymphatic.
- The fifth chakra, or throat chakra, radiates blue and holds sway over expression, helping to transmit the voice of the

Box 12-12	Color Therapy and Recognized Associations

■ **Violet**
Compassion, awareness of spiritual self, letting go

■ **Indigo**
Intuition, meditation, and spiritual awareness

■ **Blue**
Expression, relaxing, and serenity

■ **Green**
Feelings, healing, and love

■ **Yellow**
Mental energy, creativity, focus, and concentration

■ **Orange**
Joyfulness, warmth, and happiness

■ **Red**
Enthusiasm, passion, and vitality

creative soul to the physical world. Glandular system: thyroid.
- The sixth chakra, or brow chakra, sits between and slightly above the eyes. Radiating indigo, it controls internal vision, intuition, and self-realization. Glandular system: pituitary.
- The seventh chakra, or crown chakra, lies directly atop the head and corresponds to the highest vibrations.

It vibrates to the color purple and controls integration of the conscious and subconscious minds. Glandular system: pineal. It is interesting to note that the color spectrum found in rainbows is the same as that found in the chakra system.

POLARITY THERAPY

SECTION OBJECTIVES

Chapter objectives covered in this section:

11. Use the principles of polarity therapy as an energetic component of massage application.

Using the information presented in this section, the student will be able to perform the following:

- Explain the basic theory of polarity therapy
- Incorporate the principles of polarity therapy into a massage session

Polarity is a holistic health practice that encompasses some of the theory bases of Asian medicine and Ayurveda. Polarity therapy was developed by Dr. Randolph Stone in the middle 1900s. It is an eclectic, multifaceted system.

Life force energy (e.g., *chi, qi,* and *prana*) has not been a popular subject of Western scientific research. The abstract quality and esoteric nature of the concept are still primarily held in the knowledge base of "spiritual truth." Many spiritual disciplines practice the "laying on of hands." Polarity therapy is also a respectful, compassionate, and intentional laying of the hands on the body.

A physiologic explanation can be postulated as to the result of this therapeutic "laying on of hands" process. Entrainment is one of the most plausible of the physiologic responses. Because some polarity techniques involve rocking motions, all physiologic benefits of rocking apply (see Chapter 10). Gentle stimulation through application of polarity methods to joint receptors generates reflex responses to the associated muscles.

As with all methods of healing touch, something exists beyond the physiologic explanation for the benefit. This "something" is intangible but very real in the experience of it. Therein remains the mystery.

The bodywork principles of polarity blend easily with massage. The intention of the touch is the same as that of therapeutic massage, explained in Chapters 1 and 2 and as a theme throughout this text. Nothing is ever forced. The experience belongs to the client. The practitioner offers the methods not by protocol but through a practiced development of decision making guided by intuition. When the professional feels no attachment to the outcome for his or her own sense of achievement, the methods become "free" to influence the experience of the client (Figure 12-23).

As with the other methods discussed in previous sections of this chapter, the application of polarity methods is simple. However, for those interested in pursuing advanced learning, the goal is to develop the ability to deliver the methods in a purposeful and individualized way, detached from expectation but fascinated with the outcome. Eventually the practitioner learns that the more complex the client situation, the simpler the methods used. The simplicity of polarity makes it one of the gifts to bodywork.

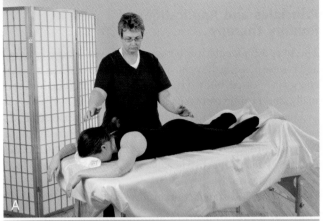
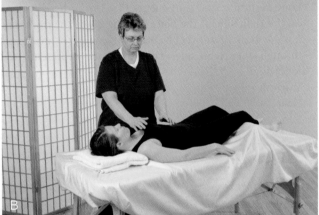
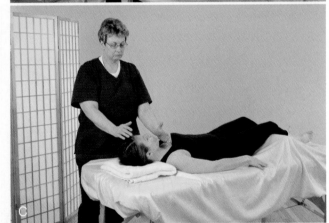
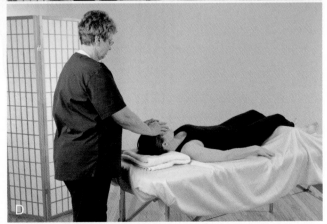

FIGURE 12-23 Energy approaches. The intention of energy-based methods is to balance the bioenergy fields of the body. The key skills are focus and intention.

Principles and Applications of Polarity Therapy

The purpose of polarity therapy is to locate blocked energy and release it, using the principles outlined here. When blocked energy is released, body systems and organs can function normally, and healing can take place naturally.

Polarity therapy does not treat illness or disease; it affects the body (life) energy, which flows in invisible electromagnetic currents through the body's organs and tissues. It stimulates the energy that is inactive in a diseased body part. The following principles apply:

1. The head and spinal column form the central neutral (0) energy axis of the body.
2. Long vertical currents of energy travel from head to foot on the right side of the body, flowing down the front and up the back. Positive (1) outward energy is expressed through the right side. The right side represents the following:
Warmth
Heat
Sun

Yang
Positive, expanding energy
3. On the left side of the body, the vertical currents flow up the front and down the back. Negative (2) inward energy is expressed through the left side. The left side represents the following:
Cooling
Contracting
Moon
Yin
Negative, receptive energy
4. Five electromagnetic currents are present on each side of the body. Each current is related to an element. The elements are ether, air, fire, water, and earth. Each current relates to the organs and functions of its area (Figure 12-24).

The Five Major Body Currents

As mentioned, the five major body currents are ether, air, fire, water, and earth.

- *Ether* is associated with hearing, the voice, the throat, and the quality of nothingness. The core current of the torso flows from north to south (head to pelvis to back). The ether

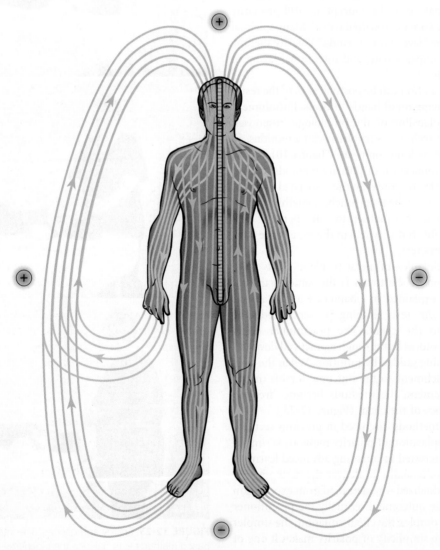

FIGURE 12-24 Electromagnetic currents traveling vertically on the body.

element represents pure vibration and responds to gentleness and love. Characteristics of the ether element are:

Color: Sky blue

Sense: Hearing

Food: Pure air

- *Air* is associated with respiration, circulation, the heart, the lungs, and speed. It flows from east to west (from front to back in a circular pattern).With a balanced air element, we are calm and relaxed. Characteristics of the air element are:

Color: Emerald green

Sense: Touch

Food: Fruits and nuts

- *Fire* is associated with digestion, the stomach, the bowels, warmth, and the heat of the body. A diagonal current found on both sides of the body, it starts at the shoulders and goes to the opposite hip. It is part of the figure-eight energy and is activated by touch, food, and exercise. Characteristics of the fire element are:

Color: Yellow

Sense: Sight

Food: Grains

- *Water* is associated with generative power, creativity, the pelvic organs, sexuality, glandular secretions, emotional drive, equilibrium, and balance. A long current that splits the body in half, it extends from the head to the foot, including the arms and legs. The right side moves clockwise, the left side counterclockwise. Characteristics of the water element are:

Color: Orange

Sense: Taste

Food: Leafy green vegetables, seaweed, watery foods

- *Earth* is associated with the elimination of solids and liquids, the bladder, the rectum, the formation of bone, structure, and support. A zigzag current is formed by solid straight lines from one side to the other. Characteristics of the earth element are:

Color: Red

Sense: Smell

Food: Tubers, meat, dairy

Each of the five electromagnetic currents passes through a corresponding finger and toe, giving its name to the finger and toe (e.g., the middle, or fire, finger; see Figure 12-24).

The polarity (positive [+] or negative [−]) of these electromagnetic currents is shown in Figure 12-25. Positive and negative are opposites. However, the use of positive and negative labels is only relative; it is a way of showing relationships.

The right side of the body is positive (+), whereas the left side of the body is negative (−). The head is positive, whereas the feet are negative. The front of the body is positive, whereas the back is negative. The top is positive, whereas the bottom is negative. Each joint is neutral and is a crossover for energy currents, which change polarity at the crossover. The neutrality of the joints allows them to be flexible. Each finger and toe has an individual polarity (see Figure 12-25).

Blocked energy usually registers as soreness, tenderness, or pain. A simple way to bring energy to an area where it is blocked is to place your left hand on the pain and your right hand opposite that area—on the back, front, or side of the body.

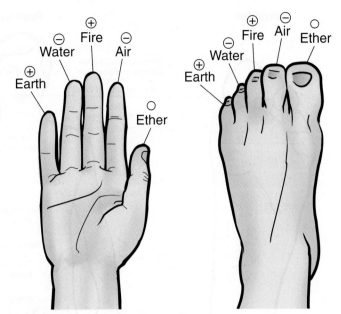

FIGURE 12-25 Finger and toe chart.

Reflexes

Reflexes are points along an energy current that connect with other points along that current. When stimulated, a reflex point can affect the other reflexes on the same energy path. Manipulations that stimulate the foot and hand poles use the reflex principles located there (Figure 12-26).

Positive and Negative Contacts

Because all polarity contacts are bipolar, both hands must be in contact with the body so that energy can move from one hand to the other through the blockage. If the energy blockage is on the front of the body, place the left hand over the painful, blocked area and the right hand on the back of the body directly opposite the left hand. This double contact draws energy through the body from front to back, side to side, and top to bottom contacts.

In practice, a positive contact (e.g., the right hand or fire finger) activates and gives energy. The opposite is also true; a negative contact (e.g., the left hand or air finger) is relaxing and receives energy.

Figure 12-26 shows the foot reflexes as they relate to the rest of the body. In addition to the feet, reflexes are present in the hands, arms, legs, and head. Alternately stimulating a reflex and then its corresponding body part can free blocked energy and allow normal functioning. The negative poles of the body are most frequently obstructed. The negative pole is stimulated first, then the positive pole, to send currents over the entire body.

The use of diagonal contacts on the body activates the serpentine brain wave currents shown in Figure 12-27.

Applying a Polarity Method

1. With most procedures, stimulate the area (rub briskly) for a few minutes, then hold and feel the energy.
2. Hold for 30 to 60 seconds. If you feel no energy after stimulating for 2 minutes, hold for 1 minute longer and then move on.

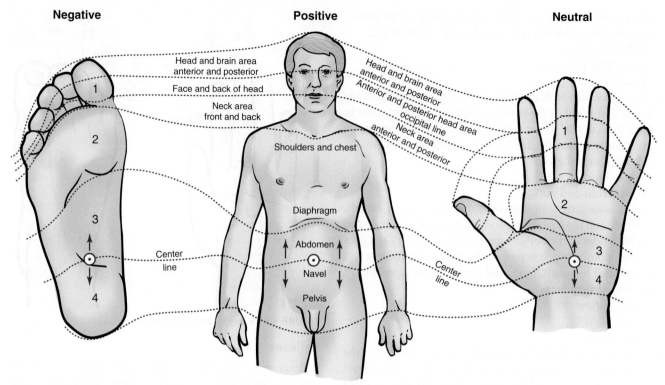

FIGURE 12-26 Reflex relationships among the hand, foot, and body.

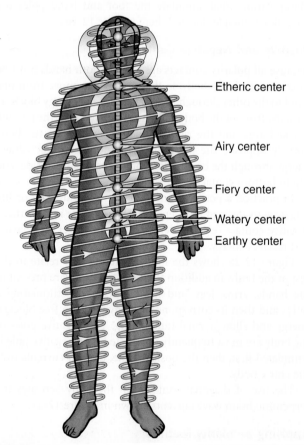

FIGURE 12-27 Brain wave currents crisscrossing the spine from the brain to the coccyx. These currents resemble the caduceus, the ancient Greek symbol for medicine. Each crossover point is known as a *chakra*, or energy center.

💡 **PROFICIENCY EXERCISE 12-7**

1. Design three original massage sessions that incorporate a principle from each topic covered in this chapter.
2. Exchange massage with three students using one of the massage sessions developed in this chapter.
3. While giving 10 general massages to "practice" clients, mentally note each time you use one of the methods in this chapter.
4. Using professional journals and massage school catalogs, find a continuing education opportunity for each method discussed in this chapter. The Internet can be a resource for finding this information.

3. When possible, keep the client's body centered between your hands.
4. Be careful not to cross your hands on your client's body.
5. When stimulating points, use the fleshy pads of your fingers.
6. Be gentle; never force. Forcing creates tension, which blocks energy. A light, gentle touch moves energy.
7. When you feel the energy, the blocked energy is released. Life energy has intelligence. After it is moving, it knows what to do and where to go.
8. People heal at different rates; do not expect a physical result after completion of a procedure. Be neutral when working with a client. Do not let your expectations be a part of the energy.
9. If the manipulations are ineffective, place your hand on your client's body and send love. Visualize energy flowing through your hands to your client (Proficiency Exercise 12-7).

2
12-7

REFLEXOLOGY

SECTION OBJECTIVES

Chapter objectives covered in this section:

12. Modify foot massage to incorporate the philosophy of reflexology.
Using the information presented in this section, the student will be able to perform the following:
• Explain the physiologic benefits of foot and hand massage
• Incorporate the principles of reflexology into a general massage session

Reflexology is the stimulation of areas beneath the skin to improve the function of the whole body or of specific body areas away from the site of the stimulation. Eunice Ingham has been credited with formalizing the system in the West, based on the theory that certain points in the foot and hand affect other body organs and areas. Historically, the approach seems to have originated in China. Foot reflexology is the most popular type of reflexology.

Another approach to reflexology is referred to as *zone therapy.* This method is based on the theory that 10 zones run through the body, and reflex points for stimulation are located within these zones.

Reflexology applies the stimulus/reflex principle to healing the body. The foot has been mapped to show the areas to contact to affect different parts of the body. Charts mapping these areas vary somewhat (Figure 12-28). Typically, the large toe represents the head, and the junction of the large toe and the foot represents the neck. The next toes represent the eyes, ears, and sinuses. The waist is about midway on the arch of the foot, with various organs above and below the line. The

reflex points for the spine are along the medial longitudinal arch. It is thought that this stimulus/response reflex is conducted through neural pathways in the body that initiate the body's electrical and biochemical activities.

The medical definition of reflexology is "the study of reflexes." Reflexotherapy is treatment by manipulation applied to an area away from the disorder. In physiologic terms, a reflex is an involuntary response to a stimulus.

This chapter's discussion of reflexology attempts to explain why foot and hand massage is beneficial in terms of standard physiology; it avoids the issue of whether actual corresponding points exist on the foot or hand that relate directly to other body areas. An explanation based on standard anatomy and physiology is better suited to the format of this textbook and may be better accepted by the public.

Research to support reflexology methods is sparse and inconclusive, and it is important to inform and educate the client about the lack of Western-based scientific validation. At the same time, when methods such as reflexology have a long and strong historical and cultural foundation, it is also wise not to completely discount the methods. Evidence-based practice does include this type of validation.

Physiologic Reflexes of the Foot

The foot is a very complex structure. The ankle and foot consist of 34 joints, with many joint and reflex patterns (Box 12-13). The nerve distribution to the feet and hands is extensive. The position of the foot sends considerable postural information from the joint mechanoreceptors through the central nervous system. The sensory and motor centers of the brain devote a large area to the foot and hand.

It seems logical to assume that stimulation of the feet activates the body-wide responses, such as gait reflexes and the autonomic nervous system. This fact alone is helpful in explaining the benefits of foot and hand massage. In addition, many nerve endings on the feet and hands correlate with acupressure points, which trigger the release of endorphins and other endogenous chemicals when stimulated. In addition, major plexuses for the lymph system are located in the hands and feet. Rhythmic compressive forces in these areas stimulate lymphatic movement.

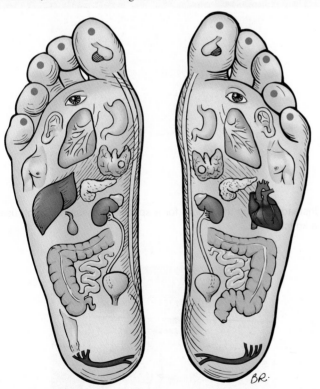

FIGURE 12-28 In traditional reflexology, thumb pressure is typically used. However, the thumb cannot withstand this amount of compressive force. Instead of using the thumbs to apply pressure, use a knuckle.

> ### Box 12-13 Reflexes Associated with the Foot
>
> *Achilles tendon reflex:* Plantar flexion/extension of the foot, resulting from contraction of the calf muscles after a sharp blow to the Achilles tendon; similar to the knee-jerk reflex.
> *Extensor thrust:* A quick, brief extension of a limb after application of pressure to the plantar surface.
> *Flexor withdrawal:* Flexion of the lower extremity when the foot receives a painful stimulus.
> *Mendel-Bekhterev reflex:* Plantar flexion of the toes in response to percussion of the dorsum of the foot.
> *Postural reflex:* Any reflex involved in maintaining posture.
> *Proprioceptive reflex:* A reflex initiated by movement of the body to maintain the position of the moved part; any reflex initiated by stimulation of a proprioceptor.
> *Rossolimo's reflex:* Plantar flexion of the second to fifth toes in response to percussion of the plantar surface of the toes.

Reflex Phenomena

Reflex phenomena must be put into perspective. Reflex points are located throughout the whole body, including the hands, head, ears, and torso. If you consider all the reflexology points, acupuncture points, neurolymphatic points, motor points, and other reflex points, the body itself can be seen as a point. Because of the reflex nature of the body and its inherent ability to self-regulate in response to stimulation, it usually is not necessary to overly focus on a particular system's name and use for a point.

More important is the ability to identify these various points during assessment procedures, to analyze the body context of the point, and to choose effective treatment for it. Assessment usually indicates an area tender to palpation if the point is hypersensitive or if the reflex structure associated with the particular point is hyperreactive. The opposite is true if the point area feels empty, numb, or disconnected from the surrounding tissue.

There are two basic treatment processes:

- If a reflexive point is tender and therefore likely to be overactive, relaxation and sedating methods are used.
- If the point is underactive, stimulation methods are applied.

If you are not sure which application is appropriate, trust the innate balancing ability of the body. Alternately use both approaches, allowing the body to choose.

Massage for the Foot

An excellent way to massage the foot is to apply pressure and movement systematically to the entire foot and ankle complex. The pressure stimulates the circulation, nerves, and reflexes. Moving all the joints stimulates large-diameter nerve fibers and joint mechanoreceptors, initiating hyperstimulation analgesia. The result is a shift in proprioceptive and postural reflexes. The sheer volume of sensory information flooding the central nervous system has significant effects in the body. The usual result is parasympathetic dominance.

Foot massage usually is boundary safe; that is, most people accept foot or hand massage when the idea of removing the clothing is objectionable. Hand and foot massage is likely to be the most effective form of self-massage. The hand and foot have similar motor cortex distribution patterns. Stimulation of the hands during the self-massage does not override the sensations to the feet being massaged. The hands are massaged while they massage the feet (Proficiency Exercise 12-8).

Often essential oils are applied to the feet (see the Aromatherapy section). The sole of the foot is highly vascular and therefore is thought to absorb the lipid (fat) in essential oils. The foot also is a safe place to apply essential oils, because the oil is not easily spread into an area of mucus membranes (e.g., the nose or eye), where it can become an irritant. See reflexology techniques demonstrated in the foot massage/reflexology protocol.

FOOT MASSAGE/REFLEXOLOGY PROTOCOL

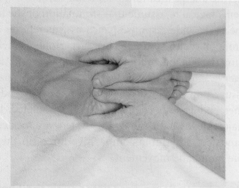

In traditional reflexology, thumb pressure usually is used. However, the thumb cannot withstand this amount of compression.

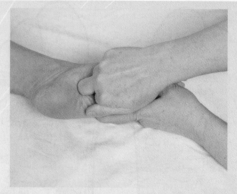

Instead of using the thumb for a specific pressure or point, use a knuckle.

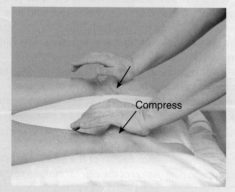

Prone compression.

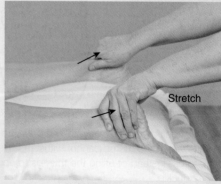

Prone stretch.

REFLEXOLOGY PROTOCOL—cont'd

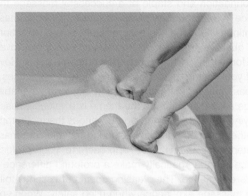

Fist compression.

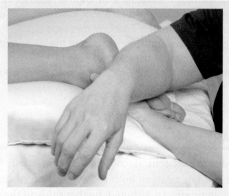

Forearm compression.

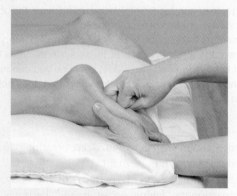

Knuckle used to compress specific reflexology points.

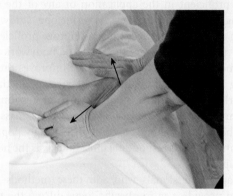

Side-lying stretch.

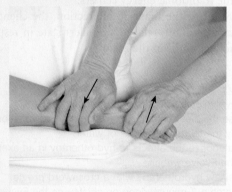

Stretch for foot, dorsal.

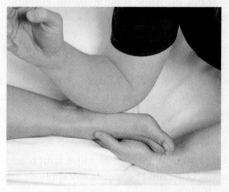

Side-lying forearm compression.

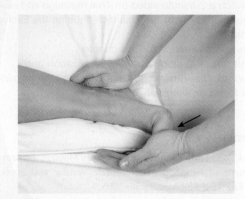

Arch and toe stretch.

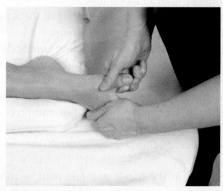

Individual toe stretch.

💡 PROFICIENCY EXERCISE 12-8

1. Exchange foot massages with another student or visit a professional reflexologist for a foot massage. Compare the effects with those of a full-body massage.
2. Using a skeletal model, move each of the joints of the foot. Then move each of the joints of your foot.
3. Massage your feet daily for 15 minutes for 2 weeks and take note of the effects.

SUMMARY

Each bodywork system is complete within itself; however, extensive overlap exists in both the application of techniques and physiologic effects. Although further study of the methods presented will benefit the massage professional, the ability to become proficient in the application of any of the systems, including therapeutic massage, is a lifelong study. Just as studying a foreign language tends to improve proficiency in a person's primary language, the study of bodywork systems complementary to therapeutic massage improves the understanding and technical application of massage methods. All bodywork systems are forms of structured professional touch that complement, not replace, each other. As massage and various bodywork methods become increasingly popular, the establishment that is responding most quickly is the health spa (see Chapter 13).

Massage professionals who add these methods to their skills can provide a more specific focus during the massage. For example, a client might enjoy a relaxing foot bath and sip a cup of hot tea while waiting for the appointment. The client and the massage therapist may drink a glass of water together.

Alternative methods also can be integrated into a massage session in many other ways.

- A cold compress could be placed on the back of the neck, the forehead, or other area of the body during the massage.
- Essential oils can be used as a room fragrance or added to the massage lubricant.
- Gliding could be focused to move lymph and blood in the veins, or it could be specifically applied in the grooves of the body to stimulate the meridians.
- Compression could be applied moving down the arteries to stimulate arterial blood flow.
- Compression, vibration, and tapping of the acupuncture points may normalize body function.
- Kneading, stretching, and friction methods applied slowly and deliberately to drag, pull, and elongate might soften and normalize the connective tissue.
- The occasional trigger point might be treated with direct pressure or frictioning, with a hot compress or stone applied afterward. An ice pack sometimes may be a better choice after frictioning to control the amount of inflammation.
- Every joint in the hands and feet may be moved, and attention may be given to compression on the bottoms of the hands and feet to stimulate the flow of lymph. The

💡 FOOT IN THE DOOR

The foundation and staple of a successful massage therapy practice is the moderate pressure, basic, full-body massage. The infinite variations in pressure levels, speed, direction, and other qualities of touch make massage valuable, in and of itself, for helping clients reach their outcome goals. However, to get your foot in the door in many massage practices, such as spas, massage franchises, and so forth, the ability to provide a little variation on the theme is a valuable asset. It is satisfying to be able to incorporate various thermotherapy and hydrotherapy methods before, during, or after the massage. An intentional and intuitive approach to your professional practice is to energetically make a profound difference in the client's experience. The pleasing scents of essential oils add to the massage experience when used safely. When you can explain to a potential employer or client how you can blend aspects of complementary bodywork methods into the massage, they can factor into your qualifications the ability to offer a variety of stress-reducing methods.

Remember to describe your skills in complementary bodywork methods ethically. Each of these systems has a unique base of knowledge and skills. Just because you can incorporate concepts of reflexology into foot massage does not mean you can claim to be a reflexologist.

client can be instructed in deep breathing to further encourage lymph movement.
- Awareness of the energy patterns of the body and the compassionate "laying on of hands" becomes part of every technique. Warm stones or seed bags can be placed on the traditional energy centers.

As a result of the massage interaction, the client should experience a pleasant, relaxed, and alert state in response to the physiologic shifts in the body

⊘volve

http://evolve.elsevier.com/Fritz/fundamentals/
12-1 Use the electronic flashcards on the Evolve website to study the therapeutic uses of water.
12-2 Categorize the effects of hydrotherapy in an exercise on the Evolve website.
12-3 Review hydrotherapy with a crossword puzzle.
12-4 Watch a 2-minute video on shiatsu on the Evolve website.
12-5 Watch a 2-minute video on Thai massage and read about the history of the Thai technique on the Evolve website.
12-6 Review new terms for this chapter.
Don't forget to study for your certification and licensure exams! Review questions, along with weblinks, can be found on the Evolve website.

References

Bernas M, Witte M, Kriederman B, et al: Massage therapy in the treatment of lymphedema: rationale, results, and applications, *IEEE Eng Med Biol Mag* 24:58, 2005.

Buchman DD: *The complete book of water therapy: 500 ways to use our oldest natural medicine*, New York, 1979, EP Dutton.

Chaitow L: *The acupuncture treatment of pain*, Rochester, Vt, 1990, Healing Arts Press.

Chaitow L: Workshop notes, trigger point assessment and treatment, Lapeer, Mich, 1988, 1991, 1992, 1993.

Chaitow L, Delany J: *Clinical application of neuromuscular techniques*, ed 2, vol 1, *The upper body*, London, 2002, Churchill Livingstone.

Cunningham S: *Cunningham's encyclopedia of crystal, gem and metal magic*, Woodbury, Minnesota, 2002, Llewellyn Publications.

Cyriax J, Coldham M: *The textbook of orthopaedic medicine treatment by manipulation massage and injection*, ed 11, vol 2, East Sussex, England, 1984, Bailliere Tindall.

Dorsher PT: Trigger points and acupuncture points: anatomic and clinical correlations, *Medical Acupuncture*, May, 2006. www.medicalacupuncture.org/aama_marf/journal/vol17_3/article_3.html, Accessed May 23, 2011.

Dorsher PT: Myofascial referred-pain data provide physiologic evidence of acupuncture meridians, *J Pain* 10:723, 2009.

Dorsher PT, Fleckenstein J: Trigger points and classical acupuncture points. Part 2. Clinical correspondences in treating pain and somatovisceral disorders, *Deutsche Zeitschrift für Akupunktur* 51:6, 2008.

Findley T: 2009 Fascia Research Congress and Scientific Background. http://structuralintegration.net/si_news/2009%20Fascia%20Research%20Congress.pdf. Accessed 1–7 2011.

Gerwin RD: (2008) The taut band and other mysteries of the trigger point: an examination of the mechanisms relevant to the development and maintenance of the trigger point, *J Musculoskelet Pain* 15(Suppl 13):115–121, 2008.

Gunn C: *Reprints on pain, acupuncture and related subjects*, Seattle, 1992, University of Washington.

Johari H: *Ayurvedic massage: traditional Indian techniques for balancing body and mind*, Rochester, Vt, 1996, Healing Arts Press.

Klingler W, Schleip MA, Zorn A: Structural integration: European Fascia Research Project Report, *Journal of the Rolf Institute*, December, 2004. Accessed July 7, 2010.www.fasciaresearch.de/ProjectInterimReport04.pdf.

Koul R, Dufan T, Russell C, et al: Efficacy of complete decongestive therapy and manual lymphatic drainage on treatment-related lymphedema in breast cancer, *Int J Radiat Oncol Biol Phys* 67:841, 2007.

Kreighbaum E, Barthels KM: *Biomechanics: a qualitative approach for studying human movement*, ed 4, New York, 1995, Benjamin Cummings.

Langevin HM: Connective tissue: a body-wide signaling network? *Med Hypotheses* 66:1074, 2006.

Langevin HM, Konofagou EE, Badger GJ, et al: Tissue displacements during acupuncture using ultrasound elastography techniques, World Federation for Ultrasound in Medicine & Biology, 2004. http://www.med.uvm.edu/neurology/TB1+BL.asp?SiteAreaID=518 accessed October 10, 2011.

Lederman E: *Fundamentals of manual therapy: physiology, neurology, and psychology*, ed 2, New York, 2005, Churchill Livingstone.

Masunaga S, Ohashi W: *Zen shiatsu: how to harmonize yin and yang for better health*, New York, 1977, Japan Publications.

Meltzer KR, Standley PR: Modeled repetitive motion strain and indirect osteopathic manipulative techniques in regulation of human fibroblast proliferation and interleukin secretion, *J Am Osteopath Assoc* 107:527, 2007.

Myers T: *Anatomy trains: myofascial meridians for manual and movement therapists*, ed 2, New York, 2008, Churchill Livingstone.

Ohashi W: *Do-it-yourself shiatsu: how to perform the ancient Japanese art of acupuncture without needles*, New York, 1993, Penguin Books.

Price S, Price L: *Aromatherapy for health professionals*, London, 2006, Churchill Livingstone.

Remvig L, Ellis RM, Patijn J: Myofascial release: an evidence-based treatment approach? *Int Musculoskel Med* 30:29, 2008.

Schleip R: An interview with Prof. Dr. Med. J. Staubesand, *Rolf Lines* 26:35, 1998. http://www.somatics.de/somatics-06.html accessed 10–11 2011.

Schnaubelt K: *Advanced aromatherapy: the science of essential oil therapy*, Rochester Vt, 1998, Healing Arts Press.

Shah JP, Danoff JV, Desai MJ, et al: Biochemicals associated with pain and inflammation are elevated in sites near to and remote from active myofascial trigger points, *Arch Phys Med Rehabil* 89:16, 2008.

Simons D: New views of myofascial trigger points: etiology and diagnosis, *Arch Phys Med Rehabil* 89:157, 2008.

Standley PR, Meltzer K: In vitro modeling of repetitive motion strain and manual medicine treatments: potential roles for pro- and anti-inflammatory cytokines, *J Bodyw Mov Ther* 12:201, 2008.

Tappan F, Benjamin P: *Tappan's handbook of healing massage techniques: classic, holistic, and emerging methods*, ed 4, New York, 2004, Appleton & Lange.

Tissarand R, Balacs T: *Essential oil safety*, New York, 1995, Churchill Livingstone.

Travell JG, Simons DG: *Myofascial pain and dysfunction: the trigger point manual*, vol 2, Baltimore, 1999, Williams & Wilkins.

Veith I, Rose K: *The yellow emperor's classic of internal medicine*, Berkeley, Calif, 2002, University of California Press.

Watt M: Plant aromatics: a data and reference manual on essential oils and aromatic plant extracts. http://atlanticinstitute.com/safety.html, Accessed May 23, 2011.

Wiseman N, Feng Y: *A practical dictionary of Chinese medicine*, Brookline, Mass, 1997, Harcourt.

Yao JH: Acutherapy, 1984, Acutherapy Postgraduate Seminars, 808 Paddock Lane, Libertyville, Ill 60048.

Yu HZ, Rose K: *Who can ride the dragon?* Brookline, Mass, 1999, Harcourt.

Zorn A: Physical thoughts about structure: the elasticity of fascia and structural integration. March, 2007. www.rolfingb.de/papers/zorn_elastic-fascia_2007.pdf. Accessed May 27, 2011.

Bibliography

Anderson SK: *The practice of shiatsu*, St Louis, 2008, Mosby.

Gold R: Thai massage: a traditional medical technique, ed 2, St Louis, 2007, Mosby.

Additional Resource

The International Medical Spa Association, 310 17th Street, Union City, New Jersey 07087.

Workbook Section

Short Answer

1. Why is continuing education required to use the methods presented in this chapter effectively?

2. What are the primary effects of hydrotherapy?

3. What are some simple hydrotherapy methods the massage practitioner can use that do not require special hydrotherapy equipment?

4. What are some important contraindications to and precautions for the use of ice?

5. What are safety precautions for incorporating stones into a massage?

6. What is systemic massage and what results can be expected from this type of massage?

7. What are the basic procedures for lymphatic massage?

8. What are the basic procedures for circulatory massage?

9. What are the physiologic mechanisms that make reflexology a valuable massage approach?

10. What are the recommended methods for foot massage?

11. Why is hand and foot self-massage beneficial?

12. What are connective tissue approaches?

13. What is the intent of connective tissue massage?

14. Why is additional education so important before using connective tissue approaches?

15. What is a trigger point?

16. How are trigger points located?

17. What methods are used to normalize trigger points?

18. What types of therapy follow treatment of a trigger point?

19. What is the Western terminology for acupuncture points, meridians, and yin and yang?

20. What wisdom is offered by the Eastern and Asian approaches for the massage practitioner?

21. Where are acupuncture points located?

22. How are acupuncture points treated?

23. How does polarity therapy combine the knowledge base of both Asian and Ayurvedic systems?

24. How is color an aspect of healing systems?

25. What are the safety precautions for including essential oils in a massage?

Matching I

Match the term to the best definition.

_____ 1. Acupressure
_____ 2. Ayurveda
_____ 3. Cryotherapy
_____ 4. Hydrotherapy
_____ 5. Myofascial release
_____ 6. Polarity therapy
_____ 7. Reflexology
_____ 8. Shiatsu
_____ 9. Systemic massage
_____ 10. Trigger point
_____ 11. Yang
_____ 12. Yin

a. In Eastern thought, the part of the whole realm of function of the body, mind, and spirit that corresponds to the parasympathetic autonomic nervous system functions

b. In Eastern thought, the part of the whole realm of function of the body, mind, and spirit that corresponds to the sympathetic autonomic nervous system functions

c. An area of local nerve facilitation that results in hypertonicity of a muscle bundle and referred pain patterns

d. Therapeutic use of various types and temperatures of water applications

e. Methods of toning or sedating acupuncture points that do not involve the use of needles

f. A system of health care that uniquely developed the tridosha system

g. The therapeutic use of ice

h. Massage primarily structured to affect one body system; an approach usually used for lymphatic and circulation enhancement massage

i. A system of bodywork that affects the connective tissue through various methods that elongate and alter the plastic component and ground substance of the connective tissue

j. An eclectic system that combines principles of Asian theory and Ayurveda

k. A massage system directed primarily at the feet and hands

l. An acupressure- and meridian-focused bodywork system

Matching II

Various reflexes are associated with the feet. Match the reflex with its description.

_____ **1.** Achilles tendon reflex
_____ **2.** Extensor thrust reflex
_____ **3.** Flexor withdrawal reflex
_____ **4.** Mendel-Bekhterev reflex
_____ **5.** Postural reflex
_____ **6.** Proprioceptive reflex
_____ **7.** Rossolimo's reflex

a. Plantar flexion/extension of the foot resulting from contraction of calf muscles after a sharp blow to the Achilles tendon; similar to the knee-jerk reflex

b. Flexion of the lower extremity when the foot receives a painful stimulus

c. Plantar flexion of the toes in response to percussion of the dorsum of the foot

d. A quick, brief extension of a limb on application of pressure to the plantar surface

e. A reflex initiated by movement of the body to maintain the position of the moved part; any reflex initiated by stimulation of a proprioceptor

f. Any reflex concerned with maintaining posture

g. Plantar flexion of the second to fifth toes in response to percussion of the plantar surface of the toes

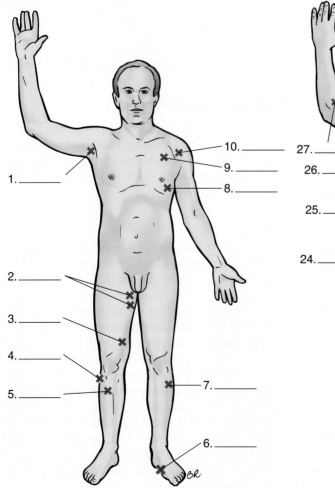
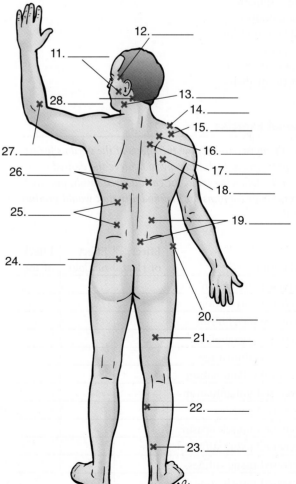

FIGURE 12-29

Labeling

Label the muscles to show the locations of common trigger points in Figure 12-29 on page 525.

A. Abductor hallucis
B. Adductor longus
C. Anterior serratus
D. Biceps femoris
E. Deltoid
F. Gastrocnemius
G. Gluteus medius
H. Gluteus minimus
I. Iliocostalis
J. Infraspinatus
K. Levator
L. Long extensors
M. Longissimus
N. Masseter
O. Multifidus
P. Pectoralis
Q. Peroneus longus
R. Soleus
S. Splenius capitis
T. Sternocleidomastoid
U. Subscapularis
V. Supinators
W. Supraspinatus
X. Temporalis
Y. Tibialis anterior
Z. Trapezius
AA. Upper trapezius
BB. Vastus medialis

Additional Exercise

Massage therapists must know the effects of the various forms and temperatures of hydrotherapy to achieve the desired results. In the following table, for each desired result, put an X in the column or columns for the modality that would produce that result.

Desired Result	Effect of Heat	Effect of Cold	Effect of Ice
1. Increased circulation			
2. Decreased circulation			
3. Increased metabolism			
4. Decreased metabolism			
5. Increased stimulation			
6. Increased inflammation			
7. Decreased inflammation			
8. Decreased pain			
9. Decreased muscle spasm			
10. Decreased tissue stiffness			
11. Increased tissue stiffness			
12. Increased muscle tone			

Problem-Solving Scenarios

1. How can you tell the difference between a trigger point and an acupuncture point?

2. A client wants a general relaxation massage but has some mild circulatory sluggishness. What style of massage would you use to best serve the client?

Assess Your Competencies

Now that you have studied this chapter, you should be able to:
- Understand the physiologic mechanisms of complementary bodywork systems
- Identify overlap in the technical skills used in the various systems and integrate concepts of these systems into therapeutic massage
- Consider a direction of interest for further study

On a separate sheet of paper or on the computer, write a short summary of the content of this chapter based on the preceding list of competencies. Use a conversational tone, as if you were explaining to someone (e.g., a client, prospective employer, coworker, or other interested person) the importance of the information and skills to the development of the massage profession.

Next, in small discussion groups, share your summary with your classmates and compare the ways the information was presented. In discussing the content, look for similarities, differences, possibilities for misunderstanding of the information, and clear, concise methods of description.

Professional Applications

1. You have been in practice as a massage therapist for about 3 years. An increasing number of your clients seem to have connective tissue problems. What types of continuing education would help you to work most effectively with these clients?

2. You have the opportunity to work in a pain management clinic with a team of health care professionals that consists of an osteopathic physician, a nurse practitioner, a psychologist, a physical therapist, an acupuncturist, and a nutritionist. Based on the information in this chapter, develop a presentation explaining the integration of complementary bodywork methods into massage therapy. (Use a separate piece of paper.) Include recommendations for additional education for yourself. Justify or explain the benefit of continuing education in one of the modalities discussed in this chapter. Explain why you think this method would offer the most benefit combined with therapeutic massage. Also, consider what other modalities the other bodywork professionals may be using in the clinic. Use the clinical reasoning model as you prepare your presentation.

Massage Career Tracks and Practice Settings

CHAPTER OBJECTIVES

After completing this chapter, the student will be able to perform the following:

1. Describe the history of the spa industry and current trends.
2. Explain the importance of branding, signature products, and services.
3. Identify types of spas.
4. Describe and demonstrate spa safety and etiquette.
5. Adapt massage for the wellness/spa practice setting.
6. Define terms and identify types of products used in the spa industry.
7. Compare a variety of spa treatments and services.
8. Define the spa franchise business model.
9. Identify cross-training recommendations for a career in the wellness/spa industry.
10. Describe a typical day at a spa.
11. Identify and demonstrate the skills and responsibilities necessary for practice in the health care environment.
12. Explain how massage therapists behave and what skills are necessary to maintain compliance with HIPAA, health insurance, record keeping, and confidentiality in the health care environment.
13. Use basic pharmacology information to practice massage safely in the health care environment.
14. Practice massage therapy as part of healthcare/complementary and alternative medicine.
15. Identify cross-training recommendations for a career in the health care environment.
16. Identify and demonstrate the skills and responsibilities necessary for massage therapy practice in the sports and fitness environment.
17. Describe and adapt massage for the sport and fitness practice setting
18. Identify cross training recommendations for a career in the sports and fitness industry.

CHAPTER OUTLINE

KEY TERMS

Best practice
Biopsychosocial model of medicine
Complementary and alternative medicine (CAM)
Franchise
Integrative medicine
Pharmacology
Recovery massage
Rehabilitative massage
Remedial massage
Spa

The three main career tracks for massage can be categorized as follows:

- Wellness/spa massage
- Health care (clinical/medical) massage
- Sports performance and fitness massage

These career tracks typically are defined more by the location where the massage is provided, common outcomes requested for the massage, and parameters that define a specific population.

The current kaleidoscope of massage practice can create much confusion for the massage student, the massage practitioner, potential employers, and the consumer. The trend is for all the outcomes, environments, and populations to overlap. Consider the following examples.

- Scar tissue management for cosmetic surgery may be combined with general full-body massage in a medical spa; this appears to be a case of clinical/medical massage, but it takes place in the spa setting.
- Restorative massage with essential oils and soft music and lighting may be provided to support relaxation and sleep for athletes after a competition; this appears to be spa focused, but the population derives from sports and fitness.
- Massage to increase flexibility, improve posture and gait, and provide lymphatic drainage may be done to address soreness after exercise for participants in a cardiac rehabilitation program; this appears to be sports and fitness targeted, but the massage is provided in the clinical/medical setting.

Think of the career situation in massage as something like a sandwich. The "filling" is always the same (i.e., the information presented in this text and in *Mosby's Essential Sciences for Therapeutic Massage*); however, each practitioner may choose different "bread" (i.e., clinical/medical massage, sports massage, or spa massage). When you graduate from a well-designed, well-implemented massage curriculum, you should have the "filling" in this professional sandwich; this chapter provides an overview of the "bread."

What determines the focus of the massage? The most obvious answers are the practice setting and individual client outcomes.

The health care/medical environment consists of health care professionals who work in various settings, such as hospitals, physical therapy clinics, and specialty centers (e.g., cancer treatment or dialysis); as private practice physicians; and in hospice and long-term care.

The sports and fitness environment consists of fitness centers, academic sports facilities (e.g., for high school track or collegiate gymnastics), and centers for professional or semi-professional athletes (e.g., golfers, football players, soccer players, baseball players). These facilities are staffed by professionals such as exercise specialists, athletic trainers, and coaches. In addition, the needs of individuals who exercise for fitness and those of recreational and mature athletes must be addressed.

The spa environment is extremely varied; it includes local day spas and chain spas in various resorts, hotel chains, and cruise ships. The focus of a massage in the spa setting can be:

- To serve as an adjunct to cosmetic procedures performed by professionals such as cosmetologists, estheticians, and nail technicians
- To serve as an adjunct to hydrotherapy treatments for the purposes of relaxation and detoxification
- To support anti-aging programs
- To serve as part of the program at a retreat center
- To support a weight management program

Regardless of the setting, the spa environment has several consistent characteristics: ambience; a peaceful, pleasant location; pampering; and multiple services that can be selected from a spa menu. The spa environment is more commercial and entrepreneurial than the sports and fitness and health care environments. The spa environment deals with strategic marketing. The spa industry is extremely innovative in creating branded (also called *signature*) products and services that identify the uniqueness of the particular spa.

Each of these three main environments has specific roles that require the various professionals, and specific ways massage fits into and supports multidisciplinary care. Regardless of the environment, each client must be addressed according to his or her unique situation. For each of the populations discussed, this chapter describes the adaptations and accommodations that may be necessary for the individual client, regardless of the environment in which the massage is provided. In each of the practice settings, the massage therapist can practice as an independent contractor, an employee, or a business owner in private practice (see Chapter 3).

THERAPEUTIC MASSAGE IN THE WELLNESS/SPA ENVIRONMENT

SECTION OBJECTIVES

Chapter objectives covered in this section:
1. Describe the history of the spa industry and current trends.
2. Explain the importance of branding, signature products and services.
3. Identify types of spas.
4. Describe and demonstrate spa safety and etiquette.
5. Adapt massage for the wellness/spa practice setting.
6. Define terms and identify types of products used in the spa industry.
7. Compare a variety of spa treatments and services.
8. Define the spa franchise business model.
9. Identify cross training recommendations for a career in the wellness/spa industry.
10. Describe a typical day at a spa.

Using the information presented in this section, the student will be able to perform the following:
- Describe various spa settings
- Describe the unique aspects of massage in the spa environment, such as brand image, safety, etiquette, and the responsibilities of the massage therapist
- List types of spa treatments and use various massage and bodywork methods in the spa environment
- Alter fundamental massage training to the specific requirements of a franchise setting

The spa industry is one of the fastest growing career options for massage therapists. Because of the increased pace and multiple stresses of modern living, people have both a need and a desire for effective relaxation to counteract or reverse life's pressures. People go to spas for fitness, stress management, peace of mind, pampering and pleasure, and health and wellness.

As mentioned, the spa industry is extremely innovative at creating signature products and services that become unique signifiers of the particular spa. Because the pressures of modern lifestyles and daily activities are becoming ever more stressful, the spa concept of a health retreat has mushroomed in popularity. Historically, American spas have not been as "cure" oriented as European spas; rather, they are more fitness and beauty oriented. However, American spas are converting quickly to an integrated system.

The massage franchise concept, although not based on the spa model, is very similar. However, the main focus is offering affordable massage in a safe, professional setting. These businesses tend to use the wellness model that encompasses the therapeutic experience of massage; it is just not provided in a medical setting.

Although the basic massage procedures in this textbook form the foundation of the various styles of massage offered in the spa environment, each spa creates its own presentation by offering different combinations of services (see Chapter 12). For example:

- Aromatherapy massage may be provided with a signature blend of essential oils developed by the spa.
- The spa may provide a signature massage style that uses aspects of Eastern and Western methods and combine it with color therapy to promote deep relaxation and support rejuvenation of the body.
- Massage with hot stones may be combined with cold hydrotherapy and meditative music created specifically for the spa to provide relaxation and introspection for self-enlightenment.
- The spa may provide historical or culturally based massage (e.g., amma, lomi lomi, Thai massage, shiatsu, or Swedish massage).

Massage students interested in the complex, ever-changing spa environment must understand the following:

- The underlying general themes of the spa industry
- How uniqueness in environment and services is developed and implemented
- The foundation of the general categories of massage application in the spa industry
- The application and benefits of spa services other than massage

With this knowledge and the appropriate skills, the massage graduate should be able to adapt easily to a specific spa and the in-house training it provides. The massage professional also needs to be able to perform to the expectations of the spa.

In addition, practitioners must understand the physical effects of hydrotherapy, the various common and safe essential oils, and the use of adjunct implements, products, and methods (e.g., stones, scrubs, muds and clays, magnets, vibration methods, color, and sound). They also must understand how these methods are combined to create the signature massage style offered by the spa. Much of this information was presented in Chapter 12.

To understand what it is like to work in a spa, it is important to understand the history of spas, the general types of spas, and the common populations drawn to various spa environments. Additionally, a knowledge of professional behavior, ethics, and business strategies characteristic of the spa environment is essential.

The History of the Spa

Although the popularity of spas seems to have sprung up overnight, people have been visiting some form of spa for thousands of years. The word spa is rooted in the Latin language and is short for *salus per aquam,* which means "health from water." The use of water as therapy can be traced back to early civilizations (see Chapter 12). Throughout history, the different time periods brought different meanings and purposes for a bath or spa. Social bathing was an important cultural process practiced by the Mesopotamians, Egyptians, Minoans, Greeks, and Romans whenever they sought health and relief from pain and disease. The natural hot springs in Bath, England, were used by the Romans and are recognized for their therapeutic properties. At Bath, the springs generate more than 1 million gallons of mineral water at a temperature of 120° F each day. This mineral water contains numerous elements, such as magnesium, potassium, sulfur, and calcium.

Native Americans also found medicinal waters and used them for regeneration and physical and spiritual health. Colonists often would build log cabins and wooden tubs for bathing near these sites. Today hot water is common; in previous centuries, hot water in nature was rare, and the process of heating water was time-consuming and labor intensive.

Eventually, baths and spas became more than just places near hot springs; they evolved into modern day resorts. During the eighteenth and nineteenth centuries, spas began to be staffed by medical professionals who prescribed and carefully monitored the treatments given to each visitor. The treatments primarily consisted of either soaking in the water or drinking it.

With the medical discoveries of the early twentieth century, hospitals replaced the spas. Existing spas changed focus and began offering luxury accommodations, and many eventually turned into vacation locations or clinics that concentrated on weight loss or catering to the wealthy.

Current trends in the spa environment indicate an interesting combination of ancient traditions from many cultures and modern scientific research. Recently many additions have been made to spa water therapies; these have come as a result of advances in technology that allow the therapeutic use of water with various types of equipment (e.g., a hot tub replaces the hot spring).

In recent years, the value of prevention, healthy lifestyles, and relaxation has been rediscovered, and the spa is again finding its place as a location uniquely qualified to address these needs. The spa industry is embracing holistic health care and wellness. Today the spa is returning to its roots; the medical spa is a growing industry.

Brand Image

A brand is a collection of products created and marketed for a specific spa business. Building a brand becomes increasingly important both for independent spa businesses and for large chains, such as branded hotel companies. The users of both day spas and resort spas rely on the strength and reputation of the brand. The challenge for spa management is to maintain brand standards internationally in the new global economy. Standardization in service delivery is essential, which is why most spas train their staff no matter what educational background the staff has coming into the spa.

The Spa Signature

Spas offer a variety of treatments along with products to meet their clients' needs and expectations. Each spa approach tends to be unique to the spa (i.e., signature treatments, or branding). Services attempt to balance scientific advances and clinical treatments with ancient wisdom and alternative approaches to total skin and body care.

A spa needs to be staffed with people who are educated, licensed, or certified as necessary and who are willing to learn and perform the spa's signature treatments. Massage professionals who are successful in the spa environment have a solid foundation both in the fundamentals of massage application and in adjunct methods such as hydrotherapy and aromatherapy. Even with this education, they are willing to undergo training to learn how to do the spa's specific treatments.

Spa Trends

An increasingly sophisticated consumer is requiring a more sophisticated spa experience. The industry is responding through a market-specific focus by creating spas with specialized services such as teen spas, men-only spas, spas for expectant mothers, and even spas that provide services for pets. A broader population is being introduced to spa services, primarily through the resort and day spa industry.

The development of clearly identifiable, branded spas will lead the way for consolidation in the spa industry. Chain spas are becoming popular; therefore, it is critical that throughout the process of brand development, companies consider targeting specific markets or appealing to a mass market. This trend is apparent with companies such as Stiener Leisure, Bliss, Starwood Spa Resorts, and Willow Stream Spas (inside Fairmont hotels). The luxury-segment market leaders, such as Mandarin Oriental, Four Seasons, and Ritz-Carlton, can expand their spas internationally by creating an additional brand to support the spa operations. As consumers develop loyalty to specific spa brands, it will become increasingly crucial for each spa to develop its signature, consistently delivered regardless of location.

Challenges of a Brand Image

With regard to massage education, the stated focus of this text is that massage application needs to be based on the client's goals and individualized for each client. In the spa environment, the massage therapist may be expected to perform standardized protocols that are based on the spa's signature approach rather than the client's goals. The massage therapist must learn these protocols and structure the massage application according to the spa's direction. At times this may be frustrating, such as when a client has chosen a specific type of massage and the massage therapist does not believe that the protocol best fits the client. The therapist may be tempted to change the protocol to meet the client's needs, only to discover that spa management expects consistency in the application of protocols.

Usually a middle ground can be found between massage-specific protocols and massage based on client outcomes. Massage therapists must be willing to modify their specific style of massage to replicate the spa-designed protocols. They must maintain a unique application for each client based on focused intent and subtle shifts in pressure, rhythm, and so on while maintaining the integrity of the spa protocol. Signature spas must be able to assure clients that regardless of who the massage therapist is, the product of massage remains consistent. Recruitment, specific on-site training for signature methods and products, and retention of massage therapists who find satisfaction in this career environment will become the ultimate challenges of the spa business.

Nevertheless, spa owners and managers realize that clients are looking for results. People expect more from their spa visits than simply being pampered. They want results, and they want to be able to integrate massage therapy into their routines for medical reasons, such as recovery from injury, pain reduction, headache control, and overall health and wellness. Spas are responding by developing menu items such as adaptive massage, targeted massage, and outcome-based massage. Massage therapists must increase their skills to provide this type of care.

Types of Spas

Many variations on the spa theme are available (Box 13-1). Therapeutic massage is one of the unifying services found in almost all spa environments.

The Medical Spa

A medical spa is a facility that operates under the full-time, on-site supervision of a licensed health care professional. The facility operates within the scope of practice of its staff (e.g., dermatology, cosmetic surgery, weight loss) and offers traditional, complementary, and alternative health practices and treatments in a spalike setting. Medical spas can be classified as integrative health and wellness spas or cosmetic medical spas. The cosmetic spa provides services related to beauty and appearance, whereas the wellness spa provides services related to education and guidance on choices affecting healthy living and longevity.

Medical spas and the use of alternative medical therapies have been increasing in popularity. Treatments at medical spas include herbal therapies, chiropractic treatments, self-help imagery, hypnosis, homeopathy, biofeedback, acupuncture, massage, and energy healing. Medical spas also are becoming very popular as adjuncts to plastic surgery, dentistry, chiropractic, dermatology, and antiaging medical practices.

Antiaging medicine is a major focus of the medical spa. It encompasses lifestyle change through education and counseling; hormone replacement therapies (as determined by a physician through laboratory testing); nutrition, antioxidants, and vitamin supplements to reduce free radical damage; and clinical tests related to antiaging.

Box 13-1 Types of Spas

Resort spas are located on the property of a hotel, normally in a resort where other activities are offered in addition to the spa program. Spa and hotel guests intermingle.

Amenity spas are similar to resort spas in that the actual goal of management is to add the spa as an amenity to the hotel. The spa therefore is not necessarily viewed as a profit center as seriously as are some resort spas.

Destination spas are a hotel property geared specifically to the spa guest and spa program. Outside guests are not normally part of the program. Everything is geared toward the spa and its program.

Blended spas are low- to high-priced spas that emphasize physical fitness, nutrition, beauty, and relaxation.

Luxury spas are high-priced spas with posh surroundings that offer an array of state-of-the-art facilities and services.

Weight loss spas cater specifically to those interested in losing weight, using a variety of methods, such as medically supervised dieting, behavioral modification, exercise, detoxification, fasting, and so on.

Medical wellness spas (described in more detail in the next section) enlist the services of physicians to assist guests in achieving optimum health and well-being. The emphasis in these spas is on prevention and lifestyle changes rather than on treatment of acute illness. Programs include back care, sports medicine, physical therapy, lifestyle education, stress management, risk reduction, smoking cessation, heart-healthy regimens, and so on.

Self-awareness spas provide a wide range of alternatives to more traditional spas and focus on such elements as spiritual awareness, the body/mind connection, holistic health, yoga, vegetarianism, acupuncture, aromatherapy, reflexology, tai chi, transcendental meditation, and so on.

Adventure spas focus on customers interested in various outdoor activities such as hiking, rafting, mountain biking, skiing, mountain climbing, and fishing.

Mineral spring spas are built around naturally occurring hot or cold water springs rich in minerals. In addition to mineral springs, some of these spas offer mud and thalassotherapy (seawater treatments), herbal wraps, saunas, and a host of other services typically found in spas.

Spas at sea or *spa cruises* are a new category that recently has been added because of the increasing popularity of cruise vacations. Some large cruise ships offer spa services and packages as part of their regular voyages.

Day (or urban) spas offer 1-day service. The client spends the day receiving various spa treatments, breakfast and lunch are provided, and activities such as aerobics and yoga are included. These are local, "in and out" spas.

Medical cosmetic procedures include cellulite treatments; Botox injections; laser hair removal; microdermabrasion; waxing and sugaring; permanent makeup application; electrolysis; hydrotherapy; sclerotherapy/vein therapy; collagen injections and fillers; chemical peels; and photorejuvenation, such as CLEARLight (a machine that uses different types of low-level lasers to treat acne) and ReLume (a machine that uses different types of low-level lasers to treat stretch marks and remove scars).

Cosmetic surgical procedures offered at some medical spas may include:

Liposuction
Liposculpture
Lipoplasty
Breast augmentation (breast implants)
Breast reduction
Gynecomastia surgery (reduction of enlarged, female-like breasts in men)
Facelift
Rhinoplasty (nose job)
Mastopexy (breast lift)
Lip augmentation
Abdominoplasty (tummy tuck)
Blepharoplasty (eyelid surgery)
Brow lifts
Forehead lifts
Facial contouring
Facial implants
Scar revision
Hair restoration
Thermage
Cosmetic dentistry

Spa services at a medical spa may include typical services and treatments, such as those presented later in this section.

Integrative Health and Wellness Centers

Another component of the medical spa environment is the integrative health and wellness center. Integrative health centers incorporate all aspects of wellness, including body therapies, fitness, yoga and meditation, nutrition, and spirituality. A guest-centered approach, rooted in education, proactive wellness, and preventive wellness, is the cornerstone of programs that address the whole person. A comprehensive program that includes both Eastern traditions and Western scientific advances provides guests with a guided approach to personal well-being. A highly trained staff, under the guidance of a physician, creates customized programs based on the needs of the individual for optimum health and wellness. These centers use a multidisciplinary approach consisting of a medical team trained in **complementary and alternative medicine (CAM)** and specialized service providers in preventive medicine, fitness, and spa services.

Massage is a very important aspect of the medical spa. It supports general healing responses and aids in the management of postprocedural pain. It also can manage postprocedural edema and support the development of supple scar tissue.

Spa Safety

Concern recently has developed about appropriate practice in the medical spa. No statistics are available on the exact number of medical spas, because no official definition of a medical spa exists, and no single licensing body regulates them. Concern has been raised that unlicensed professionals are performing medical procedures and that the environment may not be maintained in a medically appropriate, safe, and sanitary manner.

Regardless of the focus of the spa, some aspects of the spa experience should be consistent to ensure the safety and comfort of the spa client. For example, spa sanitation considerations include the following:

- Clean, unused linens and spa wear
- Sanitized, clean, and uncluttered work surfaces
- Sealed containers for implements such as cotton balls and facial pads
- Professional products that are single use or that have been taken from a larger container without coming in contact with an unsanitary or nonsterile surface
- Disposable tools and implements for any procedure that requires breaking the surface of the skin
- Cleaning of implements with a hospital-grade disinfectant, sanitization by ultraviolet (UV) light or a similar piece of equipment, or sterilization in an autoclave
- Rules requiring technicians to provide spa treatments with freshly washed and dried hands or while wearing surgical gloves
- Sealed and covered waste receptacles and laundry bins
- Tools and products that are clearly labeled and safely stored

All of the safety and sanitation requirements for massage therapists described in this text are applicable.

Health Regulations and the Spa

In April, 2003, new regulations were issued under the Health Insurance Portability and Accountability Act (HIPAA) that may affect spa practice in some cases.

Essentially, HIPAA's health information privacy rules are designed to ensure the protection and security of medical records and other personal health information and to protect an individual's right to privacy in matters involving health care. The HIPAA rules apply to all "covered entities," defined as health plans, health care clearinghouses, and health care providers that transmit any health information in electronic form in connection with a list of specified transactions. In general, if the spa company does not bill or receive payment for health care in the normal course of business, the HIPAA requirement may not apply. Regardless, privacy and client confidentiality are essential aspects of ethical professional practice.

Credentialing in the Spa Industry

Spa training and certification are in the very beginning stages. Spa Secure, introduced in July, 2004, is an international credentialing system. Spa Secure is a self-regulating organization that works in cooperation with state and federal agencies such as the Public Health Department and the Board of Barbers and Cosmetologists.

Spa Secure performs on-site inspections of spas to check for unsafe practices and to evaluate sanitation procedures, health and safety measures, and scope of practice issues. A test is administered to the management and technical staff of the

---

Box 13-2 Spa Specifics

Spa environments address the senses of sight, smell, hearing, taste, and touch. Examples include:
Sight: Use of color and light
Smell: Essential oils and flowers
Hearing: Music and wind chimes
Taste: Herbal teas and juice drinks
Touch: Massage, facials, and body wraps
    Signature spa services feature unique combinations to target the five senses:

Product Related
Smell: Product fragrance
Touch: Texture and application of product

Hydrotherapy Related
Sight: Scenery (e.g., mountain view)
Smell: Scented oils and scrubs
Hearing: Waterfall, fountain
Taste: Mineral waters, flavored waters
Touch: Whirlpool, showers

Culture Related
Sight: Plants, ethnic dress
Smell: Local flowers, incense
Hearing: Ethnic music
Taste: Ethnic food and drinks
Touch: Cultural-based bodywork (i.e., shiatsu, lomi lomi)
    Spa services and environments are targeted to populations based on:
Geography (e.g., rural, agricultural, urban, resort)
Desired outcome: Pampering, fitness, skin care, detoxification, longevity, vacation
Age: Adolescent, middle age, elderly
Gender-specific needs: Pregnancy, cosmetic surgery

---

spa. Ongoing quality is monitored through unannounced inspections of the facility to check for consistency in safety and the quality of operations (Box 13-2).

Spa Etiquette

Spa services should be provided as they are described in any promotional or informational materials and in a timely fashion. Furthermore, services should be provided in a safe, clean environment that respects privacy. Professional standards of behavior should be maintained at all times by the attending technicians, therapists, and staff. The staff must be sufficiently educated and experienced so that they can answer personal care and medical-related questions, provide guidance on appropriate treatments for specific needs, and make home care recommendations.

Spa service professionals, including massage therapists, usually are expected to wear a uniform specific to the organization. Massage therapists should always behave in an ethical and professional manner; they should be impeccably groomed, friendly, pleasant, and timely (i.e., maintain appropriate time management for sessions; see Hallmarks of a Successful Employee in Chapter 3).

Other considerations also are important:

- A guest/client is expected to give at least 24 hours' notice of a cancellation and should arrive 5 to 10 minutes before the appointment time.
- Most spas require the client to fill out a medical evaluation form designed to reveal any concerns that might be contraindications to treatments. It is the client's responsibility (and it is in the person's best interest) to fill out this form as accurately as possible.
- Dress and conduct specifications should be indicated on informational materials. In most spas, spa wear (e.g., robe, slippers) and the necessary items for enjoying the visit are all provided by the spa. If the client is particularly modest and would like to remain clothed at all times, she may want to bring a swimsuit. Jewelry and valuables should always be left at home.

The spa setting is based on client service and satisfaction. The concept of pampering is an important aspect of spa services. Some techniques for service and pampering include the following:

- Greet the client with a warm handshake and a smile. If time allows, ask if the client would like to sit in the steam room, dry sauna, or even the hot tub before the treatment. Offer the client ice water while he or she is relaxing before the treatment.
- Make sure the client is completely comfortable and at ease. The atmosphere should be warm, quiet, and comfortable, with soft music and lighting.
- Use warm towels and warm or cold eye packs during treatments.
- When the treatment is finished, meet the client outside after he or she has put on a robe. Offer tea, cookies, fresh fruit, or water. If the client accepts, the spa staff should "serve" the client the refreshment. In this way, the client feels very special. If the client declines any refreshment, walk the person to the sauna area or locker room and bid them a fond farewell (Box 13-3).

Massage Therapy in the Spa

According to the International SPA Association (ISPA), current trends include simplified spa menus, because spas are focusing on the core of their business: results-oriented treatments. Massage therapy is the number one treatment that people seek out worldwide, and the move is toward outcome-based massage.

Students who are competent in the application of the lessons in this text and in anatomy and physiology are prepared to enter spa employment upon graduation from a 500- to 1,000-hour therapeutic massage program. Although this text does not present specific spa procedures, the information prepares you to be easily and effectively trained in the signature treatments provided at individual spas.

Many spa treatments that are not related to massage are based on hydrotherapy. Therefore, students who are interested in working in a spa may want to consider spending extra time studying this information (see Chapter 12). In addition, many spa treatments target the skin; spending extra time studying

---

Box 13-3 Guidelines of the Day Spa Association

The Day Spa Association has set guidelines to help distinguish between a facility that offers spa services and a true day spa.

A true day spa has:

- A clean, safe, calming, and nurturing environment
- Private treatment rooms for each client receiving a personal service
- Separate showering and changing facilities for women and men
- Spa robes and shoes for all sizes
- Business licenses; professional, licensed estheticians and therapists on staff
- Professional spa products for which estheticians and therapists have received training in their use
- Massages: Swedish, lymphatic drainage, and reflexology (optional: shiatsu; polarity treatments; and sports, deep tissue, and deep muscle massages)
- Body treatments (one or more on the menu): body packs and wraps, exfoliation, cellulite treatments, body toning/contouring, waxing, home care program (optional: electrical impulse body toning, heat treatments, Ayurveda treatments, laser hair removal, electrolysis, hand and foot care)
- Face: Cleansing facial, home care program (optional: medical facial, electrical toning, laser hair removal, electrolysis, cosmetics, and makeup consultation)
- Aromatherapy: Personalized for body and/or face

One of the following:

- Hydrotherapy
- Steam bath and sauna

One of the following:

- Nutritional counseling/weight management
- Private trainer/yoga/meditation
- Spa cuisine

Optional:

- Hair: Full-service salon, scalp treatments, and hair packs
- Spa manicure and pedicure

Data from the Day Spa Association.

---

the integumentary system and the lymph and blood circulations, as presented both in this text and in *Mosby's Essential Sciences for Therapeutic Massage* (or a similar science text) is recommended.

Massage therapists employed by the spa industry should be licensed by the appropriate government agency and/or should have national certification from the appropriate certifying agency. Spas expect the massage therapists they employ to have educational credentials and practical experience, and they also expect their employees to pass standardized testing. A therapist's expertise typically is determined by the number of hours attended during school to obtain a license, the number of total years in practice, and the types and extent of continuing education obtained after graduation (Figure 13-1).

The Massage Practitioner's Responsibilities in the Spa or Franchise Environment

The responsibilities of the massage professional are to provide various types of massage, support other spa procedures, and

Spa Massage Therapist Part- to Full-Time Restwell Day Spa

Location: Chicago, Ill

Restwell Day Spa is in search of Massage Therapists. Duties include providing all therapeutic massages listed on our spa menu on both male and female clients, greeting clients, suggesting retail products and maintaining treatment room cleanliness. Excellent communication and customer service skills are a must!

We offer competitive pay, flexible hours, a fun and energetic environment, career advancement, FREE health club membership and more!

A minimum of one 8-hour shift per week, which may include weekends and evenings, is required. Full time is 32 hours, which creates eligibility for benefits.

Required Skills:

Attentiveness—ability to attend to member/guest needs
Massage application and adaption for client outcomes using spa menu
Good communication; must liaise with clients/staff
Time management and problem solving; will oversee day-to-day operations
Marketing, as necessary, to build clientele

Certification and Licensing:

Nationally Certified Massage Therapy License
Necessary state, county and local licensing

Education and Experience:

Graduation from licensed massage school, and 1-year minimum massage experience

PLEASE NOTE:

Only those individuals selected for an interview will be contacted. Candidates outside of the Chicago Metro area are welcome to apply, but if selected for an interview, they must be willing to travel at own cost. Relocation assistance is not offered.

FIGURE 13-1 Classified ad for a spa job.

provide education about spa services to clients. The following guidelines are important in the spa environment:

- Be punctual for appointments.
- Perform therapies and treatments in a courteous manner so that the client feels pampered and relaxed.
- Continually update your skills and education.
- Assist in educating and informing clients about spa products and services when the opportunity arises. Selling spa products and services may be expected.
- Maintain a positive attitude and a professional, personal image.
- Maintain the physical environment of the spa according to the spa's specifications.

The spa environment is a wonderful place to serve clients seeking massage. The spa industry has created one of the largest employment opportunities for massage practitioners. The spa concept is unique and requires a professional commitment to learning, as do all the career paths discussed in this chapter.

Pay Scales for Massage Therapists in the Spa Environment

Most spas and franchises hire all staff as employees, typically on a wage plus commission basis. Spas and franchises are not

---

Box 13-4 Allocation of Funds in the Spa or Franchise Business

The following are realistic expectations about guidelines and wages in the spa and massage franchise industry.

• Fee for massage with hot stones and aromatherapy	$100 (i.e., gross receipts)

The expenses that must be deducted from this $100 are as follows:

• Facility, supplies, and advertising and marketing overhead	$50
• Wages for support staff (typically $10 an hour)	$25
• Amount left for technician and therapist wages and profit margin	$25
• The minimum profit should be 50% of the $25, or $12.50 per treatment.	
• Amount left for technician's and therapist's wages	$12.50/hour

---

known for paying high wages, but they typically pay fair wages. The average is $10 to $15 an hour plus commission and gratuities. Independent contractors usually get about 50% of the charge, but they have to provide their own equipment and supplies and pay their own taxes, Social Security, and Medicare; these are not deducted from their pay.

A number of expenses that spas have must be taken into account when considering pay scales. For example, the environment of the spa or franchise is extremely important. Facility management is expensive. Marketing and advertising are essential aspects of the business plan. As a result, the overhead costs for a spa or massage franchise are high, typically at least 50% of gross income.

Employer or subcontractor wages therefore must be figured on the remaining 50% of gross receipts. In addition to the professional staff, spas and franchises require a sizable support staff, including maintenance workers, receptionists, managers, food service workers, and so on. These wages easily can account for 25% of the gross receipts left after overhead costs. Consequently, technician and therapist wages must be provided from the remaining 25%. Also, the owner needs to make a profit (Box 13-4).

The Spa Language

The spa environment has a language all its own; employees are expected to understand and use certain terms. These terms usually describe the various services and treatments, which are listed on a spa menu from which the client chooses. Some of these methods may be performed by the massage practitioner; others may fall under the scope of practice of a cosmetologist or esthetician. Clients will ask questions about various services and treatments. Employees need to understand the services, whether they perform them or not, so that they can educate the client and support the spa's business sales (Box 13-5).

| Box 13-5 | Bodywork Terms, Descriptions, and Treatments Commonly Used in the Spa Setting |

- *Bodywork exfoliation:* Exfoliation is the process by which the skin is rubbed, polished, or scrubbed or enzymes are used on it to remove dead skin cells, rancid oils, dirt, and debris.
- *Detoxification:* When the circulation and metabolism are stimulated, the body's own processing improves. This in turn improves the elimination process, helping the body to rid itself of wastes and toxins. In other words, this helps the body to detoxify itself. The end result is normally a more energetic, active individual who feels better.
- *Dry brush:* Dry brushing involves the use of a luffa, brush, washcloth, or sponge to exfoliate dead surface skin. After this process, lotion is applied. The main purpose is to stimulate circulation.
- *Salt glow:* Special salt is mixed with oil or liquid soap to exfoliate the entire body or just an area for a spot treatment. Afterward, lotion is used on the client. A dry brush tool, such as a loofah, may be used with the salt mixture for added exfoliation. If salt is used, the client should not shave for 1 to 2 days before the treatment.
- *Body polish:* Salt or any abrasive substance or granular scrub can be used as a body polish. The product used is a cream base with granules of the abrasive substance added to exfoliate and condition or soften the skin at the same time.
- *Full-body seaweed mask:* Seaweed powders normally are mixed with water to a consistency resembling pancake batter. The mixture is applied over a conditioning lotion. The entire body may be covered, or the stomach, breasts, and buttocks may be not treated, depending on the client's wishes. Essential oils are often added to full-body seaweed masks to achieve different effects on the body. The full-body seaweed mask treatment normally takes about 60 minutes.
- *Full-body mud mask:* Sea-based muds and clay muds, depending on the particular type, are said to cleanse and draw out impurities, to condition and mineralize the body, or just to soften and hydrate the skin. The mud is applied thickly to the body, which is then wrapped in plastic or foil. The client rests for 20 to 30 minutes. A full mud treatment normally takes about 60 minutes.
- *Herbal body wrap:* Linen or muslin sheets are heated and soaked in an appliance called a *hydrocollator,* in which the temperature is 150° to 175° F. Herbal pouches or bags of herbs and essential oil essences are placed in the hydrocollator to achieve the desired effects. The body is first covered with towels or rubber sheets, and the linen or muslin sheets are laid over this. The body then is wrapped in sheets and blankets, and the client is allowed to rest for 20 minutes. A cool, wet cloth is applied to the client's forehead during the treatment and changed often. This treatment can be done in 30 minutes. The sheets are very hot, and the technician must wear thick, long rubber gloves when handling them.
- *Paraffin body wrap:* When applied to the body, paraffin forms a mask with heat. This helps the body perspire, and the trapped moisture is absorbed into the skin, along with nutrients that either are put on the skin first or are in the oils in the paraffin. The paraffin may be used alone, or it may be mixed with mud or seaweed. Paraffin can be painted on the body with a paint brush. Also, large gauze strips can be dipped in the paraffin and molded to different parts of the body. Several layers are applied, because the more layers (i.e., three to five), the greater the heat and the longer it lasts. The body then is wrapped with foil or plastic, and the client is allowed to rest for 15 to 20 minutes. Paraffin commonly is used for the hands, feet, and face.

Products

Spas use many products to provide benefits, especially to treat the skin and detoxify the body (Box 13-6). *Cosmetologists* are professionals trained in cosmetic and wellness skin care; *dermatologists* are medical doctors who specialize in treating skin disease. The massage therapist needs to understand the reason a product is used and how various ingredients in the product work. Skin care products basically include cleansers, exfoliants, and moisturizers.

Massage therapists who work in spas need to understand the specific products used in their spa. This information should be provided through in-house training after the massage practitioner has been hired. Massage therapists may be required to use a certain product as a lubricant based on the spa's signature line, and they may be required to participate in the sales of products specific to the spa.

Spa Treatments

Spa treatments are the services that a spa provides. The wide range of treatments offered in spas includes wet treatments (e.g., wet table with Vichy shower and other forms of hydrotherapy), dry treatments (e.g., massage and body wraps), wellness therapies (e.g., oxygen inhalation), and health assessments, in addition to beauty treatments. Typically, a sauna, steam room, and spa pool are found at a spa. Although hydrotherapy is still regarded as an important treatment (see Chapter 12), spas no longer need to use or be near mineral water. Also, not all spas focus on hydrotherapy as a main component of treatment.

The most popular service in the spa is therapeutic massage. The second most popular service is the facial, which involves skin analysis, deep cleansing, massage, extractions (removal of blackheads and other impurities), toning, and moisturizing.

Cosmetic Treatments

The massage therapist typically does not perform cosmetic treatments. These procedures target the integumentary system (i.e., the skin), and cosmetologists, estheticians, and dermatologists are the experts in this area.

The Facial

A facial is given by a licensed esthetician or cosmetologist with special training in skin care. An *esthetician* is a skin care specialist who has undergone a professional training program similar to cosmetology. A facial, which usually lasts 50 minutes, cleanses, tones, and hydrates the skin.

A facial involves some basic steps: cleansing, skin analysis, exfoliation, massage, extraction of blackheads and other impurities, and application of products targeted to the client's

Box 13-6 Common Terminology for Spa Products

Allantoin: A substance derived from comfrey root that is believed to aid the healing of damaged skin by stimulating new tissue growth.

Aloe vera: A regenerating, soothing, softening, and reparative substance with antimicrobial and antiinflammatory properties. It is rich in more than 200 nutrients and is very healing and moisturizing.

Alpha-hydroxy acids (AHA): These acids, which include lactic acid and glycolic acid, often are used as peeling agents. Most are fruit acids. At higher concentrations they also have a descaling or keratolytic action, thinning the stratum corneum.

Alpha-lipoic acid: A powerful water- and oil-soluble antioxidant, alpha-lipoic acid is 400 times more potent than vitamin C as an antioxidant. It also increases the level of glutathione, the body's most important antioxidant, and is a powerful antiinflammatory.

Bentonite: A substance that brightens dull, lifeless skin and leaves it with a fresh, renewed texture.

Borax: A cleansing agent that helps blend water and oil. A mild alkali, it cleanses without drying the skin.

Clay, kaolin: This substance draws out impurities and is used as a deep pore cleanser. It removes excess oil, dirt, and grime.

Cleanse: To clean and remove impurities from the skin's surface.

Cleansers: Products used to remove makeup and impurities on the skin's surface. They also remove sebum (oily secretions produced by the sebaceous gland) and dead skin cells.

Cream: A cream is a more occlusive, thicker barrier on the skin. Those that contain dimethicone are particularly useful for hand dermatitis.

Emollient: An ingredient that softens and soothes the skin. Emollients are used in moisturizers to correct dryness and scaling of the skin.

Emulsion: A substance made by blending oil and water in the right proportions with an *emulsifier,* an agent that prevents the oil and water from separating.

Exfoliant: An agent used in scrubs and wraps and in some facials to remove dead skin cells from the skin's surface.

Glycerin: A humectant and emollient obtained from plants. It absorbs moisture from the air and helps keep moisture in creams and other products.

Glyceryl stearate: A substance that helps produce a neutral, stable emulsion. It is also a solvent, humectant, and consistency regulator in water-in-oil and oil-in-water formulations. It is derived from palm kernel or soy oil for cosmetic use. It also is found naturally in the body.

Humectant: A substance that increases the water-holding capacity of the stratum corneum. It is particularly important in the management of ichthyoses (inherited or acquired scaly disorders of the skin).

Lanolin: A sebum-like product obtained from washing sheep's wool. It acts as an emollient and a humectant for the skin.

Lotion: A substance that is more occlusive than an oil. Lotions are best applied immediately after bathing to retain the water in the skin and should be used at other times as necessary.

Mask: A mask draws impurities to the skin's surface. Masks also slough off dead skin cells and stimulate blood circulation, leaving the skin feeling smoother and softer. Masks are applied after cleansing but before toning and can be used once or twice a week.

Moisturizers Products that use advanced humectants to help the skin retain water; they also provide a protective barrier to prevent the evaporation of the skin's natural moisture.

Night creams: Creams that contain a higher concentration of nutrients that assist in the rebuilding of the molecular structure of the skin's underlying tissues. They also improve the skin's ability to retain moisture.

Ointments: Pure oil preparations (e.g., equal parts white, soft, and liquid paraffin or petroleum jelly), which are prescribed for drier, thicker, more scaly areas. Many clients find them too greasy.

Phospholipid: A substance derived from plants that reduces moisture loss from the skin and acts as a carrier for deep penetration.

Retinol: A vitamin A carotenoid with antioxidant and skin-renewing properties.

Rubefacient: A local irritant that reddens the skin.

Salicylic acid: A substance that softens the keratinized barrier cells, has antibacterial properties, and helps eliminate clogged pores.

Salt: A substance that is good for drying, cleansing, drawing, and soothing. It also can be used as an exfoliant. It dilates pores, allowing the skin to absorb trace minerals, and it encourages the skin to secrete its natural oil. It soothes irritated skin and aching muscles.

Serum: An intense concentration for exceptional revitalization of aging skin.

Shea butter: A moisturizing, soothing emollient fat that has cellular renewal properties.

Silicone: A substance derived from silica, a naturally occurring mineral, that has a softening effect on the skin.

Skin lighteners: Products that help reduce the production of melanin, which causes coloration of the skin. These products are used to lighten the complexion. Skin lightening regimens include their own cleansers, masks, toners, moisturizers, and serums.

Sodium bicarbonate: A highly alkaline, gentle substance that cleans, soothes, and softens the skin. It also is deodorizing, and it draws out oil and impurities.

Toner: A substance that removes any residue left by cleansers and returns the skin to its proper pH by maintaining the skin's natural acidic balance. Toners and lotions prepare the skin for the application of a moisturizer.

---

skin type (e.g., dry, oily, mixed, sensitive, or mature.) Variations on the classic European facial include the minifacial (cleansing without extractions) and specialty facials.

It is recommended that spa clients receive a facial once a month or every 6 weeks, because that is how long it takes the skin to regenerate (Box 13-7).

Peels

A peel involves the use of products to remove the surface layer of skin (dead skin) and expose the fresher tissue beneath. An enzyme peel is a special enzyme-based exfoliating treatment that breaks down and removes the dead skin layer or layers from the face. Undergoing an enzyme peel from time to time

Types of Spa Facial Treatments

- **Microdermabrasion:** A nonchemical, noninvasive procedure that removes the outermost layer of dry, dead skin cells to reveal younger, healthier-looking skin. Additional treatments encourage the production of a new layer of skin cells containing higher levels of collagen and elastin, both of which further improve the skin's appearance.
- **Facial contouring:** A combination of therapies, including deep muscle massage and acupressure, that is used to tone and tighten areas of the face and neck.
- **Facial oxygen therapy:** A combination of many different vitamins, minerals, amino acids, and enzymes, in addition to pure oxygen, which is used to cleanse, hydrate, and rejuvenate the skin.
- **European deep suction cleansing:** A very deep cleansing procedure that uses enzymes and deep suction to remove impurities from the facial pores.
- **Photofacial:** This type of facial is performed only by trained medical professionals. Photofacial is a 30-minute procedure that uses a machine that releases intense pulses of light to penetrate all layers of the skin. This causes collagen and blood vessels under the top layer to constrict. For a complete treatment, five full-face light treatments must be done, spaced at three-week intervals. Clients report minimal discomfort, and the redness and facial swelling present after treatment are short-lived. The effects are gradual and are noticed over the few weeks following the treatment.

Data from Day Spa FYI at www.dayspafyi.com/day_spa_treatments.html.

forces the body to regenerate new skin, and this process makes the skin appear stronger and healthier.

Vitamin peels (i.e., vitamins A and C) are used to repair sun damage, lighten dark spots, rehydrate the skin, and encourage elasticity.

Pedicures and Manicures
Spa pedicures and manicures moisturize the skin. The nails are trimmed, shaped, and painted.

Waxing and Hair Removal Services
Most day spas offer a variety of waxing services to remove unwanted hair, such as:
- Leg waxing
- Arm waxing
- Eyebrow waxing
- Face and lip waxing
- Bikini waxes
- Brazilian waxes
- Laser hair removal

Application of Permanent Makeup
Some day spas offer permanent makeup, a form of cosmetic tattooing.

Tanning Services
Sunless tanning services are offered by many day spas. With spray-on tanning, guests can achieve a summer tan without

exposing the skin to damaging UV rays. Some spas also offer a sunless tanning application by a spa professional, sometimes used in conjunction with an exfoliating procedure such as a salt scrub. Tanning booths may also be available.

Hair Styling
Day spas with salons offer hair styling services.

Body Treatments
Body treatments basically are facials for the whole body. The most popular body treatment is a body scrub, an exfoliating treatment in which the technician rubs off the outermost layer of dead skin cells, leaving the skin feeling soft and renewed. Medicinal salts typically are used as an abrasive to scrub the body.

A body wrap is a treatment in which products such as mud, algae, or seaweed are applied to the body, which then is wrapped in sheets, plastic, or some other covering. Wraps are thought to detoxify the body because they stimulate blood circulation and the lymphatic system. A rich cream or oil is used to soften and condition the skin and acts as a hydrating treatment.

Massage Treatments
The massage therapist must understand basic concepts related to signature services provided by spas. This section lists generic massage treatments typically found on spa menus, but you should review Chapter 12 again to better understand the types of massage services provided in the spa environment.
- *Swedish/classic massage* is general systematic massage of the soft tissues of the body to induce a state of deep relaxation. It works mainly on the muscles, ligaments, and tendons, and it increases the body's blood and lymphatic circulation. Swedish/classic massage incorporates effleurage (long gliding strokes), pétrissage (kneading), compression, vibration, and tapotement (see Chapter 10).
- *Stone therapy massage* is a combination process that uses various types and sizes of stones, which are either heated or cooled. They then are placed on the body at strategic points or are coated with oils or lotions and used to massage the client's body. The warmth and weight provided by warm stones can also be provided by rice bags.
- *Shiatsu* and *Thai massage* are Asian-based bodywork modalities involving the use of pressure and stretches that address energetic imbalances. The client wears comfortable clothes that allow for movement and lies on a futon or mat on the floor. No lubricants are used.
- *Reflexology* (zone therapy) is organized around a system of points on the hands and feet that are thought to correspond to the major joints and organs of the body.
- *Trigger point therapy* (myotherapy or neuromuscular therapy) applies concentrated finger pressure to trigger points to relax an entire area.
- *Deep muscle/connective tissue massage* releases the chronic patterns of tension in the body through slow strokes and deep pressure on contracted areas, by both following and moving across the grain of the muscles, tendons, and fascia (see Chapters 10 and 12).

- *Sports massage* is designed specifically for athletes or people who engage in a sports, exercise, or fitness program. It usually is deeper and more vigorous than an average massage. Sports massage can be used to ready the muscles for strenuous activity or to help the body recover from the aftereffects of such an activity (see Chapters 10 and 12).

Hydrotherapy Treatments

Hydrotherapy as a therapeutic modality was described in Chapter 12. Many methods of applying hydrotherapy may be available at spas, and the massage therapist may be requested to perform variations offered in the spa environment. The following sections cover the therapies commonly offered in the spa setting.

Bath Treatments

The baths typically offered at spas are:
- Plain water baths with no additives, with or without underwater massage
- Thalassotherapy (seawater) baths, with additives of seaweed, sea salts, and sometimes sea mud

Bath Additives

Additives for a bath might include the following:
- Spirulina, which is rich in vitamins and beta carotene and is effective for reducing fatigue, stimulating the metabolism, and creating a sense of focus and alertness.
- Fucus and *Ascophyllum nodosum* (a type of seaweed), which are rich in vitamins and amino acids and help relax the body and neutralize free radicals.
- *Chondrus crispus* and *Corallina officinalis,* which are both remineralizers and revitalizers.

Caution: Immersion in hot water is contraindicated for pregnant women, especially in the first trimester of pregnancy. Also, warm to hot water lowers the blood pressure. This is great for relaxation but may cause lightheadedness, which can be dangerous for a client with a heart condition.

Cleaning the Tub and Room

Although every spa has its own sanitation protocols, generally the tub must be cleaned and disinfected after each client. If the tub has jets, these must also be cleaned out. The whole tub then is rinsed and dried. The room should be sanitized and wiped down with a towel. The floors should be sanitized and dried.

Other Hydrotherapy Treatments

Vichy Shower

The Vichy shower, which originated in France, consists of a row of shower heads suspended over a massage table. The client lies on the table, and the entire body is sprayed from the head to the feet, front and back. This usually is done as part of a body mud treatment, although it is both relaxing and stimulating on its own.

Scrubs, Friction Rubs, and Ablutions

Scrubs and friction rubs help exfoliate and hydrate the skin. Scrubs usually are made of sugars, salts, and other natural ingredients and are applied by hand or with a special coarse mitten that helps remove dead, dull skin. Spas usually offer several different scrubs, such as the following types.

- *Salt glow:* Mineral-rich sea salts are used to exfoliate dry skin, revealing the healthier, younger skin beneath.
- *Aromatherapy scrubs:* These scrubs exfoliate the body and soothe the senses with therapeutic aromas.
- *Oatmeal scrubs:* Oatmeal scrubs exfoliate the body and help draw out impurities at the same time.
- *Cold rubbing (ablution):* Cold ablutions are used to invigorate, to tone up the body, to promote blood flow, to address problems of circulation, or for infections of the respiratory system. The primary effect of a cold ablution is tonic; therefore, it may be used for any condition in which a tonifying treatment is desired, such as fatigue after an illness or surgery, or after hot applications, such as saunas, whirlpools, or hot baths. Cold ablution is an excellent hydrotherapy technique when used regularly along with saunas, hot tubs, and massage. To perform a cold ablution, soak a linen cloth in cold water, wring it out, and briskly rub the upper and lower trunk or the entire body. Have the client relax until warm and dry.
- *Whole body ablution:* A whole body ablution is performed with the client lying alternately supine and prone and covered completely; care must be taken to ensure that the person does not become chilled. Using cool to cold water, dip the mitt into the water and vigorously friction a portion of the body. Depending on the cooling effect desired, the mitt may either be saturated or wrung dry before the frictioning. The body part is frictioned until it reddens. If the client is weak, dry the area using a coarse, dry towel. If the client is strong and vigorous, wait to dry the person at the end of the treatment.

The sequence for an ablution treatment is as follows (only the part being frictioned is exposed at any time):
1. Position the client supine.
2. Perform the ablution on the chest.
3. Proceed from the chest to the arms.
4. Perform the ablution on the legs.
5. Turn the client over.
6. Perform the ablution on the legs and feet.
7. Perform the ablution on the buttocks.
8. Perform, the ablution on the back.

Wraps

Body wraps help exfoliate, hydrate, and tone the skin. They also are used to detoxify the body and improve circulation. The basic body wrap is fairly simple; the body is covered with sea clay or a mineral or herbal solution and then wrapped with light sheets.

The effects of body wraps are based on two principles: absorption and compaction. Over time the body collects toxins from food, water, and air. Body wraps are believed to work first by absorbing toxins (i.e., the solution rubbed into the skin opens the pores and collects impurities) and then by compressing, or tightening, the skin to achieve a more toned look.

Different body wraps provide different results. The most common types of wraps use sea clay, seaweed, herbs, minerals, and aloe vera. Overall, sea clay is said to be the most absorbent material.

- *Enzymatic body wrap:* This wrap combines fruit acids and an invigorating scrub to exfoliate and smooth the skin and cleanse the blemish-prone skin on the back.
- *Herbal body wrap:* Special herbs are used to soothe the body and muscles as impurities are drawn away.
- *Aromatherapy wrap:* This treatment involves the use of herbs and oils.
- *Seaweed wrap:* Seaweed has healing properties that can detoxify and energize the body.

The sequence for a body wrap is as follows:

1. Place the client in a relaxed position.
2. Moisten a linen cloth of the appropriate size with cold water (warm water for respiratory diseases), wring it out well, and wrap it tightly (but not tightly enough to cause constriction) around the appropriate part of the body.
3. Wrap a dry cotton or linen cloth around the moist cloth.
4. Wrap the client in a blanket or another cloth. The client should rest for 45 to 60 minutes or, if the intention is to induce sweating, for up to 3 hours.
5. If the wrap does not feel warm after 15 minutes, apply heat in the form of a hot water bottle or by giving the client warm tea. Remove the wrap immediately if the client complains of feeling unwell.

Steam Inhalation

Some spas use steam inhalation to help break up blockages in the chest after a cold or simply to open up the air passages. Specialized inhalation equipment can be used, or make it simple with a small tub of hot water and a towel draped over the head.

Aromatherapy

Spa regimens often make use of essential oils, usually in conjunction with various hydrotherapy and massage treatments. These oils also can be diffused into the air and inhaled (see Chapter 12 for a more detailed discussion). Each spa typically has its own signature blends of essential oils, which work *synergistically* (i.e., each oil enhances the effect of the others). Often these blends are premixed in a selected carrier oil, and this, too, may be a signature blend of the spa.

Keep in mind that a single oil or blend of oils should not be used consistently every day.

Examples of blends (and individual oils) that are appropriate for massage include the following:

- *Sensual:* Ylang ylang, sandalwood, and jasmine
- *Stimulating:* Peppermint and rosemary
- *Mood lifter:* Sweet orange, rose, and geranium
- *Relaxing:* Lavender, rose
- *Soothing (for muscle aches):* Grapefruit and lemongrass

Massage Therapy Franchises

Massage therapy franchises are not marketed as spas, but the business model is very similar. Developing a career in a massage franchise environment is similar enough to the wellness/spa setting to include a description in this area.

A **franchise** is a business contract through which an individual (the franchisee) purchases the rights to sell or market the products or services (or both) of a large group that has developed a brand (the franchisor). The franchisee receives training and marketing support from the franchisor and pays a fee for ongoing support. The franchise Massage Envy was started in Arizona in 2002. It was the first massage franchise to develop a national presence, and it has grown rapidly by offering professional and affordable massage therapy services to consumers with busy lifestyles. Massage Envy offers a wide variety of treatments to customers who can buy monthly memberships. The company has largely defined the franchised market for massage, offering affordable massages at convenient locations with flexible hours. All massage therapists who work for this franchise are employees (see Chapter 3). Many different massage franchises now are available, and the market is expected to grow. Eventually some sort of blending process may occur in which the franchises offer limited spa-type services, especially skin care.

Students who commit to becoming competent in the skills provided by this text and who also are willing learners, will be well equipped to pursue successful careers in the wellness/spa and franchise environments.

Cross-Training Recommendations

If you are considering a career in the spa industry, cross-training as an esthetician/cosmetologist or esthetician may be desirable. A cosmetologist is a licensed occupation. Cosmetologists assist customers with their physical appearance. They include hair stylists who can cut, style, and color a client's hair. Some cosmetologists also are trained to provide manicures, pedicures, scalp treatments, facials, maintain hairpieces, and give a make-up analysis. Formal training and education are required. These classes are available at various community colleges, technical schools, and cosmetology schools. The length of the programs varies; most last 9 to 24 months. State education requirements vary between 1,200 and 2,100 school hours. Most are 1,500 to 1,800 hours.

Estheticians are not cosmetologists. An esthetician is a skin care specialist and performs cosmetic skin treatments such as facials, light chemical peels, body treatments, and waxing. All estheticians must be licensed in the state in which they work. They complete 250 to 600 hours of training depending on the state.

A Day at the Spa

Now that you are familiar with spa-related therapeutic massage, study the photographs in Figure 13-2, which take you through an enjoyable, safe, and sanitary day at the spa.

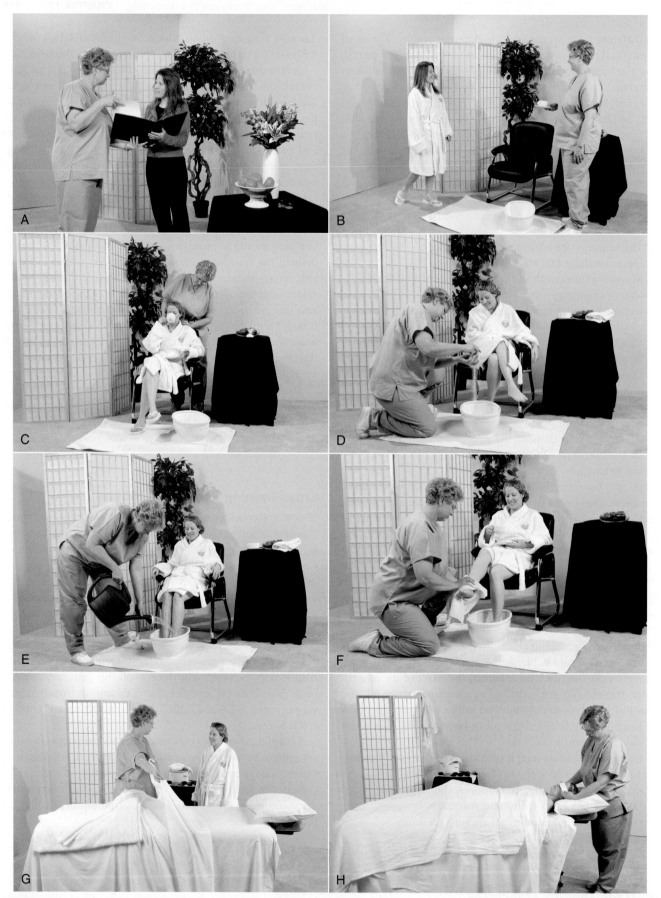

FIGURE 13-2 A day at the spa. **A,** The client is greeted warmly. The intake interview is conducted, and the client is presented with a spa menu. **B,** The client changes into spa wear and then is offered a cup of tea. **C,** The client's hair is protected with a cap. **D,** Signature aromatherapy oils and bath salts are used for the treatments. **E,** The client is encouraged to enjoy the hydrotherapy treatment. **F,** The client's feet are gently dried and then given a reflexology treatment. **G,** The client is given a relaxation-based, full-body signature massage. **H,** A compress can be placed over the client's eyes.

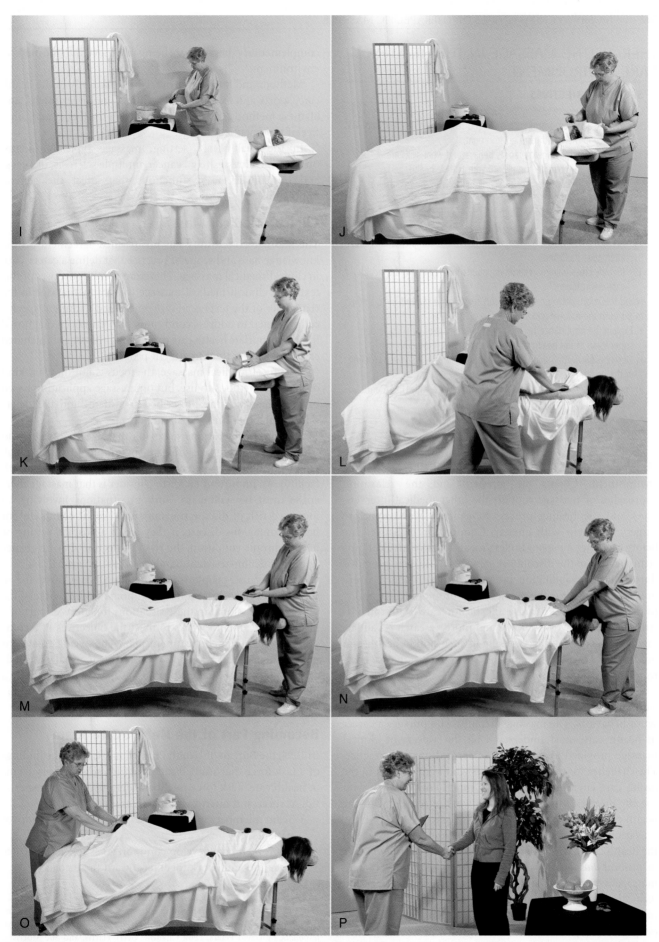

FIGURE 13-2, cont'd **I,** Hot stones are prepared for a treatment. **J,** The temperature of the stones is tested, and they then are gently placed at nodal points. **K,** A few stones can be placed on the chakras with focused energy intention. **L,** Massage can be performed with a hot stone. **M,** The massage therapist can warm the hands with the stone. **N,** The massage is given with warm hands. **O,** The massage therapist finishes and focuses (compassionate energy). **P,** The therapist says good-bye and encourages the client to visit again soon.

THERAPEUTIC MASSAGE IN THE HEALTH CARE ENVIRONMENT

SECTION OBJECTIVES

Chapter objectives covered in this section:

11. Identify and demonstrate the skills and responsibilities necessary for practice in the health care environment.
12. Explain how massage therapists behave and what skills are necessary to maintain compliance with HIPAA, health insurance, record keeping, and confidentiality in the health care environment.
13. Use basic pharmacology information to practice massage safely in the health care environment.
14. Practice massage therapy as part of healthcare/complementary and alternative medicine.
15. Identify cross-training recommendations for a career in the health care environment.

Using the information presented in this section, the student will be able to perform the following:

- Explain the importance for massage practitioners of working under supervision in the health care setting using best practices
- Describe the written and verbal communication necessary for working in the health care environment
- Perform necessary record keeping for compliance with HIPAA and health insurance billing
- Adapt massage based on prescribed medications

Therapeutic massage has much to offer in the health care environment. Clients are stressed, and the relaxation approaches of massage support the other medical interventions and the healing process in general. Massage before surgery can help with anxiety. Comfort or palliative care before and after a person undergoes an invasive medical procedure can ease the discomfort somewhat. Massage provided during drug rehabilitation programs supports the recovery process. Massage for the medical staff promotes their ability to serve effectively, because the health care staff often is stressed and overworked. More and more, research is validating the effects of massage, making its inclusion in health care possible. The possibilities for massage in the health care environment are numerous.

For massage practitioners, the health care environment is a unique place that requires a specific skill set and professional set of behaviors. The massage therapist who pursues a career in health care must understand all the aspects of clinical massage provided as part of an integrated medical practice. The challenge for massage therapists who want to work in the health care environment is not so much how to work with specific diseases, but rather how to work effectively with the health care professionals serving the patient.

Various terms are used to describe therapeutic massage in the health care environment, most commonly *clinical massage* or *medical massage*. This text is based on the premise that all massage is therapeutic and that the terms *clinical massage* and *medical massage* can be used interchangeably. Both describe massage offered within the health care environment to serve people seeking preventive care and those who have diagnosed medical conditions and are being treated at some level by a medical professional. Increasingly, massage and other complementary therapies are being integrated into the medical environment.*

Methods and knowledge overlap significantly in the health care, sports and exercise, and wellness/spa career tracks, and all these methods are solidly grounded in the theory and practice of therapeutic massage.

In the health care setting, massage typically focuses on systemic illnesses (e.g., cancer, multiple sclerosis, diabetes) and on soft tissue dysfunctions that affect the general population.

Clinical/Medical Massage

The massage community has not reached agreement on the knowledge base and scope of practice that define a career path in clinical/medical massage. Therefore, for the purposes of this textbook, clinical/medical massage (or simply massage in the remainder of the text) is an outcome-based treatment specifically targeted to address conditions that have been diagnosed by an appropriate health care professional. Massage is included as an aspect of a total treatment program.

In clinical/medical massage, the focus is not on what kind of massage methods to use, but on massage application based on the diagnosis, the prescribed treatment, and the determined outcomes for the patient.

Special considerations arise for massage therapists who work with clients in a health care environment (e.g., hospital, rehabilitation center, extended care facility, or mental health facility). An important factor to consider is that massage therapists must be willing to work in situations involving an increased risk of disease transmission. Even if clients do not have a contagious disease, if they are in a hospital setting or have a chronic condition, the risk of infection may be greater (e.g., methicillin-resistant *Staphylococcus aureus* [MRSA]).

Also, because people increasingly are being cared for in their homes by visiting nurses and home health workers, the massage professional in these situations functions as part of a health care team and works to meet the objectives of a comprehensively designed treatment plan. The overall treatment plan is supervised by a medical professional, usually a physician. The massage therapist often is supervised directly by a physician's assistant, nurse, physical therapist, occupational therapist, or some other qualified health care professional.

Becoming Part of the Health Care Team

In 1994, the Bureau of Health Professions released the findings of a task force that studied the use of interdisciplinary teams in health care. Task force members identified five characteristics of successful interdisciplinary teams.

- Team members provide care to a common group of patients.
- Team members develop common goals for performance outcomes and work together toward these goals.

---

*For specific information on how this is being accomplished, see *Integrating Complementary Therapies in Primary Care: a Practical Guide for Health Professionals*, by David Peters, Leon Chaitow, Gerry Harris, and Sue Morrison (Churchill Livingstone, 2001) and *Clinical Massage in the Health Care Setting*, by Sandy Fritz, Leon Chaitow, and Glenn M. Hymel (Mosby, 2008).

- Appropriate roles and functions are assigned to each team member.
- Members understand and respect the roles of others.
- All members contribute and share essential information about both tasks and group process.

The team also establishes a means of ensuring that plans are implemented, services are coordinated, and the performance of the team is evaluated. The interdisciplinary medical team functions as a whole and requires the understanding and involvement of all team members. Individual tasks may lend themselves to one team member or another with specialized skills, but the final outcome is a team effort. Deciding on the diagnostic and therapeutic criteria that must be met for optimum patient management is a job that typically falls to the physician.

The expectations and responsibilities of the massage therapist as part of an interdisciplinary team are still being determined. The massage therapist's role will become clearer as massage therapy becomes fully integrated into health care. The massage therapist must know the scope of practice of each of the members of the interdisciplinary team and must be able to explain his or her own role. The massage therapist must develop an understanding of various treatments used by the integrated team and must be able to contribute to the patient's care.

If you pursue a massage career in the health care stetting, you must understand the indications, necessary adaptations, and potential contraindications to massage methods in relation to each health care intervention proposed and implemented. You also must be able to adapt to the varied health care environments, equipment, and rules and regulations.

Professionalism

Professionalism is vital in the medical setting. Some characteristics of professionalism include loyalty, dependability, courtesy, initiative, flexibility, credibility, confidentiality, and a positive attitude. Behaving in a professional manner in the medical environment creates trust. Trust is one of the most important factors in preventing medical professional liability lawsuits.

Dress, attitude, and appearance all influence the credibility of the massage therapist. Typically your appearance will be generally neat and clean and will include scrubs; flat shoes with closed toes and rubber soles; little or no jewelry or makeup; short, clean, unpolished finger nails; no fragrances; and a modest hair style that is pulled away from the face. The visibility of tattoos and other forms of body art may be a concern, so make sure any you have can be concealed by the typical professional clothing.

Responsibilities of the Massage Therapist

Health care is provided in many settings, and the massage therapist must be able to adapt to the different locations. Massage is offered in hospitals, physical therapy practices, private physicians' practices, mental health facilities, chiropractic clinics, long-term care facilities, hospice care, and home health care (Figure 13-3). Each setting has policies to

---

Massage Therapist Massage Therapy

Sisters of Mercy Hospital

Washington, DC
Provide Massage Therapy services to our Hospice, chemotherapy, and specific palliative care patients. Provide one hour and half hour massages in our outpatient clinics.

REPORTS TO: Licensed Massage Therapist.

SUPERVISORY RESPONSIBILITIES: None.

SKILL AND EDUCATIONAL REQUIREMENTS:

EDUCATION:
Graduate from an approved School of Massage Therapy. Current District of Columbia license.

EXPERIENCE:
Two (2) years' experience as a Massage Therapist preferred. Must have some experience working with the public.

KNOWLEDGE, SKILLS AND ABILITY:
This position requires an individual with a great deal of sensitivity to properly interact with patients and their family members. Must be familiar with terminal illnesses and be comfortable in a hospital setting. Ability to relate to patients in various levels of care and disease processes. Strong verbal and written communication skills. Basic computer skills necessary. Some business skills needed. Very detail-oriented job. Must be able to shift from one thing to another calmly.

WORKING CONDITIONS:
The employee will be encountering patients that are diagnosed with terminal illnesses and thus the Massage Therapist must possess the emotional capacity to handle this type of patient. Will be working closely with other staff members and with supervisor; must be able to follow directions and instructions and work well with a variety of personalities. Must be willing to work off site as needed.

A

FULL-TIME LICENSED MASSAGE THERAPIST

We Care Physical Therapy

Tampa, FL

Description
The Licensed Massage Therapist develops and implements specialized massage therapy programs under the standards of the massage therapy practice act. Responsibilities include: assisting in carrying out predetermined patient-related activities in a Physical Therapy setting; performs neuromuscular, myofascial and cranio-sacral massage techniques under the direct coordination and plan of treatment established by the physical therapist. Performs other duties as assigned.

Qualifications
- ▶ *Required Education: High school or GED*
- ▶ *Preferred Education: Associate's in related field*
- ▶ *Required Experience: One year Massage*
- ▶ *Preferred Experience: One year Rehab*
- ▶ *Required Licensure: Massage therapy*
- ▶ *Required Specific Skills: Computer skills appropriate to position, customer service skills, organizational skills, written and verbal communication skills, teamwork, work independently with minimal supervision.*

B

FIGURE 13-3 A, Classified ad for hospital employment. **B,** Classified ad for a physical therapy office.

support quality care. These policies generally involve HIPAA compliance, Standard Precautions, professional conduct, supervisor hierarchy, and incident reporting procedures. Typically all professionals working in a medical setting participate in an orientation process that presents this material. As a massage therapist in the medical setting, pay close attention and always ask clarifying questions and seek assistance if you are unsure of any activity involving patients and staff. Because the medical staff members are busy, be clear and concise during all communication; however, never be afraid to ask relevant questions, so you can be a supportive team member and maintain the safety of the patients.

Massage therapists who want to work in the health care setting must be skilled and knowledgeable in the following areas:

- Infection control
- Sanitation measures
- Clinical reasoning and problem solving
- Preparation of justifications for treatment
- Setting qualifiable and quantifiable goals
- Medical terminology
- Pathology
- Medications
- Assessment
- Development of treatment plans
- Analysis of the effectiveness of methods used
- Charting/documentation and record keeping,
- Effective communication of information
- Third-party insurance reimbursement requirements

Massage therapists also must have a basic understanding of various medical tests, procedures, and treatments so that they can make safe, beneficial decisions on ways to use massage to complement the medical treatments the patient is receiving. These skills can be developed through continuing education for massage professionals or through comprehensive massage training for individuals who already have health care training (e.g., nurses and physical therapy assistants).

For professionals who already have health care training, it is unrealistic to expect that simple exposure to massage is sufficient to enable them to work effectively with the vast knowledge base of massage. It is just as unrealistic to believe that a massage professional with an entry level education can function independently in the health care environment. Supervision by a health care professional, such as a nurse, is necessary to support the entry level massage therapist. Of course, massage therapists do not diagnose; rather, they typically work from a "prescription," following treatment orders.

Massage therapists who choose to develop a career in the health care setting must be willing and able to be a team player, to accept supervision and instruction from medical professionals, to follow orders and relay information accurately (both written and verbal), and to contribute to the patient's care. Agreeing to work in this area means deference to the supervising physician, nurse, and other health care providers. They have more comprehensive education than the typical massage therapist, and they also shoulder the responsibility for the serious and even life and death decisions made during the course of health care.

In choosing a career in the health care environment, you need to understand the responsibility of providing service to those who face health challenges. This is not a decision that should be made lightly. Maintaining appropriate professional boundaries is important. The more complex a patient's condition and life circumstances are, the harder you must work to achieve a balance between empathic dedication to service and remaining neutral and objective in professional practice.

Communication Among the Health Care Team

Precise and concise exchange of information between the massage therapist and other health care professionals is important. Most communication is done in written form through treatment orders and charting. The massage professional's documentation skills must be very effective to work in the health care environment. Health care professionals, especially physicians, are very busy, and they are unlikely to be able to speak at length with you about a particular client. A balance must exist between professional exchange of information, with each member of the team carrying out his or her part of the treatment plan, and the expectation of extensive face-to-face communication.

Highly trained massage therapists are able to discuss the treatment plan intelligently with various medical professionals. They provide valid input, and if disagreement arises, they are able to state their position accurately and professionally and to justify, using evidence-based practice, their recommendations to the supervising personnel.

Pay Scales for Therapeutic Massage in the Health Care Environment

Comparing the pay scales of similar careers in the health care field is the best way to determine the pay scales for massage therapists. The emergency medical technician (EMT) provides a good example. The EMT has a similar level of education and comparable requirements in the health care setting. The basic responsibilities of an EMT are to:

- Have a high school diploma, successfully complete EMT training, register with the EMT national registry, obtain licensure from the state emergency medical services (EMS) authority, and have 2 to 4 years of related experience
- Respond to an emergency call, assesses the situation, obtain a basic medical history, perform a physical examination of the patient, and provide emergency medical care at the scene and during transit to the hospital
- Use medical equipment to treat patients and ascertain the extent of their injuries or illness
- Communicate with the medical facility receiving the patient about the patient's condition, status, and arrival time
- Be familiar with standard concepts, practices, and procedures in a particular field
- Rely on experience and judgment to plan and accomplish goals and perform a variety of tasks
- Work under the supervision of a manager

The annual salary for an EMT can range from $23,000 to $30,000.

A comparison of educational requirements for health professionals shows that those who provide direct, hands-on care to patients usually have an associate's degree (Bureau of Labor Statistics). Other health professions that have training programs similar to those for massage include phlebotomist, certified nurse's aide, dental assistant, and occupational therapy assistant. Based on these data, the annual entry level salary for massage therapy probably will range from $22,000 to $30,000. In addition, typical benefits packages, including health care, are offered. If a massage therapist has an associate's degree or higher or previous health care experience, or is dually trained (e.g., is a licensed practical nurse [LPN]), the pay rate may be as high as $35,000 a year.

Best Practice

The term *best practice* refers to the best possible way of doing something. When pursuing a massage therapy career in the health care setting, we need to determine what is best for the patient. In health care, some formal treatment procedures are considered the best way to proceed with each patient. A best practice is a technique or methodology that, through experience and research, has proven to reliably lead to a desired result. Clinical guidelines for best practices should be founded on eight key principles: validity, reliability/reproducibility, clinical applicability, clinical flexibility, clarity, multidisciplinary process, scheduled review, and documentation (Grant et al., 2008). A commitment to using the best practices in any field is a commitment to using all the knowledge and technology available to ensure success.

The term *medically fragile* sometimes is used to describe patients with serious and complicated medical conditions. One of the biggest mistakes massage therapists make is to do too much too soon; this simply exacerbates the strain on the patient's adaptive mechanisms. Because of the patient's fragile condition, continual decisions must be made on whether the person will benefit from massage treatment or be excessively stressed by it. Supervision and sharing the responsibility of patient care helps maintain this delicate best practices balance.

In 2006 the Massage Therapy Foundation began the process of developing best practice recommendations for massage therapy. Evidence-based practice guidelines are supported by systematic peer review and clinical research. The profession faces numerous challenges in establishing an evidence-based massage approach relative to health care, including ambiguous language, a multitude of massage techniques and philosophies, and lack of high-quality research. Best practice guidelines for massage therapy initially will target treatment for the most common problems clients experience, such as stress management and pain management (e.g., low back pain).

Massage therapists become contributing members of the health care team by understanding their limitations and by developing the ability to work with a physician's supervision to provide care based both on quality medical practice and on effective risk management (best practices).

Massage application in this text is presented as an outcome-based process, which is necessary to develop and follow treatment plans and work effectively in the health care setting. Best practice points to consider when offering massage in the health care environment include the following key points.

Key Points

- Typically the target population is ill or injured; however, preventive care is increasing in popularity, as is reflected in wellness programs and medical spas.
- The more injured or ill the patient, the more general the massage application.
- Massage should support, not interfere with, medical treatment.
- Healing is a body, mind, and spirit process that requires a multidisciplinary approach; this honors the roles of various professionals and respects each one's scope of practice.
- Healing does not necessarily mean cure. Successful coping is a healing process.
- Living well with hope and compassion, regardless of circumstances, is an important goal of healing.
- Massage is targeted to the body, and the appropriate scope of practice must be maintained; therefore, the massage therapist respects and honors but does not cross over into the mind and spirit aspects of treatment.
- Respect for the patient and the health care team is paramount.

Integrating Massage into the Health Care Setting

Most massage applications in the health care setting are general in nature, targeting restorative mechanisms, maintenance of homeostasis, and palliative care. Massage related to soft tissue dysfunction targets common conditions such as headaches, neck and shoulder pain, low back pain, tendinitis, bursitis, and arthritis. Pain management also is an important consideration. In addition, you must understand how the inflammatory response is connected to seemingly unrelated diseases (see Chapters 5 and 6).

Massage care is supportive, not curative, for those who are ill or injured. Massage effectively supports various forms of medical intervention (including mental health) and the body's innate ability to heal. Most diseases and injuries are cured with the medical intervention. This is especially true of acute care situations. However, many people are not necessarily cured with health care interventions such as medication or surgery; instead, their condition is managed, a situation that puts a major strain on the health care delivery system. Because most health conditions are managed and, therefore, require long-term care, treatment is expensive. Massage offers benefits for the management of many chronic health conditions in a potentially cost-effective manner.

Some health benefits of massage have been validated by research (see Chapter 5); others are based on clinical experience and/or are historically supported by the experience of many cultures over centuries of practice. The main focuses of massage in the health care environment are as follows:

- Breathing effectiveness
- Circulation support (blood and lymph)

- Comfort and pleasure
- Edema and fluid imbalance management
- Enhanced parasympathetic dominance
- Pain management
- Reduced sympathetic dominance
- Support for sleep and reduction of fatigue
- Soft tissue normalization (neuromuscular and myofascial)

These outcomes can overlap. For example, reducing sympathetic dominance should improve breathing, support sleep, and increase pain tolerance. Reducing edema could ease pain and increase circulation to an area. Neuromuscular balance allows for effective movement, and myofascial balance supports mobility and stability; together they support effective, efficient movement that encourages circulation, increases comfort, and supports productivity.

Although massage may be very beneficial to clients seen in the health care setting, it is important to remember that when people are in pain, ill, and otherwise "not well," emotions commonly are displayed.

EXAMPLE

A client with chronic pain is experiencing a flare-up. He is short-tempered because of the pain and lack of sleep. The massage seems to be irritating more than soothing. You ask whether he is comfortable and whether you can do anything to make the massage more pleasurable. His response is sarcastic. You may ask again whether there is anything you should do differently, or tell him it is okay if he wants to finish up the massage quickly. Do not try to talk the client out of the mood.

Key Points

Regardless of the setting, the following guidelines apply:

- Standard Precautions and other sanitation procedures must be followed precisely.
- The massage therapist often must work around various types of equipment and devices, such as intravenous lines.
- The massage often must be modified because the client is unable to assume the classic position of lying on a massage table.
- Many clients are confined to a bed or wheelchair.
- Privacy often is compromised, and interruptions are common.
- The environment may be noisy and busy with other activity.
- Various medications and their interaction with the effects of the massage must be considered.
- The effects of medical tests or preparation for tests can affect massage interventions.

The Health Insurance Portability and Accountability Act of 1996

The Health Insurance Portability and Accountability Act of 1996 covers a multitude of the regulatory aspects of the health care environment. As described in Chapter 2, the massage therapist should receive in-service training about procedures relating to HIPAA requirements and how they are implemented in the specific health care environment.

Medical and other health information is private and must be protected. HIPAA's Privacy Rule gives individuals rights over their health information and specifies who can look at and receive health information. The Privacy Rule applies to all forms of an individual's protected health information (PHI), whether electronic, written, or oral. The Security Rule protects health information in electronic form. It requires entities covered by HIPAA to ensure that electronic PHI is secure. Protected information includes:

- Information physicians, nurses, and other health care providers put in a medical record
- Conversations the physician has about a patient's care or treatment with nurses and others
- Information about an individual in a health insurer's computer system
- Billing information about a patient

HIPAA also seeks to limit administrative costs by supporting the use of electronic transfer of information, and it establishes guidelines for preventing fraud and abuse.

Health Insurance

Health insurance is a type of third-party payer system. This means that the consumer pays for insurance; then, when medical expenses occur, the costs are billed to and potentially covered by the insurance. Numerous third-party payers base reimbursement on what is referred to as the *allowable charge*, which has been influenced by managed care organizations and the government. *Managed care* is a broad term used to describe a variety of health plans developed to provide health care services at lower costs.

Health insurance is available to people in many ways. People can buy individual policies, but most get health insurance by being a member of a group, which pools resources to purchase health insurance. Examples of groups that provide health insurance are employees in a business (sometimes the employer offers health insurance as a benefit) or a chamber of commerce arrangement, through which small business owners can get coverage. For the massage profession, professional associations such as the American Massage Therapy Association (AMTA) and the Associated Bodywork & Massage Professionals (ABMP) offer group access to health insurance.

Insurance policies have many coverage options, from minimal coverage to maximum coverage. Some may include alternative and complementary care coverage, whereas others do not. In group coverage situations, the types and amount of coverage a person is eligible to receive may not be amendable to include certain types of treatment, such as massage therapy.

Major third-party payers with which the massage therapist should become familiar include major medical group insurance, Aetna, Blue Cross/Blue Shield, Medicaid, Medicare, CHAMPVA, TRICARE, and workers' compensation. Medicare is the largest third-party insurer in the United States, making quality health care affordable for the elderly and other select groups. Medicaid is another U.S. government-sponsored health care plan for individuals who qualify for these benefits based on income limitations and/or disability. Workers' compensation covers employees who are injured or who become ill as a result of accidents or adverse conditions in the workplace. Disability programs reimburse individuals for monetary losses incurred as a result of an inability to work for reasons other than those covered under workers' compensation.

Because of the constant rise in the cost of health insurance, growing numbers of people are uninsured and therefore do not receive some types of necessary medical care.

Health Care Reform and the Health Insurance Industry

Unlike many countries (e.g., Canada), the United States does not have a universal health care system. Instead, it has a staggeringly diverse and fragmented system of providers and payers, including (but not limited to) private insurance, out-of-pocket payment, and government-run programs (e.g., Medicare, Department of Veterans Affairs).

In March 2010, the Affordable Care Act was signed into law. All of the changes mandated by the law will not take effect at once; changes will be implemented through 2014. Although the new law does not provide a universal health care system for the United States, it does address many issues regarding the health insurance industry. (Visit the Web links section for this chapter on the Evolve website for links to the Affordable Care Act itself; also visit the website healthcare.gov, which explains the law and provides resources for finding health insurance and understanding the benefits provided under the new law.)

Health Insurance Reimbursement

Reimbursement for services by health insurance companies is a common practice in health care. Lack of reimbursement for many complementary methods, such as massage, is one of the main obstacles to their inclusion in the health care process. This situation probably will improve as more research identifies a positive risk/benefit/cost value for massage services to justify reimbursement.

In the health care environment, the infrastructure already exists for billing insurance companies for payment for services rendered. Large facilities, such as hospitals, have designated departments for health insurance billing. Small medical practices usually have a person responsible for health insurance billing. Fortunately, a major advantage of employment in the health care environment is that the massage therapist is paid a salary or fee for each massage, regardless of reimbursement.

The massage therapist with a career in health care needs to understand enough about health insurance and reimbursement to support the billing specialist (the insurance biller and coder) in this area. The massage therapist's responsibility is to maintain appropriate records to justify insurance reimbursement and to follow the preauthorized treatment plans as presented by the supervisory health care professional.

Although some massage therapists work in areas that bill directly to insurance for payment, this is not common practice. In some situations, a massage therapist may receive health insurance reimbursement outside the traditional health care setting, in the context of private practice. A physician's referral and preauthorization may be required.

Record Keeping

Record keeping in various medical settings is extremely important. It is a skill that needs to be practiced and perfected. Massage therapy training often is lax in this area, but the skill is vital for massage therapists who want a career in health care. Record keeping is the recording of relevant data. Review Chapters 4 and 11 for specific record keeping procedures relevant to massage.

Nine criteria define quality health data. The data must be:

- *Valid,* which refers to the accuracy of the information.
- *Reliable,* which means that the information can be counted on to be accurate and to support medical decisions.
- *Complete,* which simply means that the information is available in its entirety.
- *Recognizable,* which means the data can be understood by the users.
- *Timely,* which means the information allows the provider to make decisions based on the latest data about a patient or a treatment.
- *Relevant,* which means the health information is useful for the current situation.
- *Accessible,* which means the information is easily available to the provider when needed.
- *Secure,* which encompasses the effort to keep unauthorized people from accessing health information
- *Legal,* which refers to the correctness of the information and its authentication by the health care provider.

Box 13-8 provides general guidelines that must be followed in creating a credible patient record (also see Figure 13-4).

Confidentiality

Patient health care records are confidential. Most health care providers, and certainly hospitals, have policies and procedures governing the release of any information about a patient. Massage therapists must be aware of those policies. Most health care providers are in the process of implementing or have already implemented new policies and procedures incorporating the requirements of HIPAA.

Recall from Chapter 2 that all states have laws about which diseases, conditions, and events must be reported to the appropriate agencies. Some such incidents include births, deaths, gunshot wounds, communicable diseases, and evidence of child abuse. If massage therapists in the health care setting encounter any type of reportable case, they should report the situation to their supervisors. Massage therapists also should ask their supervisors whether there are any specific reportable circumstances the massage therapist should expect to encounter. When reporting is required by law, confidentiality is no longer an issue, although the format of the report

Box 13-8 Guidelines for Creating a Patient Record

The following rules help ensure that a patient's record is accurate, timely, specific, objective, concise, consistent, comprehensive, logical, legible, and reflective of the thought processes of the health care providers.

- Each page of the record should identify the patient, by name, hospital, clinic, or private physician clinical record number.
- Each entry in the record should include the date and time the entry was made and the signature and credential of the individual making the entry.
- No blank spaces should be left between entries.
- All entries should be written in ink or produced on a printer or typewriter.
- The record must not be altered in any way. Erasures, use of correction fluid, and marked-out areas are not appropriate.
- Errors should be corrected in a manner that allows the reader to see and understand the error. The following procedure is recommended:
  1. A single line is drawn through the error, and the legibility of the previous entry is checked.
  2. The correct information is inserted.
  3. The correction is dated and initialed.
  4. If there is not enough room for the correction to be made legibly at the error, a note should be made indicating where the corrected entry can be found, and the reference dated and initialed. The correct information is entered in the proper chronologic order for the date the error was discovered and corrected.

- All information should be recorded as soon as possible. Telephone contacts with the patient should be entered in the record immediately. Memories can fade, and important facts can be omitted.
- All information given to the patient before any procedures should be recorded. This ensures and verifies that the patient was properly informed of the benefits and risks before giving consent to the procedure.
- Abbreviations should be used sparingly. Only those that have been approved by the organization and that are listed in an abbreviation code on the document should be used. Otherwise, the same abbreviation can have different meanings, which can be misleading.
- All entries must be written legibly. It is embarrassing and can be expensive when caregivers cannot read their own entries in court. Because the patient record is used by so many other clinicians in providing care, it is important to the quality of patient care that the record be legible. The use of the electronic record is addressing this issue.
- All entries must be consistent with one another. The assessment must agree with the diagnostic testing, or an explanation must be given as to why it does not.
- Entries should be factual accounts. Criticisms of the patient or a colleague should never occur. Records that blame or belittle others can be damning evidence in a lawsuit.
- Some method of organizing entries, such as the SOAP format, must be used to ensure that the entries are comprehensive and reflect the thought process used in making decisions about the patient's care.

---

may or may not include the identity of the patient, so be sure to ask about the proper method for reporting. Reporting such incidents to anyone other than the responsible agency, however, is a breach of confidentiality.

Computer-Based Patient Record and the Electronic Health Record

The paper medical record is fast becoming a thing of the past. A paper record is difficult to access, often lacks information, and must be in a single location for a single user. Over the past three decades, significant strides have been made in automating the record-keeping process. The federal government is encouraging adoption of meaningful use of electronic medical records (EMRs) and other health information technology by 2014. Technology has improved, allowing the design and implementation of electronic record keeping systems that are easy to use. Automated record keeping systems have many different names, including *computer-based patient record, electronic patient record, computerized medical record,* and *electronic record.* Massage therapists must be able to use whatever electronic record-keeping system is in place in the environment where they work. The thought process is the same; the data record is the same. It may be necessary to jot paper notes while working with the patient, but eventually these notes must be entered into the electronic system (Figures 13-4 and 13-5).

Basic Pharmacology for the Massage Therapist

Pharmacology is the science of drugs and includes the development of drugs, the understanding of their mechanisms of action, and the description of their conditions of use. *Pharmacists* are the medical professionals who specialize in pharmacology. The terms *medication* and *drugs* often are used interchangeably. However, *medication* is specific to pharmaceutical agents used in the treatment of disease, whereas *drugs* can encompass a broader scope of chemical use, including substances such as cocaine and over-the-counter (OTC) medications. The following discussion typically uses the term *drug.* The focus of the section is on the possible interaction of massage influence on the body and these chemicals. Because drugs are a major treatment factor in the health care setting, it is essential that the massage therapist working in this environment understand the fundamentals of pharmacology.

Pharmacodynamics

Pharmacodynamics is the study of the effects of a drug on the body and the mode of the drug's action. The chemicals in the drug are distributed throughout the body by the blood and other fluids of distribution. Once they arrive at the proper site of action, they act by binding to receptors, usually located on the outer membrane of cells, or on enzymes located within the cell.

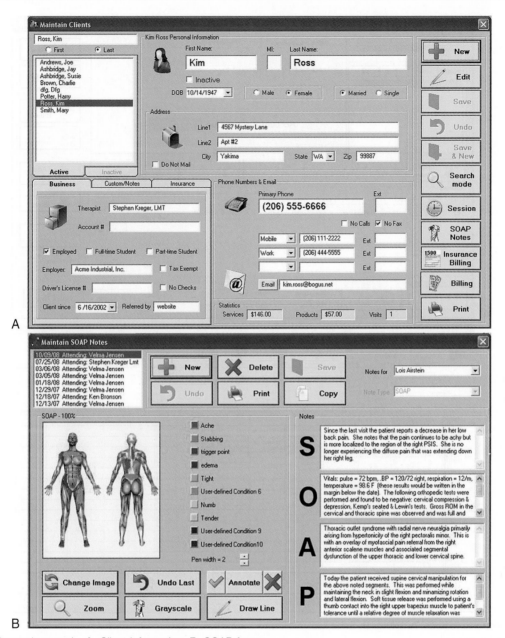

FIGURE 13-4 Electronic records. **A,** Client information. **B,** SOAP forms. (Courtesy of Island Software.)

Various drugs are designed to target specific receptors to elicit a specific response. Receptors are like biologic "switches" that turn on and off when stimulated by a drug that binds to the receptor and activates it. For example, narcotic pain relievers, such as morphine, bind to receptors in the brain that sense pain and reduce the intensity of that perception. Non-narcotic pain relievers, such as aspirin, ibuprofen (e.g., Motrin) and acetaminophen (e.g., Tylenol), bind to an enzyme located in cells outside the brain, close to where the pain is localized (e.g., the low back) and reduce the formation of biologically active substances known as prostaglandins, which cause pain and inflammation. These peripherally acting (i.e., acting outside the central nervous system) analgesics (pain modulators) also may reduce the sensitivity of the local pain nerves, meaning fewer pain impulses are sensed and transmitted to the brain.

In some instances, a drug's site of action, or receptor, may be something in the body that is not anatomically a part of the body. For example, for antacids such as Tums or Rolaids, the site of action is the acid in the stomach, which these drugs chemically neutralize. Antibiotics are another example of drugs that bind to a receptor that is not part of the body. Antibiotics bind to portions of bacteria that are living in the body and causing disease. Most antibiotics inhibit an enzyme inside the bacteria, which causes the bacteria either to stop reproducing or to die from inhibition of a vital biochemical process.

As medical science has learned more about how drugs act, pharmacologists have discovered that the body is full of different types of receptors that respond to many different types of drugs. Some receptors are very selective and specific, whereas others lack such specificity and respond to several different types of chemical molecules.

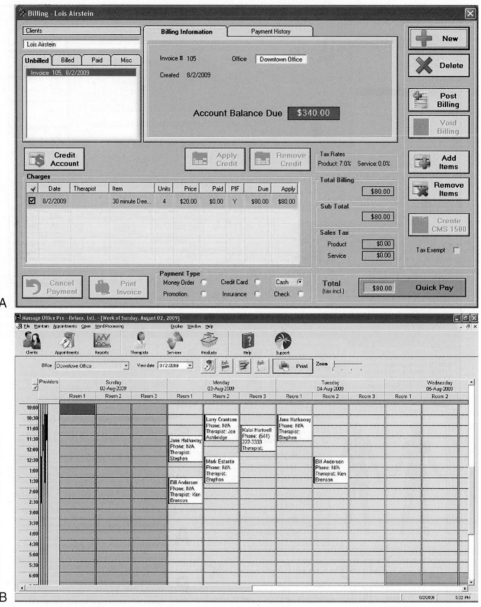

FIGURE 13-5 Electronic records. **A,** Billing. **B,** Schedule. (Courtesy of Island Software.)

The massage therapist needs to understand the action of a medication and then needs to use clinical reasoning skills to adapt the massage appropriately (see Appendix A). All chemicals taken into the body, whether medications, OTC drugs, drugs of abuse, environmental pollutants, food, vitamin supplements, herbs, or manufactured food ingredients (e.g., artificial sweeteners, colorings, and preservatives) have the potential to influence the body in both beneficial and negative ways. (Chapter 15 provides a detailed discussion of nutrition, including vitamin and herbal supplements.)

Drug Interactions

Certain foods, herbs, and vitamins can affect the action of drugs. This interaction can be supportive or detrimental. For example, patients who take certain medications (e.g., statins, which lower cholesterol) should not eat grapefruit. Serious side effects can occur if a patient taking a selective serotonin reuptake inhibitor (SSRI), such as Zoloft or Paxil, also takes St. John's wort, SAMe, or 5-HPT. Vitamins typically are best when taken with food; however, the absorption of some medications is inhibited if the drug is taken with food. The entire potential interaction process can be extremely complicated.

Using a Drug Reference

It is helpful to have a drug reference available so you can look up a particular medication to learn how it is used and the possible side effects. Then, when you apply what you know about the effects of massage on the body (see Chapters 4 and 5), you can make informed, intelligent decisions about how to adapt the massage based on the medication or medications your client is taking.

A good drug reference to add to either your book or electronic library is *Mosby's Drug Reference for Health Professions* (See Appendix C).

The Evolution of Health Care

Health care is evolving, and an emerging trend is the biopsychosocial model of medicine. This approach to health care is similar to the body/mind/spirit model of wellness. For the sake of clarity, medical practices currently derived from a biomedical Western scientific model are referred to as *conventional health care*. Many conventional health care professionals are frustrated and concerned about the inability to treat lifestyle-related illnesses effectively, particularly those that are chronic, with standard approaches using medication and surgery (Peters et al, 2002).

The term *complementary* refers to approaches or therapies that are used in addition to conventional medical treatments; for example, the use of acupuncture or massage with physical therapy and medications for patients with chronic pain syndromes. The term *alternative* refers to approaches or therapies that are used instead of or in place of conventional medicine; for example, the use of homeopathy and homeopathic remedies instead of pharmaceuticals.

Integrative Medicine

Combining conventional and complementary approaches to health care has become more accepted, because the intent is to emphasize care in a wider context of body/mind/spirit interconnectedness and the importance of supporting wellness in addition to treating pathologic conditions. This is called integrative medicine, which supports the following premises:

- The body has the power to heal itself.
- Most health problems derive from a failure of the tissues, or the individual, to adapt to the biochemical, biomechanical, and/or psychosocial stressors of life.
- Healing often requires the use of multiple techniques that involve the mind, body, and spirit to enhance the individual's adaptive capacity (self-healing) or to reduce the adaptive load, or to minimize excessive symptomatic responses.

Treatment often is individualized and depends on the patient's presenting symptoms, the context from which he or she emerged, and the processes involved.

Lifestyle illnesses (diseases of longevity) are increasing as a result of stress, fatigue, poor nutritional choices, obesity, and similar factors. Many people come to recognize the overwhelming need to change their lifestyle, and these people turn to integrative medicine as a means of change. The medical spa is a model of an integrated approach. The medical spa concept is one of relaxation, pleasure, and pampering combined with the treatment of medical conditions. The medical spa is an ideal environment for addressing health care conditions that require major lifestyle changes, such as weight management, chronic fatigue, some types of physical rehabilitation, and physical conditioning. Some medical spas also offer nutritional help to assist in a dietary lifestyle change, which in turn assists with disease, weight management, and some illnesses.

History of Conventional and Alternative Medicine

The American Medical Association (AMA) was formed in 1848. In 1900, 20% of all practitioners of medicine were considered "alternative" physicians. In the early 1900s, the AMA issued a statement to its members saying that it was unethical for physicians and members of the AMA to consult, confer, or interact with "alternative" practitioners. This began the exclusion of any medical approaches or treatments that were not considered within the mainstream of medicine.

Other factors also contributed to the near disappearance of alternative health approaches, including Rudolf Virchow's cell theory and Louis Pasteur's germ theory in the late 1800s, followed by the discovery of x-rays in the early 1900s and of penicillin in the late 1920s.

The discovery of antibiotics was a pivotal point for the emergence of conventional medicine, and the use of alternative medicine almost completely disappeared in the United States from 1920 to 1960. However, it continued as an important aspect of health care in other parts of the world, where chiropractors, naturopaths, and osteopaths remained active. For example, Dr. Leon Chaitow, who wrote the foreword to this text, qualified as a doctor of naturopathy (naturopath, or ND) and a doctor of osteopathy (osteopath, or DO) in England in 1960 and joined a thriving profession.

Beginning around 1970, alternative approaches to health and healing began to resurface in the United States. The health care culture was truly changed by the social upheaval of the 1960s. The cost of health care was becoming prohibitive. The new prominence of the field of psychology and the role of the mind in illness and disease were major influences, as was recognition of the debilitating and sometimes fatal adverse side effects of medications previously thought safe. Cardinal factors in the change were the emergence of resistant strains of bacteria, the human immunodeficiency virus (HIV) and acquired immunodeficiency syndrome (AIDS) epidemic, and the increasing inability to treat lifestyle diseases successfully with conventional medical approaches.

In 1991 Congress established the Office of Alternative Medicine (OAM) within the National Institutes of Health (NIH). (The OAM now is known as the National Center for Complementary and Alternative Medicine [NCCAM].) The purpose of the OAM was to facilitate the evaluation of alternative medical treatments and their effectiveness through research and other initiatives. The initial budget for this undertaking was $2 million.

Before it could begin the process of evaluation, the OAM needed a classification system that would allow better identification of the alternative treatments. Seven groups were established initially, but the system has since been revised to five major domains:

- *Alternative health systems:* Traditional Asian medicine, Ayurvedic (Indian) medicine, Tibetan medicine, Native American medicine, homeopathy, and naturopathy.
- *Mind/body interventions:* Meditation imagery, hypnosis, biofeedback, yoga, tai chi, Qi gong, prayer, spiritual healing, soul retrieval, and intuitive diagnosis.
- *Biologically based therapies:* Herbal medicine, special diets (Ornish, Pritikin, Weil, Atkins, macrobiotic), orthomolecular medicine, and iridology.
- *Manipulative and body-based methods:* Chiropractic, osteopathy, craniosacral therapy, massage, reflexology,

Pilates, Rolfing, structural integration, Trager body work, and Alexander technique.

- *Energy therapies:* Qigong, Reiki, polarity therapy, therapeutic touch, and electromagnetic therapies.

The focus of NCCAM is to make complementary alternative modalities safe and accessible to the American population. The agency recommended that the education of those studying conventional medicine include instruction in complementary and alternative medicine (CAM), and the education of CAM practitioners include studies in conventional medicine. The intended result is to train conventional providers who can discuss CAM with their patients, provide guidance on the use of CAM treatments, and collaborate with CAM practitioners, as well as CAM practitioners who can communicate and collaborate with conventional providers.

Some common complementary modalities that have moved into mainstream biomedical practice are massage, acupuncture, relaxation/stress management, and herbal treatments (Box 13-9). Massage is being incorporated into the conventional health care setting for three main reasons: low risk, low cost, and high patient satisfaction. Research into the physiologic mechanisms of the benefits of massage has demonstrated its efficacy (i.e., ability to produce a desired effect).

A growing aspect of integrative health care can also be seen in the increase in cosmetic surgery coupled with antiaging modalities that primarily target control of inappropriate inflammation, supporting both physical fitness and mental health.

Box 13-9   Complementary Medicine Approaches

Treatment approaches commonly considered as complementary medicine include the following health care practices:

Acupressure
Acupuncture
Alexander technique
Applied kinesiology
Aromatherapy
Autogenic training
Ayurveda
Chiropractic
Cranial osteopathy
Environmental medicine
Homeopathy
Hypnosis
Massage
Meditation
Naturopathy
Nutritional therapy
Osteopathy
Qi gong
Reflexology
Relaxation and visualization techniques
Shiatsu
Tai chi
Therapeutic touch
Yoga

From Peters D, Chaitow L, Harris G, Morrison S: *Integrating complementary therapies in primary care,* Edinburgh, 2002, Churchill Livingstone.

Beneficial and Safe Complementary Practice

People usually consult complementary practitioners with mild to moderate, long-term, painful, functional, and stress-related conditions and disorders, all of which occupy a great deal of the general medical practitioner's time. Conditions that often can be managed successfully with complementary therapies include undifferentiated illnesses and chronic structural and relapsing functional disorders. Good clinical trials suggest that for certain conditions, complementary therapies are the treatment of choice. Well-designed studies have been done on the effectiveness of complementary methods for a range of common problems, including anxiety, fibromyalgia syndrome, asthma, irritable bowel syndrome (IBS), eczema, and migraines.

The growing acceptance of complementary therapies coincides with an increased interest in lifestyle change, health promotion, and low-technology treatments. These approaches, integrated into conventional medical care, might provide inexpensive, safe ways to address conditions that currently do not respond well to conventional care.

Conventional medicine can be the best treatment for trauma and acute care. Conventional medicine can provide effective treatment for many common conditions, such as acute bacterial infection, congestive heart failure, and glaucoma. Alternative or adjunctive treatments support this care. Accepted modalities currently available in health care (e.g., nursing, physiotherapy, specialist referral, counseling, and medications) do not necessarily meet the needs of patients whose problems are not "fixable." Other people have long-term relapsing structural or functional disorders, for which medical treatment often is less than satisfactory. People with conditions that do not respond to conventional medical care alone might have better outcomes with the combined approach used in multiprofessional/multidisciplinary integrated health care. If this new type of health care approach is to succeed, those who practice complementary therapies must comply with various requirements to achieve integration into the current health care system.

The conventional health care community has concerns about the new approach, most of which are valid. If people are seen by unqualified practitioners, the risk of a missed or delayed diagnosis arises, possibly with tragic results. People may waste money on ineffective treatments and discontinue or not use effective conventional treatment. The mechanisms of benefit claimed for some complementary treatments are implausible, and many complementary therapies are scientifically unproven. Health care insurers must establish whether and how complementary therapies support health care before routine insurance coverage is authorized. Public expectation is growing that complementary therapies should be made available. Therefore it must be demonstrated that patients are being treated with a safe, effective therapy, by a qualified practitioner (Box 13-10), and that this approach is more acceptable and more cost-effective than the conventional medical alternatives.

Practitioners of complementary therapies, including massage, must comply with the logical and attainable recommendations of conventional medicine before a unified move

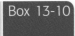

Box 13-10 Professional Requirements for Practitioners of Complementary Medicine

Qualifications: Practitioners should have a recognized qualification from a training establishment that is accredited by a suitable regulatory body.

Registration license: Practitioners must be registered with a recognized professional body that requires its members to abide by codes of conduct, ethics, and discipline.

Insurance: Practitioners must have adequate professional liability insurance coverage that applies to the period of their employment.

Consent to treatment: Patients must be fully informed about the nature of the therapy and its effects, including any side effects, and must have realistic expectations of its benefits. The informed consent of the patient or, in the case of young children, of the parent or guardian, must be gained and documented.

Medical responsibility: Practitioners should be aware that patients referred to them for treatment remain the overall responsibility of the referring clinician. Complementary and alternative medicine (CAM) practitioners should not advise the client to discontinue existing treatments without the agreement of the referring clinician.

Documentation: A written record should be kept by practitioners of the consultation and each episode of treatment. All written (and oral) information should be treated as confidential and should take into account the requirements of the Health Insurance Portability and Accountability Act (HIPAA).

Refusal to treat: Practitioners have a duty not to treat a patient if they consider the treatment unsafe or unsuitable.

Education and training: Practitioners should take responsibility for keeping abreast of developments in the practice of their therapy.

Quality standards: Practitioners, in conjunction with other health care professionals, should assist with the development of local standards and guidelines for practice.

Audits: Practitioners should undertake a clinical audit and report the results to the employing or commissioning practice/PCG. They should be responsible for monitoring the outcome of therapy; clients' opinions should be actively sought and included in any evaluation.

Research: Practitioners should be expected to agree to take part in research trials to support the evaluation and development of treatment programs.

Health and safety: Practitioners should comply with the requirements of health and safety legislation and should adhere to good practice in the protection of staff, patients, and the public.

Control of infection: Practitioners should adhere to regulations governing infection control and follow the procedure for reporting outbreaks of infection.

Modified from the Scottish Department of Health 1996 Complementary Medicine and the National Health Service: *Complementary medicine information pack for primary care groups,* June, 2000.

can be made toward integrative medicine. The main focus of this text is therapeutic massage, which is being integrated into health care, and the massage community is working to meet these recommendations. Massage has come a long way, especially in the past 5 years. Evidence-based research supports the efficacy of massage, and avenues are available for appropriate education, licensure or certification, insurance coverage, and so forth.

The biggest hurdles to integrating massage into conventional heath care are (1) finding appropriately trained massage therapists (for more information, see the textbook, *Clinical Massage in the Health Care Setting,* by Sandy Fritz, Leon Chaitow, and Glenn Hymel) and (2) identifying the source of funds to pay for massage. Currently health insurance does not routinely cover therapeutic massage. Further research must be done to show that massage treatment is more cost-effective than conventional medical treatment for various conditions and that it has the same or better benefits without an increase in risk to the patient. Research can also document whether conventional medical treatment achieves better outcomes when combined with complementary methods. When this has been shown (and the massage community is confident that it will be), the final hurdle to full integration of massage into the health care community will be overcome. Massage therapists are unlikely to work and bill health insurance companies independently. More likely, qualified massage therapists will be directly supervised by health care providers who can bill for the massage session.

Cross-Training Recommendations

If the health care setting is your career path of choice, it may be prudent also to train as a certified nursing assistant/patient care technician, licensed practical/vocational nurse, or EMT. The education in these areas will provide specific information about procedures and conduct in the health care setting and indicate that you have the skills to function in the medical setting safely as a massage therapist.

Patient care technicians, also called nursing assistants or nurse's aides, perform basic care procedures in hospitals, clinics, and nursing homes. Most programs take 1 year or less to complete and prepare students for state certification examinations. EMT training usually is a 6-month to 2-year certificate, diploma, or associate degree program depending on the level of certification. Most licensed practical/vocational nurse training programs take 1 year to complete, and a licensing examination is required.

THERAPEUTIC MASSAGE IN THE SPORTS AND FITNESS ENVIRONMENT

SECTION OBJECTIVES

Chapter objectives covered in this section:

16. Identify and demonstrate the skills and responsibilities necessary for massage therapy practice in the sports and fitness environment.
17. Describe and adapt massage for the sport and fitness practice setting
18. Identify cross training recommendations for a career in the sports and fitness industry.

Using the information presented in this section, the student will be able to perform the following:

- Provide massage in various sports and fitness environments
- Explain remedial, rehabilitative, medical, and orthopedic massage in the sports and fitness environment
- List common goals and outcomes in the sports and fitness environment
- Describe the elements of practice for a sports event

More and more sports, fitness, and rehabilitation professionals are turning to massage as part of the treatment or management of various conditions. In reality, there is no such thing as "sports massage"—only the appropriate massage application for each client. Whether the client is a runner; bowler; swimmer; surfer; golfer; or baseball, basketball, football, or soccer player, or simply a person who has just finished a treadmill stress test, he or she still needs a treatment plan designed for that person's particular needs.

Clients of sports and fitness massage present a range of different needs. Some clients are undergoing physical rehabilitation that requires an exercise program (e.g., cardiovascular and cardiorespiratory rehabilitation or physical therapy for an orthopedic injury). Other clients are taking up exercise as part of a comprehensive fitness and wellness program, including weight management. Still other clients are recreational athletes or competitive athletes, both amateur and professional.

Typically massage therapists with advanced training have some athletic clients as part of their professional practice and will modify massage for the athlete (see Chapter 14). Many massage practitioners who are interested in sports massage want to work with professional athletes. The reality is those jobs are rare, because there are not that many professional or Olympic athletes. The National Basketball Association (NBA) has fewer than 400 players, and the National Football League (NFL) has fewer than 2,500. Other team sports fall somewhere between those numbers. Individual professional athletes, such as tennis players, golfers, and bowlers, are also a small community. Most massage therapists will serve the high school, collegiate, amateur, or semiprofessional athlete and, even more, those undergoing rehabilitation or striving to maintain fitness.

Another common misconception is that professional athletes make many millions of dollars; the truth is only a few make it into that category. Most make far less, and amateurs generate no athletic income at all. Therefore justifying the cost/benefit of therapeutic massage, compared with the expense and regularity of use, is an ongoing issue. More commonly, sports fitness and rehabilitation cost money, often lots of it. If a person is going to use massage regularly, the fees have to be manageable.

Additional demands are placed on professionals who work with athletes or in physical rehabilitation because of the extraordinary circumstances of these clients. The environment of competitive sports or physical rehabilitation makes for "bigger than life" moments. There is the drama of win or lose, the trauma of injury, and the career-determining or even life or death situations of surgery and rehabilitation. Working in the sports and fitness environment can be like a roller coaster ride, but with a lot of monotony between the highs and lows.

Massage therapists in this field must be highly skilled in the massage applications appropriate for the particular type of sport or fitness activity of their individual clients. Beyond the necessary massage skills is a requirement for a host of less obvious skills: motivation, maturity, reliability, compassion, tenacity, tolerance, stamina, flexibility, commitment, faith, hope, perseverance, humbleness, self-esteem, little need for personal glory, the ability to work behind the scenes, and the ability to improvise and, above all, to problem solve.

Employment and Pay Scales

Locations and potential employers who would provide opportunities to practice sport-specific massage include fitness centers, fitness spas, sports clubs (e.g., tennis, golf, racquetball, and so on), sports training facilities (amateur and professional), gyms, sports medicine facilities, and individual athletic clients (Figure 13-6).

Because experience and additional training are necessary to work with the complexities of athletic performance demand, pay scales are somewhat higher. Instead of employment (except in fitness spas and centers), most massage therapists who specialize in massage for athletes work as independent contractors.

Remedial, Rehabilitative, Medical, and Orthopedic Massage in the Sports and Fitness Environment

The terms *remedial massage, rehabilitative massage, medical massage,* and *orthopedic massage* are all interrelated. **Remedial massage** is used for minor to moderate injuries. Methods used in remedial massage include all those presented in this text. **Rehabilitative massage** is used for more severe injuries or as part of the postsurgical intervention plan; if the injury or surgery is related to bones or joints, this type of massage can be considered orthopedic massage.

The massage methods used in rehabilitation vary. Immediately after injury or surgery, the techniques used generally are more nonspecific and focus on reducing stress and promoting healing. Attention is given to the entire body while the area of injury or surgery heals. If immobility, use of crutches, or changes in posture or gait are factors during recovery, compensation patterns are likely to develop. Massage can manage these compensation patterns while the physician, physical therapist, and athletic trainer focus on the injured area. During active rehabilitation, massage can become part of the total treatment plan for recovery when supervised by an appropriately qualified professional. The textbook *Sports and Exercise Massage: Comprehensive Care in Athletics, Fitness, and Rehabilitation,* by Sandy Fritz (Mosby, 2005), provides comprehensive information about working in this environment.

Common Goals and Outcomes for Massage in Sports and Fitness

Two primary goals of sports massage are to assist the athlete in achieving and maintaining peak performance and to support the healing of injuries. Many factors contribute to

Fitness for You

Job Title: Massage Therapist
Location: Newark, NJ

Description
Part-time Massage Therapist must be able to excel in an environment that sets goals, tracks progress, and strives for growth. Team members with our company are expected to be the most technically advanced and educated professionals, committed to positively enriching each other, our members and our guests.

Responsibilities
As a Massage Therapist for our company you will be responsible for providing sports massage as part of member services in a professional atmosphere. Massage services provide a variety of techniques targeted to support training protocols. Massage Therapists are required to provide assessment and outcome massage treatment plans in conjunction with the strength and conditioning personnel.

Qualifications
Appropriate License in massage therapy.
Additional training and experience in performance related massage therapy application.
Flexible schedule.

FIGURE 13-6 Classified ad for a fitness center position.

mechanical injuries or trauma in this environment. In sports, *trauma* is defined as a physical injury or wound, produced by an external or internal force, that was sustained as the result of a sports endeavor. Healing mechanisms manifest as the inflammatory response and resolution of the inflammatory response. The different tissues heal at different rates. For example, skin heals quickly, whereas ligaments heal slowly. Stress can influence healing by slowing the repair process. Sleep and proper nutrition are necessary for proper healing.

A massage professional should be able to recognize common sports injuries and should refer the athlete to the appropriate medical professional. Once a diagnosis has been made and the rehabilitation plan developed, the massage professional can support the athlete with general massage application and appropriate methods to enhance the healing process.

Massage professionals who intend to work with athletes must obtain additional training. Many specialized training programs for sports massage are available. Such training should include the physiologic and psychological functions of an athlete; overuse and repetitive use syndromes; the biomechanics of specific sports; the use of cryotherapy, ice massage, and other hydrotherapy methods; injury repair and rehabilitation; and education in training regimens (Arnheim and Prentice, 2005). The text *Sports and Exercise Massage: Comprehensive Care in Athletics, Fitness, and Rehabilitation* (Mosby's Massage Career Development), by Sandy Fritz (Mosby, 2006), covers these areas (Proficiency Exercise 13-1).

💡 PROFICIENCY EXERCISE 13-1

1. Look through professional journals and send for information about three different training sessions in advanced sports massage.
2. Contact a university with a sports team and speak with the athletic trainer. Find out how massage might be used to enhance athletic performance.
3. Contact a local exercise club or physical therapy department and talk with the exercise physiologist about how massage could enhance the work being done there.
4. Volunteer to work at a sponsored sports massage event held by your school or local professional massage organization.
5. With your classmates, organize a sports massage event for a local sporting function.
6. Obtain a catalog from a university that offers degrees in athletic training or exercise physiology. List the classes required to earn these degrees.

The Sporting Event as a Practice Option

Early in the 1980s the concept of sports massage was used as a public awareness and promotional activity. Representatives of massage schools and massage organizations often were present at amateur sporting events. The work was primarily based on a volunteer model, not a career setting. At that time, the AMTA offered specific sports massage testing and

| Box 13-11 | Sample Informed Consent Form for Use at Sporting Events |

Name: _____

Sporting event: _____

Date: _____

I have received, read, and understand informational literature concerning the general benefits of massage and the contraindications for massage. I have disclosed to the massage practitioner any condition I have that would be contraindicated for massage. Other than to determine contraindications, I understand that no specific needs assessment will be performed. The qualifications of the massage practitioner and reporting measures for misconduct have been disclosed to me.

I understand that the massage given here is for the purpose of stress reduction. I understand that massage practitioners do not diagnose illness or disease, perform any spinal manipulations, or prescribe any medical treatments. I acknowledge that massage is not a substitute for medical examination or diagnosis, and it is recommended that I see a health care provider for those services.

I understand that an event sports massage is limited to providing a general, nonspecific massage approach using standard massage methods but does not include any methods to address specifically soft tissue structure or function.

Participant's signature: _____ Date: _____

Participant's signature: _____ Date: _____

Participant's signature: _____ Date: _____

certification. Also during that time, sports massage was categorized by when it was given and the reasons for the massage. Some of those categories are discussed in the next paragraphs. However, if outcome-based goals are used, these categories become irrelevant. For example, if massage is used to assist a pre-exercise warm-up, it should focus on those goals.

Pre-event (Warm-Up) Massage

The pre-event, or warm-up, massage is a stimulating, superficial, fast-paced, rhythmic massage that lasts 10 to 15 minutes. The emphasis is on the muscles used in the sporting event, and the goal is to help the athlete feel that his or her body is perfect physically. Uncomfortable techniques should be avoided. The pre-event massage is given in addition to the physical warm-up; it is not a substitute. This style of massage can be used from 3 days before the event until just before the event. The massage therapist should focus on enhancing circulation and should be very careful not to overwork any area. The sports pre-event massage should be general, nonspecific, light, and warming. Neither friction nor deep, heavy strokes should be used. Massage techniques that require recovery time or are painful are strictly contraindicated. Preferably, only massage therapists who work on a continual basis with a particular athlete should give the person a pre-event massage.

Intercompetition Massage

Intercompetition massage, given during breaks in the sports event, concentrates on the muscles being used or those about to be used. The techniques are short, light, and focused.

Recovery/Post-event Massage

Recovery massage focuses primarily on athletes who want to recover from a strenuous workout or competition and who have no injuries. The method used to help an athlete recover from a workout or competition is similar to a generally focused, full-body massage and incorporates methods that support a return to homeostasis.

Promotional (Event) Massage

Promotional massages usually are given at events for amateur athletes. The massages are offered as a public service to provide educational information about massage. The sports event massage is quick-paced and lasts about 15 minutes. In this type of public, promotional environment, following a sports massage routine is important. The use of lubricants is optional, and the massage practitioner may choose not to use them because of the risk of allergic reaction, staining an athlete's uniform, or other unforeseen factors.

If a massage professional is doing promotional work at a sports event and is working with many unfamiliar athletes, the best course is to do post-event massage, because the effects of any neurologic disorganization caused by the massage are not significant. No connective tissue work, intense stretching, trigger point work, or other invasive work should be done with an athlete at a sporting event. The massage should be superficial and supportive and should be focused more on enhancing circulation. It is important to watch for swelling that may indicate a sprain, strain, or stress fracture; if any of these are noted, the athlete should be referred to the medical tent for immediate evaluation. It also is important to watch for evidence of thermoregulatory disruption, such as symptoms of hypothermia or hyperthermia; if these are noted, the massage therapist should refer the individual immediately but without using any diagnostic terms or unduly alarming the person.

It is important to have written documentation of informed consent from each person who wants to receive a massage at these events (Box 13-11). One way to do this is to provide an informed consent statement on the top of a sign-in sheet and have each participant read and sign it before receiving the massage. Each participant should be given a short brochure or pamphlet explaining the benefits, contraindications, and cautions for sports massage. If the organizer of the event allows it, the brochure could include contact information to allow participating athletes to get in touch with the massage professional at a later date.

The Sports Massage Team

Often a group of massage professionals and supervised students work an event as a team. A team leader who is familiar with the sport usually is in charge at the sporting event. All the participating massage practitioners follow a similar routine. Remember, each member of a sports massage team represents the entire massage profession. Ethical, professional behavior is essential. This is the reason the permission of the organizer is required if you intend to put contact information on a brochure about massage that you distribute at such an event.

Cross-Training Recommendations

In the sports and fitness setting, two main options exist for a massage practitioner interested in an advanced education that includes additional skills. The option most often chosen is serving as a personal trainer. A personal trainer helps people exercise. The training for this job can be obtained in a formal school format or through a series of courses, and a certification process is available. Almost all personal trainers work in physical fitness facilities, health clubs, and fitness centers, mainly in the amusement and recreation industry or in civic and social organizations.

The second option is working as an athletic trainer. Athletic training involves preventing, diagnosing, and interventions for emergency, acute and chronic medical conditions involving impairment, functional limitations, and disabilities. Athletic training is recognized by the American Medical Association (AMA) as a health care profession. To practice, individuals must complete an athletic training degree program (bachelor's degree or entry level master's degree) that is accredited by the Commission on Accreditation of Athletic Training Education.

☑ FOOT IN THE DOOR

What type of door do you want your feet in? Massage therapy is a unique career opportunity because of the spectrum of places massage can be offered. Be it a spa, franchise, hospital, chiropractors office, hospice, pain clinic, fitness center, sports team, or multiple other options, you can build a career specialization. Each career track has potential cross-training options meaning that you may need to put your feet in an additional training program such as esthetician, certified nursing assistant, or personal trainer. It is necessary for career success to be able to adapt to various practice settings, and this requires ongoing learning, whether formal (such as cross-training) or practical experience in the practice setting. Remember to keep your feet moving toward continuing education for career success.

SUMMARY

The three main career tracks described in this chapter are related to the environment in which massage is offered. Each practice setting requires professional behavior and the ability to provide excellent massage; however, the personality of the environment influences the knowledge, skills, and abilities needed to be successful in that setting. Massage practitioners newly graduated from an entry level program can work in the wellness/spa setting, as long as they are committed to expanding their skills with continuing education. The health care and sports and fitness settings typically require education beyond the entry level; therefore, if you have set your sights on a career in these areas, you must pursue a quality advanced education.

⊖volve

http://evolve.elsevier.com/Fritz/fundamentals/
13-1 Quiz yourself on hydrotherapy treatments.
13-2 Wrap yourself up in the proper sequence of the body wrap.
13-3 Review what you've learned about spas.
Don't forget to study for your certification and licensure exams! Review questions, along with weblinks, can be found on the Evolve website.

References

Fritz S, Chaitow L, Hymel G: *Clinical massage in the healthcare setting*, St Louis, 2008, Mosby.

Grant K, Balletto J, Gowan-Moody D, et al: Steps toward massage therapy guidelines: a first report to the profession, *International Journal of Therapeutic Massage & Bodywork: Research, Education, & Practice* (IJTMB) 1:19–36, 2008.

Peters D, Chaitow L, Harris G, et al: *Integrating complementary therapies in primary care*, Edinburgh, 2001, Churchill Livingstone.

Arnheim's principles of athletic training: a competency-based approach, ed 12, 2005 McGraw-Hill Humanities/Social Sciences/Languages.

Resources

Day Spa Association
    http://www.dayspaassociation.com/
    http://www.dayspaassociation.com/resources/imsa
International Spa Association
    experienceispa.com
The British Library
    St Pancras
    Euston Road
    London
    NW1 2DB
    Website: www.bl.uk/TheBritishLibrary

Workbook Section

Short Answer

1. What are the three main career tracks and practice settings in massage? Compare their similarities and differences.

2. In addition to providing therapeutic massage, what are the responsibilities of the massage professional in the spa environment?

3. What is a spa signature?

4. List five of the nine spa sanitation considerations.

5. How is the average employment wage determined for the spa and franchise settings?

6. How is the average employment wage determined for the health care setting?

7. What is a franchisee?

8. Employers in the health care environment look for what types of skills in a massage therapist?

9. What are the unique concerns of massage professionals who work in the medical environment or with people receiving home health care?

10. What is HIPAA and how is it important?

11. List eight of the 13 areas in which a massage therapist pursuing a career in the health care setting must be skilled and knowledgeable.

12. What are the nine characteristics of quality health data?

13. What are electronic record-keeping systems?

14. Describe an interdisciplinary medical team.

15. What is a best practice?

16. Explain the limitations for work with professional athletes.

17. What are two main outcome goals of massage in the sports and fitness setting?

18. Describe a sports event massage.

19. How is the average employment wage determined for the sports and fitness setting?

20. Employers in the sports and fitness environment look for what types of skills in a massage therapist?

Problem-Solving Scenarios

1. A massage therapist working in a spa finds it difficult to maintain the protocols designated by the corporation. Some clients ask her to work on their neck or back in a way that is different from the protocol. She has taken continuing education courses and would like to implement these skills with the clients when appropriate. What might she do?

2. You want to pursue a career in palliative care in a hospice setting. What additional training might be beneficial?

3. An athletic trainer tells the massage therapist to avoid stretching or deep work for a hamstring tear. The massage therapist feels he needs more direction. What questions would be helpful to ask the athletic trainer?

Assess Your Competencies

Now that you have studied this chapter, you should be able to:

- Identify the three main career tracks for massage: spas and franchises, sports and fitness, and health care
- Adapt the massage practice based on the practice setting
- Identify specific skills needed for each practice setting

On a separate sheet of paper or on the computer, write a short summary of the content of this chapter based on the preceding list of competencies. Use a conversational tone, as if you were explaining to someone (e.g., a client, prospective employer, coworker, or other interested person) the importance of the information and skills to the development of the massage profession.

Next, in small discussion groups, share your summary with your classmates and compare the ways the information was presented. In discussing the content, look for similarities, differences, possibilities for misunderstanding of the information, and clear, concise methods of description.

Professional Application

You are asked to give a presentation to a group of nurses at a local hospital. They are looking for ways to use massage in various outpatient situations. They need a general explanation of ways massage would be beneficial for many different conditions. What major points would you make during the talk?

http://evolve.elsevier.com/Fritz/fundamentals/

CHAPTER OBJECTIVES

After completing this chapter, the student will be able to perform the following:

1. Explain the benefits of massage for animals and adapt massage for cats and dogs
2. Describe indications, cautions, and contraindications for massage and appropriately adapt massage for athletes
3. Describe and apply appropriate massage in the breast area
4. Adapt for massage during pregnancy
5. Adapt massage for infants, children, and adolescents
6. Explain the aging process and adapt massage for the geriatric population
7. Recognize acute care situations and adapt massage appropriately
8. Describe the mechanisms of chronic illness and adapt massage for those with chronic conditions
9. Adapt massage to support clients undergoing oncology care
10. Adapt massage for integration into the various medical settings
11. Communicate effectively and appropriately adapt massage for individuals with physical impairments
12. Communicate effectively and appropriately adapt massage for individuals diagnosed with psychological conditions

KEY TERMS

Abuse
Acute illness
Acute injury
Anxiety
Athlete
Chronic illness
Depression
Dissociation
Hospice

Mental impairment
Pain and fatigue syndromes
Panic
Physical disability/impairment
Post-traumatic stress disorder (PTSD)
Re-enactment
State-dependent memory
Trauma

2
14-1

In this chapter we examine ways massage professionals can show respect for and accommodate those who benefit from various adaptations of the massage application, professional relationship, and massage environment. The intent is to help massage professionals focus the benefits of therapeutic massage for clients with specific needs. Each section offers a general description of the adaptive situation, the application for massage, and directions for obtaining further training and information.

Individuals (or animals) with diverse needs that require adaptation can be seen in any massage environment in which you may practice. The basic skills presented in this textbook seldom change when applied in these unique situations and sometimes unique environments. Gliding and kneading for a person (or animal), regardless of the need for adaptation, is still gliding and kneading. The difference is in the recipient of the treatment and the way the treatment is done. Working with diverse populations requires additional knowledge about the specific situations or conditions addressed. The practitioner also must keep in mind the effects of any training protocols, developmental stages, medical treatments, accommodations (e.g., barrier-free access), or counseling in conjunction with the therapeutic massage.

In the exploration of each situation, it is important always to see the individual as a person first. The language used and the approach to care require a focus on each individual person first and then on their unique needs. There are no visually impaired, hearing impaired, sick, or abused people; there are people who have visual or hearing impairments, who deal with various illnesses, or who have been abused. Basic massage skills are sufficient to serve all people, because they promote general health and increase well-being. Certainly specific rehabilitative massage requires additional education, but the most common application of therapeutic massage, in conjunction with diverse situations, is general, nonspecific support.

The massage professional's responsibility is to learn as much as possible about the client's situation and the environment in which the massage is provided. If you are working with an individual experiencing post-traumatic stress disorder (PTSD), then learn about PTSD; if you are working with children with attention deficient disorder (ADD), then you must understand ADD and its treatment protocols. If you are working with a horse in a stall, you need to understand horses. Using the clinical reasoning model, a massage professional can develop intervention plans and justifications for the benefits of therapeutic massage as part of a comprehensive care program regardless of the circumstances.

The best way to obtain information about a client's adaptive needs is to ask the person directly. It is important to understand clearly the action plans required for various environments. It is necessary to expand skills and knowledge in response to real practice challenges. There is no way a school or textbook can prepare you for every conceivable situation you may encounter in professional practice. Various research avenues are available, and the Internet is an especially wonderful source of information. When the practitioner understands the client's particular situation, the physiologic effects of massage that provide the most benefit can be identified and intervention plans can be developed (Box 14-1).

Massage can be a wonderful way to reduce stress, promote well-being, and enjoy a respite from the daily challenges of life. The ability to respond successfully and provide massage in any setting or environment, be it the rushed and hectic setting of an airport or the sacred space of the deathbed, expands your client base and ability to serve.

ANIMAL MASSAGE

SECTION OBJECTIVES

Chapter objective covered in this section:
1. Explain the benefits of massage for animals and adapt massage for cats and dogs
Using the information presented in this section, the student will be able to perform the following:
- Identify the difference between massage, grooming, and petting
- Explain the benefits of massage both for well animals and for those receiving veterinary care
- List necessary components of specific animal massage education
- Adapt a massage based on outcomes and the animal's size and species
- Recognize pain behavior and adapt massage to target pain management

Just as with humans, massage for animals is a complementary therapy that encourages the animal's own healing and wellness processes (Box 14-2). Therapeutic massage works in animals for the very same reasons that it does in humans. *Massage is more than petting.* Petting is less focused and much more general than massage. Petting animals is pleasurable and beneficial to both the animal and the person. However, massage is a deliberate, focused technique of touching. It is the manipulation of soft tissue to promote well-being at both a physical and an emotional level. The desired effect for an individual animal can be achieved by applying various mechanical forces to different areas of the body.

Each animal is assessed and treated as an individual. What works for one animal might not be right for another. Determining factors include species, age, size, activity level, injuries, and medications. Assessment identifies target areas, contraindications, and outcomes. The history is based on information from the person responsible for the animal's well-being.

The various methods used for human massage are also used for animal massage. The anatomy and physiology of animals are very similar to those of humans. However, before working with a particular species, the massage therapist should review the anatomy unique to that species (Figure 14-1).

Massage therapists who work with animals are likely to find themselves in the role of teacher. They often must demonstrate massage techniques and instruct the caretaker in their use for the specific animal. The massage therapist must be confident and comfortable with the particular animal, or the massage application will be stressful for both the massage therapist and the animal. An excellent resource for understanding animal behavior is *Animals in Translation: Using the*

Box 14-1   Use of the Clinical Reasoning Model to Determine Treatment Needs

The following example shows how the massage therapist can use the clinical reasoning model effectively in approaching a particular condition.

Example: Therapeutic massage for children with attention deficit disorder

1. **Gather facts to identify and define the situation.**
   Key questions:
   - What is the problem?

      Attention deficit disorder (ADD) is primarily an organic condition that tends to have a genetic manifestation. It is characterized by the inability to sustain focused attention, a condition called *distractibility* or *inattention*. Often one or more of the following are also present: free association to many thoughts, impulsivity, moodiness, anxiety, withdrawn or spaced-out behavior (more prevalent in females), propensity to high-stimulation activities and behavior, bad temper, impatience, poor impulse control, and hyperactivity (in attention deficit/hyperactivity disorder [ADHD]).
   - What are the facts?

      ADD tends to be a biochemical disorder of dopamine, norepinephrine, and serotonin imbalance. Stimulant medication is used to normalize the neurochemical imbalance. Stimulant medication increases sympathetic arousal, which can lead to side effects of appetite suppression, digestive upset, headache, and sleep difficulties.

      Massage affects the neurochemicals involved in ADD by increasing dopamine and serotonin levels and increasing the norepinephrine level during the first 15 minutes. Massage inhibits sympathetic arousal if it lasts approximately 30 minutes or longer and acts as a form of sensory stimulation.

2. **Brainstorm possible solutions.**
   Key question: What might I do? or What if ... ?

      If massage stimulates the same neurochemicals as the medications, the physician may find it possible to lower the dosage of medication. Because it stimulates sympathetic arousal, massage may support effective use of medication at a lower dosage. Mild cases of ADD might be controlled with massage and similar methods.

      Because massage can also inhibit sympathetic arousal, it may alleviate some of the side effects of the medication, allowing the use of a higher dosage if necessary. It may also reduce generalized stress in both child and parent.

      Possible interventions include the following:
   - Self-help methods
     - A simple hand massage routine
     - Complicated finger tapping exercises to provide sensory stimulation
     - Progressive relaxation
     - A breathing pattern consisting of a short inhalation through the nose and a long exhalation through the mouth
     - Training methods (e.g., blowing up a balloon, blowing through a flute, and blowing bubbles)
     - Stimulation of acupressure points
     - Entrainment mechanisms (e.g., rhythmic rocking)
   - Professional massage
     - Full-body, broad-based compression for 30 to 45 minutes
     - Shiatsu technique
     - Chair massage for 15 to 30 minutes
   - Massage methods taught to parents
     - Compression
     - Slow-stroke massage
     - Assisted progressive relaxation
     - Rocking

3. **Evaluate possible interventions logically and objectively; look at both sides and the pros and cons.**
   Key question: What would happen if ... ?

      Headaches and stomachaches could be helped the most by massage interventions. The interventions could help reduce stress symptoms and off-task behavior, although not every child would respond to the same type of intervention.

      Medication could be used effectively, although the dosage would need to be monitored.

      Parental involvement is necessary, because the physiologic benefits of the methods are most effective if reinforced daily. However, parental participation could be minimal and inconsistent.

      The child would usually relax with a very firm pressure. Light pressure would usually stimulate and agitate. Disrobing would be problematic.

      Drawbacks to this program include cost, parental consistency, and time factors. Also, children under age 10 may not be old enough to learn self-help methods.

4. **Evaluate the effect on the people involved.**
   Key question: How would each person involved feel?

      The child would enjoy the interventions, although a great deal of energy would be needed to keep such children focused.

      Appreciation of these children is necessary to work effectively.

      These children become bored and inattentive when required to do repetitive tasks.

5. **Develop an intervention plan and justification statements.**

      Bodywork methods clearly have much to offer in the management of behavioral difficulties and the stress faced by children with ADD/ADHD. Many interventions could be used, such as teaching self-help methods, clinical sessions, and parental teaching and coaching.

      Massage methods provided over the clothing would be emphasized to avoid the need for lubricant and disrobing. The longer 30- to 45-minute session for stress management and relaxation would be recommended for the clinical sessions. The shorter 15-minute massage would be helpful in focusing attention for task concentration, such as doing homework. This 15-minute session could be taught to the parent.

      Self-help methods could be taught to older children. A simplified version of the soothing massage could be taught to parents to encourage effective sleep and provide a calming effect. Parents could benefit from the same massage methods for stress management.

      Consistent self-massage by the child and massage by the parent to provide various forms of sensory stimulation are necessary to achieve benefits. Continuing education and encouragement for the parents, who are also stressed, are important. A supportive coaching role can be provided to complement the bodywork interventions.

Mysteries of Autism to Decode Animal Behavior, by Temple Grandin and Catherine Johnson (Grandin and Johnson, 2006; Walsh, 2009).

Although massage can be adapted for many different kinds of animals, this chapter focuses on massage for dogs, cats, and horses, which more commonly receive massage.

Box 14-2 Veterinary Care and Massage

The specialist in the health care of animals is the veterinarian. Methods such as massage should never be substituted for proper veterinary care. The American Veterinary Medical Association (AVMA) has offered the following guidelines for massage therapy in conjunction with medical care:

Massage therapy on nonhuman animals should be performed by a licensed veterinarian with education in massage therapy or, where in accordance with state veterinary practice acts, by a graduate of an accredited massage school who has been educated in nonhuman animal massage therapy. When performed by a person who is not a veterinarian, massage therapy should be performed under the supervision of or referral by a licensed veterinarian who is providing concurrent care.

Body of Knowledge for Animal Massage

Before providing massage to any animal on a professional basis, the massage therapist should obtain additional training in the following areas (Proficiency Exercise 14-1):

- *Animal behavior and handling:* Animal behavior, handling, breed characteristics, developmental periods, proper socialization, basic health routines, disease prevention, and animal communication
- *Training tools:* Clickers, collars, leashes, housetraining aids, chewing deterrents, interactive toys, and safety devices
- *Anatomy and physiology specific to the animal:* Anatomic terms, the musculoskeletal system, and comparative anatomy and physiology
- *Kinesiology and biomechanics:* Joint movements, physical structures, and gait

PROFICIENCY EXERCISE 14-1

1. Discuss with a groomer or veterinary technician what it is like to work with animals.
2. Spend time at the local Humane Society or animal rescue shelter and massage the animals to support socialization.

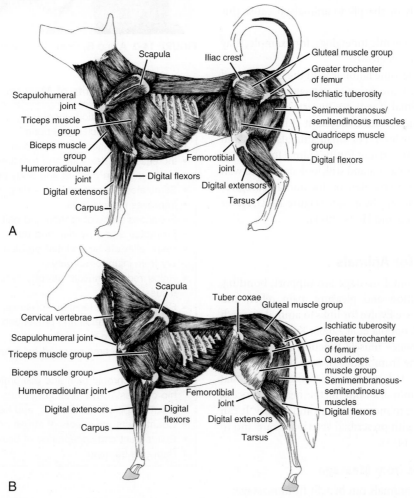

FIGURE 14-1 A, Canine musculature. **B,** Equine musculature.
(From Chistenson DE: *Veterinary medical terminology,* ed 2, St Louis, 2009, Saunders.)

- *Massage training:* Continuing education as an aspect of massage education above entry level requirements in a qualified and valid education program
- *Pathology:* Animal health, common ailments, and emergency care

Communication

With animals, just as with infants and young children, body language is an important communication process. Animals generally are very good communicators if you take the time to observe and to learn how they communicate with you.

Animals tend to interpret our movements and gestures just as if we were one of them. We should not assume that animals always understand our words and gestures the way we mean them. This is especially true for unfamiliar animals.

Some good' rules for dealing with unfamiliar animals include the following:

- Do not approach or reach for an unfamiliar animal.
- Do not make quick movements toward an animal, because they can be frightening or threatening to the animal.
- Do not stick out a hand for an animal to smell.
- Do not make direct eye contact, because this is threatening to many species of animals.
- Do not stand over most animals, because this also is threatening to them.
- Do not speak loudly or sharply to animals, because this can frighten them.
- Speak softly and in a gentle tone; dogs, for example, may interpret deep voices as growls.

The best advice is to become familiar with the gestures and signals of the animals you are going to massage. Do not risk interacting with the animal if you are uncertain how it will respond. Just as with infants and children, it is important to approach animals at their level. For small animals (dogs and cats), sit down on the floor and wait for the animal to approach you. For large animals (horses), stand still, look down and wait for the animal to approach you. Rely on the human caregiver to comfort the animal and stay by its side (Figure 14-2). Never force an interaction (Estep and Hetts, 2011).

Massage Benefits for Animals

Typical outcomes for animal massage are support, bonding, stress reduction, relaxation and pleasure, pain relief, and increased performance (see Evolve for links to animal research articles) (Porter, 2005; Coppola et al., 2006; Kathmann et al., 2006). Massage can enhance muscle function and efficiency and reduce recovery time from injury or sore muscles. Many veterinarians and respected research scientists believe that massage can assist an animal's body in the healing process. Massage has been proven to increase health and vitality. It can be used in conjunction with prescribed veterinary care and to augment that care (Box 14-3).

Animals That Benefit from Massage

Many different types of animals can benefit from massage:

- Working animals, such as dogs and horses (e.g., guide and service dogs, police horses, farm horses)

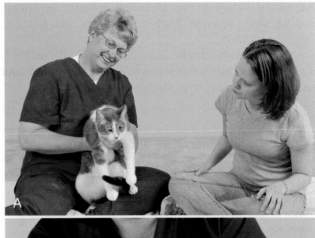
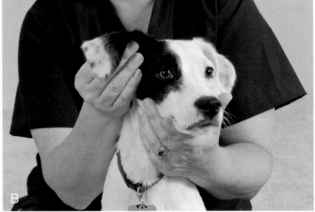

FIGURE 14-2 **A** and **B,** Examples of animal massage.

| Box 14-3 | Benefits of Massage for Animals |

- Improves circulation, increasing the supply of blood and nutrients to muscles and bone
- Aids the elimination of waste and toxins from the body
- Increases the flexibility and function of the joints
- Helps maintain posture and body balance
- Stimulates the metabolism, aiding weight loss
- Improves muscle tone
- Enhances range of motion and gait function
- Promotes a healthy skin and coat
- Helps alleviate age-related problems and assists in recovery from injury or surgery
- Helps reduce muscle atrophy resulting from inactivity or disuse
- Relieves muscle tension, soreness, and spasms
- Aids the elimination and prevention of muscular adhesions and connective tissue changes
- Shortens the time required for rehabilitation of soft tissue injuries
- Reduces chronic pain and discomfort caused by arthritis, hip dysplasia, and other conditions
- Calms hyperactive, anxious, and nervous animals
- Counteracts the effects of stress and anxiety
- Builds trust and acceptance of being touched
- Supports bonding

Box 14-4 Rehabilitative Massage for Animals

Rehabilitation therapy is any measure taken to restore maximum function after an injury, an illness, or surgery. Conditions for which rehabilitative massage may be used include the following:
- Arthritis
- Hip dysplasia
- Fractured limb (after repair)
- Cruciate ligament injury
- Intervertebral disk disease
- Muscle sprains and strains
- Scar tissue management after surgery

Rehabilitative massage for an animal should be supervised by a veterinarian and/or an experienced animal handler as part of a total treatment program.

- Entertainment and education animals
- Athletic animals (e.g., racehorses or greyhounds)
- Older animals
- Infant and adolescent animals
- Shy or recently adopted animals
- Animals recovering from injury or undergoing postoperative rehabilitation (Box 14-4)

Human Benefit

Animal massage bestows some very important benefits on the person doing the massage. Teaching those who are anxious, lonely, or depressed to massage animals can be a productive aspect of the person's treatment and care. Research has shown that when stroking an animal, people relax and their blood pressure drops.

Providing Massage for Animals

The methods of massage application presented in this text can all be adapted to animals; there are no unique modalities. However, animals generally have a more well-developed sense of smell than humans. Avoid using any scented products.

Animals comprise a population, just as do infants, the elderly, and athletes. Animals can be babies, toddlers, adolescents, parents, middle aged, and elderly. Each of these life stages presents unique circumstances that must be considered. In general, recommendations for humans can be translated to animals. For example, baby animals and baby humans act similarly, except that animals go through the stages much faster. They may be babies for only a few weeks, and then become rambunctious toddlers, and then independent adolescents. Nursing mothers can be very protective of their babies, and elderly animals have most of the characteristics of human elders.

Formal training for animal massage is varied, and opinions on the correct methods are inconsistent. A massage student who is interested in obtaining specific education in animal massage should thoroughly investigate any provider of animal massage training to make sure the individual is qualified to teach. Massage therapists who want to work with animals should obtain training in animal grooming, animal training, or some sort of veterinary assistant education. It is essential to understand the anatomy, physiology, and behavior of each species with which you intend to work. Learning grooming procedures, especially for large animals such as horses, provides the necessary skills for safety, sequence, and flow for the massage, which would follow grooming patterns and some animal behavior. The massage professional providing massage must not be tentative or afraid of the animal and must work with each animal client with confidence and respect while continually being aware of subtle communication from the animal.

Humans become very attached to their animal companions. Pets are part of the family, and the massage therapist who works with animals must be able to communicate and respect the human as much as the animal.

History and Assessment

A history and assessment are required for an animal just as they are for a human client. The massage therapist should obtain the following information from the animal's caretaker:
1. The animal's name
2. Any medical problems
3. Is the animal used to being handled?
4. Does the animal bite?
5. Is the animal easily frightened?

The massage therapist should meet the animal and become familiar with it and its human companion. Once the animal feels comfortable with the massage therapist, the next step is a visual and physical assessment to make sure the animal does not have any open wounds or sores that would be a contraindication to massage or require referral to a veterinarian.

Massage therapists need to be alert for problems that can be indicated by body temperature, texture of the skin and muscle fibers, tenderness of certain areas, and tension. The outcome for massage needs to be determined and a treatment plan established.

Massage Application

The qualities of touch previously described in this textbook also apply to massage for animals.
- **Pressure.** Just as with humans, it is important to be sure that the pressure applied is effective in achieving the determined outcomes but does not cause unnecessary pain or tissue damage. Animals do not like to be poked, prodded, or dug into. The animals with which I have worked did not have a problem communicating when the pressure was inappropriate. Animals can vocalize, attempt to move away, and nip (not bite). If the pressure is appropriately intense, the animal typically vocalizes but does not attempt to move away from the pressure and may even lean into it.

  Pressure (applied compressive force) varies with the size of the animal (e.g., a pet ferret does not need as much pressure as a horse).
- **Drag.** Hair, fur, and feathers make it difficult to apply drag to the skin surface. The superficial fascia and deeper tissues can be worked by lifting the skin (which may be quite loose)

and then using various mechanical forces to move the tissues into ease and bind.

- **Direction.** The direction of massage application, which is similar to that in human massage, varies according to the desired outcome (e.g., fluid movement or changes in muscle motor tone).
- **Duration.** The duration of a massage depends on the animal's acceptance and condition. The first session typically is an introductory meeting to allow the massage practitioner to become more familiar with the animal, to learn about its history, and to help the animal build trust and an acceptance of being touched. The first session lasts about 1 hour; the massage itself lasts 15 to 20 minutes, depending on the animal. Some animals accept a 60-minute, full-body massage at the first session, and others may take multiple sessions to learn to enjoy massage. The massage therapist works with the specific needs of each animal and teaches the person responsible for care how to perform the massage.
- **Frequency.** Therapeutic massage can be given daily for 10 to 30 minutes for healthy animals. If a disease or injury is involved, massage of different areas of the body every other day is recommended. However, the needs of each animal vary. For animals and people, a weekly massage provided as part of a well-balanced maintenance plan is recommended

Special Considerations for Horses

Massage for horses, or equine massage, is very popular. Because horses are large animals, the potential for harm to the massage therapist is greater. The following suggestions are important when massaging a horse or any large animal:

- Do not jump around or move suddenly, do not wear shiny or noisy jewelry or strongly scented products, and do not behave nervously around horses. All of these result in a nervous horse that is unsafe to work around.
- Wear hard-toed shoes or boots when working around horses. One of the most common horse-related injuries is having a foot stepped on.
- Always let the horse know what you intend to do. Quick, sudden movements startle horses and should be avoided.
- Keep all equipment away from the work area unless it is being used at the moment. This prevents the horse from stepping on it, playing with it, or chewing on it; it also prevents the massage therapist from accidentally tripping over it.
- Start massaging on the left side of the neck and work toward the rear of the horse. Then repeat on the right side. This pattern follows the standard grooming process for horses. Areas that have few muscles and bones near the surface, such as the face, legs, and hips, should be massaged carefully and gently. Stand near the horse during the massage and use fluid, rhythmic movements, not quick, jerky movements that are likely to startle the animal.
- When changing sides, either walk far enough away to avoid getting kicked or stay close to the horse's rear quarter with a hand on the rump, to break the

momentum of the kick. Never step over the lead rope or crossties. This puts you in a very dangerous position should the horse panic and pull back on the rope. Never crawl under the horse's belly. Even the most docile horse can spook and step on you.

- Be aware that some horses are ticklish and may become fidgety. During fly season, particularly, a horse often thrusts its hind leg forward to chase flies from the abdomen; therefore, it is wise to keep your head and body out of striking range when working in that area.
- When massaging the legs, bend at the hips or remain in a squat position. Do not sit on the ground or rest one or both knees on the ground. These are committed positions, which means that once you are in them, it takes longer than a split second to get out of them. In committed positions, if the horse should become frightened, the time it would take you to move away from scrambling hooves and the chance of becoming seriously injured are increased. It always helps to have your free hand resting on the horse's body while working on the legs; this way you can feel the muscles tense up and be warned that the horse is about to panic.

Pain Management

A major outcome for animal massage is pain management. Animals' behavior changes in response to pain, particularly persistent pain. The changes that occur depend on the degree of pain, the animal's tolerance of it, the animal's species, the situation in which the pain occurs, the animal's stress level, and a variety of other factors. Acute pain may produce an aversive reaction in an animal. A normally compliant, friendly animal may attempt to bite a person who is causing it pain, or the animal may try to flee from the cause of the pain.

Chronic or long-term pain (e.g., arthritis) is likely to produce more subtle behavioral changes. Animals, just like people, react to pain through coping mechanisms that are both internal and external. Descending pathways from the brain to the spinal cord inhibit neuronal activity and reduce the sensation of pain. In addition, compounds are released that have opioid effects (e.g., endorphins and enkephalins) (Cantwell, 2010).

Animals in pain often withdraw from their social group, choosing instead to remain alone, to be less active, and to be less responsive to external stimuli. Persistent pain sometimes causes an animal to traumatize the area that hurts, typically by excessively scratching, rubbing, biting, or licking the site. This behavior may actually be an attempt at pain management through counterirritation. Abnormal postures, such as a hunched back or a tiptoe gait, may also point to pain. Food and water intake often is altered when an animal is in pain, regardless of the source of the pain.

Grooming is an important activity for animals, and failure to groom is an early sign of pain. The hair or fur may be standing up rather than lying down smooth. It may be dull rather than shiny, and it may be matted or clumped, particularly around the face and mouth and the anal and genital openings.

Pain Behavior in Dogs, Cats, and Horses

Dogs

Dogs in pain generally appear quieter, less alert, and withdrawn. Their body movements are stiff, and they are unwilling to move. A dog in severe pain may lie still or adopt an abnormal posture to minimize discomfort. With less severe pain, the dog may appear restless, because the immediate response to acute but low-intensity pain may be an increased alertness. Shivering and increased respirations with panting may be seen. Spontaneous barking is unlikely; the dog is more likely to whimper or howl, especially if left unattended. It may growl without apparent provocation. A dog may lick or scratch at painful areas of its body, and the tail often is between the legs. Penile protrusion and frequent urination also may occur. A dog in pain may have an anxious look, and it may seek a cold surface on which to lie. When handled, the dog may be abnormally apprehensive or aggressive.

Cats

Cats in pain generally are quiet and have an apprehensive facial expression. The forehead may appear creased. The cat may cry or yowl, and it may growl and hiss if approached or made to move. Cats in pain have a tendency to hide or to separate from other cats. The posture usually becomes stiff and abnormal, varying with the site of the pain. A cat with head pain may keep its head tilted. If the pain is generalized in the thorax and abdomen, the cat may be crouched or hunched. With thoracic pain alone, the head, neck, and body may be extended. With abdominal or back pain, the cat may lie on its side with the back arched. If the animal is standing or walking, the back is arched and the gait is stilted. Incessant licking is sometimes associated with localized pain. With pain in one limb, the cat usually limps or holds up the affected limb.

A cat in severe pain may show frantic behavior and make desperate attempts to escape. Touching or palpating a painful area may produce an instant and violent reaction. The animal may pant, and the pulse rate may be increased and the pupils dilated. A cat in chronic pain may have an ungroomed appearance and may show a marked change from its normal behavior. The limbs are tucked, the head and neck are hunched, the ears are flattened, and the animal utters a distinctive cry or hissing and spitting sound. Cats in pain show fear of being handled and may cringe.

Horses

Periods of restlessness are typically observed in horses experiencing pain or distress. Food is held in the mouth uneaten. The horse exhibits an anxious appearance, with dilated pupils and glassy eyes. Other signs include increased respiration and pulse rate, flared nostrils, profuse sweating, and a rigid stance. With prolonged pain, the animal's behavior may change from restlessness to depression, with the head lowered. With pain associated with skeletal damage, the limbs may be held in unusual positions, the head and neck are "fixed," and the horse may be reluctant to move. Pain-induced tachycardia may be seen.

With abdominal pain, a horse may look at, bite, or kick its abdomen; it may get up and lie down frequently, walk in circles, or roll. When near collapse, the horse may stand very quietly, rigid and unmoving. Horses in pain generally show a reluctance to be handled.

Pain Medication for Animals

Opioid Agonists

Opioids used in veterinary medicine include morphine, meperidine, fentanyl, oxymorphone, etorphine (M99), and carfentanil. They are all effective analgesics that work through the central nervous system (CNS).

Implications for Massage

The side effects of the opioid antagonists in animals are similar to those in humans. These medications can depress the CNS and affect breathing and levels of consciousness. It is important to observe for these effects and immediately report them to the veterinarian.

Nonsteroidal Antiinflammatory Drugs

Nonsteroidal antiinflammatory drugs (NSAIDs) produce analgesia by reducing inflammation and peripheral sensitization. Unlike opiates, they typically do not act on the central nervous system.

Side effects of NSAIDs include gastric ulcers and interference with platelet function, anticoagulative action, and kidney function. Because cats metabolize NSAIDs slowly and toxicity can quickly occur, these pain medications are not typically used in cats. NSAIDs commonly used in dogs are aspirin, naproxen, meclofenamic acid, flunixin, phenylbutazone, dipyrone, and piroxicam.

Implications for Massage

The side effects of NSAIDs are similar to those seen in humans: altered pain perception and a tendency for increased bleeding and bruising, which would influence the amount of compressive force delivered during massage. Kidney failure is a serious condition. Signs of kidney failure include decreased appetite, increased water consumption and urination, increased sleeping, lethargy, itching, and a change in the smell of the breath. If these behaviors are noticed, the animal should be immediately referred to the veterinarian for emergency care.

Local Anesthetics

Pain relief can be obtained by using local anesthetics, which can be injected around specific nerve trunks that supply a surgical or injury site or infiltrated into the muscular and subcutaneous tissue layers around the area.

Implication for Massage

Do not massage over the area where local injections are given.

Topical Analgesics

Various ointments that act as counterirritants can be used for local pain. It is important to make sure that the ingredients are nontoxic, because animals typically lick areas that are painful.

Implications for Massage

Massage can be used to apply the ointment and to enhance its action through the use of tactile stimulation to increase the counterirritant effects.

Key Points

- Each animal is assessed and treated as an individual.
- Massage adaptation factors include species, age, size, activity level, injuries, and medications.
- Massage therapists who work with animals are likely to find themselves in the role of teacher.
- Grooming procedures provide the necessary skills for safety, sequence, and flow for the massage.

ATHLETES

14-2

SECTION OBJECTIVES

Chapter objective covered in this section:
2. Describe indications, cautions, and contraindications for massage and appropriately adapt massage for athletes
Using the information presented in this section, the student will be able to perform the following:
- List the experts in the care and training of athletes
- Identify factors to consider when adapting massage for athletes
- Identify common athletic injuries

An **athlete** is a person who participates in sports as either an amateur or a professional. Athletes require precise use of their bodies. The athlete trains the nervous system and muscles to perform in a specific way. Often the activity involves repetitive use of one group of muscles more than others, which may result in hypertrophy; changes in strength and movement patterns; connective tissue formation; and compensation patterns in the rest of the body. These factors contribute to the soft tissue difficulties that often develop in athletes. Fitness (see Chapter 15) is necessary for everyone's wellness, but the physical activity of an athlete goes beyond fitness; it is performance based.

Massage can be very beneficial for athletes if the professional performing the massage understands the biomechanics required by the sport. If the specific biomechanics are not understood, massage can impair optimum function in the athletic performance. Because of the intense physical activity involved in sports, an athlete may be more prone to injury.

The experts for athletes are sports medicine physicians, physical therapists, athletic trainers, exercise physiologists, and sports psychologists. It is especially important for athletes to work under the direction of these professionals to ensure proper sports form and training protocols. The professional athlete is more likely to have access to these professionals. Amateur athletes may not have the financial resources to hire training personnel and can be injured by inappropriate training protocols.

If a massage professional plans to work with an athlete on a continuing basis, it is important that the practitioner come to know the athlete and become part of the entire training experience.

Massage Adaptation

Typical adaptations for athletes include support for the training effect, altering the massage style for precompetition and postcompetition application, avoiding tissue damage, and complementing or taking into account the effects of medications.

Training Effect

Athletes depend on the effects of training and the resulting neurologic response for precise functioning. Because they use their bodies in specific ways to achieve performance, athletes create functional alterations in their bodies. For example, they may have increased mobility in one body area and increased muscle mass in another. It is important to understand the reasons for these changes, so that the massage can be adapted to support performance and manage problems that may occur because of the body changes based on training.

Precompetition

Adaptation of massage is especially important before competition. Without the proper training and experience, massage therapists can easily disorganize the neurologic responses if they do not understand the patterns required for efficient functioning in the sport. The effect is temporary, and unless the athlete is going to compete within 24 hours, it usually is not significant. However, if the massage is given just before competition, the results could be devastating. Any type of massage before a competition must be given carefully. Even when the massage therapist has experience with a specific athlete, caution is necessary 24 hours before competition.

Massage that focuses on enhancing circulation is appropriate (see Chapter 12). Avoid aggressive stretching, deep transverse friction, specific myofascial release, and extensive trigger point work.

Tissue Damage

An athlete often pushes the body to its limits. Although this extreme function may increase performance, it also increases the potential for tissue damage. Tissues have relative abilities to resist a particular load (force). A *load* can be one or a group of outside or internal forces acting on the body. Recall that a *force* can be defined as a push or pull. The resistance to a load is called *mechanical stress,* and the internal response is a *deformation,* or change in dimensions. Deformation also is defined as a mechanical strain. The stronger the tissue, the greater magnitude of load it can withstand.

All human tissues have viscous and elastic properties, allowing for deformation. Tissue such as bone is brittle and has fewer viscoelastic properties than soft tissue, such as muscle. The loads applied to bone and soft tissues that can cause injury are tension, compression, bend, shear, and torsion. When tissue is deformed to the extent that its elasticity is almost fully exceeded, a yield point has been reached. This is what can occur during athletic performance. When the yield point has been exceeded, mechanical failure occurs, resulting in tissue damage.

Care needs to be taken not to cause tissue damage during massage or increase tissue damage related to an existing injury. Methods with the potential to damage tissue are aggressive stretching, overpowering a client's resisting muscle contraction force, deep transverse friction, and methods often called "deep tissue massage" that involve pressure or stripping of trigger points. These same methods can increase the extent of an injury. The goal is to support healing and performance. Too often massage applied aggressively results in tissue injury. If any client is sore and stiff during movement or experiences increased pain in general or in a specific area 24 to 48 hours after a massage, tissue has been damaged and performance compromised.

The same mechanical forces that can cause tissue damage are applied therapeutically during massage to encourage tissue repair. The type of force that offers the most therapeutic value should be used during massage. In general, during the stage 1 acute and stage 2 subacute phases (see Table 11-2), the massage therapist should not use the same force as that which loaded the tissue and produced the injury. For example, if a sprain occurs from a torsion load, then kneading, which applies a torsion force, may not be the best choice until healing is progressing and stability has been restored in the area. For old injuries that have not healed in the best way possible, the massage therapist, during the massage, may need to carefully introduce the same force that caused the injury to achieve results.

Medications

Athletes commonly use medications, particularly analgesics for pain and antiinflammatory drugs, and the effects of these drugs must be considered in developing a plan of care. Pain medication reduces pain perception so that the athlete can continue to perform before healing is complete. This interferes with successful healing. Antiinflammatory drugs may slow the healing process, particularly connective tissue healing. When adapting massage, the practitioner must consider changes in sensory feedback if pain medication is used. Massage also can cause inflammation if it causes tissue damage. If the athlete uses antiinflammatory medication, healing occurs more slowly, interfering with performance potential.

Common Sports Injuries

Massage professionals working with athletes should be able to recognize common sports injuries and should refer the athlete to the appropriate medical professional. The massage therapist adapts the massage application using appropriate methods to enhance the healing process once a diagnosis has been made and the rehabilitation plan developed. Understanding sports injuries and massage application requires knowledge of tissue susceptibility to trauma and the mechanical forces involved.

Many factors contribute to mechanical injuries or trauma in sports. In sports, trauma is defined as a physical injury or wound sustained in a sport that was produced by an external or internal force. Healing mechanisms manifest as the inflammatory response and resolution of the inflammatory response. The different tissues heal at different rates. Skin heals quickly, whereas ligaments heal slowly. Stress can influence healing by slowing the repair process (see Table 11-2). Sleep and proper nutrition are necessary for proper healing.

Skin Injuries

Numerous mechanical forces can adversely affect the skin's integrity, such as friction (rubbing), scraping, compression (pressure), tearing, cutting, and penetration.

Wounds are classified according to the mechanical force that caused them:

- *Friction blister:* Continuous rubbing over the surface of the skin causes a collection of fluid below or within the epidermal layer; this is called a *blister.*
- *Abrasions:* Abrasions commonly arise from conditions in which the skin is scraped against a rough surface. The epidermis and dermis are worn away, exposing numerous capillaries.
- *Skin bruise:* When a blow compresses or crushes the skin surface and causes bleeding under the skin, the condition is identified as a bruise (also called a *contusion*).
- *Laceration:* A laceration is a wound in which the flesh has been irregularly torn.
- *Skin avulsion:* Skin torn by the same mechanism as a laceration, to the extent that tissue is completely ripped from its source, is an avulsion.
- *Incision wound:* An incision is a wound in which the skin has been sharply cut.
- *Puncture wound:* A puncture is a wound caused when a sharp object penetrates the skin.

Skin injuries are a regional contraindication to massage. Sanitation is essential, and care must be taken to prevent infection.

Muscle Injuries

Overexertion Muscle Problems

Overexertion is a problem that arises in physical conditioning and training. Even though the pattern of gradually overloading the body is the best way to achieve ultimate success, many athletes and training personnel still believe the old adage, "no pain, no gain."

Overtraining is reflected by muscle soreness, decreased joint flexibility, and general fatigue 24 hours after activity. Four specific indicators of possible overexertion are acute muscle soreness, delayed onset muscle soreness, muscle stiffness, and muscle cramps and spasms.

Acute Muscle Soreness

Overexertion in strenuous exercise often results in muscular pain. At one time or another, most people have experienced muscle soreness, usually as a result of some physical activity to which the person is unaccustomed. The older a person gets, the more easily muscle soreness seems to develop. Acute muscle soreness accompanies fatigue. This muscle pain is transient and occurs during and immediately after exercise. It is caused by a lack of oxygen to the muscles and the buildup of metabolic waste from anaerobic functions. This type of soreness dissipates as oxygen is restored and metabolic waste is removed from muscle tissue.

Delayed Onset Muscle Soreness

Delayed onset muscle soreness becomes most intense after 24 to 48 hours and then gradually subsides; usually the muscle becomes symptom free after 3 or 4 days. This type of pain is described as a syndrome of delayed muscle pain leading to increased muscle tension, swelling, stiffness, and resistance to stretching. Delayed onset muscle soreness is thought to result from several possible causes. It may arise from very small tears (microtrauma) in the muscle tissue, which result in an inflammatory process and seem to be more likely with eccentric or isometric contractions. Delayed onset muscle soreness may also arise from disruption of the connective tissue that holds muscle tendon fibers together. Another contributor is increased interstitial fluid, which results in pressure on pain-sensitive structures.

Muscle soreness can be prevented by beginning an exercise at a moderate level and gradually increasing the intensity of the exercise over time. Treatment of muscle soreness usually involves general massage with a focus on lymphatic drainage. Muscle soreness can be treated with ice applied within the first 48 to 72 hours. Antiinflammatory drugs should be avoided, if possible, because they delay healing.

Muscle Stiffness

Muscle stiffness does not produce pain. It occurs when a group of muscles has been worked hard for a long period. The fluids that collect in the muscles during and after exercise are absorbed into the bloodstream slowly. As a result, the muscles become swollen, shorter, and thicker and therefore resist stretching. Light exercise, lymphatic drainage–type massage, and passive mobilization help reduce stiffness. Stiffness also results with decreased pliability of connective tissue. This occurs when the ground substance thickens as part of an enzyme process that occurs during sympathetic dominance. Massage to restore connective tissue pliability (slow, sustained compression and kneading) plus hydration helps reduce the stiffness.

Muscle Cramps and Spasms

Muscle cramps and spasms can lead to muscle and tendon injuries. A cramp is a painful, involuntary contraction of a skeletal muscle or muscle group. Cramps often occur as a result of lack of water or other electrolytes, muscle fatigue, or interruption of the appropriate neurologic interaction between opposing muscles. A spasm is a reflex reaction caused by trauma of the musculoskeletal system. The two types of cramps and spasms are the clonic type, with alternating involuntary muscular contraction and relaxation in quick succession, and the tonic type, with rigid muscle contraction that lasts a period of time.

Cramps can be temporarily reduced with firm pressure on the belly of the cramping muscle. Cramps and spasms respond to proper hydration and rest (Arnheim and Prentice, 2005).

Muscle Guarding

When an injury occurs, the muscles that surround the injured area contract in an effort to splint the area, thus minimizing pain by limiting movement. Quite often this splinting is incorrectly referred to as a muscle spasm; however, *muscle guarding* is a more appropriate term for the involuntary

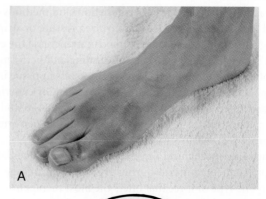

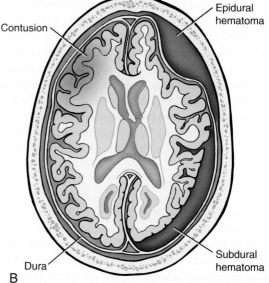

FIGURE 14-3 A, A bruised foot. **B,** Example of a brain contusion, also known as a concussion. The epidural and subdural hematomas are masses of clotted blood, resulting from broken blood vessels.

muscle contractions that occur in response to pain after musculoskeletal injury. Muscle guarding is appropriate during the acute and subacute healing processes (see Table 11-2), and massage application should not attempt to reduce it.

Contusion

A bruise, or contusion, arises from a sudden traumatic blow to the body. Contusions can range from superficial injuries to injuries involving deep tissue compression and hemorrhage (Figure 14-3).

A contusion can penetrate to the skeletal structures, causing a bone bruise. The extent to which an athlete may be hampered by this condition depends on the location of the bruise and the force of the blow. The speed with which a contusion heals, as with all soft tissue injuries, depends on the extent of tissue damage and internal bleeding. Caution is necessary when providing massage over contusions. Compressive force and depth of pressure need to be modified to prevent further injury. Lymphatic drainage–type applications are usually appropriate.

Caution: A brain contusion is a *concussion;* this is a serious condition. If bruises are seen in the muscles of the head and neck, caution and referral are necessary.

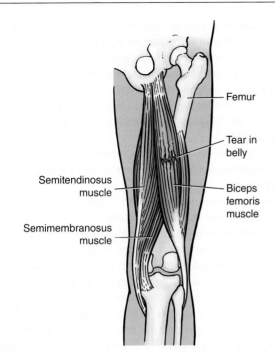

FIGURE 14-4 This example of muscle strain is located in the biceps femoris muscle of the hamstring group (in this case, a tear in the midportion of the belly of the muscle).

Strain

A *strain* is a stretch, tear, or rip in the muscle or adjacent tissue, such as the fascia or muscle tendons (Figure 14-4). The cause of muscle strain frequently is not clear. Often a strain is produced by an abnormal muscular contraction during reciprocal coordination of the agonist and antagonist muscles. Possible explanations for the muscle imbalance may be a mineral imbalance caused by profuse sweating, the collection of fatigue metabolites in the muscle itself, or a strength imbalance between agonist and antagonist muscles. Synergistic dominance of firing patterns is also crucial.

A strain may range from a tiny separation of connective tissue and muscle fibers to a complete tendinous avulsion or muscle rupture (grade 1, grade 2, or grade 3). The resulting pathologic condition is similar to that of a contusion or sprain, with capillary or blood vessel hemorrhage. The three types of strain are:

- *Grade 1 (mild) strain:* Local pain, which is increased by tension of the muscle, and minor loss of strength; mild swelling and local tenderness
- *Grade 2 (moderate) strain:* Similar to a mild strain but with moderate signs and symptoms and impaired muscle function
- *Grade 3 (severe) strain:* Severe signs and symptoms, with loss of muscle function and, commonly, a palpable defect in the muscle

Muscle strain usually causes muscle guarding. The guarding should not be reduced by massage, because it protects the area from further injury. Gentle massage over the area to encourage circulation and lymphatic drainage can support healing. During the acute and subacute phases, the soft tissue should be massaged in the direction of the fibers and crowded toward the site of the injury to promote reconnection of the ends of the separated fibers. Depth of pressure, duration, and intensity all need to be adjusted during the healing phase. Once the acute phase of healing is complete, the methods that support mobile scar formation can be introduced, including moving the tissue away from the injury site and massaging across the fibers (Cummings et al., 2009).

Tendon Injuries

Tendons have wavy, parallel, collagenous fibers that are organized in bundles surrounded by a gelatinous material that reduces friction. A tendon attaches a muscle to a bone and concentrates a pulling force in a limited area. When a tendon is loaded by tension, the wavy collagenous fibers straighten in the direction of the load; when the tension is released, the collagen returns to its original wavy shape. In tendons, collagen fibers break if the physiologic limits are exceeded. A breaking point is reached after a 6% to 8% increase in length. Because a tendon usually is double the strength of the muscle it serves, tears most commonly occur in the muscle belly, musculotendinous junction, or bony attachment.

Tendon injuries usually progress slowly over a long period. Often repeated acute injuries can lead to a chronic condition. Constant irritation caused by poor performance techniques or constant stress beyond physiologic limits eventually can result in a chronic condition. These injuries often are attributed to overuse microtrauma.

Myositis/Fasciitis

In general, the term *myositis* means inflammation of muscle tissue. More specifically, it can be considered a fibrositis, or connective tissue inflammation. Fascia that supports and separates muscle can also become chronically inflamed after injury. A typical example of this condition is plantar fasciitis.

Tendinitis

Tendinitis is marked by a gradual onset, degenerative changes, and diffuse tenderness caused by repeated microtrauma. Obvious signs of tendinitis are swelling and pain.

Tenosynovitis

Tenosynovitis is inflammation of the synovial sheath surrounding a tendon. In the acute stage, rapid onset of pain, articular crepitus, and diffuse swelling are seen. In chronic tenosynovitis, the tendons become locally thickened, and pain and articular crepitus are present during movement (Figure 14-5).

Synovial Joint Injuries

The major injuries affecting the synovial joints are sprains, subluxations, and dislocations. Sprains are among the most common and disabling injuries seen in sports. A sprain is a traumatic twisting of the joint that results in stretching or complete tearing of the stabilizing connective tissues (Figure 14-6). Ligaments, the articular capsule, and the synovial membrane all are injured.

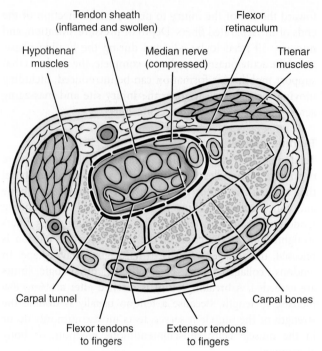

FIGURE 14-5 Tenosynovitis and carpel tunnel syndrome in cross-section view of a wrist.

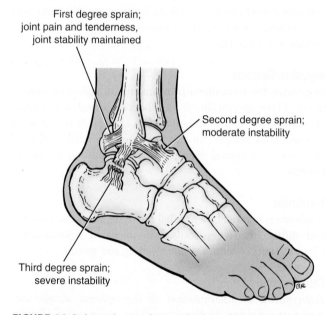

FIGURE 14-6 A sprain was the mechanism of injury to the lateral ligament complex of this ankle.

Sprains

A sprain causes the effusion of blood and synovial fluid into the joint cavity, producing joint swelling, a local temperature increase, pain or point tenderness, and skin discoloration. Ligaments and capsules, like tendons, can experience forces that completely rupture them or that produce an avulsion fracture. Ligaments and joint capsules heal slowly because of their relatively poor blood supply; however, they are plentifully supplied with nerves, and injury to these structures often causes a great deal of pain.

Like muscle strains, sprains are classified into one of three grades according to the extent of injury:

- *Grade 1 (mild) sprain:* Some pain, minimum loss of function, mild point tenderness, little or no swelling, and no abnormal motion when tested
- *Grade 2 (moderate) sprain:* Pain, moderate loss of function, swelling, and in some cases slight to moderate instability
- *Grade 3 (severe) sprain:* Extreme pain, major loss of function, severe instability, tenderness, and swelling; may also represent a subluxation

The joints most vulnerable to sprains in sports are the ankles, knees, and shoulders. Sprains occur less often to the wrists and elbows. Distinguishing between joint sprains and tendon or muscle strains often is difficult; therefore, the massage professional should expect the worst possible condition and manage it accordingly. Repeated joint twisting eventually can result in chronic inflammation, degeneration, and arthritis. Once the proper diagnosis has been made, the massage therapist can provide general full-body massage to reduce compensation patterns from changes in gait function and posture. In addition, lymphatic drainage massage can manage swelling outside the joint capsule. Massage methods that support circulation enhance healing, and hyperstimulation and counterirritation methods reduce pain. Care must be taken not to disrupt the healing tissue in the acute phase. Once the inflammation has diminished mobilization of the soft tissue promotes mobile scar formation. The duration and intensity of massage increase as healing progresses. Ligaments can take 3 to 6 months or longer to heal fully.

Dislocations and Diastasis

Dislocations are second to fractures in terms of disabling the athlete. The fingers and the shoulder joint have the highest incidence of dislocation. Dislocations result primarily from forces that cause the joint to go beyond its normal anatomic limits. The two classes of dislocations are subluxations and luxations. *Subluxations* are partial dislocations in which two articulating bones are separated incompletely. *Luxations* are complete dislocations, or a total disunion of bone apposition between the articulating surfaces.

Two types of diastases are seen: a disjointing of two bones parallel to each other (e.g., the radius and ulna or the tibia and fibula); and the rupture of a "solid" joint, such as the symphysis pubis. A diastasis commonly occurs with a fracture.

Several factors are important in recognizing dislocations:

- Limb function is lost. The athlete usually complains of having fallen or of having received a severe blow to a particular joint and then suddenly being unable to move that part.
- Deformity is almost always apparent. Because the deformity often can be obscured by heavy musculature, it is important that the injured site be evaluated by the appropriate medical professional.
- Swelling and point tenderness are immediately present.

As with fractures, x-ray examination of the dislocation sometimes is the only absolute diagnostic measure.

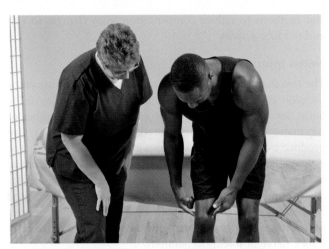

FIGURE 14-7 Joint injuries are common among athletes.

The massage practitioner needs to be aware of any history of dislocation. Increased muscle tension and connective tissue formation may occur around the dislocated joint as an appropriate stabilization process. Care must be taken to maintain joint stability while supporting mobility.

Chronic Joint Injuries

Like other chronic physical injuries or problems that arise from sports participation, chronic synovial joint injuries stem from microtrauma and overuse. The two major categories in which they fall are osteochondrosis and traumatic arthritis (*osteoarthritis,* or inflammation of surrounding soft tissues, such as the bursal capsule and the synovium). A major cause of chronic joint injury is failure of the muscles to control or limit deceleration during eccentric function. Athletes can avoid such injuries by avoiding chronic fatigue, by not training when tired, and by wearing protective gear to enhance active absorption of impact forces (Figure 14-7).

Traumatic arthritis usually is the result of accumulated microtrauma. With repeated trauma to the articular joint surfaces, the bone and synovium thicken, and pain, muscle spasm, and articular *crepitus* (grating on movement) occur. Joint wear leading to arthritis can come from repeated sprains that leave a joint with weakened ligaments. Misalignment of the musculoskeletal structure, which stresses joints, can be a factor, or arthritis can arise from an irregular joint surface or be caused by repeated articular chondral injuries. Loose bodies that have been dislodged from the articular surface can also irritate the joint and produce arthritis. Athletes with joint injuries that are improperly immobilized or who are allowed to return to activity before proper healing has occurred eventually may be afflicted with arthritis. Massage applications for chronic joint injury involve palliative care to control pain.

Bursitis

A *bursa* is a fluid-filled sac that is found in places where friction might occur in body tissues. Bursae provide protection between tendons and bones, between tendons and ligaments, and between other structures where friction occurs. Sudden irritation can cause acute bursitis. Overuse of muscles or tendons, in addition to constant external compression or

trauma, can result in chronic bursitis. The signs and symptoms of bursitis include swelling, pain, and some loss of function. Repeated trauma may lead to calcific deposits and degeneration of the internal lining of the bursa.

Bursitis in the knee, elbow, and shoulder is common among athletes. Massage can be used to lengthen the shortened structures, reducing friction. Ice applications and rehabilitative exercise are indicated. Short-term use of antiinflammatory medication may be helpful. Steroid injections at the site are a common treatment. Massage is contraindicated in the area of steroid injection until the medication has been fully absorbed by the body. Five to 7 days is a safe waiting period, after which massage may be resumed.

Bone Injuries

Because of its viscoelastic properties, bone can bend slightly. However, bone generally is brittle and a poor shock absorber because of its mineral content. This brittleness increases under tension forces more than under compression forces. Bone trauma generally can be classified as periostitis, acute bone fractures, and stress fractures.

Acute Bone Fractures

A bone fracture can be a partial or a complete interruption of the bone continuity. It can occur without external exposure or can extend through the skin, creating an external wound (open fracture). As a result of normal remodeling, a bone may become vulnerable to fracture during the first few weeks of intense physical activity or training. Weight-bearing bones undergo bone reabsorption and become weaker before they become stronger. Fractures also can result from direct trauma; that is, the bone breaks directly at the site where a force is applied. A fracture that occurs some distance from the point where force is applied is called an *indirect fracture.* A sudden, violent muscle contraction or repetitive abnormal stress to a bone also can cause a fracture. Fractures are one of the most serious hazards of sports and should be routinely suspected in musculoskeletal injures.

Stress Fractures

The exact cause of stress fractures is unknown, but a number of possibilities are likely: an overload caused by muscle contraction; altered stress distribution in the bone as a result of muscle fatigue; a change in the ground traction force (e.g., moving from a wood surface to a grass surface); or rhythmically repetitive stress.

Early detection of a stress fracture may be difficult. Because of their frequency in a wide range of sports, stress fractures always must be suspected in susceptible body areas that fail to respond to the usual management. The major signs of a stress fracture are swelling, focal tenderness, and pain. In the early stages of the fracture, the athlete complains of pain when active but not at rest. Later, the pain is constant and becomes more intense at night. Percussion (i.e., light tapping on the bone at a site other than the suspected fracture) produces pain at the fracture site. The most common sites of stress fractures are the tibia, fibula, metatarsal shaft, calcaneus, femur, lumbar vertebrae, ribs, and humerus (Figure 14-8).

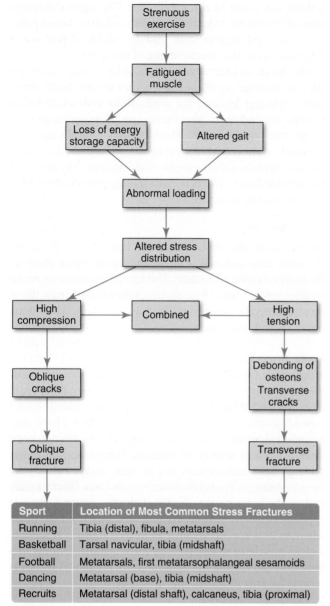

FIGURE 14-8 Sequence of events leading to stress fractures. Loss of the muscle's energy storage capacity (fatigue) leads to microscopic bone failure (stress fracture). In the text with green shading, locations of the most common sport-specific stress fractures are listed.

(Modified from Malone T, McPoil T, Nitz AJ: *Orthopedic and sport physical therapy,* ed 3, St Louis, 1997, Mosby and Miller MD, Cooper DE, Warner JJP, Cooper D: *Review of sports medicine and arthroscopy,* ed 2, Philadelphia, 2002, WB Saunders).

The management of stress fractures varies with the individual athlete, the injury site, and the extent of injury. Stress fractures that occur on the concave side of bone heal more rapidly and are managed more easily than those on the convex side. Stress fractures on the convex side can quickly produce a complete fracture. The massage practitioner needs to be aware of the potential for stress fractures and refer the athlete if necessary. The main massage approach during fracture healing is support for the whole body with general massage and methods to reduce compensation from changes in gait and reduced activity.

Nerve Injuries

The two main forces that cause major nerve injury are compression and tension. As with injuries to other tissues in the body, nerve injury may be acute or chronic. Any number of traumatic experiences that directly affect nerves can also produce a variety of sensory responses, including pain. For example, sudden stretching or pinching of a nerve can produce both muscle weakness and a sharp, burning pain that radiates down a limb. Neuritis, a chronic nerve problem, can be caused by a variety of forces that usually have been repeated or continued for a long period. Symptoms of neuritis can range from minor nerve problems to paralysis.

Pain that is felt at a point in the body other than its actual origin is known as *referred pain*. A potential cause of referred pain is a trigger point, which occurs in the muscular system. Massage applications for nerve injuries are palliative to reduce pain. If the nerve is impinged by short muscles and fascia, massage can be used to restore normal length and reduce pressure on the nerve.

Postural Changes

Postural deviations often are a major underlying cause of sports injuries. Postural misalignment may arise from unilateral (one side of the body) muscle and soft tissue asymmetries or bony asymmetries. As a result, the athlete engages in poor mechanics of movement (pathomechanics). Many sports activities, such as weight lifting, are unilateral and thus lead to asymmetries in body development. For example, a consistent pattern of knee injury may be related to asymmetries in the pelvis and legs (short leg syndrome) or reduced mobility of the ankles. A number of postural conditions are genuine hazards for athletes, making them prone to specific injuries. Some of the more important conditions are foot, ankle, and leg anomalies; spinal anomalies; and various stress syndromes.

Unfortunately, not much in the form of remedial work is usually performed. As a result, an injury often becomes chronic, sometimes to the point that the athlete must stop participating in a sport. When possible, the massage professional should try to reverse faulty postural conditions through therapy, working under the direction of an athletic trainer, orthopedist, or other qualified medical professional.

Heat Illnesses

Exercising in a hot, humid environment can cause various forms of heat illness, including heat rash, heat syncope, heat cramps, heat exhaustion, and heatstroke.

Heat Rash

Heat rash, also called *prickly heat,* is a benign condition associated with a red, raised rash that is accompanied by sensations of a prickling and tingling during sweating. It usually occurs when the skin is continuously wet with unevaporated sweat. The rash generally is localized to areas of the body covered with clothing. Massage is regionally contraindicated.

Heat Syncope

Heat syncope, or *heat collapse,* is associated with rapid physical fatigue during overexposure to heat. It is usually caused by standing in the heat for long periods or by not being accustomed to exercising in the heat. It is caused by peripheral vasodilation of superficial vessels, hypotension, or a pooling of blood in the extremities, which results in dizziness, fainting, and nausea. Heat syncope is quickly relieved by laying the athlete down in a cool environment and replacing fluids.

Heat Cramps

Heat cramps are extremely painful muscle spasms that occur most commonly in the calf and abdomen, although any muscle can be involved. The occurrence of heat cramps is related to excessive loss of water and several electrolytes or ions (sodium, chloride, potassium, magnesium, and calcium), which are essential elements in muscle contraction. Profuse sweating results in the loss of large amounts of water and small amounts of electrolytes, which destroys the balance in concentration of these elements in the body. This imbalance ultimately results in painful muscle contractions and cramps. The person most likely to develop heat cramps is one who is in fairly good condition but simply overexerts in the heat.

Heat cramps can be prevented by adequate replacement of sodium, chloride, potassium, magnesium, calcium, and, most important, water. Ingestion of salt tablets is not recommended. Sodium can be replaced by simply salting food a bit more heavily; bananas are particularly high in potassium; and calcium is present in green, leafy vegetables, milk, cheese, and dairy products. The immediate treatment for heat cramps is ingestion of large amounts of water with added electrolytes and mild stretching, with ice massage of the muscle in spasm. An athlete who experiences heat cramps generally is not able to return to practice or competition that day, because cramping is likely to recur. Massage is contraindicated and will not relieve heat cramps. Rest and hydration are indicated.

Heat Exhaustion

Heat exhaustion results from inadequate replacement of fluids lost through sweating. Clinically, the victim of heat exhaustion collapses and has profuse sweating, pale skin, a mildly elevated temperature (102° F, 39° C), dizziness, hyperventilation, and a rapid pulse.

It sometimes is possible to spot athletes who are having problems with heat exhaustion. They may begin to develop heat cramps. They may become disoriented and light-headed, and their physical performance is not up to their usual standards. In general, people in poor physical condition who attempt to exercise in the heat are most likely to suffer from heat exhaustion.

Immediate treatment of heat exhaustion requires ingestion and eventually intravenous replacement of large amounts of water. Massage is contraindicated.

Heatstroke

Unlike heat cramps and heat exhaustion, *heatstroke* is a serious, life-threatening emergency. The specific cause of heatstroke is unknown. It is characterized clinically by sudden collapse with loss of consciousness; flushed, hot skin with less sweating than would be seen with heat exhaustion; shallow breathing; a rapid, strong pulse; and, most important, a core temperature of 106° F (41° C) or higher. In the heatstroke victim, the body's thermoregulatory mechanism has broken down because of an excessively high body temperature; the body loses the ability to dissipate heat through sweating.

Heatstroke can occur suddenly and without warning. The athlete usually does not experience signs of heat cramps or heat exhaustion. The possibility of death from heatstroke can be reduced significantly if the body temperature is lowered to normal within 45 minutes. The longer the body temperature is elevated to 106° F or higher, the higher the mortality rate. Death is imminent if the body's core temperature rises to 107° F (41.7° C) or higher.

Every first aid effort should be directed toward lowering the body temperature. Get the athlete into a cool environment, strip off all clothing, sponge the person down with cool water, and fan the individual with a towel. Do not immerse the athlete in cold water. It is imperative that the victim be transported to a hospital as quickly as possible. Do not wait for an ambulance; transport the victim in whatever vehicle happens to be available. The replacement of fluid is not critical in initial first aid. Massage is contraindicated.

Hypothermia

Cold weather is a common condition in many outdoor sports in which the sport itself does not require heavy protective clothing; consequently, the weather becomes a pertinent factor in the athlete's susceptibility to injury. In most instances, the activity itself enables the athlete to increase the metabolic rate sufficiently to function normally and dissipate the resulting heat and perspiration through the usual physiologic mechanisms. If an athlete fails to warm up sufficiently or becomes chilled because of relative inactivity for varying periods, the individual is more prone to injury.

Dampness or wetness further increases the risk of hypothermia. An air temperature of 50° F is relatively comfortable, but water at the same temperature is intolerable. The combination of cold, wind, and dampness creates an environment that easily predisposes the athlete to hypothermia.

A relatively small drop in the body's core temperature can induce shivering sufficient to materially affect an athlete's neuromuscular coordination and performance. Shivering stops when the body temperature drops below 85° to 90° F (29.4° to 32.2° C). Death is imminent if the core temperature drops to 77° to 85° F (25° to 29.4° C). Treatment involves warming and drying the athlete.

Ongoing Care of the Athlete

For athletes, regular massage allows the body to function with less restriction and accelerates recovery time. There are no specific protocols for massage targeting athletes. The basic massage process presented in Chapter 10, coupled with appropriate assessment procedures (see Chapter 11) and the addition of various aspects of fluid movement, connective tissue application, and trigger point therapy (see Chapter 12), can address the needs of this population.

Key Points

- Working with athletes can be very demanding. Their schedules may be erratic, and their bodies change almost daily in response to training, competition, or injury.
- Athletes in training have reduced adaptive capacity. *Do not overmassage, cause tissue damage or assume that athletes require an aggressive approach.*
- Most athletes require varying depths of pressure, from light to very deep; consequently, the massage practitioner must make sure to use effective body mechanics.
- Athletes can become dependent on massage; therefore, commitment by the massage professional is necessary.

BREAST MASSAGE

SECTION OBJECTIVES

Chapter objective covered in this section:
3. Describe and apply appropriate massage in the breast area
Using the information presented in this section, the student will be able to perform the following:
- Determine when breast massage is appropriate
- Consider ethical principles in deciding when breast massage is performed

Note: Massage of the female breast is a controversial issue. A conservative approach is taken in this textbook. Although a body area is not a population, the topic needs to be addressed, because many women have breast health issues.

Anatomically the breast is part of the integumentary system. It becomes a functional part of the female reproductive system only during lactation. In both men and women, the breast is considered an erogenous zone. An erogenous zone is an area of the body where sexual tension concentrates and can be relieved through stimulation. Other erogenous zones are the mouth, genitals, and anus. These areas usually have some sort of erectile tissue that engorges with blood when stimulated. In the breast, the nipple is this erectile tissue. The controversy over the appropriateness of massage of the female breast centers on the breast as an erogenous area.

Considerations for Breast Massage

Breast massage can be appropriate for certain conditions, such as fibrosis and the development of scar tissue after surgery.

Surgeries

Breast Cancer

Surgery for breast cancer may involve either removal of only the cancerous tissue or a mastectomy. Often reconstructive surgery is performed. The massage practitioner must attend to contraindications and cautions in connection with treatments given after surgery. For example, radiation over the area can weaken the bones, predisposing them to fracture.

Breast Implants and Reduction

Breast implants are another consideration. Care must be taken to apply gentle pressure over the implants while still addressing the connective tissue changes that can occur when implants are used.

Breast reduction surgery is performed for both cosmetic and health reasons. The same attention is paid to scar tissue development and healing as is given in other surgical procedures.

Massage Adaptation

As for any surgery or area of healing, specific massage to the area is not provided during the acute phase. After the initial healing is complete and the attending physician has approved treatment, gentle massage that mobilizes the tissue around the surgical area can be performed. After 4 weeks, if healing is progressing well, the scar itself can be gently massaged. The most common method used is a very gentle form of skin rolling. After 3 months, myofascial methods can be used.

Scar Tissue

When the therapist works with existing scar tissue, the work progresses slowly and deliberately. Most scar tissue tends to be less pliable than the surrounding tissue. It also tends to shorten and pull. Breast surgery can result in a pulling forward of the shoulder and discomfort from taut, long tissue in the midback.

Myofascial methods (see Chapter 12) are effective for managing scar tissue. More generalized massage manipulations, such as gliding, kneading, and compression, prepare the tissue for more specific work.

Positioning the Client

Soft tissue under the breast tissue can be accessed effectively by placing the client in the side-lying position, in which the breast tissue falls away from the chest wall toward the table. In the supine position the breast tissue usually falls to the side, allowing massage over the sternum and intercostal area. These two positions provide adequate access to the soft tissue of the chest wall. For this reason, there is no reason to massage through the breast tissue proper to reach these areas (Figure 14-9).

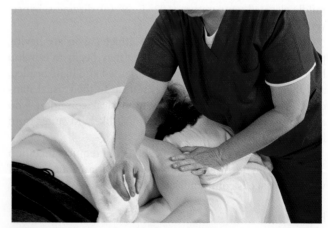

FIGURE 14-9 Using the forearm to massage around the breast tissue.

💡 PROFICIENCY EXERCISE 14-2

Investigate the surgical procedure for breast cancer, breast augmentation with implants, or breast reduction. Write an intervention plan and justification statement for the use of therapeutic massage. Use the model in Box 14-1 as an example.

Example: Therapeutic massage for _____

1. **Gather facts to identify and define the situation.**
   Key questions: What is the problem? What are the facts?
2. **Brainstorm possible solutions.**
   Key question: What might I do? or What if … ?
3. **Evaluate possible interventions logically and objectively; look at both sides and at the pros and cons.**
   Key question: What would happen if … ?
4. **Evaluate the effect on the people involved.**
   Key question: How would each person involved feel?
5. **Develop an intervention plan and justification statements.**

Ethical Considerations

The ethical principles discussed in Chapter 2 serve as the basis for decision making regarding the appropriateness of breast massage for either men or women. The massage professional should particularly consider the following:

- *Proportionality:* The benefit must outweigh the burden of treatment.
- *Nonmaleficence:* The practitioner must do no harm and must prevent harm from occurring.
- *Beneficence:* The treatment must contribute to the client's well-being.

Breast examination and the teaching of breast self-examination are adequately undertaken by other health care professionals. It is not necessary for the massage professional to provide such services.

Breast massage as part of a general massage serves no specific physiologic purpose that cannot be achieved in ways other than breast massage; therefore, the concerns may outweigh the benefit (Proficiency Exercise 14-2).

Key Points

If breast massage for a specific condition is deemed appropriate by a health care professional and the client is referred to the massage professional, the following measures are recommended:

- Work with specific written informed consent for breast massage.
- Work with another professional in the room, much as a male gynecologist has a female nurse present during examinations. If this is not possible, male therapists should refer a female client to a female therapist.
- Use careful draping. Do not expose the entire breast unless absolutely necessary. Do not expose both breasts.
- Work gently, professionally, and confidently.
- Avoid the nipple area.

PREGNANCY

SECTION OBJECTIVES

Chapter objective covered in this section:

4. Adapt for massage during pregnancy

Using the information presented in this section, the student will be able to perform the following:

- List the three stages of pregnancy and describe the physical and emotional changes associated with each
- List common disorders of pregnancy and determine the need for referral
- Design a general massage session to meet the needs of a pregnant woman
- Teach a support person basic massage methods to use during labor

Pregnancy is divided into three distinct segments: the first, second, and third trimesters. A pregnant woman undergoes extensive physical and emotional changes during each of these stages.

First Trimester

During the first 3 months (the first trimester), the woman's body must adjust to tremendous hormonal changes, which are likely to cause mood swings. This is also a very vulnerable time for the developing baby. The following changes are common during the first trimester.

- *Nausea,* or the sensation of feeling sick, and vomiting are commonly referred to as *morning sickness.* Morning sickness tends to be most severe in the early morning but can occur in the evening and may last all day and night. Symptoms usually diminish by the tenth week of pregnancy and usually are gone by the end of 14 weeks. Only rarely does this last through the entire pregnancy.
- *Frequent urination* occurs because of the presence of the hormone progesterone, which causes relaxation of the smooth muscle of the bladder. This tendency diminishes by the second trimester. The therapist should offer the use of the restroom to the client before beginning the massage.
- *Constipation* occurs because the hormone progesterone causes relaxation of the smooth muscle of the large intestine. This results in slow movement of the fecal matter through the system and increased water absorption from the colon. Constipation may continue throughout the pregnancy. Mechanical pressure from the enlarging uterus contributes to the problem.
- *Blood pressure* often falls in early pregnancy, specifically the diastolic pressure. This is also the result of the presence of progesterone, which relaxes the muscular wall of the blood vessels. The expectant mother may be fatigued and may feel light-headed or faint, especially during prolonged standing. Blood pressure usually returns to normal during the fourteenth week of pregnancy. The therapist may want to offer to help the client off the massage table in case she has light-headedness on sitting up or standing.
- *Breast changes* begin during this stage, including a sense of increased fullness, tenderness, and heightened sensitivity. These changes may continue throughout the pregnancy.

- *Musculoskeletal changes* are caused by the influence of estrogen, progesterone, and relaxin. Relaxin is produced as early as 2 weeks into the pregnancy and is at its highest levels in the first trimester; it then falls 20% and remains at that level until labor. Relaxin affects the composition of collagen in the joint capsules, ligaments, and fascia to allow greater elasticity. This enables more movement in the joints and creates more yield in the abdomen. Although all joints are affected, the most vulnerable are those of the pelvis, such as the symphysis pubis and sacroiliac joint, and those that bear weight, such as the ankle and the joints of the foot.
- *Taste* and *smell* are altered in the early stages of the pregnancy. Certain smells and foods become disagreeable to the woman. The client should be asked before any scented oils or other fragrances are used.

Massage given during the first trimester is general wellness massage, which may help balance the mother's physiologic responses. Positioning is not a concern unless the breasts are tender. Deep work on the abdomen is avoided so as not to disrupt the attachment of the baby to the uterine wall. Surface stroking can be pleasurable to the client.

Second Trimester

The second trimester usually brings a leveling of the hormones, and the woman feels better. During this time she may start to "show" and feel the first movements of the baby. If the pregnancy was planned, this is a joyful time. If not, the physical evidence of the growing baby may cause additional stress for the mother.

Toward the end of the second trimester, the connective tissue, under the influence of relaxin, begins to soften to allow the pelvis to spread. The following are common considerations during the second trimester.

- *Joint looseness* develops because of the softening of the connective tissue, and the muscles of the legs, gluteals, and hip flexors must provide joint stabilization and tension; as a result, pain can develop. Overstretching must be avoided.
- *Carpal tunnel syndrome*, caused by fluid retention, is common among pregnant women and may be perpetuated even after the birth as a result of caring for the infant.
- *Edema* is common at any time during the pregnancy as a result of the retention of fluid. As the pregnancy advances, edema of the legs occurs in up to 40% of women. The mechanical obstruction created by the uterus and its contents causes an increase in venous pressure distally, resulting in edema. Although edema may be caused by excessive weight gain, it may also be a symptom of pre-eclampsia. In the latter case, the midwife or physician should be informed.
- *Pre-eclampsia* is a very serious complication that requires medical attention. The diagnosis of pre-eclampsia is made when the patient has elevated blood pressure, generalized edema, and a high concentration of protein in the urine. Some common elements that may predispose women to pre-eclampsia are:
  - First pregnancy
  - Multiple pregnancies
  - Chronic hypertension or long-term hypertension

- Chronic renal disease
- Malnutrition
- Diabetes

Supine hypotension occurs as the fetus grows and compresses the aorta and inferior vena cava against the lumbar spine. This may cause the woman to feel faint when she is lying on her back.

Shortness of breath is also common. This is the result of a combination of mechanical changes in the thorax and the position of the diaphragm and physiologic changes.

During massage in the second trimester, support for the abdomen is important. The side-lying position is most comfortable, and lying on the left side produces the least amount of abdominal congestion for the expanding uterus. Be attentive for strain in the back muscles during positioning. Keep the head in alignment with the spine. Using a support so that the shoulder lies comfortably and does not fall forward or toward the ear is helpful. Support between the knees helps keep the hips in the neutral position and relieves stress in this area. A support under the top arm may also be comfortable. Allow the client to change position often. As in the first trimester, deep work on the abdomen must be avoided.

Third Trimester

During the last (third) trimester, the weight of the growing baby, the postural shifts, and the movement of the internal organs may cause discomfort for the pregnant woman. Because many of the internal organs are pushed up and back, the diaphragm does not work as efficiently. The mother uses her neck and shoulder muscles to breathe, possibly causing discomfort or thoracic outlet symptoms. Breathing pattern disorders may develop. Massage offers temporary relief of these symptoms.

About 2 weeks before birth (in the first pregnancy), the baby turns head down and drops into the birth canal. This provides more space for the diaphragm to work and breathing becomes easier, but pressure on the bladder causes frequent urination. Impingement on lymph vessels may cause the legs and feet to swell. Edema or fluid accumulation may be a symptom of more serious complications, and the client should be referred to a physician immediately if these are noted. The low back may ache from the postural shift. The breasts have enlarged in preparation for lactation. A woman may not feel very attractive at this point and most likely is not very comfortable physically. Fatigue and sleep disturbances may result. Massage is gentle, supports comfort, and assists circulation. If a comfortable position cannot be found, allow the client to change position often and use the restroom as needed. General massage may help the woman feel better for a little while and support comfortable sleep.

Disorders of Pregnancy

Although pregnancy and delivery are considered normal physiologic functions, problems can occur. Early recognition and referral are important (McKinney et al., 2009). Warning signs of a pregnancy at risk that require immediate referral include the following:

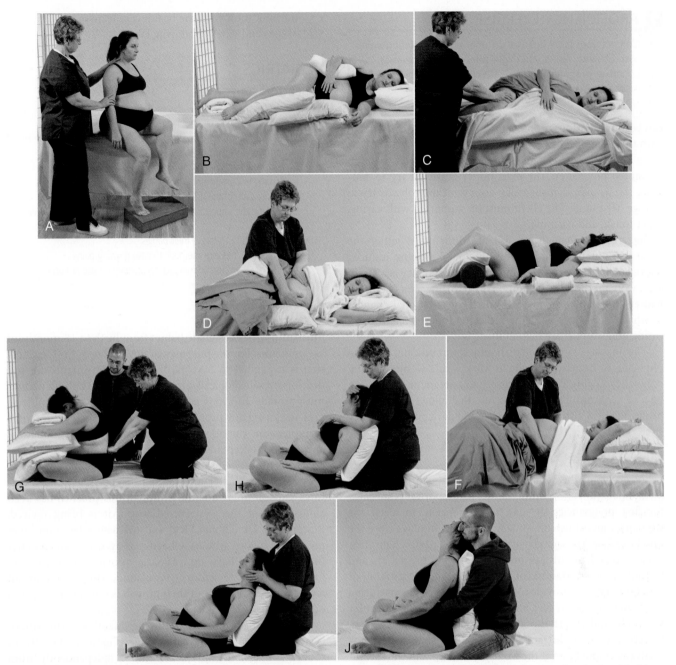

FIGURE 14-10 Prenatal massage. **A,** Assist the client onto the table. **B,** Bolster. **C,** Perform the massage with the client in the side-lying position. **D,** Gentle massage of the baby. **E,** Client bolstered in the supine position. **F,** Massage of the lower back. **G,** Client in seated position while support person is taught technique. **H,** Effective seated positioning. **I,** Massage the face with focus and intention. **J,** Client's partner performs supportive massage.

- Vaginal bleeding
- Severe, continuous abdominal pain
- Breaking of water (rupture of membranes)
- Pre-eclampsia, edema, dizziness, elevated blood pressure, severe headache
- Fever, frequent and painful urination (may indicate a urinary tract infection)
- Excessive vomiting of such severity and frequency that no food or fluids can be retained
- Excessive itching (occasionally may suggest a liver or kidney dysfunction [cholestasis])

Recommendations for Massage During Pregnancy

Unless specific circumstances or complications are involved, massage for pregnant women should be a general massage (Figure 14-10). Do not massage vigorously or extremely deeply, do not overstretch, and do not massage the abdomen other than with superficial stroking. Avoid massage on the inside of the ankle, because a reflex point in that area can stimulate uterine contractions (this area is located on the spleen meridian). Watch for fever, edema, varicose veins, and severe mood swings. After birth, postpartum depression

PROFICIENCY EXERCISE 14-3

1. Contact your local hospital or other agency offering child-birth classes. Ask if you might attend as an observer.
2. Locate a pregnant dog or cat. While giving the animal a massage, gently palpate the abdomen.

can become a serious problem for some women. Refer a client with these conditions to her physician immediately.

In some cases pregnancy is not a joyous event, as in an unwanted pregnancy. The practitioner must not try to convince the woman that she really does want the baby or try to change her mood. The client must be supported with caring, quiet touch, and listening.

Interrupted pregnancies also are difficult. Whether the cause is spontaneous abortion in the first 3 months, induced abortion, or miscarriage, an interrupted pregnancy is a strain on a woman's body and emotional well-being. If a client has had an interrupted pregnancy, watch for emotional changes at what would have been the projected time of birth. Extra caring and support are helpful then.

The massage professional should communicate with the physician or licensed midwife to work with a woman during pregnancy. Giving a general massage to a pregnant woman can be a very rewarding experience, one that allows the massage professional to watch the miracle of life develop (Proficiency Exercise 14-3).

Labor

Labor occurs as the baby moves down the birth canal before birth. Education and birthing classes are important, especially for first pregnancies. It may be appropriate to teach the woman's support person some massage techniques before the onset of labor. Massage given by the support person helps that person to feel useful and involved with the pregnancy and birthing process. Massage of the lower back and stroking of the abdomen may provide comfort and a point of focus during labor. Massaging the feet often is helpful. Massage can relax the body and divert the attention of the nervous system, thereby providing distraction during early labor. Labor proceeds easier and faster if the woman is relaxed and works with her body.

During a phase of labor called *transition,* the woman often does not want to be touched. Transition occurs just before the second stage of labor, with the actual movement of the baby down the birth canal. The contractions at this time are very hard and have not yet been replaced by the urge to push.

After delivery, massage may help the woman's body return to normal, it may reduce the stress of taking care of a new baby, and it may give the client some time to take care of herself.

Key Points

- Each trimester of pregnancy typically requires unique massage adaptation.
- Pregnancy is not an illness, but disorders occur, and the massage therapist needs to monitor for referral.

- Communication with the health care team is important.
- Massage can be helpful during labor.

PEDIATRICS

SECTION OBJECTIVES

Chapter objectives covered in this section:
5. Adapt massage for infants, children and adolescents
Using the information presented in this section, the student will be able to perform the following:
- Explain the infant stage from birth to 3 years old
- Explain the importance of adapting massage to the physical and emotional state of the infant
- Understand the importance of a confident touch when working with infants
- Teach parents to massage their babies
- Apply general massage methods to ease growing pains
- Train family members in massage techniques for use at home

Infants

Most authorities designate babies from birth to 18 months of age as infants. For the purposes of this textbook, the classification is expanded to 3 years of age because infants are still developing neurologically until that time. One or both parents must provide informed consent for the massage and must be present during any professional interaction with the infant.

Protection, nutrition, connection, bonding, stimulation, and soothing acceptance are crucial for human infants. Infants are born with a need for sociability, along with the more basic needs for food, shelter, and so forth. The people of most cultures massage their infants. Although this practice has been almost lost in the westernized world, it is being revived. Research by Dr. Tiffany Field and her associates shows that premature infants who have been massaged fare much better than those who have not. Massage provides an organized, logical approach to sensory stimulation, which is important for infants because part of their growth is learning to sort and organize sensory stimulation.

As mentioned, physiologically the infant's growth pattern is not complete until 3 years of age (Figure 14-11). By 12 months of age, the infant can move independently from place to place but still is utterly dependent on the protection of a parent or family group. Two-year-olds are still babies. Three-year-olds are quite different in both function and body form. By the time a child can control bladder and bowel functions reliably (about age 3), cognitive functions are better able to be organized. When learning the meaning of "no," picking up toys, and sharing, the infant is ready to pass into childhood.

Understanding the limitations of these walking infants is important. How many 2-year-olds have been spanked for not sharing toys or putting toys away, when physically and developmentally they are incapable of understanding the concept? Touch then becomes negative in connotation. Lots of hurts happen at this age. The parents' expectations can be too high, resulting in frustration on the part of both parents and child. These wonderful and challenging twos are a great time to take time out and give the baby a massage. If the child is approached

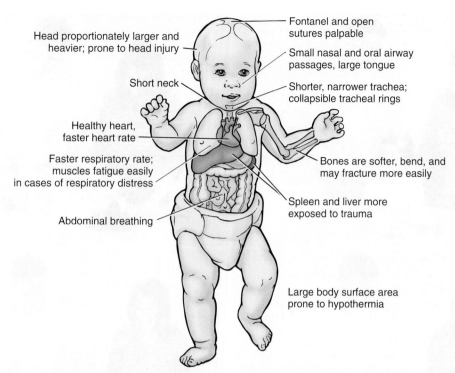

FIGURE 14-11 The unique anatomic and physiologic features of infants and young children.

Labels in figure:
- Head proportionately larger and heavier; prone to head injury
- Short neck
- Healthy heart, faster heart rate
- Faster respiratory rate; muscles fatigue easily in cases of respiratory distress
- Abdominal breathing
- Fontanel and open sutures palpable
- Small nasal and oral airway passages, large tongue
- Shorter, narrower trachea; collapsible tracheal rings
- Bones are softer, bend, and may fracture more easily
- Spleen and liver more exposed to trauma
- Large body surface area prone to hypothermia

appropriately, this experience can be calming for both the parent and the child, and touch then becomes a very positive experience.

When working with anyone, the massage professional needs to "meet" the person where he or she is at that moment. This is most important when working with infants. A fussy baby or a 2-year-old in a tantrum is caught up in the physiologic process. It takes time for both the nervous and endocrine systems to calm down. When verbal skills are not sufficient to express the problem, crying may be a way to burn off internal agitation that has built up through the day.

A parent or massage practitioner who expects the infant to settle into the massage immediately may be disappointed. Relaxing takes time. Repetitive long strokes and rhythmic movement of the limbs can initiate a calming response in an infant (Figure 14-12). Bilateral (on both sides) pressure is calming. Swaddling provides this type of consistent, even pressure that reduces neural activity. If the baby stiffens with the massage, the tactile stimulation most likely is too intense, too light, uneven, or painful. The infant nervous system is very sensitive. Confining the massage to the feet or rhythmic rocking may be preferable to stroking for infants who seem highly tactile sensitive. In well-baby care, a shorter massage of 15 to 30 minutes is sufficient. A confident touch is important; babies can detect nervousness immediately. To them this is not a "safe" touch, and they will not respond and may even try to withdraw. When just the right combination of methods is found, the infant responds calmly to the touch.

Teaching parents to massage their own babies is appropriate. Massage may be especially helpful for parents who have trouble bonding with their infants. Bonding is the attachment process that occurs between parent and child. Although bonding is considered primarily an emotional response, it is

PROFICIENCY EXERCISE 14-4

1. Using professional journals, investigate resources for learning more about infant massage.
2. Find a litter of puppies or kittens and massage these "babies."

theorized that some biochemical and hormonal interaction may support the process. The hormone oxytocin is present in both the mother and the father and may be a factor in the bonding process. Massage, through skin stimulation, increases the oxytocin level.

Other than in a hospital-type setting, the massage practitioner is unlikely to develop a clientele of infants. However, teaching infant massage can be an exciting career addition. Classes and various books and videos are available to help the massage therapist develop infant massage classes for caregivers. Learning massage is an excellent way for parents to become confident with their touch.

The nervous system of an infant born to a mother addicted to drugs or alcohol is especially challenged (Figure 14-13). Research is under way to determine whether the gentle, organized, tactile approaches of massage can help these special babies. The initial findings are promising. Babies, especially babies of drug-addicted mothers, sometimes are abandoned, and hospitals place these infants in what is called a *boarder nursery*. A hospital may be open to the volunteer efforts of a massage therapist, which could provide a great learning experience for both the massage professional and the hospital staff.

Remember, each baby is different. "Listen" to these little bodies and structure the massage to best meet the baby's needs (Proficiency Exercise 14-4).

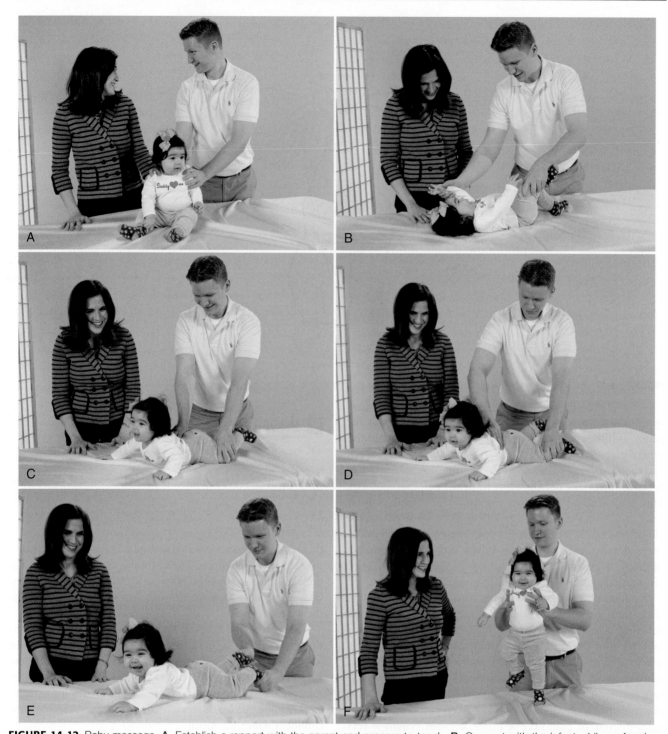

FIGURE 14-12 Baby massage. **A,** Establish a rapport with the parent and prepare to teach. **B,** Connect with the infant while performing assessments. **C,** Make sure the massage is pleasurable to the baby. **D,** Even babies have tender points; keep alert for changes in expression. **E,** After treating tender points, return to pleasurable massage. **F,** A happy baby and an educated mom.

Children

Providing massage services for children is not much different from providing massage for adults. For the purposes of this textbook, children are people ranging from 3 to 18 years of age. Children love physical contact. It is interesting that the horsing around and wrestling that occur during play look a lot like massage.

From age 3 to puberty, physical growth is seen mostly in height. At adolescence, growth in height accelerates under the influence of increased hormone levels, and sexual maturation occurs. Both physical and emotional growing pains are common. Physical growing pains occur because the long bones grow more rapidly than the muscle tissue, resulting in a pull on the periosteum, or connective tissue bone covering, which is a very pain-sensitive structure. Massage can help by gently lengthening the muscles, stretching the connective tissue, and providing symptomatic relief of pain through the effects of counterirritation, hyperstimulation analgesia, gait

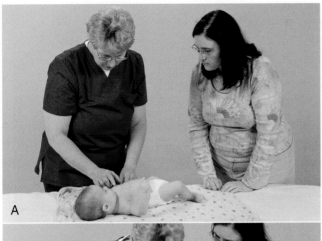

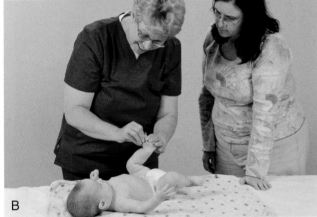

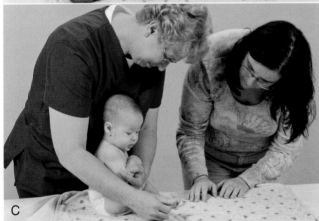

FIGURE 14-13 Massage for an ill or injured infant. **A,** Assess the infant and explain to the parent or caregiver what you intend to do. Always follow the treatment plan provided by a physician. **B,** Take time to connect with the baby. **C,** Showing care and concern, teach the parent or caregiver how to massage the baby.

control, and release of endorphins. Because children may have shorter attention spans than adults, a 30-minute massage usually is sufficient.

Adolescents

Adolescents live in bodies that are changing every second. Hormone levels fluctuate constantly, and mood swings occur regularly. Growth is accelerated, and natural sleep-wake patterns often are disrupted. It is not uncommon for a teenager

PROFICIENCY EXERCISE 14-5

1. Give massages to three children or adolescents of various ages. Make sure the parent or guardian is present.
2. Develop a one-page handout with five massage techniques that families can share.

to be up all night and want to sleep all day. Massage may help an adolescent become more comfortable with this ever-changing body. It certainly helps with physical growing pains. Use special caution when working with adolescent boys. The reflexive physical sexual response is sensitive, and almost anything can trigger an erection. The therapist should be sensitive to this by not using a smooth sheet over the groin area when working with male adolescents. Instead, keep the sheet bunched in this area to disguise any physical response to the massage.

It also is important that the practitioner never work with children or adolescents unless a parent or guardian is present. Part of the massage time can be used to teach the parent or guardian some massage methods to help the child and to teach the child some massage methods for use on the parent. Massage provides a structured approach to safe touch. It may help families stay connected during both good and difficult times (Figure 14-14) (Proficiency Exercise 14-5).

Key Points

- The permission of a parent or guardian is required to work with minors.
- Parents can be taught to massage their infants and children.

GERIATRICS

SECTION OBJECTIVES

Chapter objectives covered in this section:
  6. Explain the aging process and adapt massage for the geriatric population
Using the information presented in this section, the student will be able to perform the following:
- Provide a rationale for the benefits of massage for the elderly
- Describe the physical, mental, and emotional changes associated with the aging process and adapt massage methods accordingly
- Understand the need for fee and time adjustments when working with the elderly

In the industrialized societies, the fastest growing segments of the population are those over age 80. People in their advanced years can benefit greatly from massage. Although the massage methods are no different, elderly individuals do present specific concerns, and appropriate adjustments are required in massage application.

The age range for the category "elderly" is flexible. Some 60-year-olds have the problems of the aged, and some 85-year-olds are in better physiologic condition than some 60-year-olds. Because of this, the wiser course with people over age 65 is to consider the physiologic condition rather than the

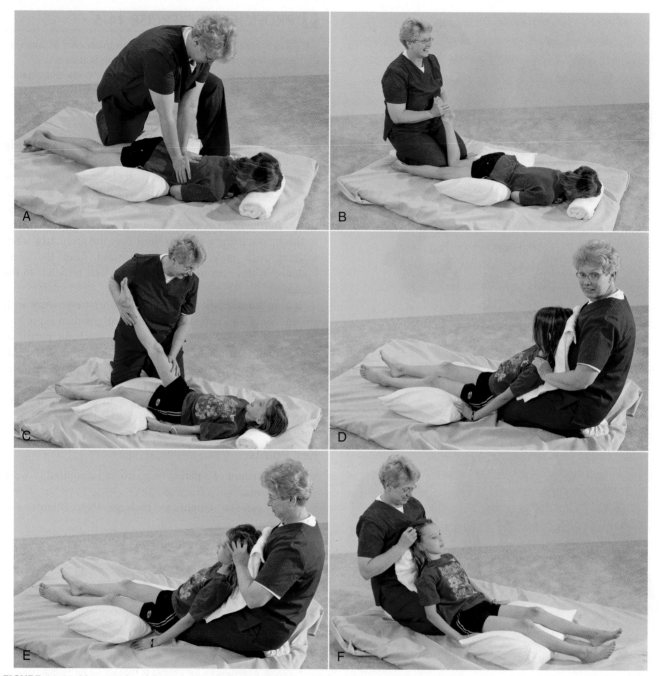

FIGURE 14-14 Massage for children and adolescents. **A,** Most children prefer to keep their clothes on and like a mat. **B,** Interact with the parent or guardian (not pictured). **C,** Maintain your focus on the child. **D,** Continue to connect with the parent or guardian and explain your massage methods. **E** and **F,** Relax, nurture, and remember to teach the parent or guardian.

chronologic age. Specific care for the aging population is called *geriatrics.*

Massage practitioners who plan to work with elderly individuals may need more training to learn about their special needs. In most cases a general massage session using the skills presented in this text and an attentive, caring attitude are sufficient for interacting professionally with the elderly (Figure 14-15) (Proficiency Exercise 14-6).

PROFICIENCY EXERCISE 14-6

1. Volunteer to give massages at a local senior citizens center for at least 4 weeks or a total of 32 hours.
2. Contact a local nursing home and ask whether a resident who has few visitors might appreciate receiving a massage. Commit to a minimum of two massages a month for 6 months.

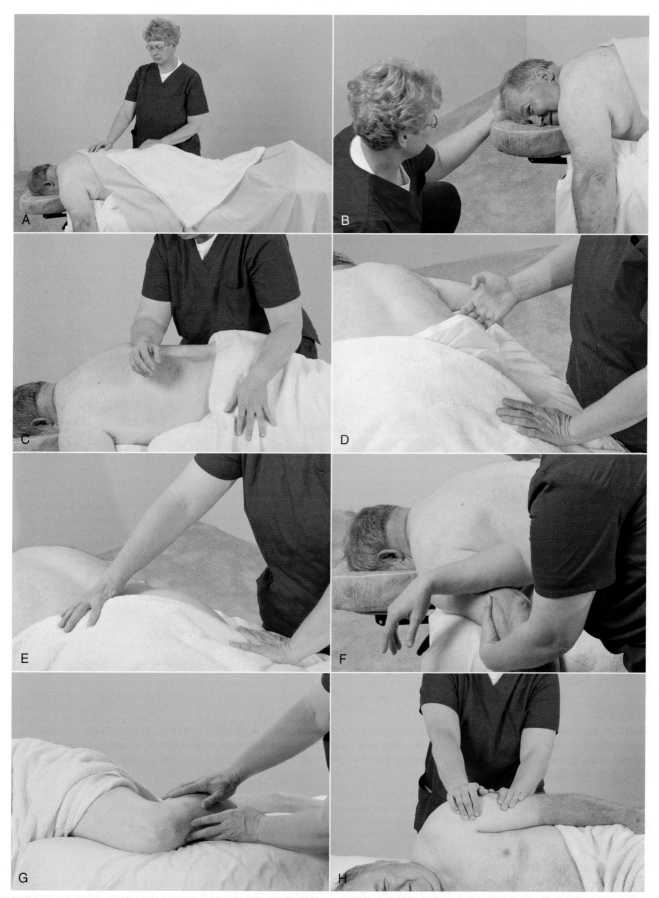

FIGURE 14-15 Massage procedure for an elderly client. **A,** Drape the client for modesty and warmth. **B,** Interact appropriately with the client. **C,** Be cautious but confident in providing the massage. **D,** Respectfully move underclothing. **E,** Maintain secure draping. **F,** Use broad-based contact and be cautious about depth of pressure and degree of drag. **G,** Be vigilant in observing the client's reactions and adapt the massage as appropriate. **H,** The side-lying position often is most comfortable for elderly clients.

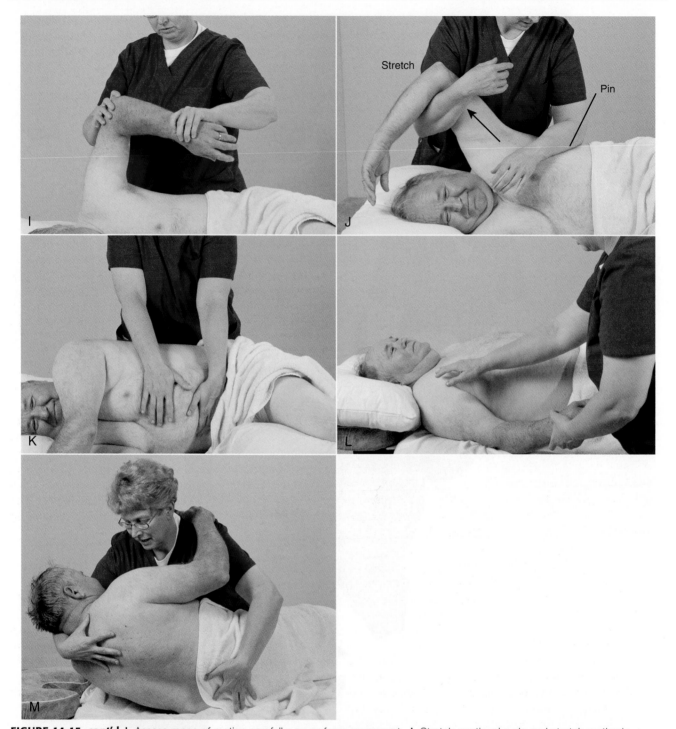

FIGURE 14-15, cont'd I, Assess range of motion carefully: never force movement. **J,** Stretch cautiously; pin and stretch methods increase tension on tissue while protecting joints. **K,** Abdominal massage supports digestive and elimination functions. **L,** Gentle oscillation (shaking and rocking) is effective for supporting joint function. **M,** If necessary, assist the client in getting off the massage table and donning clothing.

Massage Adaptation

Physical Effects of the Aging Process

The aging process is normal. Muscle tissue diminishes, as do fat and connective tissue. Connective tissue becomes less pliable, reproduces more slowly, and forms fibrotic tissue more easily. Bones are not as flexible and are more prone to breaking. Joints are worn, and osteoarthritis is common. The

skin is thinner, circulation is not as efficient, and fluid in the soft tissue is reduced.

The body tends to collapse a bit during aging. The spaces provided for the nerves are reduced, and bones and soft tissue structures can put pressure on the nerves, resulting in sciatica and thoracic outlet syndrome. Feet hurt because the intricate joint structure of the foot has broken down. Circulation to the

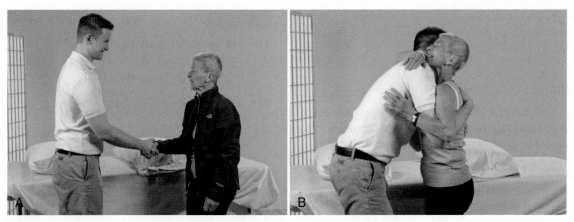

FIGURE 14-16 Physical contact with an elderly client. **A,** A proper handshake. **B,** A professional hug.

extremities is diminished, often resulting in a burning pain (Schmidt Luggen and Hill, 2004; Keene Elkin et al., 2007). These conditions are not life-threatening, but they may cause a person to feel miserable. If only temporarily, massage can help ease the discomfort of these conditions.

Dehydration, lack of appetite, and weight loss can be problems with advanced age, but the parasympathetic stimulation produced by massage can increase appetite and improve digestion for elderly clients. Proper hydration is very important. Sleep also can be improved. Many elderly people have periods of insomnia or disrupted sleep patterns. Improved sleep supports restorative mechanisms and increases vitality.

Medications

Many elderly people take several medications. The elderly also are more sensitive to the dosage level of medication and less able to self-regulate homeostatic processes. The massage professional must be attentive to the physiologic interactions between the effects of massage and the medications. Regular massage may allow reduction of the dosages of some medications, although this is a decision that needs to be made between the client and his or her physician.

Depression and Dementia

Elderly people are sometimes depressed. This frequently is both a chemical depression and a situational condition. Massage stimulates neurochemicals that can lift mild depression temporarily. Dementia, such as Alzheimer's disease, has shown temporary improvement after massage. Wandering behavior has decreased, and an increased awareness of the current environment has been observed (Sierpina et al., 2005; Suzuki et al., 2010).

If a person does not have adequate cognitive functioning skills, as in cases of dementia caused either by the aging process or by medications taken for other conditions, they will be unable to give informed consent for the massage. The guardian, physician, or other health care professional must intervene to give the necessary permission.

Social Interaction

Many elderly people are alone. Their spouses have passed away, and their families are busy with their own lives. We all need stimulation. If a person is not physically and emotionally stimulated, neurologic function begins to deteriorate. The interaction with a massage therapist can provide both physical and emotional stimulation for the elderly. If nothing else, the physical contact with another human being provides sensory stimulation, with beneficial results (Figure 14-16).

Because some elderly clients are alone or have a limited income (or both), the massage therapist should take into consideration not only the fees charged but also the amount of time spent with the elderly client. The social interaction of talking with an elderly client may be just as important as the physical interaction of the massage. If the massage professional listens attentively, much can be learned from the elderly, who have many years of experience to share. The time should be given willingly. However, professional boundaries need to be maintained, including boundaries around the time spent for the appointment.

Key Points

- The age range for the category "elderly" is flexible. Physiologic age is a better indicator than chronologic age.
- Adaptations are based on the physiologic changes of aging, such as thinner skin, less efficient circulation, and sleep disturbances.
- Medication use is common in the elderly.
- Depression and dementia may interfere with the client's ability to provide informed consent for care.

ACUTE CARE

SECTION OBJECTIVES

Chapter objective covered in this section:

7. Recognize acute care situations and adapt massage appropriately
Using the information presented in this section, the student will be able to perform the following:
- Define acute illness and injury
- Determine the appropriate massage application for the acute healing phase
- Use a specific massage sequence to support wound healing
- Adapt massage application to manage scar tissue
- Adapt massage application to manage acute pain

Acute care assumes that an individual has a current injury or illness. Combining pain management strategies and palliative care provides a framework for massage for acute care situations.

Acute Illness

Application of massage differs for acute illness and acute injury. Acute illness follows palliative massage care guidelines. One concern when working with individuals experiencing illness is whether the illness is contagious and how it is spread. If the individual is experiencing a fever, the body is actively involved in fighting the disease and adaptive ability is strained. Avoiding massage or working only in a limited manner, such as providing a foot massage, may be prudent. If massage is used during an acute illness, it should be a general approach involving moderate pressure that is not painful, and it should be limited to 30 to 45 minutes.

Acute Injury

Acute injury indicates that damage to the body has occurred, such as a fracture, wound, sprain, strain, burn, contusion, and so on. It is important to know both the cause and outcome to understand the nature of the injury (e.g., a fracture caused by a fall in a person who has osteoporosis). Massage therapists working in the medical setting, especially hospitals, often encounter surgically created wounds, such as an incision site; surgical procedures may include various types of microsurgery or minimally invasive surgery, in which tiny incisions are used to enable faster healing.

Wound Healing

Surgical incisions are performed in a sterile environment, which helps reduce the risk of infection. Wounds that occur from accidents are more prone to infection. With any type of wound, infection control is essential. Massage in the area of a wound in the acute stage is contraindicated to prevent infection. Massage can occur once the protective skin barrier has healed.

Infection is not as much of a concern with forms of injury that do not involve wounds; however, the process of healing still needs to be understood so that massage supports healing. These types of injuries include sprains, strains, contusions, and so forth. (Recall that the section on athletes earlier in this chapter describes the care of these types of injuries, because they are common occurrences in that special population.) However, anyone can sprain an ankle or fall and strain a muscle or get hit and end up with a contusion.

Box 14-5 lists recommendations for massage during various stages of healing. Massage during wound healing also targets functional scar development (Box 14-6). Methods to address old scars that may be problematic are also described in Box 14-6.

Acute Pain Management

Massage is very effective at managing acute and chronic pain and supports other pain treatments, such as medication,

---

Box 14-5 Massage Approach During Healing

Massage During the Acute Phase
- Manage pain
- Support sleep

Massage During the Early Subacute Phase
- Manage pain
- Support sleep
- Manage edema
- Manage compensation patterns

Massage During the Later Subacute Phase
- Manage pain
- Support sleep
- Manage edema
- Manage compensation patterns
- Support rehabilitative activity
- Support mobile scar development
- Support tissue regeneration process

Massage During the Remodeling Phase
- Manage irreversible compensation patterns
- Restore tissue pliability
- Support rehabilitation activity
- Encourage appropriate scar tissue development
- Manage adhesions
- Restore firing patterns, gait reflexes, and neuromuscular responses
- Eliminate reversible compensation patterns

---

ultrasound, hydrotherapy, and so on. A common error is to think of massage targeting pain reduction as therapeutic change. It is palliative. Massage that is so aggressive it creates inflammation and excessive pain during application is incorrect, as is massage that produces inflammation and pain afterward, except in very rare situations in which methods to introduce therapeutic inflammation are indicated. Pain management massage strategies are presented in Box 14-7.

Key Points

- Acute care assumes that the person has a current injury or illness.
- Pain management strategies and palliative care provide a framework for massage in acute care situations.

CHRONIC ILLNESS

SECTION OBJECTIVES

Chapter objectives covered in this section:
8. Describe the mechanisms of chronic illness and adapt massage for those with chronic conditions
Using the information presented in this section, the student will be able to perform the following:
- Explain the basic cause of chronic illness
- Explain the difference between acute illness and chronic illness
- Develop realistic expectations for working with people who have a chronic illness

Box 14-6 Therapeutic Massage Application for Wounds, Scars, Sprains, and Strains

Days 1-3
- Sanitation and prevention of infection are essential.
- Avoid the area during massage to protect the wound from contamination.
- Lymphatic drainage can be used above and below the wound. Do not drain if any signs of infection are present, such as heat, swelling, redness (especially any type of streaking), pus, or sour smell.

Day 3-4
- Use bend, shear, and tension forces around the wound far enough away to prevent any chance of contamination. The goal is to gently drag the skin in multiple directions to prevent adhesions from forming. The connective tissue formation is random at this time. The wound edges should not be disturbed.

Days 5-6
- Increase the intensity and depth of the forces in the area that has been treated and move closer to the wound. Reduce the intensity and gently apply bend, shear, and stretch (tension) force to the tissue. The wound edges should not be disturbed.

Day 7
- Again increase the intensity in the previously treated areas and then move closer to the wound. At this point the wound should be moving a bit from the forces loading the adjacent tissue, but the wound edges must not be disturbed. Progressively increase the intensity daily by moving closer and closer to the wound.
- As soon as the wound has healed completely (14 days is typical, but it can take longer) begin to bend and shear the scar tissue and stretch it using tension forces.
- To prevent infection, make sure the wound is completely healed before working on it directly. Before working on the scar formation in the healing tissue, work on the tissue surrounding the wound; this can be addressed after the acute phase has passed (usually after 2 to 3 days). Maintain attention to the scar for at least 6 months. These methods can be taught to the client or family member.

Old and Problematic Scars
- Old scars that have adhered to underlying tissue can be softened and stretched. All mechanical forces are used in multiple directions on the scar each session until the scar tissue and the tissue at least 1 inch away from the scar become warm and slightly red. The intensity should be enough that the client feels a burning, stretching sensation. A small degree of inflammation is desirable, and after the massage the area may be a bit tender to the touch but should not be painful to movement. Ideally the area would be treated every other day, allowing the tissue to recover on the alternate days. These methods can be taught to the client or family member.

Box 14-7 Massage Strategies for Pain Management

1. General full-body application with a rhythmic, slow approach for 45 to 60 minutes as often as feasible.
   Goal: Parasympathetic dominance with reduced cortisol production and increased production of pain-modulating neurochemicals.
2. Typically a moderate pressure depth is used, with enough compressive force to move through the superficial fascia to deeper tissue using a broad-based application. No poking, frictioning, or application of pain-causing methods should be done. In some cases light pressure should be used, especially for patients undergoing radiation therapy and those who are especially fragile.
   Goal: Support serotonin and gamma amino-butyric acid (GABA) production and reduce substance P and adrenaline.
3. Drag is slight unless connective tissue is targeted. Drag is targeted to lymphatic drainage (unless contraindicated) and skin stimulation.
   Goal: Reduce swelling and create counterirritation through skin stimulation.
4. Nodal points (e.g., in the feet, hands, head, and along the spine) have high concentrations of neurovascular components. They are the locations of cutaneous nerves, trigger points, acupuncture points, reflexology points, and so on. When these points are massaged with a sufficient depth of pressure that does not cause pain, a "good hurt" sensation is created without eliciting defensive guarding or withdrawal; this may help relieve pain.
   Goal: Elicit gate control response and release of endorphins and other pain-inhibiting chemicals.
5. Direction of massage varies but deliberately targets fluid movement unless contraindicated.
   Goal: Support circulation.
6. Mechanical forces of shear, bend, torsion, and so on are introduced with an agitation quality to "stir" the ground substance without creating inflammation.
   Goal: Increase tissue pliability and reduce tissue density.
7. Mechanical forces of shear, bend, and torsion are used to address adhesions or fibrosis; however, these forces must be specifically targeted and limited in duration.
   Goal: Reduce localized nerve irritation or circulation.
8. Muscle energy methods and lengthening are applied rhythmically and gently and are targeted to shortened muscles.
   Goal: Reduce nerve and proprioceptive irritation and improve circulation.
9. Stretching to introduce tension force is applied slowly, without pain, and targeted to shortened connective tissue.
   Goal: Reduce nerve and proprioceptive irritation.
10. Massage therapists are focused, attentive, and compassionate but maintain appropriate boundaries.
    Goal: Support entrainment, bioenergy normalization, and palliative care.

Chronic illness is defined as a disease, an injury, or a syndrome that shows either little change or slow progression. Acute illness or injury is a short-term condition that resolves through normal healing processes and, if necessary, supportive medical care. Compared with chronic illness, acute conditions can be dealt with relatively easily, because healing produces measurable results. Dealing with chronic illness is difficult for the person who has it, for the physician and the health care team, and for the massage therapist. In many situations little can be done except to make day-to-day living with the illness more tolerable. Healing is an option in some situations, but even then total recovery is a long process that requires work, commitment, and support.

The dynamics of family relationships, work situations, emotions, and coping skills play an important role. This process may be subconscious and therefore difficult for the client to recognize or change. The dynamics required to support chronic illness patterns reach far beyond the physiology of the disease, and professional counseling may be required.

Working with chronic illness does not often produce measurable improvements. More often a slowed deterioration or, at best, stabilization is seen. For this reason, the treatment of chronic illness does not easily fit into the current medical system, which is geared mostly toward acute and traumatic care.

Massage Adaptation

Massage therapists who work with people with a chronic illness should understand as much as possible about the illness. By using this information and conferring with the physician and other health professionals involved in the client's care, the massage practitioner can integrate the effects of massage into the comprehensive treatment plan, helping the client achieve the highest quality of life possible.

Long-term debilitating diseases such as Parkinson's disease, multiple sclerosis, systemic lupus erythematosus (SLE), rheumatoid arthritis, fibromyalgia, chronic fatigue syndrome, asymptomatic infection with the human immunodeficiency virus (HIV), acquired immunodeficiency syndrome (AIDS), and disk problems that cause back pain respond well to the short-term symptomatic relief massage provides. Massage also can reduce general stress, helping the individual to cope better with the condition (see Chapters 5 and 6). Treatment plans focus on therapeutic change, condition management, or palliative care. Because of the nature of chronic illness, the emotional factors involved, and possible secondary gain, the treatment most often chosen is condition management, with palliative care provided during acute episodes of the illness. This recommendation does not mean that an actual therapeutic change plan is not possible; it simply is not as common.

Often additional training is required just to understand chronic illness patterns, the effects of the medications involved, and the skill necessary to work in conjunction with other health care professionals.

Medications

People with chronic illnesses usually are under a physician's care and may be taking medications. The massage practitioner must work closely with these medical professionals to understand the effects of the various treatments and medications (See Appendix C).

The Chronic Illness Cycle

Chronic illness follows an uneven cycle, with good and bad periods. On good days the person may overexert herself and deplete an already weakened energy source. The immune system may be compromised, making the person with a chronic illness more susceptible to infections such as colds and influenza. Because most chronic illness patterns have good days and bad days, the intensity of massage sessions must be geared to the client's condition that day. When symptoms are more active, the better course may be to give massages more often for shorter periods.

Encouraging Hardiness

One approach to rehabilitating chronically ill individuals is a hardening or toughening program. Hardiness is the physical and mental ability to withstand external stressors. Individuals with chronic illnesses often reduce their activity levels, isolate themselves, and become less hardy. Massage, hydrotherapy, specially designed hardening programs, and exercise can increase a person's hardiness.

Alternative Approaches to Healing

Mind/body approaches, behavior modification, relaxation techniques, spiritual healing, and other types of interventions and alternatives may be helpful to those with chronic illnesses. All these approaches tend to empower the client, rallying the powerful internal resources that human beings have. It is important not to discount a method that a person may use for self-help.

Goals and Expectations for Massage
The Massage Therapist

The massage professional who wants to work with the chronically ill must have realistic expectations. Instead of developing a massage approach to bring about a cure for the illness, which is out of the scope of massage practice anyway, the focus should be on helping the client feel better for a little while. There is value in knowing that massage may be the only care of this type the client is receiving, that not getting worse is an improvement for the client, that some people need their illness to cope, and that massage eases their suffering in the illness pattern.

Often the client's present situation is the best that can be achieved under the existing circumstances. If each pattern presented by a client is seen as a solution to a pre-existing condition, it is easier to understand why approaches that relieve the symptoms and support healing often are met with resistance. For example, a client with a chronic fatigue syndrome pattern consumes four or five cups of coffee

PROFICIENCY EXERCISE 14-7

1. Choose one chronic illness and investigate it thoroughly.
2. Develop an educational brochure explaining the benefits of massage as part of a plan for coping with the chronic illness you have investigated. Share the brochure with fellow students.

after noon and finds that she cannot sleep at night because caffeine is known to disturb sleep. Massage has been ineffective in supporting sleep. The client will not stop drinking coffee in the afternoon, because she cannot function at work if she does. So what does the massage therapist do? There is no easy answer, and survival mechanisms reinforce short-term solutions even if the behaviors create long-term problems.

The Client

A resourceful goal for working with people with chronic illness is helping a client rediscover the fact that each person is in charge of his or her own life, and the illness is not. The illness may have been allowed to take over the person's life and personal power. "Healing" may be the act of reasserting control over one's life, not getting rid of the disease. The benefits of massage may provide enough relief to enable the client to find the necessary inner resources for dealing constructively with the effects of chronic illness, enhancing the client's quality of life and the lives of those around him or her (Proficiency Exercise 14-7).

Key Points

- Dealing with chronic illness is difficult for the person who has it and the health care team.
- A clinical reasoning process is used to determine the type of care most beneficial for a client with a chronic illness.
- The massage practitioner must work closely with medical professionals to understand the effects of the various treatments and medications.
- Complementary and alternative forms of health care may be helpful to those with chronic illnesses.

ONCOLOGY CARE

SECTION OBJECTIVES

Chapter objective covered in this section:
9. Adapt massage to support clients undergoing oncology care
Using the information presented in this section, the student will be able to perform the following:
- Define cancer and oncology
- List the types of cancer treatments
- Adapt massage application for patients undergoing cancer treatment
- Describe the use of palliative-based massage as part of cancer treatment

The treatment of cancer, called *oncology*, combines disease-specific scientific knowledge, public health awareness, and psychosocial sensitivity. *Cancer* refers to any one of a large number of diseases characterized by the development of abnormal cells that divide uncontrollably and have the ability to infiltrate (metastasize) and destroy normal body tissue. Tumors are cell masses that are either benign or malignant and cancerous. Not all tumors are cancerous, and not all cancers form tumors. For example, leukemia is a cancer that involves blood, bone marrow, the lymphatic system, and the spleen, but it does not form a single mass or tumor. Not only do cancerous cells invade and destroy normal tissue, they also can produce chemicals that interfere with body functions. For instance, some lung cancers secrete chemicals that alter the levels of calcium in the blood, affecting nerves and muscles and causing weakness and dizziness.

Cancer occurs with increasing incidence throughout the middle years of life and later. The American Cancer Society (ACS) estimates that half the men and one third of the women in the United States will develop cancer during their lifetimes. The three most commonly diagnosed cancers in women are expected to be cancers of the breast, lung, and bronchus. Colon cancer and rectal cancer are expected to be the most commonly diagnosed cancers in men. The most common cause of cancer death among men and women is cancer of the lung and bronchus. The most common cause of death in patients with cancer is infection, followed by respiratory failure, hepatic failure, and renal failure. Usually, many months pass between the diagnosis of metastatic cancer and the development of these complications.

Treatment

Until recently, cancer was considered incurable. However, it is no longer an automatic death sentence. More than half the people diagnosed with cancer survive 5 years or longer after diagnosis. One key to survival is early detection of cancer, and many screening tests are available. Massage therapists should know some of the most common nonspecific symptoms, such as fatigue, pain, anorexia, insomnia, and nausea. Occasionally the massage therapist may find that a client has a palpable mass. It is important for the massage therapist to support regular physician screening care and to refer clients when symptoms indicate the need.

Once cancer has been diagnosed, the care of the oncology patient begins with a detailed history and physical examination. Most patients with cancer receive some type of therapy once a histologic diagnosis has been made. Treatment for cancer can be curative or palliative. *Staging* is the process of finding out how much cancer there is in the body and where it is located. Accurate staging provides a basis for both the provider and the patient to weigh individual benefits and risks associated with a treatment.

Whether treatment has a curative or a palliative intent, success depends on the patient's disease stage and acceptance of the treatment plan. If the intent of therapy is curative, both the oncology team and the patient are more apt to accept the harshness and toxicities of treatment. Massage intervention spans the time of treatment, recovery, and return to health.

Multidisciplinary Care

Over the past few years, the value of a multidisciplinary and integrative approach to the care and treatment of individuals with cancer has been increasingly recognized. Increasingly, it is common to use several treatment modalities together (concurrently) or in sequence with the goal of preventing recurrence. This is referred to as *multimodality treatment* of the cancer. In many health care environments, multidisciplinary cancer clinics offer people the opportunity to be evaluated by the medical oncologist, surgical oncologist, radiation oncologist, nutritionist, physical therapist, and social worker at the time of their first or second clinic visit. Therapeutic massage is fast becoming an important aspect of multidisciplinary care in these settings.

Other complementary therapies, such as meditation, yoga, and aromatherapy, are incorporated into the multidisciplinary care centers. The spiritual needs of individuals are also considered and supported. In the multidisciplinary approach to patient management, each discipline performs a complementary function. In this regard cancer care, like hospice care, is becoming a model for effective integrative medical care with many professionals working together to achieve the best possible outcome.

Surgery

Surgery is performed to diagnose cancer, determine its stage, and treat the cancer. The primary care physician most often refers the person to a surgeon for biopsy and pathologic diagnosis; therefore, the surgical oncology team often is the first to see an individual with a newly diagnosed or suspected cancer.

A biopsy involves taking a tissue sample from the suspected cancer for examination by a specialist in a laboratory. A biopsy often is performed in the physician's office or in an outpatient surgery center. A positive biopsy result indicates the presence of cancer; a negative biopsy result may indicate that no cancer is present in the sample.

When surgery is used for treatment, the cancer and some tissue adjacent to the cancer typically are removed. In addition to locally treating the cancer, surgery may yield information useful for predicting the likelihood of cancer recurrence and whether other treatment modalities will be necessary.

Radiation Therapy

Radiation therapy, or radiotherapy, uses high-energy rays to damage or kill cancer cells by preventing them from growing and dividing. Similar to surgery, radiation therapy is a local treatment used to eliminate or eradicate visible tumors. Radiation therapy is not typically useful in eradicating cancer cells that have already spread to other parts of the body. Radiation therapy may be delivered externally or internally. With external radiation, high-energy rays are delivered directly to the tumor site from a machine outside the body. Internal radiation, or brachytherapy, involves the implantation of a small amount of radioactive material in or near the cancer.

Radiotherapy has both curative and palliative indications in the treatment of cancer. Radiation often is given in conjunction with surgery and chemotherapy. Radiotherapy is an integral and indispensable modality for pain relief and palliation of other symptoms, such as metastatic disease to bone or obstructing bronchial lesions. Individuals undergoing radiation experience varied symptoms, most often related to the organs that are within the direct radiation field. Radiation dermatitis and skin breakdown can occur, and patients often have associated fatigue and nausea.

Patients receiving brain radiation, whether for a primary CNS tumor or a metastatic lesion, can experience myriad symptoms, including severe fatigue, disequilibrium, nausea, vomiting, confusion or short-term memory loss, and hair loss.

Chemotherapy

Chemotherapy is any treatment involving the use of drugs to kill cancer cells. More than half of all people diagnosed with cancer receive chemotherapy. For millions of people who have cancers that respond well to chemotherapy, this approach helps treat their cancer effectively, enabling them to enjoy full, productive lives. Although surgery and radiation therapy destroy or damage cancer cells in a specific area, chemotherapy works throughout the body. Chemotherapy can destroy cancer cells that have metastasized or spread to parts of the body far from the primary tumor.

More than 100 chemotherapy drugs are used in various combinations. Cancer chemotherapy may consist of single drugs or combinations of drugs. A single chemotherapy drug can be used to treat cancer, but these drugs generally are more powerful when used with other drugs.

Chemotherapy can be administered through a vein, usually throughout a line that stays in place; injected into a body cavity; or delivered orally in the form of a pill. Chemotherapy is different from surgery or radiation therapy in that the cancer-fighting drugs circulate in the blood to parts of the body where the cancer may have spread and can kill or eliminate cancers cells at sites great distances from the original cancer. As a result, chemotherapy is considered a systemic treatment. Unfortunately, most chemotherapy drugs cannot distinguish between a cancer cell and a healthy cell. Therefore, chemotherapy often affects the body's normal tissues and organs, which results in complication of treatments or side effects.

Side Effects of Chemotherapy

Side effects of chemotherapy cause inconvenience and discomfort and occasionally may be fatal. In addition, and perhaps more important, side effects may prevent delivery of the prescribed drug dose at the specific time scheduled by the treatment plan. Because the expected outcome of therapy is based on the delivery of treatment at the dose and according to the schedule prescribed in the treatment plan, a change from the treatment plan may reduce the chance of achieving the optimum outcome. In other words, side effects not only cause discomfort and unpleasantness, they also may compromise the chances of cure by preventing the delivery of therapy at its optimum dose and time.

All chemotherapy is associated with a wide variety of side effects. However, some side effects occur more frequently than others. How the individual receiving chemotherapy experiences side effects, which ones, and their severity depend on a variety of factors, including the type of cancer, the type of chemotherapy drug or regimen used, the person's physical condition and age, and other such factors. The following side effects typically associated with chemotherapy are most pertinent to the massage therapist's understanding and to the development of a massage treatment plan:

- Anemia
- Fatigue
- Infection/neutropenia
- Nausea/vomiting
- Mouth sores
- Hair loss
- Constipation
- Diarrhea
- Pain
- Reproductive/sexual dysfunction
- Low platelet count (thrombocytopenia)

Fortunately, over the past 20 years a great deal of progress has been made in the development of treatments to help prevent and control the side effects of cancer therapy. Many side effects once associated with chemotherapy now can be easily prevented or controlled, allowing many people to work, travel, and participate in many of their other normal activities while receiving chemotherapy. For example, modern drugs to prevent vomiting (called *antiemetics*) have reduced the severity of nausea and vomiting with chemotherapy. In addition, blood cell growth factors can protect patients from infection, reduce the fatigue associated with anemia, and ensure that treatment can be delivered according to the planned dose and schedule.

Fatigue is one of the most common complaints of people with cancer and is also increased in some cancer survivors. Fatigue exists in 14% to 96% of people with cancer, particularly in individuals actively undergoing treatment. Fatigue is difficult to describe, and patients express it in a variety of ways, using terms such as tired, weak, exhausted, weary, worn-out, heavy, or slow.

For many people diagnosed with cancer, fatigue may become a critical issue in their lives. Fatigue may influence a person's sense of well-being, daily performance, activities of daily living, relationships with family and friends, and compliance with treatment. Therapeutic massage is beneficial for managing some side effects, such as fatigue and pain. Hospice care also provides an extraordinary service for cancer patients and their families.

Palliative Care

Many patients are understandably concerned about the possibility of experiencing pain and discomfort during treatment for cancer. Palliative care is aimed at relieving suffering and improving quality of life in patients undergoing treatment for the primary condition. Such care addresses physical symptoms, such as pain, shortness of breath, and nausea, but also nonphysical causes of pain, such as sadness, depression, and anxiety. Palliative care is not the same as hospice, which provides end of life care for patients who no longer want to pursue more aggressive therapy. A major priority of palliative care is to incorporate the principles of palliative care into the care of all patients with cancer from the time of diagnosis, not only in the setting of advanced or terminal disease. Palliative care focuses on the whole person, encompassing body and mind to enhance comfort and preserve dignity.

Therapeutic Massage Strategies During Cancer Treatment

Massage is accepted as part of a multidisciplinary approach to cancer treatment. The benefits of massage are obvious: stress management, preoperative and postoperative pain management, management of treatment side effects, and more. There are no specific protocols for massage and cancer care. The person undergoing cancer treatment must be evaluated each session, and the massage treatment must be based on the individual's status at that time.

The concern that massage increases metastasis is unfounded. However, it is prudent not to massage over any type of tissue masses. Specific, extensive, full-body lymphatic drainage may task already compromised immune function and should not be used. The areas of radiation treatment need to be avoided, because the skin is damaged by the treatment.

> **Caution**
> - Avoid all sources of heat (hot water bottles, heating pads, and sun lamps) on the treatment field.
> - Avoid exposing the treatment area to cold temperatures (ice bags or cold water treatment).
> - Avoid any form of salt water treatment.
> - Avoid the use of all lotions or oils on the skin in the treatment field and use only approved lotion during massage.
> - Avoid direct massage of the treatment area other than light application of approved lotion (Mantik Lewis et al, 2006).

Bones under areas of radiation treatment can be brittle; therefore, massage pressure levels need to be monitored carefully. Do not use any massage methods that may cause tissue damage, because chemotherapy reduces the body's ability to repair tissues. The general protocol may be too intense during cancer treatment, but the modified palliative protocol is appropriate.

Key Points

- Cancer treatment can be curative or palliative.
- Massage as part of an oncology treatment plan targets palliative care as part of symptom management, especially the side effects of treatment.
- Survival rates for cancer patients are steadily increasing as a result of early detection and advances in treatment.
- Cautions for massage typically arise from changes in the client's skin as a side effect of treatment.

HOSPITAL, LONG-TERM CARE, AND HOSPICE PATIENTS

SECTION OBJECTIVES

Chapter objectives covered in this section:

10. Adapt massage for integration into the various medical settings
Using the information presented in this section, the student will be able to perform the following:
- Explain the importance of comfort measures
- Adapt massage application based on the circumstances of hospital care
- Adapt massage application for individuals in long-term medical care
- Define hospice care
- Adapt massage for end of life care

Use of massage therapy in hospitals is becoming more common. Some of the reasons it is used include:
- Pain management
- Relief for cancer patients
- Pregnancy massage
- Adjunct to physical therapy
- Mobility/movement training
- Palliative care

A common theme in hospital-based massage is pain management. Massage is very effective at managing acute and chronic pain and supports other pain treatments, such as medication, ultrasound, and hydrotherapy. As mentioned, although massage targeting pain reduction commonly is thought of as therapeutic change, in reality it is palliative (see Chapter 6). Massage for the hospital patient is not targeted specifically to the pathologic condition or injury; rather, it is intended to provide comfort care and symptom management (Box 14-8; also see Box 14-7).

The Importance of Palliative Care

The purpose of palliative care is to reduce suffering and create comfort. Massage offers pleasure, comfort, and relief from aching, all of which can reduce suffering. The massage used in palliative care is based on pleasure and compassion, and the focus is on reducing discomfort and providing comfort. Gentle, nonspecific massage application is used. As a reminder, gentle does not necessarily mean light pressure. Gentle means slow, focused, and pleasurable. Pressure typically is not deep, but most patients enjoy a sense of pressure that feels good.

| Box 14-8 | Benefits of Massage for Hospital Patients |

1. *Pain:* Through the use of massage, the subjective experience of pain is diminished, even when the use of analgesics is reduced.
2. *Anxiety:* Anxiousness caused by the hospital stay and fear of procedures is reduced.
3. *Nausea:* The subjective experience of nausea and the use of antiemetics are reduced.
4. *Stress:* Physiologic indicators of stress (e.g., raised cortisol level) are diminished, and indicators of reduced stress (e.g., improved serotonin level) are increased.
5. *Sleep:* The ability to sleep more easily and for longer periods increases with massage.

Recommendations for a gentle, soothing, palliative massage include the following:
- Make sure the client is in a comfortable position and is physically supported.
- Use lotion when massaging to reduce friction and add moisture to the skin.
- Target areas that have the most discomfort (i.e., have limited movement). Massage is helpful in areas of prolonged pressure from sitting or lying. Often the neck, shoulders, low back, and calves ache as a result of immobility.
- Determine what pressure or movement is the most helpful and adjust the level and focus of pressure in response to feedback.
- Give a hand and foot massage, which can provide a sense of comfort and well-being. Gentle yet firm movements can be used.
- Encourage the person to continue to tell you what is most helpful and to let you know right away if any method causes discomfort.
- Maintain the intention of reducing suffering by focusing attention on what feels good.

Typically the massage lasts no longer that 45 minutes, and 15 to 30 minutes in targeted areas may be sufficient.

Adapting to the Hospital Room

Maintaining Proper Body Mechanics

One of the biggest challenges massage therapists face in the hospital or long-term care setting is providing massage when individuals are unable to lie on a massage table. Often massage is provided in the hospital bed or a standard chair (Figure 14-17). In these situations, massage therapists must pay special attention to their body mechanics. Fortunately, deep pressure requiring a lot of leverage is not usually needed.

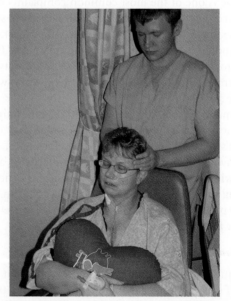

FIGURE 14-17 Providing massage in a hospital chair. (From Fritz S, Chaitow L, Hymel G: *Clinical massage in the healthcare setting*, St. Louis, 2007, Mosby. Courtesy of Laura Cochran.)

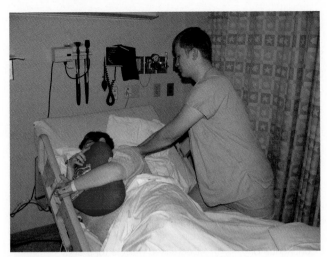

FIGURE 14-18 Working around medical devices. (From Fritz S, Chaitow L, Hymel G: *Clinical massage in the healthcare setting*, St. Louis, 2007, Mosby. Courtesy of Laura Cochran.)

Maintain the basic principles of body mechanics as presented in Chapter 8 as much as possible. If the hospital bed can move up and down, adjust the height to a comfortable level. When possible, avoid reaching and instead stay as close to the patient as possible. If the patient's mobility is limited, placing one knee on the bed or sitting on the bed may be helpful. However, before doing this, clear it with the individual who is supervising; in some cases this is not allowed. If you sit or kneel on the bed, use a clean towel as a sanitary barrier. Place it on the bed then sit or kneel on it. Do not get into uncomfortable positions and keep changing your position. It may not be possible to access all body areas.

Working Around Medical Devices

Working with individuals in hospital beds means that you must know how to operate the bed's controls. It also is important to be able to operate the nurse call buttons. Another challenge is working around various medical devices such as monitors, intravenous (IV) lines, and so on. Be cautious when moving around in the hospital room to avoid disturbing equipment (Figure 14-18).

Avoid all areas where something enters or exits the body, such as IV lines, catheters, drains, respiratory devices, and so forth. Avoid all surgical sites. Do not disturb or remove any bandaging. If this should occur, inform the nurse so that infection control is maintained. Be cautious when working around monitoring leads and do not dislodge them. If this should occur, call the nurse. Do not attempt to replace them, because proper placement is required for accurate information.

Use only the lotion provided or approved by the hospital. Do not add anything to the lotion.

The Massage Therapist's Responsibilities to the Patient and Medical Personnel

- Do not attempt to help a patient out of bed to use the restroom or other activity. Do not assist a patient to move into various positions. It is better to let the person move, because he or she will be protective of sensitive areas.

- Be courteous to other patients who may be sharing a hospital room. However, do not provide massage if asked unless authorized to do so.
- Leave the room when the physician, nurses, or other hospital personnel are providing care.
- Massage therapy is almost always provided in the hospital or similar medical setting as optional care. If a patient is sleeping or does not want a massage, do not insist. Report the situation to the supervising personnel.

Long-Term Care

Although not the same as a hospital, a long-term care facility is similar, because a variety of medically based services are provided to care for people with a chronic illness or disability. In addition, long-term care helps meet personal needs. Most long-term care provides people with support services for activities such as dressing, bathing, and using the bathroom. Long-term care can be provided at home, in the community, in assisted living, or in nursing homes.

According to the Center for Medicare and Medicaid Services (CMS), by 2020, 12 million older Americans will need long-term care. A study by the U. S. Department of Health and Human Services says that people who reach age 65 will likely have a 40% chance of entering a nursing home. About 10% of the people who enter a nursing home will stay 5 years or longer. The remaining elderly will be cared for at home. The need for home-based long-term care will increase as the elderly population grows (CMS, 2011).

Assisted living facilities offer housing alternatives for individuals who may need help with dressing, bathing, eating, and toileting but who do not require the intensive medical and nursing care provided in nursing homes. Assisted living facilities may be part of a retirement community, nursing home, or senior housing complex or may be stand-alone facilities. Assisted living provides 24-hour supervision, assistance, meals, and health care services in a homelike setting. Residents of assisted living facilities usually have their own units or apartments.

Massage therapy can be integrated into long-term care services. The adaptations used for hospital patients also can be used for long-term care residents.

Terminal Illness, End-of-Life Care, and Hospice Care

When nothing further can be done to prolong life, care focuses more on comfort measures. Hospice is a philosophy of care, not a place. Hospice care can be provided in a hospital or long-term care setting, a specific residential hospice setting or, most commonly, in the home (Box 14-9).

The experts in terminal illness are the dedicated hospice nurses and staff members who treat death with dignity. It has been said that the staff members of hospices are midwives to the dying.

To work successfully with those dealing with a terminal illness, the massage practitioner must be aware of his or her

Box 14-9 Providing Massage in the Home

It is important to move efficiently into and out of the area without disrupting the natural rhythm of the environment. It is important to respect the client's environment. Examples include removing shoes to protect the carpet and carrying special rubber-soled shoes to wear during the massage or wiping up water splashes in the restroom after washing your hands. It is important to make sure the massage equipment and lubricants do not damage the client's floors or walls. Place a sheet on the floor under the massage table to protect the flooring.

Confidentiality is extremely important. The intimacy of the environment makes it more difficult to maintain professional boundaries and time management without seeming distant and hurried. It takes longer to enter and exit the on-site environment, not just because of the equipment setup and breakdown, but also because of the need to be respectful of the area and polite. The personal safety of the massage professional is a concern because the on-site massage environment has fewer safeguards than an office setting. Get to know those living in the home ahead of time, make sure someone always knows where you are, and check in with that person. Always carry a cell phone with you.

Table 14-1 Signs and Symptoms of the Final Stages of Death

Signs and Symptoms	Reason
Coolness, color, and temperature change in hands, arms, feet, and legs; mottling of the legs; perspiration	Peripheral circulation diminishes as blood shunts to vital organs. Patient may feel cool to touch, but core temperature is normal.
Increased sleeping	Conservation of energy, psychological withdrawal, medications.
Disorientation, confusion about time, place, person	Metabolic changes, medications, changing sleep/wake cycles, decreased oxygenation.
Incontinence of urine and/or bowel	Decreased muscle tone and consciousness.
Upper airway secretions; noisy respirations	Decreased cough reflex, inability to expectorate secretions or clear throat, relaxation of glottis, decreased muscle tone.
Restlessness	Metabolic changes and decrease in oxygen to the brain.
Decreased intake of food and fluids, nausea	Blood shunted away from gastrointestinal (GI) tract, causing decreased GI motility and anorexia; ketosis.

Modified from Ebersole P, Touhy TA, Hess P, Jett KF: *Toward healthy aging: needs and nursing response*, ed 7, St Louis, 2007, Mosby.

personal feelings about death. Massage professionals who want to work with clients during this very important, challenging, and special time of life are strongly encouraged to become hospice volunteers and to take the training that hospices offer.

No one knows when a person is going to die (Table 14-1). However, two very powerful psychological forces influence living and dying: hope and the will to live. Attitudes about death vary. Adults usually have more fears about death than children do. They fear pain, suffering, dying alone, the invasion of privacy, loneliness, and separation from family and loved ones. They worry about who will care for and support those left behind. Elderly people usually have fewer of these fears than younger adults. They may be more accepting that death will occur and have had more experience with dying and death. Many have lost family members and friends. Some welcome death as freedom from pain, suffering, and disability.

Dr. Elisabeth Kübler-Ross wrote about death, and her works have much to offer. Bernie Siegal's books also are excellent. Massage professionals interested in working with the terminally ill would benefit from reading their works.

Massage Adaptation

Massage has much to offer in comfort measures for the terminally ill. Being bedridden and immobile is painful. Massage can distract the sensory perception and provide temporary comfort measures. It provides continued human contact and can give caregivers something useful, rewarding, and positive to do for their loved one who is dying.

Massage can become an important stress reduction method and a means of support for family members and caregivers. Caring for someone who is terminally ill can be very stressful. The support person may need to receive massage simply to have someone take care of him or her for an hour. Teaching

PROFICIENCY EXERCISE 14-8

1. Plan your funeral. List all plans and details regarding final arrangements.
2. Talk with an attorney about living wills.
3. Volunteer to provide massage for hospice staff members (devote a minimum of 32 hours to this).
4. Write about how you wish to be taken care of when it is your time to die. How much intervention do you want? Do you want to die in a hospital or at home? When do you want hospice services?

simple massage methods to caregivers provides them with a means of meaningful and structured interaction with their loved one, in addition to a means of connecting with and supporting each other.

The massage professional should be an integral part of the team that works to make this time of passage as gentle as possible. This means that once the decision to work with someone who is terminally ill has been made, it is important to stay with the process until the client dies, if possible. The therapist probably will grow to care for the person and will mourn and grieve when death comes.

As always, it remains the client's choice as to what is wanted, and he or she must give informed consent. A client who is dying needs to retain as much personal empowerment as possible. It should not be discouraging if all that is done during a massage session is to stroke a client's hands. At this time, especially, it is crucial to "listen" and "allow" (Proficiency Exercise 14-8).

Key Points

- A major outcome for hospital patients is pain management.
- Adaptation for individuals in the hospital or other medical facility is required because of the presence of medical equipment (e.g., the hospital bed) and devices such as catheters and intravenous lines.
- Infection control is a priority.
- Clients receiving long-term care may require adaptations similar to those for patients in the hospital.
- Hospice care is a way of providing care, not a place where care is provided.
- Hospice is an integrated care approach.
- The goals of hospice care are to ensure that individuals needing care are as free of pain and symptoms as possible, yet still alert enough to enjoy the people around them and make important decisions for themselves.

INDIVIDUALS WITH PHYSICAL IMPAIRMENT

SECTION OBJECTIVES

Chapter objectives covered in this section:

11. Communicate effectively and appropriately adapt massage for individuals with physical impairments

Using the information presented in this section, the student will be able to perform the following:

- Communicate more effectively with people who have a physical impairment
- Become aware of subtle discrimination
- Adjust the massage environment to better support those with a physical impairment

According to the guidelines of the Americans with Disabilities Act, a **physical disability/impairment** is any physiologic disorder, condition, cosmetic disfigurement, or anatomic loss that affects one or more of the following body systems: neurologic, musculoskeletal, special sense organs, respiratory (including speech organs), cardiovascular, reproductive, digestive, genitourinary, hemic and lymphatic, skin, and endocrine. Extremes in size and extensive burns also may be considered physical impairments (McGladre and Pullen, 1994).

People with physical impairments can benefit from massage for all the same reasons that any other individual can. The client's body may develop compensation patterns in response to the disability. For instance, a person who uses a wheelchair could have increased neck and shoulder tension from moving the chair. In addition, dealing with a physical impairment daily can make routine functions more stressful. The following sections present guidelines that may help the massage therapist provide services for clients with a variety of physical and sensory impairment.

A therapist must never presume to know, understand, or anticipate a client's need. *It is important to ask!* A concerned therapist does not try to pretend that the client's unique situation does not exist, but rather responds professionally. After the client has provided the necessary information about the disability, the therapist should accept the impairment as part of how the person functions.

Personal Awareness

Feeling uncomfortable is common in any new situation. This discomfort comes from not knowing what to do or say or from various other causes. Sometimes we are uncomfortable and cannot move beyond these feelings. The client will sense our discomfort. Simple disclosure of feelings allows communication and understanding, though communicating these types of feelings and accepting their personal limitations may be difficult for professionals. Sometimes referral to a practitioner who is not affected by a particular situation is the best choice for both the massage professional and the client.

Often the type of impairment is put first rather than the person. If the impairment is first in the massage therapist's mind, the person is not. Lack of knowledge is a huge contributing factor to this form of subtle discrimination. The massage professional is responsible for acting professionally and communicating effectively with all clients, including those who have disabilities. The best source of information is the person with the impairment:

- Ask your client to explain his or her situation.
- Ask what assistance, if any, might be needed.
- Ask how that assistance should be given if requested.

The practitioner should use good judgment when deciding whether to ask if assistance is needed and then should wait until the person accepts the offer before providing assistance. The client can give the best directions on how to proceed. For example, in offering assistance, it may be best to say, "If you need any assistance, I am glad to help. Tell me what you need." If the offer is declined, no offense should be taken.

If another person is present, all remarks should be directed to the client and not to the companion.

Barrier-Free Access

All massage facilities must be barrier free. Commercial buildings usually are required by law to have barrier-free access and elevators, in addition to restroom facilities accessible to individuals with a handicap (Proficiency Exercises 14-9 and 14-10).

💡 PROFICIENCY EXERCISE 14-9

1. Obtain a course catalog from a college and compare your current massage education with the curriculum required for a nurse, a physical therapy assistant, an occupational therapist, a respiratory therapist, or other similar health care professional.
2. Discuss with a physician, chiropractor, physical therapist, or psychologist the skills he or she would want to see in a massage professional who would work with the person in the professional setting.

💡 PROFICIENCY EXERCISE 14-10

Contact your local building department and speak with the person in charge of the barrier-free code requirements. Find out the requirements and the reason for each.

Massage Adaptation

Supporting Clients Who Are Blind or Have Low Vision

Many people with a visual impairment have some type of sight. Comparatively few people have no vision at all.

The therapist should begin the conversation by using the client's name so that the person is aware of being addressed. The therapist then should state his name; he should not touch the client until the person is aware of his presence in the room. When assisting a client with a visual impairment, the therapist should never push or pull on the person. Instead, if guiding is necessary, the therapist should stand just in front and a bit to the left of the client, who can then touch the therapist's right elbow when following.

Useful directions should also be given to a person with a visual impairment. If asked where something is, the therapist should not point and say "over there." Instead, terms such as *left, right, about 10 steps,* and so on are much easier to follow. You may also use the example of time on a clock for some clients to indicate where things are located. For example, "The massage table is at 12 o'clock, and a chair for your belongings is at 3 o'clock." It is not necessary to speak more loudly to individuals with a visual impairment; they usually can hear just fine.

If a person with a visual impairment places anything anywhere, it should not be moved. If a door is opened, the direction of the opening (toward or away from the person) and the location of the hinges (left or right) should be explained. It is best to let the client open the door to become better oriented to its position.

If a service dog is harnessed and working, whether it is a guide dog for someone with a visual impairment or any other support service, the therapist must not pet, feed, or in any other way interact with the dog. This distracts the dog and makes its job difficult.

Supporting Clients with a Speech Impairment

Understanding a person with a speech problem can be difficult. The therapist should ask the person to repeat anything that was unclear until it is understood and then should repeat what was said so that the person can clarify if necessary. If the therapist cannot understand what is being said, the client should be informed of this. If necessary, a notepad can be used to put communication in writing. Although speaking with an accent is not a speech impairment, it can make communication difficult. Not speaking the same language also hinders communication.

Supporting Clients Who Are Deaf or Hard of Hearing

To gain the attention of a client who is deaf or hard of hearing, the therapist should lightly tap the person once on the shoulder or discreetly wave a hand. If no interpreter is present, all talking should be done in a normal tone and rhythm of speech.

If a client can lip read, the massage therapist should always face the person and not cover her own mouth when talking.

A normal voice tone and speed should be used. If the therapist normally speaks quickly, the speed should be slowed a bit. If necessary, a notepad can be used to put communication in writing.

Hearing aids amplify sound; they do not make sound clearer. Reducing background noise helps the hearing impaired to hear better. With this in mind, it may be wise to ask before using any music during the massage session. Getting too close to a hearing aid can cause the device to make high-pitched noises; take care when massaging near the ears.

Supporting Clients with a Mobility Impairment

There are many types of mobility impairment and many reasons for it. For example, a person who uses a wheelchair may not be paralyzed.

When speaking to a client who uses a wheelchair, the therapist should do so from eye level, so sitting down or squatting may be the best option. Looking up strains the client's neck. A wheelchair must never be pushed unless the person gives permission. The individual also will give directions for pushing the wheelchair over barriers.

When a client must be transferred from a wheelchair to the massage table, the client can give the best directions on how to proceed. A transfer to a mat on the floor may be easier to accomplish, in which case the massage should be given there. The most efficient transfer is a lateral transfer to a table that is the same height as the wheelchair. This entails a shift in body mechanics by the massage therapist to accommodate a lower table (Figure 14-19).

Special care must be taken in giving a massage to a person with paralysis, because normal feedback mechanisms are not functioning. The client's tissues can be injured by inappropriate pressure or drag. Clients with catheters or other equipment must instruct the therapist in the handling of the devices. In most cases the catheter can be ignored.

If the client has undergone amputation and uses a prosthesis, he or she may or may not want the device removed during the massage. Ask permission before massaging near the amputated area. If the client is comfortable with this, massage can be especially beneficial if a prosthesis is used. Although no scientific validation is available, professional experience has shown that massage strokes carried the full length of the amputated limb seem to feel good to the client.

Supporting Clients with Brain Injuries

Brain injuries can result from external trauma, such as a blow to the head, or internal trauma, such as a cerebrovascular accident (CVA), loss of oxygen to the brain, or tumor.

Each individual who suffers a brain injury experiences different effects, depending on the part of the brain injured. Brain injury can cause cognitive, physical, behavioral, and personality changes. In addition, the effects often change over time. Some impairments are permanent, whereas others improve slowly or may also fluctuate from day to day.

Depending on the client's needs, the massage therapist must adapt the massage. If the client has altered mobility, provide barrier-free access and offer assistance on and off the massage table. Adapt communications skills to meet any

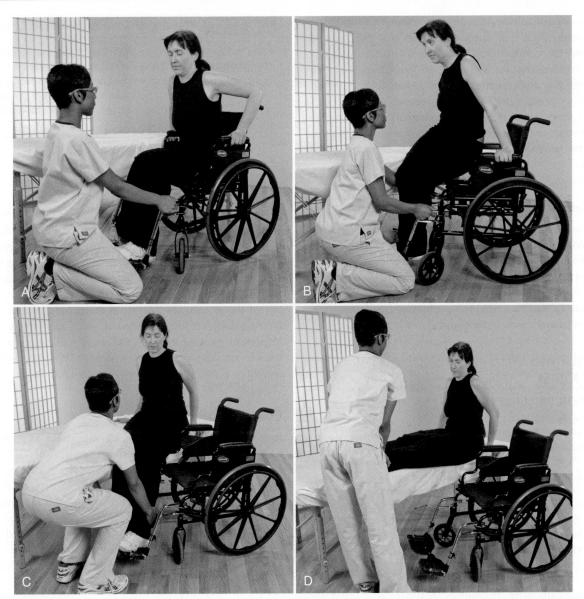

FIGURE 14-19 Transfer of a client from a wheelchair to the massage table. **A,** Place the wheelchair close to the massage table and stabilize the chair (i.e., lock the wheels). **B,** Carefully monitor the client's movements as he or she transfers to the table. **C,** After the client is seated on the table, prepare to assist by lifting the legs. **D,** Transfer the legs to the massage table.

cognitive, behavioral, and personality challenges presented by the client.

Supporting Clients with Size Considerations

If the client is short, a stool may be needed to help him or her reach the massage table, clothing hangers, or restroom fixtures. The massage professional should casually sit down to establish eye contact with the client so that the person does not have to look up, which strains the neck.

A very large person (in height or weight or both) may not trust the massage table and may be more comfortable on a floor mat. Getting up and down from the floor may be difficult. Sometimes seated massage is the better option. Ask the client what is preferable. If the practitioner is nervous about doing the massage on the massage table, the client must be told, because the therapist's anxiety will affect the quality of the massage.

Supporting Clients with Burns and Disfigurements

People who have been burned may face an assortment of challenges ranging from impaired mobility to disfigurement. As burns heal, scar tissue replaces functional epithelial tissue. All the functions of the skin are compromised, including excretion, sensation, and protection. Scar tissue tends to contract and pull, which can make the area of the healed burn feel shortened or tight. Severe contractures sometimes develop and must be treated medically. Myofascial release and other connective tissue techniques can soften and gently stretch connective tissue. Massage of this type may reduce the effect of this shrinkage somewhat. Professionals who want to serve clients who have been burned need additional training in these methods.

Many disfigurements tend to draw our attention, because the mind is designed to notice differences. Although many disfigurements do not limit function in any way, they can create social difficulties. Attempting not to notice a disfigurement usually fails. The client recognizes that the situation exists and has various levels of comfort with the condition. Honest communication is effective in redirecting the attention from the disfigurement to the person over time. The practitioner might offer a simple statement, such as, "I can't help but notice (the particular disfigurement). I'm not uncomfortable, but the difference naturally draws my attention. Please be patient with me until I become more familiar with you."

Key Points

- Use people-first language when working with clients who have some sort of disability.
- The client is the best source of information about what assistance, if any, and what accommodation, if any, may be needed.
- All massage facilities need to have barrier-free access.
- Do not interact with service animals.

INDIVIDUALS WITH A PSYCHOLOGICAL DIAGNOSIS

SECTION OBJECTIVES

Chapter objectives covered in this section:

12. Communicate effectively and appropriately adapt massage for individuals diagnosed with psychological conditions

Using the information presented in this section, the student will be able to perform the following:

- Define mental impairment based on the provisions of the Americans with Disabilities Act
- Understand the importance of verifying informed consent when working with individuals who have a psychological diagnosis
- Structure a massage to support psychological interventions

The Americans with Disabilities Act defines **mental impairment** as any mental or psychological disorder, such as mental retardation (developmental disabilities), organic brain syndrome, emotional or mental illness, and specific learning disabilities. The conditions considered in this section include:

- Chemical addictions
- Chemical imbalances in the brain
- Intellectual disabilities
- Cognitive disabilities
- Psychiatric disorders
- Post-traumatic stress disorder

It is important to understand how our minds work and the interaction that constitutes the mind/body connection. It now is well accepted in the scientific community that the mind, the body, and the spirit are linked to a person's health and well-being. A dedicated student of massage will seriously consider taking some psychology courses at a community college or other educational center and will keep up-to-date on new research findings. Massage will continue to have a very important place in mind/body medicine and treatments, along with other forms of mental health services.

| **Box 14-10** | The Importance of Informed Consent |

Informed consent is an important concern when working with clients with chemical imbalances, developmental disabilities, or who are under the influence of drugs (both prescribed and not). Special care must be taken to ensure that the client is able to provide informed consent. When doubt exists, the massage should not be given.

The actual massage approach is no different when the therapist works with individuals with a psychological diagnosis than if the condition did not exist. The important factor is the person receiving the massage. Practitioners who want to work with clients with psychological diagnoses need additional training to be able to understand the physiology and psychology of the various disorders and the challenges these clients face. An understanding of psychotropic pharmacology also is important, because massage and these medications affect the body in similar ways. This type of work should be supervised closely by a psychologist or psychiatrist (Box 14-10).

Chemical Addictions

Individuals withdrawing from chemical and alcohol addictions may find that massage helps reduce stress levels. The type of chemical to which the person is addicted determines the types of stressful experiences incurred. The massage therapist assesses the client to decide whether the massage could calm an anxious client or give a boost to a depressed client. Heavy connective tissue massage should be avoided during withdrawal phases. Toxins released from this type of massage may overtax a system already burdened with withdrawal detoxification.

Chemical Imbalances in the Brain

Certain types of mental disorders arise from an imbalance of brain chemicals. Hyperactivity, ADD, bipolar (manic-depressive) disorder, schizophrenia, seasonal affective disorder, obsessive-compulsive disorder, and clinical depression are just a few brain chemical disorders.

Medications

Medication is important in helping these individuals. The massage professional should never make the client feel guilty for taking medication or suggest that medication is not necessary. Medication must be monitored carefully by a physician, with the smallest effective dosage given to prevent side effects. Massage cannot replace medication, but regular massage may allow the client's physician to reduce the dosage and duration of some types of medication in some situations. In other situations the side effects of certain medications can be managed with massage. It is very important to work with the client's physician and chart the client's response to the massage carefully (See Appendix C).

Intellectual Disabilities

Massage for those with intellectual disabilities has the same effect as for everyone else. Care must be taken to communicate at the client's level of understanding, but not below functioning level. Adults with intellectual disabilities are not children and should not be treated as such. People with intellectual disabilities may become frustrated and anxious during a day of challenges. If accepted by these clients, massage is soothing, calming, and beneficial. However, remember, not everyone likes to be touched, and the individual's needs must be respected.

Cognitive Disabilities

Autism Spectrum Disorder

Autism spectrum disorder is believed to be characterized by impaired social interaction and communication and a restricted repertoire of interests. Contrary to popular belief, most children and adults with autism spectrum disorder do want to be touched. A very reliable, structured touch with firm, consistent pressure usually is preferred. Massage applied in a very deliberate way within the client's comfort level has been shown to increase social interaction somewhat and reduce anxiety.

Learning Disabilities

Difficulties with processing sensory input, which occurs in some learning disorders, may be helped by the organized, systematic, sensory stimulation of massage. Having a learning difficulty is stressful, and stress from dealing with the environment aggravates the learning difficulty. Self-esteem is hard to maintain when a person has been made to feel stupid in school because he or she could not write, spell, or read. People with learning disabilities are not stupid; they just need to learn differently. Massage helps reduce their stress, thereby facilitating learning and enabling them to feel more positive about themselves.

Psychiatric Disorders

Psychiatric disorders, such as anxiety, panic, depression, and eating disorders, interplay in a combination of autonomic nervous system functions and hormone neurotransmitters, neuropeptides, and other brain chemicals.

Anxiety, Panic, and Depression

Anxiety is an uneasy feeling usually connected with increased sympathetic arousal responses. Panic is an intense, sudden, and overwhelming fear or feeling of anxiety that produces terror and immediate physiologic change that results in paralyzed immobility or senseless, hysterical behavior. A panic attack is an episode of acute anxiety that occurs at unpredictable times with feelings of intense apprehension or terror. It may be accompanied by a feeling of shortness of breath that leads to hyperventilation, dizziness, sweating, trembling, and chest pain or heart palpitations. Most symptoms can be directly related to overactivation of the sympathetic autonomic nervous system.

Depression is characterized by a decrease in vital functional activity; mood disturbances of exaggerated emptiness, hopelessness, and melancholy; or unbridled periods of high energy with no purpose or outcome.

Anxiety and depressive disorders are commonly seen with fatigue and pain syndromes. Pain and fatigue syndromes are multicausal and often chronic, nonproductive patterns that interfere with well-being, activities of daily living, and productivity. Some such syndromes are fibromyalgia, chronic fatigue syndrome, infection with the Epstein-Barr virus, sympathetic reflex dystrophy, headache, arthritis, chronic cancer pain, neuropathy, low back syndrome, idiopathic pain, somatization disorder, and intractable pain syndrome. Acute pain and "episodes" of chronic conditions can be factors in these syndromes. Panic behavior, phobias, and the sense of impending doom, along with a sense of being overwhelmed and/or hopelessness, are common with these conditions. Symptoms of these conditions and syndromes include mood swings, breathing pattern disorders, sleep disturbance, concentration difficulties, memory disturbances, outbursts of anger, fatigue, and changes in habits of daily living, appetite, and activity levels.

A breathing pattern disorder often is a significant underlying factor with anxiety and panic. Massage can normalize the breathing muscles, which must be done to correct a breathing pattern dysfunction.

Eating Disorders

Eating disorders involve mood disorders, physiologic responses to food, and control issues. They are complicated situations that usually require professional intervention. The job of the massage therapist is to be aware of the possibility of an eating disorder and to refer the client. Any substantial weight loss must be referred to a physician. Individuals with anorexia nervosa (a starving disorder) lose a great deal of weight. Recognizing bulimia, which involves binge eating and purging using vomiting and laxatives, is more difficult. The teeth and gums are affected by the stomach acids, and the massage professional may notice this. Referral should be made because of symptoms, not because the therapist is attempting to diagnose the disorder.

Massage Adaptation

When working with clients with psychiatric disorders, the most common massage approach is general stress reduction. This type of massage may take the edge off the mood through the influence of massage on the autonomic nervous system. The type of massage given can be adjusted to be a little more stimulating or a little more relaxing. The key is to begin where the person is at the time of the massage. Someone who is anxious initially may resist long, slow strokes and instead may do better with a strategy that begins with active joint movement, postisometric relaxation, lengthening and stretching, and rapid compression and then gradually shifts into a calming, rocking massage with long, slow strokes. The person who is a little depressed may not initially want to join in with an active participation massage. Instead, the work might begin with rocking and long, slow strokes and end with stimulating active joint movement, rapid compression, and tapotement.

Massage affects the brain chemicals by encouraging the release of serotonin, dopamine, and the endorphins, which alter mood. It also affects the release of various hormones that influence mood. Massage has a strong normalizing effect on the autonomic nervous system and can support other interventions for psychiatric disorders.

Post-Traumatic Stress Disorder

Post-traumatic stress disorder (PTSD) is the re-experiencing of flashback memory, in addition to state-dependent memory, somatization, anxiety, irritability, sleep disturbance, concentration difficulties, times of melancholy or depression, grief, fear, worry, anger, and avoidance behavior. Excessive stress can manifest as a number of disorders, such as cardiovascular problems, including hypertension; digestive difficulties, including heartburn, ulcer, and bowel syndromes; respiratory illness; susceptibility to bacterial and viral illnesses; endocrine dysfunction, particularly adrenal or thyroid dysfunction; delayed or diminished cellular repair; sleep disorders; and breathing pattern disorders, to mention just a few. PTSD can have long-term effects.

Trauma occurs as a result of physical injury by violent or disruptive action or by a toxic substance or as a result of psychic injury caused by a short-term or long-term severe emotional shock. Military personnel who have experienced trauma are a special concern.

Because therapeutic massage works well in normalizing the effects or physiologic manifestations of stress on the body, it can be an effective tool in the management of or recovery from PTSD.

Adrenaline is the key to solidifying events into memory. If adrenaline is blocked through the use of the medication propranolol, memory is impaired. When traumatic events occur, adrenaline is secreted. The more adrenaline and the longer the exposure to the elevated levels, the stronger the memory. PTSD may be a manifestation of memories that were encoded in the presence of increased and sustained adrenaline exposure. These memories are literally too strong. If the adrenaline levels are reduced as soon as possible after a traumatic event, lingering post-traumatic stress symptoms are not as permanent. Therapeutic massage can influence adrenaline levels by reducing sympathetic dominance and supporting parasympathetic dominance.

Researchers, including Tiffany Field, have found that massage is effective in calming individuals with PSTD. The military is investigating the use of multiple interventions, including massage, to treat military personnel exposed to trauma. The drug propranolol can be used to weaken old memories. Old memory patterns are recalled, and the medication (which interferes with adrenaline) is administered. The memory is not lost; it is just reduced in intensity. Treatment of this debilitating condition continues to advance, but in the meantime, therapeutic massage appears to be beneficial.

Abuse

People who have experienced various forms of abuse often experience PTSD. When people are abused, whatever the form

of abuse, they must learn to survive as best they can at the time of the abuse. These survival mechanisms take many forms, such as dissociation, hypervigilance, aggressive behavior, learning to "disappear," low self-esteem, and withdrawal. As mentioned, PTSD is common. These patterns may generalize into many life situations.

If the abuse happens to a young child, the victim's coping mechanisms develop around a twisted reality. The younger the child, the more difficult effective survival will be, and possibly the more magnified the inappropriate survival mechanisms that develop. The older we are, the more inner resources we have to support effective coping. The effects of the abuse should not be judged by their intensity or context.

Trauma, State-Dependent Memory, and Dissociative Behavior

The body remembers trauma in some way. The technical term for this is state-dependent memory. This type of memory is encoded in the brain in a manner that includes the position, emotion, and chemicals, in addition to the nervous system activation and all other combined physiologic effects that influence the internal functions, at the time the experience occurred. Later, when the physical and emotional states change, the memory of the incident may be vague or forgotten.

State-dependent memory functions in all life experiences. When a person gets ready to hit a baseball or drive a car, the individual assumes the appropriate position and the body remembers what is required. In a traumatic experience, this mechanism locks in all the factors that coincide with the experience. In the future, this repressed memory may be triggered by any one of the sensations or physiologic factors involved in the state-dependent memory. For example, the sense of smell often triggers a memory. With massage, the pressure, location of the touch, and position or movement of the client may trigger the client's memory.

A person who experiences trauma during the formative years may have difficulty sorting it all out in adulthood. The memories may be spotty or piecemeal, or only one of the sensations (e.g., smell, touch, position) may be encoded in the memory. It is important not to discount this memory pattern simply because all the pieces do not fit together to form a whole picture. It may be affirming to know that all the pieces do not have to fit together for the person to have enough information to resolve and integrate past experiences and develop more resourceful behavior for the present and future.

Sexual abuse in an older child often is laden with mixed signals, role confusion, and secrecy.

Physical abuse (e.g., beatings, neglect) and emotional abuse (e.g., criticism, unrealistic expectations, brain washing, indoctrination) ravage a person's self-esteem.

Some life experiences that may affect a person in a manner similar to deliberate abuse are illness, medical procedures, hospitalization, accidents, or other trauma, such as that experienced by military personnel or survivors of natural disasters. This process is also common in the training and development of athletes, dancers, and musicians. Developing these skills is difficult and often physically painful. The success of the individual's coping skills depends on the type of support received during and soon after the traumatic event, in addition to the dynamics surrounding the situation. A child who attempts to hide the pain during a medical procedure so as not to upset the parents is being denied full emotional and physical expression in the situation. If the medical staff does not explain the procedure so that the child comprehends or if the child is too young to understand, this, too, may become a difficult situation to integrate into a person's life experiences. If a parent or support person is physically separated from or emotionally unavailable to a child or adult during a crucial time, this can have a lasting effect.

Abuse of an adult, such as occurs with rape, violent crime, stalking, spouse beating, and abuse of the elderly, also must be considered. Typically, adults feel powerless in the situation and may feel as though the abuse is deserved or that they somehow did something to cause it. If elderly individuals are also mentally impaired, such as with Alzheimer's disease, they may become childlike in their reasoning and survival mechanisms. Those who have experienced upheaval in their environment, war-torn areas, or areas of disaster can develop feelings of powerlessness and devastation even when the person is no longer in the environment and is now safe.

The touch of the massage therapist may remind the body of the trauma. As the body remembers, it may somehow resolve and integrate the experience. Often the client does not remember the details or recall who, what, where, when, or how. Instead, a vague uneasiness, or **dissociation** (i.e., detachment, discontentedness, separation, isolation), develops. One mechanism for surviving physical, sexual, and emotional trauma is to "leave the body" and therefore not feel the abuse or to believe that the abuse is happening to someone else.

Many types of appropriate dissociative coping mechanisms are valuable in times of performance, demand, emergency, or survival. This is sometimes called "entering the zone" or "zoning out." However, if the pattern of dissociation becomes repetitive and generalized, coping becomes strained. One way to relearn appropriate touch is through giving and receiving massage.

The massage professional should be aware of a client dissociating during a massage. It is not our job to change the dissociative pattern by reminding the client to remain aware of his or her body unless the client specifically requests it. More specialized training is required to deal effectively with all the ramifications of a client's shift in coping style. This frequently involves professional counseling.

The process must happen gently, at the client's pace, and must never be hurried. The client leads, and the therapist follows that lead. As this happens, the practitioner can begin to recognize the pattern of the dissociation and the massage techniques or positions that seem to trigger the pattern. With this information the therapist can alter the approach to the massage, providing the client with the opportunity to stay with the body more easily.

For example, if the therapist notices that every time the client's left knee is bent the client's body becomes unresponsive, the eyes become distant, or the breathing shifts, it is best to work with the knee in a different position. Also, rather than moving the client, the practitioner can have the client move himself into the position, which is more empowering for the individual. Over time, it becomes easier to notice these little steps, which will reacquaint the client with his body.

Some people who have been traumatized may also self-abuse, which can take many forms, such as a destructive lifestyle, addictive processes, and self-inflicted trauma. Self-abuse may be calming for the person. Endorphins and other chemicals are released during self-abuse. The mechanisms of counterirritation and hyperstimulation analgesia come into play. The massage professional may notice bruises, cuts, burns, or other injuries on the client's body. In a professional manner, the practitioner should bring these areas to the client's attention and note them in the client's record. Acknowledging an injured area to a person who abuses herself may cause the person to feel guilty or ashamed, tell a cover story, or ignore the question. This behavior indicates potentially serious underlying conditions and referral is indicated.

Occasionally a client demands or requests very deep massage when the soft tissue condition does not indicate the need for this type of invasive work. Self-abuse mechanisms may be involved in this situation. It is important not to become involved in a situation that perpetuates an abuse pattern. The therapist needs to trust his or her intuition about appropriate care but should not force the client to face the situation by confronting the person with the possibility of self-abuse mechanisms. The decision to deal actively with an abusive history requires commitment and time from the client. Professional help and/or support groups often are needed. Also, some individuals do not want to recover their memories of abuse; this is a valid response for these clients. The practitioner must not suggest that a client was abused or that the client needs to deal with his or her situation. Our job is to honor, respect, consider, regard, protect, defend, preserve, praise, value, safeguard, shelter, sustain, support, tolerate, appreciate, approve, recognize, understand, and accept and never to harm.

Boundaries are very important. Review the importance of respect for personal boundaries (see Chapter 2).

Listening and believing what the body and the client say are significant. The client may personalize the nurturing touch of the therapist (transference) and may want to involve the therapist in the experience. Referral for appropriate counseling is important. When a person is actively exploring personal trauma and its results, it is important that the massage therapist not take on the client's problems (countertransference).

Re-enactment and Integration: Dealing with Flashbacks

Re-enactment means reliving the event as though it were happening again right now. Integration involves remembering the event, yet being able to remain in the present moment, with an awareness of the difference between then and now, to bring some sort of resolution to the event.

Re-enactment does not necessarily provide the awareness and understanding necessary to integrate the physical response and emotional feelings into the client's experience in an empowering way. Instead, with re-enactment the client repeats an abusive pattern and feels disempowered and lost. The massage professional must be aware of the potential for harm to a client by deliberately triggering a re-enactment response. Without the additional and necessary support of qualified counselors and other support personnel to provide for an integration process, a re-enactment is undesirable.

If a client should respond during the massage by crying, shaking, becoming ticklish, agitated, or fearful or demonstrating another emotional pattern, it is important for the massage professional to be quiet and let the person experience the emotion. If needed, provide tissues in an unobtrusive way. Changes in breathing are common. For example, the client may cough, hold the breath, increase the breathing rate, or yawn. It is wise during these situations to avoid telling the client how to breathe. Breathing patterns are usually directly linked to experiences. Unless a client has high blood pressure and is holding the breath, the massage therapist should only observe the breathing and identify changes. In some instances it is best to continue to massage the area the same way that triggered the response but to slow down, allowing the body to integrate the information. The client should be asked no questions other than, "Do you want me to continue?" The practitioner should be calm and accepting of the response and should never try to encourage or stop the response.

It is important not to interfere with the person's experience by interjecting suggestions. At other times it is appropriate to stop the massage and wait for the response to dissipate. The therapist needs to stay connected with the client but distanced from the client's experience. The emotional experience belongs to the client, not to the practitioner, who works as a support in a quiet, simple way. When the emotional response has dissipated, the massage can be continued. If the client asks what happened, a simple explanation based on state-dependent memory is sufficient. Similar explanations, as previously mentioned, help the client understand what happened. A client who seems unsettled and needs additional help coping should be referred to a qualified counselor.

Confidence, respect, and trust are necessary to provide the type of massage that enhances the well-being of those who have been or are being traumatized. Always remember that confidentiality is a sacred trust; the therapist does not talk about clients or any experience with clients to anyone else.

Working with those who have been traumatized is rewarding, but it can be very difficult. Additional training is needed to serve clients who have a history of trauma. The actual techniques of massage are no different, but an understanding of coping mechanisms and somatic (body) memories requires additional study. Bodywork in some form may be a valuable tool for some individuals who want to resolve these issues, whereas for others it is not the best choice. Effective decision-making skills and support and supervision by qualified professionals determine the appropriateness of massage interventions for this population (Proficiency Exercises 14-11 and 14-12).

Key Points

- An understanding of psychotropic pharmacology is important, because massage and these medications affect the body in similar ways.

PROFICIENCY EXERCISE 14-11

Based on the information presented in this section, choose one psychological challenge and design an intervention plan and justification statement for the use of therapeutic massage. Use the model in Box 14-1 as an example.

Student note: Here is the clinical reasoning process again. If you have been practicing by doing the exercises in the beginning of this chapter, you should be starting to understand the process.

Example: Therapeutic massage for _____

1. **Gather facts to identify and define the situation.**
   Key questions: What is the problem? What are the facts?
2. **Brainstorm possible solutions.**
   Key questions: What might I do? or What if ... ?
3. **Evaluate possible interventions logically and objectively; look at both sides and the pros and cons.**
   Key question: What would happen if ... ?
4. **Evaluate the effect on the people involved.**
   Key question: How would each person involved feel?
5. **Develop an intervention plan and justification statements.**

PROFICIENCY EXERCISE 14-12

1. Find and read three books that deal with surviving trauma, or research PubMed (www.pubmedcentral.nih.gov) for the treatment of trauma.
2. Visit a safe house or shelter for abused women and talk with the volunteers who work there.
3. Contact the child protection agency in your community and obtain information on recognizing child abuse and reporting suspected cases.
4. Investigate methods used by the military to help soldiers deal with stress.
5. Describe an incident in which you felt abused. Also describe an incident in which you feel you abused someone.
   I felt abused when:

   I abused someone when:

FOOT IN THE DOOR

When you are able to adapt massage to meet the unique needs of individuals, your foot more easily gets into the doors to a variety of massage careers. Do you have a specific area of passion and compassion? For example, do you feel drawn to specialize in hospice care? Maybe you want to work with athletes or infants. Do you have a specific understanding of what it is like to be deaf or blind? Maybe you have cultural experience or are bilingual, which can help you better interact with a specific group of people. When you are competent and passionate about your career goals, others can begin to believe in you. What a great way to get your foot in the door, by serving a group of clients who share an experience, activity, condition, or time of life!

- Informed consent may be difficult to obtain.
- It is necessary to understand the signs, symptoms, and treatments for any condition a client may have.
- A team approach for assisting those with psychological disorders is important.

SUMMARY

Respect is important in any interaction with another person or with an animal. In all situations, remember to see and address the person first and then to accommodate the individual's specific needs by offering assistance and following the directions provided by the client. Massage therapists who want to focus their professional skills to best meet a client's specific needs will seek out training and information pertinent to the client's therapeutic needs. Often the knowledge required to provide massage to many diverse populations becomes too extensive, and specialization becomes necessary. When this is the case, such as when a massage professional obtains additional training for pregnancy, labor, and delivery massage, the information is integrated into the fundamentals of massage, and the additional training focuses on the application of the massage fundamentals for the special situation.

The wise professional recognizes when less intervention is more appropriate. Considerable learning, great skill, and patiently developed empathy are required to therapeutically hold a person's hand.

⊜volve

http://evolve.elsevier.com/Fritz/fundamentals/
14-1 Review what you've learned about common sports injuries.
14-2 Quiz yourself on massage and the pregnent client.
14-3 Read the author's personal thoughts on hospice care.
Don't forget to study for your certification and licensure exams! Review questions, along with weblinks, can be found on the Evolve website.

References

Arnheim DD, Prentice WE: *Principles of athletic training: a competency based approach*, ed 12, Boston, 2005, McGraw-Hill.

Cantwell SL: Traditional Chinese veterinary medicine: the mechanism and management of acupuncture for chronic pain, *Top Companion Anim Med* 25:53, 2010.

Center for Medicare and Medicaid Services (CMS): What is long-term care? www.medicare.gov/LongTermCare/Static/Home.asp. Accessed May, 2011.

Coppola CL, Grandin T, Mark Enns R: Human interaction and cortisol: can human contact reduce stress for shelter dogs? *Physiol Behav* 87:537, 2006.

Cummings NH, Stanley-Green S, Higgs P: *Perspectives in athletic training*, St Louis, 2009, Mosby.

Estep D, Hetts S: Proper etiquette with animals. www. AnimalBehaviorAssociates.com. Accessed April, 2011.

Grandin T, Johnson C: *Animals in translation: using the mysteries of autism to decode animal behavior*, Fort Washington, Penn, 2006, Harvest Books.

Kathmann I, Cizinauskas S, Doherr MG, et al: Daily controlled physiotherapy increases survival time in dogs with suspected degenerative myelopathy, *J Vet Intern Med* 20:927, 2006.

Keene Elkin M, Griffin Perry MA, Potter PA: *Nursing interventions and clinical skills*, ed 4, St Louis, 2007, Mosby.

Lewis SL, Heitkemper MM, Ruff Dirksen S, et al: *Medical-surgical nursing in Canada: assessment and management of clinical problems*, St. Louis, 2006, Mosby.

McGladre Y, Pullen R: *The Americans with Disabilities Act (rev)*, New York, 1994, Panel Publishers.

McKinney ES, Rowen James S, Smith Murray S, et al: *Maternal-child nursing*, ed 3, St Louis, 2009, Elsevier.

Porter M: Equine rehabilitation therapy for joint disease, *Vet Clin North Am Equine Pract* 21:599, vi, 2005.

Schmidt Luggen A, Hill C: Mobility. In Ebersole P, Hess P, Schmidt Luggen A, editors: *Toward healthy aging: needs and nursing response*, ed 6, St Louis, 2004, Mosby.

Sierpina VS, Sierpina M, Loera JA, et al: Complementary and integrative approaches to dementia, *South Med J* 98:636, 2005.

Suzuki M, Tatsumi A, Otsuka T, et al: Physical and psychological effects of 6-week tactile massage on elderly patients with severe dementia, *Am J Alzheimers Dis Other Demen* 25:680, 2010.

Walsh F: Human-animal bonds. I. The relational significance of companion animals, *Fam Process* 48:462, 2009.

Bibliography

American Psychiatric Association: *Diagnostic and statistical manual of mental disorders*, rev. ed., Washington, DC, 2000, APA.

American Veterinary Medical Association: Colloquium on recognition and alleviation of animal pain and distress, *J Am Vet Med Assoc* 191:1184, 1987.

Association of Veterinary Teachers and Research Workers (Working Party): Guidelines for the recognition and assessment of pain in animals, *Vet Rec* 118:334, 1986.

Australian Council for the Care of Animals in Research and Teaching (ACCART): Proceedings of the animal pain conference, *ACCART Newsletter* 3:11, 1990.

Bateson P: Assessment of pain in animals, *Anim Behav* 42:827, 1991.

Canadian Council on Animal Care (CCAC): Ottawa, Ontario, CCAC.

Corydon V, Clark G: *ADHD throughout the life span*, Las Vegas, 1997, Random Clark Publications.

Gentle MJ: Pain in birds, *Animal Welfare* 1:235, 1992.

Horacek HJ Jr: *Brainstorms: understanding and treating the emotional storms of attention deficit/hyperactivity disorder from childhood through adulthood*, New Jersey, 2000, Aronson.

Short CE, Van Poznak A, editors: *Animal pain*, New York, 1992, Churchill Livingstone.

Silverman J: How much is enough? *Lab Animal* 20:20, 1991.

Wall PD: Defining pain in animals. In Short CE, Van Poznak A, editors: *Animal pain*, New York, 1992, Churchill Livingstone.

Workbook Section

All Workbook activities can be done electronically online as well as here in the book. Answers are located on ⊜volve

Short Answer

1. What is the single most important factor in effective communication with individuals who have a disability or for whom age or health is a factor?

2. What special massage skills are needed to work with people who have a disability and those for whom age or health is a factor?

3. What is the best source of information about any situation, condition or disability?

4. What factors must be considered when massaging animals?

5. What adjustment to a massage session may be required when working with children?

6. Why do children like massage?

7. What is a major benefit of massage for children and adolescents?

8. Why is it important to teach parents and children some basic massage methods to share with each other?

9. Who gives informed consent for massage for individuals under 18 years of age?

10. What is a realistic goal for the massage professional when working with people who have a chronic illness?

11. What is the importance of hardiness and how does massage encourage it?

12. Why is close supervision by the physician or another health professional important when the massage professional is working with people who have a chronic illness?

13. What can the massage therapist learn from working with the elderly?

14. What special physical conditions are common among the elderly?

15. Are special skills required for working with the elderly?

16. Why is massage beneficial for infants?

17. Who is the best person to massage a baby?

18. What key elements are important when massaging an infant?

19. What is the recommended approach to massage for a person being treated for cancer? Why?

20. What important points should the massage professional remember when working with clients who have a physical disability?

21. When working with people who have an psychological or a intellectual impairment, the massage therapist must keep in mind what important factor?

22. How can massage be beneficial for withdrawal from addiction, for learning disabilities, and for intellectual disabilities?

23. Are special massage skills required for working with pregnant women? Explain.

24. What part can teaching massage to the expectant father or other support person play?

25. What can the massage therapist learn from providing massage for a person who is dying?

26. What is the best source of information about working with the dying?

27. What can massage offer to someone who is dying?

Problem-Solving Scenarios

1. A client begins to shake and to breathe very deeply during the massage. What do you do?

2. A client has been hospitalized and has requested that you come to the hospital and give him a massage. What do you need to do to be able to give the client a massage in the hospital?

3. An elderly client wants you to stay after the massage and have a cup of coffee. What do you do?

4. A young father is having trouble holding his newborn baby. What can you do?

5. A client with a speech difficulty needs to provide informed consent. How could this be accomplished?

6. A client is near death. She does not want a full massage but needs to be touched. What can you do?

Assess Your Competencies

Now that you have studied this chapter, you should be able to:

- Develop a massage environment that best serves clients, including barrier-free access and support services when necessary
- Demonstrate the communication skills that are important for working with a client with a disability and for people-first communication
- Gather information on additional training that can help you better serve clients with specific conditions, age-related needs, performance demands, and a variety of disabilities.

On a separate sheet of paper or on the computer, write a short summary of the content of this chapter based on the preceding list of competencies. Use a conversational tone, as if you were explaining to someone (e.g., a client, prospective employer, coworker, or other interested person) the importance of the information and skills to the development of the massage profession.

Next, in small discussion groups, share your summary with your classmates and compare the ways the information was presented. In discussing the content, look for similarities, differences, possibilities for misunderstanding of the information, and clear, concise methods of description.

Professional Application

You are asked to give a presentation to a group of nurses at a local hospital. They are looking for ways to use massage in various outpatient situations. They need a general explanation of ways massage would be beneficial for many different conditions. What major points would you make during the talk?

Research for Further Study

A major approach in massage is generalized, nonspecific, body-supportive care. This approach does not seek to intervene, but rather tries to provide support and to nurture health. Brainstorm the various applications for massage in diverse situations and then do some research to find sources that support some of the concepts.

CHAPTER OBJECTIVES

After completing this chapter, the student will be able to perform the following:

1. List and describe challenges individuals face that interfere with wellness.
2. Describe the importance of diet to a wellness lifestyle and plan a healthy diet.
3. Explain physical exercise as part of a wellness program.
4. Identify and define relaxation and restorative activities.
5. Explain how the mind and body connection affects wellness.
6. Implement and respect the importance of an individualized spiritual approach to wellness.

KEY TERMS

Aerobic exercise
Challenge
Commitment
Control
Deep inspiration
Defensive measures
Denial
Endurance
Fitness
Forced expiration
Forced inspiration
Overload principle
Quiet expiration
Quiet inspiration
Stressors
Training stimulus threshold

CHAPTER OUTLINE

Massage is an important part of any wellness program, because it restores body balance and provides a connection with other human beings. As a massage professional, you must understand the components of wellness. With this information, you can explain to clients how massage fits into the overall wellness plan. In addition, you can use this same information to create your own wellness plan.

Everyone would benefit by developing a personal wellness plan. Just as in designing a massage, there is no right way or wrong way to formulate this plan. However, by following a few basic guidelines, each of us can discover what works for us as individuals, and that is the best plan. Massage practitioners need to remember that as wonderful as massage is, it addresses only a part of the person. Wellness is about the whole person. The empathetic massage professional realizes that during a client's search for wellness, the time spent with the massage practitioner provides focused attention, acceptance, and effective listening, which are as important as the massage methods used.

As with massage, often the simpler the overall wellness program, the better. Box 15-1 provides attributes around which a wellness program can be built. A wellness program also needs to change as the individual changes. We are supposed to be well, and our bodies will recognize the best process for achieving wellness. Wellness has a domino effect. Simple alterations in lifestyle produce a chain reaction throughout a person's life. Therefore, people need to commit to only a few carefully planned lifestyle changes and then allow the rest of the pieces of their lives to fall into place. When an effective wellness program is carried out, a person looks forward to getting back to living life to the fullest and, at the appropriate time, to dying with dignity.

Box 15-1 Elements of a Wellness Program

Body
Nutrition
Light and dark exposure
Sleep
Breathing
Physical fitness
Sensory stimulation

Mind
Relationships with oneself and others
Communication
Beliefs
Intellectual stimulation

Spirit
Sense of purpose
Connection
Faith
Hope
Love

We are considered well/healthy when the body, mind, and spirit are in ideal balance.

We are not well when imbalance exists; balance must then be restored.

CHALLENGES TO WELLNESS

SECTION OBJECTIVES

Chapter objectives covered in this section:
1. List and describe challenges individuals face that interfere with wellness.
Using the information presented in this section, the student will be able to perform the following:
- Explain the meaning of vertically ill
- Identify Dr. Hans Selye
- List common stress responses
- Explain the basic concept of stress management
- Relate excessive demands to increased stress
- Explain loss and how it relates to wellness
- Describe the role of intuition and wellness
- Explain the importance of qualified professional help and personal relationships for maintaining wellness

In the words of a renowned nutrition scientist, Professor Jeffrey Bland, many people are "vertically ill" (Chaitow, 1991). Such people are not sick enough to lie down, but they are certainly not well. More than just the type of stress is involved in this condition; it is the amount of stress that accumulates until the breakdown begins. It is only a matter of time before physical health, the mind, or the quality of life simply falls apart under the accumulation of multiple stressors.

Resistance usually occurs when an adjustment is necessary. Initially we may resist change, which can come from our own bodies or coping patterns or from family and friends who interact with us. Remember, if our behavior changes, the people around us also must change. Changes should be made slowly, if possible, to allow the "pieces" (your own body, family, friends, or coworkers) to comment, complain, support, and

resist; but do not give in and quit. Persist with the wellness program and give your body, family, and friends time to get used to your new lifestyle.

Making a change leading to wellness takes determination. Letting go of behavioral patterns is difficult. It is very hard to do this alone; therefore, relationships with those who are supportive and believe in us (e.g., support groups, professional therapy) are helpful. The massage professional can be an important support person for the client making wellness changes.

Stress

Stress is our response to any demand on the body or mind to respond, adapt, or alter. It is a state of readiness to survive, one that requires hypervigilance by the body and mind. A person's emotional reaction to stress may be the difference between positive action and destructive breakdown, especially if many of the stressors seem beyond control (Chaitow, 1991). Dr. Hans Selye (1978), an expert on stress, said:

> The ancient Greek philosophers clearly recognized that with regard to human conduct, the most important but perhaps also most difficult thing was "to know thyself." It takes great courage to attempt this honestly. Yet it is well worth the effort and humiliation, because most of our tensions and frustrations stem from compulsive needs to act the role of someone we are not.

Before any wellness program can be developed, a person needs to at least "explore thyself." The next step is to analyze and explore the stressors that we all encounter in our daily lives. The three major elements of stress are:
- The stressor itself
- Defensive measures
- Mechanisms for surrender

Recall from Chapters 5 and 6 that **stressors** are any internal perceptions or external stimuli that demand a change in the body. The **defensive measures** are the ways our bodies defend against the stressor, such as the production of antibodies and white blood cells or behavioral and emotional defenses. However, sometimes defending is not the best way to deal with stress. It is important and resourceful to know when to quit, or surrender. Hormonal and nervous stimuli encourage the body to retreat and ignore stressors. On an emotional level this sometimes is called **denial**, which can be an important method of coping with stress (Selye, 1978).

Mental excitement and physical stressors cause an initial exhilaration followed by a secondary phase of depression. A law of physics states that for every action, there is an equal and opposite reaction. Certain chemical compounds, such as the hormones produced during the acute alarm reaction phase of the general adaptation syndrome (see Chapters 5 and 6), are able first to key up the body for action and then to cause depression (Box 15-2). Both effects may have great protective value for the body. It is necessary to be "keyed up" for peak accomplishment, but it is equally important to relax and restore in the secondary phase of depression. This prevents us from carrying on too long at top speed. As Selye (1978) wrote:

| Box 15-2 | Common Stress Responses |

- General irritability, hyperexcitation, or depression
- Pounding heart
- Dry throat and mouth
- Impulsive behavior and emotional instability
- Overpowering urge to cry, run, or hide
- Inability to concentrate
- Weakness or dizziness
- Fatigue
- Tension and extreme alertness
- Trembling and nervous tics
- Intermittent anxiety
- Tendency to be easily startled
- High-pitched, nervous laughter
- Stuttering and other speech difficulties
- Grinding the teeth
- Insomnia
- Inability to sit still or physically relax
- Sweating
- Frequent need to urinate
- Diarrhea, indigestion, queasiness, and vomiting
- Migraine and other tension headaches
- Premenstrual tension or missed menstrual cycles
- Pain in the neck or lower back
- Loss of appetite or excessive appetite
- Increased use of chemicals, including tobacco, caffeine, and alcohol
- Nightmares
- Neurotic behavior
- Psychosis
- Proneness to accidents

These signs of stress are produced by fluctuations in the autonomic nervous system and resulting shifts in endogenous chemicals.

The fact is that a person can be intoxicated with his own stress hormones. I venture to say that this sort of drunkenness has caused much more harm to society than the alcoholic kind. We are on our guard against external toxicants, but hormones are parts of our bodies; it takes more wisdom to recognize and overcome the foe which fights from within. In all our actions throughout the day, we must consciously look for signs of being keyed up too much, and we must learn to stop in time. To watch our critical stress level is just as important as to watch our critical quota of cocktails and even more so. Intoxication by stress is sometimes unavoidable and usually insidious. You can quit alcohol and, even if you do take some, at least you can count the glasses; but it is impossible to avoid stress as long as you live, and your conscious thoughts often cannot gauge its alarm signals accurately. Curiously, the pituitary is a much better judge of stress than the intellect. Yet, you can learn to recognize the danger signals fairly well if you know what to look for.

We all respond differently to general stress because of our individual conditioning and genetic makeup. As a whole, each person tends to respond consistently, with one set of signs, in individualized patterns caused by the malfunctioning of whatever happens to be the most vulnerable part in his or her physiology (genetic weak link). When warning signs appear, it is time to stop, change the activity, and divert the body's attention to something else.

Stress Management

Stress has many different causes, and many methods of stress management can be used. In general, if proportionately too much stress occurs in any physical or emotional area of the body, the energy needs to be diverted to a different area. If a person is thinking too much, then he or she should use the larger muscles of the body (e.g., work in the garden, take a brisk walk, exercise). If too much exercise is causing stress, balance can be restored by reading a novel, watching a movie, or listening to soft music. If too much stress occurs in the body as a whole, rest is required. If we do not rest of our own accord, the body may become ill so that we rest for awhile.

Life Demands

Today, many of the demands placed on us are outside the design of the body: too much information, too much to know, too much to do, too many responsibilities, and too many places to be. Our lives have become hurried, marked by a constant battle for time. We have too many options and too many choices, and it all costs too much.

Wellness often revolves around simplification of a person's lifestyle. Simplification requires choices, boundaries, discipline, and "letting go" in many dimensions. For example, to simplify life it may be necessary to let go of a few volunteer activities and concentrate on only one or two that are especially meaningful. It may mean letting go of many acquaintances and instead cultivating a few supportive friends. Simplification may mean letting go of belief systems (e.g., family gatherings tend to be complex affairs) and cultivating easy relationships without the fuss. Letting go may involve a sense of relief, but also a feeling of loss that must be resolved.

Loss and Grief

Sometimes an event in life removes some part of us. It could be a body part, a body function, a relationship, a member of our family, or a job. Loss heals through grieving. Grief is a physiologic response that includes stimulation of the sympathetic autonomic nervous system. The emotional response is alarm first, then disbelief and denial, progressing to anger and guilt. This process continues toward finding a source of comfort and finally adjusting to the loss. To heal, we need to reconstruct that part or learn to live resourcefully without it. We also need to give ourselves the time we need to work through the process of grieving.

Intuition: Recognizing When Wellness Is Off Balance

Many of us have been sick, or at the very least vertically ill. It may take extraordinary effort to reverse these situations. That is when we realize maybe we should have taken better care of ourselves in the first place. This realization does not always come at once, though. We all have that "voice in the back of our head" and that feeling when something "just isn't right." Learning to recognize our intuition and actually *listen* to it is an important component of maintaining wellness in our lives.

🔔 PROFICIENCY EXERCISE 15-1

Identify something in your life that is interfering with your self-concept. For example, do you have an acquaintance who makes you feel inferior, or are you ashamed of some habit, such as nail biting? Often the identification is the beginning of the process of change.

🔔 PROFICIENCY EXERCISE 15-2

Begin to build a library about wellness. Take inventory of the books and magazines you already have. Categorize them and commit to adding one new book at least every 3 months. Explore your public library and the Internet to become familiar with the wellness resources they offer.

A balance exists between intuition and scientific research in wellness (i.e., what science knows and what we know we need). In developing a wellness program, it is important to consider these two very important sources of information. Science and intuition are both needed to maintain wellness.

Seeking Help
Professional Help

Wellness training requires an extensive amount of information about diet, exercise, lifestyle, and behavior patterns. It is important to consult those with experience to obtain that information. Do not depend on only one information source. For each topic, talk with experts and read as many books or high-quality websites as possible (e.g., WebMD or the website of the Centers for Disease Control and Prevention [CDC]) before making decisions about what could be done to benefit or improve your wellness. Remember, only a few symptoms combine to create a huge array of illness and disease patterns. Fortunately, a combination of only a few lifestyle changes is required to redirect a disease pattern toward a more resourceful and healing pattern (Proficiency Exercise 15-1).

Many professionals can help us with specific therapeutic interventions as the wellness program is developed. Physicians, counselors, other health care providers, educators, and religious and spiritual advisors all play an important part in helping us become well again or maintain our wellness. Ultimately, each of us must do the work and take responsibility for our life, but it is important to use the help that is available. For example, if someone wants to increase his or her wellness by losing weight, a certified personal trainer would be helpful. Other examples include seeking education to better manage finances, becoming involved in a support group for addictive behaviors, and obtaining guidance from a spiritual advisor to walk a path of faith.

Supportive Relationships

Our sense of self in relation to others is also important. If this connection with others is not respected and nurtured, the wholeness of our life is strained. This strain may interfere with our spiritual, emotional, and physical health.

When we have developed a healthy relationship with ourselves, we can also develop and sustain healthy relationships with others. Supportive relationships are important to wellness. If a relationship continues to generate messes in your life, maybe it is not a resourceful relationship. This does not mean that effort and concern are not required for family and friends or even global concern for a population. What is important is that we are empowered in a relationship and free to give and

receive with a balance of energy exchanged. Sometimes one gives more and other times one receives more, but the total outcome is mutual support for one another's highest good that supports wellness (Proficiency Exercise 15-2).

THE BODY: NUTRITION

SECTION OBJECTIVES

Chapter objective covered in this section:

2. Describe the importance of diet to a wellness lifestyle and plan a healthy diet.

Using the information presented in this section, the student will be able to perform the following:

- Describe the main food groups
- Identify nutrition that supports wellness by planning a healthy diet
- Explain the importance of proper hydration in the diet
- List the components of an antiinflammatory diet
- Explain how nutritional supplements and herbs influence wellness

Our bodies are our dwelling places in this life. They are the most concrete aspects of our being. The care of our bodies is an important part of any wellness program.

According to the National Cancer Institute, poor nutrition is the reason three out of four people develop a disease or illness. Given these statistics, it is clear that good nutrition means more than just choosing certain foods; it is about wanting to live a life without the complications of disease and illness. Therefore, people need to educate themselves about proper nutrition.

Proper nutrition is easy to explain. However, because of our fast-paced lifestyle and the food that is advertised to our population, people do not always follow healthy nutritional recommendations. This is because nutrition involves more than just eating. Eating affects the mood, mood influences feelings, and behavior supports feelings. Food, therefore, becomes an emotional issue.

The Main Food Groups
Proteins

Proteins are the chief structural components of the body. Enzymes, some hormones, muscle tissue, and a substantial proportion of chromosomes are proteins. Proteins are essential components of the cell membrane. They break down into amino acids, which the body then absorbs and uses to meet its metabolic requirements, including growth and development. Important compounds such as epinephrine and acetylcholine are derived from amino acids. Dietary proteins include animal products and bean and grain combinations.

Carbohydrates

The term *carbohydrate* often means any food that is rich in either complex carbohydrates (starches, as found in grains such as brown rice) or simple carbohydrates (sugars, as found in candy, soda, and desserts). Carbohydrates (saccharides) are divided into four groups: monosaccharides, disaccharides, oligosaccharides, and polysaccharides. Monosaccharides and disaccharides are commonly referred to as sugars.

Carbohydrates perform many important jobs in the body, especially in storing and providing energy. Complex carbohydrates are long chains of glucose molecules, which is the main fuel for the manufacture of adenosine triphosphate in the cell. The liver converts sugars to glucose.

Fats

Fats, or lipids, are triglycerides that break down into fatty acids and glycerol. A fatty acid is a molecule consisting of a chain of carbons with no double bonds (saturated) or several double bonds (unsaturated). The unsaturated fats most closely resemble body fat and are more easily assimilated and used. Saturation (the addition of hydrogen molecules) makes fat a solid and less desirable in the diet. Linoleic acid is an example of a fatty acid that is essential to human nutrition. In addition to serving as a reservoir of stored energy, fats are essential components of many hormones, the cell membrane, and the myelin sheath of the nerve fibers. Dietary fats are found in nuts, seeds, oils, and animal products.

Vitamins

Vitamins are growth factors needed in small amounts for daily body metabolism. They are classified as fat soluble or water soluble. Many vitamins act as enzyme activators (coenzymes). The fat-soluble vitamins are more toxic, because excess amounts are stored in the fat tissue and are not excreted readily. Water-soluble vitamins are absorbed and excreted more easily.

Minerals

The body uses two kinds of minerals, macrominerals and trace minerals. It needs larger amounts of macrominerals than trace minerals. The macromineral group is made up of calcium, phosphorus, magnesium, sodium, potassium, chloride, and sulfur. The body needs just a tiny bit of each trace mineral. Trace minerals include iron, manganese, copper, iodine, zinc, cobalt, fluoride, and selenium.

Planning a Healthy Diet

The basics of balanced nutrition are explained in the Department of Agriculture's new guide to good eating. These newer recommendations have reconfigured the previous six-section MyPyramid guide into MyPlate (www.ChooseMyPlate.gov). MyPlate supports a diet that is high in fruit, vegetables, whole grains, and fat-free or low-fat milk and milk products, but that also includes lean meats, poultry, fish, beans, eggs, and nuts. Saturated and transfats should be avoided, along with extra sodium and sugars.

| Box 15-3 | Functions of Water in the Human Body |

- Provides a medium for chemical reactions
- Plays a crucial role in regulating chemical and bioelectric distributions within cells
- Transports substances such as hormones and nutrients
- Aids oxygen transport from the lungs to body cells
- Aids carbon dioxide transport from body cells to the lungs
- Dilutes toxic substances and waste products and transports them to the kidneys and liver
- Distributes heat around the body

From Fritz S: *Mosby's essential sciences for therapeutic massage: anatomy, physiology, biomechanics, and pathology,* ed 4, St Louis, 2013, Mosby.

MyPlate urges the general public to make the most sensible choices from every food group, to find a healthy balance between food consumption and physical activity, and to understand the amount of calories a food has and its impact on general calorie counts.

Cycles of high and low blood sugar are produced by unbalanced diets, aggravated by improper spacing between meals, and promoted by substances such as coffee, alcohol, and soft drinks. These fluids stimulate the production of adrenaline, which forces the release of sugar into the bloodstream. The body then releases insulin to lower the sugar level again.

Adequate fiber and water in the diet promote bladder and bowel habits that support wellness. Eating on a regular schedule is important to support body rhythms that in turn support wellness (Figure 15-1).

Hydration

Drinking enough plain water is very important to a wellness program (Box 15-3). A healthy diet requires adequate hydration. The total amount required varies from person to person and depends on multiple factors, including the individual's physical condition, diet, age, activity level, and even where the person lives (Table 15-1).

Fruits and Vegetables

Fruits and vegetables reduce the risk of cardiovascular disease. Folic acid and potassium appear to contribute to this effect, which has been seen in several epidemiologic studies. Inadequate consumption of folic acid also is responsible for higher risks of serious birth defects, and a low intake of lutein, a pigment in green, leafy vegetables, has been associated with greater risks of cataracts and degeneration of the retina. Fruits and vegetables also are the primary source of many vitamins needed for good health; if these foods are eaten raw, the nutrients are not diminished, such as occurs with cooking or processing. Only a few vegetables provide better nutrient absorption when cooked.

Red Meat

High consumption of red meat has been associated with an increased risk of coronary artery disease, probably because of meat's high saturated fat content. Excessive consumption of

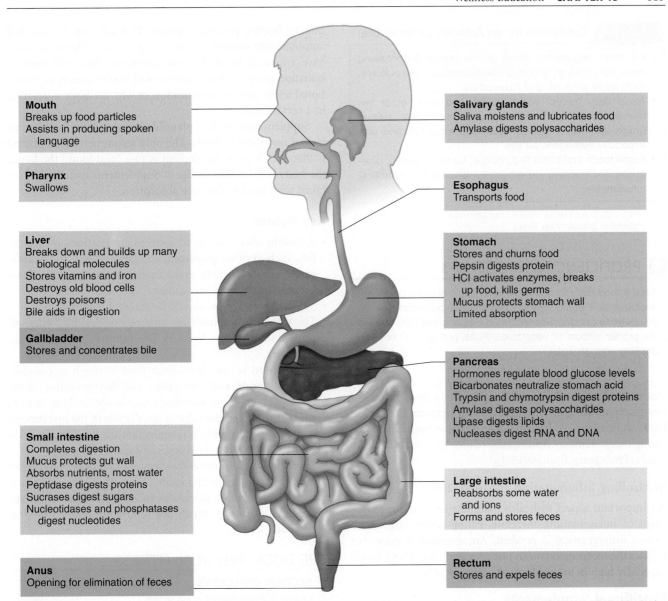

Mouth
Breaks up food particles
Assists in producing spoken
    language

Pharynx
Swallows

Liver
Breaks down and builds up many
    biological molecules
Stores vitamins and iron
Destroys old blood cells
Destroys poisons
Bile aids in digestion

Gallbladder
Stores and concentrates bile

Small intestine
Completes digestion
Mucus protects gut wall
Absorbs nutrients, most water
Peptidase digests proteins
Sucrases digest sugars
Nucleotidases and phosphatases
    digest nucleotides

Anus
Opening for elimination of feces

Salivary glands
Saliva moistens and lubricates food
Amylase digests polysaccharides

Esophagus
Transports food

Stomach
Stores and churns food
Pepsin digests protein
HCl activates enzymes, breaks
    up food, kills germs
Mucus protects stomach wall
Limited absorption

Pancreas
Hormones regulate blood glucose levels
Bicarbonates neutralize stomach acid
Trypsin and chymotrypsin digest proteins
Amylase digests polysaccharides
Lipase digests lipids
Nucleases digest RNA and DNA

Large intestine
Reabsorbs some water
    and ions
Forms and stores feces

Rectum
Stores and expels feces

FIGURE 15-1 Summary of digestive function. (From Patton KT, Thibodeau GA: *Anatomy and physiology,* ed 7, St Louis, 2010, Mosby.)

Table 15-1	Water Composition of Different Body Tissues
Tissue	Water Composition (%)
Blood	83.0
Kidneys	82.7
Heart	79.2
Lungs	79.0
Spleen	75.8
Muscle	75.6
Brain	74.8
Intestine	74.5
Skin	72.0
Liver	68.3
Skeleton	22.0
Adipose tissue	10.0

From Fritz S: *Mosby's essential sciences for therapeutic massage: anatomy, physiology, biomechanics, and pathology,* ed 3, St Louis, 2009, Mosby.

fatty red meat also increases the risk of type 2 diabetes and colon cancer, can aggravate the inflammatory response, and increases pain sensitivity. The elevated risk of colon cancer may be partly related to the carcinogens produced during cooking and the chemicals found in processed meats such as salami and bologna.

Poultry and Fish

Poultry and fish have less saturated fat and more unsaturated fat than red meat. Fish also is a rich source of the essential omega-3 fatty acids. Eggs do not appear to increase the risk of heart disease (except among diabetics), probably because the effects of a slightly higher cholesterol level are counterbalanced by other nutritional benefits, especially with eggs from chickens fed special vegetarian diets to increase nutritional value.

Nuts and Healthy Fats

Many people have avoided nuts because of their high fat content, but the fat in nuts, including peanuts, is mainly

Box 15-4 Guidelines for an Antiinflammatory Diet

- Eat fruits, vegetables, whole grains, omega-3–containing eggs, fish, chicken, yogurt (unsweetened) with live cultures, extra virgin olive oil, and flaxseed oil.
- Avoid dairy (except yogurt, keifer, and some other fermented products), pork, beef, processed meat, refined grains and sugar, artificial food, and most fats and oils, especially hydrogenated oils.
- Some foods and herbs (e.g., ginger, turmeric, cumin, pineapple, and papaya) are especially valuable for controlling inflammation.

From Fritz S: *Sports and exercise massage: comprehensive care in fitness, athletics, and rehabilitation*, St Louis, 2006, Mosby.

 PROFICIENCY EXERCISE 15-3

Keep a food diary for 2 days. If your diet is not well balanced, decide what it would take to achieve a well-balanced diet. Do you need to cut down on saturated fats or sugar? Do you eat the proper amount of vegetables, fruits, and grains? Are you drinking enough water?

unsaturated, and walnuts in particular are a good source of omega-3 fatty acids. Also, people who eat nuts are actually less likely to be obese. Perhaps because nuts are more satisfying, eating them seems to significantly reduce the intake of other foods (Proficiency Exercise 15-3).

Controlling Inflammation Through Diet

An important aspect of health maintenance is the management of inflammation; therefore, eating a diet targeted to reduce inflammation is prudent. An antiinflammatory diet follows the recommendations just provided (Box 15-4). Foods especially high in antioxidants also are valuable.

Nutritional Supplements

Food sources of vitamins and minerals are compromised by depleted soil and artificial fertilizers and tainted by pesticides and other chemicals. The nutritional value of food also is compromised by long-term storage and preservation. Obtaining optimum nutritional value from the food we eat is difficult without extraordinary attention to our diet, which requires time, dedication, and discipline.

Many people take nutritional supplements to help achieve optimum nutrition. Experts disagree on the value of all vitamins, but many recommend a quality multivitamin. The U.S. Food and Drug Administration (FDA) does not regulate the nutritional supplement industry, so caution should be exercised when choosing any nutritional supplement, including multivitamins. Choosing supplements verified by the U.S. Pharmacopeia (USP) may help ensure safety. Herbs, which are very powerful substances that also are not regulated by the FDA, should not be used as nutritional supplements or medicines without knowledge of their effects.

More and more research is showing that many people are lacking in vitamin D, along with other nutrients. As doctors become more educated in the nutritional aspect of

human health, patients' vitamin D levels will be checked automatically during a visit to a physician. Physicians who have educated themselves on nutrition likely will order a nutrition panel for their patients with health concerns. Nutritional levels can be an indication of why the body is reacting in a certain manner.

Supplementation is a plausible answer to the problem of lack of nutrition in foods. The only recommendation offered is that the closer a supplement is to a "real food," the better the body will be able to use it. Supplements usually are best taken with food to enhance absorption.

Key Points

- A healthy diet consists of appropriate portions of healthy fats, such as olive, grapeseed, and flaxseed oils, and healthy carbohydrates (whole grain foods), such as whole wheat bread, oatmeal, and brown rice.
- Vegetables and fruits should be eaten in abundance.
- The diet includes moderate amounts of healthy sources of protein such as nuts, legumes, fish, poultry, lean meat, eggs, and dairy.
- People need to eat clean, fresh food as much as possible. Organic foods and free-range and hormone-free meat, poultry, and fish are becoming easier to obtain. Even though the cost is higher, the value is usually worth the investment.
- A high-quality multiple vitamin that breaks down quickly in the digestive system is suggested for most people.
- A healthy diet minimizes the consumption of fatty red meat; refined grains, including white bread, white rice, and white pasta; and sugar. It eliminates foods made with trans fats, which eliminates as much fast food and prepared food as possible.

THE BODY: PHYSICAL FITNESS

SECTION OBJECTIVES

Chapter objective covered in this section:
3. Explain physical exercise as part of a wellness program.
Using the information presented in this section, the student will be able to perform the following:
- Describe the importance of exercise and stretching
- Explain aerobic exercise
- Implement a self-care exercise program
- Describe the physiologic changes that occur with exercise
- Explain the metabolic rate
- Explain flexibility
- Demonstrate safe stretching methods

Fitness is a general term used to describe the ability to perform physical work. Performing physical work requires cardiorespiratory functioning, muscular strength and endurance, and musculoskeletal flexibility. To become physically fit, individuals must participate regularly in some form of physical activity that challenges all large muscle groups and the cardiorespiratory system and promotes postural balance.

Our bodies are designed for purposeful movement toward a goal, such as gathering food for the day or running for safety. The body still functions as though this were the reality, even though we do not need to work as hard to gather our food in

Evolve Activity 15-2

2
15-1

💡 PROFICIENCY EXERCISE 15-4

Locate an exercise and stretching program taught by a qualified instructor at your local community center or health club. Eastern examples of exercise include tai chi, martial arts, and yoga; Western examples include spinning, dance, aerobics, and swimming. You also can buy an exercise and stretching video. Participate in the program for 6 weeks, monitoring all movements for correctness and comfort.

Remember that endurance is a measure of fitness. It is the ability to work for prolonged periods and the ability to resist fatigue. It includes muscular endurance and cardiovascular endurance. Muscular endurance refers to the ability of an isolated muscle group to perform repeated contractions over a period of time; cardiovascular endurance refers to the ability to perform large muscle dynamic exercise, such as walking, swimming, or biking, for long periods.

the grocery store, and seldom do we have to run or fight for our lives.

Exercise and stretching programs are important parts of any wellness program, because they provide the activity our body was designed to have. Now we run in place and ride stationary bikes. Exercise has become an essential purpose unto itself. Fitness programs need to be appropriate; it is important to modify exercise systems and stretching programs to fit the individual. Many resources are available for studying exercise and stretching programs.

Frequent 5-minute stretches and breathing breaks should be built into everyone's day, especially those who spend prolonged periods in static positions. Such breaks may increase productivity, and people may feel less fatigue at the end of a busy day.

Any exercise and stretching program must begin slowly. Activity levels can be increased gradually each week. It takes about 7 to 8 weeks for those new to movement to reach a level of comfort. More activities may be added slowly once the body has adapted (Proficiency Exercise 15-4).

Deconditioning

Deconditioning occurs with prolonged bed rest, and its effects are frequently seen in someone who has had an extended illness. Deconditioning is marked by a decrease in maximum oxygen consumption, cardiac output, and muscular strength, which occurs very rapidly. These effects are also seen, although possibly to a lesser degree, in an individual who has spent some time on bed rest without any accompanying disease process and in an individual who is sedentary because of lifestyle or increasing age.

Aerobic Exercise Training

Aerobic exercise training is an exercise program that focuses on increasing fitness and endurance. A training response requires exercise of sufficient intensity, duration, and frequency to produce both cardiovascular and muscular adaptation in a person's **endurance**. This is different from training for a particular sport or event, by which the individual improves in the exercise task used for training and may not improve in other tasks or in whole body conditioning.

Adaptation

Adaptation results in increased efficiency of body function and represents a variety of neurologic, physical, and biochemical changes in the cardiovascular, neuromuscular, and myofascial systems. Performance increases as a result of these changes, and these systems adapt to the training stimulus over time. Significant changes in fitness can be measured in 10 to 12 weeks.

A person with a low level of fitness has more potential to improve than one who has a high level of fitness. This is reflected in the **training stimulus threshold**, or the stimulus that elicits a training response. Training stimulus thresholds vary, depending on the individual's health, level of activity, age, and gender. The higher the initial level of fitness, the greater the intensity of exercise needed to elicit a significant change.

Energy Expenditure

Energy is expended by individuals engaging in physical activity. Activities can be categorized as light or heavy by determining the energy cost. Most daily activities are light activity and are aerobic (oxygen based), because they require little power but occur over prolonged periods. Heavy work usually requires energy supplied by both the aerobic and anaerobic systems (non–oxygen based).

Conditioning

The rapid increase in energy requirements during exercise requires equally rapid circulatory adjustments. The adjustments are essential to meet the increased need for oxygen and nutrients; to remove the end products of metabolism, such as carbon dioxide and lactic acid; and to dissipate excess heat. The shift in body metabolism occurs through a coordinated activity of all the systems of the body: neuromuscular, respiratory, cardiovascular, metabolic, and hormonal.

Effective endurance training must produce a conditioning or cardiovascular response. Conditioning depends on three critical elements of exercise: intensity, duration, and frequency.

Intensity

The intensity of exercise is based on the **overload principle**; that is, to achieve improvement, a stress on an organism must be greater than the one regularly encountered during everyday life. To improve cardiovascular and muscular endurance, an overload must be applied to these systems.

The exercise intensity load must be just above the training stimulus threshold for adaptation to occur. Once adaptation to a given load has occurred, the training intensity (exercise load) must be increased for the individual to achieve further improvement. Increasing intensity too quickly can result in injury.

Duration

The optimum duration of exercise for cardiovascular conditioning depends on the total work done, the intensity and frequency of the exercise, and the person's fitness level. Generally speaking, the greater the intensity of the exercise, the shorter the duration needed for adaptation. The lower the intensity of the exercise, the longer the duration needed. A 20- to 30-minute session at 70% of the maximum heart rate generally is optimal. The maximum heart rate can be determined in a number of ways. For example, it can be estimated by subtracting a person's age from 220 (this is only an approximate guide). For most individuals, the maximum heart rate declines with age, and values usually are 150 to 200 beats per minute.

When the intensity is below the heart rate threshold, a 45-minute continuous exercise period may provide the appropriate overload. With high-intensity exercise, 10- to 15-minute exercise periods are adequate. Three 5-minute daily periods may be effective in someone who is deconditioned. Exercising for longer than 45 to 60 minutes increases the risk of musculoskeletal injury and soreness, and the risk does not justify the benefit.

Frequency

The optimum frequency for fitness training generally is three to four times a week. Frequency varies, depending on the person's health and age. If training is done at low intensity, greater frequency may be beneficial. A frequency of two times a week does not generally evoke cardiovascular changes, although individuals who are deconditioned initially may benefit from a program of that frequency. As frequency increases beyond the optimum range, the risk of musculoskeletal injury and soreness increases. For individuals who are in good general health, exercising 30 to 45 minutes at least three times a week appears to protect against coronary heart disease.

Maintaining Fitness

The frequency or duration of physical activity required to maintain a certain level of aerobic fitness is less than that required to improve it. The beneficial effects of exercise training are reversible. The process of deconditioning occurs rapidly when a person stops exercising. After only 2 weeks of reduced activity, significant reductions in work capacity can be measured, and improvements can be lost within several months.

The Exercise Program

Because the components of an exercise program can be accomplished in many ways, a person can engage in many activities that support health. One day you might walk for about an hour, and the next day you might strengthen the core muscles with activities on exercise balls or a movement program, such as tai chi. Yoga supports flexibility. Climbing stairs is a great exercise.

An appropriate exercise program can result in higher levels of fitness for a healthy individual, slow the decrease in functional capacity of the elderly, and recondition those who have been ill or who have chronic disease or a sedentary lifestyle. The three components of an exercise program are (1) the warm-up, (2) aerobic exercise, and (3) the cool-down.

The Warm-Up

The purpose of the warm-up period is to enhance the numerous physiologic adjustments that must take place before physical activity. Physiologically, a time lag exists between the onset of activity and the adjustments the body must make to meet the physical requirements.

A warm-up raises the muscle temperature. The higher temperature increases the efficiency of muscular contraction by reducing connective tissue viscosity and increasing the rate of nerve conduction. More oxygen is extracted from hemoglobin at higher muscle temperatures, which supports the aerobic process. Dilation of constricted capillaries, resulting in increased circulation, increases oxygen delivery to the active muscles and minimizes oxygen deficit and the formation of lactic acid. Venous return also increases. Adaptation in the sensitivity of the neural respiratory center increases the respiratory rate.

Warm-up activities include rhythmic movement of the large muscles of the body. An increasingly brisk walk is an excellent warm-up activity.

Aerobic Exercise

The aerobic exercise period is the conditioning part of the exercise program. Attention to the intensity, frequency, and duration determines the effectiveness of the program. In choosing a specific method of training, the exerciser's main consideration is intensity; it should:
- Be sufficient to stimulate increased cardiac output
- Enhance local circulation
- Increase aerobic metabolism within the appropriate muscle groups
- Not cause injury
- Be weight bearing, to support bone health
- Exceed the threshold level, to allow adaptation
- Not evoke fatigue symptoms

In aerobic exercise, submaximal, rhythmic, repetitive, dynamic exercise of large muscle groups is emphasized. The four types of training that condition the aerobic system are continuous, interval, circuit, and circuit-interval methods.

Continuous Training

Continuous training involves a submaximal energy requirement sustained throughout the exercise period. Once the steady state is achieved, the muscle obtains energy by means of aerobic metabolism. Stress is placed primarily on the slow-twitch muscle fibers. The activity can be prolonged for 20 to 60 minutes without exhausting the oxygen transport system. The work rate is increased progressively as training improvements are achieved; overload can be accomplished by increasing the exercise duration. In a healthy individual, continuous training is the most effective way to improve endurance. Brisk walking and swimming laps are excellent examples of continuous training.

Interval Training

In interval training, the exercise period is interspersed with relief or rest intervals. Interval training is generally less demanding than continuous training. In a healthy individual, interval training tends to improve strength and power more than endurance. The relief interval is either a rest relief (passive recovery) or a work relief (active recovery), and it ranges in duration from a few seconds to several minutes. Work recovery involves continuing the exercise but at a reduced level from the work period. During the relief period, a portion of the muscular stores of adenosine triphosphate (ATP), the source of energy for muscle, and the oxygen associated with myoglobin, both of which were depleted during the work period, are replenished by the aerobic system.

The longer and more intense the work interval, the more the aerobic system is stressed. With a short work interval, the duration of the rest interval is critical if the aerobic system is to be stressed. A rest interval equal to one-and-a-half times the work interval allows the succeeding exercise interval to begin before recovery is complete and stresses the aerobic system. An example would be a 5-minute work interval followed by a 7-minute rest interval.

A significant amount of high-intensity exercise can be achieved with interval or intermittent work if the work-relief intervals are spaced appropriately. An example would be lap swimming with rest periods or race walking or sprinting short distances with slower periods of walking interspersed.

Circuit Training

Circuit training uses a series of exercise activities. At the end of the last activity, the individual starts from the beginning and again moves through the circuit. The series of activities is repeated several times. Several exercise modes can be used involving large and small muscle groups and a mix of static or dynamic effort. Use of circuit training can improve strength and endurance by stressing both the aerobic and anaerobic systems. Often a combination of aerobic activities and weight training is included in the exercise program. Core training that strengthens the postural muscles of the torso can be included in circuit training. Activities using various sizes of exercise balls promote postural balance and core strength.

Circuit-Interval Training

A combination of circuit and interval training is effective because of the interaction of aerobic and anaerobic production of ATP. In addition to the aerobic and anaerobic systems being stressed by the various activities, the relief interval allows a delay in the need for anaerobic processes and the production of lactic acid, because the rest period allows the blood oxygen levels to replenish.

The Cool-Down

A cool-down period is necessary after the aerobic exercise period. The cool-down period prevents pooling of the blood in the extremities, because the exerciser continues to use the muscles to maintain venous return. The cool-down enhances the recovery period through oxidation of metabolic waste and replacement of the energy stores and prevents myocardial ischemia, arrhythmias, or other cardiovascular conditions.

The characteristics of the cool-down period are similar to those of the warm-up period. Total body exercises, such as calisthenics or brisk walking, that decrease in intensity are appropriate. The cool-down period should last 5 to 10 minutes and should be followed by a flexibility regimen.

Physiologic Changes That Occur with Exercise

Changes in the cardiovascular and respiratory systems and in muscle metabolism occur with endurance training. These changes happen at rest and with exercise. It is important to note that all of the following training effects cannot result from one training program. A regular regimen of exercise with a variety of activities is necessary to achieve and maintain fitness.

Cardiovascular Changes

Changes at rest involve a reduction in the resting pulse rate with a decrease in sympathetic dominance and lower levels of norepinephrine and epinephrine. Parasympathetic restoration mechanisms increase, and a decrease in blood pressure can occur. Blood volume and hemoglobin often increase, which facilitates the oxygen delivery capacity of the system.

Changes during exercise include an increase in the pulse rate and a decrease in norepinephrine and epinephrine. Cardiac function increases, as does extraction of oxygen by the working muscle.

Respiratory Changes

Changes at rest include larger lung volumes as a result of improved pulmonary function. Changes during exercise occur as a result of a larger diffusion capacity in the lungs because of the larger lung volumes and a greater alveolar-capillary surface area. Breathing is deeper and more efficient.

Metabolic Changes

Muscle hypertrophy and increased capillary density are observed at rest and during exercise after endurance training. Also, the number and size of mitochondria increase significantly, which increases the capacity to generate ATP aerobically. The rate of depletion of muscle glycogen decreases, and blood lactate levels during submaximal work are lower because of an increased capacity to mobilize and oxidize fat, in addition to an increase in fat-mobilizing and metabolizing enzymes (Box 15-5).

Other System Changes

Changes in other systems that occur with exercise training include a decrease in body fat, blood cholesterol, and triglyceride levels and an increase in heat acclimatization and the breaking strength of bones, ligaments, and tendons.

Flexibility

Flexibility is the ability to move a single joint or series of joints through a normal, unrestricted, pain-free range of motion.

Box 15-5   Metabolic Rate

The metabolic rate is the rate of energy release. The basal metabolic rate (BMR) is not the minimum metabolic rate and does not indicate the smallest amount of energy that must be expended to sustain life. The BMR is the smallest energy expenditure that can sustain life and also maintain the waking state and a normal body temperature in a comfortably warm environment. It is the rate of energy expenditure under basal conditions; that is, when the individual is (1) awake but lying down and not moving; (2) in a comfortably warm environment; and (3) 18 to 23 hours have passed since the last meal.

The BMR is not the same for all individuals because of the following factors:

- *Size:* The BMR is calculated from an individual's height and weight. A large individual has more surface area (and a higher BMR) than a small individual.
- *Gender:* Men oxidize their food approximately 5% to 7% faster than women. Therefore, even if a man and a woman are the same size, the man has a higher BMR. This gender difference probably results from the difference in the proportion of body fat determined by sex hormones. Women tend to have a higher percentage of body fat (and thus a lower total lean mass) than men. Fat tissue is less metabolically active than lean tissue, such as muscle.
- *Age:* The younger the individual, the higher the BMR for a given size and sex.
- *Thyroid hormones:* Thyroid hormones (triiodothyronine [T_3] and thyroxine [T_4]) stimulate the basal metabolism. Without a normal amount of these hormones in the blood, the body cannot maintain a normal BMR.
- *Body temperature:* An increase in body temperature increases the BMR. A decrease in body temperature (hypothermia) has the opposite effect.
- *Drugs:* Stimulants increase the BMR, and depressants reduce the BMR.
- *Other factors:* Other factors, such as emotions, pregnancy, and lactation (milk production), also influence the basal metabolism.

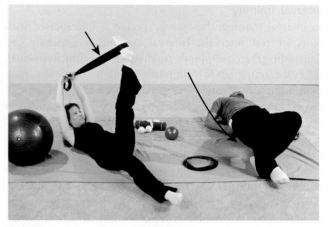

FIGURE 15-2 Examples of self-stretching.

tissue, particularly connective tissue structures, to increase joint range of motion. The end result is increased flexibility. Stretching methods should not increase joint flexibility beyond the normal range of motion.

Passive stretching involves an external force, applied either manually or mechanically, that lengthens the shortened tissues while the person is relaxed. Active inhibition uses various muscle energy methods in which the person participates in the stretching maneuver. The result is an increased tolerance to the sensation of stretch.

Stretching methods should increase pliability in fascia and not stretch ligaments unless some sort of contracture exists. Stretching should increase efficient mobility but not create instability or strain the joint. . Increased tissue temperature increases fascial pliability and can make stretching more effective. Many types of flexibility programs are available. Yoga is an excellent example. Massage is an excellent way to support flexibility programs, especially if the methods used address both the elasticity and pliability of the soft tissue. When the body gets the movement it needs, relaxation activities are more effective (Figure 15-2).

THE BODY: RELAXATION

SECTION OBJECTIVES

Chapter objective covered in this section:
4. Identify and define relaxation and restorative activities.
Using the information presented in this section, the student will be able to perform the following:
- Describe the relationship of relaxation to the autonomic nervous system
- Define mindfulness
- Describe the relationship of breathing to wellness
- Explain the phases of breathing
- Demonstrate relaxed breathing
- Perform and teach basic breathing exercises
- Explain the importance of restorative sleep to wellness

Flexibility depends on the extensibility of muscle tissue, which allows muscles that cross a joint to relax, lengthen, and yield to a stretch force. The arthrokinematics of the moving joint and the ability of connective tissues associated with the joint to deform also affect joint range of motion and an individual's overall flexibility.

Dynamic flexibility refers to the active range of motion of a joint. This aspect of flexibility depends on the degree to which a joint can be moved by a muscle contraction and the amount of tissue resistance met during the active movement.

Passive flexibility, the degree to which a joint can be passively moved through the available range of motion, depends on the extensibility of muscles and connective tissues that cross and surround a joint. Passive flexibility is a prerequisite for but does not ensure dynamic flexibility.

Stretching

Stretching is a general term used to describe any therapeutic technique designed to lengthen (elongate) shortened soft

Relaxation methods initiate a parasympathetic response. Because muscle tension patterns are habitual, most successful relaxation methods combine the movements of moving, stretching, tensing, and then releasing the muscles (progressive relaxation). The heart and breathing rates are synchronized (entrainment) while the individual focuses on a quiet or neutral topic, event, or picture (visualization). Slow, rhythmic music can be a beneficial component of a relaxation program. Most meditation and deliberate relaxation processes are built around this pattern.

The focus of relaxation is to quiet the physical body, not necessarily to create a spiritual experience; however, many prayer systems use similar patterns, which also are beneficial for relaxation.

Almost any type of pleasurable, simple, repetitive activity that requires focused attention induces the relaxation response. Gardening, needlepoint, knitting, playing music, and watching fish in an aquarium or birds at a bird feeder are all forms of relaxation if there is no need to achieve, compete, or produce results in a specific period. Knitting a sweater for pleasure and having to finish one in a week are two different activities. Relaxation takes time, and when something is urgent, it usually interferes with the ability to relax.

Mindfulness

Mindfulness is a concept of relaxation. Being mindful is similar to the centering or focusing methods presented in Chapter 9. Mindfulness is being attentive to the moment, secure that we have learned from and then have let go of the past, and that we are planning for the future without worry. A human "doing" is not mindful; mindfulness is about a human "being."

Just as tension patterns are habitual, relaxation can become a habit. Typically, it takes 8 to 10 weeks of consistent reinforcement to build a habit pattern.

Unlike exercise, which can be varied to prevent boredom, a relaxation sequence needs to be the same each time to reinforce the conditioned response to the habit structure. It is important to use the same location, music, time of day, smells (e.g., essential oils), colors, position, and breathing pattern in the sequence. Any of the components of the relaxation program can soon become triggers to relaxation.

A person should experiment with relaxation methods until the right program is found, then consistently use it every day for at least 15 minutes. (It takes this long for the physiology to make a shift from an aroused state to a relaxed one.) Many audio programs provide progressive relaxation and self-hypnosis and pull together all the components of a relaxation program. This type of resource can be very useful. Self-massage can also support relaxation (Figure 15-3) (Proficiency Exercise 15-5).

Breathing

Breathing provides us with essential air. Breathing patterns are a direct link to altering autonomic nervous system patterns,

which in turn affect mood, feelings, and behavior. Almost every meditation or relaxation system uses breathing patterns. Other ways to modulate breathing are through singing and chanting.

Proper breathing is important, yet most of us do not breathe efficiently. For many the air quality is poor. The rest of us may be in too big a hurry to breathe deeply. Slow, deep breathing takes time. Recall from Chapter 6 that the simple bellows breathing mechanism is a bodywide coordination of muscle contraction and relaxation. The shoulders should not move during normal relaxed breathing. The accessory muscles of respiration in the neck area should be activated only when a demand exists for increased oxygen and increased physical activity. If the accessory muscles activate without an increase in physical activity, the body resorts to the sympathetic dominance breathing pattern. If the person does not balance the oxygen and carbon dioxide levels through increased activity

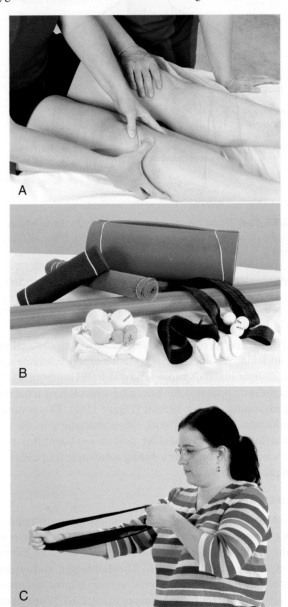

FIGURE 15-3 Self-massage. **A,** Teaching self-massage to a client. **B,** Products for use in self-massage. **C,** Self-applied muscle energy technique using a resistance band.

💡 PROFICIENCY EXERCISE 15-5

Design a daily 15-minute relaxation program especially for you.

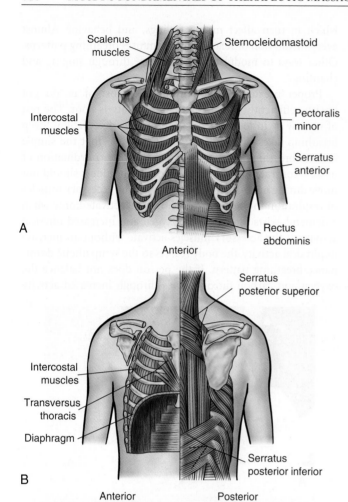

FIGURE 15-4 Breathing muscles. (Modified from Seidel HM et al: *Mosby's guide to physical examination*, ed 5, St. Louis, 2003, Mosby.)

levels, breathing dysfunction (hyperventilation) occurs in the extreme. Breathing pattern disorders can perpetuate anxiety states and many disturbing physical symptoms (see Box 5-9, p. 190).

The accessory muscles of respiration (e.g., the scalenes, sternocleidomastoid, serratus posterior superior, levator scapulae, rhomboids, abdominals, and quadratus lumborum) may be constantly activated for breathing when forced inhalation and expiration are not needed (Figure 15-4). This results in dysfunctional muscle patterns. Often shortening in the quadratus lumborum or shoulder pain is not identified as an inefficient breathing pattern during assessment by the massage professional.

Phases of Breathing

Breathing comprises three phases of inspiration (bringing air into the body) and two phases of expiration (moving air out of the body). Quiet inspiration takes place when an individual is resting or sitting quietly. The diaphragm and external intercostals are the prime movers. As deep inspiration occurs, the actions of quiet inspiration are intensified. When people need more oxygen, they breathe harder. Any muscles that can pull the ribs up are called into action. Forced inspiration occurs when an individual is working very hard and needs a

great deal of oxygen. Not only are the muscles of quiet and deep inspiration working, but also the muscles that stabilize and/or elevate the shoulder girdle to elevate the ribs directly or indirectly.

Quiet expiration is mostly a passive action. It occurs through relaxation of the external intercostals and the elastic recoil of the thoracic wall and tissue of the lungs and bronchi, with gravity pulling the rib cage down from its elevated position. Essentially no muscle action is involved. Forced expiration brings in muscles that can pull down the ribs and muscles to compress the abdomen, forcing the diaphragm upward.

Normal breathing consists of a shorter inhale in relation to a longer exhale. The ratio of inhale time to exhale time is one count inhale to two to four counts exhale. The ideal pattern is two to four counts for the inhale and at least eight counts for the exhale. The reverse of this pattern, in which the exhale is shorter and the inhale is longer, is the basis for breathing pattern disorders. Bodywork and breathing retraining methods seek to restore normal breathing.

Massage to Support Breathing Function

Consider breathing mechanisms during the assessment. One way to determine whether a client uses the accessory muscles for relaxed breathing is to place your hands on the person's shoulders while they breathe; the shoulders should not move up and down (Figure 15-5).

Another method to detect the use of accessory muscles is to observe the client; if the accessory muscles are used, movement is concentrated in the upper chest instead of in the lower ribs and abdomen.

If the breathing pattern is dysfunctional, the accessory muscles show increased tension and a tendency to develop trigger points. These conditions can be identified through palpation. Also, connective tissue changes are common, because breathing dysfunction often is chronic.

Therapeutic massage can normalize many of these conditions and support more effective breathing. Breathing well is very difficult if the mechanical components are not working efficiently. Many who have attempted breathing retraining have become frustrated by their inability to accomplish the pattern. They may be more successful after the body and the mechanism of breathing have become more normal.

The breathing exercises presented in Box 15-6 can be taught to clients. Three common activities can help normalize a breathing pattern: yelling, crying, and laughing, because all three support an extended exhale. Each of these activities is sustained for 3 to 5 minutes, and they can be valuable in any breathing retraining program (Proficiency Exercise 15-6).

Sleep

Restorative sleep is necessary for wellness. Lack of quality sleep is becoming a major health concern. Many people do not get enough sleep. An absolute minimum of 6 hours of uninterrupted sleep is necessary, and most people require 8 to 9 hours.

During sleep the body renews, repairs, and generally restores itself. Growth hormone is an important factor in this process, with more than half of its daily secretions taking place

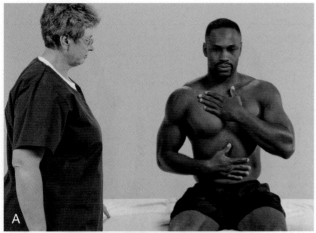

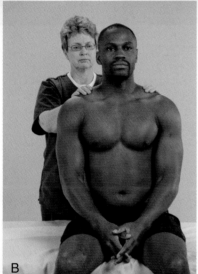

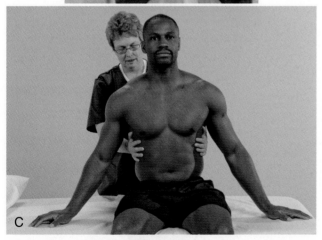

FIGURE 15-5 Breathing assessment. **A,** Observe the client's breathing. **B,** Place your hands on the client's shoulders. They should not move up and down unless the client is using accessory muscles inappropriately during normal, relaxed breathing. **C,** Place your hands on the client's lower ribs. These areas should move if the client is breathing properly.

during sleep. If the deeper stages of sleep are not sustained, the body's restorative mechanisms are compromised. Sleep and dreaming are when we seem to repair, sort, and restore emotionally. Dreaming is still a mystery, but research indicates that it is essential for emotional well-being. Sleep disturbances

PROFICIENCY EXERCISE 15-6

1. This exercise helps you understand how normalizing breathing affects the entire body. Begin by doing a simple physical assessment: move yourself into forward trunk flexion, side-bending lateral trunk flexion, trunk extension, neck flexion, extension, and lateral flexion. Identify the areas of your body that seem most restricted. Now yell or howl as loud as you can for 1 minute. Next, pretend to cry and sob for 1 minute. Finally, belly laugh as hard and as long as you can.
   Now perform the simple physical assessment again. In the space provided, describe the results.

2. Develop a "how to breathe" handout to give to clients. Include at least three different breathing patterns.

PROFICIENCY EXERCISE 15-7

In the space provided, analyze your personal sleep pattern using the information in this section. Identify three activities that support restorative sleep and three activities that can be improved.
   My current sleep pattern is as follows:

   Three current activities that support sleep are:
   1.
   2.
   3.
   Three activities that could improve sleep are:
   1.
   2.
   3.

are, in fact, a major factor in many chronic fatigue and pain syndromes.

Many things can interrupt sleep, such as pain that repeatedly awakens the person, external random noise (e.g., traffic noise), tending to infants and children, varied work schedules, a restless or snoring bed partner (including pets), sinus or other respiratory difficulties (e.g., coughing), and urinary frequency. Others have disrupted sleep patterns because of insomnia, sleep apnea, hormone fluctuations, high cortisol (stress hormone) levels, medications, and stimulant intake, such as caffeine. Regardless of the perpetuating factors, sleep is compromised, and the deep sleep stage is seldom achieved.

Light/dark cycles regulate sleep patterns. For effective sleep we need adequate exposure to daylight, which stimulates serotonin. We also need adequate exposure to darkness. Absence of light supports the release of melatonin, a pineal gland hormone that is involved with the sleep pattern. With the advent of artificial lighting, we have spent less and less time in the dark, which disturbs sleep. Methods to support effective sleep are presented in Box 15-7 (Proficiency Exercise 15-7).

Box 15-6 Breathing Exercises

The following breathing exercises should be taught to clients in an instructional format that addresses the client's specific needs for better breathing.

Exercise 1 (Figures A and B)
1. Sit in a relaxed position.
2. Place your hands in your lap and interlace the fingers.
3. Firmly press your fingers and thumbs into the tops of your hands.
4. Hold this position as long as possible without discomfort as you breathe normally.

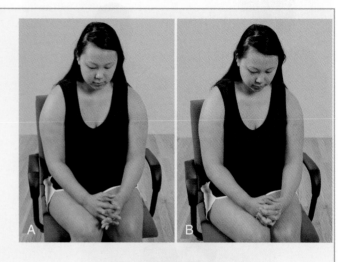

Exercise 2 (Figure C)
1. Place your hands behind your head.
2. Point your elbows up and back.
3. Hold this position as long as it is comfortable while breathing normally.

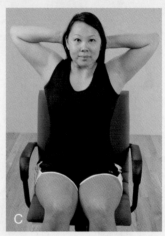

Exercise 3 (Figure D)
1. Interlace your fingers behind your back.
2. Pull your shoulder blades together.
3. Hold this position as long as possible while breathing normally.

These exercises inhibit the accessory breathing muscles. Essentially, in these positions the client cannot use the accessory muscles to breathe, and the intercostal muscles and diaphragm are supported in breathing function. Clients should do these exercises as often as possible throughout the day. They should try to accumulate 30 minutes of exercise per 24-hour period.

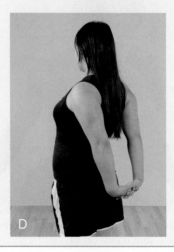

Box 15-6 Breathing Exercises—Cont'd

Exercise 4 (Figures E and F)
1. Sit in a relaxed, upright position in a chair with arms.
2. Place your arms on the arms of the chair.
3. Firmly press the part of your forearms that is closest to the elbow into the arms of the chair.
4. Hold this position as long as it is comfortable and breathe normally.

Exercises for Controlled Breathing
1. Lift your chin into the air and relax your shoulders.
2. Slowly exhale through your mouth, similar to blowing out a candle, and at the same time pull in your abdomen. Then exhale until you have expelled as much air as possible without straining.
3. At the bottom of the breath (i.e., when no further air can be exhaled without strain), stop breathing. This is different from holding your breath, which requires effort. Remain in this resting phase for 3 to 5 seconds.
4. Before inhaling, relax all muscles, drop your chin to your chest, and keep your shoulders relaxed.
5. Inhale slowly through your nose until your lungs are comfortably full, allowing your abdomen to expand.

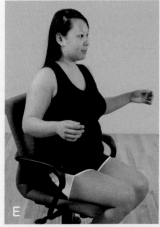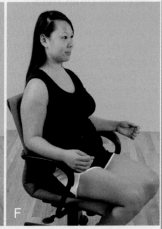

6. Stop breathing for 3 to 5 seconds. Then repeat the entire sequence, beginning with step 1.
   The exhalation should take two to four times as long as the inhalation.
   Many additional resources are available for retraining breathing patterns. Find one that is comfortable and use it regularly.

Box 15-7 Supporting Restorative Sleep

Therapeutic massage supports restorative sleep in the following ways:
- It reduces the activity of the sympathetic autonomic nervous system and also cortisol levels.
- It promotes parasympathetic autonomic nervous system dominance.
- It relieves or reduces pain and discomfort that may interrupt sleep.

Self-help measures for supporting restorative sleep include the following:
- Maintain a regular sleep/wake cycle. Get up and go to bed at the same time every day, including days off.
- Get at least 30 minutes of daylight exposure by being outside or by placing yourself in front of an open window.
- Exercise moderately on a regular basis but do not exercise aerobically 4 hours before sleeping.
- Reduce stimulant intake substantially and ingest no stimulants 10 hours before sleeping. If you go to bed at 11 PM, do not drink caffeinated beverages (e.g., energy drinks, colas, or coffee) after 1 PM.
- Concentrate protein food intake 6 hours before going to sleep. Eat carbohydrates after this time. Do not eat a heavy meal before going to bed. Do not go to bed hungry. Eat a small snack of complex carbohydrates without sugar with some dairy product (e.g., yogurt) 30 minutes before bed if hungry. Although a protein, turkey is high in tryptophan, which encourages sleep. A small turkey sandwich is a possible bedtime snack.
- Stretch gently 1 hour before retiring. A slow, rhythmic pattern is best.
- Stay in a dark room or one that has soft lighting (only enough light for safe movement) 1 hour before bedtime.

Stretching in the dim light is an excellent way to begin the winding down process to prepare for sleep.
- Develop a bedtime ritual that you follow consistently. The ritual should begin 30 minutes before going to bed. Make sure to stay in dim lighting. This ritual should be 15 minutes long. It can include hygiene (e.g., washing up and brushing your teeth) but should not consist of full body application of water, because both hot and cold application can stimulate the body. (A warm bath 1 hour before sleep is relaxing.) Meditating or reading something that is gentle and can be finished in 5 or 10 minutes may be helpful. Listening to soft and gentle music is soothing. Various aromas are considered relaxing and are available in such forms as scented candles, incense, and essential oil diffusers. Drinking a cup of relaxing herbal tea is soothing. Meditate, pray, and review your day in a thankful way. After you develop this ritual, it needs to be reinforced. Do it the same way every night. Eventually the ritual will signal the body into a sleep pattern.
- When drowsiness occurs, immediately relax into sleep. The drowsy pattern known as the *sleep window* lasts only about 15 minutes, and then a new body rhythm cycle begins, which lasts about 90 minutes.
- If you miss the sleep window, continue with calm activities until the sense of drowsiness again occurs. Then go to bed.
- Sleep in the dark. Especially, do not sleep with the television on.
- Get up at the same time in the morning regardless of when you went to bed.
- Avoid long naps. A short 15- to 30-minute nap usually is all right for midday fatigue.

THE MIND

SECTION OBJECTIVES

Chapter objective covered in this section:

5. Explain how the mind and body connection affects wellness.

Using the information presented in this section, the student will be able to perform the following:

- Define mind
- Relate mind, emotions, feelings, and behavior as a pathway to stress or wellness
- Define emotions
- Explain how emotions relate to maladaptive learned behavior
- Relate feelings to emotions
- Describe how massage therapy interacts with the physiologic feelings related to emotions
- Explain addictive behavior
- Describe a wellness expression of a full range of emotion
- Define self-concept and self-worth
- Define resourceful coping

The mind is the part of us that reasons, understands, remembers, thinks, and adapts. It coordinates the conscious and subconscious parts of us that influence and direct mental and physical behavior. The mind processes what we believe; it involves emotions and feelings, behavior, self-concept, and coping.

We can change our mind (beliefs) fairly quickly, although habitual belief patterns are difficult to overcome. Belief changes need to be supported over time to be reflected in lifestyle and wellness programs. The body responds to mind changes, but more time may be required for the effects of that response to manifest in the organic form of the body's anatomy and physiology. Patience is required to objectively identify body changes in response to mind changes. This interaction between mind and body is the basis for current approaches to mind/body medicine.

Emotions

Emotions begin or end in our mind. Feelings, the actual physical sensations, can be caused by emotions, and feelings can in turn cause emotions. Physical sensations that occur in our body need to be understood. If our body experiences a sensation, our mind tries to understand the meaning. For example, if a medication is taken that increases the heart rate, the mind may interpret the increase in heart rate as a threat to safety and the person becomes fearful. Fear is an emotion. If a person is afraid, the heart rate increases and the person feels anxious. The emotions lead to actions that represent the consequences of how we think and what we do. What we think and feel and how we live are all inextricably linked.

As human beings, we learn to be helpless, to be addictive, and to have low self-esteem. We learn to hate. The important point to remember is that if we learned the maladaptive behavior in the first place, we can also learn a more resourceful behavior to use instead. Emotions can be very powerful. If used resourcefully, they can provide us with the empowerment to reach our goals. Many good things have come from an emotion turned into resourceful behavior.

Box 15-8 **Immunity and the Mind**

The immune system is controlled directly by the mind. The science of psychoneuroimmunology has clearly established that unresolved emotions and thought patterns of hate, fear, anger, and jealousy reduce the efficiency of the body's defenses (Chaitow, 1991).

In 1975 Dr. Robert Adder conditioned rats to dislike sweetened water by injecting them with a chemical to make them feel ill whenever they drank it. After the injections had been stopped for some time, some rats began dying. On investigation, Adder found that the chemical he had used was a suppressor of immune function. The rats not only had become conditioned to feeling ill whenever they drank sweet water, they also were mimicking the chemical's other effects and depressing their immune systems. This ability to depress the immune function was proof of nervous system control over the immune system. Many subsequent tests have confirmed this finding in human beings (Chaitow, 1991).

💡 PROFICIENCY EXERCISE 15-8

List any emotions that gave you the motivation to complete this educational program in therapeutic massage.

Wellness encompasses a full range of emotion. Some pride themselves on not feeling certain emotions, but if we can experience an emotion in a resourceful way, it is not healthy to deny its expression. For example, if something as powerful as anger is turned inward, it does not lead to positive outcomes. However, if expressed resourcefully, to the person or in the situation involved, a sense of resolution takes place, and we can get on with our lives, free of the anger.

Wellness comes from using the emotion instead of the emotion using us. Used resourcefully, emotions can provide the motivation to achieve wellness. When used in a negative manner, they can make us ill and can be destructive to those who share our lives (Box 15-8) (Proficiency Exercise 15-8).

Feelings

Feelings are the body's physical interpretation of emotions. They occur as a response to the effect of hormones, neurotransmitters, and other endogenous chemicals. Behaviors such as the need to create crises, eating disorders, accident proneness, hypervigilance, panic, illness, and codependent relationships generate the physical sensations we call feelings. Behaviors such as gentle caregiving, giving presents, and appreciating beauty generate feelings of compassion, nurturing, and belonging.

People use chemical substances such as food, nicotine, alcohol, and drugs to create or dampen feelings. Often if a person's physiology can be changed, his or her feelings can also be changed. The easiest way to change the physiology is to move, as in exercising or breathing. A massage also changes

💡 PROFICIENCY EXERCISE 15-9

Honestly identify two personal behaviors that have a repetitive pattern, one resourceful and one unresourceful. What feelings are generated by these behaviors? For the unresourceful behavior, identify one alternative resourceful behavior to generate similar feelings.

Example

Resourceful behavior: Watching uplifting human interest movies
Feelings: Empowerment, security, connectedness
Unresourceful behavior: Overeating at night
Feelings: Being connected, fulfilled, cared for
Replacement behavior: Playing with my dog

Your Turn

1.
- Resourceful behavior:
  Feelings:
- Unresourceful behavior:
  Feelings:
- Replacement behavior:
2.
- Resourceful behavior:
  Feelings:
- Unresourceful behavior:
  Feelings:
- Replacement behavior:

💡 PROFICIENCY EXERCISE 15-10

List three addictive behaviors. For each, list three alternative behaviors that are less damaging yet may generate similar feelings.
Addictive behavior:
Alternative behaviors:
1.
2.
3.
Addictive behavior:
Alternative behaviors:
1.
2.
3.
Addictive behavior:
Alternative behaviors:
1.
2.
3.

the physiology. This is perhaps why massage "feels" so good. Being touched in a resourceful way supports wellness. Sensory stimulation is essential for the body to thrive. Many people are deprived of touch, and many adults exchange touch only in the context of a sexual relationship. Touch is essential for wellness. Touching generates and expresses feelings. The power of touch was explored in the very beginning of this text.

When feelings are detrimental to wellness, an opposing response must be activated to restore a balance. For example, if you are weighed down with too much thinking, moving around and pulling some weeds in the garden creates a balance. If you feel angry, find a way to laugh. If you feel down, help someone. If you feel anxious and alone, get a hug or a massage (Proficiency Exercise 15-9).

Behavior

Behavior is what we do in response to emotion, to trigger thoughts and feelings, and occasionally to avoid feelings. Resourceful behavior results in feeling good about what has happened. Detrimental behavior still results in a good feeling (or we would not do it), but often we feel bad about what happened, and/or others feel bad.

Addictive Behavior

Addictive behavior creates physical sensations that feel pleasant and bypass the conscious experience of emotion. A person who is addicted to food, drugs, alcohol, exercise, pain, crisis, or loss develops a lifestyle that both protects and supports the substance or behavior of choice. Addictions require a great

deal of time and energy. Addictive behavior throws the balance of wellness off course. It takes hard work and lots of support to change an addictive behavior. Sometimes a less damaging addiction is replaced by a more damaging one, and vice versa (Chaitow, 1991). For example, a person may use a food habit to bypass the emotion of loneliness and then alter the food habit by creating an exercise dependency. Whichever is the more damaging addiction needs to be evaluated. Behavior changes that are at least steps in the resourceful direction should not be discouraged. To truly alter behavior, a person must evaluate his or her sense of self (Proficiency Exercise 15-10).

Self-Concept

What we think about ourselves and how we talk to ourselves are aspects of self-concept. They are very important contributors to wellness. Most of us want a purpose and a sense of achievement, success, and self-confidence.

A positive self-concept is achievable when we stop comparing ourselves with one another. Misjudging our worth threatens our well-being. Rather than basing their personal value on an external standard, healthy people develop internal standards of self-worth. Everyone is good at something; no one is good at everything. Measure success and self-worth by how good you feel about your accomplishments, instead of by money or fame. Especially with massage, an inner sense of accomplishment is important. Massage is a quiet, unpretentious profession. It does not usually receive a lot of public glory. Massage is an important and needed service, and its benefits often cannot be measured objectively.

Coping

An aspect of wellness is the ability to live each day and feel we did our jobs well. How we lived that day influences our mind's perception of how we feel, and sometimes the simplest things can make a difference. For example, when we are stressed and preoccupied by our responsibilities in the day, stopping for a moment to notice the sun shining and feeling the warmth on our faces may be a simple way to regain our balance and cope with all that daily stress. This mind exercise is an example of a resourceful coping mechanism. Resourceful coping consists of commitment, control, and challenge.

Commitment

Commitment is the ability and willingness to be involved in what is happening around us, to have a purpose for being. This purpose is more than what we do; it is how we serve. It is possible to serve in many ways. A career in massage can be a path of service or just a job. Purpose and service have nothing to do with the task. Picking up garbage is as much a service as is being a doctor. Cleaning house, cutting hair, building houses, and packing cartons all can be paths of service. The commitment to support wellness contributes to the greater good.

Control

Control is characterized by the belief that we can influence events by the way we feel, think, and act. This is internal control, not external control. Internal control involves adjusting ourselves to the situation and looking for ways to respond resourcefully. Those who exert external control attempt to control circumstances and people. It is impossible to control the weather, most circumstances, and most people. Relying on external control is a poor coping mechanism.

The eternal wisdom in the saying, "Grant me the serenity to accept the things I cannot change, the courage to change the things I can, and the wisdom to know the difference," speaks to self-concept and internal versus external control.

The saying, "If given lemons, make lemonade," speaks to internal control. Finding the humor in life helps support internal control. Not all life events have humor, but most have something that can bring a smile if not a laugh. For instance, one day while I was staring out the window grieving the death of a loved one, a chipmunk jumped up on the sill with so many sunflower seeds stuffed in his little cheeks that they were sticking out of his mouth and he was trying to stuff more in. This is an example of what I like to call a "chuckly" blended with the tears.

Challenge

Living each day as a challenge supports wellness. A challenging day is filled with things to learn, skills to practice, tasks to be accomplished, and obstacles to overcome. Beginning each day with the affirmations, "I greet the day and all that it holds" may generate an attitude of challenge. Those who see change as a challenge cope much better than those who do not. Using available, resourceful coping mechanisms to cope with change in life allows the individual to welcome changes as leading to personal development.

Poor stress-coping skills in the form of attempted external control and unproductive emotions, such as unresolved anger, suppress our immune systems and predispose us to infection and poor health. The individual's response to the stress, not the stress itself, determines the effect on the person's immunity (see Box 15-8) (Chaitow, 1991). Wellness includes

⬤ PROFICIENCY EXERCISE 15-11

In the space provided, take inventory of yourself to see what coping mechanisms you have. List three effective coping mechanisms and three that are not as effective. Choose one of these ineffective coping mechanisms and develop a plan to change it.

Effective coping mechanisms:
1.
2.
3.
Ineffective coping mechanisms:
1.
2.
3.
Plan for change of one ineffective coping mechanism:

learning more efficient ways to cope with life, such as through counseling and behavior modification programs if needed.

To improve coping skills, pay attention to people who cope well and ask them to share how they manage. Attending seminars and reading books on effective coping, assertiveness, and development of internal control provide additional resources. Professional counseling can be helpful. Remember, we learned the coping mechanisms we currently have, and we can learn even better ways to cope (Proficiency Exercise 15-11).

THE SPIRIT

SECTION OBJECTIVES

Chapter objective covered in this section:
6. Implement and respect the importance of an individualized spiritual approach to wellness.

Using the information presented in this section, the student will be able to perform the following:
• Identify a personal approach to spirituality
• Consider a personal meaning of faith, hope, and love
• Describe the relationship of spirituality to wellness
• Respect an individual's spiritual path

Our spirit is the part of us that transcends. Our spiritual selves "know our truth." Spiritual wellness consists of faith, hope, and love.

Faith

Faith is the ability to believe, trust, and know certain things that science cannot prove. It is the strength of wellness and involves the expression of that connecting strength each day through faith in ourselves, our partners, our families, and humanity as a whole. Faith is essential to wellness (Proficiency Exercise 15-12).

Hope

Hope is the belief, assurance, conviction, and confidence that our future will somehow be okay. It is the belief that the

💡 PROFICIENCY EXERCISE 15-12

On a separate sheet of paper, write a poem, story, or song or draw a picture about your source of faith. This piece of art is just for you, so do not be concerned that anyone else will see it.

💡 PROFICIENCY EXERCISE 15-13

Complete the following sentence 10 different ways.
I hope
I hope
I hope
I hope
I hope
I hope
I hope
I hope
I hope
I hope

💡 PROFICIENCY EXERCISE 15-14

During a learning experience, one or two people may emerge who teach us more than we expected to learn. Often the learning has nothing to do with the courses we are studying. This is a love sharing. Go to those who have shared their love with you and say "Thank you."

choices we make now will be the most resourceful choices as we create our future. Without hope, no sense of continuity exists. Temple Grandin, an admirable woman with autism, said, "I like to hope that even if there is no personal afterlife, some energy impression (of me) is left in the universe. I do not want my thoughts to die with me" (Sacks, 1996) (Proficiency Exercise 15-13).

Love

Love has no concrete explanation. It is a prerequisite for wholeness, and wholeness is necessary for wellness. This is not romantic love; it is bigger, stronger, more empowering, and mightier. It is quiet, gentle, forgiving, and nonjudgmental.

A teenage boy was struggling to put these most important issues into perspective. He came to his mother and said, "I have figured out the meaning of life." Wondering this herself, she asked her son what he had discovered. The son replied, "When I play my music and I feel great and those who listen to me feel great, then I have shared my love, and my power gets bigger and so does theirs. But if I play my music and only I feel great and those who listen feel bad and weak, then I have taken their power, and this is evil. This is the meaning of life." This type of love celebrates the irrepressible process of life. This is the love of wellness (Proficiency Exercise 15-14).

Spiritual health is essential to wellness. Each individual has a unique belief and experience of faith, hope, and love. Just as with all aspects of wellness, these beliefs and behaviors can be resourceful and adaptive or unresourceful and maladaptive.

🚪 FOOT IN THE DOOR

The massage professional needs to walk the talk. To get and keep your foot in the career environment you desire, your feet first need to walk your way through your own wellness journey. Wellness is a process. How do you determine your own body, mind, and spiritual health status? What do you do to maintain and increase your wellness profile? Would you do the same activities you recommend to clients? The broad spectrum of wellness maintenance directly influences your career. If you are not supporting your own wellness, how you provide massage will be affected. Stamina will reduce, fatigue will increase, clear and concise thinking will be influenced, and mood altered. Why would a client walk in your door to receive a massage from an un-well massage therapist? Maintaining your wellness will get your foot in the door and keep it there.

However, unlike the body and mind, for which the information relating to wellness has been well researched and somewhat standardized, our spiritual path is beyond hard science and concrete suggestions. It is a sacred place created by each individual and is to be respected. There are some right ways to a healthy body and mind as previously described. There also are healthy expressions of spirituality, but they are much more varied and less concrete. Resourceful spirituality provides us with faith and hope and love. These elements strengthen us and protect us from becoming faithless, hopeless, and loveless.

When we nourish faith, we find strength to survive, thrive and help others.

When we nourish hope, we can endure, create, and plan for our future.

When we nourish love, we care, have empathy, and support vibrant life in all its forms and bring respect and strength to support what is right and good.

Faith, hope, and love combined have far more strength than fear, destruction, and hate. The coming together of those who live a life based on faith, hope, and love—regardless of culture, religion, or past experience—forms the spiritual strength of our universal present and potential future.

SUMMARY

Wellness encompasses more than the components discussed in this chapter. Wellness is living life in a simple, gentle, respectful way for ourselves, with others, and in the environment. Wellness is the result of the healing that takes place on multiple levels when we take care of ourselves; this, then, extends to caring for others and the planet in general. A competent massage professional practices self-care and educates clients about the basic components of wellness. This chapter has addressed methods for managing the physical, emotional, and spiritual stress in our lives.

It has been said, "When half the world is receiving a massage and the other half is giving a massage, we shall have peace." Wellness is peace within and sharing that peace in simple ways. Sharing this peace consistently with respect and compassion can support the wellness of us all, and with faith, hope, and love provide peace for our world.

ⓔvolve

http://evolve.elsevier.com/Fritz/fundamentals/

15-1 Challenge yourself with questions on challenges to wellness

15-2 Review vocabulary on nutrition

15-3 Work out your memory with this exercise

Don't forget to study for your certification and licensure exams! Review questions, along with weblinks, can be found on the Evolve website.

References

Chaitow L: *The body/mind purification program*, New York, 1991, Fireside.

Sacks O: *An anthropologist on Mars: seven paradoxical tales*, New York, 1996, Vintage Books.

Selye H: *The stress of life*, ed 2, New York, 1978, McGraw-Hill.

Workbook Section

Short Answer

1. What are the basic components of a wellness program?

2. List common stress responses.

3. How are communication, demands, loss, seeking help, and intuition interrelated?

4. List the components of a balanced diet.

5. List the steps for efficient, relaxed breathing.

6. What are the main components of a physical fitness exercise program?

7. What are the main components of an exercise program?

8. List the changes that occur with exercise.

9. Define flexibility and stretching.

10. Explain how entrainment and mindfulness support relaxation.

11. Explain the interrelationship of self-concept, behavior, and emotions.

12. How can spiritual fitness support resourceful coping?

Assess Your Competencies

Now that you have studied this chapter, you should be able to:

- Define stress
- Identify the basic components of a wellness program
- Implement a body approach to wellness
- Implement a mind approach to wellness
- Implement a spiritual approach to wellness
- Provide general wellness guidelines to clients

On a separate sheet of paper or on the computer, write a short summary of the content of this chapter based on the preceding list of competencies. Use a conversational tone, as if you were explaining to someone (e.g., a client, prospective employer, coworker, or other interested person) the importance of the information and skills to the development of the massage profession.

Next, in small discussion groups, share your summary with your classmates and compare the ways the information was presented. In discussing the content, look for similarities, differences, possibilities for misunderstanding of the information, and clear, concise methods of description.

CHAPTER OBJECTIVES

After completing this chapter, the student will be able to perform the following:

1. Use clinical reasoning to integrate the information from science studies and this text to complete a comprehensive history, assessment, and care/treatment plan.
2. Write comprehensive case studies.
3. Analyze care/treatment plans and offer and justify alternate approaches to care.
4. Pick out three of the case studies in this chapter, develop a treatment plan that differs from the one presented, and be able to justify the appropriateness of your approach for the condition.

CHAPTER OUTLINE

This chapter integrates the information from this textbook and your science studies. The recommended textbook for anatomy, physiology, pathology, and kinesiology is *Mosby's*

Essential Sciences for Therapeutic Massage: Anatomy, Physiology, Biomechanics, and Pathology, although other texts can be used successfully. Competency in therapeutic massage practice is reflected both in a solid understanding of the content of your science studies and an ability to apply the information practically for individual clients. DVD 1 at the back of this book contains three additional video case studies showing the process through pretreatment interviews, assessment, and the massage session.

The following 20 case studies cover the most common outcome goals of clients. These cases cover at least 80% of the common conditions seen by massage professionals in day and destination spas and in wellness, health, fitness, sports, and medical settings. If you carefully study the process of clinical reasoning exemplified in these cases, you should be able to address almost all other conditions you encounter in your professional practice.

Each case study is presented in the following format:
- Case narrative
- Assessment
- Clinical reasoning
- Treatment plan development

The cases present an integrated approach to goal-oriented and outcome-based individual client care. Each case study attempts to describe real situations with complicating factors in addition to the main issues. For example, seldom can you use massage to enhance athletic performance or manage low back pain without having to consider other factors, such as coexisting conditions, work activities, stress tolerance, medications, and client compliance. The massage work environment is a factor; massage on a cruise ship is different from massage in a rehabilitation center. If the client cannot justify the cost or does not show up for regular appointments, even the best treatment plan is meaningless. Skills and knowledge also are factors. What a massage professional with 2 years of experience and an entry level education is able to accomplish is far different from what a professional with 15 years of experience and hundreds of hours of advanced education can achieve.

This textbook is designed as an entry level text and the assumption that you do not have professional experience. One purpose of these case studies is to model the use of a critical thinking process. As a massage therapy student and soon to be a graduate, you can use these case studies as patterns for how to develop massage treatment plans even when experience is minimal. If you challenge yourself to study the process of each case study, you will begin the habit of thinking in this fashion. The story form for each case is an effective method for learning. Each case can provide a platform for common situations you may encounter in your professional practice. This can be helpful for you as a new massage therapist, so that you do not feel overwhelmed at the beginning of your professional practice. These case studies provide you with examples that you can follow and modify.

Because clients' situations vary so much, writing massage protocol recommendations for an individual condition is almost impossible. For example, the pathology related to irritable bowel syndrome (IBS) is understood in terms of signs and symptoms; however, the issue becomes how that generic information relates to an individual client who seeks help through massage, especially in light of the multiple influences in a client's life. Consequently, recommendations for massage for IBS are very limited; although the information may help a massage professional begin to think about how best to serve an individual client, this is only the beginning. The treatment plan for massage must address each client's entire set of circumstances, not just a single condition the person may have.

The treatment plans presented here have been developed accordingly. Based on many years of professional experience, the author has found that the recommendations provided in the case studies have a good expectation of meeting realistic goals for clients. Each case study has a primary goal, with numerous influences that make clinical reasoning and decision making the only effective ways to evaluate and develop appropriate massage treatment plans.

Research is necessary with every new client. If the client has a diagnosed condition, it is important to look up information about that medical condition and any treatment being done for it. For example, if a client has been burned (as in one of the case studies), the massage professional must understand the different categories of burns, the types of scar development, the treatments used to support burn healing, the expected changes in the tissue even after healing, and other related factors.

This type of research begins during the interview with the client, because he or she has useful knowledge, and continues in the fact-gathering portion of the clinical reasoning process. This text and *Mosby's Essential Sciences for Therapeutic Massage: Anatomy, Physiology, Biomechanics, and Pathology,* provide information on the most common conditions encountered by massage professionals and serve as important places to begin the research process. In addition to textbooks, medical dictionaries, texts on pharmacology and pathology, and the Internet have been used to gather pertinent information to support appropriate treatment plan development.

For example, a client might come in for massage to reduce aching caused by playing tennis. The client requests massage that has sufficient depth of pressure and drag to address the second, third, and fourth layers of muscle tissue and to increase the pliability of the connective tissue ground substance. If muscle aching were the only condition detected, those methods would be appropriate. However, this same client is taking an anticoagulant medication because of a heart condition—and

suddenly, the entire treatment plan changes. The question becomes, how does the massage professional meet the main goal of the client—reduction of deep muscle aching—without causing bruising or other complications arising from the heart condition and the medication taken to treat it? To further complicate the issue, the client wants only a 30-minute massage. To serve the client competently, the massage professional must understand tennis, the training effects that support tennis playing, performance-connected muscle soreness, anticoagulant medication (how and when it is used and the effects and side effects), the client's heart condition and any therapies besides medication used to treat it, and any other pertinent facts. All this information influences the types of massage applications chosen and assists with the decisions on how deep or superficial, how fast or slow, how rhythmic, or how frequent the massage application should be.

The case studies attempt to give examples of ways to meet common but complicated massage client goals in the context of the bigger picture. As you study each case, evaluate it to see whether a variation of the recommended treatment plan might be effective. Also, consider all the other conditions that would benefit from a similar treatment plan. For example, one of the cases discusses a client with asthma; however, a similar massage process would be appropriate for someone with emphysema or chronic bronchitis.

When you study the cases, follow this rubric:

1. Identify the main goal and all the conditions and complicating factors.
2. Identify the overlapping issues that alter the treatment process or the superimposed cautions for massage application.
3. Brainstorm about what you agree with in the presented treatment plan and what you might do differently.
4. Dissect the assessment processes.
5. With the physical assessment information, actually put yourself in the positions described and experience what they feel like.
6. Relate those postures and sensations to the goals of the client and the recommendations for massage application.

CASE 1 GENERALIZED STRESS AND ANXIETY WITH BREATHING PATTERN DISORDER SYMPTOMS

Note: Generalized stress and anxiety with breathing pattern disorder symptoms is the most common stress condition seen by the massage therapist. This condition also is common in pain and fatigue syndromes and in post-traumatic stress disorder.

The client is a 37-year-old male. Friends and the client's primary care physician recommended massage to help him deal with stress-induced physical symptoms. Three weeks ago he had a complete physical, because he was required to purchase a life insurance policy to cover the mortgage on a new home. The family had outgrown their smaller home with the recent birth of their third child. Although the physical indicated that all signs were within normal parameters, the man's blood pressure was slightly elevated. It was recommended that he see his family doctor, who did not find anything medically out of the norm but who did notice that the client was impatient and irritable. The client told the doctor that he was not sleeping well and said that he was experiencing some heartburn about once a week, occasional constipation, and neck and shoulder stiffness. He had also gained 10 pounds since his last visit 2 years ago. The doctor felt that stress was the main cause of the man's problems and suggested that he exercise more often, reduce the caffeine in his diet, and lose some of the extra weight. In addition, therapeutic massage was suggested for the muscle stiffness and for relaxation.

The client arrives at a fitness center for his first visit. He has never had a massage before, and he is visibly nervous and in a hurry. The massage professional introduces himself and explains that the first massage visit is primarily an initial assessment process that will take 90 minutes. The cost of the first session is $75. Each massage session after the initial session will last 60 minutes, and the cost will be $50 per session. The client states that he understands the arrangement and agrees to the assessment and treatment plan process.

Assessment

Observation

The massage professional observes the way the client moves about the office, how he breathes, and the rate of his speech. It is evident that the client is feeling rushed, because he looks at his watch many times during the interview and the massage and makes it clear that he has to be at an appointment by 4 PM. The client's shoulders move up and down during breathing. The inhale-to-exhale ratio indicates that the client routinely inhales longer than he exhales. He seems to swallow air when he talks, and he belches a couple of times during the interview. He chews gum, rolls his shoulders back, and often attempts to stretch his neck to the left. He also pulls at his right shoulder and neck area with his left hand. His eyes dart about when he talks, his voice is a bit too loud for the environment, and he cannot sit in the chair for longer than a few minutes without fidgeting or getting up and walking around. When he does sit still, his fists are clenched. He smiles often and jokes about being stressed. His weight is proportional to his height, although he has early evidence of a "pot belly." He is right-handed. The client seems a bit uneasy with the idea of a male giving him a massage.

Interview and Goals

The interview process consists of casual conversation supported by a client information form. The client information form and conversation indicate that the client is 37 years old, married, and an advertising executive and that he recently had moved to the city from a small town. The client has three children, ages 9, 6, and 8 months. He has a family history of maturity-onset diabetes, hypertension, and stroke. He has not had any symptoms other than slightly higher than normal blood pressure. He had one surgery as a child for appendicitis. He ran track in high school and college but has not exercised

regularly since then. Occasionally he enjoys playing basketball and racquetball but has not found a new group of people with whom to play since moving to the city. He occasionally takes aspirin for a headache and Tums for heartburn. He does not take any vitamins or herbs. He drinks coffee and cola beverages. He does not smoke. He was in a car accident 3 years ago and suffered a mild whiplash-type injury. He has difficulty falling asleep at night. His wife tells him that he tosses and turns in his sleep and grinds his teeth. Currently, he feels tired in the morning, and he gets only about 5 hours of sleep a night. The baby still wakes up at night, and he gets up with the child every other night. When asked about his stress load, he lists the new job, the large mortgage, and the fact that he is now concerned about his health. He says that he has always been a bit high-strung. He also discloses that he is worrying a lot. The long hours required at the new job are making his wife angry, because he is not keeping up with his tasks at home as he did before they moved. He sits at a desk, is on the phone a lot, and has to attend and run business meetings twice a week.

To allow the client to become more comfortable with the idea of a male therapist, the benefits of massage are explained in relation to therapeutic goals rather than relaxation and pleasurable sensation.

The client's main goals for the massage are to sleep better, to be more relaxed and less irritable, to lower his blood pressure, and to reduce the stiffness in his neck and shoulder.

Physical Assessment

Posture

Right shoulder is high and anteriorly rotated. Head is slightly forward, and lumbar curve is slightly flattened. Right leg is moderately externally rotated, and right arm is slightly internally rotated. Left knee is hyperextended.

Gait

Stride and arm swing are shortened on the right, and client rolls to the outside of the left foot during the heel strike and toe-off phase.

Range of Motion

Lateral bending of the neck to the left is reduced to 30 degrees. Rotation is equal on both sides but painful during the last few degrees when rotation is to the right. External rotation of the right arm is limited to 75 degrees and internal rotation of the right hip to 40 degrees. Trunk extension is limited to 15 degrees. Eversion of the left foot is slightly limited. Ribs are resistant to being sprung, more so on the left, indicating rigidity in the thorax.

Palpation

Near Touch. Upper shoulder on the right is warm.
Skin. Skin on the right shoulder, pectoralis bilaterally, lateral ribs, neck, and lumbar region has damp areas that redden when stroked. Skin of upper chest bilaterally, right shoulder, and entire lumbar region is taut. Tissue is restricted inferiorly and diagonally to the left on chest and produces a smaller skin fold in lumbar area on the left.

Superficial Connective Tissue. Neck tissue shows mild edema and a sensation of bogginess, as well as a bind resistance to movement toward the left. Connective tissues of the lumbar area and both of the lateral legs palpate shortened and thick. Surgical scar on the abdomen appears bound to underlying structures when moved.

Vessels and Lymph Nodes. No palpable differences.

Muscles. Lumbar and posterior thorax muscles in the second layer are tight but long. Pectoralis major on the right is short. Occipital base muscles are painful to moderate pressure. Abdominals and gluteus maximus are soft and reduced in tone. Hamstrings are short bilaterally. Gastrocnemius and soleus on the left are tight and short. Deep lateral hip rotators on the right are tight and short. Subscapularis on the right is short, and infraspinatus is tight but long. Anterior serratus palpates bilaterally as tender, with tender points corresponding to damp, red areas on the skin. Pectoralis minor on the right is short. Psoas is short bilaterally. Muscles of mastication are tight and short.

Tendons. Subscapular tendon on the right is tender to moderate pressure.

Deep Fascia. Lumbar dorsal fascia, iliotibial band, and abdominal fascia are thick and have reduced pliability.

Ligaments. No apparent changes.

Joints. No observable changes, but some heat, edema, and pain with moderate palpation pressure are noted in the right glenohumeral joint.

Bones. No apparent changes.

Abdominal Viscera. Abdomen is generally soft. Some rigidity is present in the large intestine at the splenic flexure.

Body Rhythms. Heart rate fluctuates from 65 to 80 beats per minute. Breathing rhythm is fast and uneven and does not appear entrained to heart rhythm. Peripheral circulation is good and even. Craniosacral rhythm is fast and uneven, similar to breathing pattern.

Muscle Testing

Strength
Pectoralis muscles and adductor muscles test strong, with inhibition in the gluteus medius, which tests weak. Muscles that retract the scapula are weak. Gluteus maximus bilaterally tests weak.

Neurologic Balance
Antagonists to pectoralis and internal shoulder rotators are inhibited. Abdominals and gluteus are inhibited.

Gait
Shoulder and hip flexors on the right are not inhibited in the normal reflex pattern. When arm flexors are activated, hip flexors do not inhibit as they should.

Interpretation and Treatment Plan Development
Clinical Reasoning
What Are the Facts?
The main contributing factors are generalized stress with episodes of anxiety and breathing pattern disorder symptoms.

(These conditions are discussed in Chapters 5, 6, and 15 of this text.) To work effectively with a client who has these conditions, the massage professional must research them. The general experience of stress is sympathetic dominance in the autonomic nervous system when fight-or-flight or fear mechanisms are detrimental instead of beneficial. When the energy is rallied for these high-activity demands but the body stays still, such as with this client, the physiologic activity manifests internally, resulting in the symptoms of increased heart rate, high blood pressure, digestive disturbances, and changes in breathing. The muscles also assume either the flight or attack position, but movement does not occur, therefore generalized tension builds. When the respiratory mechanism is functioning with auxiliary breathing muscles, oxygen intake may exceed the physical demand, and sympathetic arousal occurs. A vicious cycle begins, with internal and external stimuli increasing sympathetic arousal, which increases breathing and muscle tension, which in turn increases sympathetic arousal. Anxiety with an increase in vigilance (looking for what is wrong) perpetuates. Mood is altered, and physical symptoms manifest in a strange collection of seemingly unrelated symptoms. Because a breathing pattern disorder is a functional process (i.e., the activity is normal but occurs at inappropriate times), no diagnosable pathologic condition is present. The most common and measurable symptom is elevated blood pressure, which fluctuates situationally, unlike with primary hypertension, in which the blood pressure is constantly high. Because physical distress symptoms are present but medical tests indicate nothing wrong, people become frustrated. Management of a breathing pattern disorder requires that the individual make lifestyle changes. However, because of the stress syndrome and the sympathetic activation, people often look for causal factors outside themselves and can become irritable and restless. This is a very common pattern presented by many clients seeking massage.

For this client, stress is professional, personal, and financial. Time urgency is apparent. The client is generally in good health. He has mildly elevated blood pressure that is not being treated medically. There is evidence of sympathetic autonomic nervous system arousal, constipation, heartburn, disrupted sleep, and upper chest breathing and a history of high-pressure jobs. The client talks fast and is restless, admits to being irritable, grinds his teeth at night, and chews gum during the day. This physiologic state is supported by an intake of caffeine. Assessment indicates shortening and tenderness in the auxiliary breathing muscles, with the beginning of second-degree functional stress in both the posture (stability) and phasic (movement) muscles.

What Are the Possibilities in Both Function and Dysfunction and the Massage Intervention Options?
The client seems to display breathing pattern disorder symptoms in response to sustained sympathetic arousal. The client has sufficient postural distortion to interfere with the mechanics of breathing, which would cause the symptoms and perpetuate the increase in sympathetic activity.

The client's activity levels are not in balance with the level of sympathetic nervous system arousal. Increased aerobic exercise with a stretching program would be appropriate.

The client is clearly stressed and has some mild anxiety. Causal factors could be the physical changes in posture resulting from extended sitting and talking on the phone, the decrease in physical activity, or the buildup of internal pressure from work and family. If this is primarily a cognitive problem, referral to a psychologist is indicated. If the indication is more physical, massage and exercise would be helpful. It is likely that all elements are involved.

Possibilities

1. The massage intervention can be structured to deal with the postural alterations and the shortening in muscle and connective tissue structures that are causing the breathing dysfunction.
2. Massage would support a moderate exercise program by managing postexercise muscle soreness.
3. The client should experience some benefit; however, it is likely that some sort of cognitive or psychological intervention is needed. A combination of the two approaches would be most satisfactory.

What Are the Logical Outcomes of Each Possible Intervention?

Massage application should reduce the sympathetic arousal, but the effect would be temporary. Adding exercise and stretching would prolong the effects of massage. The breathing function would improve, and the breathing pattern disorder symptoms should diminish, but these results also would be temporary. The client would need to change his stress perception or reduce the stress load for symptom reversal. Massage application could help manage the physical stress response if lifestyle changes are deemed impossible at this time or if counseling is avoided. Massage would have to be given often—twice a week at minimum—to be effective.

Cost and time commitments would be required for all interventions. Massage alone twice a week would require 4 hours of total time commitment (massage and travel time), and the cost would be $100 per week. The financial burden for this client is not a concern for a short-term intervention process, but the time commitment is. If the client seeks counseling, massage could be reduced to once a week. The time would be about the same, but the cost would be higher for the counseling appointments. Some of the cost for counseling would be offset by insurance reimbursement.

What Is the Impact on the People Involved for Each Possible Intervention?

The massage therapist is familiar with dealing with these conditions, because the fitness center is affiliated with the local hospital's wellness and prevention program. The physician is favorable. The wife is a bit resistant, because the increase in exercise and massage further reduces the client's time at home. If his mood improves, she would be more supportive. The client is supportive of exercise and willing to try massage but is resistant to any type of counseling.

Decision Making and Treatment Plan Development

Quantifiable Goals

1. Reduce shortening of breathing muscles by 75%
2. Reduce postural distortion by 50% and increase range of motion in restricted areas by 75%
3. Increase connective tissue pliability by reducing bind in short areas by 75%
4. Reduce edema in shoulder by 90%
5. Normalize blood pressure to appropriate range (under 120/80 mm Hg)

Qualifiable Goals

1. The distressful stress symptoms will diminish, resulting in improved sleep and reduced irritability at work and at home.
2. The client will have a more relaxed demeanor, resulting in improved relationships at work and home.

The goal is to calm the sympathetic autonomic nervous system and introduce a normal balance between the parasympathetic and sympathetic functions. When this is achieved, the client's sleep should improve as a result of a drop in cortisol levels, and tossing and turning should diminish because muscle tension will have lessened. The teeth grinding and need to chew gum during the day should decline, which would reduce the strain in the mastication and neck muscles.

Breathing should move from an upper chest breathing pattern to more normal diaphragmatic breathing, with the inhale phase being shorter than the exhale phase in a ratio of 1:4. As the auxiliary breathing muscles relax, posture improves, and air swallowing declines, the belching and heartburn should improve. The neck and shoulder stiffness should diminish when these muscles are no longer used for breathing. Mood should also improve.

Appointments would be scheduled in the evening so that the client can go home and go to bed.

Treatment Regimen

Therapeutic Change

This is a therapeutic change process in the short term with realistic expectations of a condition management treatment program for the long term.

The client decides to join the lunchtime basketball game for local businessmen 3 days a week. He will commit to a massage twice a week for 6 weeks and then re-evaluate, hoping to reduce the massage frequency to once a week.

A general full-body massage session will be used, with a depth of pressure sufficient to elicit the relaxation response and generate an increase in endorphins and serotonin. All massage manipulations will be used except friction and tapotement, because friction causes pain, and tapotement is generally a stimulating method. The rhythm will be slow and even, meeting the client's body rhythms and then slowing over the course of the session. The direction of massage will be primarily toward the heart but with changes as necessary to address the connective tissue bind. Lymphatic drainage methods will be used on the right shoulder. Muscle energy methods will be used, especially to address the eye and neck reflexes and to lengthen all short muscles identified during the assessment.

Because the major tension is in the neck and shoulders, having the client roll his eyes in large circles or his head in small circles while broad-based compression is applied to the tender areas, especially the occipital base muscles, will be helpful. Kneading and skin rolling with myofascial techniques, coupled with lymphatic drainage, will increase pliability in the areas of thick and short connective tissues. Active trigger points in muscles will be addressed with the least invasive measures possible to reduce the guarding response and pain behaviors, because pain increases sympathetic arousal. Positional release will be the primary choice and will be applied to the indicated areas in the serratus anterior and intercostal muscles.

Muscles that are inhibited will be encouraged to function through the use of limited tapotement (i.e., not so much as to arouse the nervous system) at the origin and insertion of these muscles.

Range-of-motion methods will focus on reducing the internal rotation of the right arm and the external rotation of the left leg. The integrated muscle energy methods will be the primary application combining these patterns so that the muscle imbalances can be treated in sequence. The abdominal massage sequence will ease constipation.

Teaching the client simple breathing and relaxation exercises, as described in Chapter 15, is appropriate.

CASE 2 MUSCLE TENSION HEADACHE

A 26-year-old female is in good health except for frequent headaches that radiate pain from the back of her skull around her ears and over her eyes. Migraine and cluster headaches have been ruled out. The diagnosis is muscle tension headaches. Because no medical reason has been found for the headaches, they are assumed to be related to stress. They do not follow any cyclic pattern. A relationship to the menstrual cycle has not been indicated.

The client has a temporary job as a waitress while she finishes college. She spends a lot of time sitting, reading, and working at the computer. She notices increased tension in her neck, shoulders, and lower back when she has to spend a lot of time with her studies. She swims three times a week for exercise and is careful with her diet. She has a moderate intake of caffeine and alcohol, and she smokes. She is not under any medical care.

Because common over-the-counter analgesics such as aspirin and acetaminophen bother her stomach, she is seeking an alternative to manage the pain. She has tried chiropractic care, with limited success, and often experiences a headache right after an adjustment. She has heard that massage can help these types of headaches. The client has completed an informed consent process and has agreed to treatment.

Assessment
Observation

The client is nearsighted and wears glasses. She repositions her glasses often, and she squints in the bright light. She is very polite and soft-spoken. She appears frustrated and tired of the inconvenience of the headaches. She is neatly groomed and very organized; she provides a list of all the treatments that have been tried for the headaches, including a food diary and schedules attempting to identify the cause of the headaches. Her weight is normal for her height. She has long, thick hair that she wears in a ponytail.

Interview and Goals

The client's history reveals that she has had headaches for as long as she can remember. She has a headache severe enough to interfere with daily activities about 10 days out of a month. The headaches last about 12 hours, and the pain is a 7 on a scale of 1 to 10 (1 being slight, 10 being extreme). She does not remember any injury or surgery or any childhood diseases other than the normal ones. She had the headaches during adolescence. She generally ignores the headaches, but they are becoming draining. The family history provides no insight. There is a family history of cancer. She wore braces for 3 years and recently had them removed. She has worn glasses and has had long hair since her early teens. She admits to being a perfectionist.

Her goals for the massage are to reduce the frequency and intensity of the headaches.

Physical Assessment
Posture
No obvious postural asymmetry.

Gait
No obvious gait distortions.

Range of Motion
Slightly limited in all directions in the neck with moderate reduction of capital flexion. Temporomandibular joint (TMJ) opens only to two fingers' width (three is normal).

Palpation
Near Touch. Neck near the occipital base and the lower back are warm.
Skin. All areas are normal except for goose bumps and dampness at the occipital base and lower back. Tissue texture is symmetric and normal. Unable to lift a skin fold over the entire length of the spinal column.
Superficial Connective Tissue. Superior and inferior binding of connective tissue is present at the occipital base, sacrum, forehead, and calves.
Vessels and Lymph Nodes. Normal
Muscles. Tender points are noted in the masseter, frontalis, temporalis, and occipital base muscles. Moderate pressure on these points results in pain that mimics the headaches. Neck extensors are short and tight. Surface muscle tone seems generally high. Calf muscles are tight and short bilaterally.

Tendons. Normal

Deep Fascia. Fascia from the skull to the sacrum binds. Scalp is tightly bound to the skull.

Ligaments. Normal

Joints. TMJ palpates tender to mild pressure and has reduced range of motion.

Bones. Normal

Abdominal Viscera. Normal

Body Rhythms. Rhythmic but fast

Muscle Testing

Strength

Normal except that head and neck extensors are overly strong. Head and neck flexors are inhibited.

Neurologic Balance

Tonic neck reflexes and eye-righting reflexes are overactive; consequently, limb and back extensors do not inhibit when client looks down toward navel.

Gait

Normal except that head seems to be held stiffly when client walks.

Interpretation and Treatment Plan Development

Clinical Reasoning

What Are the Facts?

Muscle tension headaches are a common and recurring problem for many people. They are benign, although all other causes of headaches need to be ruled out. The headaches occur because muscle and connective tissue exerts pressure on the nerves and blood vessels in the face, skull, neck, and shoulders. Trigger point activity that refers pain into the headache pain pattern is common. Individuals who are light sensitive and/or who have visual problems that result in squinting are prone to muscle tension headaches. Heavy headgear or hair that is heavy or styled tightly against the skull presses on pain-sensitive structures. Stress that causes sympathetic arousal, resulting in the attack posture, is a common contributor to muscle tension headaches. Pain of any type can cause the muscles of the head, neck, and face to tighten and can perpetuate muscle tension headaches; in this way, a vicious cycle develops. Headaches often "layer," so that even if a migraine is the primary headache type, the pain of the migraine causes an accompanying muscle tension headache.

Postural strain, such as sitting at a computer or driving, or static positions, such as reading a book, result in muscle tension and pressure on pain-sensitive structures, causing a muscle tension headache. Postural strain that attempts to keep the eyes level affects the righting and ocular pelvic reflexes of the neck, eyes, and trunk. Head, neck, and torso flexors should facilitate and head, neck and torso extensors inhibit when the eyes and head move down toward the midline of the body; the process should reverse when the eyes and head move up, as in looking at the ceiling. Looking right and rotating right cause the muscles on the right to contract concentrically and the muscles on the left to be inhibited and in eccentric function, and vice versa for the left side.

Upper chest breathing is often a contributing factor, because the auxiliary breathing muscles can cause headaches if they are tense or short or have trigger points.

Low back tension and lower leg tension are also common and need to be addressed in conjunction with the more obvious muscle tension pattern near the head. Connective tissue bind from the occipital base to the sacrum can fix the head, putting pressure on pain-sensitive structures. Poor air quality and noisy environments with uneven or fluctuating lighting can cause headaches. Smoking often contributes to muscle tension headaches.

A muscle tension headache is usually a functional condition, and no obvious pathologic condition can be diagnosed. With the client in this case, no pathologic reason has been found for the headaches. However, stress is implicated; the client is a self-admitted perfectionist, which supports the stress diagnosis. Shortening of the fascial connection between the skull, occipital base, and sacrum is present. The muscles of the base of the skull and the face, as well as the muscles of mastication, are tender to moderate pressure and reproduce headache pain. The head and neck extensors are short, as are the calf muscles.

What Are the Possibilities in Both Function and Dysfunction and the Massage Intervention Options?

Eye strain, the weight and position of the glasses, and the heavy hair in a ponytail all may be contributing causal factors. Eye strain from extended sitting, coupled with the stress of studying, could be contributing to the low back and calf tension.

The clenched jaw and tight arms and legs are components of the attack posture. This posture is part of the sympathetic response and could be part of the symptoms. The noisy environment of the restaurant where the client works could be making the situation worse. Smoking is also a contributing factor. Muscle tension probably is interfering with circulation. No one significant factor appears to be causing the headache pattern; rather, the cause may be the cumulative effect of many small contributing factors, which would explain the random pattern of occurrence. If stress and strain reach a certain level, the headache occurs, such as when the client wears a tight ponytail, has to read in bright light, smokes more than normal, or is stressed by a tight work schedule or a school paper due. The cumulative effect is a headache.

Possibilities

1. Massage and a stretching program, such as yoga, would be helpful.
2. The heavy hair, eye strain, and ill-fitting glasses may be causes, and referral to the client's optometrist is prudent. A different hair style would reduce the weight and strain on the scalp and the muscles in that area.

What Are the Logical Outcomes of Each Possible Intervention?

Some soft tissue factors make muscle tension headaches likely, and these can be addressed with massage. If the muscle tension is reduced and the connective tissue bind is normalized (conditions noted in the assessment), more external stress may be required to cause the headaches.

Yoga-type activity would provide stress reduction, help retrain breathing, stretch short muscles, and introduce pliability to the binding connective tissue structures.

A change in glasses to improve the client's eyesight may diminish a causal factor, as might a new hair style.

Cost and time are issues. The client is on a limited budget and very busy. Weekly massage sessions would be the minimum required for measurable results.

What Is the Impact on the People Involved for Each Possible Intervention?

The client does not want to cut her hair but is willing to make her ponytail less tight. She will see the optometrist for a checkup. She is not interested in yoga. She will get massages and seems excited about the possibilities for improvement. She is concerned about finances and can afford only two massage sessions a month.

Decision Making and Treatment Plan Development

Quantifiable Goals

1. Reduce headache pain by 75%
2. Reduce frequency and duration of headaches by 50%

Qualifiable Goal

The headaches will decline in number, reducing interference with the client's daily life activities.

Treatment Regimen

Therapeutic Change/Condition Management

The massage sessions will be standard 60-minute appointments at $40 per session, every other week, with time allocated to teach the client self-massage methods. Full-body relaxation massage, using sufficient depth of pressure to increase serotonin and endorphins and produce a parasympathetic effect, will be the main intervention. The primary methods will be compression, gliding, and kneading. Myofascial methods will be used on the areas of connective tissue bind, primarily in the occipital and lumbar areas. The short calf muscles will be addressed with muscle energy methods to lengthen the muscles. The trigger point areas that refer into the headache pain pattern will be addressed with positional release methods, if possible, and with tense-and-relax or reciprocal inhibition and lengthening if necessary. The pulsed muscle energy or integrated muscle energy method will be used for areas more resistant to lengthening. Trigger point areas that do not respond to the more conservative methods will be addressed with direct compression and stretching of the local tissue, which will be achieved by introducing bending and torsion forces into the affected soft tissue structure. Massage of the face, scalp, and neck is necessary.

The client will be taught self–positional release on the areas of trigger point activity. She will be shown how to apply muscle energy methods, particularly using the position of the eyes or the head to activate a tensing or inhibition of muscles. The main self-help method demonstrated will be to move the soft tissue area restricted by shortened muscles in the position of the tension and then to roll the eyes in slow circles. With this technique, the muscles will move into a facilitated and inhibited neurologic pattern. The area then will be gently stretched when the breath is exhaled.

Breathing exercises, as described in Chapter 15, will also be taught as self-help.

CASE 3 GENERALIZED PAIN SYNDROME: SUBCLINICAL FIBROMYALGIA

The client is a 46-year-old female. She works as an administrative assistant for a demanding boss. She has a random work schedule that often involves working into the evening; however, she enjoys the challenges of her job. She has been divorced for 7 years and has two children, who are both in college. Her finances are stable. She is 25 pounds overweight, does not exercise, and does not smoke. She is susceptible to upper respiratory infections. Her sleep and eating cycles are erratic.

She is experiencing generalized muscle and joint aching. She has had symptoms for 5 years, but this past year has been the most difficult. The pain is not constant and fluctuates in intensity and duration. Bad days are beginning to outnumber good days. Medical testing has not revealed any pathologic condition. She has seen a rheumatologist and does not quite fit the profile for fibromyalgia syndrome, although she has many of the symptoms and some of the history. Over-the-counter pain medication upsets her stomach.

The client had a severe bout of flu and pneumonia 8 years ago. Her last physical was 6 weeks ago. Her thyroid-stimulating hormones were a bit elevated, indicating that there may be a thyroid hormone deficiency. Currently she is not being treated with medication, but she will be retested in 6 months. She is menopausal but still has an occasional menstrual cycle marked by sporadic, heavy bleeding. She is not undergoing hormone replacement therapy at this time. She has mild stress and urinary incontinence. The excess weight is a concern, as is her bone density to some degree. A bone scan indicated some bone loss but not sufficient for a diagnosis of osteoporosis. Her cholesterol level is a bit high but still in the normal range.

Her physician recommended an exercise and weight loss program and referred her to the affiliated fitness center, where she saw a brochure for therapeutic massage.

Assessment

Observation

The client is restless, changes position often, and sighs frequently. Movement in the shoulders is noted during normal relaxed breathing. She is neatly groomed and wears high heels. She has a pleasant, even speaking voice. She provides extensive detail in answering all questions. She asks many questions, looking for specific answers. She looks bloated, with indications of swelling in the extremities. Her fat distribution is in the abdomen, creating the "apple shape," which is an indicator of an increased risk of heart disease and diabetes.

Interview and Goals

The client does not drink much water; she usually drinks tea or juice. Her client information form shows a family history of autoimmune problems. She has a sister with multiple sclerosis, and her grandmother had lupus. The client had one vaginal birth, and the other child was born by emergency cesarean section because of a breech presentation. She takes a multivitamin but no other medications. She has tried various nonsteroidal antiinflammatory drugs (NSAIDs) for pain, but they did not help. Cymbalta was recommended. This medication is thought to work by correcting an imbalance of serotonin and norepinephrine, two brain chemicals known to influence mood. It belongs to a class of antidepressants called *selective serotonin and norepinephrine reuptake inhibitors* (SNRIs). This medication is also used to treat peripheral neuropathy. The client used the medication for 3 months but did not experience enough relief to justify some of the side effects that occurred.

She indicates that she is stressed but not overwhelmed. She gets a cold every year in the fall, has intestinal gas, and has chronic pain in her muscles and joints. She is restless more than fatigued. She does not participate in exercise and says that she really hates it. She has always been clumsy. She enjoys singing. On a 1 to 10 pain scale (1 being slight, 10 being extreme), she indicates that her pain is usually a 6 with episodes of 8.

Her goals for the massage are to manage the pain and to relax.

Physical Assessment

Posture

Mild lordosis is present, likely functional from wearing high heels. Protruding abdomen, moderate forward head position, and elevated and winged scapula on the left are noted. Shoulders are bilaterally rounded forward, with both arms internally rotated. Legs are externally rotated, more so on the right. Calves are short, and most of the body weight is carried on the balls of the feet.

Gait

Counterbalancing movement of the arms is awkward and reduced. Hips move up and down instead of in a rotational pattern. Most movement occurs at the hips, and client has a short stride. Weight is carried on the ball of the foot, with little heel strike.

Range of Motion

Client is stiff, and her movements are awkward. External rotation and horizontal abduction of the arms are limited by 25%, and dorsiflexion is reduced by 50% bilaterally. Muscle guarding is apparent during passive range of motion, and the client cannot let the body areas go limp.

Palpation

Near Touch. No unusual areas noted.

Skin. Skin feels dry, and pliability is reduced, with binding; skin will not easily lift in a skinfold throughout the body, more so in the lumbar area. Skin shows a reddening, histamine response with light stroking. The effect is most apparent in fleshy areas and less apparent around the joints.

Superficial Connective Tissue. Generally feels boggy and shows nonpitting edema. Edema is more apparent in the legs, which show slight pitting.

Vessels and Lymph Nodes. Normal

Muscles. Surface layer muscles generally feel soft and nonresilient. Abdominals and gluteus maximus bilaterally are flaccid and long. Second and third layers of muscles (stabilizers and fixators) are short, but client is intolerant of moderate pressure and tenses surface muscle layer so that palpation is difficult. Client is deconditioned as a result of a sedentary lifestyle. Postural muscles (layer three) in lumbar and cervical regions are short. Calves are short, with connective tissue changes resulting in fibrosis, increased tissue density, and ropiness. Muscles of the forearm are tender to palpation with moderate pressure, probably from computer work.

Tendons. Tender points activated by moderate pressure are common in musculotendinous regions body-wide.

Deep Fascia. Occipital and cervical fascia, lumbar dorsal fascia, and plantar fasciae are short and bind in all directions.

Ligaments. Joint structure generally is stiff.

Joints. End-feel of joints is stiff and binding. Client guards all range of motion and cannot relax to allow passive range of motion. Light palpation over sacroiliac (SI) and sternoclavicular joints is surprisingly painful.

Bones. Palpation is normal, but caution is indicated because of loss of bone density.

Abdominal Viscera. Difficult to palpate. Surface of abdomen is lumpy. Deeper palpation is uncomfortable to client.

Body Rhythms. Slightly slow and sluggish. Rhythms seem out of sync with each other. Breathing is labored.

Muscle Testing

Strength

Client resists muscle testing, indicating that it hurts to maintain the testing positions. She attempts to cooperate but feels everything is weak and sore. Calves and pectoralis muscles are too strong, with inhibition in antagonist patterns.

Neurologic Balance and Gait

Unable to perform.

Interpretation and Treatment Plan Development

Clinical Reasoning

What Are the Facts?

A strain on the adaptive capacity of the body can manifest as pain syndromes. Generalized pain syndromes are multicausal, and good medical care is required to rule out serious underlying causes. Once a diagnosis of chronic pain syndrome has been made, pain medication and muscle relaxers often are prescribed; however, these are not very successful for long-term treatment. Symptoms that go undiagnosed are especially difficult to treat. In this case the client has not been diagnosed with fibromyalgia, but she displays many of the symptoms. Fibromyalgia is a condition characterized by aching and pain in the muscles, tendons, and joints all over the body but especially along the spine. Measurable changes in body chemistry and function occur in some people who have fibromyalgia, and these changes may be responsible for certain symptoms. However, fibromyalgia is not associated with muscle, nerve, or joint injury; inadequate muscle repair; or any serious bodily damage or disease. Also, people who have fibromyalgia are not at greater risk for any other musculoskeletal disease. The underlying pathology appears to be related to central nervous system sensitization where normal sensation is interpreted as pain.

The pain of fibromyalgia usually seems worse when a person is trying to relax and is less noticeable during busy activities or exercise. Other symptoms are often associated with the pain, including sleep disturbance, depression, daytime tiredness and headaches, alternating diarrhea and constipation, numbness and tingling in the hands and feet, feelings of weakness, memory difficulties, and dizziness.

The exact cause of fibromyalgia is unknown. However, many theories attempt to explain why people develop fibromyalgia. Stress contributes to the onset of the condition. Other possible causes include conscious or subconscious tension, disordered sleep, abnormal production of pain-related chemicals in the nervous system, deficient production of growth hormone, a lower pain threshold, a heightened perception of pain, and tenderness in certain areas, such as the upper back and forearms.

The onset of fibromyalgia occurs when the stress in a person's life is prominent. Stress often results in disturbed sleep patterns, a lack of restful sleep, and disruption of the production of chemicals necessary to control or regulate pain. Physical and emotional factors may also contribute to the onset of fibromyalgia. For example, a physical illness (e.g., an infection) can cause changes in body chemistry that lead to pain and sleeplessness.

This case describes a typical history pattern of fibromyalgia, including a bad bout of flu and the accumulation of internal and external stressors over many years. Cumulative trauma and age-related changes, deconditioning from lack of exercise, and a reduction in hardiness are contributing factors. Hormone changes are common. Irregular sleep and eating patterns disrupt the body's sleep/wake cycle. The pain is usually the aching, somatic type. Often any increase in activity results in increased pain over the next 48 hours. This increases the likelihood that the client will remain inactive, which contributes to the problem.

What Are the Possibilities in Both Function and Dysfunction and the Massage Intervention Options?

The client may be slowly deteriorating toward full-blown fibromyalgia. Thyroid deficiency or menopausal symptoms also may be present.

Possibilities

1. General constitutional massage may be helpful, with caution regarding the intensity because the pain can be aggravated by massage that is too aggressive.
2. Application of reflexology and polarity would be appropriate and would have little likelihood of increasing the current symptoms.
3. Lymphatic drainage massage is indicated, and light pressure and rhythmic application are appropriate. The deeper muscles that are short and the connective tissue changes should be addressed once pain tolerance has increased and the client can tolerate deeper pressure.
4. An exercise program was recommended by the physician. Hydrotherapy, with a focus on alternating hot and cold applications, is supported both for relaxation and for hardening. Mineral salt soaks can alleviate some edema and aching. Massage would be needed regularly, at least once a week.

What Are the Logical Outcomes of Each Possible Intervention?

Exercise and massage, with the integration of reflexology and polarity, may increase the pain symptoms in the short term. Hydrotherapy application of alternating hot and cold with mineral salt soaks would be well tolerated if introduced gradually. Massage is less likely to cause discomfort if given carefully. The client is able to schedule the time and has the finances.

What Is the Impact on the People Involved for Each Possible Intervention?

The client is not supportive of exercise, and compliance does not seem likely. She is lonely and indicates that the idea of massage and how it feels is comforting to her. She says she would do hydrotherapy but does not like to be cold.

The massage professional realizes that the client has implicated boundary issues and that this is a long-term professional commitment. Without some exercise, the condition will not improve. The client needs to be encouraged to work with a medical exercise professional to support compliance with an exercise program.

Decision Making and Treatment Plan Development

Quantifiable Goals

1. Reduce aching pain from a 6 to a 4 on a 1 to 10 pain scale
2. Reduce constant aching to intermediate aching with more good days per week (4 good and 3 bad)

Qualifiable Goal

The client will be able to perform daily living and work activities more efficiently and participate in a moderate exercise program without intensifying the current symptoms.

Treatment Regimen

Condition management will be pursued, with moderate applications affecting therapeutic change in a three-stage treatment plan.

Some clear soft tissue dysfunctions must be addressed. The lordosis, forward head, rounded shoulders with internally rotated arms, and immobile pelvis with externally rotated legs strain the adaptive mechanisms. This posture puts extreme pressure on the SI joints and neck stabilizers and restricts the mobility of the thorax, resulting in shallow, upper chest breathing. The shortened calf muscles and plantar fasciae, the result of wearing high heels for so many years, have body-wide implications. Reduced lymphatic movement, strain caused by maintenance of posture, control of postural sway, and restricted breathing all were indicated in the assessment. All these factors must be addressed, but caution is necessary. This client, although not sick, seems to have reached the end of her adaptive capacity. Therapeutic change must be introduced very gradually. Slowing the degeneration and managing the current symptoms are initially most important. Attempting too many adaptations likely would make matters worse.

The three phases of the treatment plan are as follows:

- *Phase One:* The first phase will focus on general relaxation and hyperstimulation analgesia for pain control. The duration of the massage will not exceed 45 minutes. The massage will be rhythmic and repetitive, using primarily gliding and kneading, with a pressure and depth that the client identifies as pleasurable. Parasympathetic activation and an increase in serotonin are the goals; therefore, the massage will have a compressive quality but will not cause pain. Lymphatic drainage and circulation enhancement are appropriate. Simple polarity methods will be used to comfort the client and support relaxation. Foot massage, with reflexology points in mind, will have a more intense quality, bordering on "good hurt," in an attempt to encourage endorphins and other endogenous pain-killing chemical activity, as well as hyperstimulation analgesia and counterirritation. Localization of this type of intensity to the feet prevents any other delayed muscle soreness from developing. The client will be encouraged to drink water; take hot, relaxing Epsom salt baths; and be consistent with the mild water aerobics program, set up by an exercise physiologist, that she has agreed to try. This phase could last 12 weeks.
- *Phase Two:* Massage pressure and depth will increase to address the short muscles and introduce the concept of "good hurt" into the areas that are short and tight in the second and third layer of muscles. Myofascial methods will address the areas of connective tissue bind. Muscle energy, primarily positional release, will be used on tender points identified by the deeper massage. Foot massage of sufficient pressure and intensity to cause a good hurt will continue. The client should be only mildly sore the next day and only in a couple of areas. The exercise program will be supported by a focus on water aerobics and mild training with light weights. Self-help will include a splash of cold water after a warm bath and daily cool water foot soaks. The temperature of the foot baths should be decreased to cold within a 2-week period. This phase could last up to 12 weeks.
- *Phase Three:* The goal now is to introduce small, incremental structural and functional shifts to the postural

distortion. The massage quality will increase in depth of pressure and drag to address the connective tissue bind in the deeper postural muscle layers and the underlying muscle tension. The massage will remain relaxing, rhythmic, and pleasurable but will take on the quality of an adjunct to the exercise program. Muscle energy methods, particularly the integrated methods, can address body-wide muscle interaction patterns. More aggressive connective tissue methods to restore pliability will be introduced with muscle energy methods and muscle lengthening, but this must be coupled with strengthening of the weakened and inhibited muscle patterns. Trigger point activity, particularly in the muscle belly of concentrically short muscles, can be gradually addressed one area per session. Alternating hot and cold showers, beginning with hot and ending with cold, should replace the baths and soaks. This phase will last 12 to 24 weeks.

The entire process could take 1 year.

If the client does not maintain an exercise program, condition management would be more appropriate treatment and would level out at the first phase of the long-term plan. After 6 months the less invasive applications described in phase two could be introduced to see how the client responds. Without a corresponding exercise program, phase three would be too aggressive.

CASE 4 NECK AND SHOULDER PAIN WITH LIMITED RANGE OF MOTION

The client is a 34-year-old male truck driver. He is right-handed but drives primarily with his left hand. Three years ago he took a hard fall while riding his mountain bike. He suffered a mild concussion and remembers that his neck was stiff for about a month. He is in good health, active, and exercises regularly. He eats a moderate diet and does not abuse caffeine or alcohol, nor does he smoke.

The client is experiencing radiating pain into his left scapula and upper deltoid and down his left arm to the elbow. The pain was sudden in onset, and it has an aching, throbbing quality. The pain grows worse as the day progresses, and it is interfering with his sleep, because he cannot find a comfortable position. He also complains of a stiff neck, especially if he tries to turn his head to the right. This has been occurring for about 6 months. He had an upper respiratory infection and a severe cough a month before the current pain symptoms began. He was referred to chiropractic care by his medical doctor. The chiropractor has had limited success and suspects muscle involvement. Heat provides temporary relief, and cold makes the condition worse. Aspirin helps, as do muscle relaxers, but medications are not the best long-term solution. The client is single, financially stable, and available for appointments on a regular basis.

Assessment
Observation

Client frequently rubbed the left side of his neck, left shoulder, and upper arm in a line pattern that followed the brachial plexus distribution. He is frustrated with his situation but seemed happy in general. He joked about his condition and that it was an excuse to get a massage.

Interview and Goals

Nothing out of the ordinary is seen on the client information form other than the information given in the case. Referral information from the chiropractor indicates generalized soft tissue restriction in the neck and shoulder area. In answering a question, the client says that he was on vacation in Mexico for 3 weeks before he got the cold and cough. The cough lasted for a week, and he used over-the-counter cough suppressants. For years the client has ridden a bike at least three times a week for 10 miles. The head injury from his fall was considered minor and was not treated other than with the initial evaluation. He was told the neck stiffness was normal for this type of injury and would dissipate, which it did. He looks over his left shoulder while backing up the truck he drives. He cannot remember doing anything unusual, but he woke up with the stiffness in his neck and pain in his shoulder. He thinks he "slept funny."

The client's goal is to get a massage for a few weeks, but he wants only the neck and shoulder pain addressed. He understands that full-body massage is necessary to address localized problems successfully, but he says that nothing else bothers him. He intends to keep seeing the chiropractor.

Physical Assessment

Posture

Basically symmetric with minor rotation of the head to the left. Right leg is moderately externally rotated. Lumbar curve is flat. Chin juts forward with corresponding tilt of the head back and a slight forward head position.

Gait

Head is held stiffly during walking. Arm and leg swing appears normal. Weight is carried on outside of right foot instead of evenly distributed between both feet.

Range of Motion

Right rotation and lateral flexion of the head are limited by 15%. Internal rotation of the right leg is limited by 10%.

Palpation

Near Touch. Client flinched before the neck area on the left was actually touched. Heat is noted in the area.

Skin. Surface is damp with goose bumps from the base of the head to midarm on the left. When rubbed, the area shows increased reddening and itching from histamine response. Resilience is reduced over the area of skin surfaces that are damp and red. Most superficial connective tissue binds in the caudal and diagonal directions to the right. Bilateral bind is seen on the chest from the superior to midsternal area and to the shoulder.

Superficial Connective Tissue. Skin folds between the scapulae are uneven, with the left side more restricted. Connective tissue bind in all directions exists in the right lumbar area.

Vessels and Lymph Nodes. Normal

Muscles. The neck extensors, particularly at the occipital base, and the arm horizontal adductors are short. Scalenes on the left are short, with trigger point activity and typical referred pain patterns into the symptom area. All serratus muscles are tight, with the anterior serratus short (concentric) and the posterior superior and inferior serrati long (eccentric). Eccentric muscles display attachment trigger points, and concentric muscles exhibit muscle belly trigger points. Calf muscles are short.

Tendons. Mild tenderness in response to moderate pressure is seen at the subscapular and pectoralis major arm attachments bilaterally.

Deep Fascia. Mild caudal binding (tissue moves up but binds when moving down) occurs in all superficial fascial regions: thorax, abdomen, lumbar area, iliotibial band, calves, and plantar fasciae.

Ligaments. Normal

Joints. Functional range-of-motion limitations are seen where short muscles reduce extension, horizontal abduction, and internal rotation. No specific joint problems are identified.

Bones. Normal

Abdominal Viscera. Normal

Body Rhythms. Breathing rhythm is fast in relation to other rhythms. Client has a tendency for upper chest breathing.

Muscle Testing

Strength

Muscles identified as short tested overly strong, with an exaggerated contraction response. Client had difficulty applying a gradual increase in pressure against resistance and instead responded by quickly jerking and pushing with full strength. These same muscles would not inhibit when the antagonists were contracted. Weakness was noted in the neck flexors. Movement of the eyes downward did not increase neck flexor strength, as would be expected. Movement of the eyes upward, as in looking over the head, increased flexor weakness and significantly increased tension in the neck extensors. Shoulder and hip firing patterns show synergistic dominance.

Gait

Opposite hip flexor and extensor patterns did not inhibit as expected (when the right hip flexors were activated, the left did not inhibit but maintained strength, and vice versa). Arm and leg patterns also were out of sync, with flexion bilaterally and lack of inhibition regardless of direct activation of antagonist or expected inhibition pattern in gait. The hip flexors on the same side, when activated, would be expected to inhibit the arm flexors (i.e., left inhibits left and right inhibits right), but this did not occur. Arm flexors stayed activated and tested strong regardless of the muscle pattern activated.

Interpretation and Treatment Plan Development

Clinical Reasoning

What Are the Facts?

Neck and shoulder stiffness and pain are among the most common complaints a massage professional encounters. These can have many causal factors. Postural distortion from a rotated or elevated shoulder girdle is common. This condition is often a compensation pattern that develops in response to postural distortion somewhere else in the body. Because the eyes must be positioned forward and level with the horizontal plane, muscle tone, firing patterns, and joint functions commonly shift in this region. To correct this, the entire body pattern needs to be addressed. A common cause of the problem is eye strain, especially combined with a static seated position, such as occurs with desk and computer work or extended periods of driving. Distorted sleep patterns, often coupled with nasal congestion, add to the situation. Upper chest breathing, such as is found with breathing pattern disorders, almost always involves neck and shoulder compensation. A forward head position strains the neck and shoulder structure. The brachial plexus and cervical plexus are often impinged, because the space through which these nerves travel is crowded, and any increase in muscle tension, changes in the joint position in the area, shortening of the connective tissue, or increases in fluid may result in pressure on nerves and blood vessels. The scalene and pectoralis minor muscles often are involved. (*Note:* Muscle aching gets worse as the day goes on. Joint pain is worse in the morning, gets better during the day, and then increases as the body fatigues.)

The client is young and generally in good health. He has a history of head trauma, along with occupational and recreational activities that have resulted in postural distortion. The anterior flexors and adductors are shortened, and the posterior extensors are inhibited, long, and locked into an eccentric contraction pattern. The generalized connective tissue binding is consistent with repetitive use and the activities that require static positions. Trigger point referred pain patterns are consistent with the symptoms.

What Are the Possibilities in Both Function and Dysfunction and the Massage Intervention Options?

Repetitive strain should be suspected with the static position of truck driving (i.e., looking left and arm positions that shorten the brachial space). The effects of biking also should be considered, given its static position of arms forward, torso bent forward with back rounded, and head forward and extended at the occipital base. Calf shortening and general fascial shortening, attributable to the client's occupational and recreational activities, may be other factors.

Both biking and driving have the arms forward and in a bent forward position with the trunk flexed; this would disrupt gait reflexes over time.

The client displays the typical muscle patterns of a person who has had an extended cough (serratus involvement).

An ongoing adaptive process over the past few years likely has finally caught up with the client, and the coughing bout probably further shortened the muscles that surround the brachial nerve plexus. Soft tissue impingement has likely irritated the brachial plexus on the left.

The head trauma and resulting stiff neck may have caused an adaptive process that has deteriorated, resulting in nerve pain in the symptom area. A trigger point referral pain pattern in the scalenes is implicated.

In situations like this, all the stated possibilities probably are involved in the pattern.

Possibilities

1. Massage intervention would need to reduce trigger point activity in all identified areas and increase the pliability of all binding and short connective tissue structures.
2. Muscle energy methods and massage manipulations to lengthen shortened muscles, plus exercise and stretching activities that balance the repetitive posture of driving and biking, should be introduced.
3. Yoga would be a valid option.

What Are the Logical Outcomes of Each Possible Intervention?

Massage and a stretching program would be effective in reducing symptoms.

What seems like a simple problem is actually quite complex, and effective intervention would take longer than the client indicates he is willing to commit in time. Because the situation is likely a cumulative adaptive process, the condition may become worse before it improves.

What Is the Impact on the People Involved for Each Possible Intervention?

The client resists the complexity of the situation, believing it is a localized issue, and does not want long-term intervention.

He is not interested in yoga but would read a book about stretching and incorporate some of the stretches.

Decision Making and Treatment Plan Development

Quantifiable Goals

1. Restore normal resting length to concentrically contracted short muscles
2. Increase right rotation and lateral flexion of the head by 10%
3. Increase external rotation of the right leg by 10%
4. Reverse connective tissue bind

Qualifiable Goal

The client will be able to use his arm and turn his head without pain during normal daily work and recreational activities.

Treatment Regimen

Therapeutic Change/Condition Management

The treatment plan will consist of 12 weekly sessions. Each session will include a generalized massage with a myofascial drag component, coupled with muscle energy and trigger point approaches to lengthen the short muscles that are directly contributing to the brachial plexus impingement. This will include the lateral neck flexors on the left and the horizontal arm adductors and internal arm rotators bilaterally. Six weekly sessions will be scheduled, and the results will then be evaluated. Gait reflex and firing patterns will be monitored to identify any improvement. Self-help stretching education will be presented to the client. With the client's permission, information will be provided to the chiropractor on massage intervention methods for long-term chiropractic support.

CASE 5 GENERALIZED LOW BACK PAIN WITH LIMITED RANGE OF MOTION

The female client is 28 years old. She is a cashier and bagger at a large grocery store chain and has been on the job for 1 year. She is 40 pounds overweight, with fat distribution primarily in the breasts and abdomen. She has been experiencing low back pain for a few years. The pain is sporadic but worse during her menstrual period, which is also marked by moderately severe menstrual cramps. Since she started working at the store, the menstrual cramps have grown steadily worse.

A general physical indicated no apparent pathologic condition. A physical examination ruled out disk and nerve problems and indicated muscle tension and strain. Her doctor said the probable cause is her excess weight. On her doctor's recommendation, she started a walking program and has been reducing her food portions to support gradual weight loss.

The doctor also prescribed muscle relaxants, to be taken as needed. Lately the client has been taking the medication daily in the evening. The pain worsens as the day goes on; it is relieved initially when she lies down but becomes worse if she lies or sits still for an extended period. She was referred to a physical therapist who designed a rehabilitation exercise program and recommended massage intervention under the physical therapist's supervision.

Assessment

Observation

The client is restless; she is in and out of her chair during the entire interview because she is unable to sit for longer than about 10 minutes before her back begins to hurt. Each time she gets up, she places her hands on her knees and pushes herself up. She places her hands behind her back and rubs the lumbar area frequently. When she stands, she distributes her weight evenly on both feet, locks the knees back, and crosses her arms across her chest. She then paces, putting her hand on her left hip. She sighs, as if movement is labored. She also appears to be retaining fluid. Her face is strained. Her manner is pleasant, but her conversation is peppered with negatives and frustration.

Interview and Goals

The history indicates that the client has worked as a cashier since high school and is a student studying computer science. She either stands at the counter, moving groceries and packing bags, or sits in class or at the computer. She has always been a bit overweight, as are her mother and father. She has never been active, and the only sports activity she enjoys is bowling. Nothing unusual shows up on the history form other than painful menstrual cramps, use of muscle relaxants, and typical childhood diseases. A sharp pain occurs in her back when she coughs or sneezes. Rolling over in bed is uncomfortable. When asked to place her hands on the pain area, she presses across the lumbar area as she moves the pelvis into anterior and posterior rotation. She also specifically points at the sacroiliac (SI) joints. She is single and has a small circle of friends. Her parents and sister live in the next town. She is in a bowling league in the winter.

The client's goals for the massage are to reduce her low back dysfunction substantially and to increase her general well-being.

Physical Assessment

Posture

Moderate lordosis, slight kyphosis, and an increased cervical curve with a forward head and a tendency for hyperextended knees are seen. Posture is bilaterally symmetric from the anterior and posterior views. Postural distortion is most apparent when client is viewed from the side.

Gait

Client walks stiff-legged, with little movement at the SI joints. Contralateral arm swing is minimal.

Range of Motion

Trunk flexion in the lumbar area is restricted, and most forward movement occurs at the hips; it is limited by short hamstrings. Muscle spasm pain limits side bending of the torso to 20 degrees bilaterally. Rotation at lumbar area is limited to the right.

Palpation

Near Touch. Heat is noted in the lumbar area.

Skin. Damp areas are noted in the lumbar area lateral to the spine near the sides of the body, and the skin is generally tight in the areas where symptoms occur. The fingernails have some horizontal ridges and hangnails. Adherence of the skin with binding is palpated in the lumbar area, more lateral and adjacent to the iliac crest.

Superficial Connective Tissue. Bogginess and a mild tendency for surface edema are noted.

Vessels and Lymph Nodes. Normal

Muscles. Abdominals and gluteus maximus are long, weak, and flaccid. Neck flexors, latissimus dorsi, psoas, hamstrings, quadratus lumborum, and all calf muscles are short.

Tendons. Musculotendinous junction of the hamstrings is tender at the ischial hamstring attachment and taut at the knee attachment.

Deep Fascia. Lumbar dorsal fascia is short and binding, with influence extending up into the cranial base and along the lateral aspect of the legs and bottoms of both feet. The abdominal fascia is loose, nonelastic, and nonresilient.

Ligaments. Reduced pliability is noted around the SI joint.

Joints. SI joint is restricted bilaterally; the knees are hyperextended. Lumbar vertebrae seem compressed. Symphysis pubis is up-slipped on the left with a bilateral anterior pelvic rotation, more so on the right.

Bones. Normal

Abdominal Viscera. Abdomen is soft with no palpable abnormalities.

Body Rhythms. Fast with mild dysrhythmia.

Muscle Testing

Strength

Difficult to access because client experiences pain in low back during testing. Abdominals and gluteus maximus are weak, back extensors are too strong, and psoas bilaterally appears weak.

Neurologic Balance

Difficult to test because client experiences pain. Generally client seems deconditioned.

Gait

Muscle interaction pattern has shifted from the normal opposite arm/leg flexor/flexor-extensor/extensor facilitation pattern to a same-side arm/leg flexor and arm/leg extensor pattern. As a result, the contralateral arm swing has been lost, and a substantially reduced, same-side arm swing pattern is noted. Gluteus maximus does not fire in the normal sequence. Hamstrings fire first during leg extension.

Interpretation and Treatment Plan Development

Clinical Reasoning

What Are the Facts?

Low back pain in the absence of disk dysfunction is very common in both males and females. Causal factors vary, but common elements exist. Client histories include either standing or sitting in static positions, coupled with upper torso twisting or some sort of trauma, such as a car accident or strain during lifting or pushing. Medication is not very effective in the management of low back pain. Some sort of pelvic rotation distortion usually is present, as is an upper body compensation pattern of rotated shoulder girdle, altered head position, or change in the thoracic or cervical spinal curvature. Sternoclavicular joint dysfunction is often seen with SI joint dysfunction.

The three most common causes of low back pain are:

- Muscle/connective tissue shortening with some nerve entrapment.
- Trigger point activity in the psoas, quadratus lumborum, and hamstrings, which causes a more generalized, aching pain with painful spasm on sudden movement or coughing and sneezing. This pattern is aggravated by any type of static position, including prolonged lying down, and often results in restless activity, such as changing positions frequently.
- SI joint dysfunction, which has a more localized pain pattern. The pain normally gets worse as the day progresses and eases when the person lies down.

The three forms are often found in conjunction, which further complicates the issue.

The client in this case fits the profile of combined muscle, connective tissue, and SI joint dysfunction. She does not like exercise and movement, especially because walking is labored and awkward. She stands, twists, and lifts weight with her arms as she bags groceries, which puts strain on her low back. She is overweight, with the "apple type" fat distribution that shifts the center of gravity forward, requiring the back extensors to work harder to maintain an upright posture.

She has menstrual cramping, and the low back pain is worse during menstruation. This makes sense, because psoas tightening is common during menstruation. Stress tends to lower pain tolerance and increase muscle tension. The ridges in her nails and the hangnails indicate both long-term and current stress influence. The physical therapist has instituted a rehabilitation exercise program, and the client is following a walking program. Medication has not been identified as a long-term option.

What Are the Possibilities in Both Function and Dysfunction and the Massage Intervention Options?

The client has common symptoms of general low back pain with SI joint involvement. Her job activities are common causes of activities that can aggravate an existing situation. In her case, the job seems to be aggravating the symptoms, which range from occasional and bearable to constant and distressing.

She could likely be helped by mobilization of the SI joint, with recommendations provided to the physical therapist.

Because of the edema, some subclinical kidney dysfunction may be present that would result in low back aching; the patient should be referred for diagnosis of this condition. Menstrual difficulties are part of the history and might be an underlying factor.

Stress levels are increased and are likely contributing to the increase in pain perception. Chronic pain is disempowering emotionally and draining on the neurochemical functions of the body. All the endogenous opioids, such as endorphins and serotonin, and other mood-elevating neurochemicals may be insufficient for the current demands in her life, and the results of this insufficiency are sporadic mood difficulties and increased pain perception. Referral to the physician with a recommendation for counseling and possible trial of one of the serotonin-modulating medicines is prudent.

The client's generally inactive lifestyle has resulted in deconditioning and a predisposition to muscle aching. This, combined with her excess weight and the abdominal fat distribution, is likely a main causal factor.

Possibilities

1. General massage can be provided with a focus on restoring pliability to shortened connective tissue structures and reducing trigger points activated in the short muscles, accompanied by muscle energy methods to lengthen the short muscle groups and restore normal firing patterns.
2. Lymphatic drainage massage is indicated to manage the edema.
3. Reflexology may be effective, especially when combined with full-body massage, because it is well tolerated and the client shows shortening of the plantar fasciae.
4. Stress levels could be managed with massage and some sort of gentle movement activity, such as walking or yoga or both.
5. Aromatherapy is an option in conjunction with massage and as a self-help measure.

Recommendations are indicated for an increased intake of water, fresh fruits, and vegetables, in addition to mineral salt soaking baths, to support normal fluid balance in the interstitial space; this would reduce the edema. A combined, multidisciplinary approach offers the greatest likelihood of sustained benefit.

What Are the Logical Outcomes of Each Possible Intervention?

Cost is a factor in all the massage applications. Time is limited, as is the client's stamina. Too much intervention would tend to overwhelm her, and compliance would decrease. She is already seeing a physical therapist and walking.

Massage may provide the most benefit, with little energy requirement from the client. Aromatherapy and hydrotherapy are self-maintaining and pleasant and have low cost and time factors.

What Is the Impact on the People Involved for Each Possible Intervention?

The client likes the massage, mineral salt bath, and aromatherapy ideas but is resistant to yoga. She seems a bit desperate, and the massage therapist will have to monitor boundary issues and maintain a supportive relationship with other caregivers.

Decision Making and Treatment Plan Development

Quantifiable Goals

1. Increase mobility of the lumbar region by 75%
2. Reduce pain-affected days by 50%
3. Restore normal gait and firing patterns

Qualifiable Goal

The client will be able to perform work and school activities without limitations caused by low back pain 5 of 7 days a week. She will experience less fatigue when walking.

Treatment Regimen

Condition management will be pursued, with moderate expectations of therapeutic change.

A 1-hour massage will be provided twice a week for the first 4 weeks or until improvement is noted and indicated by reduced pain perception and an increased range of motion. The frequency then will be reduced to once a week. This may be the maintenance schedule, because ongoing massage intervention is probably in order to maintain a stable condition after physical therapy is complete.

The massage will consist of full-body application with reflexology and lymphatic drainage.

The focus is to increase mood-elevating chemicals with a broad-based, deep but not painful, compressive force and rhythmic application. Once the stress levels have dropped, the decreased pliability of shortened connective tissue structures can be addressed with myofascial methods. Reduction of trigger point activity in the short muscles is indicated, using positional release and direct pressure. Trigger point work will be combined with muscle energy methods and lengthening for the short muscle groups.

The client will be referred to an aromatherapist for consultation and recommendation regarding essential oils to be used during the massage and for self-application.

The client will be taught self-help measures, including hydrotherapy consisting of soaking baths, heat on the aching muscles, and cold on the joint pain. The client will be taught self foot massage and how to use softballs, baseballs, and foam rollers to massage painful areas in her back.

Close contact with the physical therapist will be necessary to achieve effective treatment for the client. The client will also be referred to her physician for recommendations regarding counseling and medication for mood regulation.

CASE 6 ATHLETIC DELAYED ONSET MUSCLE SORENESS

The client is a 22-year-old rookie cornerback professional football player. It is the second week of training camp, and the weather is hot and humid. The training regimen includes various running and sprinting segments, position-dependent drills, and strengthening and conditioning with a weightlifting program. The team's warm-up includes stretching activities. Maximum performance is required to secure a position on the team, and the competition is fierce. During the past 5 days, the team has been practicing in full equipment for the morning practice and in pads, helmet, and shorts for the afternoon practice. The training staff has been diligent about keeping all players hydrated, and ice baths are available. The client has been regularly soaking his legs in the ice water tubs.

One afternoon the client reports to the trainer that he aches all over and has some cramping in his hamstrings and calves. The leg cramping goes away with increased hydration and ingestion of electrolytes. He has been referred to the team massage therapist for management of delayed onset muscle soreness. The client does not want the massage during the afternoon break, because he is afraid it will affect his afternoon practice; therefore, he is requesting evening sessions after team meetings.

Assessment

Observation

The client is emotionally pumped but seems fatigued. His movements are generally a bit stiff. He keeps trying to stretch out while talking. He shows upper chest breathing, he is talking fast, and the exhale is shorter than the inhale. His phasic (movement) muscles appear bulked up.

Interview and Goals

When asked how well he is sleeping, he reports that he is tossing and turning and cannot get comfortable. He also reports a 5-pound weight gain and an increase in thigh, arm, and chest measurements. His history indicates a grade 2 groin pull on the right the last year of college. It healed well but continues to get stiff. He has to keep the area stretched out or he feels the pulling. He has been playing football since high school. Nothing unusual is disclosed in the history form except a recent tendency for constipation. On a pain scale of 1 to 10, he says he feels like a 12.

His goals for the massage are to reduce the aching and stiff feelings and to enhance his athletic performance. The trainer's goal is management of delayed onset muscle soreness.

Physical Assessment

Posture
Appropriate for football positional demands.

Gait
Slightly reduced stride on the right.

Range of Motion
Abduction of the right leg is reduced by 10% compared with the left leg and has a binding end-feel. Elbow and knee flexion bilaterally are reduced slightly because of soft tissue approximation (muscle tissue bumping into itself).

Palpation
Near Touch. Client generally is giving off heat.
Skin. Generally taut and damp with axillae, feet, and hand sweating. Binding at clavicles; may interfere with lymph flow. Tissue in general feels dense but boggy.
Superficial Connective Tissue. Dense
Vessels and Lymph Nodes. Difficult to palpate, because they seem buried in tissue.
Muscles. Muscle tone is appropriate for training effect. General tone is increased from client's first visit a month ago, indicating a response to training effects during training camp. Gluteus maximus is short and tight.
Tendons. General tenderness at musculotendinous junction in the phasic (movement) muscles of the arms and legs.
Deep Fascia. Mild binding during both superior and inferior movement in the sheath that runs from the cranial base to the sacrum and continues down the iliotibial band into the calves. Bind also is noted in the abdominal muscles and the pectoralis fasciae.
Ligaments. Normal
Joints. Aching increased with traction, indicating a soft tissue problem as a primary causal factor.
Bones. Normal
Abdominal Viscera. Abdominal muscle development makes palpation difficult; appears normal, with some fullness over the descending colon.
Body Rhythms. Fast upper chest breathing pattern.

Muscle Testing

Strength
All muscles test strong, but excessive synergistic recruitment is evident.

Neurologic Balance
Generalized hypersensitivity, evidenced by a fast, jerky contraction pattern and inability to contract muscles slowly.

Gait
Normal, but inhibition pattern for the arms is slow to engage (it takes a few seconds for muscles to let go).

Interpretation and Treatment Plan Development

Clinical Reasoning

What Are the Facts?
Delayed onset muscle soreness is a complicated response to increased physical and muscular activity demands. It can be local or generalized, depending on the activity. Although the term *delayed onset muscle soreness* indicates a muscle problem, the situation more likely involves the circulatory, lymph, and autonomic nervous systems and breathing functions. Simple delayed onset muscle soreness in local areas results when a muscle moves repetitively in eccentric contractions. This is common in any type of weight-training program intended to bulk up, or create hypertrophy, in muscles. Inflammation occurs and possibly some microtearing of muscle fibers. Inflammatory mediators (primarily histamine), which are released during physical activity, increase capillary permeability; as a result, interstitial fluid accumulates, causing simple edema. The increased fluid pressure in the tissue stimulates pain receptors, making the person feel stiff and achy.

In addition, the buildup of metabolic byproducts (not lactic acid) from exercise irritates nerve endings. Increased muscle tone can result in pressure on lymphatic vessels, interfering with the normal lymphatic flow and further stressing the lymphatic system. In addition, increased sympathetic arousal, which is part of athletic function, especially in contact sports, increases arterial pressure and blood flow. If the normal expansion in the capillary bed of the muscle is restricted because of increased muscle tension and connective tissue thickening, more plasma flows out of the capillaries but cannot return, requiring the lymphatic system to handle the increased interstitial fluid volume. When the body is in a sympathetic state, the ground substance of the connective tissue thickens to provide more resistance to impact. This process should reverse itself when arousal diminishes and parasympathetic dominance takes over, but often with athletes the arousal levels do not reverse and the connective tissue remains thicker, placing pressure on pain receptors and contributing to stiffness. The combination of fluid pressure and connective tissue thickening makes the tissue feel taut and dense. More complex patterns result with sustained sympathetic arousal. Upper chest breathing patterns and a tendency for breathing pattern disorders are common and perpetuate the underlying sympathetic arousal.

Management of this condition requires the reduction of any muscle tension interfering with circulation and lymphatic flow, mechanical drainage of interstitial fluid, support for arterial and venous circulation, reduction of the sympathetic arousal pattern, and an increase in ground substance pliability. The process must be accomplished without adding any inflammation to the tissues. Frictioning and any other methods that would cause tissue damage are contraindicated.

The delayed onset muscle soreness seen in planned training programs is to be expected. Each sport (in this case football) position places specific demands on certain movement patterns. It is essential that massage applications support the training effect and not interfere with it. Although symmetry in form is ideal, specific sport demand causes hypertrophy in certain muscle groups, and body-wide compensation occurs during a normal training regimen. This has to be considered during the assessment and the application of massage.

This particular client has symptoms of combined delayed onset muscle soreness and sustained sympathetic arousal. His breathing is appropriate to training activity but is not reversing during down time; consequently, his sleep is disturbed, and he is constipated. Tissues are filled with fluid, and thickened ground substance makes the tissue feel dense. Connective tissue binding exists in the back and the groin, especially on the right, and in the chest in the area of the right and left lymphatic ducts. Reduced abdominal movement, resulting from the upper chest breathing and the overdeveloped abdominal muscles (primarily the rectus abdominis), does not support movement of the lymph in the abdominal cavity. The muscle strength, with synergistic recruitment and slow response to inhibition patterns, can be attributed to overtraining and sympathetic arousal.

What Are the Possibilities in Both Function and Dysfunction and the Massage Intervention Options?

The client probably is excited about being in professional football and trying to prove himself in camp. He may have some anxiety about making the team, because competition is fierce for his position. This all contributes to the sympathetic arousal. He may be overtraining, especially in the weight room, because he is quickly bulking up.

The training regimen in general is a cause of a delayed onset muscle soreness pattern and stress. The weight of equipment worn during practice (about 20 pounds) is a new strain on the system, and adjusting to it can increase soft tissue soreness. Needing to learn all the plays in the playbook can add to the stress.

Possibilities

In combination with the athletic trainer's support and proper hydration, massage can be focused to achieve the following:
1. Reduce the sympathetic arousal
2. Soften the connective tissue ground substance
3. Increase lymphatic flow

Stretching could be increased and weight training intensity reduced to more appropriate levels.

What Are the Logical Outcomes of Each Possible Intervention?

The massage will likely help but needs to be done in the evening before the client goes to bed. This will make scheduling difficult.

The player must stay hydrated, and increased urine production may awaken him at night, interfering with sleep.

If the massage intervention is too intense, he may be sluggish the next day and his performance will be compromised.

Sleep would improve, which would reduce the recovery time. Reflexes should be more appropriate, and coordination and timing should improve, which supports performance.

What Is the Impact on the People Involved for Each Possible Intervention?

Training personnel referred the client; therefore, they are supportive. The position coach does not like rookies "babied" and feels that the client should "tough it out" a bit and not look like a whiner. The player has had massage before and liked it but is worried about anything that could affect his performance. The massage therapist feels that it is important to deal with the situation but does not enjoy beginning massage at 9:30 PM. The player is likely to respond to the nurturing and to notice a reduction in anxiety.

Decision Making and Treatment Plan Development

Quantifiable Goals

1. Reduce pain sensation to a tolerable 5 (on a scale of 1 to 10)
2. Ease feelings of stiffness by 50%
3. Normalize breathing

Qualifiable Goals

The player will be able to perform at or near optimum levels and will be able to participate in all training activities without excessive soreness.

Treatment Regimen

Condition Management

Daily massage will be given for 5 days just before bed for 45 minutes. The frequency then will be reduced to two times per week. Lymphatic drainage and circulation enhancement massage with rhythmic, broad-based compression deep enough to spread muscle fibers in all muscle layers and to increase serotonin and endogenous opiate (endorphin) availability will be provided. Application of all methods should not create any inflammation or alter the training effect. The focus will be on reducing sympathetic arousal and normalizing muscle tension, reflex patterns, and fluid dynamics in the body. Limited use of myofascial release in the binding tissue of the back, groin, and chest, along with controlled used of kneading, primarily to squeeze out the capillary beds and soften the ground substance, is appropriate. Abdominal massage to encourage peristalsis, with a specific focus on the large intestines to move fecal matter, is indicated. Breathing, muscle tone, firing pattern, reflexes, and sleep patterns will be monitored as indicators that the player is responding to massage.

CASE 7 THIRD TRIMESTER PREGNANCY

The client is 34 years old and in the eighth month of her second pregnancy. She has a 9-year-old son. The pregnancy has progressed normally, and the client has had the usual minor complaints of nausea, swelling in the ankles, low back ache, and shoulder and neck pain. She has noticed that her breathing has become more labored in the past 2 weeks. She feels pressure on her bladder, but bowel function is normal. She has been receiving massage on and off during the pregnancy. Now that her posture is changing with the increase in the size of the baby, she is more uncomfortable and wants to begin a more frequent and regular schedule of massage until the baby is born. She lives in the country, and the weather has been snowy and icy. Because she feels clumsy and is concerned about falling, she has been staying home and would prefer on-site massage sessions.

Assessment

Observation

The client's movement is awkward, and she often places her hands on the lumbar area for support. She breathes with her neck and shoulder muscles and is at times short of breath. The baby looks as if he or she has taken up all available abdominal space and is still being carried high in the abdomen.

Interview and Goals

The baby has a normal activity level and has not settled into the head-down position. Nothing on the history form indicates problems with the pregnancy or cautions for massage. The client takes a prenatal vitamin but no other medications. Her obstetrician is an osteopath who supports massage. The doctor did some joint manipulation earlier in the pregnancy but would prefer that other methods be used until after the baby's birth.

The client's goals for the massage are to be more comfortable in general, to reduce the edema, to sleep better, and to ease the muscle and joint aching in both her low back and neck. She realizes that the effects of massage are temporary, but at this point, even a few hours of relief would be welcome.

Physical Assessment

Posture

Functional lordosis as a result of the pregnancy.

Gait

Normal contralateral gait pattern is evident, but the increased weight in the front, coupled with the change in the center of gravity, makes movement awkward and labored.

Range of Motion

Forward flexion of the trunk is limited by the pregnancy. Lateral bending is limited in both directions and is linked to the client feeling as if she is losing her balance. Range of motion in the ankles and wrists is mildly limited by the edema. Lateral flexion of the head is reduced to 30 degrees bilaterally.

Palpation

Near Touch. Increased heat is noted in the upper shoulders. Over the abdomen, a sense of an increase in the density of the air is noted, and the baby moves during this palpation.

Skin. Skin is generally dry and a bit flaky but shows no abnormal color changes. It is slightly rough, and stretch marks are present in the lower abdomen. The skin is mobile over the connective tissue except in areas of edema. Hair is a bit dry, and some has fallen out.

Superficial Connective Tissue. Pliable and resilient

Vessels and Lymph Nodes. Normal

Muscles. Neck and shoulder muscles that function as breathing muscles are short, as are the back extensors.

Tendons. Tenderness at abdominal attachments.

Deep Fascia. Normal for this stage of pregnancy; abdominal fascia is stretched.

Ligaments. General laxity, normal for this stage of pregnancy.

Joints. Joint play is increased in all major joints. Symphysis pubis is up-slipped on the right. SI joint is mobile but compressed, as are the lumbar vertebrae. Rib movement is restricted by the baby.

Bones. Normal

Abdominal Viscera. Unable to palpate

Body Rhythms. Even and slightly slow. Breathing is labored and occasionally out of sync with the other body rhythms. Pulse points are even in the legs.

Muscle Testing

Not performed.

Interpretation and Treatment Plan Development

Clinical Reasoning

What Are the Facts?

Normal pregnancy is a healthy state, with caution implicated for massage. In the first trimester, the main concern is not to overstress the mother in any way that would interfere with normal development of the baby. Deep abdominal massage is avoided, as are any invasive and painful massage or bodywork approaches.

Consideration is necessary for the hormonal changes that may result in increased sensitivity to odors or mood changes. Breasts enlarge and are tender, and fatigue is common. During the second trimester, the hormonal changes result in connective tissue changes, and joint stability may become somewhat loose. The abdomen begins to expand, and lying on the stomach is uncomfortable unless support is provided. The body's response to hormonal changes evens out. In the third trimester, strain is put on the postural muscles, because the center of gravity shifts forward. Pressure from the growing baby compresses the abdominal contents; this interferes with normal diaphragmatic breathing and can increase the urgency or frequency of urination. Edema is common in the ankles and wrists. Getting comfortable becomes difficult. Backaches and neck and shoulder aching are common. Backache results from the shift in the center of gravity and from the intraabdominal pressure; neck and shoulder pain arises from the use of accessory muscles for breathing. The breasts continue to change and enlarge, preparing for lactation. All these conditions reverse themselves over time after the baby's birth.

Management and comfort care (palliation) are the goals at this stage of pregnancy.

This client shows the normal third trimester adaptations of the body.

What Are the Possibilities in Both Function and Dysfunction and the Massage Intervention Options?

The SI joint pain and lumbar area aching are likely caused by the functional lordosis and joint laxity. The short shoulder and neck muscles are attributable to the use of accessory breathing muscles. The mild edema in the ankles and wrists is common in the third trimester because of the increased strain on the lymphatic system and because some of the lymph pathways are obstructed by the baby and by postural shifts.

Possibilities

1. Full-body massage can provide hyperstimulation analgesia to reduce the aching. It also can lengthen the shortened neck and shoulder muscles and assist in movement of the lymphatics, with caution.
2. Caution is indicated with stretching and joint movement, because hypermobility is noted in the joints. The up-slipped symphysis pubis is consistent with the posture shifts and compression of the SI joints; this condition increases the sensation of pelvic instability.
3. Because the client's obstetrician is an osteopath, referral for manipulation of the SI joints and symphysis pubis could bring short-term relief. This could be continued until the baby has been born and the pelvis stabilizes.

What Are the Logical Outcomes of Each Possible Intervention?

The client wants massage at home; therefore, the cost is higher to cover travel and set-up time. Her husband and son can be taught basic massage methods so that they can help during the final weeks of pregnancy.

Positioning on the side will require alteration of some massage applications and can strain the massage practitioner's body mechanics somewhat, because the ideal positioning for leaning uphill in some areas may not be available. The side-lying position is generally supportive and is effective for body mechanics. Additional bolsters are necessary.

What Is the Impact on the People Involved for Each Possible Intervention?

The massage therapist is supportive of home visits for a short time.

Decision Making and Treatment Plan Development

Quantifiable Goal

Increase comfort levels, as self-reported by the client

Qualifiable Goals

The client will be supported, her stress will be reduced in the final stages of pregnancy, and she will be prepared for effective delivery.

Treatment Regimen

Palliative Care/Some Condition Management

Full-body massage will be provided twice a week for 1 hour at an in-home rate of $50 per hour plus a $30 travel and set-up fee. The massage position will be altered to side-lying, with the client lying primarily on the left side as long as she is comfortable.

Pressure will be broad based and applied to a depth that is comfortable, and the focus will be on supporting the circulation but not specifically on performing full-body lymphatic drainage. Broad-based compression will be used for the short muscles of the neck, shoulders, and upper chest while the client moves her head or arm in circles to relax the accessory breathing muscles. Gentle traction of the SI joint and lumbar vertebrae to ease compression will be incorporated into the general massage session. Full-body rhythmic massage will create counterirritation and hyperstimulation analgesia, reducing the perception of discomfort for a short time.

Note: For these massages, special attention should be given to atmosphere, such as soft music and lighting, with a parasympathetic focus. Scentless massage lubrication should be used, because the client is sensitive to odors. It is important to entrain the body rhythms of the mother and baby. Care must be taken to match but not superimpose any rhythm patterns. Gentle, soothing, circular stroking of the abdomen can increase the pliability of the stretched skin in the area. Foot massage is comforting and balancing. Pressure on the inside of the ankle and up the calf should be avoided. If the client's breasts are aching, she can be taught a circular gliding massage technique for the breast area.

CASE 8 PREMENSTRUAL SYNDROME

The client is a single, 29-year-old female with a 5-year-old child. She has been diagnosed with premenstrual syndrome (PMS). After ovulation she is increasingly irritable and anxious. She experiences general swelling and some bloating. Often, but not always, she gets a migraine headache about a week before her menstrual period. Her weight is within normal range for her height, but she can increase half a clothing size during the menstrual period.

She takes ibuprofen as needed for pain, and she is taking a multivitamin and additional B vitamins. She is weaning herself off coffee by switching to green tea, which also has caffeine but not as much as coffee. On weekends she rides her bike and roller-blades for exercise. She has not changed her diet. She recently joined a PMS support group.

The client has a stable income, but the days off work and the mood fluctuations during her premenstrual period are beginning to disturb her employer. Currently, she is 3 days past ovulation and just beginning to experience symptoms.

Assessment

Observation

The client is clearly distressed about her mood swings, as indicated by her emphatic voice tone and her facial expression. She appears bloated.

Interview and Goals

The history form indicates that the client has migraine headaches and that she uses a barrier method for birth control. She has had one pregnancy. She severely sprained her right ankle 3 years ago. She experiences digestive bloat and low back ache just before her period. She appears fatigued, and she says she suffers from sleep difficulties and nervous tension the second half of her menstrual cycle. She falls asleep but wakes up frequently and cannot get back to sleep.

The client is intent on management of the premenstrual syndrome and indicates that her goals for the massage are to focus on and deal with the fluid retention and chemical imbalance that accompany PMS.

Physical Assessment

Posture

Posture is symmetric, with the shoulders slightly rolled forward. Weight is dispersed to the inside of the right foot, and the right knee is mildly hyperextended.

Gait

Normal except for flat-foot loading, in which the weight is on the inside rather than the outside of the right foot.

Range of Motion

Within normal range except for moderate hypermobility in the right ankle.

Palpation

Near Touch. No perceivable abnormality

Skin. Oily and smooth with binding noted in the superior (cranial) direction (tissue moves down, binds when moved up) around the right ankle and upper chest.

Superficial Connective Tissue. Evidence of fluid retention, with pitting edema in the ankles.

Vessels and Lymph Nodes. Lymph node areas in the axillae display tenderness to moderate pressure.

Muscles. Trigger point activity is present in the right medial gastrocnemius.

Tendons. Right Achilles tendon is slightly short.

Deep Fascia. Sheath between the gastrocnemius and the soleus on the right seems bound together.

Ligaments. Deltoid ligament on the right ankle is unstable and lax.

Joints. Right ankle is hypermobile and has increased joint play.

Bones. Normal

Abdominal Viscera. Abdomen is boggy and moderately distended. Lower abdomen is tender to moderate pressure.

Body Rhythms. Breathing is uneven and slow, with no current evidence of upper chest breathing. Cardiac pulses are normal but changeable from 55 to 70 beats per minute without change in activity. Craniosacral undulation is reduced, which is common with static lymphatic movement.

Muscle Testing

Strength

Not performed.

Neurologic Balance

Not performed.

Gait

Normal except for the gastrocnemius and the soleus on the right, which do not inhibit when appropriate.

Interpretation and Treatment Plan Development

Clinical Reasoning

What Are the Facts?

Premenstrual syndrome is a collection of symptoms that include fluid retention, bloating, headache, backache, changes in balance mechanisms and coordination, food cravings, irritability, anxiety, depression, and decreased ability to concentrate. Women may experience a few or many of the symptoms, and this is changeable from cycle to cycle. All of the causal factors for premenstrual syndrome have yet to be discovered. Imbalances in serotonin and dopamine are evident. The increase in progesterone during the postovulation period supports fluid retention. Prostaglandins seem to be a factor in the pain and cramping, and aspirin and other nonsteroidal antiinflammatory drugs are often prescribed because they interfere with prostaglandin synthesis.

This client shows common premenstrual symptoms, especially bloating, fluid retention, irritability, food cravings, and headache. The symptoms are severe enough to compromise her work situation. She also has mild postural distortion and ankle hypermobility.

What Are the Possibilities in Both Function and Dysfunction and the Massage Intervention Options?

Serotonin imbalance is evidenced by the chocolate and carbohydrate cravings, and dopamine imbalance by the irritability. Because ibuprofen helps the pain and cramping, prostaglandins are likely to be involved. The progesterone increase during the postovulation period can contribute to the fluid retention, bloating, and breathing changes. The distress from the symptoms could be increasing the sympathetic fight-or-flight response, creating a self-perpetuating cycle.

Possibilities

1. Massage would promote fluid and neurochemical balance and reduce sympathetic arousal.
2. Recommendations for meditative movement activity, such as tai chi or yoga, and referral to an herbalist and aromatherapist for evaluation are viable options.

What Are the Logical Outcomes of Each Possible Intervention?

Massage is cost-effective, and the closeness of the massage practitioner's office to the client's work place makes it convenient. The appointment schedule may vary, depending on the symptoms. Massage once a week is appropriate during the preovulatory phase; more frequent sessions should be scheduled during the symptom phase.

The only herbalist and aromatherapist is a 2-hour drive away, but because frequent appointments are not required, this should not be a limiting factor. These products can be expensive. A tai chi class is available through the support group.

What Is the Impact on the People Involved for Each Possible Intervention?

The client is motivated and indicates compliance with keeping appointments. The support group also recommends tai chi and yoga and other therapies, such as aromatherapy.

Decision Making and Treatment Plan Development

Quantifiable Goals

1. Reduce self-reported PMS symptoms by 50%
2. Reduce by 75% the number of days the client takes off work because of PMS symptoms

Qualifiable Goal

The client will experience increased well-being and reduction of mood swings.

Treatment Regimen

Condition Management

Massage appointments will be made weekly until the symptoms appear and then twice weekly until the symptoms dissipate. One-hour sessions are indicated at $40 per session. The sessions will include general massage to reduce sympathetic arousal, with a broad-based compressive force that has pressure depth but that does not cause any guarding or pain. Sufficient pressure will be necessary to increase serotonin and endorphin availability. An increase in these chemicals should reduce food cravings and pain perception and hopefully level the mood fluctuations. Lymphatic drainage will be used to reduce tissue fluid. Because the pressure of superficial lymphatic drainage is very light (just moving the skin), this will be the last method used during the massage.

The client also displays compensation patterns from the ankle sprain and a rolled shoulder pattern, likely from the biking. Because these areas have no direct effect on premenstrual syndrome management and the client's goals, they will not be addressed specifically during the initial treatment plan massage, although improvement may be noted with general massage application. The ankle compensation patterns may become an issue in future sessions, and the treatment plan can be amended at that time.

CASE 9 REPETITIVE STRAIN/OVERUSE INJURY: BURSITIS

The client is a 48-year-old man who has been diagnosed with bursitis of the left elbow. He is a manager of a retail center, and most of his day involves phone and computer work. The bursa at the olecranon around the attachment of the triceps has become irritated and inflamed. The client fell and hit the elbow 6 months ago. The bursa was injured but healed with no apparent problems. The client recently began a

weight-training program that includes biceps and triceps toning. He admits that he overtrained, doing both upper body and lower body exercises every day instead of following an alternate-day pattern. In addition, he used more weight than was necessary.

The client was given a cortisone injection at the inflamed site and is taking aspirin. He has been told to rest the area and maintain range of motion but not to lift weight with the arm. The client expresses concern about losing recently acquired muscle tone and bulking. He had become overweight and deconditioned in his early 40s after being very fit in his 20s and 30s. He is determined to reclaim a fit body. He is already receiving massage on a weekly basis with the goal of managing stress and the muscle soreness caused by exercise. He is now specifically focused on reversing the bursitis.

Assessment

Observation

The client is a bit restless and impatient. Frustration is evident in his voice over what seems to him to be a delay in his training program. He rubs the sore elbow often.

Interview and Goals

The client is taking a muscle-building supplement that contains various vitamins and amino acids. He slipped on the ice and severely bruised the left elbow. It was speculated that he may have ruptured the bursa at the olecranon. The bursitis is in the acute, possibly subacute, stage. The history indicates a family tendency for cardiovascular problems, primarily arteriosclerosis. The death of a relative prompted the client to begin a diet and exercise program. His blood pressure is slightly elevated but is not being treated medically, and his doctor expects that it will fall into the normal range with weight reduction, stress management, and exercise.

Physical Assessment

Posture

Mild anterior rotation of the left shoulder and moderate anterior rotation of the left pelvis are seen. The left elbow is carried in a flexed, loose-packed position.

Gait

Client's stride is short when he moves forward on the right leg and counterbalances, with the right arm moving into extension instead of the left arm.

Range of Motion

Pain limits flexion and extension of the left elbow to 100 degrees. External rotation of the left arm is limited to 70 degrees.

Palpation

Near Touch. Area of the bursa in the left arm is warm.
Skin. Skin is damp and slightly red near the bursal inflammation. Goose bumps are seen with light skin stroking over the bursal inflammation, and skin binding at the triceps attachment.

Superficial Connective Tissue. Adherent at the triceps attachment at the elbow.

Vessels and Lymph Nodes. Normal

Muscles. Triceps and biceps are short on the left. Quadriceps are long and taut and hamstrings are short on the right. Muscle mass of biceps seems out of proportion to triceps. Internal rotators of the left arm are short, with inhibition of the external rotators. Gluteus maximus on the left is inhibited and flaccid and not firing appropriately during hypertension.

Tendons. Tendons are tender to moderate pressure at the right hamstring attachment at the pelvis and at all attachments of the left triceps.

Deep Fascia. Iliotibial band is binding in all directions on the right leg.

Ligaments. No palpable problems

Joints. Compression of the left elbow joint does not cause additional pain, but traction does; the problem likely is in the primary soft tissue.

Bones. Normal

Abdominal Viscera. Normal

Body Rhythms. Fast, with some indication of sympathetic arousal and upper chest breathing.

Muscle Testing

Strength

Triceps on the left is inhibited, and biceps is too strong; quadriceps is inhibited, and hamstring is too strong on the right. Left gluteus maximus is weak. Trigger point activity is found in these same muscle groups, with the trigger point in the belly of the short, concentrically contracted muscles and at the attachments of the inhibited, long, eccentrically contracted muscles.

Neurologic Balance

Client is unable to increase resistance gradually against pressure; he uses maximum force, and movement is abrupt and jerky. Abdominal muscles are not firing appropriately.

Gait

Gait patterns are normal, even though local inhibition and increased tone are noted with individual strength testing of direct antagonist and antagonist patterns.

Interpretation and Treatment Plan Development

Clinical Reasoning

What Are the Facts?

Bursitis is an inflammation of the synovial fluid–filled sacs around joints, tendons, and ligaments. Bursitis develops with impact trauma, sustained compression (it is often found in the knees of carpet layers, carpenters, and others who do a lot of work on their knees), and repetitive strain. Repetitive movement causes both friction and a tendency for shortening of the muscle and connective tissue structures, which further increases the tendency for rubbing, causing inflammation. Bursitis can also occur if the position of the bones of the joint

and ligament alignment changes, or if the muscles pull unevenly on the joint structures.

This type of inflammation responds to applications of ice, nonsteroidal antiinflammatory drugs (e.g., aspirin) and, if necessary, localized injection of a steroid. The medication, especially aspirin, thins blood. Massage pressure needs to be altered to prevent bruising during massage. Areas where the steroid was injected must be avoided, because the medication exerts its effect on the local tissues, and massage may disperse the steroid. Recently, transdermal patches of antiinflammatory and analgesic drugs have been used successfully instead of injection, but the same cautions exist. The muscle and connective tissue elements around the inflamed bursa are usually short, and lengthening and stretching of this soft tissue are necessary. If the problem is localized and not the result of a more general postural shift, spot work may be helpful. However, as soon as the body begins to compensate for the condition, full-body effects develop, therefore even localized bursitis is best addressed in the context of full-body massage.

This client shows connective tissue shortening around the olecranon, with both the agonist and antagonist for elbow flexion short and tight on the affected side. A corresponding pattern that does not show symptoms is present in the opposite leg.

What Are the Possibilities in Both Function and Dysfunction and the Massage Intervention Options?

The previous injury may have caused some scar tissue and shortening of the triceps tendon. The rotational pattern of the shoulder and hip also increases the likelihood of the triceps rubbing at the attachment on the elbow. The short, tight muscles with trigger points may be changing the joint angle and orientation of the connecting bones, increasing the likelihood of friction at the bursa. The repetitive strain of the weight lifting for the biceps and triceps is partly causal and likely aggravating the scar tissue from the previous injury. The client admits to overtraining, and he also may be training the flexors more than the extensors of the affected elbow, setting up the muscle imbalance. Massage is indicated, and better results would be obtained if the sessions were scheduled for every other day.

Possibilities

1. Friction and myofascial release are options in the areas of connective tissue adhesion.
2. Direct pressure combined with muscle energy methods is indicated for the trigger points in the concentrically short muscles.
3. Lengthening and stretching of the short muscles, with stimulation of the eccentric and inhibited muscles, could be effective.

What Are the Logical Outcomes of Each Possible Intervention?

Massage to lengthen the shortened muscles and ease the connective tissue dysfunction would reduce the tendency for rubbing. If eccentrically activated muscles are further inhibited and become longer, the situation can worsen. Connective tissue binding is at the triceps, and further complications of the situation would need to be addressed in combination with muscle stimulation of the triceps and reduction of excessive shortening of the biceps.

Massage directly over the site of the steroid injection is contraindicated for at least 7 more days, which interferes with application of scar tissue release in the area. The client is taking aspirin and therefore may bruise with direct application of compression to trigger points. Alternate methods are needed to address the trigger point problem. The client needs to ice the area frequently.

Because this is a regular client, an increase in massage frequency is a time and cost burden. The massage therapist will have to find available scheduling to accommodate the more frequent appointments.

What Is the Impact on the People Involved for Each Possible Intervention?

Because the client is already receiving massage, the additional appointments are acceptable as long as results are readily apparent within a month. The client's expectations are a bit unrealistic. He resists ice application.

The massage therapist is willing to accommodate the increase in the number of appointments for a short time.

Decision Making and Treatment Plan Development
Quantifiable Goals

1. Restore range of motion of the left elbow and arm to normal
2. Reverse any compensation caused by postural changes

Qualifiable Goal

The client will be able to resume work and moderate, appropriate exercise and weight training without causing irritation of the bursa or elbow.

Treatment Regimen

Therapeutic Change/Return to Condition Management
Full-body massage appointments will be increased from once a week to three times per week for 1 month. The focus will be on generalized massage to address the compensation patterns in the opposite leg and the rotational pattern of the shoulder and pelvis. Compression, gliding, and kneading will be applied to the short biceps and hamstrings with tense-and-relax and lengthening techniques.

Tapotement and pulsed muscle energy methods will be used after general gliding and kneading to stimulate inhibited muscles and to focus on reducing trigger point activity and lengthening short muscles. In 1 week, connective tissue work will begin on the elbow, with myofascial approaches and skin rolling used to soften the ground substance for the first four sessions of connective tissue application. No additional inflammation will be introduced.

After this application, if heat and other indicators of inflammation are reduced in the area, very controlled use of friction and bending and shearing of adhered tissue can begin. This process needs to be monitored carefully to ensure that

the bursitis symptoms do not recur. Aspirin should be discontinued before the introduction of therapeutic inflammation, or the methods will not be as effective, because it is the inflammatory process that changes the connective tissue fiber structure. Depth of pressure will elicit a "good hurt" sensation, and all layers of the short and tight tissues need to be addressed, especially synergists and fixators in the deeper muscle layers.

CASE 10 JOINT SPRAIN WITH UNDERLYING HYPERMOBILITY AND LAX LIGAMENT SYNDROME

The client is a 16-year-old female cheerleader. She has been involved in dance and gymnastics since she was 5 years old. The client is generally in good health but has a history of various sprains and strains.

The current injury occurred when her leg tangled in a fellow cheerleader's leg, resulting in a grade 1 sprain of the lateral collateral ligament of the right knee. The deltoid ligament on the lateral aspect of her right ankle received a second-degree sprain when she landed on the outside of her foot. This same ankle was sprained last year.

Appropriate first aid was administered, and follow-up medical care included external stabilization and passive and active movement without weight bearing to promote healing with pliable scar tissue formation. Antiinflammatory and pain medications were used for the first 3 days and then withdrawn because these medications can slow healing. The client was on crutches for a few days until she could bear weight on her foot. Weight bearing has been allowed for the past 5 days. It has been 10 days since the accident.

The client's mother cleared the massage with her doctor, who supports the intervention to manage some of the compensation from using crutches and to promote healing of the injured area. The client complains of neck, shoulder, and low back stiffness and pain.

Assessment
Observation

The client is limping slightly. Discoloration is present around the ankle but not the knee. The ankle still appears swollen, but the knee looks normal. The client fidgets during the interview. Her mother is concerned but not overbearing, letting the client answer most questions and adding information where pertinent. The right ankle is wrapped with an elastic support.

Interview and Goals

The history notes multiple sprain injuries and a tendency for generalized hypermobility. The client hopes to participate in a cheerleading competition in 2 months. Her mother is more realistic, thinking it will be at least 3 months before the ankle is strong enough for competition. The client complains of being stiff all over. No unusually pertinent information is indicated on the history form.

The client's goals for the massage are to support healing of the injured ankle and knee, reduce the general stiffness, and reverse the compensation from limping and the use of crutches.

Physical Assessment

Posture

Client is not fully weight bearing on the injured leg. Her posture is very good except for a slight lordosis and hyperextension of her knees, which is common in gymnasts.

Gait

Limited by limping, pain, and a sense of instability.

Range of Motion

Client is generally hypermobile, most likely because of training effects from dance training, gymnastics, and cheerleading.

Palpation

Near Touch. Heat is detected at the ankle and knee injury sites and in the shoulders.

Skin. Drag and dampness are present in areas of heat. Bruising surrounds the area of ankle injury. Skin is smooth and pliable with no areas of bind noted.

Superficial Connective Tissue. Connective tissue is resilient. Localized swelling remains at lateral right ankle.

Vessels and Lymph Nodes. Normal

Muscles. Muscles feel elastic but generally shorter in the belly, especially the calves, hamstrings, and adductors. Trigger point activity is evident in the belly of the adductors, hamstrings, and quadriceps in the injured leg. Supraspinatus, upper trapezius, and pectoralis major and minor are short bilaterally, with tenderness in the axillae where the crutches contact. Psoas is short bilaterally. Muscles of the right leg have increased tone, most likely because of normal guarding of the injured joints. Quadratus lumborum and the gluteal group on the left are tender to moderate pressure. A very tender area near the musculotendinous junction of the lateral head of the right gastrocnemius palpates like a grade 1 muscle tear.

Tendons. Tendons in the muscles of the right leg are tender to moderate pressure.

Deep Fascia. Resilient but seem too long.

Ligaments. Generally loose

Joints. End-feel is not identified until the joint is in hyperextension. Increased joint play is noted in major mobility joints.

Bones. Normal

Abdominal Viscera. Normal

Body Rhythms. Normal

Muscle Testing

Strength and Neurologic Balance

Muscles test normal except for those guarding the injured knee and ankle, which is expected. These muscles are displaying increased tone and are not inhibited as expected. Left quadratus lumborum is firing before tensor fasciae latae and gluteus medius.

Gait

Gait is disrupted by limping and crutches. Flexor patterns in the arms are facilitating together instead of following contralateral patterns. Flexors and extensors of the left leg do not inhibit when tested against the arms.

Interpretation and Treatment Plan Development

Clinical Reasoning

What Are the Facts?

Ligament sprains and muscle strains are common injuries and are diagnosed as slight (first degree), moderate (second degree), or severe (third degree). When a joint shows a sprain (i.e., rupture of some or all of the ligament fibers), there is usually accompanying muscle strain with the possibility of muscle fiber tears. It is important not to stretch muscle tears in the acute phase. Protective spasm (guarding) is intense and painful in first- and second-degree tears. If a total breach of a muscle or tendon has occurred, the person may feel very little pain. First- and second-degree injuries are more painful and have a greater tendency for swelling than a third-degree injury. When a joint is sprained, strain in the muscles that are extended during the injury is common. Spasm around the tear (tiny microtears to more severe tears) acts to approximate (bring torn fibers together to support healing), protect, and guard the area. In general, all the muscles that surround the joint increase in tone to stabilize and reduce movement. This should dissipate as the injury heals but can become chronic, limiting range of motion of the area. Ligaments begin repair immediately, and the inflammatory response is an important part of this process. Some inflammatory mediators are vasodilators, which help blood reach ligaments. This is important, because ligaments do not have a good blood supply. Muscle tears heal much easier because of the high vascular component of the tissue. It takes 3 to 6 months or longer for a grade 2 sprain to heal fully. Repeated injury contributes to ligament laxity and joint instability.

Sprains are common in people with joint hypermobility. The hypermobility can occur in only one joint that has a recurring injury or can be more general, appearing in most joints of the body. Some disorders (e.g., Marfan's syndrome) are characterized by lax connective tissue. Most ligament laxity is functional, such as an increased range of motion required in many sports or dance activities. Once the plastic range of a ligament has been increased, it does not return to the previous range but remains long and lax. Joint play is increased, and instability results.

The client fits this profile. She will likely remain hypermobile, with increased compensating muscle tone to provide stability. This situation leads to general stiffness, especially if activity is reduced. Depending on the degree of laxity, the client may find that stretching does not reduce muscle tightness, because joint end-feel and longitudinal tensile force do not occur until the joint is hyperextended or reaches an anatomic barrier.

What Are the Possibilities in Both Function and Dysfunction and the Massage Intervention Options?

The client's gait changes seem to arise from the use of crutches. Because the injury is recent and the crutches are no longer used, gait dysfunction should easily reverse with massage and general activity.

The low back pain may stem from a dermatome distribution referring back from the knee combined with postural changes from limping and the use of crutches. The tendency for low back pain may exist because the client's psoas muscles are short.

Possibilities

1. Massage can support the healing process in the acute, subacute, and final healing stages by increasing circulation to the area, maintaining normal and appropriate muscle tone, and supporting mobile scar formation.
2. Referral for diagnosis of the suspected muscle tear is recommended.
3. Referral to a physical therapist or exercise physiologist for a sequential strengthening program for the vulnerable joints is indicated.

What Are the Logical Outcomes of Each Possible Intervention?

Massage intervention would need to be long term to meet the client's goals, with an incremental treatment plan for the current acute and subacute healing stages.

Cost and time are factors, and the mother or father needs to be with the client because she is a minor.

What Is the Impact on the People Involved for Each Possible Intervention?

The client has unrealistic healing expectations and likely will be frustrated with a 6-month intervention plan.

Decision Making and Treatment Plan Development

Quantifiable Goals

1. Reduce generalized stiffness by 75%
2. Reverse compensation caused by the use of crutches
3. Support circulation and scar formation in injured areas

Qualifiable Goals

The client will be able to resume normal daily activities, but not sports activities, within 2 weeks. She will be able to resume limited cheerleading activities within 6 weeks and full use of the area in 6 months.

Treatment Regimen

Condition Management/Therapeutic Change

Condition management consists of two phases. Therapeutic change is targeted for phase three.

- *Phase one: Acute phase (current).* One-hour massage will be provided three times for the first week. Full-body massage will be used to support circulation and reverse the muscle tension in the shoulders and chest caused by the use of crutches. Specific application of gliding will be used along the sprained ligament and associated strained tendons in the fiber direction of the muscle and toward the injury to help align the scar tissue. Lymphatic drainage in the swollen areas will support healing. Passive range of motion with rocking

and gentle shaking to all adjacent joints will encourage mobility and healing in the injured areas.

Ongoing ice application will encourage circulation as a secondary effect of the cold. The injured areas would benefit from ice application for 20 minutes two or three times a day.

- *Phase two: Subacute phase.* Ice applications will be valuable for 1 or 2 more weeks. Massage applications will be provided for full-body sessions twice a week for 6 weeks and then reduced in frequency to once a week for 3 months if healing is progressing well. Very gentle gliding across the fiber configuration of the tissue will support mobile scar formation. The intensity of gliding and cross-fiber friction on the injured tissues will gradually increase as healing continues. Trigger points and general tone in the muscles that are guarding will be addressed with muscle energy methods, lengthening, and broad-based compression. Kneading can restore the pliability of the connective tissue ground substance. The area of the gastrocnemius that may have been torn will be treated with caution. No deep pressure will be used, but localized stroking across the grain of the muscle can support mobile scar formation. Because self-stretching is not effective without moving into hyperextension patterns, the client's muscle tissue can be manually stretched and lengthened during massage with compression and kneading that introduce bending and torsion forces into the soft tissue. The psoas muscles can be lengthened with muscle energy methods.
- *Phase three: Therapeutic change.* Six months of weekly full-body massage will be provided. Once healing of the injury is complete, the underlying hypermobility can be addressed. Systematic frictioning can be applied to lax ligaments to introduce therapeutic inflammation and encourage increased connective tissue fiber formation. This will be applied to the injured lateral collateral ligament and deltoid ligament, as well as the rest of the connective tissue stabilizing units of the ankle and knee. This needs to be done in small increments, and the area should not be excessively painful the next day. Pain to the touch with moderate pressure is appropriate, but pain should not occur with movement. This is a painful intervention and needs to be done frequently. It is appropriate to teach a family member to perform the technique. Antiinflammatory drugs should not be used, nor should ice be applied to the area, because the goal is creation of controlled inflammation to encourage collagen formation. Full-body massage with direct tissue stretching should continue. At the end of the 6-month period, the frequency of massage intervention could be reduced to a maintenance schedule of every other week. The client will be encouraged to maintain a strengthening and stretching program and to reduce exaggerated joint movements to support restabilization of the joints.

CASE 11 OSTEOARTHRITIS AND ARTHROSIS

The client is a 67-year-old male with osteoarthritis and arthrosis in both knees. He is a sales manager, financially stable, and has a flexible schedule. He has always been active and has a history of participating in high school and college sports. He ran track and played basketball. During that time, he had various minor to moderate injuries, including knee trauma. In his words, "I would just tough it out and play anyway." To compound the problem, he was in a car accident when he was 36 and broke his left ankle. He also spent 12 years in the U.S. Marine Corps as a sergeant.

Currently he enjoys golf and racquetball. He does not want to use a golf cart, because he enjoys the walking, and he needs the exercise because of a cardiac condition. He plays racquetball for 1 hour on Tuesdays and Saturdays but really suffers with knee pain between times. His condition is worst at his early morning Sunday golf game. Initially, he is very stiff, which interferes with his golf swing, but he warms up as time goes on.

He uses topical capsicum cream and takes aspirin for the arthritis and for the cardiac condition. He is currently 20 pounds over what his doctors would like him to weigh. The extra weight bothers his knees. He thinks that he has gained some of the weight because the knee pain has slowed him down.

The left knee is more painful than the right. In the future he may undergo joint replacement surgery, but for now he is exploring any methods that will allow him to remain active.

He has never had massage and has the support of his physicians. Admittedly, he is skeptical about massage. He says he is not one to be "fussed over" and just wants the job done.

Assessment

Observation

The client is tall; 6 feet, 4 inches. He has long legs, a short torso, broad shoulders, and a bit of a pot belly. His center of gravity is high, which would place strain on the knees. He carries himself like a Marine. He is loud and gruff but seems kind underneath the facade. He seems a bit nervous about massage therapy. His shoulders move when he breathes.

Interview and Goals

The client says he aches all over but that he has lived hard and should expect to be creaky. The joint pain is worse in the morning, gets better as he moves around, and then gets worse again. He has had various and numerous joint injuries and soft tissue trauma. Four years ago his blood pressure rose, and he had angioplasty to unclog two coronary arteries. He takes aspirin to keep his blood thin and to manage the arthritis. He says that he does not seem to bruise easily. He was taking blood pressure medication but did not like the sexual side effects and insisted he go off it. The doctor agreed as long as the client could keep his blood pressure down with diet and exercise. He has done a good job of this. Nothing else of concern is indicated on the history form. He quit smoking 10 years ago. He used to drink heavily but now drinks only a glass or two of red wine two to three times a week. His sleep is restless, because his knees ache. Heat application helps.

The client's goal for the massage is management of his knee pain.

Physical Assessment

Posture

Overall, client has decent postural symmetry. Cervical curve is flat. Left foot is a bit flat. Ribs are held tight and rigid.

Gait

Client walks stiffly with reduced knee flexion and extension.

Range of Motion

Range of motion in most jointed areas is in the acceptable range for mild daily activities but stiff and resisting for any exercise. The left ankle is moderately restricted in eversion and inversion.

Palpation

Near Touch. Heat is noted at the knees and between the scapulae. Client has a presence of high energy that is felt as the air pressure–type of resistance noted when the same poles of a magnet are held together.

Skin. Rough and binding almost everywhere, with edema at the knees; there is evidence of many traumas (i.e., various scars in many body areas).

Superficial Connective Tissue. Reduced pliability body-wide —almost an armor-like feel, with edema at the knees.

Vessels and Lymph Nodes. Seem normal, but ability to palpate is restricted by tissue density.

Muscles. Well developed but dense and inflexible. Trigger point activity is evident in quadriceps and gluteals. Muscles that surround the knees have increased tone and isometric contraction in both antagonist and agonist patterns. These muscles obviously are attempting to guard the knee joints.

Tendons. Tender to moderate pressure around the knees and scapular attachment.

Deep Fascia. Thick and inflexible.

Ligaments. Mild laxity at injured ankle and knees.

Joints. Most are within the normal range of motion, but crepitus is common, as is a tendency for leathery or hard end-feel. Knees hurt with compression and traction. Most other joints show resistance to traction, indicating binding. Client indicates that most joints are stiff but not painful. Most of the pain is in the knees.

Bones. Increased bony development around the area of the ankle break. Bump noted in the right clavicle (client had forgotten he had broken it falling out of a tree when he was a child).

Abdominal Viscera. Difficult to palpate because of internal abdominal fat distribution.

Body Rhythms. Strong and fast. Client breathes with his chest but does not necessarily display breathing pattern disorder symptoms other than talking loudly and mild evidence of sympathetic arousal. Pulses are even, and cranial rhythm displays a strong, even undulation.

Muscle Testing

Strength

Client pushes hard against resistance and finds it difficult to use 50% effort. No areas of weakness are noted. Client was unable to isolate a muscle pattern and continually recruited and contracted muscles in areas other than the test area during assessment.

Neurologic Balance

Antagonist balance at knees is lost. All muscles around joint have a tendency for isometric contraction with uneven pull on the knee joint. Synergistic dominance is noted with knee firing patterns.

Gait

Leg muscles do not inhibit as they should against arm activation. Eye reflex patterns do not inhibit movement (phasic) muscles when appropriate. Hip extension and abduction firing patterns are activating in unison instead of in normal sequence.

Interpretation and Treatment Plan Development

Clinical Reasoning

What Are the Facts?

Osteoarthritis and arthrosis are common and have a number of causes. A genetic tendency to develop this condition is one factor. The most common cause is wear and tear on the joint structure, in addition to past trauma and increased weight. The pain is caused by irritation of the synovial membrane and joint capsule and by muscle contraction, which attempts to guard the area. Osteoarthritis has no cure, but it can be managed to improve the quality of life. Joint replacement surgery is a last option. Advances in technology have greatly improved the outcomes of this surgery.

Muscle guarding involves shortening of muscle groups to protect an area. It usually occurs in all the muscles that cross the joint. Because flexors, adductors, and internal rotators have more mass, when tone increases, the pull is greater from these muscles than from the extensors, abductors, and external rotators. The bone fit at the joint can be pulled out of alignment, creating further irritation in the joint capsule. Also, muscles that cross the joint pull the joint space together. This, coupled with weight bearing at the hips, knees, and ankles, reduces the joint space and increases the potential for rubbing of the bony structures, increasing the inflammation, swelling, and pain. This type of muscle guarding is very different from muscle spasms and cramps, which are spontaneous, painful muscle contractions caused by certain mechanisms in the brain.

Arthritic joints often are unstable and have a lax ligament structure. Because the client's knees are affected (closed kinetic chain—hip/knee/ankle), disruption of the knees affects the hips and ankles.

Management includes easing mechanical strain on the knee joint by normalizing the muscle tone without reducing stability and resourceful muscle guarding. Corresponding muscle shortening and weakening in the hips and ankles also must be addressed. Lymphatic drainage–type methods work well if the fluid is outside the capsule. Edema can increase stiffness and reduce range of motion. Sometimes needle aspiration is necessary if excess fluid builds up inside the capsule. Some increase in synovial fluid in the capsule can be beneficial, because an increase in hydrostatic pressure can separate the bone surfaces, easing the rubbing.

Correcting any posture deviation that contributes to the joint irritation may be possible in younger clients, but in older clients, especially after age 75, this becomes more difficult. Pain management is supported with counterirritation and hyperstimulation analgesia applications, a reduction in sympathetic arousal, and an increase in the pain-modulating chemicals in the system, such as serotonin and enkephalins. The joints must be kept moving or the condition worsens. Massage that incorporates passive and active joint movement supports pain management, allowing the client to move with less pain. Joint tractioning can offer temporary relief. Application of hot and cold hydrotherapy to manage pain and encourage circulation is appropriate. Cold can be applied after activity, and heat can be used to warm up before activity or as a counterirritation at night to promote sleep.

This client's history and posture give strong indications of the development of osteoarthritis and arthrosis. His body type (long legs with upper body mass) strains the knees in general. In addition, he has used his body hard for a long time.

What Are the Possibilities in Both Function and Dysfunction and the Massage Intervention Options?

The client is still relatively young and in good health. He is motivated to change, as indicated by his previous diet and exercise alterations. The knee joints and left ankle are likely damaged beyond regeneration.

Possibilities

1. Massage can be beneficial for management of pain, stiffness, and muscle pain related to guarding of the painful joint. Also, deterioration may be slowed, prolonging the time before replacement surgery is required. Generally, increasing tissue pliability and circulation, combined with management of sympathetic arousal, could help this client. Short-term symptomatic pain relief or pain reduction is a reasonable expectation, but the massage effects will wear off, and an ongoing appointment schedule is needed.

2. Racquetball may not be the best activity, because the constant running in different directions in short bursts and the starting and stopping are hard on the knees. Swimming could be an option.

3. Gradual introduction of a conservative flexibility program would be helpful.

What Are the Logical Outcomes of Each Possible Intervention?

The recreation center where the client plays racquetball has a swimming pool; therefore, access is convenient. A senior yoga class also is available at the recreation center, as is massage. Cost and scheduling are not primary concerns.

Massage has a good likelihood of successful management of conditions as long as the client has regular appointments and realizes that this is a long-term care program. Cardiac medication may alter the amount of pressure tolerated by the client. Regular reports should be sent to his doctor.

What Is the Impact on the People Involved for Each Possible Intervention?

Swimming does not meet the client's desire for competition. He may try anyway but will not commit. Yoga does not thrill the client, but he is willing to try it as long as the class is not full of "old fogies." He is willing to play less racquetball and more golf but says golf does not make him sweat like racquetball does, and he needs something to make him sweat.

Patience is necessary for everyone. The progress from the massage will most likely be slow, and the effectiveness wears off. The massage therapist needs to realize that under the gruffness is likely an individual who is afraid and vulnerable. Awareness of and respect for boundary issues are necessary to keep the client empowered.

Decision Making and Treatment Plan Development

Quantifiable Goal

Reduce sensation of stiffness and pain by 50% as long as regular appointments are scheduled

Qualifiable Goal

The client will be able to participate in moderate, low-impact sports exercise activities without being hindered by arthritic pain and joint stiffness.

Treatment Regimen

Condition Management

A long-term massage program is required with an initial schedule of twice a week right after racquetball. This will help reduce some of the strain on the client's knees from racquetball. Because of the client's size and the complex application of massage, 1½-hour sessions are needed. The cost is $70 per session. The appointment schedule will be reduced to weekly as soon as improvement is noted and the client's condition stabilizes.

Full-body massage with multiple goals is needed. The fibrotic and binding connective tissue structure noticed bodywide will need to be systematically but slowly addressed. The focus is on increasing the pliability of the ground substance to reduce muscle density and fascial shortening and maintain more flexibility of the body. Effective methods could be myofascial release plus broad-based application of compression with the forearm, and possibly the knee and foot, against the tissue to compress the soft tissue and carry it away from the bone, with the client actively moving the adjacent joint. Sidelying positioning for the legs and working on a floor mat would facilitate this type of application.

The client will likely require varying degrees of pressure and depth of application. The sensation should be on the edge of "good hurt," sufficient to trigger the release of endorphins, endocannabinoids, and serotonin but not enough to elicit guarding or bracing. Caution for bruising is indicated because of his use of aspirin. Gliding with drag can stretch the soft tissue. Until the client's muscle tone normalizes, use of active resistance for muscle energy methods may be counterproductive. Direct manipulation of the spindle cell and tendon

responses or having the client make circles with his eyes and head to initiate muscle facilitation and inhibition in the limbs is likely to be more effective. Kneading can introduce shear, bending, and torsion forces to increase ground substance viscosity, especially around all the scars.

The knees can be a primary focus after muscle tone and tissue density normalize a bit. The trigger point activity can be addressed, specifically the ones in the quadriceps and gastrocnemius that refer pain into the knees. Traction of the knees can temporarily separate joint surfaces. Surface edema can be moved with lymphatic drainage.

Application of ice and heat between massage sessions will be encouraged. The client can also use one of the many counterirritant ointments and gels which contain menthol as the primary cooling ingredient.

CASE 12 NERVE IMPINGEMENT SYNDROME

The client is a 34-year-old female. She has been a cosmetologist for 12 years and maintains a very busy practice. The client has been self-employed for the past 4 years and has two employees. The business specializes in hair weaving and various types of braiding.

She has been experiencing right arm and wrist pain for the past 2 years. She was diagnosed with carpal tunnel syndrome (median nerve impingement), but surgery is not recommended until more conservative interventions have been exhausted. There are also indications of brachial plexus impingement from a minor whiplash injury 3 years ago. Another contributing factor is the client's use of birth control pills.

She is experiencing the typical symptoms of pain in the wrist and hand with numbness in the thumb and first two fingers. The muscles in the hand show no signs of atrophy. Her right arm feels heavy, and she has aching and numbness from her upper arm down into the right scapular area. Tapping the wrist makes the hand tingle, and reaching for the floor with the right hand and lateral flexing of the head to the left increase the symptoms. She wakes up at night with her arm feeling numb. Heat applications help. She also takes an over-the-counter pain medication, Aleve (naproxen).

Assessment

Observation

The client's height and weight appear to be normal. She seems a bit swollen. She is a pleasant, energetic, and accommodating person. She draws a distinct line pattern of pain down her arm and hand and across the shoulder under the scapula.

Interview and Goals

The client information form does not indicate any contributing factors other than stress and fatigue from long working hours. She uses birth control pills. The client is "not complaining" because she has worked so hard for her business success. She rates her pain a 7 on a 1 to 10 scale. She indicates that she begins her day at a pain level of 3 and that the pain worsens as the day progresses. She can tolerate the pain in the morning but finds that by the afternoon, her capability is adversely affected.

The client's goal for the massage is to reduce the arm pain.

Physical Assessment

Posture

Right shoulder is high and anteriorly rotated. Right arm is internally rotated. Head is tilted to the right.

Gait

Arm swing is short on the right.

Range of Motion

External rotation is limited to 60 degrees. Client resists lateral flexion of the head to the left, because it feels tight and makes the arm ache.

Palpation

Near Touch. Anterior triangle of the neck on the right is warm.

Skin. Dampness is noted in the upper right shoulder region, which corresponds with an area of heat. Skin is smooth and resilient. Tissue binds around the right wrist and up into the forearm.

Superficial Connective Tissue. Generally boggy

Vessels and Lymph Nodes. Normal

Muscles. Scalenes on the right are short, and scalenes on the left are inhibited and long. Sternocleidomastoid is short and fibrotic on the left, right rhomboids are inhibited and long, anterior serratus is short on the right, right subscapularis is short, and pectoralis minor is short on the right. Wrist flexors are bilaterally short, with trigger point activity in the flexor pollicis longus, pronator teres, brachioradialis, and supraspinatus on the right.

Tendons. Tender at insertion of right flexor digitorum group bilaterally. Subscapular tendon on the right is tender to moderate pressure.

Deep Fascia. Palmar fasciae bilaterally are short. Retinaculum on the right is short, with reduced pliability compared with the left hand.

Ligaments. Retinaculum at the right wrist is thick.

Joints. Normal

Bones. Normal

Abdominal Viscera. Normal

Body Rhythms. Normal; respiratory circulation is craniosacral.

Muscle Testing

Strength

Short muscles with trigger point activity test strong but cannot sustain the resistance because of an increase in symptoms.

Neurologic Balance

Normal

Gait

Muscles in the right arm are not inhibiting appropriately, as indicated in the gait testing protocol.

Interpretation and Treatment Plan Development

Clinical Reasoning

What Are the Facts?

Nerve impingement (entrapment) syndromes are a common cause of pain. The distribution of pain depends on the nerve impinged. Impinged cervical plexus nerves usually refer pain up into the head. Brachial plexus nerve impingement refers pain into the shoulder and down the arm. Lumbar plexus impingement refers into the gluteals and groin or down the side of the leg to the knee. Sciatic nerve pain radiates down the back of the leg. The pain of individual nerve impingement, such as the median nerve in carpal tunnel syndrome, follows the distribution of the nerve. Trigger point pain patterns can follow similar distribution patterns and are a common component of nerve-type pain. The person usually has a history of trauma or repetitive strain with resulting muscle guarding. Fluid retention in vulnerable areas, such as the wrist, can be causal. This can happen with pregnancy or the use of birth control pills. Often the condition has multiple causal factors. Soft tissue impingement of nerves is the easiest of these types of syndromes to manage, and surgery should be avoided if possible because scar tissue formation after the surgery can cause future problems. If surgery is performed, scar development needs to be managed in the acute, subacute, and remodeling stages. Bony impingement usually requires referral to a chiropractor, an osteopath, a physical therapist or, in extreme cases, a surgeon. Tight muscles, both concentric and isometric (short) and eccentric (long), can press on nerves. Connective tissue shortening and adhesions are common causes of impingement. Women are somewhat more vulnerable to impingement syndromes such as carpal tunnel syndrome.

This client has multiple causal factors. Her job and increased demands for her service are increasing the amount of repetitive strain in the affected area. The whiplash injury can predispose the scalenes and other muscles of the neck and shoulder girdle to shortening. She is also retaining fluid, likely from the birth control pills.

What Are the Possibilities in Both Function and Dysfunction and the Massage Intervention Options?

The client probably has brachial plexus impingement, in addition to trigger point activity that is referring into the wrist area. Edema at the wrists is adding to the impingement. The connective tissue at the carpal tunnel is also thick. The source of most of the symptoms is unclear.

Possibilities

1. Massage intervention would need to address each area: short muscles; trigger points in the belly of the muscles; short, thick connective tissue; and edema.

2. Spot work is possible but usually unsuccessful, because areas of compensation, although not currently noticed, are likely developing. The client indicates that she is stressed, therefore full-body massage is most beneficial.

3. The client would benefit from a moderate exercise and flexibility program.

What Are the Logical Outcomes of Each Possible Intervention?

Massage is likely to reduce symptoms and prevent the condition from getting worse. It at least would slow the deterioration. Long-term care is probable.

Time is the biggest issue. Also, repetitive strain injury benefits from rest, which the client cannot easily do because of work demands. Early morning weekday appointments are available, and this is the best time for the client.

Because the massage therapist is an employee of the pain clinic the client has chosen for treatment, the clinic may be able to receive some reimbursement from the client's insurance company for the acute care. Insurance probably will not pay for maintenance massage care.

What Is the Impact on the People Involved for Each Possible Intervention?

The client is compliant but unwilling to reduce her work schedule. She says she will begin a regular stretching program, but compliance seems unlikely because of time constraints.

Decision Making and Treatment Plan Development

Quantifiable Goal

Reduce pain to a 3 on a 1 to 10 pain scale without pain increasing throughout the workday

Qualifiable Goal

The client will be able to work a 40-hour week without limiting pain.

Treatment Regimen

Therapeutic Change/Condition Management

A 1-hour full-body massage with a lymphatic drainage component will be given twice a week. Methods to increase natural pain-modulating mechanisms (e.g., endorphins and serotonin) and to support the parasympathetic process for stress management are appropriate.

Acute phase treatment will proceed as follows:

- Short muscles will be addressed with general massage and muscle energy and lengthening methods. All layers of muscles will be worked, because synergists and fixators are involved. Inhibited antagonists will be stimulated.
- Trigger point activity that refers symptoms in short muscles will be addressed with positional release or integrated muscle energy methods and lengthening. The results will be evaluated before connective tissue methods are introduced.
- Self-help methods will be taught to the client. Pulsed muscle energy and lengthening for short muscles and positional release for more active trigger points will be demonstrated.

This phase could take 6 weeks.

After the acute phase, connective tissue methods will be introduced to restore pliability to the thick fascial areas of the right forearm and wrist. Careful use of friction to create therapeutic inflammation is necessary. Monitoring will ensure that the methods do not aggravate the symptoms.

The client will be observed for posture improvement and the development of symptoms in the areas of compensation, such as the low back. Should such symptoms develop, she will be reassessed for short muscle imbalance and connective tissue shortening. Also, trigger points that refer to areas experiencing symptoms will be identified and treated.

When the client's condition is stable, appointments will be reduced to a maintenance schedule of once a week.

CASE 13 GENERAL RELAXATION

The client is a 44-year-old male who is on a vacation cruise. He has a high-stress job and has been having problems in his personal relationship. He will be on the cruise for 2 weeks and would like to schedule four massage sessions, two each week. Although he knows he has numerous minor musculoskeletal issues, he is not interested in addressing any of them. His goal is relaxation and pampering. He has no contraindications for relaxation massage.

Assessment

Observation

The client appears fatigued and frazzled. His weight appears normal for his height, and he looks moderately physically fit.

Interview and Goals

The client does not state anything on the client information form that would indicate contraindications. He indicates that he is stressed and that he gets an occasional tension headache. He takes no medication, although he takes a daily general multivitamin.

He wants general massage with firm pressure that does not hurt. He does not want to participate; in fact, he hopes that he falls asleep.

When asked what type of relaxation sensation he would like and his goal for the massage, he replies that he wants to feel loose, sleepy, and calm.

Physical Assessment

Note: The client did not want to participate in an extensive physical assessment process. Assessment information is gathered during the general observation and the first massage.

Posture

Slight forward head position and hyperextended knees when standing in symmetric stance.

Gait

Somewhat rigid

Range of Motion

Within normal range

Palpation

Near Touch. Skin is warm; client has a slight sunburn.

Skin. Skin is normal. Binding is seen in the lumbar and occipital base areas. Client has extensive body hair.

Superficial Connective Tissue. Fibrotic at iliotibial band bilaterally.

Vessels and Lymph Nodes. Normal

Muscles. Muscle tissue is dense. Hamstrings are short, and abdominals are long and weak.

Tendons. Normal

Deep Fascia. Plantar and lumbar fasciae are short.

Ligaments. Normal

Joints. Knee flexion bilaterally is limited by 10 degrees.

Bones. Normal

Abdominal Viscera. Normal

Body Rhythms. Upper chest breathing pattern.

Muscle Testing

Not performed

Interpretation and Treatment Plan Development

Clinical Reasoning

What Are the Facts?

This case falls into the category of palliative care. The focus is on relaxation in a vacation environment, but similar treatment plans would be indicated for individuals having surgery before and after the procedure, acute care, and for care of the terminally ill.

Relaxation and pleasurable sensation are important functions of therapeutic massage. Massage is used to balance the autonomic nervous system functions and usually provides support for a reduction in sympathetic arousal, in addition to the potential for a more parasympathetic balance. Relaxation can mean different things to different people. For most clients, relaxation is an experience of parasympathetic dominance with serotonin, dynorphin, enkephalin, and endorphin responses. For those who would like to be alert but relaxed, the focus must be on stimulating norepinephrine and dopamine production. It is important to determine what the client means by "being relaxed." Asking questions that help the client clarify his or her interpretation of the relaxation experience can provide information on what the physiologic outcomes should be.

Entrainment is an important aspect of relaxation because it coordinates body rhythms. Soft, rhythmic music and indirect lighting can be helpful in achieving a parasympathetic result. Aromatherapy is an advanced intervention requiring specialized training, but simple, safe application of some common essential oils may be calming. Lavender is one of the most calming. Various applications of heat are also comforting. A warm hot water bottle at the feet or behind the neck may be pleasurable.

What Are the Possibilities in Both Function and Dysfunction and the Massage Intervention Options?

The client has numerous areas of short and long muscles actively coupled with connective tissue dysfunction, but addressing these areas would not meet the client's goal. The upper chest breathing pattern could be addressed, because that should result in a calming effect.

Possibilities

1. The massage practitioner can offer the client a selection of aromas and music, and he could pick the ones he prefers.
2. Warm compresses can be placed over the client's eyes, and a warm pack can be provided for his feet. An alternative would be a warm foot bath before the massage.

What Are the Logical Outcomes of Each Possible Intervention?

Because of his sunburn, the client may not want the hot water application.

He may be allergic to the volatile oils in the essential oils.

The massage environment must be quiet, and the massage professional must limit conversation so that the client can fall asleep if he wishes and is not required to engage in conversation.

What Is the Impact on the People Involved for Each Possible Intervention?

The massage professional must remain focused on the client's goal and not address the other musculoskeletal issues identified.

Decision Making and Treatment Plan Development

Quantifiable Goal

Induce the relaxation response and support parasympathetic dominance, indicated by slowing of breathing and what the client experiences and reports.

Qualifiable Goal

The client will feel relaxed, sleepy, and calm.

Treatment Regimen

Palliative Care

A full-body massage will be given with gliding, kneading, compression, and rocking for 90 minutes, with a rhythmic approach used to match the music selected by the client. The pressure level will be moderate to deep but will not elicit discomfort. Sufficient nonirritating lubricant will be used to prevent pulling of the body hair or irritation of the sunburn. The client will be offered a warm, damp towel to remove the lubricant after the massage. The massage professional can do this for the client as a way of gently waking him up after the massage. A massage focused on the feet, hands, head, and face sends the most signals into the central nervous system for relaxation. Attention to the thorax, shoulders, neck, and midback muscles provides inhibition and lengthening of the auxiliary breathing muscles to support relaxed breathing. The client will be positioned in the prone, side-lying, and supine positions, and he will be moved unobtrusively. The scent selected will be placed in a diffuser or mist bottle to prevent any skin irritation.

The massage practitioner will stay focused and calm, intent on creating a quiet space with empathy and compassion, no expectations, and no interruptions for the client.

CASE 14 SLEEP DISTURBANCE

The client is a 52-year-old female. She is married and has three children: two grown and one in high school. She is satisfied with her personal and professional life most of the time. Currently, she works part-time as a nurse, but is considering returning to school to advance her career options.

The client is menopausal; she had a hysterectomy when she was 46, but she still has her ovaries. She is taking a low-dose hormone replacement (estradiol) and uses a topical progesterone cream. The estrogen and progesterone, plus the addition of soy to her diet and vitamin E supplementation, have controlled her hot flashes. However, she is still moody and restless, and she is experiencing sleep problems. She is also mildly hypertensive but is not taking medication for it. She is 15 pounds above her ideal weight. She is active; she plays golf and tennis and bowls. For the past 6 months she has been on a very low fat diet and has lost 12 pounds. She loves coffee, and she quit smoking 9 years ago.

She has minor aching in her knee joints and is generally stiff in the morning but loosens up with a hot shower and some stretching. She has had an occasional massage while on vacation but has never had massage that focused on a specific outcome goal. She became aware of the benefits of massage in a book she was reading about managing menopause.

Assessment

Observation

The client's appearance is appropriate for her age. She has some wrinkling, which is explained by the smoking and by the greater susceptibility of Caucasian skin to sun damage. Because she colors her hair, the color and texture will not provide reliable information on stress response. She is a bit overweight, with fat distribution in the lower abdominal area, which is typical for menopause. The fat helps convert body chemicals to estrogen-like substances, replacing the estrogen production of the ovaries. The fat appears to be between the abdominal wall and the skin, which is of much less concern than fat distribution in the abdominal cavity, which is an indication of stress and increased cortisol secretion, with implications for cardiovascular problems. Her mood seems even, although she is a bit intense in her conversation. She yawns and sniffs frequently, which may indicate a tendency for a breathing pattern disorder.

Interview and Goals

The client information form indicates that she uses reading glasses; has minor sinus congestion, especially in the fall; and has urge incontinence, which causes a need to urinate frequently, including at night. She has a tendency to bloat and has the aching knees and generalized morning stiffness previously mentioned. She has had three pregnancies and a hysterectomy. She has mild hypertension and is fatigued from lack of sustained sleep. When questioned, she reports that just as she is falling asleep, she has to get up to urinate. Then she has difficulty falling asleep again. During the night she either wakes up and then feels the urge to use the restroom, or bladder pressure wakes her up. She feels as if she is up and down all night. In an attempt to reduce bladder frequency, she has restricted her fluid intake. She is also having some vivid dreams with the themes of running, looking for things, or trying to find people in a crowd.

She is undergoing hormone replacement therapy and takes a multivitamin supplement for menopausal women that includes some herbs, particularly black cohosh, gingko biloba, and extra vitamin E. She also takes a calcium/magnesium with vitamin D supplement. She had her appendix and tonsils out as a child. She is involved with various sports for leisure and exercise.

Her main goal for the massage is to sleep better. After the effects of massage on mood-regulating neurochemicals and the morning stiffness and joint aching in her knees were explained to her, she also became interested in addressing those goals. However, she is mainly concerned about her sleep quality and will base her evaluation of the effectiveness of the massage on this outcome.

Physical Assessment

Posture

Generally symmetric, but the shoulders are held a bit high and bilaterally rotate forward; this is so slight at this time that no compensation pattern is noted in any other body area.

Gait

Normal

Range of Motion

Knees are restricted in flexion, and range of motion is reduced by 10%. External rotation of both shoulders results in a minor reduction in mobility.

Palpation

Near Touch. Slightly increased heat in the upper thorax.
Skin. Surface texture is dry; hair is brittle; nails are well formed, but cuticles are dry and cracked. Elasticity is reduced in upper thorax around clavicles and at sacrum and on the bottoms of the feet. Skin is somewhat tight against the subcutaneous layer and does not lift easily.
Superficial Connective Tissue. Generally reduced pliability, with indications of minor dehydration (pinched skin fold holds its shape longer than normal).
Vessels and Lymph Nodes. Normal
Muscles. No obvious neuromuscular issues or trigger point activity.
Tendons. Normal
Deep Fascia. Short and binding
Ligaments. Slightly dense
Joints. Minor stiffness with soft but binding (leathery) end-feel. Knees are moderately painful with both compression and traction.

Bones. Normal with reservations; family history indicates possible tendency for osteoporosis.

Abdominal Viscera. Moderate bloat

Body Rhythms. Breathing is a bit irregular and has an upper chest quality. Heart rate has moments of increased rhythm. Cranial rhythm seems inhibited (sluggish lymphatic movement is likely responsible).

Muscle Testing

Strength
Normal

Neurologic Balance
Normal

Gait
Normal

Interpretation and Treatment Plan Development

Clinical Reasoning

What Are the Facts?

The client is menopausal and has typical manifestations of that stage of life; she is taking measures to manage the uncomfortable mood and circulatory changes. She has a family history of osteoporosis and cancer, and she herself has a history of smoking.

Menopause is a normal process that begins as a woman's hormonal patterns change and ovarian production and menstruation cease. Changes in urinary and sleep patterns are common. The urinary stress and urge incontinence can be related to changes in membranes in the urinary tract in response to reduced estrogen levels. Sleep changes are related to urinary urge, hot flashes, and changes in the serotonin level in relation to the estrogen level.

Breathing function is mechanically altered with the connective tissue changes, causing an upper chest breathing pattern; this results in oxygen levels in the blood that support sympathetic nervous system arousal.

Connective tissue changes and dry skin indicate mild dehydration and insufficient dietary fat intake. Estrogen also helps tissues maintain proper hydration, and with a reduction in estrogen, connective tissue ground substance does not hydrate as easily.

Evidence of osteoarthritis is present in the client's knees (pain on compression), and soft tissue involvement is noted (pain on traction).

What Are the Possibilities in Both Function and Dysfunction and the Massage Intervention Options?

The client may be predisposing herself to connective tissue changes by restricting water and an appropriate healthy fat intake. She is doing this because of the weight gain and urinary urge. The reduction in estrogens may have altered the serotonin balance; this affects the production of melatonin, which controls aspects of the sleep cycle. Also, the bladder urgency is disturbing her sleep.

Breathing changes may be increasing the tendency for sympathetic dominance with increased cortisol levels; these higher levels would interfere with deep sleep and contribute to the type of dreams the client is having.

Possibilities

1. A general full-body massage is indicated, with deep but not painful compression to encourage parasympathetic dominance and to support levels of serotonin, endorphins, dynorphins, and enkephalins and other mood-regulating neurochemicals for mood and sleep. This massage approach, coupled with a drag quality to increase the pliability of the superficial connective tissue, should address the client's major and minor concerns, including the knee pain. The mechanics of breathing also must be addressed, but the major anatomic reason for upper chest breathing seems to be connective tissue binding with sympathetic arousal.
2. The client needs to increase her intake of fluids and essential fatty acids (e.g., olive oil) to support proper tissue hydration and hormone and neurotransmitter function.
3. She should be referred to her doctor for the urinary urgency. However, reducing cortisol levels and supporting deep sleep should help with the nighttime urgency.
4. A slow stretching program with a meditative quality would be helpful.

What Are the Logical Outcomes of Each Possible Intervention?

The massage should result in management of the conditions of concern. Regular ongoing appointments are required, and this creates a time and cost burden for the client. Referral to the doctor is necessary to rule out more serious reasons for the urinary problem.

Increasing fluid may temporarily aggravate the urinary stress. The stretching program may temporarily increase stiffness if the client is too aggressive, but moderate stretching would help maintain relaxation, joint mobility, and connective tissue pliability.

The client is self-seeking massage, and this type of client often is the most compliant in terms of keeping appointments and following through with self-help education.

What Is the Impact on the People Involved for Each Possible Intervention?

The massage professional needs to be committed to a regular appointment schedule.

Some emotional undertones to the client's case, especially the restlessness, wanting to return to school, and tension with her daughter, may surface during the sessions. The massage professional must maintain appropriate boundaries and make the appropriate referrals. The client likely does not realize the emotional nature of the situation and may be confused if these issues surface. Redirection to the massage process and the referral will be helpful.

Decision Making and Treatment Plan Development

Quantifiable Goals

1. Improve sleep quality, as self-reported by client
2. Balance mood and physical stress levels, as self-reported by client
3. Reverse upper chest breathing pattern, as measured by therapist

Qualifiable Goal

The client will be less fatigued and stiff, which will allow her to perform her desired daily exercise activities.

Treatment Regimen

Condition Management/Therapeutic Change

A weekly 1-hour massage will be provided on an open-ended, ongoing basis. The cost will be $50, and every tenth massage will be free.

The massage methods used will include gliding with moderate to deep but not painful pressure to increase the levels of serotonin and other mood-regulating neurochemicals and to reduce sympathetic arousal. Gliding also will be done with sufficient drag to cause connective tissue creep in binding areas and to increase viscosity in areas that show reduced pliability. Kneading also will be done, with localized use of skin rolling at the thorax and sacrum to increase connective tissue water binding. Rhythmic rocking with entrainment to the client's selected soft, slow music will encourage parasympathetic dominance. The range of motion of the knees and shoulders will be normalized with muscle energy methods and lengthening. Binding connective tissue will be stretched by means of bending and torsion forces applied with compression and kneading.

The client will be taught breathing exercises as presented in Chapter 15 of this textbook. The information in Chapter 15 also will be used to teach her methods of maintaining a supportive sleep cycle.

She will be educated in the importance of drinking water and of appropriate fat intake and will be referred to her physician and nutritionist for confirmation of this information for her specific needs and for diagnosis of the bladder urgency.

She will be referred to a slow stretching program, such as yoga, to address the connective tissue stiffness and to support sleep and relaxation.

CASE 15 CIRCULATION IMPAIRMENT

The client is a 57-year-old male with type 2 diabetes mellitus. He is non-insulin-dependent at this point and is taking an oral hypoglycemic medication that stimulates the secretion of insulin. He is 40 pounds overweight, and part of his diabetic management is weight loss. He lost 25 pounds initially but has not lost any weight in 3 months.

His exercise is closely monitored to minimize blood sugar fluctuations. He walks and uses a rowing machine. He has begun to notice some impaired circulation in his legs and some burning in his feet. He reports that he has developed minor symptoms of vascular insufficiency and diabetic neuropathy, a common complication of diabetes. His doctors are exploring all options to manage the condition.

The nurse on the diabetic management team has recommended massage, because recent studies have shown benefit in both supporting circulation and better insulin regulation. The client is willing to try anything that can help, and because the massage therapist is affiliated with the medical team, he feels confident that the nurse who is responsible for the management of his program will supervise the process.

The client is in a long-term relationship and has a good support system.

Assessment

The following information was provided by the medical team:

> The client is a 57-year-old male with moderate type 2 diabetes mellitus. He is being treated with Glucotrol, diet, exercise, and education in diabetes and stress management. Renal function is good. Recent developments include vascular impairment and diabetic neuropathy in the feet. The massage prescription is for stress reduction with secondary support for peripheral circulation. The frequency and duration are two times per week for 1 hour per session.

Note: This case study is an example of the way a massage therapist responds to a massage prescription. The goals for the massage are determined by the physician. The assessment that follows is done to determine how best to meet those goals and achieve the treatment plan provided.

Observation

The client is visibly nervous and fidgety. He prefers to stand to complete the intake process. He wrings his hands often and regularly sighs deeply. The client's excess weight is carried in his abdomen and gluteal area.

Interview and Goals

The client reports that he has never had a massage. He is ticklish and is concerned about taking off his clothing. He was in a car accident 10 years ago and had a whiplash injury and a concussion. He experiences aching after exercise. Other than the diabetes, he is in good health. He works as a maintenance supervisor and trouble-shooter for a local manufacturing firm. He used to drink beer, but alcohol is no longer part of his diet. He also quit smoking 3 years ago. He still misses smoking, especially the morning coffee and cigarette, but he is determined to do whatever it takes to manage the diabetes. His mother died of complications of the same disease.

He understands that the goal for the massage is to help him relax, which will help regulate insulin levels. Additional outcomes would be to increase circulation and reduce the numbing and prickling sensation in his feet caused by the neuropathy.

Physical Assessment

Posture

Moderate lumbar lordosis and forward head position.

Gait

Clumsy, with a flat-foot landing on his feet rather than the normal heel strike–toe off pattern.

Range of Motion

Trunk flexion is inhibited by the abdominal fat mass. Plantar flexion and dorsiflexion are decreased by 20% bilaterally.

Palpation

Near Touch. No noticeable difference

Skin. Normal except for a bluish cast in the feet. Lower extremities are cool. Binding is present in the lumbar area and at the base of the neck. Palpable fat layer is present under the skin, with excessive accumulation in the abdomen and gluteals.

Superficial Connective Tissue. Bind in the lumbar area, thorax, and calves.

Vessels and Lymph Nodes. Lymph circulation appears normal, but pulses are weaker in the feet, and vessels seem constricted.

Muscles. Somewhat decreased in tone overall, with evidence of the exercise effect increasing muscle tone in the legs and arms but not in the abdomen or gluteal region.

Tendons. Right Achilles tendon is nonpliable.

Deep Fascia. Binding in the lumbar and anterior thoracic sheaths and nonresilience in the abdomen. Plantar fasciae are short bilaterally.

Ligaments. Normal

Joints. No evidence of arthritis or pain on compression or traction. Lumbar curve is exaggerated. Knees and feet ache.

Bones. Normal

Abdominal Viscera. Difficult to palpate because of internal and external fat distribution.

Body Rhythms. Slow, uneven breathing rate.

Muscle Testing

Not performed

Interpretation and Treatment Plan Development

Clinical Reasoning

What Are the Facts?

Diabetes is caused by impaired release of insulin by the pancreas, by inadequate or abnormal insulin receptors on the cells, or by destruction of insulin before it can become active. Type 2 diabetes is a maturity onset form often found in adults who are overweight, especially if a family history of the disease is a factor. Diabetes symptoms include increased thirst and appetite. The high blood glucose levels have detrimental effects on most body systems; these effects include impaired eyesight, neuropathy, impaired circulation, a tendency for thrombosis and emboli, and diminished resistance to infection. Wounds heal slowly, and kidney function is strained. The individual also is susceptible to atherosclerosis. All this must be taken into account when massage is applied.

The client in this case has impaired peripheral circulation with neuropathy in the lower legs. Kidney function is normal.

The client has no history of blood clots. He is taking medication that has common side effects of diarrhea, dizziness, fatigue, headache, heartburn, loss of appetite, upset stomach, sun sensitivity, vomiting, and weakness. Serious side effects of medication that require referral include blood disorders, breathing difficulties, dark urine, itching, jaundice, light-colored stools, low blood sugar, muscle cramps, rash, sore throat, fever, tightening in the hands and feet, and unusual bleeding or bruising. The massage practitioner needs to pay particular attention to dizziness, weakness, breathing, jaundice, itching, and symptoms of low blood sugar (besides dizziness and weakness, these include pallor, a rapid heart rate, and excessive sweating). Diabetic clients should always have their medications with them, and fruit juice or another quick-acting carbohydrate should be available. Muscle cramps, rash, and bruising also need to be considered. Cautions and accommodations are necessary. The skin can become thin and fragile in areas of impaired circulation.

This client is also anxious, indicating sympathetic dominance. He is ticklish and uncertain about taking off his clothes. He is overweight and experiences muscle aches after exercise. His knees bother him. He was in a car accident that injured his neck. He has fascial shortening in the feet, lumbar area, and thorax.

What Are the Possibilities in Both Function and Dysfunction and the Massage Intervention Options?

The possibilities for intervention are limited by the treatment plan provided by the physician. The physician has ordered relaxation massage and support for peripheral circulation with a schedule of biweekly 1-hour sessions.

Of more concern is how to follow the treatment plan when the client is ticklish and nervous about taking his clothes off. The client could be introduced to massage through use of a seated massage format over the clothing until he is more comfortable and then could be transferred to the more traditional massage on the table with draping.

What Are the Logical Outcomes of Each Possible Intervention?

The chair massage over the clothing would address the issue of the client not wanting to take off his clothes. However, this type of massage may not provide enough relaxation response to support the goals of the physician. Also, addressing the problem of impaired circulation in the legs would be more difficult.

Tickling can be managed by using more pressure. Because the client's skin is in good shape and he has no history of thrombosis or embolism, broad-based compression would be a good method.

What Is the Impact on the People Involved for Each Possible Intervention?

The client would be more comfortable with the chair massage initially, and over time he would be able to move from the chair to the table. Once he realizes that he enjoys the massage and is not being tickled, he should relax.

Decision Making and Treatment Plan Development

Quantifiable Goals

As determined by the physician

Qualifiable Goals

As determined by the physician

Treatment Regimen

In accordance with treatment orders, the client will be given a 1-hour massage twice a week. The fees will be billed through the physician's office. Massage intervention will begin in the chair, with education provided about the effects of massage. Demonstration of the type of massage used to prevent tickling will be included, and draping methods also will be demonstrated.

While the client is using the seated position, the main focus of the massage will be to reduce sympathetic dominance and support normal breathing. Compression will be applied over the clothing, with shaking and rhythmic rocking of the arms and wrists and passive and active range of motion of the neck.

Once the client's apprehension about getting on the table and taking off his clothing has eased, a general full-body massage will be used to promote parasympathetic dominance. The connective tissue shortening will be addressed with myofascial release, always with an awareness of skin fragility. With the increase in connective tissue pliability, circulation and breathing should improve. The short, tight calf muscles will be addressed with slow gliding strokes, accompanied by monitoring for bruising. The calf muscle must have sufficient contractile capacity to promote circulation.

Circulation in the lower extremities will be encouraged with general full-body massage, with compression over the arteries moving proximal to distal. Caution will be used so that any evidence of thrombosis can be detected.

Addressing any areas of discomfort related to past injury or causes other than the diabetes will be cleared with the physician before the treatment plan is altered.

Recommendations to the physician will include massage application to reduce postexercise aching, which will support compliance with the exercise program; alteration of the exercise program to include some resistance exercises targeting the gluteal and abdominal areas; and normalization of the posture to support optimum energy expenditure. Evidence of an altered upper chest breathing pattern also is seen; because this perpetuates sympathetic arousal, it would be beneficial to address the problem by having the client participate in a breathing retraining program.

CASE 16 FATIGUE CAUSED BY CANCER TREATMENT

The client is a 46-year-old female with early detected, stage I breast cancer. The cancer was detected by mammography 12 months ago. She had a lumpectomy and radiation therapy. The outcome looks good. She is currently undergoing treatment with tamoxifen. All medical test results, including those from thyroid and bone density tests, are within normal parameters.

Two years ago the client married for the first time. She managed a branch bank for many years but retired from that job and is seeking a more meaningful career. She loves restoring antiques and hopes to pursue this as both a hobby and a money-making enterprise. Although money is a concern for her, she is willing to commit both time and resources to those things that increase the quality of her life. She heard about massage at a support group meeting and was intrigued by the studies that showed that massage supports the immune function and helps with the anxiety and depression that can accompany the diagnosis and treatment of cancer.

Her main concern is fatigue. After a year of focusing on treatment, she wants to get on with her life, but the fatigue keeps her motivation suppressed. She experienced fatigue during radiation treatment but expected to resume her normal energy level once treatment was over. In addition to the benefits mentioned in the studies, she hopes that massage will help her regain her energy. Her doctor is very supportive of massage but wants to speak to the massage practitioner before sessions begin to review the proposed treatment plan.

Assessment

Observation

The client is soft spoken but direct and does not avoid eye contact or difficult topics. Her body motions seem slow, and she appears tired. Her body fat is evenly distributed.

Interview and Goals

Information from the client history form indicates a slight family history of breast cancer but not in her immediate family. She has always been a bit overweight. She had her first menstrual period at 10 years of age, and she still has regular menstrual periods. She has taken birth control pills on and off for years. Birth control is not an issue at this point, because her husband has had a vasectomy. She gets an occasional headache but nothing significant. She has had the normal childhood illnesses. She feels as if she is not sleeping deeply.

Her goal for the massage is an improved energy level.

Physical Assessment

Posture

Concave upper chest and bilaterally internally rotated arms. Slight kyphosis. Jutting chin with slight forward head position. Flattened lumbar curve with bilateral posterior pelvic rotation. Left knee is hyperextended.

Gait

Weight is carried on the heels, with shortened stride and arm swing.

Range of Motion

Capital and cervical flexion combined allow only 10 degrees of motion. External rotation of arms is limited to 75 degrees. Abduction and extension of shoulders are limited to 20 degrees. Trunk extension at lumbar region is limited to 15 degrees. Hip extension is limited to 20 degrees and dorsiflexion to 15 degrees.

Palpation

Near Touch. Energy field seems uneven and erratic.

Skin. Skin is dry and shows obvious effects of radiation in treatment area. Two large moles are present on left shoulder. Bind is present in the thorax between the scapulae and in the lumbar area. Bind also is noted in the hamstrings and calves. Connective tissue seems dense in the lumbar area and hamstrings but thin in the thorax and abdomen.

Superficial Connective Tissue. Scar tissue at the surgical site is pliable, with a small area of bind near the axilla.

Vessels and Lymph Nodes. Normal, although caution is indicated in the left axilla adjacent to the treatment area.

Muscles. Occipital base, arm external rotator and adductor, and hamstring muscles are short. Gluteal group and abdominals are weak and almost flaccid. Calves are short.

Tendons. Pain reported on palpation of the subscapular tendon bilaterally. Achilles tendons are short.

Deep Fascia. Nonpliable and short in the cervical and lumbar areas and in the plantar fasciae. Abdominal fascia is nonresilient.

Ligaments. Normal

Joints. Minor pain with direct compression over the SI joints. Joints of the foot seem immobile.

Bones. Probable fragility over the radiation site.

Abdominal Viscera. Abdomen is soft and has no detectable masses or abnormalities.

Body Rhythms. Uneven and erratic; client feels out of sync with herself. Rhythms fluctuate often.

Muscle Testing

Strength

General muscle strength is fair, with excessive tone in calves and occipital base muscles.

Neurologic Balance

Normal

Gait

Normal contralateral pattern but labored. Gluteus maximus does not fire effectively.

Interpretation and Treatment Plan Development

Clinical Reasoning

What Are the Facts?

The client has received successful treatment for breast cancer. The causes of breast cancer are not fully known. However, health and medical researchers have identified a number of risk factors that increase a woman's chances of getting breast cancer. Risk factors are not necessarily causes of breast cancer, but they are associated with an increased risk of developing the disease. It is important to note that some women have many risk factors but do not develop breast cancer, whereas other women have few or no risk factors but do get the disease.

Being a woman is the number one risk factor for breast cancer. (*Note:* Males also get breast cancer.) For this reason, it is important for females to perform regular breast self-examinations, have clinical breast examinations, and have routine mammograms to detect any problems at an early stage. Massage therapists need to understand the risk factors for cancer in general and in this case for breast cancer specifically.

Factors that can be controlled include the following:
- Having more than one alcoholic drink per day
- Taking birth control pills for 5 years or longer (slightly increases the risk of breast cancer)
- Not getting regular exercise
- Currently using or having recently used some forms of hormone replacement therapy for 10 years or longer (may slightly increase the risk of breast cancer)
- Being overweight or gaining weight as an adult
- Being exposed to large amounts of radiation (e.g., having frequent spinal x-rays during scoliosis treatment)

Factors that cannot be controlled include the following:
- Aging
- Having a mother, daughter, or sister who has had breast cancer
- Having the mutated breast cancer genes BRCA-1 or BRCA-2
- Previously having had breast cancer
- Being young (under 12 years of age) at the time of the first menstrual period, starting menopause later than usual (over 55 years of age), never being pregnant, or having the first child after 30 years of age

Breast cancer can recur at anytime, but many recurrences happen within the first 2 years after diagnosis.

Breast cancer may recur locally within the breast or chest area, in areas adjacent to the breast (underarm lymph nodes), or at distant locations (metastatic type). The most common sites for metastatic breast cancer are the lungs, liver, bones, and brain.

This client is 1 year postdiagnosis and has multiple risk factors for cancer development. She is currently taking tamoxifen. The most common side effect of the medication is hot flashes similar to those experienced during menopause. Tamoxifen may induce menopause in a woman who is close to menopause; however, it rarely does in young women. Other common side effects are vaginal dryness, irregular periods, and weight gain.

The surgical procedure used for breast cancer depends on the stage of the disease, the type of tumor, the woman's age and general health, her preference, and the physician's recommendation. Surgery is a form of local treatment for breast cancer, as opposed to systemic treatment that involves the entire body, such as chemotherapy. Studies have shown that most women with early-stage disease (stage I or stage II) who are treated with breast conservation measures (procedures that preserve the breast) and irradiation have the same survival rate as women treated with mastectomy.

This client had a lumpectomy, which is appropriate treatment for her stage of cancer, and underwent radiation therapy. Radiation therapy uses high-energy x-rays to destroy cancer cells in the treated area (local treatment). It is most often used with breast-conserving surgery but may also be recommended after a mastectomy for women who have four or more lymph nodes that test positive for cancer cells. The purpose is to destroy any cancer cells that may be left after breast surgery. Radiation therapy may also be used palliatively to relieve symptoms, shrink tumors, and reduce pressure, bleeding, pain, or other symptoms of advanced cancer.

Cancer cells grow and divide rapidly, and they are very sensitive to the effects of radiation. Normal cells grow and divide less rapidly and recover more fully from the effects of radiation. The side effects of radiation are the result of temporary damage to the normal cells. It is important to remember that the side effects of radiation are directly related to the dose and the area treated. Common side effects include:

- *Local skin reactions:* Itching, redness, or dryness and scaling of the skin. The degree of skin reaction is very individualized. Skin irritation continues for approximately 2 weeks after the end of treatment. Healing then begins.
- *Fatigue:* This resolves gradually after treatment.

The client in this case also has a stage 2 postural distortion; this indicates functional stress that is causing a nonoptimum movement pattern characterized by fatigue with moderate activity.

What Are the Possibilities in Both Function and Dysfunction and the Massage Intervention Options?

The main goal for the massage is management of the fatigue, which could be residual from the radiation treatment and the stress of the past year. The medication also could be causing fatigue or an interrupted sleep pattern. Another factor that is contributing to the fatigue might be the postural changes that make movement labored and tiring, especially so since the client began a moderate exercise program.

Possibilities

1. Massage could act as a stress management method, supporting effective sleep patterns and restoring a more normal movement pattern. This massage approach would be a general constitutional approach with specific but cautious focus on the postural distortion.
2. Because the client's body rhythms seem out of sync, a rhythmic focus and approach to massage with music she enjoys could support entrainment.
3. The short muscles and connective tissue could be addressed with various massage, muscle energy, lengthening, and stretching methods.

What Are the Logical Outcomes of Each Possible Intervention?

The general massage, focused on quieting the stress response and supporting sleep and well-being, would help with the cancer recovery process in general but would not specifically address the postural changes that may be contributing to the fatigue. The approach should bring about some entrainment to disordered body rhythms.

A more aggressive massage approach to increase range of motion and make movement in general easier may be too aggressive this soon after cancer treatment.

What Is the Impact on the People Involved for Each Possible Intervention?

The doctor supports a more moderate approach that begins with the general massage and introduces the shift in muscle tension and posture gradually.

The client wants to address the problem more aggressively.

The massage therapist agrees with the slower, more cautious approach recommended by the doctor.

Decision Making and Treatment Plan Development

Quantifiable Goal

Increase restorative sleep by 80% as reported by client

Qualifiable Goal

The client will be able to participate in reasonable daily activities without fatigue.

Treatment Regimen

Condition Management

One-hour massage sessions will be given on a weekly basis at the massage office for $40 per session.

General full-body massage with sufficient pressure to increase serotonin levels will be given. The application will feel comfortably intense but not painful. The main methods will include variations in the depth, drag, direction, speed, and rhythm of gliding strokes. Caution will need to be observed over the irradiated site, where a decrease in pressure over the bony structure is appropriate. Rhythmic rocking and gentle shaking of the joints of the extremities will support relaxation and may increase range of motion. The two moles will be watched for changes, and any changes in the breast or axillae will be referred immediately. Gentle myofascial release methods, primarily skin stretching, can be used over the areas of connective tissue bind. Caution is required over the irradiated skin because of sensitivity and likely skin changes arising from the treatment.

The massage application will be rhythmic and relaxing. Polarity and reflexology concepts can be incorporated into the massage to support the process. Music of the client's choice that is soothing and has a rhythm of about 60 beats per minute can be used. Entrainment will be supported.

Once the client shows positive, sustained results from the methods described, positional release and pulsed muscle energy methods and lengthening can be introduced to address the postural distortion. Because the client is taking yoga classes, some postural change should occur that the massage can support. Heavy connective tissue work and invasive methods that introduce any sort of inflammation will be avoided. Any major change in the treatment plan will be approved by the physician.

CASE 17 BREATHING DISORDER: ASTHMA

The client is a 14-year-old male. His parents are exploring support care to help him manage his asthma. The client has been managing his asthma since he was 6 years old. Asthmatic triggers include smoke, perfumes, dust allergy, and exercise. The client has just entered high school and wants to be involved in sports. He shows a talent for golf and is frustrated when his breathing problems interfere with his game.

The client uses a combined medication program that includes Singulair and Ventolin. He does well on the medication, and side effects are minimal. When using the inhaler, he occasionally gets a headache or stomachache, a racing heart, and feels agitated.

Massage therapy was suggested to help with stress and with relaxation of the breathing muscles. The young man is not so sure about the massage therapy. He does not want to take off his clothes, and he does not want his parents in the room watching. He thinks he is doing fine with the medications, but there has been some indication that he has been overusing his inhaler. The medical team would like him to try relaxation methods before they try adjusting his medication.

Assessment

Observation

The client slouches in the chair and looks disgusted. He fidgets. The parents are a bit overpowering and do not let the client speak for himself.

The use of auxiliary breathing muscles is evident. The client is a bit short for his age but appears normal in adolescent development. He is right-handed.

Interview and Goals

In addition to asthma, the client information form indicates headaches and a digestive disturbance (nausea) that is related to the medication he is taking. The client broke his left collarbone 5 years ago. He has typical adolescent stress and difficulty falling asleep. He is allergic to dust, and his asthma is triggered by sensitivity to scent and smoke. He has some acne on his back, chest, and face.

He takes a multivitamin daily.

He does not want to talk about massage for the asthma, but as a goal, he is interested in a sports massage application for enhancing his golf game.

Physical Assessment

Posture

Slight kyphosis (common in asthma). Slight anterior rotation and elevation of the left shoulder with a lateral head tilt to the left.

Gait

Normal; arm swing is a bit short bilaterally.

Range of Motion

Arm extension and external rotation are slightly limited bilaterally, more so on the left.

Palpation

(Palpation examination was limited because client would not take off his clothes.)

Near Touch. Heat is evident in the upper chest and shoulder.

Skin. Normal (as identified on the arm). Bruise is noted on the right forearm.

Superficial Connective Tissue. Unable to assess

Vessels and Lymph Nodes. Unable to assess

Muscles. Breathing muscles are short, tight, and tender to moderate palpation. Tender points in the intercostals and anterior serratus are very sensitive to pressure. Trigger point activity is evident in the sternocleidomastoid muscles.

Tendons. Subscapularis and supraspinatus tendons bilaterally are tender to moderate pressure. Muscle attachments at the occipital base are tender to moderate pressure.

Deep Fascia. Short in the cervical area; unable to assess other areas.

Ligaments. Appear normal

Joints. Acromial clavicular and sternal clavicular joints on the left are tender to compressive force. Facet joints of the upper ribs are fixed and rigid.

Bones. Healing of broken clavicle noted.

Abdominal Viscera. Unable to assess

Body Rhythms. Breathing is strained, particularly the exhale phase; strain was exaggerated when parents were speaking for client.

Muscle Testing

Strength

Left arm extensors are weak. Rhomboids are weak. Pectoralis major is overly strong and would not inhibit.

Neurologic Balance

Reactive muscle twitching occurs with light touch on neck and chest. Shoulder muscles misfire.

Gait

Left arm extensors do not hold when facilitated by the left hip flexors.

Interpretation and Treatment Plan Development

Clinical Reasoning

What Are the Facts?

Asthma is a lung disease that affects 12 million to 15 million Americans, including approximately 10% to 12% of children under age 18. Asthma is a disease of the bronchial tubes characterized by tightening of these airways. It is one of the chronic obstructive pulmonary diseases (others are chronic bronchitis and emphysema.) Common symptoms include shortness of breath, coughing, wheezing, and tightening in the chest.

When a person breathes, air is taken into the body through the nose and then passes through the windpipe into the bronchial tubes. At the end of the tubes are tiny air sacs, called *alveoli,* that deliver oxygen to the blood. These air sacs also collect unusable carbon dioxide, which is exhaled from the body. During normal breathing, the bands of muscle that surround the airways are relaxed, and air moves freely. In people with asthma, allergy-causing substances and environmental triggers, such as smoke and scents, cause the bands of muscle surrounding the airways to tighten, and air cannot move freely. Less air causes a person to feel short of breath, and the air moving through the tightened airways causes a whistling sound known as *wheezing*.

Asthma can be controlled but not cured. It is not commonly fatal, but it can become life-threatening if it is not treated or controlled. Medications are used to prevent and control asthma symptoms, to reduce the number and severity of asthma episodes, and to improve airflow.

Asthma is treated with two kinds of medicines: quick-relief medicines to stop asthma symptoms and long-term control medicines to prevent symptoms. Inhaled corticosteroids are the preferred medicines for long-term control of asthma. One common side effect from inhaled corticosteroids is a mouth infection called *thrush*.

In rare cases leukotriene modifiers, such as Singulair (montelukast), can have serious side effects involving psychological reactions such as agitation, aggression, hallucinations, depression, and suicidal thinking.

The client is not interested in massage for the asthma but will discuss massage for his golf game. The restriction in arm mobility and the rotated and elevated shoulder are implicated as disturbing the golf swing.

What Are the Possibilities in Both Function and Dysfunction and the Massage Intervention Options?

The client has compensated for labored breathing since he was 6 years old. This has likely resulted in the postural shift and muscle tenderness identified during the assessment.

Playing golf may be straining the compensation patterns, making his breathing seem more labored. However, golf is a good sport choice, because the activity can be controlled and calming, as long as the performance remains relaxed and competition stays within reason.

Possibilities

1. A stretching program may be as beneficial as massage and may be more comfortable for the client. Adolescents commonly are very body aware and will assert their need for privacy and independence. The client may be embarrassed about the acne.
2. The initial suggestion for the massage would be for the client to experience a massage over the clothing in a seated position in the massage chair. Because he is a minor, the parents must be present for supervision; however, this could be accomplished by leaving the treatment room door open and having the parents seated just outside the door. Massage could then progress to a mat and still be done over the clothing.
3. Massage on a weekly basis has shown benefit for those with asthma. As the client becomes more comfortable, additional methods could be used. The palpation assessment could be completed when the client has become tolerant of his skin being touched.

What Are the Logical Outcomes of Each Possible Intervention?

Medication side effects of headache and gastrointestinal distress could be reduced by the massage.

Medication influence on the sympathetic autonomic nervous system may reduce the parasympathetic influence of the massage, reducing the benefits.

A stretching program may not address some of the shortening in the auxiliary breathing muscles that are most affected by the asthma.

What Is the Impact on the People Involved for Each Possible Intervention?

The client will accept massage better if he notices improvement in his golf game. If concrete benefits are seen, his compliance should increase.

The massage professional is uncomfortable talking the client into massage but confident that a focus on golf improvement would also gain beneficial results for the asthma. The massage professional is also uncomfortable with the overbearing parents and would have to establish appropriate working boundaries that respect the client's and the parents' rights.

The client is resistant. The parents are frustrated.

The medical team is very supportive.

Decision Making and Treatment Plan Development

Quantifiable Goal

To manage the side effects of medications and reduce sympathetic dominance

Qualifiable Goal

The client should be able to increase his performance in sports.

Treatment Regimen

Condition Management

A series of 10 weekly, 45-minute sessions of massage that begin in the chair over the clothing and focus on the respiratory function and golf swing will be provided. Broad-based compression, shaking, rocking, tapotement, vibration, joint movement (both active and passive), and various forms of muscle energy methods will be used to effectively lengthen short areas in both muscles and connective tissue. Positional release can be used on the tender points identified during assessment and can be taught to the client. Initially the focus will be on the upper body and arms, but gradually it will be extended to a more full-body approach if the client becomes willing.

A referral will be made to a flexibility program, an option that may be more comfortable for the client and that suggests that he choose the intervention he feels is most beneficial. The methods suggested for the massage sessions could be demonstrated on one of the parents so that the client can observe and become more comfortable with the process.

One of the parents must be present during the massage, and he or she can observe quietly from the open door during the session. All questions will be addressed before or after the session, but during the session the interaction must be between the client and the massage practitioner unless the client indicates otherwise.

The client and parents will monitor the effects of massage on both the asthma and the golf game and will report to the massage practitioner each session.

The golf pro where the client practices has indicated a willingness to work with helping people understand the benefits of massage and a flexibility program for good golf play. A referral for a meeting with the golf pro is appropriate.

A report will be sent monthly to the client's doctor.

CASE 18 SEASONAL AFFECTIVE DISORDER (SAD)

The client is a 32-year-old female. She is married and has two children, 6 and 9 years old. She is a teacher but has chosen to stay home while her children are young. She has been diagnosed with a form of depression called *seasonal affective disorder (SAD)*. She experiences moderate symptoms, including an increased appetite and a carbohydrate craving, and she gains about 20 pounds every winter. She loses some of the weight in the summer, but over the years she has become overweight. She wants to be alone and has lost all interest in sex. She is fatigued, she says she feels as if she weighs 1,000 pounds, and she cannot get enough sleep. She does not want to do anything, but manages to drag herself through the day to meet her major responsibilities. She has a hard time remembering details and is impatient with unexpected demands on her time. Her muscles ache, and she continually has a dull headache.

She is taking Prozac, a selective serotonin reuptake inhibitor (SSRI), and has recently begun using light therapy. Both seem to help.

She is interested in complementary methods, especially aromatherapy and homeopathy. She has also read that massage can have a positive effect on depression. She loves massage and has treated herself to massage when on vacation. A holistic health center with a massage clinic just opened in her hometown, and the rates are affordable with a package plan. Her doctor is supportive, especially if massage will help her be more compliant with an outdoor walking program.

Assessment

Observation

The client appears fatigued and has circles under her eyes. She carries the excess weight in her hips. She wants to sit down immediately when she enters the office, and when she gets up from the chair, she appears to have to exert an extraordinary amount of effort. Her demeanor is pleasant, but she seems to have to work at it. She does not offer information but does respond to questions.

Interview and Goals

The client history form indicates that she has headaches, wears contact lenses, has bouts of diarrhea, uses birth control pills, and has some abdominal bloating when she eats ice cream (likely a dairy sensitivity). Muscle aching is described as all over the body, with more stiffness than pain. She has had two pregnancies and one miscarriage. There is a history of heart problems on her father's side of the family. She is fatigued and depressed and has periods of anxiety. Even though she sleeps more than 10 hours a day, she feels as if that is not enough and that she is not rested in the morning. She has been attempting to lose weight with a low-fat diet. She fell down some stairs a few years ago. She was shaken up and had a slight concussion but was fine in a few days.

The client's goals for the massage are to reduce her depressive symptoms and to support her efforts at relaxation and exercise.

Physical Assessment

Posture

Generally bilaterally symmetric with no obvious postural distortions.

Gait

Slow and labored with reduced arm swing.

Range of Motion

Within normal range but guarded at the end-range.

Palpation

Near Touch. Body dissemination of energy seems low. The sense of same magnetic poles placed together is absent.
Skin. Normal but dry. Hair is dry, and fingers have hangnails.
Superficial Connective Tissue. Very slight bogginess
Vessels and Lymph Nodes. Normal
Muscles. Normal; no obvious tender areas or shortened muscles.
Tendons. Normal
Deep Fascia. Mild bind in the plantar fasciae.
Ligaments. Normal
Joints. End-feel is normal and soft, but client seems to guard and stiffen before physiologic end-range of joint movement is reached.
Bones. Normal
Abdominal Viscera. Soft with evidence of gas.
Body Rhythms. Entrainment seems off. Breathing is slow, with an even inhale-to-exhale ratio and some sighing. Heat rate is within normal range, but pulses are hard to feel. Full-body undulation (craniosacral or lymphatic, depending on the structure) is difficult to palpate.

Muscle Testing

Strength

Muscles test strong, but client exerts extraordinary effort during assessment.

Neurologic Balance

Client does not want to sustain pressure against resistance. She says she is tired. Gluteus maximus firing is off. Synergistic dominance is evident.

Gait

Shoulder and hip flexors on the opposite side inhibit instead of facilitate, whereas on the same side, they facilitate. Normal gaiting reflexes appear to be reversed. When client looks down, extensors twitch and flexors and adductors are inhibited rather than facilitated. When client looks up over her head, flexors and adductors inhibit as appropriate.

Interpretation and Treatment Plan Development

Clinical Reasoning

What Are the Facts?

Temporary depression is a normal reaction to loss, life's struggles, or injured self-esteem. However, feelings of sadness that become hopeless and intense, last for long periods, and prevent a person from leading his or her everyday life are not normal. A mental illness left untreated can worsen, lasting for years and causing untold suffering, and can possibly even lead to suicide. It is important for massage professionals to recognize the signs of depression and refer appropriately (Box 16-1).

Seasonal depression, or SAD, is a depression that occurs each year at the same time, usually starting in the fall or winter and ending in the spring or early summer. It is more than just "the winter blues" or "cabin fever." A rare form of SAD known as *summer depression* begins in late spring or early summer and ends in the fall.

People who suffer from SAD have many of the common signs of depression: sadness, irritability, loss of interest in their usual activities, withdrawal from social activities, and inability to concentrate (Box 16-2). Symptoms of winter SAD differ from symptoms of summer SAD (Box 16-3).

In the United States, 4% to 6% of the population suffers from SAD, and 10% to 20% may suffer from a milder form of winter blues. Three fourths of the sufferers are women, most of whom are in their 20s, 30, or 40s. Although SAD is most common during these ages, it also can occur in children and adolescents. Older adults are less likely to experience SAD.

The illness is more commonly seen in people who live at high latitudes (geographic locations farther north or south of the equator), where seasonal changes are more extreme.

To achieve effectiveness and to prevent a relapse of depression, medications generally are prescribed for 6 to 12 months for people treated for first-time depression. These medications usually must be taken regularly for at least 4 to 8 weeks before their full benefit takes effect.

The client in this case is taking Prozac. The side effects of Prozac, an SSRI, can include the following:
- Agitation
- Nausea or vomiting

Box 16-2	Common Symptoms of Seasonal Affective Disorder (SAD)*

Anxiety: Tension, inability to tolerate stress, phobias.
Social problems: Irritability, loss of pleasure in being with others and a desire to avoid contact, which could even turn into unwillingness to leave the home or bed.
Loss of libido: Decreased interest in sex.
Sleep problems: Tendency to sleep for longer periods; sleep is restless and less satisfying.
Mood swings: In the spring, when SAD lifts, some sufferers experience a dramatic swing in mood and a short period of hypomania, a sudden surge of energy and enthusiasm that brings problems of its own.
Menstrual difficulties: During the winter, premenstrual tension may be worse than in other seasons, causing irritability, sleep problems, appetite changes, and a low energy level.
Hopelessness: Feelings of desperation, which sometimes lead to overdependence on relationships, work, or home.
Excessive eating and drinking: Carbohydrates, alcohol, and coffee.
Increased sensitivity to pain: Headaches, muscle and joint pain.
Other physical ailments: Constipation, diarrhea, heart palpitations.

*Not all people with SAD have these symptoms.

Box 16-1	Signs and Symptoms of Depression

- Sadness (lingering)
- Loss of energy
- Feelings of hopelessness or worthlessness
- Loss of enjoyment of things that were once pleasurable
- Difficulty concentrating
- Uncontrollable crying
- Difficulty making decisions
- Irritability
- Increased need for sleep
- Insomnia or excessive sleep
- Unexplained aches and pains
- Stomachache and digestive problems
- Decreased sex drive
- Sexual problems
- Headache
- Change in appetite, causing weight loss or gain
- Thoughts of death or suicide
- Attempt at suicide

Box 16-3	Symptoms of Winter SAD and Summer SAD

Symptoms of Winter SAD
The symptoms of winter SAD include the seasonal occurrence of the following:
- Fatigue
- Increased need for sleep
- Decreased levels of energy
- Weight gain
- Increased appetite
- Difficulty concentrating
- Increased desire to be alone

Symptoms of Summer SAD
The symptoms of summer SAD include the seasonal occurrence of the following:
- Weight loss
- Trouble sleeping
- Decreased appetite

- Diarrhea
- Sexual problems, including low sex drive or inability to have an orgasm
- Dizziness
- Headaches
- Insomnia
- Increased anxiety
- Exhaustion

The client's gait reflex patterns are disrupted. Also, she is restricting her fat intake.

What Are the Possibilities in Both Function and Dysfunction and the Massage Intervention Options?

The client might not have enough fat in her diet. There is evidence of lactose intolerance with the gas and bloating. Referral to her doctor with a recommendation that she see a nutritionist would be wise.

The client's fall could have disrupted her normal gait patterns. Although not causal to the SAD, walking reflexes are nonoptimal and require increased energy expenditure, which is contributing to the fatigue. Working to re-establish a normal gait may be helpful. A wobble board and large gym ball activities could support massage, and if improvement is not noted with general intervention, referral to an exercise physiologist would be indicated.

Although medication seems to help, some of the symptoms indicate side effects of the medication, and referral back to the physician for re-evaluation of the medication and dosage would be prudent.

Possibilities

1. General constitutional massage has been shown to help those with various types of depression. Massage with sufficient pressure affects the serotonin and dopamine levels, and both neurotransmitters are implicated in SAD.
2. The normal gait reflex patterns can be stimulated with massage, which may make walking less fatiguing.
3. The client could be referred to an aromatherapist and a homeopath but not until approval is obtained from her physician.

What Are the Logical Outcomes of Each Possible Intervention?

Referral to the physician for further evaluation seems a cautious and prudent choice to clarify the client's symptom pattern. This does involve time and cost factors, as do referrals to other professionals. Introducing too many interventions at one time can be confusing as to what is having beneficial or detrimental effects.

Working with the gait reflexes is a simple and safe intervention during the massage, but the consequences of the fall could be more complicated, and specific protocols for retraining the walking pattern would need to be provided by a specialist, such as an exercise physiologist.

General, nonspecific massage is likely to provide quick, observable benefits but might not be sustaining if underlying factors exist that need to be determined. The cost for massage is reasonable, and the location is convenient.

Gym balls and wobble boards are easy to locate and inexpensive. The wobble board would require a person to spot during use to prevent falling. The exercise gym ball is safe to use alone.

What Is the Impact on the People Involved for Each Possible Intervention?

The client likes massage and is interested in homeopathy and aromatherapy. She is open to returning to her physician for further evaluation. The physician is supportive of massage but not of homeopathy.

The massage practitioner feels confident providing the massage but believes that as yet unidentified factors need to be resolved.

Decision Making and Treatment Plan Development

Quantifiable Goals

1. 50% improvement in gait
2. Support body's natural defenses against depression

Qualifiable Goal

The client will be able to exercise without pain and fatigue.

Treatment Regimen

The client will be referred back to her physician with the proposed treatment plan for massage and the following recommendations:

- The client may benefit from a nutritional evaluation. Medication side effects concur with the symptoms described on the client history form, and re-evaluation of the medication type or dosage may be indicated. The medication dose should be monitored, because massage does increase available levels of serotonin. Gait seems disrupted, and further evaluation from a physical therapist or exercise physiologist may be beneficial. Referral to the aromatherapist is recommended, because the client has expressed an interest in this complementary method.
- The client will receive a weekly 1-hour massage, and the schedule will be increased to twice a week if her symptoms worsen. The massage will be a general full-body approach with sufficient pressure for the client to feel the intensity of the session but with no pain or guarding. A general intervention to improve gait patterns will be to have the client roll her eyes in large, slow circles while the legs and arms are massaged. After six sessions of the general massage, pulsed muscle energy methods for the arm and opposite leg flexors will be introduced to encourage normal facilitation patterns.
- The client could benefit from a daily session of bouncing and stretching on a large exercise gym ball.

CASE 19 SPORTS PERFORMANCE ENHANCEMENT

The client is a 22-year-old female college student studying exercise science and athletic training. She is also a competitive marathon runner. Four years ago, she lost her left leg below the knee in an automobile accident. She has rehabilitated successfully and has been fitted with both a running prosthesis and a prosthesis for general use.

She is currently training for a marathon. She is determined to commit herself to the best performance possible. As an amateur athlete, she coordinates her own training program and works with a running coach. She had a first-degree ankle sprain 2 years ago, experiences generalized cramping if she overtrains, and has had one experience of shin splints. These symptoms improve when she drinks enough water or sports drinks and stretches. She occasionally gets side stitches.

She is a student of the sport and is constantly studying the effects of diet and training protocols to enhance her performance. She is interested in incorporating massage into her program to support recovery and flexibility and to reduce the potential for injury. Finances are secure as a result of an insurance settlement from the accident. She has determined that she can afford $150 per month to pay for massage and wants the maximum benefit from the investment.

Assessment

Observation

The client is a slim, muscular, fit female. Unless she is carefully observed, there is little evidence of the amputation. The client does not attempt to conceal the prosthesis and speaks freely about the accident. She is more concerned about total body performance than the loss of the leg.

Interview and Goals

The client information form indicates minor muscle pain related to training. She experiences mild episodes of phantom pain, usually in response to an increase in training. The pain is managed with rest, massage of the stump, and stretching. Her calf gets tight, she had shin splints in her right leg 8 months ago, and she sprained her right ankle 2 years ago.

She has occasional fatigue and restless sleep if she overtrains or experiences the phantom pain. She has athlete's foot and is currently being treated for that. She takes performance-based supplements in a well-balanced formula.

The client's goal for massage is support for a training regimen to enhance performance and help prevent injury.

Physical Assessment

Posture

Symmetric except for highly developed thigh muscles, with increased development on the left and a slightly elevated iliac crest on the left.

Gait

Normal with the prosthesis except for increased arm swing on the right. She indicates that she has experienced extensive rehabilitation to support normal gait after the amputation.

Range of Motion

Normal

Palpation

Near Touch. Energy sensation off the body is high and even. Heat is present at the amputation site.

Skin. Damp areas are noted at the amputation site and on the medial calf on the right. There are no areas of inflammation, abrasion, or skin irritation from the prosthesis. Skin is smooth and resilient. Small area of bind is noted just under the right clavicle in the chest.

Superficial Connective Tissue. Small bind and increased tissue density in the legs.

Vessels and Lymph Nodes. Normal

Muscles. Normal with hypertrophy in the legs. Decreased pliability with slight increase in density and shortening of the hamstrings. Tenderness and pain radiate to three areas on the stump, two in the vastus lateralis and one in the vastus medialis, indicating trigger point activity.

Tendons. Normal except for some shortening in the right Achilles tendon.

Deep Fascia. Plantar fascia is slightly short on the right.

Ligaments. Normal

Joints. No evidence of inappropriate end-feel or bind. Slight decrease in dorsiflexion on the right.

Bones. Normal

Abdominal Viscera. Normal

Body Rhythms. Normal

Muscle Testing

Strength

Normal

Neurologic Balance

Normal

Gait

Higher degrees of facilitation between extensors and flexors on the right arm and left leg seem to be appropriate compensation for amputation.

Interpretation and Treatment Plan Development

Clinical Reasoning

What Are the Facts?

An understanding of the basic physical concepts involved in exercise and training protocols is important to a massage professional who works with athletes in conditioning, performance enhancement, and injury rehabilitation. To increase a sustainable power output, the athlete must follow a carefully designed training program that will improve the individual's ability to (1) produce metabolic energy by both aerobic and anaerobic means; (2) sustain aerobic energy production at high levels before lactic acid accumulates excessively in the blood; (3) recruit more of the efficient slow-twitch muscle fibers in muscle groups used in competition; and (4) become more skillful by recruiting fewer nonessential muscle fibers during competition. Careful attention to maintaining a sufficient intake of fluids and carbohydrates before, during, and after strenuous competition and training sessions is also important (see Chapter 15).

Shin splints (medial tibial stress syndrome), side stitches, plantar fasciitis, muscle cramps, muscle strains, dehydration, and hyponatremia can quickly make running a painful experience. This client is experiencing shin splints, one of the most common running injuries. This is an inflammation of the tendons along the inside of the shinbone. Shin splints result when too much stress is put on tired calf muscles, as occurs with running on hard surfaces. Changing surfaces (from hard to soft) also tends to aggravate the calf muscles. The symptoms of shin splints include aching, throbbing, or tenderness of the shin. Pain is felt when the inflamed area is pressed. The best preventive measure is to stretch the calf muscles. Proper warm up and stretching before a run helps develop flexibility, which is a key factor in avoiding shin splints.

What Are the Possibilities in Both Function and Dysfunction and the Massage Intervention Options?

The client is in good physical condition, with minor changes that seem appropriate compensation for amputation and use of the prosthesis.

Trigger point activity in the leg with the amputation may be causing the phantom pain. An aggressive training program may be contributing to fatigue and muscle aching.

Possibilities

1. Massage is indicated for support of sports training programs. It can facilitate fluid exchange in the muscles, manage symptoms of delayed onset muscle soreness, and maintain appropriate pliability in soft tissue structures.
2. Massage can help reduce trigger point activity in the client's left leg, support restful sleep, and encourage well-being.

What Are the Logical Outcomes of Each Possible Intervention?

The client has specific and realistic expectations for sports massage and goals that are achievable.

She has determined that funds are available for massage, but the frequency of massage needed to achieve the desired results might exceed her funds. Massage two to three times per week would be optimal, with more frequent intervention during intensive training periods. The client's funds support one massage per week.

The massage therapist is aware of the time commitment required to serve a client with these goals effectively.

What Is the Impact on the People Involved for Each Possible Intervention?

All parties involved are supportive of massage, and the massage therapist is qualified to work with this level of athletic performance.

The massage therapist is willing to commit to the time necessary to support this athlete but is concerned about feeling taken advantage of, because fee reductions may be required. The client is very independent and a bit demanding but realistic and understanding of the massage therapist's concerns.

Decision Making and Treatment Plan Development

Quantifiable Goals

1. Reduce episodes of phantom pain by 50%
2. Reduce postexercise aches by 50%
3. Increase sleep effectiveness to support recovery time

Qualifiable Goal

The client will be able to participate in a training program with minimal discomfort.

Treatment Regimen

Condition Management

The massage therapist is an instructor at a massage school. The client will receive a 1-hour massage twice a week for $150 per month and will allow students to observe and participate in the sessions as part of a sports massage internship program. The athlete will be supported at various preliminary events by the students.

The massage will be a performance-based, full-body application and will be structured to meet the daily needs of the training regimen. Ongoing contact with the coach is requested. The massage will support rather than seek to change compensation patterns in gait in response to the amputation, because overall posture and performance are good.

Trigger points will be addressed with a variety of methods, and the results will be monitored to see if the phantom pain episodes decrease. The massage will be scheduled in the evening so the client can go to bed afterward. Sleep will be supported through encouragement of parasympathetic activation.

Appropriate methods that affect the neuromuscular/connective tissue and fluid dynamics of the body will be chosen each session. The client requires various levels of pressure, from very light pressure for lymphatic drainage to deep pressure to address the muscles of stabilization in the layer closest to the bone. Care will be taken not to increase inflammation in any area.

CASE 20 SCAR TISSUE MANAGEMENT

The client is a 28-year-old male computer technician who works 50 hours per week. He is in good health, active in a variety of outdoor activities, and concerned about maintaining the quality of his life.

Six years ago, while burning leaves, he was burned on his chest. He had first- and second-degree burns, in addition to small areas of third-degree burns. He was fortunate to be treated in a major burn center and received the best of care. The scarring was managed very well. Only one area had to be grafted, and the donor site was on his thigh; scarring also is present in that area.

Although the areas with a first-degree burn healed with no scarring, the areas with a second-degree burn did scar, with what is called *hypertrophic scars*. The client feels as if these scars are causing tightness across his chest and finds the sensation a nuisance.

The client has had massage a few times before and found that it lessened the tightness in his chest for a short time. He has read about various forms of connective tissue massage and the effect on scars. In the context of general massage, he would like to explore the possibility of using massage to make himself more comfortable and for general stress management. Because he just received a raise, he has $100 per month to spend for massage care.

Assessment

Observation

The client is of average height and weight. He looks fit and walks with an energetic flair. He is talkative and likes to tell jokes. He is left-handed. He sits calmly during the interview and fills out the necessary paperwork without difficulty.

Interview and Goals

The client information form indicates that the client has some numbness in the burn area. He had various childhood injuries, such as a broken wrist and sprained ankles, but he cannot remember just when it all happened. None of the injuries bother him. The burn has been his most serious injury. He was anxious for a time after the accident and had some nightmares, but that has passed. The surgeries he underwent were for the skin grafts on the third-degree burn area and for removal of skin from the donor site. He does not take medication or vitamins. His diet is adequate for a bachelor who lives with two other guys. He does drink and party on the weekends.

The client's goals for massage are general stress management and reduction of stiffness in his burn scars.

Physical Assessment

Posture

Symmetric with evidence of slight concavity of the chest. Knees are slightly hyperextended.

Gait

Normal

Range of Motion

Horizontal abduction of the arm is restricted to 80 degrees. Shoulder flexion on the left is restricted to 130 degrees.

Palpation

Near Touch. No observable problems.
Skin. Skin on the chest has areas of flat scars and areas of scar development that are somewhat rough and raised, with identifiable bands of scar tissue. Areas of pigment change are noted in the scarred region. Skin on the chest and between the scapulae on the back is binding. Skin fold cannot be lifted on burn scars. Skin fold can be lifted on the back with difficulty, and it is uncomfortable for the client.
Superficial Connective Tissue. Moderate adherence in the area of the scars on both the chest and donor area.

Vessels and Lymph Nodes. There is concern over pressure on the vessels in the chest and at the clavicle. There is no evidence of edema.
Muscles. Quadriceps are short, and rhomboids are long. Trigger point type activity is noted in the supraspinatus and occipital base, but no recognizable referred pain pattern is experienced
Tendons. Normal
Deep Fascia. Pliability of the lumbar dorsal fascia and iliotibial bands is reduced.
Ligaments. Normal
Joints. Horizontal abduction of the shoulder is limited by soft tissue bind. Sternoclavicular joint on the left is restricted.
Bones. Bone changes in the right wrist indicate healing of a bone break.
Abdominal Viscera. Normal
Body Rhythms. Full expansion of the thorax is somewhat restricted during deep inhalation. Body rhythm is even, and pulses are in the normal range.

Muscle Testing

Strength

Left arm flexors are weak to moderate resistance.

Neurologic Balance

Normal

Gait

Normal

Interpretation and Treatment Plan Development

Clinical Reasoning

What Are the Facts?

The client appears to have a restricted sternoclavicular joint on the left; referral to a chiropractor or osteopath is indicated. Treatment for this condition should correct the weak muscles of arm flexion.

Mild to moderate connective tissue binding is present, causing a concavity in the chest and reduction of horizontal abduction of the shoulder. The area corresponds with the burn scars. Corresponding areas of connective tissue bind are noted between the scapulae. The muscles in this area are also tight and long.

The short quadriceps muscles correspond with the hyperextension of the knees.

Trigger points do not refer a recognizable pain pattern. Burn scars are evident, with reduced tissue pliability and some adhesion.

A burn that causes blisters is a second-degree burn. Typically this type of burn is characterized as superficial or deep. A superficial second-degree burn involves only the most superficial dermis. It manifests as blistering or sloughing of overlying skin, causing a red, painful wound. Typically, the burn blanches but shows good capillary refill. Hairs cannot be pulled out easily. Healing occurs within 14 days, usually without scarring and without requiring surgical intervention.

A deep second-degree burn involves more of the dermis. It may manifest as blisters or a wound with a white or deep red base. Sensation is usually diminished, and healing takes longer than 14 days. Hypertrophic scarring occurs when the healing phase lasts longer than 2 weeks. Débriding and grafting, therefore, are recommended by 2 to 3 weeks.

Studies have shown that stretching the connective tissue with sufficient force creates an elastic response in scar tissue. The most common causes of contractures are scarring and lack of use because of immobilization or inactivity. Severe contracture in this client is not evident, but scar shortening is.

Scar tissue from burns and grafts can be sensitive, and work needs to proceed with caution to ensure that the area is not damaged by the tissue stretching.

What Are the Possibilities in Both Function and Dysfunction and the Massage Intervention Options?

The connective tissue shortening of the burn scars on the chest probably is binding and restricting both range of motion of the arm and upper chest motion.

Possibilities

1. Massage that exerts a drag on the skin and superficial fascia could increase pliability in the area.
2. General massage on a weekly basis could support stress management, relaxation, and an active lifestyle.

What Are the Logical Outcomes of Each Possible Intervention?

Massage is indicated for the stated goals, but the finances allocated are insufficient to support massage on a weekly basis to address goals.

What Is the Impact on the People Involved for Each Possible Intervention?

The client and massage professional are both supportive of massage and the realistic outcome of the goals, but the finances are difficult. The client has to reassess priorities in terms of where he spends his money. He is willing to invest some of his weekend partying money to cover the cost of massage on a weekly basis if he sees enough value in his progress, and he is willing to commit to a 3-month, 12-session trial period.

Decision Making and Treatment Plan Development

Quantifiable Goals

1. Reduce stress symptoms by 75% as reported by the client
2. Increase connective tissue pliability in burn scars by 30%

Qualifiable Goal

The client should be able to perform work and daily activities with minor tension on the scar tissue and be less irritated by the tissue changes in the burn scars.

Treatment Regimen

Condition Management

Weekly massage will be provided at $45 per hour session. The massage will consist of myofascial techniques with sufficient

drag to increase pliability of the scar tissue in the burn and donor areas. Caution will be needed to ensure that the intensity of the work is sufficient to address the connective tissue binding but does not damage the tissue in the area. The connective tissue work will be done before the general massage session, because generating a pulling sensation is likely to be intense and somewhat uncomfortable. The pressure used will exert force in the horizontal plane to stretch the area of the scars. Tensile and shear forces will be used first, then bend and torque as the tissue becomes more pliable. The intensity of the work will progress slowly.

When the skin and superficial fascia can be lifted, skin rolling methods will be introduced. The client will not have to endure this work for longer than 10 minutes, and frequent breaks will be included. Because mild inflammation will be introduced into the area, lymphatic drainage will be used to support movement of any restricted lymphatic flow away from the burned area. The possible trigger points will be monitored only, with no direct intervention other than what occurs during massage of the area.

General massage will be given, with methods used as needed to address range of motion and stress management; these methods will be determined at each massage session. Pressure levels will need to be sufficient to stimulate an increase in serotonin and enkephalin blood levels to achieve the relaxation and stress management goals. The massage rhythm, speed, and duration will address the shift from the stress response to parasympathetic dominance. The massage will be rhythmic and will support entrainment, with sufficient pressure exerted to address the deeper layers of soft tissue without causing pain or guarding.

SUMMARY

Each of the case studies in this chapter should challenge the student to continue to develop clinical reasoning skills and perfect assessment and technical therapeutic massage skills (Proficiency Exercise 16-1). More important, each case study told a story about a person who was seeking assistance. Remember, the most proficient application of massage is not competent practice until compassion, respect, and desire for the highest good of the client are the motivating intent of the massage. Each client you serve has the potential to be a great teacher if you are willing to learn. Knowledge needs experience to support your development as a therapeutic massage professional. Congratulations on your accumulation of knowledge as presented in this text. My hope is that each one who has learned from this text persists with the accumulation of knowledge and experience to serve and be served in this humble and important profession.

🚪 FOOT IN THE DOOR

This final chapter provides examples of 20 common scenarios you will encounter as a massage professional. If you expect to convince employers or potential clients that you are a competent massage therapist, you will need to be able to function as described in the case studies. When you study and practice and if you are taking your education seriously, these skills will get your foot in the door. Ultimately, it is your responsibility to be excellent.

You probably have had a teacher you thought was not effective, or maybe you feel that a classmate has interfered with your education. No excuse. This textbook, especially when paired with *Mosby's Essential Sciences for Therapeutic Massage,* and the accompanying online course can prepare you for career success. Remember, the cases presented in this chapter reflect entry-level education. That means that you still need lots of experience and more education, especially self-teaching.

Remember, each client you work with will be a teacher. When you are attempting to get your foot in the door as a new massage therapy graduate, admit that you are a beginner. However, make sure to communicate your commitment to excellence and passion for massage. You have the foundation to build upon if you have been a committed and excellent student. If you have some weakness in your career foundation because you did not devote your energy and time to your massage education, then fix it. Read your books, watch your DVDs, and practice giving massages. Ask (and if necessary pay) for help. Your efforts will get your foot in the door for a massage career, and your skills will keep you there.

Workbook Section

Assess Your Competencies

Now that you have studied this chapter, you should be able to:

- Use clinical reasoning to integrate the information from science studies and this text to complete a comprehensive history, assessment, and care/treatment plan.
- Write comprehensive case studies.
- Analyze care/treatment plans and offer and justify alternate approaches to care.
- Pick out three of the case studies in this chapter, develop a treatment plan that differs from the one presented, and be able to justify the appropriateness of your approach for the condition.

A

Indications and Contraindications to Massage

Indications are determined by evidence provided by research and expert consensus when research is not available. Indications for massage are reviewed in this textbook in Chapter 6. Determining contraindications is more difficult. When intelligent decision making and experience are coupled with appropriate adaptation, the result is very few contraindications, and most conditions fall into the caution category. However, because this is an entry-level textbook, it is assumed that the reader does not have experience and is still learning the process of critical thinking. Therefore, the recommendations in this appendix are conservative. Because each situation is different, making recommendations on when to give a massage and when not to give one is difficult. Each individual situation must be evaluated to determine whether massage is indicated or contraindicated. The existence of contraindications does not always mean that therapeutic massage is inappropriate. What most contraindications require is caution, which may call for modification of the massage treatment and, in some cases, supervision by and cooperation with the health care team. The clinical reasoning model is a valuable tool for making decisions about contraindications. This appendix presents two models of a guideline system for determining the indications and contraindications for massage. Specific conditions, symptoms, indications, and contraindications for massage follow. Use a medical dictionary to look up unfamiliar terms.

THE ONTARIO MODEL

The following are absolute contraindications (CI) to massage (i.e., massage treatment should not be given).

General

1. Acute-stage pneumonia
2. Advanced kidney failure (modified treatment may be possible with medical consent)
3. Advanced respiratory failure (modified treatment may be possible with medical consent)
4. Diabetes with complications (e.g., gangrene, advanced heart or kidney disease, very high or unstable blood pressure)
5. Eclampsia-toxemia in pregnancy
6. Hemophilia
7. Hemorrhage

8. Liver failure (modified treatment may be possible with medical consent)
9. Postcerebrovascular accident (CVA, stroke), condition not yet stabilized
10. Postmyocardial infarction (MI, heart attack), condition not yet stabilized
11. Severe atherosclerosis
12. Severe hypertension (if unstable)
13. Shock (all types)
14. Significant fever (higher than 101° F [38.3° C])
15. Some acute conditions that require first aid or medical attention:
    - Anaphylaxis
    - Appendicitis
    - CVA
    - Diabetic coma, insulin shock
    - Epileptic seizure
    - MI
    - Pneumothorax, atelectasis
    - Severe asthma attack, status asthmaticus
    - Syncope (fainting)
16. Some highly metastatic cancers not judged to be terminal
17. Systemic contagious/infectious condition

Local (Regional): Avoid or Modify Massage in the Indicated Area

1. Acute flare-up of inflammatory arthritis (e.g., rheumatoid arthritis, systemic lupus erythematosus, ankylosing spondylitis, Reiter's syndrome); may be general CI, depending on case
2. Acute neuritis
3. Aneurysms deemed life-threatening (e.g., of the abdominal aorta); may be general CI, depending on location
4. Ectopic pregnancy
5. Esophageal varicosities (varices)
6. Frostbite
7. Local contagious condition
8. Local irritable skin condition
9. Malignancy (especially if judged unstable)
10. Open wound or sore
11. Phlebitis, phlebothrombosis, arteritis; may be general CI if located in a major circulatory channel

12. Recent burn
13. Sepsis
14. Temporal arteritis
15. Twenty-four to 48 hours after antiinflammatory treatment (target tissue and immediate vicinity)
16. Undiagnosed lump

General

The following conditions require an awareness of the possibility of adverse effects from massage therapy. Substantial treatment adaptation may be appropriate. Medical consultation often is needed.

1. Any condition of spasticity or rigidity
2. Asthma
3. Cancer (including finding appropriate relationships to other current treatments)
4. Chronic congestive heart failure
5. Chronic kidney disease
6. Client taking antiinflammatory drugs, muscle relaxants, anticoagulants, analgesics, or any other medications that alter sensation, muscle tone, standard reflex reactions, cardiovascular function, kidney or liver function, or personality
7. Coma (may be absolute CI, depending on cause)
8. Diagnosed atherosclerosis
9. Drug withdrawal
10. Emphysema
11. Epilepsy
12. Hypertension
13. Immunosuppressed client
14. Inflammatory arthritides
15. Major or abdominal surgery
16. Moderately severe or juvenile-onset diabetes
17. Multiple sclerosis
18. Osteoporosis, osteomalacia
19. Pregnancy and labor
20. Post-MI
21. Post-CVA
22. Recent head injury

Local (Regional)

1. Acute disk herniation
2. Aneurysm (may be general CI, depending on location)
3. Any acute inflammatory condition
4. Any antiinflammatory treatment site
5. Any chronic or long-standing superficial thrombosis
6. Buerger's disease (may be general CI if unstable)
7. Chronic arthritic conditions
8. Chronic abdominal or digestive disease
9. Chronic diarrhea
10. Contusion
11. Endometriosis
12. Flaccid paralysis or paresis
13. Fracture (while casted and immediately after cast removal)
14. Hernia

15. Joint instability or hypermobility
16. Kidney infection, stones
17. Mastitis
18. Minor surgery
19. Pelvic inflammatory disease
20. Pitting edema
21. Portal hypertension
22. Prolonged constipation
23. Recent abortion/vaginal birth
24. Trigeminal neuralgia

Other Important Considerations

1. Massage therapists are expected to know how and when to consult with physicians and other health care professionals.
2. Most emotional or psychiatric conditions affect massage treatment. Individual decisions must be made according to case circumstances and, in many instances, medical advice. Medications may be a factor.
3. The client may be allergic to certain massage oils and creams or to cleansers or disinfectants used on sheets and tables.
4. The presence of pins, staples, or artificial joints may alter treatment indications.
5. The massage therapist should be aware of the role of common chronic conditions that affect public health (e.g., cardiovascular disease, cancer, substance abuse, chronic mental diseases). The local health department can provide additional information on public mental health services, environmental hazards, occupational health, or various health care organizations available in the community.

THE OREGON MODEL: INDICATIONS AND CONTRAINDICATIONS BY BODY SYSTEM

This extensive list was developed by the Oregon Board of Massage. However, no specific recommendations regarding indications or contraindications for massage were made. The descriptions of the disease processes and the massage recommendations were added by this author, using a very conservative approach. If an indication for massage is not listed for a disease process, massage has no direct benefit; such cases are designated N/A. Again, this textbook covers basic massage. Advanced training in the clinical application of massage, in addition to direct supervision by a physician, chiropractor, physical therapist, psychologist, dentist, podiatrist, or other health care professional, greatly expands the application of massage in rehabilitative situations.

The Integumentary System

Assessment parameters include color (e.g., pallor, jaundice, cyanosis, erythema, mottling), texture (e.g., dry, moist, scaly), scars (normal and keloid), vascularity (e.g., dilated veins, angiomas, varicosities, ecchymoses, petechiae, purpura),

...es, lesions, nail condition, hair condition, ...n, and edema.

...s that suggest the need for evaluation and referral ...umps or masses, rashes of unknown origin, lesions, ...s, urticaria, itching of unknown origin, cyanosis, jaun-...ice, ulcerations, multiple bruises, and petechiae.

Specific Disease Processes and Bacterial Conditions

Acne
Definition/symptoms: Inflammation of the skin affecting the sebaceous gland ducts

Indications: Massage increases systemic circulation; may assist healing

Contraindications: Regional; avoid affected area; do not use ointments that clog pores

Carbuncle
Definition/symptoms: Mass of connected boils

Indications: Massage may increase systemic circulation and may assist healing

Contraindications: Refer client to physician; regional; avoid affected area

Cellulitis
Definition/symptoms: Inflammation of the subcutaneous tissue with redness and swelling

Indications: Avoid

Contraindications: Regional; may be associated with erysipelas, a contagious condition; refer client to physician

Folliculitis
Definition/symptoms: Inflammation of the hair follicles

Indications: Massage may increase systemic circulation and assist healing

Contraindications: Regional; refer client to physician; avoid affected area

Furuncle (Boil)
Definition/symptoms: Pus-filled cavity formed by infection of a hair follicle

Indications: Massage may increase systemic circulation and assist healing

Contraindications: Regional; refer client to physician; avoid affected area

Impetigo
Definition/symptoms: Highly contagious bacterial skin infection that occurs most often in children; begins as a reddish discoloration and develops into vesicles with a yellow crust

Indications: Massage may increase systemic circulation and assist healing

Contraindications: Regional; refer client to physician; avoid affected area

Syphilis
Definition/symptoms: Primary stage: a usually painless lesion (chancre) present on exposed skin; secondary stage: begins

about 2 months after chancre disappears and produces a variety of symptoms, including skin rash

Indications: N/A

Contraindications: General; rash is contagious; refer client to physician

Viral Conditions

Bell's Palsy
Definition/symptoms: Infection of the seventh cranial nerve; primary symptom is paralysis of facial features, including the eyelids and mouth

Indications: Relaxation massage may facilitate healing

Contraindications: Regional; refer client to physician for diagnosis

Herpes Simplex
Definition/symptoms: Acute viral disease marked by groups of watery blisters on or near mucous membranes

Indications: Recurrence is stress induced; massage may reduce stress levels

Contraindications: Regional; contagious; avoid affected area

Herpes Zoster (Shingles)
Definition/symptoms: Viral infection that usually affects the skin of a single dermatome; produces a red, swollen plaque that ruptures and crusts

Indications: Condition is painful; general massage may ease pain

Contraindications: Regional; avoid affected area; may need to refer client to physician

Warts
Definition/symptoms: Usually benign excess cell growth of the skin

Indications: N/A

Contraindications: Regional; avoid affected area; contagious; may become malignant; if any changes in wart occur, refer client to physician

Fungal Conditions

Ringworm, Athlete's Foot, Fungal Infection of the Nails
Definition/symptoms: Scaly and crusty cracking of the skin

Indications: Keep area dry; do not use lubricants

Contraindications: Regional; do not use lubricants near the area because fungi thrive in a moist environment

Allergic Reactions

Atopic Dermatitis (Eczema)
Definition/symptoms: Common inflammation of the skin marked by papules, vesicles, and crusts

Indications: Symptom of an underlying condition; refer client to physician for diagnosis

Contraindications: Regional; avoid affected area

Contact Dermatitis
Definition/symptoms: Inflammation that occurs in response to contact with an external agent

Indications: Use unscented lubricants (scents often cause allergic reactions)

Contraindications: Regional; avoid affected area

Urticaria (Hives)

Definition/symptoms: Red, raised lesions caused by leakage of fluid from the skin and blood vessels; primary symptom is severe itching

Indications: Do not use scented products; hives may have an emotional component

Contraindications: Regional; avoid affected area

Benign Conditions

Mole

Definition/symptoms: Pigmented, fleshy growth of skin

Indications: Watch for any change in a mole; refer client to physician if a change is noted

Contraindications: Regional; avoid mole

Psoriasis

Definition/symptoms: Chronic inflammation of the skin; probably genetic; symptoms include scaly plaque and excessive growth rate of epithelial cells

Indications: May be stress-induced; massage reduces stress

Contraindications: Regional; avoid affected area

Scleroderma

Definition/symptoms: Autoimmune disease that affects blood vessels and connective tissue of the skin; primary symptom is hard, yellowish skin

Indications: N/A

Contraindications: Regional (except in systemic cases); refer client to physician

Malignant Conditions

Skin Cancer

Definition/symptoms: Squamous cell carcinoma, basal cell carcinoma, melanoma, Kaposi's sarcoma

Indications: N/A

Contraindications: Watch for any change in a mole or existing skin condition; if this occurs, refer client to physician immediately

The Skeletal System, Muscular System, and Articulations

Assessment parameters include range of motion, swelling, masses, deformity, pain or tenderness, temperature, crepitus, spasm, paresthesia, pulses, skin color, paralysis, atrophy, and contracture.

Deviations that suggest the need for evaluation and referral include malalignment of an extremity, asymmetry of musculoskeletal contour, progressive or persistent pain, masses or progressive swelling, numbness and/or tingling with loss of function, diminished or absent peripheral pulses, pallor and/or coolness of one extremity, redness and/or increased temperature of one extremity, and difference in size of extremities.

Specific Disease Processes

Atonicity (Flaccidity)

Definition/symptoms: Reduced ability or inability of the muscle to contract (hypotonicity)

Indications: Massage to tone; relaxation of opposing muscle groups

Contraindications: Regional; refer client to physician for diagnosis before proceeding

Contracture

Definition/symptoms: Fixed resistance to passive stretching of muscles; usually the result of fibrosis or tissue ischemia

Indications: Massage and stretch

Contraindications: Do not stretch past fixed barrier

Convulsion

Definition/symptoms: Sudden, involuntary series of muscle contractions, sometimes called a *seizure*

Indications: N/A

Contraindications: Refer client to physician immediately

Fibrillation

Definition/symptoms: A small, local contraction of muscle that is invisible under the skin; results from spontaneous, synchronous activation of single muscle cells

Indications: Massage, direct pressure

Contraindications: If continuous, refer client to physician for diagnosis

Hypertonicity

Definition/symptoms: Increased muscle tone

Indications: Massage and stretch

Contraindications: Recurrence without explanation; refer client to physician for diagnosis

Spasms (Cramp)

Definition/symptoms: Sudden, painful onset of a muscle contraction

Indications: Use reciprocal inhibition; push muscle belly together and slowly stretch

Contraindications: If recurring and transient, refer client to physician

Tic

Definition/symptoms: Spasmodic twitching; often occurs in the face

Indications: May be stress-induced; massage is beneficial in reducing stress

Contraindications: Refer client to physician for diagnosis to rule out underlying pathologic condition

Soft Tissue Injuries

Dislocation

Definition/symptoms: Displacement of a bone within a joint

Indications: N/A

Contraindications: Immediately refer client to physician

...oms: Traumatic injury of ligaments that ...al joint; may involve injury (strain) of muscles or

...dications: PRICE (protection, rest, ice, compression, ...levation), first aid, gentle massage, and range of motion facilitate healing

Contraindications: Regional; all traumatic injuries should be evaluated by a physician

Strains

Definition/symptoms: Traumatic injury caused by overstretching or overexertion of muscle or tendon tissue

Indications: PRICE, first aid, gentle massage, and range of motion may facilitate healing

Contraindications: Regional; all traumatic injuries should be evaluated by a physician

Subluxation

Definition/symptoms: Any deviation from the normal relationship in which the articular cartilage is touching any portion of its mating cartilage

Indications: Massage may help relieve muscle spasm

Contraindications: Refer client to physician

Infectious Processes

Osteomyelitis

Definition/symptoms: Bacterial infection of the bone; symptoms include deep pain and fever

Indications: N/A

Contraindications: General; immediately refer client to physician; difficult to diagnose and treat

Inflammatory Processes

Ankylosing Spondylitis

Definition/symptoms: Chronic inflammatory disease; can be progressive; usually involves the sacroiliac joint and spinal articulations; cause is unknown, appears to be genetic; if progressive, calcification of the joints and articular surfaces occurs; begins with feelings of fatigue and intermittent low back pain; synovial tissue around the involved joints becomes inflamed; heart disease also may occur

Indications: Massage may be helpful under direct supervision of a physician

Contraindications: General; refer client to physician; avoid any area of inflammation

Bursitis

Definition/symptoms: Inflammation of a bursa

Indications: Massage may take pressure off the joint by relaxing and normalizing surrounding musculature; ice

Contraindications: Regional; avoid affected area; work above and below jointed area

Fibromyalgia

Definition/symptoms: General disruption in connective tissue muscle component; symptoms include tender point activity; vague symptoms of pain and fatigue

Indications: Massage may be beneficial; work with physician

Contraindications: General; refer client to physician for diagnosis; do not use therapeutic inflammation methods

Gouty Arthritis

Definition/symptoms: Metabolic condition in which sodium urate crystals trigger a chronic inflammatory process

Indications: Dietary adjustment necessary

Contraindications: Regional; avoid area of inflammation

Lupus Erythematosus

Definition/symptoms: Chronic inflammatory disease that affects many body tissues; common symptom is a red rash on the face

Indications: Massage may be beneficial under physician's close supervision

Contraindications: General; systemic disease

Osgood-Schlatter Disease

Definition/symptoms: Osteochondrosis (inflammation of bone and cartilage) of the tibial tuberosity

Indications: N/A

Contraindications: Regional; avoid affected area

Rheumatoid Arthritis

Definition/symptoms: Autoimmune inflammatory joint disease characterized by synovial inflammation that spreads to other tissues

Indications: Stress responsive; massage can be helpful under medical supervision

Contraindications: General; work closely with physician

Tendinitis

Definition/symptoms: Inflammation of tendon and tendon-muscle junction

Indications: Massage may assist healing; ice

Contraindications: Regional; avoid affected area; work above and below the area

Tenosynovitis

Definition/symptoms: Inflammation of a tendon sheath, usually from repetitive movement

Indications: Massage may relieve muscle hypertension and assist healing of area; ice

Contraindications: Regional; avoid affected area; work above and below the area

Compression Processes

Carpal Tunnel Syndrome

Definition/symptoms: Inflammation in tendon sheaths in the carpal tunnel that creates pressure on the median nerve; symptoms include weakness and tingling in the hand

Indications: Symptoms often are confused with thoracic outlet syndrome; massage is proving to be beneficial

Contraindications: Regional; refer client to physician for diagnosis

Degenerative Processes

Muscular Dystrophy

Definition/symptoms: A group of muscle disorders characterized by atrophy of skeletal muscle without nerve involvement

Indications: Massage is beneficial; work closely with supervising physician

Contraindications: General

Osteoarthritis

Definition/symptoms: Degenerative joint disease of the articular cartilage; age and joint damage are risk factors

Indications: Massage is beneficial

Contraindications: Regional; avoid area of inflammation

Osteoporosis

Definition/symptoms: Loss of minerals and collagen from bone matrix, resulting in reduced volume and strength of skeletal bone

Indications: Gentle massage is beneficial; use care and caution

Contraindications: General

Abnormal Spinal Curve

Kyphosis

Definition/symptoms: Abnormal increased convexity of the thoracic spine

Indications: Massage is beneficial as part of the treatment plan

Contraindications: Regional; in severe cases proceed after obtaining physician's recommendation

Lordosis

Definition/symptoms: Abnormal increased concavity in the curvature of the lumbar spine

Indications: Massage is beneficial as part of the treatment plan

Contraindications: Regional; in severe cases proceed after obtaining physician's recommendation

Scoliosis

Definition/symptoms: Lateral curve of the vertebral column

Indications: Massage is beneficial as part of the treatment plan

Contraindications: Regional; in severe cases proceed after obtaining physician's recommendation

Disordered Muscular Processes

Low Back Pain

Definition/symptoms: May be of many varieties: muscular, nerve entrapment, or disk problem

Indications: Massage can be beneficial as part of the treatment plan

Contraindications: Regional; important to refer client to physician to rule out serious condition of the spine or viscera

Spasmodic Torticollis

Definition/symptoms: A contracted state of the cervical muscles that causes pain and rotation of the head

Indications: Massage is beneficial

Contraindications: Regional; refer client to physician for diagnosis to rule out serious disease

Temporomandibular Joint (TMJ) Dysfunction

Definition/symptoms: Disorder in functioning of the TMJ; pain and muscle contraction

Indications: Massage is beneficial; work closely with dentist and physician

Contraindications: Regional if painful

Neurologic Conditions

Assessment parameters include mental status, the presence of involuntary movements, coordination and balance, muscle tone and strength, changes in sensory perception (i.e., touch, pain, temperature, vibration, position sense, hearing, vision).

Deviations that suggest the need for evaluation and referral include inequality of pupil size; diplopia; abnormal Babinski's sign (extensor plantar response); seizures (partial or generalized); significant personality changes; changes in sensorium; progressively worsening or persistent headache; temporary loss of speech, vision, or motion; triad of fever, headache, and nuchal rigidity; vomiting; and change in pupil size with head injury.

Specific Disease Processes

Dyskinesia

Definition/symptoms: Impairment of the power of voluntary movement, resulting in fragmentary or incomplete movement and possibly pain

Indications: Massage is beneficial as part of a physician-directed treatment plan

Contraindications: General; refer client to physician for diagnosis and treatment plan

Dystonia

Definition/symptoms: Disordered, random tonicity of muscles

Indications: Massage is beneficial as part of a physician-directed treatment plan

Contraindications: General; refer client to physician for diagnosis and treatment plan

Insomnia

Definition/symptoms: Inability to sleep or interrupted sleep

Indications: Massage is beneficial

Contraindications: Regional; refer client to physician for specific diagnosis to rule out serious underlying condition

Peripheral Neuropathy

Definition/symptoms: General functional disturbances and/or pathologic changes in the peripheral nervous system caused by diabetic neuropathy, ischemic neuropathy, or traumatic neuropathy; symptoms include numbness, burning, and pain

...ssage is beneficial as part of the treatment

...ations: General; refer client to physician for
...o determine underlying condition

...nitus

Definition/symptoms: Noise in the ear; symptoms include ringing, buzzing, roaring, or clicking

Indications: N/A

Contraindications: Regional; refer client to physician for specific diagnosis

Vertigo

Definition/symptoms: Sensation of movement, not to be confused with dizziness

Indications: N/A

Contraindications: General; usually symptomatic of underlying condition; physician's diagnosis required

Vascular Processes

Cerebrovascular Accident (CVA)

Definition/symptoms: Stroke; a disturbance in cerebral circulation; major causes include atherosclerosis (thrombosis), embolism, hypertensive intracerebral hemorrhage or ruptured saccular aneurysm; symptoms differ, depending on where the disturbance in circulation occurs; general symptoms include weakness or paralysis of the arm or leg, headache, numbness, blurred or double vision, and confusion or dizziness; often only one side is affected; symptoms persist for at least 24 hours, usually much longer

Indications: Massage may be beneficial during recovery under physician's supervision and during long-term care for continued support

Contraindications: Refer client to physician for diagnosis

Headache

Definition/symptoms: Pain or dull ache in the head and upper neck; can have a variety of causes, such as muscle tension, sinus pressure, pinched nerve, vascular disruption (e.g., migraine headache, cluster headaches), and toxins

Indications: Massage may be beneficial

Contraindications: Refer all clients with a persistent, severe headache to physician for specific diagnosis

Head Injury

Definition/symptoms: Contusion (bump on the head); laceration (cut or break in the skin); subdural and epidural injury may produce disorientation, nausea, and uneven pupil dilation

Indications: Immediately refer client to physician if any of the signs listed above are noted

Contraindications: General; all traumatic injuries must be evaluated by a physician

Transient Ischemic Attack (TIA)

Definition/symptoms: Episodes of neurologic dysfunction that usually are of short duration (a few minutes) but may persist for 24 hours; reversible; symptom pattern is the same

with each attack, because the same vessel is involved; small strokes, seizures, migraine symptoms, postural hypotension, and Stokes-Allen syndrome may be misdiagnosed as TIAs

Indications: Massage may be beneficial under physician's supervision

Contraindications: Refer client to physician for diagnosis

Infectious Processes

Conjunctivitis

Definition/symptoms: Inflammation and/or infection of the mucous membranes of the eye

Indications: N/A

Contraindications: Regional; refer client to physician; may be contagious; avoid affected area

Parkinson's Disease

Definition/symptoms: Nervous disorder characterized by abnormally low levels of the neurotransmitter dopamine, resulting in involuntary trembling and muscle rigidity

Indications: Massage is beneficial as part of a physician-directed treatment plan

Contraindications: General

Poliomyelitis

Definition/symptoms: Viral infection of the nerves that control skeletal muscles

Indications: Massage is beneficial as part of a physician-directed treatment plan

Contraindications: General

Postpolio Syndrome

Definition/symptoms: Symptoms of fatigue and general muscle weakness that appear years after resolution of poliomyelitis

Indications: Massage is beneficial as part of a physician-directed treatment plan

Contraindications: Regional; refer client to physician for specific diagnosis

Neuromuscular Processes

Multiple Sclerosis

Definition/symptoms: Primary disease of the central nervous system marked by degeneration of myelin

Indications: Massage is beneficial as part of a physician-directed treatment plan

Contraindications: General

Spinal Cord Injury

Definition/symptoms: Traumatic injury or degenerative process of the spinal cord; may result from compression, cut, or tissue replacement in scarring

Indications: Massage is beneficial as part of a physician-directed treatment plan

Contraindications: Regional

Trigeminal Neuralgia (Tic Douloureux)

Definition/symptoms: Compression or degeneration of the fifth cranial nerve; primary symptom is recurring episodes of stabbing pain in the face

Indications: Avoid entire area of trigeminal nerve innervation; massage may trigger pain response

Contraindications: Regional

Miscellaneous Disorders

Seizure Disorders

Definition/symptoms: Sudden bursts of abnormal neuronal activity that cause temporary changes in brain activity; may vary from mild, affecting conscious motor control or sensory perception, to severe, resulting in convulsion

Indications: Massage may be beneficial

Contraindications: General; follow physician's recommendation for massage

Sleep Apnea

Definition/symptoms: Cessation of breathing during sleep

Indications: Stress may be a factor; massage is beneficial in reducing stress

Contraindications: Regional

Thoracic Outlet Syndrome

Definition/symptoms: Compression of brachial nerve plexus; primary symptom is pain that radiates to the shoulder and arm

Indications: Massage is beneficial as part of the treatment plan

Contraindications: Regional; refer client to physician for specific diagnosis

Endocrine System

Assessment parameters include fatigue, depression, changes in energy level, hyperalertness, sleep patterns, and mood. These can affect the skin, hair, and personal appearance.

Deviations that suggest the need for evaluation and referral include cold, clammy skin; numbness of fingers, toes, or mouth; rapid heartbeat, a feeling of faintness; vertigo; tremors; dyspnea (difficulty breathing); thyroid nodule; unusually warm hands and feet; and lethargy.

Specific Disease Processes

Diabetes Mellitus

Definition/symptoms: Metabolic disorder; body loses the ability to oxidize carbohydrates because of faulty pancreatic activity, especially of the islets of Langerhans, which affects insulin production; symptoms include thirst, hunger, and acidosis; severe symptoms include difficulty breathing and changes in blood chemistry that lead to coma

Indications: Massage is given under supervision of the primary care physician; it is beneficial for circulation enhancement and stress reduction; exercise also is beneficial

Contraindications: General; work only under physician's supervision

Hyperglycemia

Definition/symptoms: High blood sugar, resulting from inadequate insulin in the blood; symptoms are the same as those for diabetes mellitus

Indications: See Diabetes mellitus

Contraindications: See Diabetes mellitus

Hypoglycemia

Definition/symptoms: Low blood glucose, resulting from an excess of insulin in the blood; symptoms include lightheadedness, anxiety, and forgetfulness

Indications: Dietary changes; massage is helpful and may relieve stress

Contraindications: Refer client to physician to determine the cause of low blood sugar

Hyperthyroidism

Definition/symptoms: Overproduction of thyroid hormone; can be caused by a tumor or by problems with the self-regulatory mechanism in the pituitary gland; symptoms include anxiety, bulging eyes, high metabolic rate, and nervousness

Indications: Massage is beneficial for relaxing the client

Contraindications: General; work within physician's recommendations

Hypothyroidism

Definition/symptoms: Underproduction of thyroid hormone; symptoms include sensitivity to cold, weight gain, fatigue, and dullness

Indications: Massage is beneficial for stimulating metabolic function

Contraindications: General; work within physician's recommendations

Neuropathy

Definition/symptoms: Functional disturbance or pathologic change in the peripheral nervous system; symptoms include numbness, burning, and tingling pain

Indications: Massage is beneficial under medical supervision; may calm hypersensitive nerves

Contraindications: General; work under physician's direction

Cardiovascular System

Assessment parameters include skin color and appearance, respiratory rate and effort, condition of nails and nail beds (e.g., clubbing, cyanosis), pain or tenderness and points of radiation, swelling, and symmetry of chest cavity.

Deviations that suggest the need for evaluation and referral include pulse over 90 or under 60 beats per minute; dyspnea; pitting edema; distended neck veins; glossy appearance of the skin; positive Homans sign (calf tenderness with dorsiflexion of the foot); asymmetry of limb circumference; red, warm, tender, and hard veins; edema, pain, and tenderness of extremity; clubbing of nail beds; chest pain (especially if radiating to left arm); central or peripheral cyanosis; pallor; mottling or cyanosis of a limb; stasis ulcers; and splinter hemorrhages (small red to black streaks under the fingernails).

cesses

...ptoms: Reduced red blood cell count or hemo-
...mptoms include fatigue and pallor
...ications: Massage can be beneficial as part of the treat-
...ent plan
Contraindications: General; refer client to physician for
diagnosis and proceed under physician's direction

Aneurysm

Definition/symptoms: Abnormal widening of the arterial wall;
tends to form thrombi and also to burst; a pulsating bulge and
pressure are felt with accompanying symptoms of pain
Indications: N/A
Contraindications: Regional; immediately refer client to
physician; avoid direct heavy pressure into arterial vessels

Angina Pectoris

Definition/symptoms: Chest pain caused by inadequate oxygen to the heart (usually because of blocked coronary arteries)
Indications: Massage is beneficial as part of a lifestyle
change
Contraindications: General; massage is performed under
physician's supervision

Arteriosclerosis and Atherosclerosis

Definition/symptoms: Hardening of the arteries; a type of
coronary heart disease; symptoms may be mild to severe; may
be mistaken for other problems
Indications: Massage is beneficial as part of a lifestyle
change
Contraindications: General; perform massage under physician's supervision

Congestive Heart Failure

Definition/symptoms: Left heart failure; inability of the left
ventricle to pump effectively; one symptom is increased fluid
retention
Indications: Massage is beneficial in helping diuretics
remove excess fluid
Contraindications: General; must work under physician's
supervision; client may have difficulty breathing in a supine
position

Deep Vein Thrombosis

Definition/symptoms: Blood clot in deep veins; risk factor for
pulmonary embolism (blood clot in the heart); often asymptomatic; symptoms may include swelling, edema, and pain
described as aching and throbbing
Indications: N/A
Contraindications: Regional to general, depending on the
severity of symptoms; always refer client to physician for
unexplained pain; never massage over such areas

Hemophilia

Definition/symptoms: Blood clotting disorder; primary
symptom is spontaneous bleeding resulting from an inability
to form clots

Indications: Extremely light energy type of massage given
only under physician's direction
Contraindications: General; work only under physician's
supervision

Myocardial Infarction (MI)

Definition/symptoms: Death of cardiac muscle cells, usually
from inadequate blood supply, often from coronary thrombosis or coronary artery disease; symptoms include severe
pain in the chest or left arm, difficulty breathing, and
weakness
Indications: During rehabilitation, massage can be beneficial when supervised by a physician
Contraindications: General; refer client to physician
immediately

Mononucleosis

Definition/symptoms: Induced by Epstein-Barr virus; symptoms include fever, fatigue, and swollen glands
Indications: Massage is beneficial as part of the treatment
plan; care must be taken with contagious conditions
Contraindications: General; refer client to physician for
specific diagnosis

Phlebitis

Definition/symptoms: Inflammation of a vein; may be caused
by a blood clot; symptoms include edema, stiffness, and pain;
veins may streak red
Indications: N/A
Contraindications: Regional to general; see Deep Vein
Thrombosis

Raynaud's Syndrome

Definition/symptoms: Arteriospastic condition caused by
vasospasms of the small cutaneous and subcutaneous arteries
and arterioles; usually activated by cold but can be emotionally triggered; symptoms include skin pallor and pain
Indications: Care must be taken to avoid triggering the
symptoms; interview client carefully; massage may be beneficial for stress reduction
Contraindications: Refer client to physician for specific
underlying diagnosis; condition may be symptomatic of
serious disorder

Syncope

Definition/symptoms: Sudden loss of strength; fainting; may
be caused by a cardiac spasm resulting from closure of coronary arteries
Indications: N/A
Contraindications: General; immediately refer client to
physician

Varicose Veins

Definition/symptoms: Enlarged veins in which blood
pools; caused by collapse of valve system; tend to form
thrombi
Indications: N/A
Contraindications: Regional; avoid affected area

Lymphatic and Immune Systems

Assessment parameters include skin color and condition, evidence of eye irritation, lymph nodes, and nasal discharge/irritation.

Deviations that suggest the need for evaluation and referral include client history of chronic fatigue or recurrent physical ailments (e.g., skin, respiratory, gastrointestinal) in the absence of general illness; history of food intolerance; failure to gain weight; unexplained weight loss; rashes of unknown origin; urticaria; enlarged, tender nodes; and excessive or persistent dryness and scaliness of skin.

Specific Disease Processes

Allergy

Definition/symptoms: Hypersensitivity of immune system to relatively harmless environmental antigens; symptoms include increased mucous membrane inflammation, occasionally spastic bladder

Indications: Massage is beneficial

Contraindications: Refer client to physician for specific diagnosis

Autoimmune Disease

Definition/symptoms: Disease in which the immune system attacks the body's own tissues; symptoms include inflammation, fatigue, and allergy

Indications: Massage is beneficial with physician's recommendation

Contraindications: General; refer client to physician for specific diagnosis

Chronic Fatigue Syndrome

Definition/symptoms: May be induced by a virus; symptoms include swollen glands, low-grade fever, muscle and joint aches, headache, and fatigue

Indications: Massage is beneficial

Contraindications: General; refer client to physician for specific diagnosis

Human Immunodeficiency Virus (HIV) Infection

Definition/symptoms: Viral infection transmitted by means of body fluids; causes immunosuppression

Indications: Massage is beneficial with physician's recommendation; follow antiviral precautions for control of virus; 10% bleach solution; avoid body fluid contact

Contraindications: General; work with physician

Lymphedema

Definition/symptoms: Swelling of tissue caused by partial or complete blockage of lymph vessels

Indications: Massage is beneficial as part of the treatment plan and is given under the supervision of the primary care physician

Contraindications: Refer client to physician for diagnosis

The Respiratory System

Assessment parameters include the rate and pattern of respiration, chest movement, color, nodes, chest configuration, ease of chest excursions, fremitus, and pain.

Deviations that suggest the need for evaluation and referral include inspiratory flaring of the nostrils; use of accessory muscles; intercostal retractions or bulging; pursed lips on exhalation; splinting; uneven chest movement; altered tactile fremitus/crepitus (increased or decreased); cyanosis or pallor; enlarged, tender nodes; pain with breathing; and a respiratory rate over 20 respirations per minute in the absence of exertion or strong emotion.

Specific Infectious Disease Processes

Asthma

Definition/symptoms: Recurring muscle spasms in the bronchial wall accompanied by fluid retention and production of mucus; stress-specific condition

Indications: Massage is beneficial; monitor breathing closely

Contraindications: Work under direction of primary care physician

Tuberculosis

Definition/symptoms: Infectious disease caused by *Mycobacterium tuberculosis;* early stage requires testing to reveal infection; advanced cases are marked by lung destruction, coughing, fatigue, weakness, and weight loss; may be confused with bronchitis and pneumonia

Indications: Droplet transmission; contagious; be aware of sanitation

Contraindications: General; work only if physician recommends and clears for contagious condition

Upper Respiratory Infection (Bronchitis, Common Cold, Sinusitis, Pneumonia)

Definition/symptoms: Viral or bacterial in origin; symptoms include increased production of mucus, fever, body aches, and headaches

Indications: Light massage may be beneficial to ease body ache; avoid heavy pressure; watch for contamination

Contraindications: Refer client to physician if symptoms are severe or persist longer than 2 weeks

The Gastrointestinal System

Assessment parameters include skin (see earlier section, The Integumentary System); contour of abdomen (flat, rounded, concave, protuberant, distended); symmetry; observable masses; palpable masses; movement; tenderness or pain; and location and contour of umbilicus.

Deviations that suggest the need for evaluation and referral include a history of persistent or recurring nausea or vomiting; abdominal pain of unknown origin; rebound tenderness; epigastric pain that occurs 1 to 3 hours after meals; rigid or boardlike abdomen (unrelated to calisthenic exercise);

...sing abdominal or epigastric pain; history ... vomitus; difficulty swallowing; masses or ...ed, tender nodes; bulge or swelling in abdomen; ... location or inversion/eversion of umbilicus; and ...s in oral cavity or on lips or tongue.

Specific Disease Processes

Constipation

Definition/symptoms: Slow movement of bowels; hard, compacted, dry stool

Indications: Massage is beneficial; increase fiber and water consumption and moderate exercise; may be drug related

Contraindications: Refer client to physician if severe or persistent or if a mass is felt in the large intestine

Diarrhea

Definition/symptoms: Loose bowels; excessive loss of water in stool; can be caused by a virus or bacterium or can be a symptom of other disease processes

Indications: Loose stool is not uncommon 24 hours after vigorous massage

Contraindications: Refer client to physician if symptoms persist or if dehydration is present

Flatulence

Definition/symptoms: Intestinal gas

Indications: May be diet or stress related; massage may reduce stress

Contraindications: Refer client to physician if intestinal tract is painfully distended or to rule out severe underlying condition

Halitosis

Definition/symptoms: Bad breath; may indicate digestive problems or sinus infection

Indications: N/A

Contraindications: Refer client to physician for specific diagnosis

Inflammatory Processes

Appendicitis

Definition/symptoms: Inflammation of the mucosal lining of the appendix, caused by trapped food or fecal matter; more common in individuals under age 25; symptoms include mild periumbilical pain, nausea, vomiting, increasing pain in the lower right quadrant, muscle spasm, and rebound tenderness

Indications: N/A

Contraindications: Immediately refer client to physician

Cholelithiasis and Cholecystitis

Definition/symptoms: Gallstones formed as a result of inflammation; primary symptom is severe pain in upper abdomen radiating to back and right shoulder

Indications: N/A

Contraindications: Immediately refer client to physician

Cirrhosis of the Liver

Definition/symptoms: Chronic disease that replaces liver tissue with connective tissue; major cause is alcohol consumption; early symptoms include gas, change in bowel habits, slight weight loss, nausea in the morning, and a dull, heavy ache in the right upper quadrant of the abdomen; advanced symptoms include jaundice, peripheral edema, bleeding, and red palms

Indications: Massage is beneficial in stress reduction and drug withdrawal

Contraindications: Refer client to physician for diagnosis; work under physician's supervision

Colitis

Definition/symptoms: Inflammatory condition of the large intestine; one type (irritable bowel syndrome) is brought on by stress

Indications: Painful condition; massage may be helpful in general stress and pain reduction

Contraindications: Immediately refer client to physician; work with chronic conditions under direct supervision of physician

Crohn's Disease (Regional Enteritis)

Definition/symptoms: Chronic relapsing inflammatory disease of the intestinal tract; symptoms include intermittent diarrhea, colicky pain in lower abdomen, fatigue, low-grade fever

Indications: Painful condition; massage may be helpful in general stress and pain reduction

Contraindications: Refer client to physician immediately; with chronic conditions, work under physician's direct supervision

Diverticulosis

Definition/symptoms: Formation of small pockets in the large intestine, caused by herniation of the mucosa; if pockets become inflamed, condition is called *diverticulitis;* symptoms include gas, diarrhea, and pain

Indications: Diet may need adjustment to include more fiber

Contraindications: Refer client to physician if pain or symptoms persist

Duodenal Ulcer

Definition/symptoms: Ulcer caused by hyperacidity in duodenal bulb; stress related; symptoms include burning pain that feels better after eating

Indications: Massage is beneficial for reducing stress; lifestyle and diet changes may be necessary

Contraindications: Refer client to physician for specific diagnosis; support physician's treatment plan

Hepatitis

Definition/symptoms: Infectious disease that has generalized effects in the body but that predominantly affects the liver; type A is common in children and in people living in institutions; it is transmitted by fecal matter, orally through contaminated food and water; usual symptoms are mild and flulike; types B and C affect all age groups and are transmitted through blood, needles, the fecal/oral route, and sexual contact

Indications: Careful use of aseptic procedures

Contraindications: General; refer client to physician and work only with physician's recommendation and guidelines concerning contagious condition

Gastritis

Definition/symptoms: Acute inflammation of the stomach; a common condition usually caused by irritants such as alcohol or aspirin; symptoms include pain, nausea, and belching

Indications: Massage is beneficial, because gastritis sometimes is stress related and massage may reduce stress

Contraindications: Refer client to physician for specific diagnosis

Hernia

Definition/symptoms: Protrusion of a loop or piece of an organ or tissue through an abnormal opening; hiatal—protrusion of any structure (usually the esophagus or end of the stomach) through the hiatus of the diaphragm; inguinal—protrusion through the inguinal ring, causing swelling of the scrotum and possibly a medical emergency; umbilical—protrusion at the umbilicus; in inguinal and umbilical hernias, weakness may be felt in the abdominal wall

Indications: N/A

Contraindications: Refer client to physician; avoid area

Pancreatitis

Definition/symptoms: Inflammation of the pancreas; may be present with diabetes and is aggravated by consumption of alcohol; one symptom is severe abdominal pain

Indications: Painful condition; massage may be helpful in general stress and pain reduction

Contraindications: Refer client to physician immediately; with chronic conditions, work under physician's direct supervision

Stress Ulcer

Definition/symptoms: Ulcer related to severe stress (e.g., trauma, burns, long-term illness); symptoms similar to those seen in gastritis

Indications: Massage is beneficial for reducing stress; lifestyle and dietary changes may be necessary

Contraindications: Refer client to physician for specific diagnosis; support physician's treatment plan

Ulcer

Definition/symptoms: Peptic ulcer—break or open sore not covered by protective mucus in the gastrointestinal wall that is exposed to pepsin and gastric juice; often caused by alcohol, pepsin, bile salts, and stress

Indications: Massage is beneficial to reduce stress levels; lifestyle and dietary changes may be necessary

Contraindications: Refer client to physician for specific diagnosis; support physician's treatment plan

The Metabolic System

Assessment parameters include eating patterns, skin, hair, nails, weight and height data, and general health status.

Deviations that suggest the need for evaluation and referral include significant underweight or overweight, evidence of nutritional deficiencies (e.g., dry hair or skin, fatigue), and respiratory problems.

Specific Disease Processes

Cystic Fibrosis

Definition/symptoms: Inherited disorder that disrupts cell transport and causes exocrine glands to produce thick secretions; thick pancreatic secretions may block the pancreatic duct

Indications: Massage is beneficial with specific training to loosen mucus with percussive techniques

Contraindications: General; work under direct care of physician

Malnutrition

Definition/symptoms: Deficiency of calories in general and often in protein; malnutrition may be caused by increased nutrient demand on the body without sufficient food intake (e.g., severe burns, illness, or lack of food, especially protein); symptoms include flaking skin, brittle hair, hair loss, slow-healing sores, bruising, susceptibility to infection, and fatigue; more common in children and the elderly and with drug and alcohol abuse; be aware of eating disorders. (*Note:* Malnutrition also can be caused by insufficient or improper digestion and absorption of food.)

Indications: With anorexia or bulimia, massage may be beneficial for stress reduction

Contraindications: Refer client to physician for diagnosis and treatment plan

Obesity

Definition/symptoms: Excess body fat (over 30% of normal body weight); risks of obesity include diabetes, stroke, heart attack, gallstones, and high blood pressure

Indications: Morbid obesity (over 60% of normal body fat) may cause difficulty positioning client; fluid retention, risk of blood pressure fluctuation, and interference with breathing are other possible problems; may need to alter massage position

Contraindications: Refer client for nutritional and dietary consultation

The Genitourinary System

Assessment parameters include pain (groin, periumbilical, flank, abdominal, dysuria), patterns of urination and output, urine consistency (color, concentration, or hematuria), edema (facial, ankle), weight changes, skin changes, discharge, and masses.

Deviations that suggest the need for evaluation and referral include a history of unusual vaginal, urethral, or nipple discharge; breast, penile, scrotal, or inguinal masses or lumps;

...ions, or growths; changes in urinary fre-
...control or in urine characteristics; sudden
...bnormal periods, edema, skin abnormalities,
...nderness (costovertebral angle, abdominal area, or
...ack), masses or lumps, and tender or enlarged nodes.

Specific Disease Processes

Breast Cancer

Definition/symptoms: Abnormal, malignant tissue growth on
or in the breast; most common cause of cancer in women;
encourage monthly breast self-examination and regular
checkups

Indications: Be aware of changes in tissue around axillary
region

Contraindications: If changes are noted, refer client to physician; early diagnosis is important

Dysmenorrhea

Definition/symptoms: Painful menstruation; may be caused
by endometriosis (abnormal growth and distribution of
uterine lining); symptoms include heavy periods and clotting

Indications: Massage is beneficial for stress reduction and
pain

Contraindications: Refer client to physician for diagnosis

Pelvic Inflammatory Disease

Definition/symptoms: Inflammation of the uterus, fallopian
tubes, ovaries, and surrounding tissue; infection often is introduced by intercourse; symptoms include pain and tenderness
in the lower abdomen, backache, pain during intercourse,
heavy periods, and vaginal discharge

Indications: N/A

Contraindications: Refer client to physician for diagnosis

Premenstrual Syndrome (PMS)

Definition/symptoms: Occurs approximately 1 week before
onset of period; symptoms include breast tenderness and
swelling, fluid retention, headache, irritability, anxiety, depression, and poor concentration

Indications: Massage is beneficial

Contraindications: Refer client to physician if symptoms
are severe

Testicular Cancer

Definition/symptoms: Malignant growth in the testicle;
usually a slow-growing lump

Indications: N/A

Contraindications: Refer client to physician immediately if
he mentions such a symptom

Toxic Shock Syndrome

Definition/symptoms: Staphylococcal bacterial infection that
can arise from the use of tampons; can be life-threatening;
initial flulike symptoms with red rash; can be prevented by
changing tampons several times a day. (*Note:* This condition
also has occurred in women who do not use tampons.)

Indications: N/A

Contraindications: Immediately refer client to physician

Urinary Tract Infection

Definition/symptoms: Acute pyelonephritis—inflammation
of the kidney and pelvis; usually occurs in women with abrupt
onset of fever, chills, malaise, and back pain, also tenderness
on palpation over the costovertebral region; cystitis—affects
men and women, usually caused by transmission of bacteria
through the urethra because of improper cleansing after bowel
movement; may cause pain in lower abdomen above pubic
bone and low back ache

Indications: N/A

Contraindications: Refer client to physician for diagnosis
and treatment

Sexually Transmitted Diseases

Genital Herpes

Definition/symptoms: Viral infection; primary symptom is
blisterlike lesions

Indications: N/A

Contraindications: Refer client to physician; follow sanitation requirements

Gonorrhea

Definition/symptoms: Bacterial infection; may be asymptomatic, or symptoms may include painful urination and pus or
cloudy discharge

Indications: N/A

Contraindications: Refer client to physician; contagious;
follow sanitation requirements

Human Immunodeficiency Virus (HIV) Infection

Definition/symptoms: Viral infection transmitted by blood
and body fluids

Indications: Massage is beneficial with physician's recommendation; follow antiviral precautions for control of virus
with 10% bleach solution; avoid body fluid contact; immediately wash area thoroughly with antiviral agent should body
fluid contact occur

Contraindications: Refer client to physician for treatment;
follow sanitation requirements

Syphilis

Definition/symptoms: Bacterial infection; in stage one, red
sore (chancre) appears; in stage two, flulike symptoms develop;
in stage three, the disease attacks the brain and nervous tissue

Indications: N/A

Contraindications: Refer client to physician; contagious;
follow sanitation requirements

Psychiatric Disorders

Assessment parameters include general appearance and
behavior, sensorium, mood and affect, thought content, and
intellectual capacity.

Deviations that suggest the need for evaluation and referral
include marked changes in posture, dress, hygiene, motor
activity, speech, or facial expression; lack of orientation
to time, place, or person; inappropriate manifestation of
anxiety, agitation, anger, euphoria, or depression; presence of

hallucinations, delusions, paranoia, and illusions; changes in usual intellectual capacity; or suicidal or homicidal ideation.

Specific Disease Processes

Anxiety, Depression (Bipolar or Manic/Depressive Disorders)

Definition/symptoms: All types of emotionally erratic or unusual behavior may be symptomatic; listen to conversation carefully; often symptoms are subtle, and client may try to hide discomfort; symptoms may include anorexia (self-starvation); bulimia (eating and vomiting and/or laxative abuse); addictive disorders; chemical and compulsive behavior; somatization disorder; manifestation of physical pain or symptoms from emotional causes; and post-traumatic stress disorders, often associated with sexual and physical childhood abuse

Indications: Massage is beneficial under the direction of a psychiatrist or psychologist; always work within the physician's or counselor's treatment parameters

Contraindications: Refer client to physician for counseling care; client often will dissociate from the body or will be hypersensitive to stimulation; the therapist must be sensitive to psychiatric issues, because often the massage therapist is the first person with whom the client shares these issues; it is important to refer the client for competent counseling and psychiatric care

Skin Pathology: Common Skin Disorders

The following photos depict commonly encountered skin disorders. Please note that skin problems may result from various causes, such as parasitic infestations; fungal, bacterial, or viral infections; reactions to substances encountered externally or taken internally; or new growths. Many skin manifestations have no known cause, and others are hereditary.

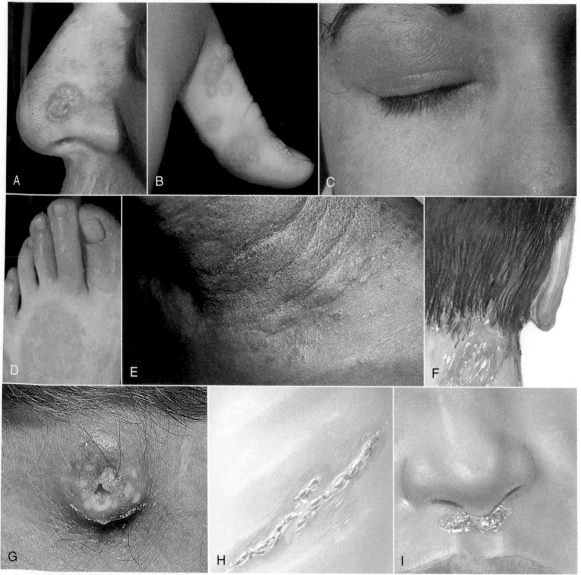

A, Basal cell carcinoma (from Habif TP: *Clinical dermatology: a color guide to diagnosis and therapy*, ed 3, St Louis, 1996, Mosby). **B,** Common warts (from Habif TP: *Clinical dermatology*, ed 2, Mosby). **C,** Contact dermatitis (reprinted with permission from the American Academy of Dermatology, © 2011, all rights reserved). **D,** Contact dermatitis from shoes (reprinted with permission from the American Academy of Dermatology, © 2011, all rights reserved). **E,** Contact dermatitis from application of Lanacane (from Zitelli BJ, Davis HW: *Atlas of pediatric physical diagnosis*, ed 5, Philadelphia, 2007, Mosby). **F,** Dermatitis (from Bork K, Brauninger W: *Skin diseases in clinical practice*, ed 2, Philadelphia, 1998, WB Saunders). **G,** Furuncle (boil) (from Jaime A. Tschen, MD, Department of Dermatology, Baylor College of Medicine, Houston). **H,** Herpes zoster (shingles) (from Bork K, Brauninger W: *Skin diseases in clinical practice*, ed 2, Philadelphia, 1998, WB Saunders). **I,** Impetigo contagiosa (from Bork K, Brauninger W: *Skin diseases in clinical practice*, ed 2, Philadelphia, 1998, WB Saunders).

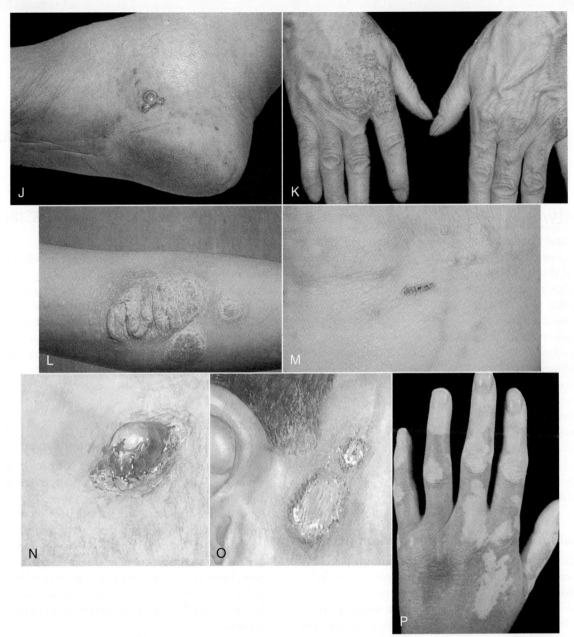

J, Kaposi's sarcoma (from Habif TP: *Clinical dermatology: a color guide to diagnosis and therapy*, ed 3, St Louis, 1996, Mosby).
K, Nummular eczema (reprinted with permission from the American Academy of Dermatology, © 2011, all rights reserved). **L,** Psoriasis (reprinted with permission from the American Academy of Dermatology, © 2011, all rights reserved). **M,** Scabies (from Habif TP: *Clinical dermatology*, ed 2, Mosby). **N,** Squamous cell carcinoma (from Bork K, Brauninger W: *Skin diseases in clinical practice*, ed 2, Philadelphia, 1998, WB Saunders). **O,** Tinea corporis (ringworm) (from Bork K, Brauninger W: *Skin diseases in clinical practice*, ed 2, Philadelphia, 1998, WB Saunders). **P,** Vitiligo (reprinted with permission from the American Academy of Dermatology, © 2011, all rights reserved).

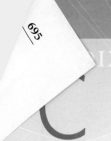

Basic Pharmacology for the Massage Therapist

MaryAnne Hochadel, PharmD

OVERVIEW

Any chemical that affects the physiologic processes of a living organism can broadly be defined as a drug. The study or science of drugs is known as *pharmacology*. Pharmacology encompasses a variety of topics, including the following:

- Absorption
- Biochemical effects
- Biotransformation (metabolism)
- Distribution
- Drug history
- Drug origin
- Drug receptor mechanisms
- Excretion
- Mechanisms of action
- Physical and chemical properties
- Physical effects
- Therapeutic (beneficial) effects
- Toxic (harmful) effects

Information to Help Clarify Medication Actions

A massage therapist must understand the reason a patient is taking a medication and the action of that medication to be able to determine the potential interaction of the drug with the physiologic effects of massage and the adjustments to massage that may be necessary. The following information must be gathered. Most of it can be obtained in a drug consult before the massage. The patient may be able to supply information, and supervising medical personnel also can explain the actions of medications. Many reputable drug compendia are available online that can provide information on medications and dietary supplements. A trusted community pharmacist also may be a great resource for information about a specific drug or therapy.

- Drug name (generic name and brand name)
- Reason the patient is taking the drug
- What does the medicine do?
- When and how is the medication taken?
- What are the possible side effects (reactions of the body to the medicine)?
- Will the medicine react with any other medicines, food, or drinks?
- Should any activities be avoided?
- Are there any signs indicating that the medicine is working?

COMMON MEDICATIONS AND POSSIBLE IMPLICATIONS FOR MASSAGE

The information in the following sections can help the massage practitioner determine what interaction, if any, massage may have with a pharmaceutical. General categories and examples are given for each classification. This is not meant to be an exhaustive list, but rather a general guide for the more commonly prescribed drugs and their brand names. It is important to research any medication, vitamin, dietary supplement, or herb a client takes for its action in the body and possible interaction with massage.

Cardiovascular Medications

Vasodilators (Including Antianginal Drugs)

Examples: nitroglycerin (Nitro-Dur, Nitrostat), isosorbide dinitrate (Isordil) or isosorbide mononitrate (Monoket), hydralazine, minoxidil

Vasodilating medications cause the blood vessels to dilate (widen). Some of the antihypertensive agents lower blood pressure by dilating the arteries or veins. Other vasodilators are used in the treatment of angina (chest pain), hypertension, heart failure, and diseases characterized by poor circulation. Nitrates, which are often used to treat angina, act by increasing the amount of oxygen that reaches the heart muscle.

Implications for massage: Massage has a mild peripheral vasodilatory effect. The action of the medications may increase the effect of the massage. The blood pressure–lowering effect of massage may result in dizziness after the massage. Have the client contract and relax the leg muscles for 1 to 2 minutes before getting off the massage table.

Beta Blockers

Examples: atenolol (Tenormin), bisoprolol (Zebeta), carvedilol (Coreg), labetalol (Normodyne, Trandate), metoprolol (Lopressor, Toprol-XL), propranolol (Inderal)

Beta-blocking medications block nerve stimulation of the heart and blood vessels, slowing the heart rate and reducing high blood pressure. They are used in the treatment of a wide range of diseases, including angina, hypertension, migraine headaches, heart failure, and arrhythmias.

Implications for massage: These drugs may distort the expected effect of the massage. Caution is warranted, and the massage therapist should watch for any exaggerated effects. The client may be susceptible to cold. Massage may help with the constipation that can be a side effect of these drugs. The blood pressure–lowering effect of massage may result in dizziness after the massage. Have the client contract and relax the leg muscles for 1 to 2 minutes before getting off the massage table.

Calcium Channel Blockers

Examples: amlodipine (Norvasc), Diltiazem (Cardizem LA, Tiazac), nifedipine (Adalat CC, Procardia XL), verapamil (Calan, Verelan, Covera HS)

Calcium channel blockers are thought to prevent angina and arrhythmias by blocking or slowing calcium flow into muscle cells, which results in vasodilation (widening of the blood vessels) and greater oxygen delivery to the heart muscle.

Implications for massage: The expected effect of the massage may be distorted. Care must be taken to watch for any exaggerated effects. Massage may help with constipation. The blood pressure–lowering effect of massage may result in dizziness after the massage. Have the client contract and relax the leg muscles for 1 to 2 minutes before getting off the massage table.

Antiarrhythmics

Examples: amiodarone (Cordarone, Pacerone), digoxin (Lanoxin), dronedarone (Multaq), propafenone (Rythmol), sotalol (Betapace, Betapace AF), quinidine, and some beta blockers or calcium channel blockers (see above)

Antiarrhythmics are prescribed when the heart does not beat rhythmically or smoothly (a condition called *arrhythmia*). The broad class is composed of many pharmacologically different types of agents, all with varying effects on electrical impulse conduction and the rate and force of contraction of the heart.

Implications for massage: The client may complain of joint and muscle pain and swelling in the extremities that are medication related. If this occurs, refer the client to the prescribing physician. Massage may help with constipation. The client may experience dizziness after the massage. Have the client contract and relax the leg muscles for 1 to 2 minutes before getting off the massage table.

Antihypertensives and Diuretics

Examples of antihypertensives: beta blockers, calcium channel blockers, angiotensin-converting enzyme (ACE) inhibitors (including benazepril, captopril, enalapril, lisinopril, quinapril), angiotensin receptor blockers (ARBs) (including candesartan, irbesartan, losartan, olmesartan, telmisartan, valsartan), prazosin, terazosin, clonidine, and minoxidil.

Examples of diuretics: chlorothiazide; chlorthalidone; hydrochlorothiazide; budesonide; furosemide; torsemide.

Examples of potassium-sparing diuretics: spironolactone, triamterene, amiloride.

Combinations of antihypertensives: Patients commonly are prescribed a medication that is a combination of two antihypertensives, including diuretic combinations.

High blood pressure, or hypertension, occurs when the pressure of the blood against the walls of the blood vessels is higher than what is considered normal; this condition eventually can damage the brain, eyes, heart, and kidneys. Diuretics are used in antihypertensive therapy. Many diuretics may deplete the body of potassium unless they are the potassium-sparing kind, and a potassium supplement or food source high in potassium may be recommended by the physician.

Implications for massage: The expected effect of the massage may be distorted. Care must be taken to watch for any exaggerated effects. Massage may help with constipation. The blood pressure–lowering effect of massage may result in dizziness after the massage. Have the client contract and relax the leg muscles for 1 to 2 minutes before getting off the massage table. The stress-reducing effect of massage may affect the dosage of these medications. Have clients monitor themselves carefully and ask their physicians to watch for a possible need to reduce the dosage or change the medication. Massage has the effect of increasing fluid movement and may enhance the diuretic effect temporarily.

Cardiac Glycosides (Digitalis Glycosides)

Examples: digoxin (Lanoxin)

Cardiac glycosides slow the heart rate but increase contraction force. Their uses include regulating irregular heart rhythm, increasing the volume of blood pumped by the heart, and medicating congestive heart failure.

Implications for massage: Monitor the client's heart rate, because massage tends to slow the heart rate. If the rate falls below 50 beats per minute, stop the massage and refer the client immediately to the physician. Regular use of massage may affect the dosage of this medication. Have the client monitor the dose carefully with the physician.

Anticoagulants and Medications That Inhibit Platelets

Examples: warfarin (Coumadin, Jantoven), dabigatran (Pradaxa), ticagrelor (Brilinta), clopidogrel (Plavix), heparin, enoxaparin (Lovenox), dalteparin (Fragmin), aspirin

Anticoagulants and platelet inhibitors are medications that prevent blood clotting (blood thinners). They may be used in the treatment of conditions such as stroke, heart disease, embolism (blood clots), and abnormal blood clotting. Warfarin acts by preventing the liver from manufacturing the proteins responsible for blood clot formation.

Implications for massage: The response to stress levels can affect the action of anticoagulants. Massage alters the body's response to stress and may interact with the dosage of this medication. Avoid any massage methods that may cause bruising, including compression, friction, tapotement, and skin rolling. Do not massage an injection site. Watch for bruising and report any bruising to the client. Joint swelling and aching may result from the use of these medications. Refer clients who have any joint symptoms to the physician.

...mics

...amine (Questran), colestipol, ezetimibe, ...(Lipitor), lovastatin, simvastatin (Zocor), ...in (Pravachol), rosuvastatin (Crestor), gemfi- ...il, fenofibrate (Lipofen, Lofibra), omega-3 fatty acids (Lovaza)

Antihyperlipidemics are used to reduce the serum levels of cholesterol and/or triglycerides, which form plaque on the walls of arteries. The statins reduce the body's internal production of cholesterol. Some antihyperlipidemics bind to bile acids in the gastrointestinal tract, reducing the body's absorption of cholesterol.

Implications for massage: Occasional muscle pain and joint pain can occur when statin or fibrate medications are used. Refer clients who complain of these conditions to a physician. Massage may help constipation. Some people experience occasional dizziness. Watch clients carefully as they get up from the massage table.

Gastrointestinal Medications

Anticholinergics

Examples of anticholinergics: dicyclomine (Bentyl), hyoscyamine (Levsin, Levbid, NuLev, Symax)

Examples of opioid with anticholinergic: diphenoxylate, atropine (Lomotil, Lonox)

Anticholinergic medications slow or block nerve impulses at parasympathetic nerve endings, preventing muscle contraction and glandular secretion in the organs involved. Because these medications slow the action of the bowel by relaxing the muscles and relieving spasms, they are said to have an antispasmodic action. They also can help alleviate diarrhea.

Implications for massage: The client's response to relaxation effects may be altered as a result of alteration of parasympathetic action.

Antiulcer Medications

Examples: cimetidine (Tagamet), famotidine (Pepcid), ranitidine (Zantac), omeprazole (Prilosec) , lansoprazole (Prevacid), sucralfate (Carafate)

These medications relieve symptoms and promote healing of gastrointestinal ulcers. They also relieve gastrointestinal reflux of stomach acid, which may cause chronic heartburn. Most work by suppressing the production of excess stomach acid. Sucralfate works by forming a chemical barrier over an exposed ulcer, protecting the ulcer from stomach acid.

Implications for massage: The stress reduction capacity of massage may enhance the effectiveness of these medications.

Hormones

A hormone is a substance produced and secreted by a gland. Hormones stimulate and regulate body functions. Most often hormone medications are used to replace naturally occurring hormones that are not being produced in amounts sufficient to regulate specific body functions. This category of medication includes oral contraceptives and certain types of medications used to combat inflammatory reactions.

Antidiabetic Medications

Examples: glipizide, glyburide

The treatment of diabetes mellitus may involve the administration of insulin or oral antidiabetic medications. Glucagon is given only in emergencies (e.g., insulin shock or when blood sugar levels must be raised quickly). Oral antidiabetic medications are used for the treatment of type 2 diabetes (adult onset, insulin resistant). Early medications in this category induced the pancreas to secrete more insulin by acting on small groups of cells in the pancreas that make and store insulin. Newer oral agents often help increase the insulin sensitivity of the tissues. Individuals with insulin-dependent (juvenile onset, or type 1) diabetes must control their blood sugar levels with insulin injections.

Implications for massage: Changes in stress levels may affect the dosage. The client's physician should monitor the dosage if massage is used on a regular basis. Do not provide vigorous massage, because it may put undue stress on the system, requiring the blood sugar level to adjust. Avoid massaging injection or infusion sites.

Sex Hormones

Examples: estrogens (Estradiol, Premarin, Cenestin), oral contraceptives, progesterones (medroxyprogesterone [Provera]), androgens (testosterone, Androgel)

Estrogens are used as replacement therapy to treat symptoms of menopause in women whose bodies are no longer producing sufficient amounts of estrogen. Medroxyprogesterone is used to treat uterine bleeding and menstrual problems. Most oral contraceptives (birth control pills) combine estrogen and a progesterone, but some contain only a progesterone. Testosterone stimulates cells that produce male sex characteristics, replace hormone deficiencies, stimulate red blood cells, and suppress estrogen production. Athletes sometimes take medications called *anabolic steroids* (chemicals similar to testosterone) to reduce the elimination of protein from the body, which results in an increase in muscle size. This use of these medications is dangerous; anabolic steroids can adversely affect the heart, nervous system, and kidneys.

Implications for massage: Estrogens can change the body's blood clotting ability. Watch for bruising and adjust pressures as needed. Be aware of any symptoms of blood clots and refer the patient to the physician immediately if these are noted. Most hormones can increase fluid retention. Massage may temporarily increase fluid movement, reducing swelling. Unusual fluid retention should be referred to the prescribing physician immediately. Hormones have a widespread effect on the body and mood. Emotional states may fluctuate, and the ability to handle stress changes with the hormonal fluctuations. Massage can reduce stress levels, help even out mood, and promote a sense of well-being.

Steroids

Examples: dexamethasone (Decadron), methylprednisolone (Medrol), prednisolone (Orapred), prednisone

Examples of common steroid hormone creams or ointments: triamcinolone, hydrocortisone

Oral steroid preparations may be used to treat inflammatory diseases such as arthritis, or conditions such as poison ivy, hay fever, or insect bites. Steroids also may be applied to the skin to treat certain inflammatory skin conditions.

Implications for massage: Changes in stress levels may affect the dose. The client's physician should monitor the dosage if massage is used on a regular basis. Avoid any massage methods that may create inflammation, such as friction, skin rolling, or stretching methods that pull excessively on the tissue.

Thyroid Medications

Example: levothyroxine (Synthroid, Levoxyl, Levoxine), thyroid (Bio-throid)

Implications for massage: Changes in stress levels may affect the dosage. The client should monitor the dosage if massage is used on a regular basis.

Antiinfective Medications

Antibiotics

Examples: aminoglycosides, cephalosporins, macrolides (erythromycin, clarithromycin, azithromycin), penicillins (including ampicillin and amoxicillin), quinolones (ciprofloxacin, levofloxacin), tetracyclines

Antibiotics are used to treat a wide variety of bacterial infections. There are many different classes of antibiotics. Antibiotics do not destroy viruses, such as those that cause the common cold.

Antivirals

Example: acyclovir (Zovirax), valacyclovir (Valtrex), medications used to treat HIV infection

Antiviral medications are used to combat viral infections; however, they do not eliminate or cure viral infections. Medications for HIV may predispose an individual to accumulation of lactic acidosis and muscle soreness; be alert to possible medication side effects, and if lactic acidosis may be present, refer the client to the physician before proceeding with the massage.

Antifungals

Example: nystatin, fluconazole (Diflucan), itraconazole (Sporanox), ketoconazole (Nizoral)

Fungal infections are treated to prevent the growth of fungi and to cure the condition. Many topical antifungals are used to treat fungal skin conditions such as athlete's foot or groin itch.

Pediculicides and Scabicides

Example: lindane, permethrin (Elimite), pyrethrins (Pronto Plus), benzyl alcohol (Ulesfia), spinosad (Natroba)

Pediculicides and scabicides are used to treat lice and scabies infestations. Lindane can cause serious neurotoxicity and must be carefully applied and handled.

Implications for massage for antiinfective medications: A person who is taking an antiinfective medication may have a stressed immune system or may be truly immunocompromised. They may also have an infection that is considered contagious to others. Therefore, it is important to avoid overstressing the system when providing massage and to take care not to expose clients to contagious diseases, such as colds, the flu, or infestations. Postpone appointments if necessary. Gastrointestinal side effects are common with many antibiotics. Massage may calm symptoms temporarily. Universal precautions are required when dealing with any bacterial, viral, or other condition caused by infectious pathogens.

Antineoplastic Medications

Examples: tamoxifen (Nolvadex), flutamide, etoposide, Gleevec, Sprycel, Sutent, Tarceva, Votrient

Antineoplastic medications are used in the treatment of cancer. Most of the medications in this category prevent the growth of rapidly dividing cells, such as cancer cells. Antineoplastics are without exception extremely toxic and can cause serious side effects. Many more cancer drugs now are supplied in oral form, and the number of treatments is expanding rapidly.

Implications for massage: Individuals undergoing chemotherapy are physiologically stressed because of the toxicity of the medications. Work gently and under the direct supervision of the client's physician.

Central Nervous System Medications

Antianxiety Drugs/Sedatives

Examples: benzodiazepines diazepam (Valium), lorazepam (Ativan), alprazolam (Xanax), temazepam (Restoril); buspirone (Buspar); diphenhydramine (Unisom); hydroxyzine (Atarax); zaleplon (Sonata); zolpidem (Ambien); eszopiclone (Lunesta); barbiturates (phenobarbital, secobarbital).

Antianxiety drugs and sedatives are used in the treatment of anxiety, panic disorder, and insomnia. They selectively reduce the activity of certain chemicals in the brain.

Implications for massage: These medications generally act as central nervous system (CNS) depressants. Massage can increase or decrease the effect of these medications, depending on whether the massage is structured to have a more stimulating or relaxing effect. The dosage of these drugs needs to be carefully monitored when they are used in conjunction with massage. Watch for excessive drowsiness. The physician may be able to reduce the dosage if massage is used on a regular basis. Work in conjunction with the prescribing physician.

...azines haloperidol, risperidone (Risp-...azole (Abilify), olanzapine (Zyprexa), que-...eroquel), clozapine (Clozaril, Fazaclo)

...anquilizers or antipsychotic agents usually are pre-...ribed for patients with psychoses (certain types of mental disorders) or for bipoloar illness. These medications calm certain areas of the brain but permit the rest of the brain to function normally.

Implications for massage: These medications generally act as CNS depressants. Massage can increase or decrease the effect of these medications, depending on whether the massage is structured to have a more stimulating or relaxing effect. Because of the potential effects on blood pressure or dizziness, the client should avoid sudden positional changes after the massage. The dosage of these drugs needs to be monitored carefully when they are used in conjunction with massage. These medications are used to treat severe mental disorders. Work only with direct supervision from the prescribing physician. Massage can help with constipation in individuals taking these drugs.

Antidepressants

Examples: tricyclic antidepressants (amitriptyline), selective serotonin reuptake inhibitors (SSRIs; e.g., fluoxetine [Prozac, Sarafem], sertraline [Zoloft], paroxetine [Paxil]), serotonin/norepinephrine reuptake inhibitors (SNRIs; e.g., venlafaxine [Effexor]), and monoamine oxidase inhibitors (MAOIs; e.g., phenelzine)

Antidepressants are used to combat depression. They also are used as preventive therapy for migraine headaches, severe premenstrual syndrome, and neuropathic types of pain, although the manner in which they help relieve pain is not clearly understood. They work mostly by increasing the concentration of certain chemicals necessary for proper nerve transmission in the brain.

Implications for massage: Massage nonspecifically causes a shift in neurotransmitters and other brain chemicals. Massage has a stimulating effect on the CNS even when used for relaxation. The relaxation effect is a secondary result of the nervous system stimulation. Massage can increase serotonin levels. Watch carefully for any increase or decrease in the effect of the medications. Work with the supervision of the prescribing physician to adjust the dosage when massage is used as part of therapy. Massage can help with constipation.

Amphetamines and Related Stimulants

Examples: methylphenidate (Ritalin, Concerta, Metadate, Daytrana), dexmethylphenidate (Focalin), amphetamine salts (Adderall)

Amphetamines are adrenergic medications that are nervous system stimulants. They commonly are used to treat attention deficit disorders and occasionally may be used as anorectics (medications used to reduce the appetite). These medications temporarily quiet the part of the brain that causes hunger, but they also keep a person awake, speed up the heart, and raise blood pressure. After 2 to 3 weeks, these medications begin to lose their effectiveness as appetite suppressants. They also are used to treat narcolepsy. Amphetamines stimulate most people, but they have the opposite effect on hyperkinetic children and adults. When hyperkinetic children and adults take amphetamines or adrenergic medications, their level of activity is reduced. Most likely, amphetamines selectively stimulate parts of the brain that control activity.

Implications for massage: Massage nonspecifically causes a shift in neurotransmitters and other brain chemicals. Massage has a stimulating effect on the CNS even when used for relaxation. The relaxation effect is a secondary result of the nervous system stimulation. Watch carefully for any increase or decrease in the effect of the medications. Work with supervision from the prescribing physician, who may need to adjust the dosage when massage is used as part of therapy. Massage can help with constipation.

Anticonvulsants

Examples: phenobarbital, phenytoin (Dilantin), carbamazepine (Tegretol), lamotrigine (Lamictal), levatiracetam (Keppra), divalproex (Depakote), gabapentin (Neurontin), pregabalin (Lyrica).

Anticonvulsants are used to control seizures and other symptoms of epilepsy. They selectively reduce excessive stimulation in the brain. Some of these medications are used as mood stabilizers for bipolar illness or to treat neuropathic pain syndromes.

Implications for massage: Massage has a stimulating effect on the CNS even used for relaxation. The relaxation effect is a secondary result of the nervous system stimulation. Watch carefully for any increase or decrease in the effect of the medications. Work with supervision from the prescribing physician when massage is used as part of therapy.

Antiparkinsonism Agents

Examples: carbidopa-levodopa (Sinemet), bromocriptine (Parlodel), benztropine (Cogentin), trihexyphenidyl, ropinirole (Requip), pramipexole (Mirapex), entacapone (Comtan)

Parkinson's disease is a progressive disorder that is caused by a chemical imbalance of dopamine in the brain. Antiparkinsonism drugs are used to correct the chemical imbalance, thereby relieving the symptoms of the disease. Benztropine and trihexyphenidyl also are used to relieve tremors caused by other medications. Ropinirole and pramipexole may be used to treat restless leg syndrome at night.

Implications for massage: Massage nonspecifically causes a shift in neurotransmitters and other brain chemicals, including dopamine. Massage has a stimulating effect on the CNS even when used for relaxation. The relaxation effect is a secondary result of the nervous system stimulation. Watch carefully for any increase or decrease in the effect of the medications. Watch for excessive drowsiness. Work with supervision from the prescribing physician, who may adjust the dosage when massage is used as part of therapy. Massage can help with constipation.

Analgesics

Analgesics are used to relieve pain. They may be either narcotic or nonnarcotic. Narcotics act on the brain to cause deep analgesia and often drowsiness. Narcotics relieve pain and give the patient a feeling of well-being. They also are addictive.

A number of analgesics contain codeine or other narcotics combined with nonnarcotic analgesics (e.g., aspirin or acetaminophen). Tylenol #3 and Vicodin are examples.

Nonnarcotic pain relievers include the following:

- Salicylates, such as aspirin (relieve pain, antiinflammatory, and treat fever)
- Acetaminophen (relieves pain and fever but does not reduce inflammation)
- Nonsteroidal antiinflammatory medications (NSAIDs; e.g., celecoxib, ibuprofen, naproxen, oxaprozin) (inhibit prostaglandins, reducing pain and inflammation; some agents [ibuprofen] also relieve fever)

Implications for massage: Massage reduces pain perception in several ways: through gate control hyperstimulation analgesia and counterirritation and by stimulating the release of pain-inhibiting or pain-modifying chemicals in the body. Massage supports analgesics and has the potential to reduce the drug dosage and the duration of treatment. Aspirin thins the blood. Watch for bruising. Timing of the massage in relation to the analgesic dosage may be important. Pain perception is inhibited when a person is taking analgesics. Feedback mechanisms for pressure and massage intensity are not accurate. Reduce the intensity of massage and avoid methods that cause inflammation. Narcotics are constipating, and massage can help with constipation. Dizziness may result with the use of these medications. Have the client relax and contract the muscles of the legs for a few minutes before getting off the table.

Antiinflammatory Medications

Antiinflammatory medications reduce the body's inflammatory response. Inflammation is the body's response to injury, and it causes swelling, pain, fever, redness, and itching. Examples of antiinflammatory medications include:

- NSAIDs: See Analgesics.
- Steroids: corticosteroids (e.g., prednisone, methylprednisolone, prednisolone, dexamethasone).

Note: Skeletal muscle relaxants often are given in combination with an antiinflammatory medication such as aspirin. However, some doctors believe that aspirin and rest are better for alleviating the pain and the inflammation of muscle strain than are skeletal muscle relaxants. When sore muscles tense, increasing muscle tone, they cause pain, inflammation, and spasm. Skeletal muscle relaxants (e.g., orphenadrine, cyclobenzaprine, meprobamate, and chlorzoxazone) can relieve pain and these symptoms.

Implications for massage: Massage therapists should not perform any techniques that create inflammation or damage tissue. Mood may be altered in addition to pain perception. Feedback mechanisms for pressure and massage intensity are not accurate. The intensity of the massage should be reduced. Massage can reduce muscle spasm, reducing the need for muscle relaxants. Muscle spasm often is a protective response acting to immobilize an injured area. Use massage to reduce but not remove these protective spasms. Many antiinflammatory medications are available over the counter (OTC), and the client may neglect to report their use to the massage therapist. Ask clients whether they are taking any OTC medications.

Respiratory Medications
Antitussives

Examples: dextromethorphan, codeine, hydrocodone

Antitussives control coughs. Dextromethorphan is available in OTC products; narcotic antitussives are available by prescription.

Expectorants

Examples: guaifenesin

Expectorants are used to change a nonproductive cough to a productive one (one that brings up phlegm). Expectorants are supposed to increase the amount of mucus produced. However, drinking water or using a vaporizer or humidifier is probably as effective for increasing the production of mucus.

Decongestants

Examples: phenylephrine. Restricted sale: pseudoephedrine. Removed from U.S. market: ephedrine, phenylpropanolamine hydrochloride

Decongestants constrict blood vessels in the nose and sinuses to open air passages. Adrenergic agents (decongestants) are available as oral preparations, nose drops, and nose sprays. Oral decongestants are slow acting but do not interfere with the production of mucus or the movement of the cilia (special hairlike structures) of the respiratory tract. They can increase blood pressure; therefore, they should be used cautiously by patients with high blood pressure. Topical decongestants (nose drops or sprays) provide fast relief. They do not increase blood pressure as much as oral decongestants, but they do slow cilia movement. Topical decongestants should not be used for more than a few days at a time.

Implications for massage: Avoid the prone position, because it increases congestion

Bronchodilators

Examples: theophylline, aminophylline, albuterol, salmeterol, formoterol

Bronchodilators (agents that open the airways in the lungs) and agents that relax smooth muscle tissue, such as that found in the lungs, are used to improve breathing. Inhalant bronchodilators are most commonly prescribed for asthma and chronic obstructive pulmonary disease (COPD; e.g., emphysema) and act directly on the muscles of the breathing tubes. Theophylline and aminophylline have limited use.

Antihistamines

Examples: Nonsedating or low sedating: loratadine (Claritin), fexofenadine (Allegra), cetirizine (Zyrtec)

Traditional (sedating): diphenhydramine (Benadryl), clemastine (Tavist-1), dimenhydrinate (Dramamine)

Histamine is a body chemical that, when released, typically causes swelling and itching. Release of histamine is often a response to exposure to an allergen. Antihistamines counteract these symptoms of allergy by blocking the effects of histamine. Antihistamines are commonly used for mild respiratory or skin allergies, such as hay fever (seasonal allergies) or hives. Some types of antihistamines are also used to prevent or treat the symptoms of motion sickness.

Implications for massage for respiratory medications: Bronchodilators are sympathomimetic and act on sympathetic nerve stimulation. Because some respiratory agents can reduce sweating, heat hydrotherapy should be avoided. Antihistamines can excite or depress the CNS. Most of these medications can cause drowsiness. Because they act on the CNS, the expected results of the massage can be distorted. The client may be unable to relax or may be excessively drowsy and dizzy after the massage. Many massage methods produce reddening of the skin caused by the release of histamine. This reaction may be altered and feedback may be inaccurate in clients taking antihistamines. Avoid this type of work with such clients. Codeine can cause constipation. Massage may prove beneficial. Many of these medications are available over the counter, and clients may neglect to report their use to the therapist. Make sure to ask clients if they are taking any OTC medications.

Vitamins and Minerals

Vitamins and minerals are chemical substances that are vital to the maintenance of normal body function. Many people take supplemental vitamins and minerals. Multivitamins, calcium, vitamin C, and vitamin D supplements are especially common. A high intake of supplements, especially individual vitamins, can cause adverse reactions or may have implications for massage. The practitioner needs to investigate further to determine any suspected interaction. At this point, specific research has not been done to determine what the specific interactions might be. It is necessary to compare the effects of the vitamin and/or mineral with the type of massage application to determine whether the two together are inhibitory or synergistic.

Dietary Supplements and Herbs

Herbs and other dietary supplements are agents used to support certain functions of the body. None of these agents are regulated in the same manner as drugs, and unlike drugs, they are not intended to be used to diagnose, treat, cure, or prevent any disease. However, their action may be similar to that of pharmaceutical medications. Some medications are derivatives of plants. Ask clients whether they are taking herbs or other dietary supplements, and if so, the names and their reasons for taking them. The practitioner needs to investigate further to determine any suspected interactions. At this point, specific research has not been done to determine what the specific interactions might be. It is necessary to compare the effects of the supplement with the type of massage application to determine whether the two together are inhibitory or synergistic.

Bibliography

Clinical Pharmacology (online database). www.clinicalpharmacology.com. Accessed August 15, 2011.

Consumers Guide editors: *Prescription medications*, Lincolnwood, Ill, 1995, Signet.

Corey G, et al: *Issues and ethics in the helping professions*, ed 6, Belmont, Calif, 2002, Brooks/Cole.

Griffith H, Moore SW: *Complete guide to prescription and non-prescription drugs*, Los Angeles, 2002, The Body Press Division of Price Stern Sloan.

Hochadel M, et al: *Mosby's drug reference for health care professionals*, ed 3, St Louis, 2012, Mosby.

Smith WD, Lai LS: Massage therapy: implications for pharmaceutical care, *US Pharmacist* 34(5):Epub, 2009. uspharmacist.com. Accessed October 14, 2011.

Glossary

abbreviation: Shortened forms of words or phrases.

absolute risk: The chance a person will develop a specific disease or potential injury over a specified period.

abuse: Exploitation, misuse, mistreatment, molestation, or neglect.

acquired immunodeficiency syndrome (AIDS): A disease of the immune system, which is caused by the human immunodeficiency virus (HIV).

active assisted movement: Movement of a joint in which both the client and the therapist produce the motion.

active joint movement: Movement of a joint through its range of motion by the client.

active listening: Clarifying a feeling attached to a message but not adding to or changing the message.

active range of motion: Movement of a joint by the client without any type of assistance from the massage practitioner.

active resistive movement: Movement of a joint by the client against resistance provided by the therapist.

acupressure: Methods used to tone or sedate acupuncture points without the use of needles.

acupuncture: Stimulation of certain points with needles inserted along the meridians (channels) and ah shi ("ouch") points outside the meridians.

acupuncture point: An Asian term for a specific point that correlates with a neurologic motor point.

acute: A term that describes a condition in which the signs and symptoms develop quickly, last a short time, and then disappear.

acute illness: A short-term illness that resolves by means of the normal healing process and, if necessary, supportive medical care.

acute injury: Indication that damage to the body has occurred such as a fracture, wound, sprain, burn, or contusion.

acute pain: A symptom of a disease condition or a temporary aspect of medical treatment. Acute pain acts as a warning signal, because it can activate the sympathetic nervous system. It usually is temporary, has a sudden onset, and is easily localized. The client frequently can describe the pain, which often subsides without treatment.

adaptation: A response to a sensory stimulation in which nerve signaling is reduced or ceases.

aerobic exercise: An exercise program focused on increasing fitness and endurance.

allied health: A division of medicine in which the professional receives training in a specific area of medicine to serve as support for the physician.

altruistic love and kindness: The assertion of a common humanity in which other people are worthy of attention and affirmation for no utilitarian reasons but rather for their own sake.

anatomic barriers: Anatomic structures determined by the shape and fit of the bones at the joint.

antagonism: The process by which massage produces the opposite effect.

antagonistic: When massage produces the opposite effect sought.

antagonists: The muscles that oppose the movement of the prime movers.

anxiety: A feeling of uneasiness, usually connected with an increase in sympathetic arousal responses.

applied kinesiology: Methods of evaluation and bodywork that use a specialized type of muscle testing and various forms of massage and bodywork for corrective procedures.

approximation: The technique of pushing muscle fibers together in the belly of the muscle.

aromatherapy: A healing discipline involving the use of essential oils.

art: Craft, skill, technique, and talent.

arterial circulation: Movement of oxygenated blood under pressure from the heart to the body through the arteries.

arthrokinematic movement: Accessory movements that occur as a result of inherent laxity or joint play that exists in each joint. The joint play allows the ends of the bones to slide, roll, or spin smoothly on one another. These essential movements occur passively with movement of the joint and are not under voluntary control.

aseptic technique: Procedures that kill or disable pathogens on surfaces to prevent transmission.

aspirational ethics: Ethical behavior motivated by a professional's desire to provide the highest possible benefit and welfare for the client.

Asian approaches: Methods of bodywork that have developed from ancient Chinese methods.

assessment: The collection and interpretation of information provided by the client, the client's family and friends, the massage practitioner, and referring medical professionals.

asymmetric stance: The position in which the body weight is shifted from one foot to the other while standing.

asymmetric standing: Standing with one foot in front of the other; the most efficient standing position.

athlete: A person who participates in sports as an amateur or a professional. Athletes require precise use of their bodies.

attention: The direction of awareness to any object, sense, or thought for the sake of gaining clarity.

attunement: The process by which the phases of attention among two or more people and the environment come into harmony through resonance or cohesion (union) of their interpersonal brain activity, especially from physical touch.

autonomic nervous system: The body system that regulates involuntary body functions using the sympathetic fight-flight-fear response and the restorative parasympathetic relaxation response. The sympathetic and parasympathetic systems work together to maintain homeostasis through a feedback loop system.

autoregulation: The control of homeostasis through alteration of tissue or function.

Ayurveda: A system of health and medicine that grew from East Indian roots.

bacteria: Primitive cells that have no nuclei. Bacteria cause disease by secreting toxic substances that damage human tissues, by becoming parasites inside human cells, or by forming colonies in the body that disrupt normal function.

balance: The ability to maintain the body's center of gravity within the base of support.

balance point: The point of contact between the practitioner and the client.

beating: A form of heavy tapotement involving use of the fist.

benign tumor: A term that describes a tumor that remains localized within the tissue from which it arose and does not undergo malignant changes. Benign tumors usually grow very slowly.

best practice: A technique or methodology that through experience and research has proven to reliably lead to a desired result.

biomechanics: Body motions and the muscular forces used to complete tasks.

biopsychosocial model of medicine: An approach to medicine the recognizes that biologic, psychological, and social factors all play a significant role in human functioning.

body mechanics: Use of the body in an efficient and biomechanically correct way.

body segment: The area of the body between joints that provides movement during walking and balance.

body supports: Pillows, folded blankets, foam forms, or commercial products that help contour the flat surface of a massage table or mat.

body/mind: The interaction between thought and physiology that is connected to the limbic system, hypothalamic influence on the autonomic nervous system, and the endocrine system.

body/mind/spirit: The three primary, interrelated, interacting, and integrated layers that comprise a healthy, balanced, and unified human being.

bodywork: A term that encompasses all the various forms of massage, movement, and other touch therapies.

boundary: Personal space that exists within an arm's length perimeter. Personal emotional space is designated by morals, values, and experience.

burnout: A condition that occurs when a person uses up energy faster than it can be restored.

breathing pattern disorders: A complex set of behaviors that lead to overbreathing in the absence of a pathologic condition. These disorders are considered a functional syndrome, because all the parts work effectively, and the condition therefore is not caused by a specific pathologic condition.

care/treatment plan: The plan used to achieve therapeutic goals. It outlines the agreed objectives; the frequency, duration, and number of visits; progress measurements; the date of reassessment; and massage methods to be used.

career: A chosen pursuit; a life's work.

caution: Condition that requires the massage therapist to adapt the massage process so that the client's safety is maintained.

centering: The ability to pay attention to a specific area of focus.

center of gravity: The average position of an object's weight distribution.

certification: A voluntary credentialing process that usually requires education and testing; tests are administered either privately or by government regulatory bodies.

chakra: Energy fields or centers of consciousness within the body.

challenge: Living each day knowing that it is filled with things to learn, skills to practice, tasks to accomplish, and obstacles to overcome.

charting: A systematic form of documentation.

chemical effects: The effects of massage produced by the release of chemical substances in the body. These substances may be released locally from the massaged tissue, or they may be hormones released into the general circulation.

chronic: A term that describes disease that develops slowly and lasts for a long time, sometimes for life.

chronic illness: A disease, injury, or syndrome that shows little change or slow progression.

chronic pain: Pain that persists or recurs for indefinite periods, usually for longer than 6 months. It frequently has an insidious onset, and the character and quality of the pain change over time. It frequently involves deep somatic and visceral structures. Chronic pain usually is diffuse and poorly localized.

circulation: The flow of blood through the vessels of the body.

circulatory: A term that describes systems that depend on the pumping action of the skeletal muscle (i.e., the arterial, venous, lymphatic, respiratory, cerebrospinal fluid circulatory systems).

client: A recipient of service, be it from a wellness or a health care professional, regardless of his or her health status. All patients are clients, but not all clients are patients.

client information form: A document used to obtain information from the client about health, pre-existing conditions, and expectations for the massage.

client outcome: The results desired from the massage and the massage therapist.

client/practitioner agreement and policy statement: A detailed written explanation of all rules, expectations, and procedures for the massage.

client records: All information related to the client.

clinical massage: Massage therapy practice involving more extensive use of assessment and specific focused techniques and applications with the intention of achieving clinical treatment or functional outcomes and remediation of symptoms.

clinical reasoning: Form of critical thinking that targets a specific therapeutic practice.

coalition: A group formed for a particular purpose.

code of ethics: An agreed-upon set of behaviors developed to promote high standards of practice.

cognition: Conscious awareness and perception, reasoning, judgment, intuition, and memory.

comfort barrier: The first point of resistance short of the client's perceiving any discomfort at the physiologic or pathologic barrier.

commitment: The ability and willingness to be involved in what is happening around us so as to have a purpose for being.

communicable disease: A disease caused by pathogens that are easily spread; a contagious disease.

compensation: The process of counterbalancing a defect in body structure or function.

complementary and alternative medicine (CAM): A group of diverse medical and health care systems, practices, and products that are not generally considered part of conventional medicine.

compression: Pressure into the body to spread tissue against underlying structures. (This massage manipulation sometimes is classified with pétrissage.) Also, the exertion of inappropriate pressure on nerves by hard tissue (e.g., bone).

compressive force: Pressure exerted against the surface of the body to apply pressure to the deeper body structures; pressure directed in a particular direction.

concentric isotonic contraction: Application of a counterforce by the massage therapist while allowing the client to move, which brings the origin and insertion of the target muscle together against the pressure.

condition management: The use of massage methods to support clients who are unable to undergo a therapeutic change but who wish to function as effectively as possible under a set of circumstances.

confidentiality: Respect for the privacy of information.

conflict: An expressed struggle between at least two interdependent parties who perceive incompatible goals, scarce resources, and/or interference from the other party in achieving their goals.

connective tissue: The most abundant tissue type in the body; it provides support, structure, space, and stabilization and is involved in scar formation.

conservation withdrawal: A parasympathetic survival pattern that is similar to "playing 'possum" or hibernation.

contamination: The process by which an object or area becomes unclean.

contraindication: Any condition that renders a particular treatment improper or undesirable.

control: The belief that a person can influence events by the way he or she feels, thinks, and acts.

cortisol: A stress hormone produced by the adrenal glands that is released during long-term stress. An elevated level indicates increased sympathetic arousal.

counterirritation: Superficial stimulation that relieves a deeper sensation by stimulating different sensory signals.

counterpressure: Force applied to an area that is designed to match exactly (isometric contraction) or partly (isotonic contraction) the effort or force produced by the muscles of that area.

countertransference: The personalization of the professional relationship by the therapist in which the practitioner is unable to separate the therapeutic relationship from personal feelings and expectations for the client.

craniosacral and myofascial approaches: Methods of bodywork that work both reflexively and mechanically with the fascial network of the body.

cream: A type of lubricant that is in a semisolid or solid state.

credential: A designation earned by completing a process that verifies a certain level of expertise in a given skill.

cross-directional stretching: Tissue stretching that pulls and twists connective tissue against its fiber direction.

cryotherapy: Therapeutic use of ice.

culture: The arts, beliefs, customs, institutions, and all other products of human work and thought created by a specific group of people at a particular time.

cupping: The type of tapotement that involves the use of a cupped hand; it often is used over the thorax.

cutaneous sensory receptors: Sensory nerves in the skin.

database: All the information available that contributes to the therapeutic interaction.

deep inspiration: The movement of air into the body by hard breathing to meet an increased demand for oxygen. Any muscles that can pull the ribs up are called into action.

deep tissue: The tissues beneath the superficial structures being treated.

deep tissue work: A generic term commonly used to describe a variety of techniques to address specific deep tissues and structures, regardless of the force or pressure exerted or the level of discomfort or pain experienced during or after the application.

deep transverse frictioning: A specific rehabilitation technique that creates therapeutic inflammation by producing a specific, controlled reinjury of tissues through the application of a concentrated, therapeutic movement that moves the tissue against its grain over only a very small area.

defensive climate: An atmosphere characteristic of competition that inhibits the mutual trust required for effective conflict management.

defensive measures: The means by which the body defends itself against stressors (e.g., production of antibodies and white blood cells or through behavioral or emotional means).

denial: The ability to retreat and to ignore stressors.

depression: A condition characterized by a decrease in vital functional activity and by mood disturbances of exaggerated emptiness, hopelessness, and melancholy or of unbridled high energy with no purpose or outcome.

depth of pressure: Compressive stress that can be light, moderate, deep, or varied.

dermatome: The cutaneous (skin) distribution of spinal nerve sensation.

diagnosis: The process of identifying the disease or syndrome a person is believed to have.

direction: The flow of massage strokes from the center of the body outward (centrifugal), or from the extremities inward toward the center of the body (centripetal). Direction can be circular motions; it can flow from origin to insertion of the muscle, following the muscle fibers, or can flow transverse to the tissue fibers.

direction of ease: The position the body assumes with postural changes and muscle shortening or weakening, depending on how it has balanced against gravity.

discipline: An area of study involving particular concepts, a specific vocabulary, and so on.

disclosure: Acknowledging and informing the client of any situation that interferes with or affects the professional relationship.

disinfection: The process by which pathogens are destroyed.

dissociation: A state of detachment, discontentedness, separation, or isolation.

documentation: The process of creating and maintaining client records.

dopamine: A neurochemical that influences motor activity involving movement (especially learned fine movement, such as handwriting), conscious selective selection (what to pay attention to), mood (in terms of inspiration), possibility, intuition, joy, and enthusiasm. If the dopamine level is low, the opposite effects are seen, such as lack of motor control, clumsiness, inability to decide what to attend to, and boredom.

drag: The amount of pull (stretch) on the tissue (tensile stress).

drape: Fabric used to cover the client and keep the individual warm during the massage.

draping: The procedures of covering and uncovering areas of the body and turning the client during the massage.

draping material: Coverings that provide the client with privacy and warmth. The most commonly used coverings are standard bed linens, because they are large enough to cover the entire body and are easy to use for most draping procedures.

dual role: Overlap in the scope of practice, with one professional providing support in more than one area of expertise.

duration: The length of time a method lasts or stays in the same location.

dysfunction: An in-between state in which one is "not healthy" but also "not sick" (i.e., experiencing disease).

centric isotonic contraction: Application of a counterforce while the client moves the jointed area, which allows the origin and insertion of the muscle to separate. The muscle lengthens against the pressure.

effleurage (gliding stroke): Horizontal strokes applied with the fingers, hand, or forearm that usually follow the fiber direction of the underlying muscle, fascial planes, or dermatome pattern.

electrical-chemical functions: Physiologic functions of the body that rely on or produce body energy; often called *chi, prana,* or meridian energy.

electromyography (EMG): Used to evaluate and record electrical activity of skeletal muscles.

empathy: The ability to identify with the feelings and experience of another.

employee: A person who works for another for a wage.

end-feel: The perception of the joint at the limit of its range of motion. The end-feel is either soft or hard (see *joint end-feel*).

endangerment site: Any area of the body where nerves and blood vessels surface close to the skin and are not well protected by muscle or connective tissue; therefore, deep, sustained pressure into these areas could damage these vessels and nerves. The kidney area is included, because the kidneys are loosely suspended in fat and connective tissue, and heavy pounding is contraindicated in that area.

endocannabinoids: A group of neuromodulatory chemicals involved in a variety of physiologic processes including appetite, pain sensation, mood, memory, motor coordination, blood pressure regulation, and combating cancer.

endogenous: Made in the body.

endurance: A measure of fitness. The ability to work for prolonged periods and the ability to resist fatigue.

energy: The capacity to carry out an action, whether it is moving the limbs or thinking.

energetic approaches: Methods of bodywork that involve the subtle body responses.

enkephalins, endorphins, and dynorphins: Neurochemicals that elevate mood, support satiety (reduce hunger and cravings), and modulate pain.

entrainment: The coordination of movements or their synchronization to a rhythm.

entrapment: Pathologic pressure placed on a nerve or vessel by soft tissue.

environmental contact: Contact with pathogens found in the environment in food, water, and soil and on various surfaces.

epinephrine (adrenaline): A neurochemical that activates arousal mechanisms in the body; the activation, arousal, alertness, and alarm chemical of the fight-or-flight response and all sympathetic arousal functions and behaviors.

ergonomics: The study of the design of equipment, the working environment, and the workload with the goal of reducing musculoskeletal stress on the body.

essential oils: Distilled extracts from aromatic plants.

essential touch: Vital, fundamental, and primary touch that is crucial to well-being.

ethical behavior: Right and good conduct that is based on moral and cultural standards as defined by the society in which we live.

ethical decision making: The application of ethical principles and professional skills to determine appropriate behavior and resolve ethical dilemmas.

ethics: The science or study of morals, values, or principles, including ideals of autonomy, beneficence, and justice; principles of right and good conduct.

evidence-based practice: Use of current best evidence in making decisions about the care of patients

exemption: A situation in which a professional is not required to comply with an existing law because of educational or professional standing.

experiment: A method of testing a hypothesis.

expressive touch: Touch applied to support and convey awareness and empathy for the client as a whole.

external sensory information: Stimulation from an origin exterior to the surface of the skin that is detected by the body.

facilitation: The state of a nerve in which it is stimulated but not to the point of threshold; the point at which it transmits a nerve signal.

fascial sheath: A flat sheet of connective tissue used for separation, stability, and muscular attachment points.

feedback: A method of autoregulation to maintain internal homeostasis that interlinks body functions; a noninvasive, continual exchange of information between the client and the professional.

fitness: A general term used to describe the ability to perform physical work.

focus/centering: The ability to focus the mind by screening out sensation.

forced expiration: The movement of air out of the body, produced by activating muscles that can pull down the ribs and muscles that can compress the abdomen, forcing the diaphragm upward.

forced inspiration: Movement of air into the body that occurs when an individual is working very hard and needs a great deal of oxygen. This involves not only the muscles of quiet and deep inspiration, but also the muscles that stabilize and/or elevate the shoulder girdle to directly or indirectly elevate the ribs.

franchise: A business contract through which an individual (the franchisee) purchases the rights to sell or market the products or services (or both) of a large group that has developed a brand (the franchisor).

frequency: The number of times a method repeats itself in a time period.

friction: Specific circular or transverse movements that do not glide on the skin and that are focused on the underlying tissue.

fungi: A group of simple parasitic organisms that are similar to plants but that have no chlorophyll (green pigment). Most pathogenic fungi live on tissue on or near the skin or mucous membranes.

gait: A walking pattern.

gate control theory: A term that refers to a hypothetical gating mechanism that functions at the level of the spinal cord; a "gate" through which pain impulses reach the lateral spinothalamic system. Painful impulses are transmitted by large-diameter and small-diameter nerve fibers. Stimulation of large-diameter fibers prevents the small-diameter fibers from transmitting signals. Stimulating large-diameter fibers (e.g., through rubbing or massaging) helps suppress the sensation of pain, especially sharp pain.

general adaptation syndrome: The process that calls into play the three stages of the body's response to stress: the alarm reaction, the resistance reaction, and the exhaustion reaction.

general contraindications: Factors that require a physician's evaluation to rule out serious underlying conditions before any massage is indicated. If the physician recommends massage, the physician must help develop a comprehensive treatment plan.

gestures: The way a client touches the body while explaining a problem. These movements may indicate whether the problem is a muscle problem, a joint problem, or a visceral problem.

goals: Desired outcomes.

Golgi tendon receptors: Receptors in the tendons that sense tension.

growth hormone: A hormone that promotes cell division; in adults it is implicated in the repair and regeneration of tissue.

guarding: Contraction of muscles in a splinting action, surrounding an injured area.

hacking: A type of tapotement in which the surface of the body is alternately struck with quick, snapping movements.

hardening: A method of teaching the body to deal more effectively with stress; sometimes called *toughening.*

hardiness: The physical and mental ability to withstand external stressors.

healing: The restoration of well-being.

health: Optimum functioning with freedom from disease or abnormal processes.

heart rate variability: A physiologic phenomenon in which the interval between heart beats varies.

heavy pressure: Compressive force that extends to the bone under the tissue.

hepatitis: A viral inflammatory process and infection of the liver.

histamine: A chemical produced by the body that dilates the blood vessels.

history: Information from the client about past and present medical conditions and patterns of symptoms.

homeostasis: Dynamic equilibrium of the internal environment of the body through processes of feedback and regulation.

hormone: A messenger chemical in the bloodstream.

hospice: A philosophy and practice for end-of-life care.

human immunodeficiency virus (HIV): The virus responsible for AIDS.

hydrotherapy: The use of various types of water applications and temperatures for therapy.

hygiene: Practices and conditions that promote health and prevent disease.

hyperstimulation analgesia: The process of diminishing the perception of a sensation by stimulating large-diameter nerve fibers. Some methods used are application of ice or heat, counterirritation, acupressure, acupuncture, rocking, music, and repetitive massage strokes.

hyperventilation: Deep or rapid breathing in excess of physical demands.

hypothesis: The starting point of research; it is based on the statement, "If this happens, then that will happen."

impingement syndromes: Conditions that involve pathologic pressure on nerves and vessels; the two types of impingement are compression and entrapment.

indication: A therapeutic application that promotes health or assists in a healing process.

inflammatory response: A normal mechanism, characterized by pain, heat, redness, and swelling, that usually speeds recovery from an infection or injury.

informed consent: The client's authorization for any service from a professional based on adequate information provided by the professional. Obtaining informed consent is a consumer protection process that requires that clients have knowledge of what will occur and that their participation is voluntary; they also must be competent to give consent. Informed consent is an educational procedure that allows clients to make knowledgeable decisions about whether they want to receive a massage.

inhibition: A decrease in or the cessation of a response or function.

initial treatment plan: A plan that states therapeutic goals, the duration of the sessions, the number of appointments necessary to meet the agreed goals, costs, the general classification of intervention to be used, and the objective progress measurement to be used to identify attainment of goals.

insertion: The muscle attachment point that is closest to the moving joint.

integrated approaches: Combined methods of various forms of massage and bodywork styles.

integration: The process of remembering an event while being able to remain in the present moment, with an awareness of the difference between then and now, to bring some sort of resolution to the event.

integrative medicine: The combination of different types of treatments to emphasize care in a wider context of body/mind/spirit interconnectedness and the importance of supporting wellness in addition to treating pathologic conditions.

intercompetition massage: Massage provided during an athletic event.

interoceptive awareness: The conscious ability to be aware of proprioception, equilibrium or balance, and visceral sensations in the body, such as the heart and respiratory rates.

intersubjectivity: The nonverbal sense of being with another person, a direct result of the interpersonal resonance that occurs during co-regulation of movements, sensations, and emotions.

·imacy: A tender, familiar, and understanding experience ·tween beings.

intuition: Knowing something by using subconscious information.

isometric contraction: A contraction in which the effort of the muscle or group of muscles is exactly matched by a counterpressure such that no movement occurs, only effort.

isotonic contraction: A contraction in which the effort of the target muscle or group of muscles is partly matched by counterpressure, allowing a degree of resisted movement.

job: An activity performed regularly for payment.

joint end-feel: The sensation felt when a normal joint is taken to its physiologic limit (see *end-feel*).

joint kinesthetic receptors: Receptors in the capsules of joints that respond to pressure and to acceleration and deceleration of joint movement. The two main types of joint kinesthetic receptors are type II cutaneous mechanoreceptors and pacinian (lamellated) corpuscles.

joint movement: The movement of the joint through its normal range of motion.

joint play: The inherent laxity present in a joint.

kinesiology: The science of the study of movement and the active and passive structures involved, including bones, joints, muscle tissues, and all associated connective tissues.

kinetic chain: The process by which each individual joint movement pattern functions as part of an interconnected aspect of the neurologic coordination pattern of muscle movement.

language: Made of socially shared rules that involve sounds and symbols, definitions, ability to make up new words, and grammar.

law: A scientific statement that is true uniformly for a whole class of natural occurrences.

lengthening: The process in which the muscle assumes a normal resting length by means of the neuromuscular mechanism.

legend drug: Any medication that requires a prescription.

leverage: Leaning with the body weight to provide pressure.

license: A type of credential required by law; licenses are used to regulate the practice of a profession to protect the public's health, safety, and welfare.

longitudinal stretching: A stretch applied along the fiber direction of the connective tissues and muscles.

lubricant: A substance that reduces friction on the skin during massage movements.

lymph system: A specialized component of the circulatory system that is responsible for waste disposal and immune response.

lymphatic drainage: A specific type of massage that enhances lymphatic flow.

malignant tumor: The type of tumor (cancer) that tends to spread to other regions of the body.

mandatory ethics: Ethical behavior that is motivated only by compliance with the law.

manipulation: Skillful use of the hands in a therapeutic manner. Massage manipulations focus on the soft tissues of the body and are not to be confused with joint manipulation using a high-velocity thrust.

manual lymphatic drainage: Methods of bodywork that influence lymphatic movement.

marketing: The advertising and other promotional activities required to sell a product or service.

massage therapy: The scientific art and system of assessment of and manual application of certain techniques to the superficial soft tissue of skin, muscles, tendons, ligaments, and fascia and the structures that lie within the superficial tissue. The hand, foot, knee, arm, elbow, and forearm are used for the systematic external application of touch, stroking (effleurage), friction, vibration, percussion, kneading (pétrissage), stretching, compression, or passive and active joint movements within the normal physiologic range of motion. Massage includes adjunctive external applications of water, heat, and cold for the purposes of establishing and maintaining good physical condition and health by normalizing and improving muscle tone, promoting relaxation, stimulating circulation, and producing therapeutic effects on the respiratory and nervous systems and the subtle interactions among all body systems. These intended effects are accomplished through the physiologic energetic and mind/body connections in a safe, nonsexual environment that respects the client's self-determined outcome for the session.

massage chair: A specially designed chair that allows the client to sit comfortably during the massage.

massage environment: An area or location where a massage is given.

massage equipment: Tables, mats, chairs, and other incidental supplies and implements used during the massage.

massage mat: A cushioned surface that is placed on the floor.

massage routine: The step-by-step protocol and sequence used to give a massage.

massage table: A specially designed table that allows massage to be done with the client lying down.

massage therapist: A term that means the same thing as massage practitioner; also includes massage technologist, massage technician, masseur, masseuse, myotherapist, massotherapist, bodyworker, bodywork therapist, somatic therapist, or any derivation of these terms.

mechanical effects: These occur when various types of mechanical force (tension, bending, shear, torsion, and compression) are applied directly to the body and directly affect the soft tissue through techniques that normalize the connective tissue or move body fluid and intestinal contents.

mechanical methods: Techniques that directly affect the soft tissue by normalizing the connective tissue or moving body fluids and intestinal contents.

mechanical response: A response based on a structural change in the tissue. The tissue change is caused directly by application of a technique.

mechanical touch: Touch applied with the intent of achieving a specific anatomic or physiologic outcome.

medical massage: A synonym for clinical massage.

medications: Substances prescribed to stimulate or inhibit a body process or replace a chemical in the body.

mental impairment: Any mental or psychologic disorder, such as mental retardation, developmental disabilities, organic brain syndrome, emotional or mental illness, and specific learning disabilities.

mentoring: Career support provided by a more experienced practitioner.

meridian: Nerve tracts in the tissue, located in the fascial grooves, along which energy flows.

metastasis: The migration of cancer cells.

methicillin-resistant *Staphylococcus aureus* (MRSA): A potentially dangerous type of bacteria that is resistant to certain antibiotics and may cause skin and other infections.

mobilization: The process of making a fixed part movable or releasing stored substances, as in restoring motion to a joint, freeing an organ, or making substances held in reserve in the body available.

modality: A method of application or the employment of any physical agents and devices. The term is commonly misused to describe forms of massage (e.g., NMT, myofascial, Swedish).

moderate pressure: Compressive pressure that extends to the muscle layer but does not press the tissue against the underlying bone.

motivation: The internal drive that provides the energy to do what is necessary to accomplish a goal.

motor point: The point where a motor nerve enters the muscle it innervates and causes the muscle to twitch if stimulated.

motor tone: The nervous system's control of how long or short a muscle is by regulating the degree of muscle fiber contraction.

movement cure: A term used in the nineteenth and early twentieth centuries for a system of exercise and massage manipulations focused on treating a variety of ailments.

multiple isotonic contractions: Movements of the joint and associated muscles by the client through a full range of motion against partial resistance applied by the massage therapist.

muscle energy techniques: Neuromuscular facilitation; specific use of active contraction in individual muscles or groups of muscles to initiate a relaxation response; activation of the proprioceptors to facilitate muscle tone, relaxation, and stretching.

muscle spindles: Structures located primarily in the belly of the muscle that respond to both sudden and prolonged stretches.

muscle testing procedures: An assessment process that uses muscle contraction as a test element. Strength testing is done to determine whether a muscle responds with sufficient strength to perform the required body functions. Neurologic muscle testing is designed to determine whether the neurologic interaction of the muscles is working smoothly. Applied kinesiology uses muscle strength or weakness as an indicator of body function.

muscle tone: Determination of the shape and location of a muscle and the density and pliability of all the fluid, fibers, and connective tissue of the muscle.

musculotendinous junction: The point where muscle fibers end and the connective tissue continues to form the tendon; a major site of injury.

myofascial approaches: Styles of bodywork that affect the connective tissues; often called *deep tissue massage, soft tissue manipulation,* or *myofascial release.*

myofascial release: A system of bodywork that affects the connective tissue of the body through various methods that elongate and alter the plastic component and ground matrix of the connective tissue.

needs assessment: History taking using a client information form, and physical assessment using an assessment form. The information is evaluated to develop a care plan.

nerve impingement: Pressure against a nerve by skin, fascia, muscles, ligaments, or joints.

neurologic muscle testing: Testing designed to determine whether the neurologic interaction of the muscles proceeds smoothly.

neuromuscular mechanism: The interplay and reflex connection between sensory and motor neurons and muscle function.

neuromuscular re-education: Therapeutic exercise techniques used to develop and restore balance, movement, coordination, kinesthetic sense, posture, proprioception, muscular tone and activity by way of activation of both nerves and muscles.

neuromuscular therapy: An umbrella term that encompasses a variety of treatment approachs, many of which can be used for addressing trigger points.

neurotransmitter: A messenger chemical in the synapse of the nerve.

nomenclature: A system of names.

norepinephrine (noradrenaline): A neurochemical that functions in a manner similar to epinephrine but is more concentrated in the brain.

occupation: A productive or creative activity that serves as a regular source of livelihood.

oil: A type of liquid lubricant.

open-ended question: A question that cannot be answered with a simple, one-word response.

opportunistic invasion: An infection caused by potentially pathogenic organisms that are found on the skin and mucous membranes of nearly everyone. These organisms do not cause disease until they have the opportunity, such as with impaired immunity.

origin: The attachment point of a muscle at the fixed point during movement.

orthopedic tests: Assessments for bone, joint, ligament, and tendon injuries.

oscillation: Any effect that varies in a back-and-forth, or reciprocating, manner.

osteokinematic movements: The movements of flexion, extension, abduction, adduction, and rotation; also known as *physiologic movements.*

overload principle: A stress on an organism that is greater than the one regularly encountered during everyday life.

oxytocin: A hormone that is implicated in pair or couple bonding, parental bonding, feelings of attachment, and care giving, along with its more commonly known functions in pregnancy, delivery, and lactation.

pain and fatigue syndromes: Multicausal and often chronic nonproductive patterns that interfere with well-being, activities of daily living, and productivity.

pain-spasm-pain cycle: Steady contraction of muscles, which causes ischemia and stimulates pain receptors in muscles. The pain, in turn, initiates more spasms.

palliative care: Care intended to relieve or reduce the intensity of uncomfortable symptoms but that cannot effect a cure.

palpation: Assessment through touch.

panic: An intense, sudden, and overwhelming fear or feeling of anxiety that produces terror and immediate physiologic change, resulting in immobility or senseless, hysterical behavior.

parasympathetic autonomic nervous system: The restorative part of the autonomic nervous system. The parasympathetic response often is called the *relaxation response.*

passive joint movement: Movement of a joint by the massage practitioner without the assistance of the client.

passive range of motion: Movement of a joint in which the therapist, not the client, effects the motion.

pathogenic animals: Large, multicellular organisms sometimes called *metazoa.* Most metazoa are worms that feed off human tissue or cause other disease processes.

pathologic barrier: An adaptation of the physiologic barrier that allows the protective function to limit rather than support optimum functioning.

pathology: The study of disease.

patient: Recipient of care.

patterns: The product of the replication of structures and functions that entwine and influence each other.

peak performance: Maximum conditioning and functioning in a particular action.

peer support: Interaction among those involved in the same pursuit. Regular interaction with other massage practitioners creates an environment in which both technical information and dilemmas and interpersonal dilemmas can be sorted out.

person-to-person contact: The transmission of pathogens from one person to another through contact or often by airborne transmission.

pétrissage (kneading): Rhythmic rolling, lifting, squeezing, and wringing of soft tissue.

pharmacology: The science of drugs; it includes development of drugs, understanding of their mechanisms of action, and description of their conditions of use.

phasic muscles: The muscles that move the body.

physical agents: Tools or materials used in the application of therapeutic modalities; they consist of energy and materials applied to the client or patient to assist in the achievement of therapeutic goals.

physical assessment: Evaluation of body balance, efficient function, basic symmetry, range of motion, and ability to function.

physical disability/impairment: Any physiologic disorder, condition, cosmetic disfigurement, or anatomic loss that affects one or more of the following body systems: neurologic, musculoskeletal, special sense organ, respiratory (including speech organs), cardiovascular, reproductive, digestive, genitourinary, hemic and lymphatic, skin, and endocrine. Extremes in size and extensive burns also may be considered physical impairments.

physiologic barriers: The result of the limits in range of motion imposed by protective nerve and sensory functions to support optimum performance.

piezoelectricity: The production of an electrical current by application of pressure to certain crystals (e.g., mica, quartz, Rochelle salt) or to connective tissue.

placebo effect: Improvement in a patient's disease or condition even if the treatment is not specifically validated.

polarity: A holistic health practice that encompasses some of the theory base of Asian medicine and Ayurveda. Polarity is an eclectic, multifaceted system.

positional release: A method of moving the body into the direction of ease (the way the body wants to move out of the position that causes the pain); the proprioception is taken into a state of safety and may stop signaling for protective spasming.

positioning: Placing the body in such a way that specific joints or muscles are isolated.

postevent massage: Massage provided after an athletic event.

postisometric relaxation (PIR): The state that occurs after isometric contraction of a muscle; it results from the activity of minute neural reporting stations called the *Golgi tendon bodies.*

post-traumatic stress disorder: A disorder characterized by episodes of flashback memory, state-dependent memory, somatization, anxiety, irritability, sleep disturbance, concentration difficulties, times of melancholy or depression, grief, fear, worry, anger, and avoidance behavior.

postural muscles: Muscles that support the body against gravity.

powder: A type of lubricant that consists of a finely ground substance.

power differential: A term that describes the difference in knowledge and skills between the client and the professional; it exists because one is placed in the position of controlling the situation.

prefix: A word element placed at the beginning of a root word to change the meaning of the word.

premassage activity: Any activity included in the preparation for a massage, including setting up the massage room, obtaining supplies, and determining the temperature of the room.

prescription: An oral or written direction or order for dispensing and administering a healthcare intervention.

pressure: Compressive force.

PRICE first aid: A treatment regimen for an injury that includes *p*rotection, *r*est, *i*ce, *c*ompression, and *e*levation.

prime movers: The muscles responsible for movement.

principle: A basic truth or rule of conduct.

profession: An occupation that requires training and specialized study.

professional: A person who practices a profession.

professionalism: The adherence to professional status, methods, standards, and character.

professional touch: Skilled touch delivered to achieve a specific outcome; the recipient in some way reimburses the professional for services rendered.

progress (or session) notes: The use of a charting process to record each massage with the client.

prone: Lying face down.

proprioceptive neuromuscular facilitation (PNF): Specific application of muscle energy techniques that uses strong contraction combined with stretching and muscular pattern retraining.

proprioceptors: Sensory receptors that detect joint and muscle activity.

protozoa: One-celled organisms that are larger than bacteria. They can infest human fluids and cause disease by parasitizing (living off) or directly destroying cells.

pulsed muscle energy: Procedures that involve engaging the comfort barrier and using minute, resisted contractions (usually 20 in 10 seconds), which introduces mechanical pumping in addition to PIR or RI.

qualifiable: A term that describes goals measured by criteria determined by the practitioner that indicate when the goal is achieved.

quantifiable: A term that describes the measurement of goals by objective criteria (e.g., time, frequency, 1 to 10 scale) that can demonstrate an increase or a decrease in the ability to perform an activity or an increase or a decrease in a sensation, such as relaxation or pain.

quiet expiration: Movement of air out of the body through passive action. This occurs through relaxation of the external intercostals and the elastic recoil of the thoracic wall and tissue of the lungs and bronchi, with gravity pulling the rib cage down from its elevated position.

quiet inspiration: Movement of air into the body while resting or sitting quietly. The diaphragm and external intercostals are the prime movers.

range of motion: The movement of joints.

rapport: The development of a relationship based on mutual trust and harmony.

reciprocal inhibition (RI): The effect that occurs when a muscle contracts, obliging its antagonist to relax to allow normal movement.

reciprocity: The exchange of privileges between governing bodies.

recovery massage: Massage structured primarily for the uninjured athlete who wants to recover from a strenuous workout or competition.

re-enactment: Reliving an event as though it were happening at the moment.

referral: Sending a client to a health care professional for specific diagnosis and treatment of a disease.

referred pain: Pain felt in an area other than the source of the pain.

reflective listening: The ability to restate information in a way that indicates the listener has received and understood the message.

reflex: An involuntary response to a stimulus. Reflexes are specific, predictable, adaptive, and purposeful. Reflexive methods work by stimulating the nervous system (sensory neurons), and tissue changes occur in response to the body's adaptation to the neural stimulation.

reflexive effects: When various mechanical forces are introduced into body tissues during massage with the intent to stimulate the nervous system, endocrine system, and the chemicals of the body.

reflexive methods: Massage techniques that stimulate the nervous system, the endocrine system, and the chemicals of the body.

reflexology: A massage system directed primarily to the feet and hands.

refractory period: The period after a muscle contraction during which the muscle is unable to contract again.

regional contraindications: Contraindications that relate to a specific area of the body.

rehabilitation massage: Massage used for severe injury or as part of interventions after surgery.

relative risk: The chance of occurrence as expressed in comparative terms by describing the outcome rate for people exposed to the factor in question, compared with the outcome rate for those not exposed to the factor.

remedial massage: Massage used for more severe injuries or as part of the postsurgical intervention plan.

research literacy: The knowledge and understanding of scientific concepts and processes required for personal and professional decision making.

resonance: The alignment of psychobiologic states between a client or patient and a therapist.

resonator: A device or system that has resonance or shows resonant behavior.

resourceful compensation: Adjustments made by the body to manage a permanent or chronic dysfunction.

resting position: The first stroke of the massage; the simple laying on of hands.

rhythm: The regularity of application of a technique. If the method is applied at regular intervals, it is considered even or rhythmic. If it is choppy or irregular, it is considered uneven or not rhythmic.

right of refusal: The right of either the client or the professional to stop the massage session.

rocking: Rhythmic movement of the body.

root word: The part of a word that provides its fundamental meaning.

safe touch: Secure, respectful, considerate, sensitive, responsive, sympathetic, understanding, supportive, and empathetic contact.

sanitation: The formulation and application of measures to promote and establish conditions favorable to health, specifically public health.

science: The intellectual process of understanding through observation, measurement, accumulation of data, and analysis of findings.

ientific method: A means of objectively researching a oncept to determine whether it is valid.

of practice: The knowledge base and practice param- of a profession.

loyed: Working for oneself rather than another.

serotonin: The neurochemical that regulates mood in terms of appropriate emotions, attention to thoughts, calming, quieting, and comforting effects; it also subdues irritability and regulates drive states.

service: An action performed for another person that results in a specific outcome.

severe acute respiratory syndrome (SARS): A respiratory illness marked by symptoms such as headache, fever, aches and, commonly, pneumonia.

sexual misconduct: Any behavior that is sexually oriented in the professional setting.

shaking: A technique in which the body area is grasped and shaken in a quick, loose movement; sometimes classified as rhythmic mobilization.

shiatsu: An acupressure- and meridian-focused bodywork system from Japan.

side-lying: The position in which the client is lying on his or her side.

signs: Objective abnormalities that can be seen or measured by someone other than the patient.

skin rolling: A form of pétrissage that lifts the skin.

slapping: A form of tapotement for which a flat hand is used.

SOAP notes: A problem-oriented method of medical record keeping; the acronym SOAP stands for *s*ubjective, *o*bjective, *a*ssessment (analysis), and *p*lan.

soft tissue: The skin, fascia, muscles, tendons, joint capsules, and ligaments of the body.

somatic: A term that means pertaining to the body.

somatic pain: Pain that arises from stimulation of receptors in the skin (superficial somatic pain) or in skeletal muscles, joints, tendons, and fascia (deep somatic pain).

spa: From the Latin for "health from water."

special tests: Methods used to assess the presence and degree of a client's or patent's condition. These assessments commonly involve specific stressing of particular structures.

speed: The rate of application (i.e., fast, slow, varied).

spindle cells: Sensory receptors in the belly of the muscle that detect stretch.

stabilization: Holding the body in a fixed position during joint movement, lengthening, and stretching.

Standard Precautions: Procedures developed by the Centers for Disease Control and Prevention (CDC) to prevent the spread of contagious diseases.

standards of care: Treatment guidelines developed by the profession for a given condition, which identify the appropriate treatment based on scientific evidence and clinical experience.

standards of practice: The principles that form specific guidelines to direct professional ethical practice and quality care, including a structure for evaluating the quality of care. Standards of practice are an attempt to define the parameters of quality care.

start-up costs: The initial expenses involved in starting a business.

state-dependent memory: The encoding and storing of a memory based on the effects of the autonomic nervous system and the resulting chemical levels of the body. The memory is retrievable only during a similar physiologic experience in the body.

sterilization: A process that destroys all microorganisms.

stimulation: Excitation that activates the sensory nerves.

strain/counterstrain: The use of tender points to guide the positioning of the body into a space where the muscle tension can release on its own.

strength testing: Testing intended to determine whether a muscle is responding with sufficient strength to perform the required body functions. Strength testing determines a muscle's force of contraction.

stress: Any substantial change in routine or any activity that forces the body to adapt.

stressors: Any internal perceptions or external stimuli that demand a change in the body.

stretching: Mechanical tension applied to lengthen the myofascial unit (muscles and fascia); two types are longitudinal stretching and cross-directional stretching.

stroke: A technique of therapeutic massage that is applied with a movement on the surface of the body, whether superficial or deep.

structural and postural integration approaches: Methods of bodywork derived from biomechanics, postural alignment, and the importance of the connective tissue structures.

subtle energies: Weak electrical fields that surround and run through the body.

suffering: An overall impairment of a person's quality of life.

suffix: A word element placed at the end of a root word to change the meaning of the word.

superficial fascia: The connective tissue layer just under the skin.

superficial pressure: Pressure that remains on the skin.

supervision: Support from more experienced professionals.

supine: The position in which the client is lying face up.

supportive climate: A collaborative environment that leads to mutual trust and to an atmosphere conducive to managing differences.

symmetric stance: The position in which body weight is distributed equally between the feet.

sympathetic autonomic nervous system: The energy-using part of the autonomic nervous system, the division in which the fight-or-flight response is activated.

symptoms: Subjective abnormalities that are not objectively detectable and can only be felt by the patient.

syndrome: A group of different signs and symptoms that usually arise from a common cause.

synergistic: The interaction of medication and massage to stimulate the same process or effects.

system: A group of interacting elements that function as a complex whole.

systemic massage: Massage structured to affect one body system primarily. This approach usually is used for lymphatic and circulation enhancement massage.

tapotement: Springy blows to the body at a fast rate to create rhythmic compression of the tissue; also called *percussion*.

tapping: A type of tapotement that uses the fingertips.

target muscle: The muscle or groups of muscles on which the response of the methods is specifically focused.

taxonomy: The science of classification according to a predetermined system.

techniques: Methods of therapeutic massage that provide sensory stimulation or mechanical change of the soft tissue of the body.

tendon organs: Structures found in the tendon and musculotendinous junction that respond to tension at the tendon. Articular (joint) ligaments contain receptors that are similar to tendon organs and adjust reflex inhibition of the adjacent muscle when excessive strain is placed on the joints.

tensegrity: An architectural principle, developed in 1948 by R. Buckminster Fuller, that underlies the structure of the geodesic dome. A tensegrity system is characterized by a continuous tensional network (in the body, tendons, ligaments, and fascial structures) connected by a discontinuous set of compressive elements, or struts (bones).

terminology: Language specific to a specialized field of knowledge.

Thai massage: A combination of elements from yoga, shiatsu, and acupressure that work with the energy pathways of the body and the therapy points located along these lines.

therapeutic applications: Healing or curative powers.

therapeutic change: Beneficial change produced by a bodywork process that results in a modification of physical form or function that can affect a client's physical, mental, and/or spiritual state.

therapeutic process: The capacity of the musculoskeletal system (and other systems) of the body to self-correct, come into balance, and achieve equilibrium through the skillful normalization of tissue tone by a massage therapist.

therapeutic relationship: The interpersonal structure and professional boundaries between professionals and the clients they serve.

thermotherapy: The application of heat and cold, often used for rehabilitation purposes.

tonic vibration reflex: Reflex that tones a muscle with stimulation through vibration methods at the tendon.

touch: Contact with no movement.

touch technique: The basis of soft tissue forms of bodywork methods.

toughening/hardening: The reaction to repeated exposure to stimuli that elicit arousal responses.

traction: Gentle pull on the joint capsule to increase the joint space.

training stimulus threshold: The stimulus that elicits a training response.

transference: The personalization of the professional relationship by the client.

trauma: Physical injury caused by violent or disruptive action, toxic substances, or psychic injury resulting from a severe long- or short-term emotional shock.

trigger point: An area of local nerve facilitation; pressure on the trigger point results in hypertonicity of a muscle bundle and referred pain patterns.

tuberculosis (TB): A bacterial infection that usually affects the lungs but may invade other body systems.

vibration: Fine or coarse tremulous movement that creates reflexive responses.

viruses: Microorganisms that invade cells and insert their genetic code into the host cell's genetic code. Viruses use the host cell's nutrients and organelles to produce more virus particles.

wellness: The efficient balance of body, mind, and spirit, all working in a harmonious way to provide quality of life.

yang: The portion of the whole realm of function of the body, mind, and spirit in Eastern thought that corresponds with sympathetic autonomic nervous system functions.

yin: The portion of the whole realm of function of the body, mind, and spirit in Eastern thought that corresponds with parasympathetic autonomic nervous system functions.

Index